MEDICAL
immerse yourself
LANGUAGE

second edition

Susan Turley

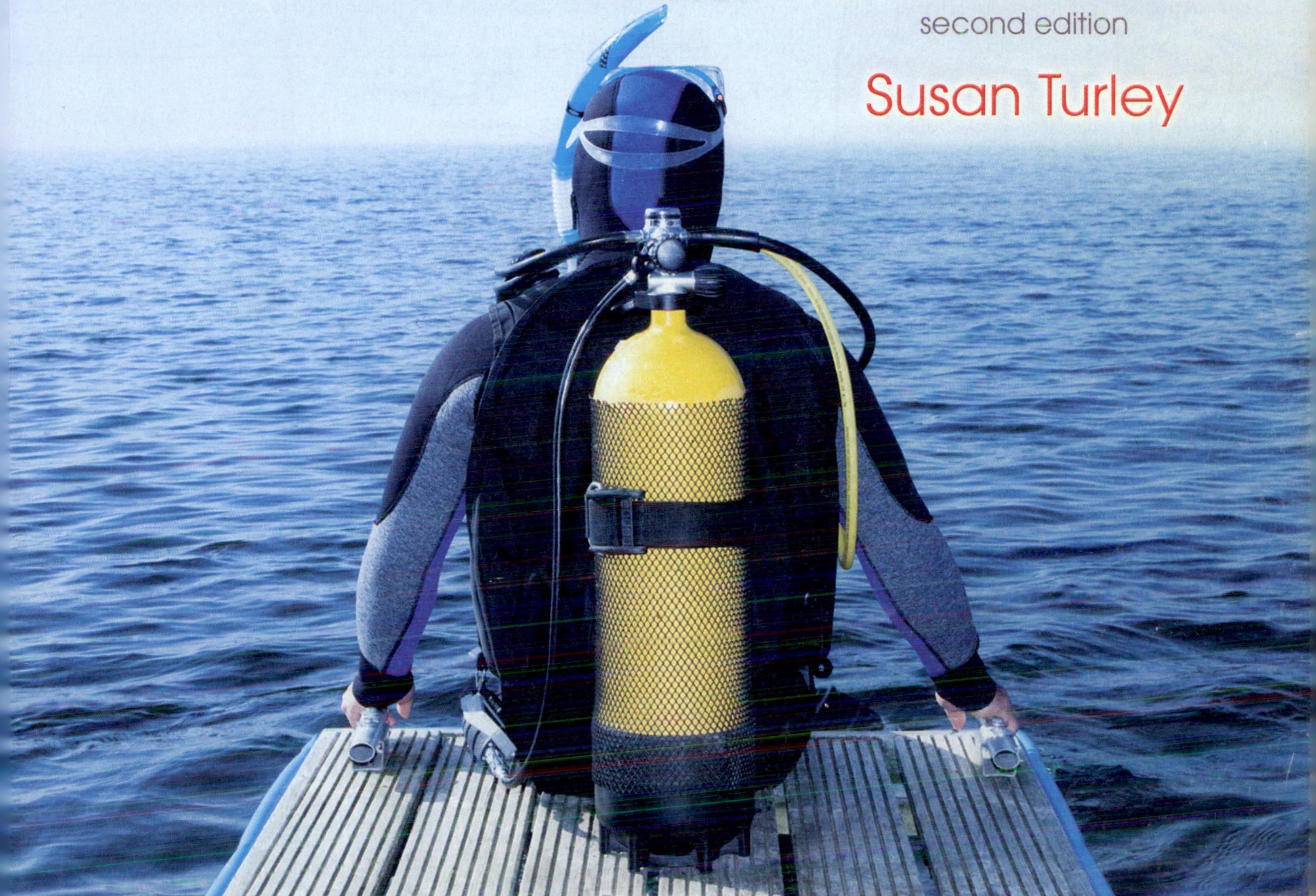

Pearson

Boston Columbus Indianapolis New York San Francisco Upper Saddle River
Amsterdam Cape Town Dubai London Madrid Milan Munich Paris Montreal Toronto
Delhi Mexico City Sao Paulo Sydney Hong Kong Seoul Singapore Taipei Tokyo

Library of Congress Cataloging-in-Publication Data

Turley, Susan M.
  Medical language / Susan M. Turley. — 2nd ed.
     p. ; cm.
  Includes index.
  ISBN-13: 978-0-13-505578-6
  ISBN-10: 0-13-505578-4
 1. Medicine—Terminology. I. Title.
  [DNLM: 1. Terminology as Topic—Problems and Exercises. W 18.2 T941m 2011]
  R123.T87 2011
  610.1'4—dc22

                                                         2009045786

Publisher: Julie Levin Alexander
Assistant to Publisher: Regina Bruno
Editor-in-Chief: Mark Cohen
Associate Editor: Melissa Kerian
Assistant Editor: Nicole Ragonese
Development Editor: Cathy Wein
Senior Media Editor: Amy Peltier
Media Project Manager: Lorena Cerisano
Managing Production Editor: Patrick Walsh
Production Liaison: Christina Zingone
Production Editor: Kate Boilard, Laserwords Maine
Manufacturing Manager: Ilene Sanford
Manufacturing Buyer: Pat Brown
Senior Art Director: Maria Guglielmo
Cover/Interior Designer: Christine Cantera

Medical Illustrator: Anita Impagliazzo
Cover Image: Getty Images, Inc.—Lifesize Royalty Free
Director of Marketing: David Gesell
Executive Marketing Manager: Katrin Beacom
Marketing Specialist: Michael Sirinides
Marketing Assistant: Judy Noh
Manager, Rights and Permissions: Zina Arabia
Manager, Visual Research: Beth Brenzel
Manager, Cover Visual Research and Permissions: Karen Sanatar
Image Permission Coordinator: Annette Linder
Composition: Laserwords, Maine
Printer/Binder: Quebecor Worldcolor, Versailles
Cover Printer: Lehigh-Phoenix Color/Hagerstown

10 9 8 7 6 5 4 3 2 1

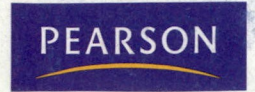

www.pearsonhighered.com

ISBN-13: 978-0-13-505578-6
ISBN-10: 0-13-505578-4

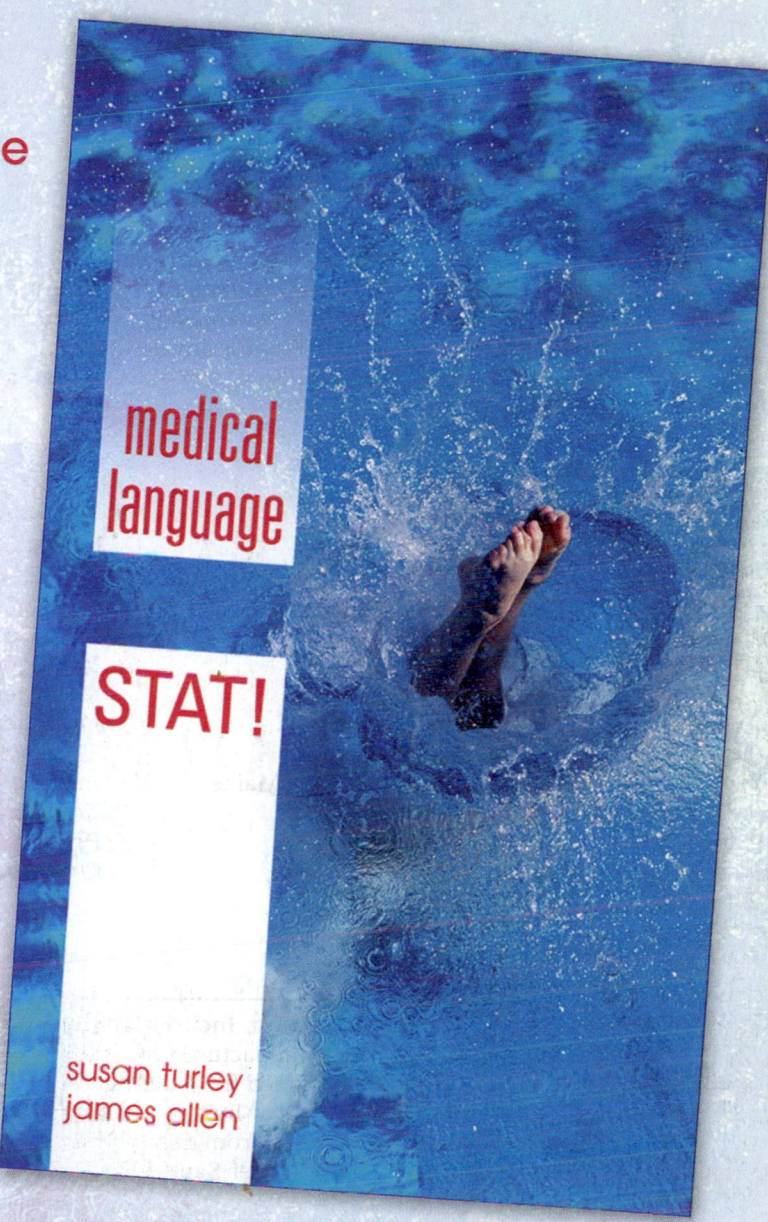

CUSTOMIZE THIS BOOK?

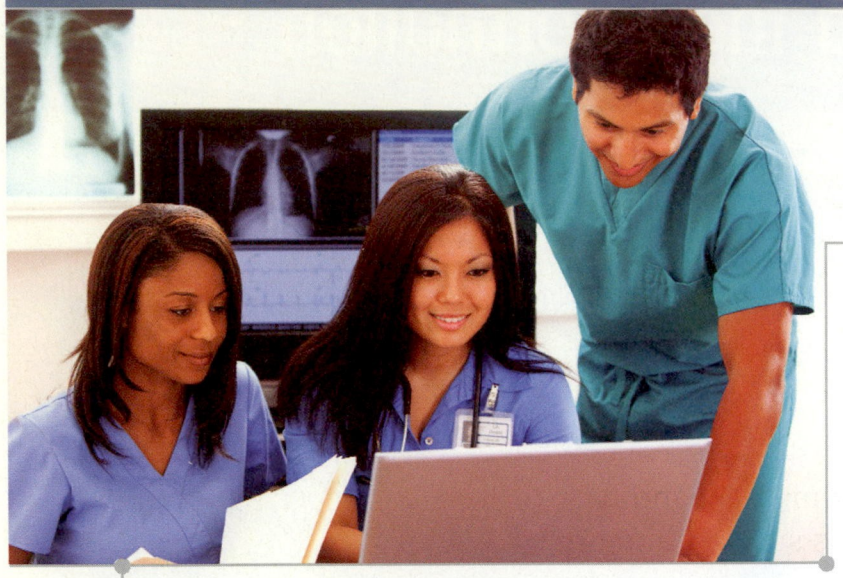

NOW the Power is in Your Hands

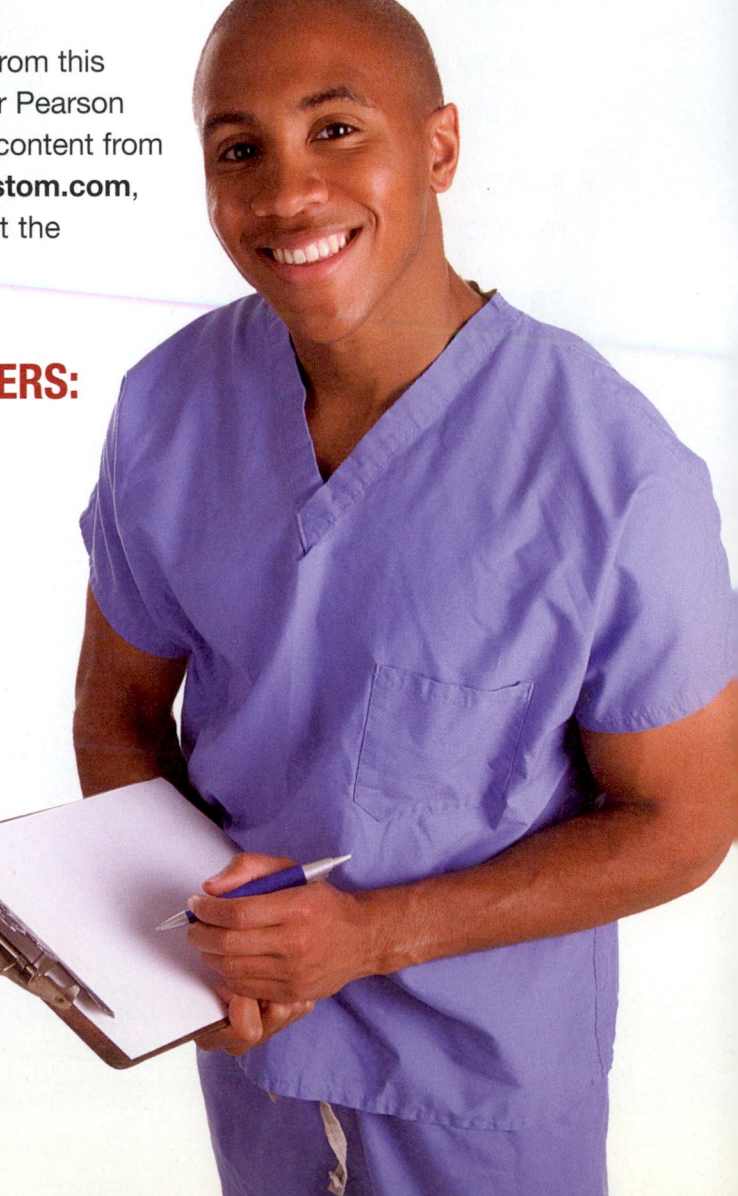

Create your ideal text by assembling content from this book or combining content from this and other Pearson titles. You can even add your own material or content from other sources! Just click on **www.pearsoncustom.com**, type in the keyword "allied health," and select the Custom Library.

PEARSON CUSTOM LIBRARY OFFERS:

- **FLEXIBILITY** Choose only the content you need from one or more titles. Sequence them based on your course syllabus.

- **USE OF OUTSIDE MATERIALS** Up to 20% can come from outside sources. We'll secure the permissions.

- **COST SAVINGS** Students pay only for the content you choose.

- **QUALITY FINISHED PRODUCT** Your book wil be professionally designed and will have sequential pagination and an index.

- **PERSONALIZATION OPTIONS** You may wish to have your name, your course, and your school printed on the cover.

- **COMPLIMENTARY PREVIEWS** See your book before you decide to adopt! Build your book and then you can request a preview copy.

DEDICATION

To my husband Al
for his support and love

To our children, Daniel,
Minh, and Lien

CONTENTS IN BRIEF

Two Journeys

In August 2000, I began two journeys—the adoption of children into our family and the writing of this textbook. Although very different, these two journeys shared a common thread of language and communication.

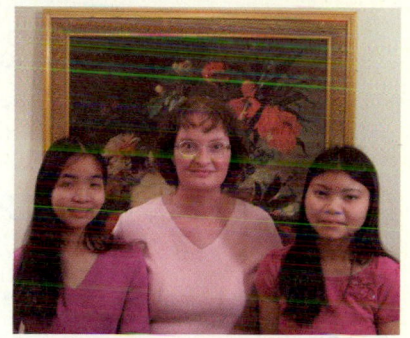

The first journey was the adoption of two beautiful children, Minh and Lien (ages 8 and 9), who joined our family from an orphanage in Vietnam in 2001. This journey of adoption involved completing much paperwork and research, learning a new language and culture, and traveling to an exotic land.

For many months prior to the adoption, nearly everything I did on a day-to-day basis was, in some way, affected by the decision to adopt. I purchased a Vietnamese dictionary, an English/Vietnamese dictionary, and a Vietnamese-language CD-ROM and began to spend at least an hour each day studying. A Vietnamese-American friend tutored me, teaching me Vietnamese phrases and laughing with me when I unknowingly said something I didn't intend to say. My studies were rewarded, however, when I was able to communicate with my new daughters in their own language, even as they quickly learned to speak English. As I write this page now in mid-2009, our family is preparing to travel to Vietnam and Cambodia as a homecoming visit and for a mission trip, and I am ever-mindful of the many children in need of help and homes.

The second journey was the process of writing this textbook. This journey also involved paperwork and research, but I did not need to learn a new language or culture. Because of my many years of experience in the healthcare field, I already understood medical language and culture.

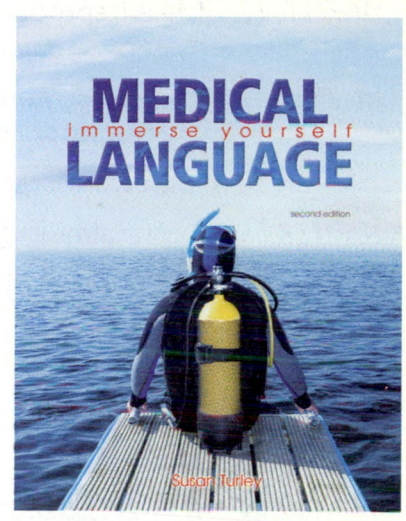

I did, however, need to determine the best way to convey that knowledge to each student who studies this textbook. And so, as I wrote, I drew on my own efforts and struggles to learn a new language during the adoption process. Those insights helped me identify with students who are learning medical language for the first time and enabled me to include textbook features that would support and strengthen students' efforts as they learned.

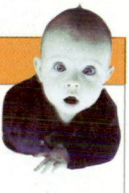

Did You Know?

The royalties from this textbook are given to provide ongoing financial support to orphanages and programs for street children in various countries around the world.

Dive Into Something Different

No new medical terminology book has touched the lives of so many people as profoundly as *Medical Language*. We credit the astounding success of the award-winning first edition to its special ability to meet the needs of students and educators. This new edition only builds upon our commitment, and so we have once again challenged our development team (see page xviii) to critique every feature, every page, every word—all to help enhance the teaching and learning process. The result has been an integration of features that "you," the customer, have asked for and will not find in other books.

CHAPTER FORMAT

Each medical specialty chapter follows a consistent organization designed for student success.

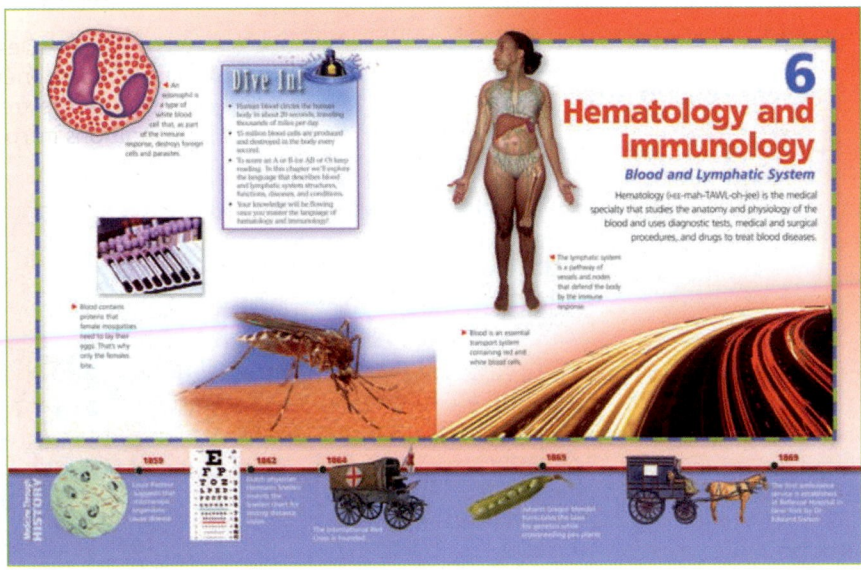

1 **Visual Introduction**—Engages readers with a stimulating collection of fun facts and images that help "launch" the chapter.

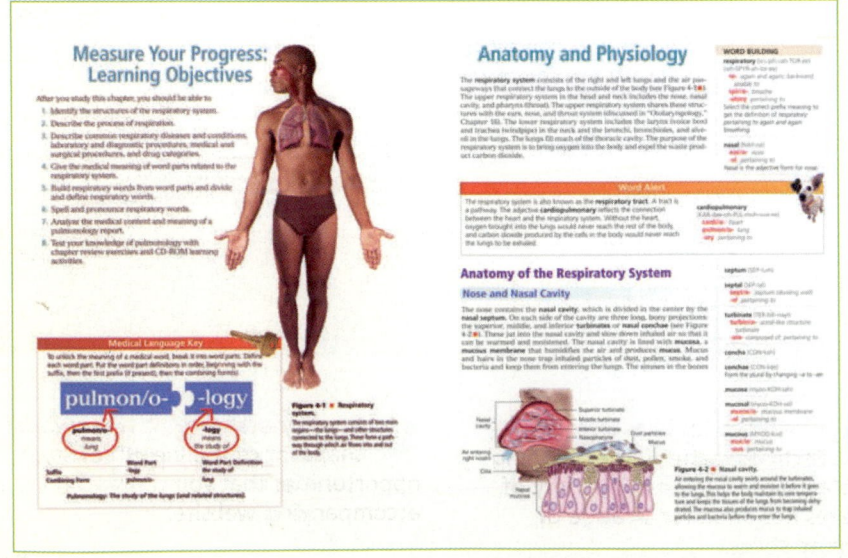

2 **Objectives/Medical Language Key**— Focuses readers on the goals of each chapter and provides a word analysis of the chapter title.

3 **Anatomy and Physiology**— Presents fundamental information about relevant body systems—reflecting the level of detail that the vast majority of educators told us they need.

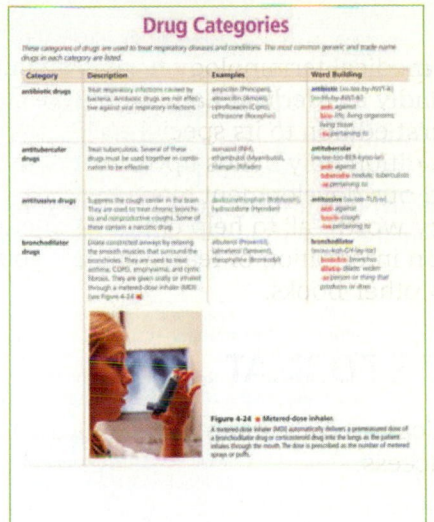

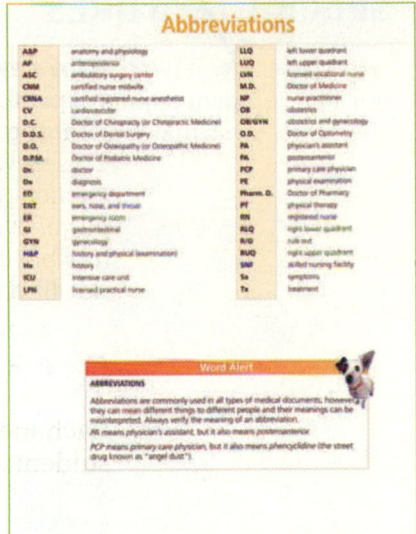

4 **Vocabulary Review**—Reinforces understanding with an at-a-glance review of each key term, a description, and an analysis of its word parts. A self-study quiz section follows with a heavy emphasis on word construction.

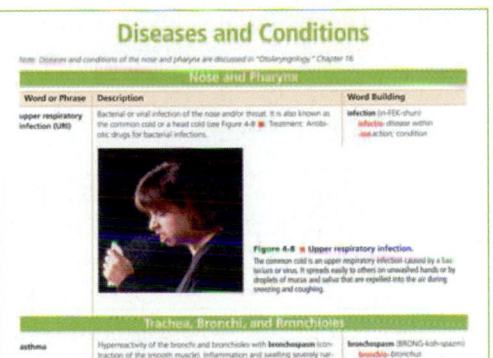

6 **Drug Categories**—Describes the most common generic and trade name drugs used to treat the diseases and conditions introduced.

7 **Abbreviations**—Provides a quick-reference listing of the most common abbreviations related to each medical specialty.

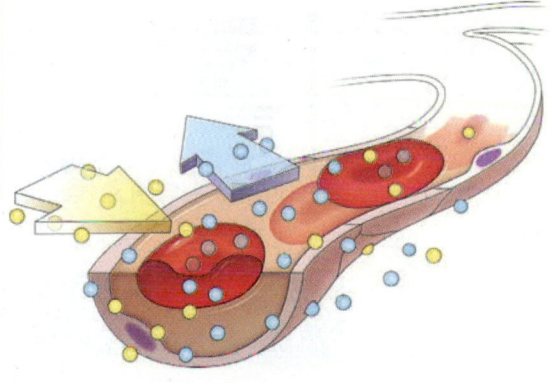

5 **Terms Related to Pathologies and Procedures**—Provides word analysis, descriptions, rich visuals, and fun facts about diseases and conditions and diagnostic and medical procedures.

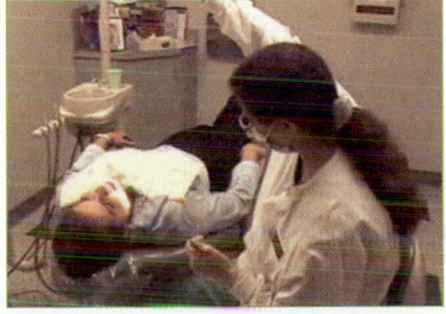

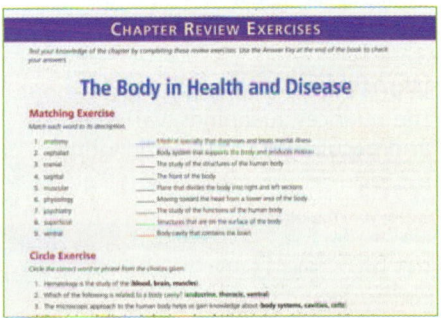

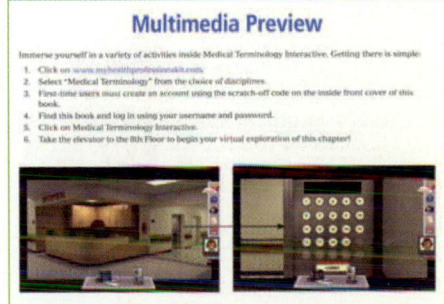

8 **Career Focus**—Orients readers to a career option in each medical specialty. Videos for each career are at www.myhealthprofessionskit.com inside of Medical Terminology Interactive.

9 **Chapter Review Exercises**—Fortifies reader understanding with a fun and extensive variety of quizzes designed for a range of learning styles.

10 **Multimedia Preview**—A visual snapshot of the wealth of study opportunities that you can find on the accompanying website.

SPECIAL FEATURES

"How would you describe the ideal medical terminology textbook?" That is the question we asked our development team of students and instructors. Their responses helped us craft this array of special features that make this book unique.

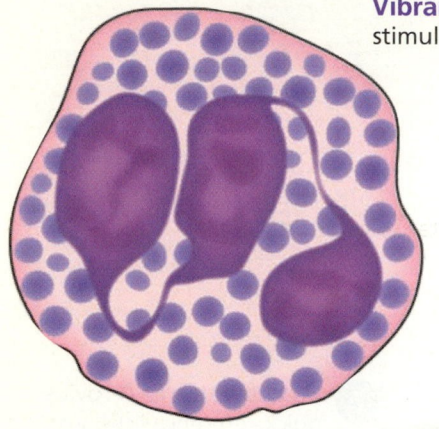

Vibrant Illustrations and Photographs—Brings medical language to life and stimulates understanding, especially for visual learners.

> Neutrophils are blood cells, but they are also part of the immune response of the lymphatic system because they are (**phagocytes** that specifically engulf and destroy bacteria. This process is known as **phagocytosis**.) Neutrophils only live a few days or even just a few hours if they are actively destroying bacteria. One neutrophil can destroy about 10 bacteria before it dies.
>   2. **Eosinophils** make up just 1–4% of the leukocytes in the blood. An eosinophil has large, red-pink granules in its cytoplasm, and its nucleus has two lobes (see Figure 6-6 ■ and Table 6-1). Eosinophils are also known as eos.

WORD BUILDING
myelocyte (MY-eh-loh-site)
myel/o- *bone marrow; spinal cord; myelin*
-cyte *cell*
phagocyte (FAG-oh-site)
phag/o- *eating; swallowing*
-cyte *cell*

Word Building—A section in the margins and within various tables throughout, this appears whenever a new word is introduced. It gives readers the tools to understand unfamiliar words on their own—reinforcing that word building is an ongoing process.

Special Boxes—Spark reader interest with key details relating the material to the real world of medicine.

Across the Life Span

Pediatrics. The first food for many babies is colostrum from the mother's breast. Colostrum is rich in nutrients and contains maternal antibodies. For the first few days of life, the newborn's intestinal tract is permeable and allows these antibodies to be absorbed from the intestine into the blood, where they provide passive immunity to common diseases.

Geriatrics. Older adults often complain that food does not seem as flavorful as when they were younger. The aging process causes a very real decline in the ability to smell and taste food as the number of receptors in the nose and on the tongue decreases.

Across the Lifespan—An infusion of relevant information related to pediatrics and geriatrics.

A Closer Look

The large intestine is inhabited by millions of beneficial bacteria that produce vitamin K to supplement what is in the diet. These bacteria also change the yellow-green pigment in bile to the characteristic brown color of feces. Bacteria in the large intestine feed on undigested materials and produce intestinal gas or **flatus**.

A Closer Look—A quick, focused glance at a pertinent detail related to material being covered.

Did You Know?

The appendix or vermiform appendix can be up to 8 inches in length. *Vermiform* is a Latin word meaning wormlike. The appendix plays no role in digestion. It is part of the lymphatic system and the immune response (discussed in "Hematology and Immunology," Chapter 6).

Did You Know?—Fun, interesting information designed to stimulate reader curiosity.

Clinical Connections

Immunology (Chapter 6). Some parts of the gastrointestinal system are also part of the body's immune response. Saliva contains antibodies that destroy microorganisms in the food we eat. Small areas on the walls of the intestines (Peyer's patches) and in the appendix contain white blood cells that destroy microorganisms. However, ingested microorganisms can still cause gastrointestinal illness.

Clinical Connections—Examples of the relationships and synergies between medical specialties.

Word Alert

SOUND-ALIKE WORDS

The prefix *intra-* means within. The prefix *inter-* means between.

interventricular	(adjective)	Pertaining to between the two ventricles *Example: The interventricular septum is the dividing wall between the right and left ventricles.*
intraventricular	(adjective)	Pertaining to within the ventricle *Example: Intraventricular blood is found within the right and left ventricles.*

Word Alert—Important notes about the nuances, meanings, variations, and peculiarities of selected words.

It's Greek to Me!

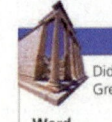

Did you notice that some words have two different combining forms? Combining forms from both Greek and Latin languages remain a part of medical language today.

Word	Greek	Latin	Medical Word Examples
breathe, breathing	spir/o- pne/o-	hal/o-	respiration, inspiration, inhalation, exhalation eupnea, bradypnea, tachypnea
chest	thorac/o- pector/o-	steth/o-	thoracic, stethoscope expectorant
lung	pneum/o- pneumon/o-	pulmon/o-	pneumococcus, pneumoconiosis, pulmonary pneumonia, pneumonectomy
pus	py/o-	purul/o-	pyothorax, empyema, purulent

It's Greek to Me!—Useful reminders about how Greek and Latin combining forms remain part of medical language today.

MEDICAL TERMINOLOGY INTERACTIVE

With purchase of this book students have access to an immersive media study experience. Click on www.myhealthprofessionskit.com, select the Medical Terminology discipline, and log on to this book using the access code inside the front cover. You will soon be transported to Medical Terminology Interactive—a virtual world of fun quizzes, word games, videos and other self-study challenges.

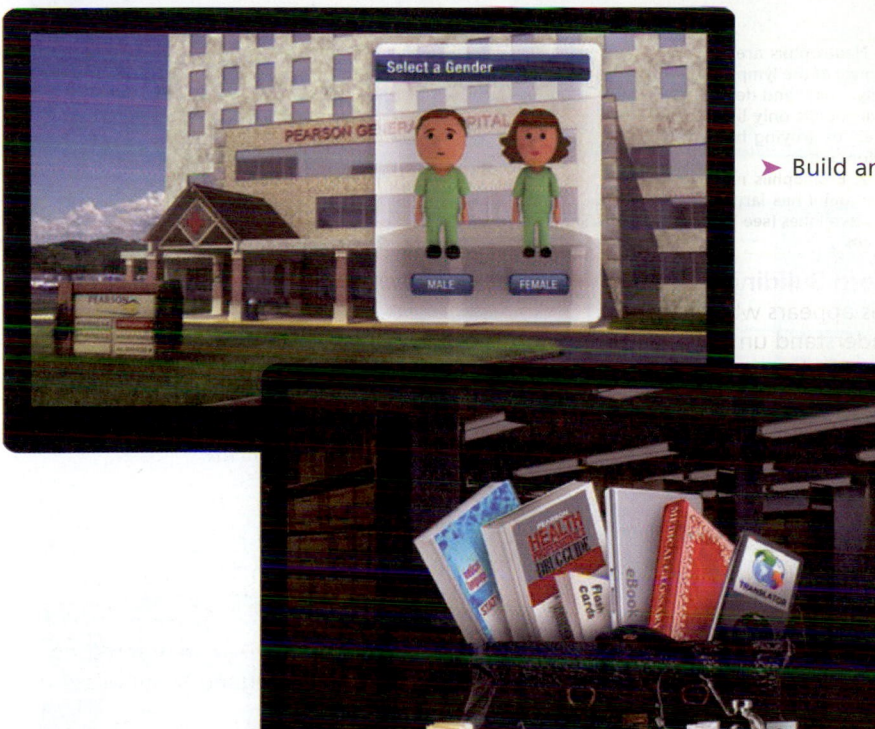

➤ Build an avatar to get started

➤ Explore your medical bag where you'll find reference materials, Spanish translations, flashcards and more.

➤ Start in the lobby and navigate to the elevator where you'll select a floor correlated to the chapter you wish to study.

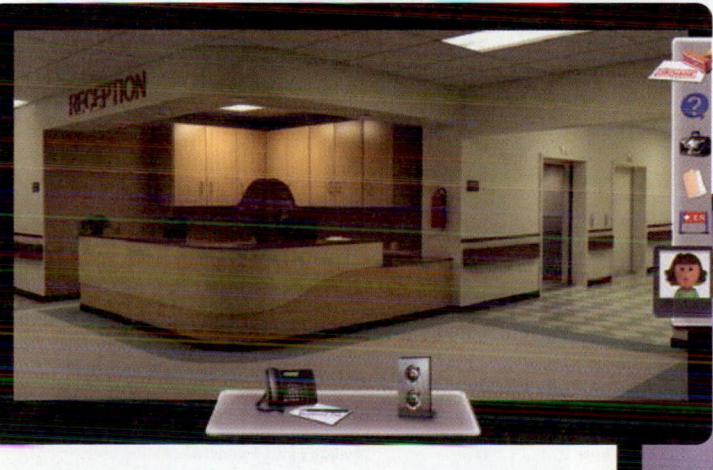

➤ When you arrive on a floor you'll have the opportunity to enter one of three rooms. Each room has clickable objects that will activate a different activity.

Medical Records Room. Here you will find exercises related to spelling, pronunciation, and transcription. Plus you'll explore a variety of learning modules.

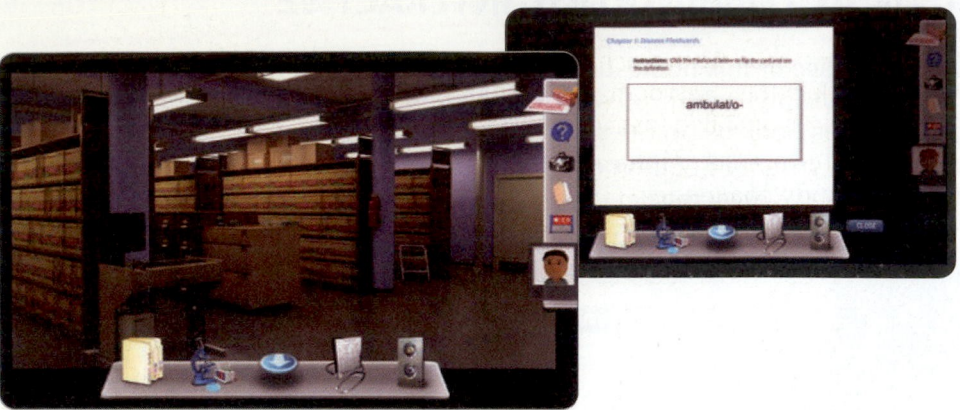

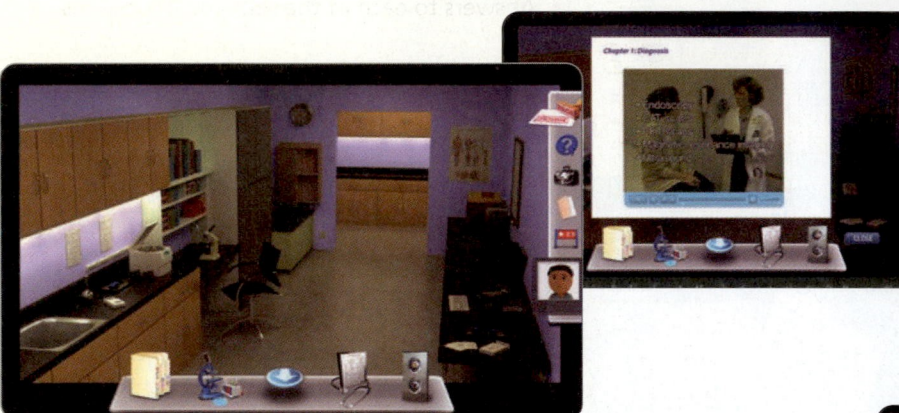

Laboratory. This is where you will be able to watch a variety of videos and also practice with flashcards to help you study.

Examination Room. This is the place to play a variety of educational games and quizzes such as Word Surgery, Racing Pulse, and Beat the Clock.

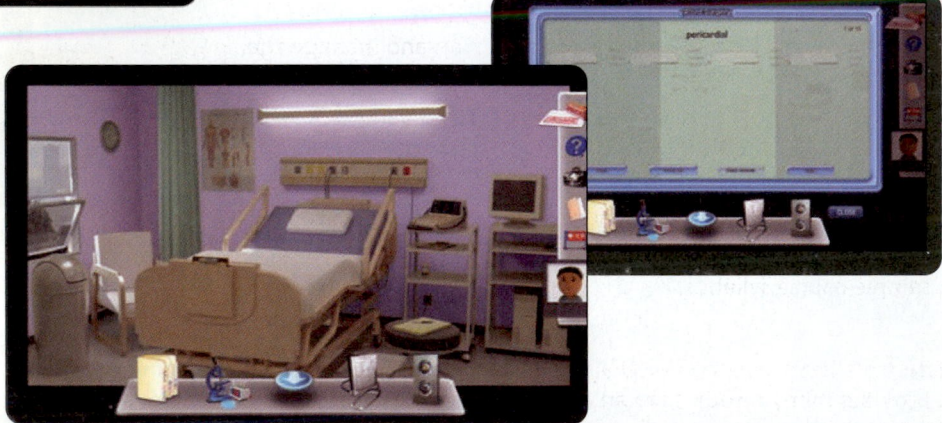

ER. Finally, if you're ready for the ultimate challenge in our virtual hospital, visit the ER. This stands for Exam Review and here you'll be transported to the set of a medical terminology quiz show where you can customize your gaming experience. Practice and enjoy as you become an ER champ!

The Medical Terminology Interactive experience allows you to track your progress chart as you proceed through the various floors and rooms. It also allows you to email the results of your work to your instructor.

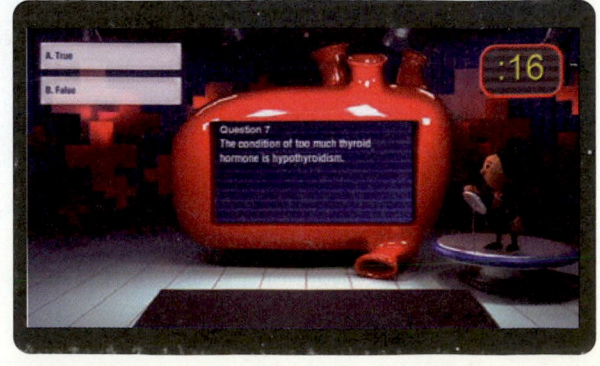

COMPREHENSIVE LEARNING PACKAGE

Medical Language offers a rich array of ancillary materials for instructors and helps infuse a spark in the classroom. The full complement of supplemental teaching materials is available to all qualified instructors from your Pearson sales representative.

Annotated Instructor's Edition (ISBN: 0-13-510657-5)— This is an annotated version of the book that contains every page of the student edition but with margin material to help enrich the instructional experience. It includes:

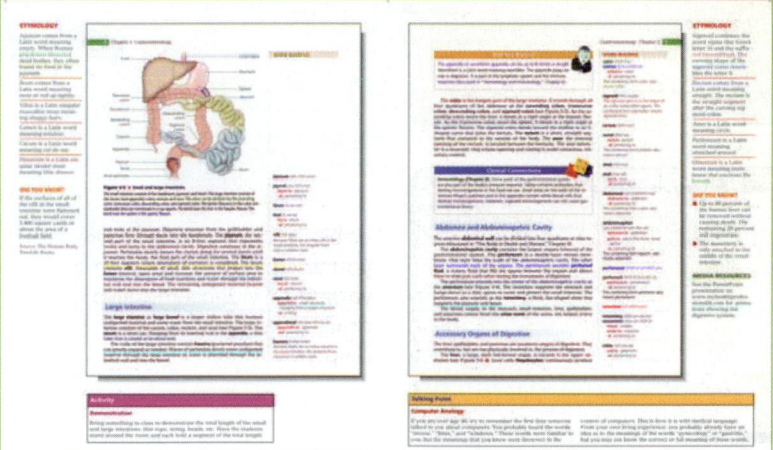

- An array of teaching pearls and tips
- Interesting facts and anecdotes
- Extra content, such as word derivations, not covered in the book
- Answers to each of the self-study questions

Instructor's Resource Manual (ISBN: 0-13-505766-3)—This contains a wealth of material to help faculty plan and manage the course. It includes:

- Articles with useful ideas such as classroom management tips, how to construct test questions, and how to put students at ease on the first day of class.
- Nearly 100 ready-made worksheets which can be used for quizzes or homework assignments.
- A sample course syllabus.

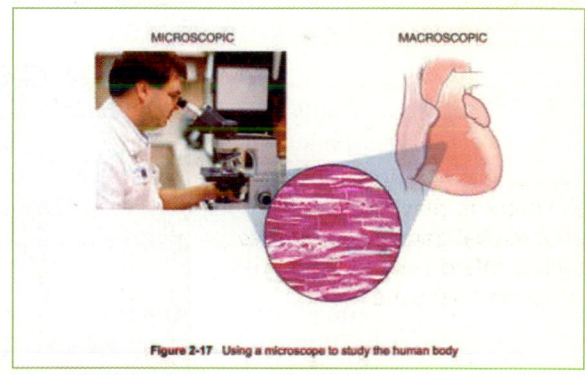

Figure 2-17 Using a microscope to study the human body

Instructor's Resource DVD-ROM (ISBN: 0-13-505805-8)—This disk provides many resources in an electronic format. It includes the following:

- The complete 4,800-question test bank that allows instructors to generate customized exams and quizzes
- A comprehensive, turn-key lecture package in PowerPoint format containing discussion points and a powerful library of images, animations, and videos.
- PowerPoint content to support instructors who are using Personal Response Systems ("clickers").
- A complete image library that includes every photograph and illustration from the textbook.

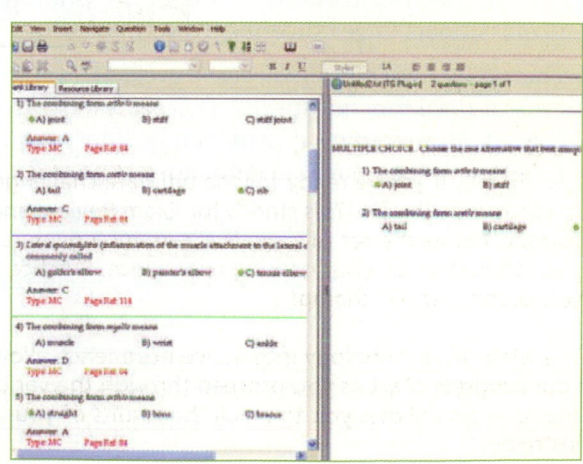

Preface

Something Different

You may have already noticed that there is something different about this book. Perhaps by examining the cover and thumbing through the pages, you have taken note of the abundance of real-world medical images. Maybe you have discovered some of the practice exercises that abound within these pages, many of which place you in the hypothetical role of a healthcare professional. Or perhaps you have already begun exploring the revolutionary student media materials that are rich with highly engaging and interactive activities that add a unique dimension to your learning. As you begin this exciting and important journey into the world of medical language and medicine, we offer you a single promise—that you will soon become immersed in a new, exciting learning experience.

As a soon-to-be healthcare professional, your knowledge, hard work, and interpersonal skills will have a direct impact in health care throughout your career. Therefore, we wish to do everything in our power to help you learn and to empower you as you then affect others with the fruits of your learning. And so, we encourage you to immerse yourself in this book and the rich variety of resources it offers to help you learn medical language.

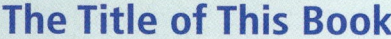

The Title of This Book

Let us start at the beginning by examining the title of this book, *Medical Language.*

Medical

Medicine is the drama of life and death, and few subjects are as compelling, profound, or worthy of study. This book is about real medicine. As you know, real medicine affects real patients—their lives, their families, and their futures. As a healthcare professional, no matter which aspect of patient care you touch, you will have great responsibilities. Therefore, we feel it is our responsibility to provide you with as realistic a view as possible of medicine today. Here are some examples of how we have done this:

- The majority of the images in this book incorporate medical illustrations and photographs that include a diverse array of real people, instead of cartoon-like illustrations. Many of the photographs are of real healthcare professionals in real healthcare settings.

- The chapter review exercises present real medical reports with related critical-thinking questions. There are also exercises where you play the role of the healthcare provider in interpreting a patient's condition and rephrasing it as medical language.

- The student media will immerse you in the virtual world of Medical Terminology Interactive, where you will explore a variety of fun study opportunities. In one of them, you will listen to real doctors dictating real medical sentences for you to interpret.

- Within Medical Terminology Interactive you will find the video library *Real People, Real Medicine,* which was filmed in association with this book to profile a variety of healthcare workers on the job.

Language

A language is a method of communicating and an expression of the people, events, and culture it represents. This book is about medical language. As opposed to simply memorizing vocabulary words, the complete experience that this book offers is the opportunity to embrace the world of medicine, just as if you were learning a foreign language. Like traveling to Tokyo for a year to learn Japanese, the goal here is for you to become immersed in the sights and sounds of the new culture of medicine. This book surrounds you with context that brings the medical words to life.

A Living Language

You will not be a passive reader of this book. Instead, you will be challenged to listen, speak, write, watch, respond, examine, think, and make connections. You should consume this book by writing notes in it and filling in your answers. By being an active participant in your own learning process, the concepts presented here will come alive in vibrant color and full texture. This book is a *living* document about a *living* language. Through the features of this book and the accompanying multimedia resources, you will get a true taste of the world of medicine in *living* color.

You will notice that, unlike most other medical terminology books, the chapters in this book are titled by medical specialties, as well as by body systems. This reflects the real world of medicine. For example, people with skin conditions visit a dermatologist, not an "integumentary system specialist." That's why the related chapter in our book is titled "Dermatology." A patient with heart problems is treated in a hospital's cardiology department and not in a "cardiovascular system department." Our decision to present the chapters of the book in this manner is an example of our commitment to make this book a realistic reflection of actual medicine as practiced in the real world. This distinction from conventional books was tested extensively during development of this book, and we are gratified that instructors and students have overwhelmingly supported and validated this form of presentation.

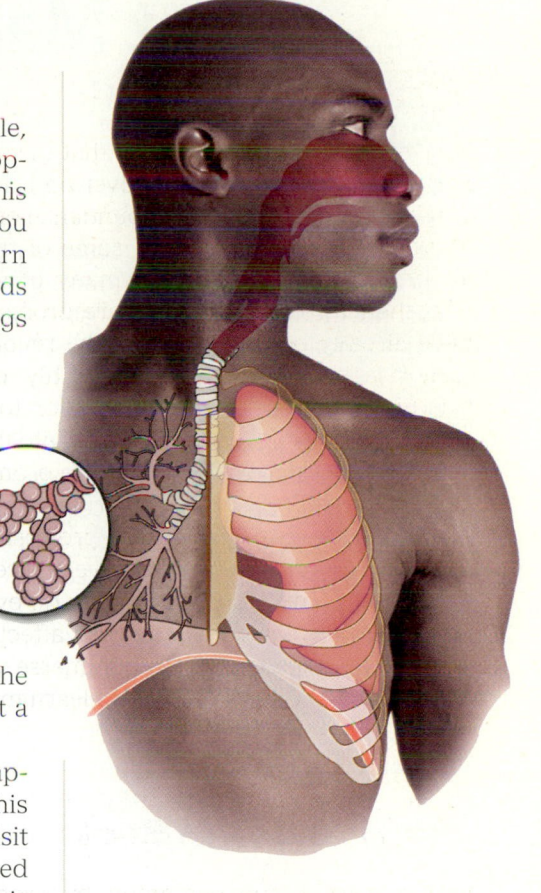

Immerse Yourself!

You are about to begin an interactive learning experience between you, this book, and your instructor—one that will equip you with a vital tool and inspire you to become a true consumer of medical language. The goal of this book is to connect with you, to engage your visual, auditory, and kinesthetic senses, to stimulate you, and to fuel your complete understanding of the topic. So as you engage in the multisensory experience within these pages, remember that we are not encouraging you to merely *discover*, *learn*, *know*, or even *understand*, the information. Instead, we want you to **live it**! So dig in, dive in, and immerse yourself!

What Makes This Book Different

We Listened

In developing this book over the past two editions, we have immersed ourselves in the perspective of you, our readers. We have strived to make **Medical Language** a customer-driven text by aggressively and comprehensively researching the needs and desires of current medical terminology students and instructors. We aimed to guarantee that we were "speaking the same language" as the people who would ultimately be using this book. To this end, we formed a highly qualified development team of 150 reviewers, with a collective 2,250 years of teaching experience, four physician specialists, as well as 11 students across the United States whom we called upon to help steer us toward success.

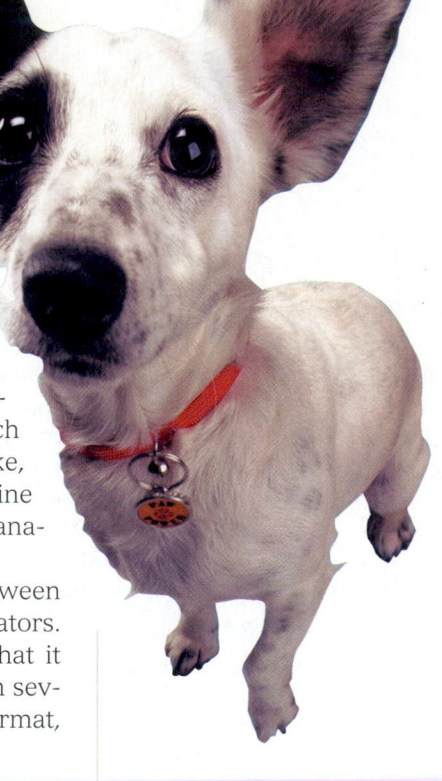

Over the past 7 years we have sat in classrooms, hosted focus groups, and conducted thorough manuscript reviews. We asked for blunt and uncompromising opinions and insights. We also commissioned dozens of detailed reviews from instructors, asking them to analyze and evaluate each draft of the manuscript. They not only told us what they did and didn't like, but they identified, page by page, numerous ways in which we could refine and enhance our key features. Their invaluable feedback was compiled, analyzed, and incorporated throughout **Medical Language,** 2nd edition.

The text you now see is truly the product of a successful partnership between the author, the publisher, and our development team of students and educators. We asked our team to imagine their ideal medical terminology book—what it should include, how it should look. We had the author meet personally with several instructors to discuss the specifics of the book's organization, layout, format, and features. We asked question after question. We listened.

And We Learned

Here are some of the recommendations that we heard from our team and responded to as we created this book:

- **Design** Students and instructors alike told us they wanted an appealing, uncluttered design with lots of rich images and enough white space to allow for notetaking.

- **Exercises** Both students and instructors suggested that we provide a greater quantity and variety of exercises than any other book, thus providing maximum opportunities to reinforce learning.

- **Illustrations** Students and instructors alike suggested that we display colorful and interesting illustrations as large as possible on the page, with opportunities to label those images as practice opportunities.

- **Special Boxed Features** Students asked for highlighted boxes that would help break up the reading and also provide them with opportunities to learn something new or interesting, thereby providing additional context.

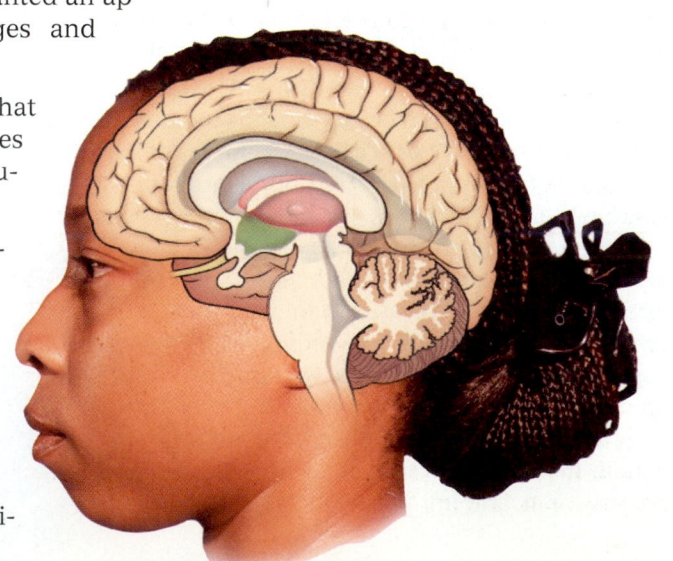

- **Medical Specialties Approach** A substantial majority (75%) of instructors told us that they prefer a medical specialties approach, rather than just an anatomical body systems organization.

- **Focus on Word Building** Another substantial majority of instructors (over 70%) asked for a focus on word building and suggested that we present the analysis of combining forms, suffixes, and prefixes throughout each chapter and not simply at the end of each chapter or in isolated boxes.

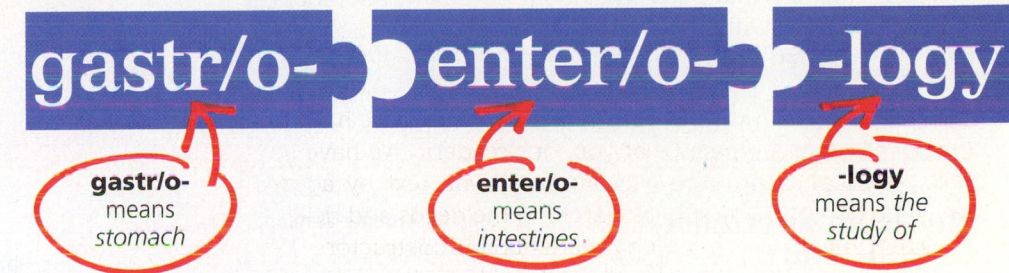

gastr/o- means *stomach*

enter/o- means *intestines*

-logy means *the study of*

- **Medical Report Activities** Instructors suggested that we include an activity in each chapter that challenges students to analyze an actual medical report.

- **Lecture Support Materials** Instructors told us about the increased challenge of creating interesting, dynamic lectures and suggested that we create a fully loaded PowerPoint presentation system that is complete with ready-to-use lectures that include a multitude of illustrations and photographs, plus animations and real-world videos.

- **Tools for Testing** Instructors asked for a complete testing package that is customizable to fit their needs. Additionally, they asked for these test items to be available in online course formats.

A Commitment to Accuracy

As part of our respect for real medicine, and the importance of getting it right the first time, we have made a commitment to accuracy. It was important to us to attain the highest level of accuracy possible throughout this educational package in order to match the requirement for precision in today's healthcare environment. The author draws on her 30 years of experience as a nurse, medical transcriptionist, health information manager, and educator to provide accurate and complete information throughout. Our thorough manuscript review process charged members of our development team to read every page, every test question, and every vocabulary word. No less than 12 content experts have read each chapter for accuracy and analyzed every bit of content that comprises the ancillary resources. We have also engaged the technical editing services of four physician specialists who have carefully reviewed the chapters that correspond to their respective practices.

While our intent and actions have been directed at creating an error-free text, it is still possible for some mistakes to occur. Pearson takes this issue seriously and therefore welcomes any and all feedback that you can provide along the lines of helping us enhance the accuracy of this text. If you identify any errors that need to be corrected in a subsequent printing, please send them to: Pearson Health Science Editorial, Medical Terminology Corrections, 1 Lake Street, Upper Saddle River, NJ 07458.

Our Development Team

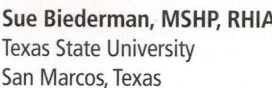

We can truly say that each individual on our development team has infused this book with ideas, vision, and passion for medical language. Our team crafted the blueprints for this book and has contributed to the birth of a landmark educational tool. Their influence will continue to have an impact for decades to come. Let us introduce the members of our team.

Physician Specialist Consultants

Stephen Caldwell, MD
Director of Hepatology
Digestive Health Center of Excellence
Charlottesville, Virginia

John H. Dirckx, MD
Former Medical Director
University of Dayton
Student Health Center
Dayton, Ohio

Joseph Gibbons, MD
Internal Medicine Physician
Centennial Medical Group
Elkridge, Maryland

James Michelson, MD
Professor of Orthopedic Surgery
George Washington University School of Medicine
Washington, D.C.

Instructional and Editorial Consultant

James F. Allen, Jr., RN, BSN, MBA/HCM, JD
Lansing Community College
Lansing, Michigan

Expert Accuracy Reviewer

Duane A. Dreyer, PhD
Miller-Motte College
Cary, North Carolina

Ancillary Content Providers

James F. Allen, Jr., RN, BSN, MBA/HCM, JD
Lansing Community College
Lansing, Michigan

Michael Battaglia, MS, Ed
Greenville Technical College
Greenville, South Carolina

Dale Brewer, BS, MEd, CMA, (AAMA)
Pensacola Junior College
Pensacola, Florida

Angela M. Corio, PT, MPT
Carolinas Rehabilitation
Charlotte, North Carolina

Jean M. Krueger-Watson, PhD
Clark College
Vancouver, Washington

Garnet Tomich, BA
San Diego, California

Katherine Twomey, MLS
Greenville Technical College
Greenville, South Carolina

Manuscript Reviewers
(*Reviewer conference attendee)

Betsy Adams, AAS, BS, MSBE
Alamance Community College
Graham, North Carolina

Denise M. Abrams, PT, MASS
SUNY Broome Community College
Appalachian, New York

Mercedes Alafriz-Gordon, BS
High Tech Institute
Phoenix, Arizona

Diana Alagna, RN, AHI, CPT
Branford Hall Career Institute
Southington, Connecticut

Jana Allen, BS, MT*
Volunteer State Community College
Gallatin, Tennessee

Ellen Anderson, RHIA
College of Lake County
Northfield, Illinois

Judy Anderson, MEd
Coastal Carolina Community College
Jacksonville, North Carolina

Wendy Anderson
MTI College
Sacramento, California

Lori Andreucci, MEd, CMT, CMA
Gateway Technical College
Racine, Wisconsin

Debbie Bedford, CMA, AAS
North Seattle Community College
Seattle, Washington

Tricia Berry, OTR/L
Hamilton College
Urbandale, Iowa

Sue Biederman, MSHP, RHIA
Texas State University
San Marcos, Texas

Richard Boan, BS, MS, PhD
Midlands Technical College
Columbia, South Carolina

Jennifer Boles, MSN, RN, NCSN
Cincinnati State Technical and Community College
Cincinnati, Ohio

Julie E. Boles, MS, RHIA
Ithaca College
Ithaca, New York

Annie M. Boster, PT
Bishop State Community College
Mobile, Alabama

Susan A. Boulden, RN
Mt. Hood Community College
Aloha, Oregon

Beth Braun, MA, PhD
Truman College
Chicago, Illinois

Shannon Bruley, BAS, AEMT-IC
Henry Ford Community College
Dearborn, Michigan

Juanita R. Bryant, CMA-A/C
Sierra College
Penn Valley, California

Thomas Bubar, BA, MS
Erie Community College
Williamsville, New York

Susan Buboltz, RN, MS, CMA
Madison Area Technical College
Madison, Wisconsin

Patricia Bufalino, MA, MN, RN, FNP
Riverside Community College
Moreno Valley, California

Mary Butler, BS
Collin County Community College
McKinney, Texas

Toni Cade, MBA, RHIA, CCS, FAHIMA
University of Louisiana at Lafayette
Lafayette, Louisiana

Cara L. Carreon, BS, RRT, CMA, CPC
Ivy Tech Community College
Lafayette, Indiana

Rafael Castilla, MD
Ho Ho Kus School
Ramsey, New Jersey

Julia I. Chapman, BS
Stark State College of Technology
North Canton, Ohio

Kim Christmon, BS, RRT
Volunteer State Community College
Gallatin, Tennessee

Paula-Beth Ciolek
National College of Business and Technology
Richmond, Kentucky

Deresa Claybrook, MS, RHIT
Oklahoma City Community College
Oklahoma City, Oklahoma

Mike Cochran, BA, RT(R)(CT), ARRT, VSRT, SWDSRT
Southwest Virginia Community College
Richlands, Virginia

Christine Cole, CCA
Williston State College
Williston, North Dakota

Ronald Coleman, EdD
Volunteer State Community College
Gallatin, Tennessee

Bonnie Crist
Harrison College
Indianapolis, Indiana

Cathleen Currie, RN, BS
College of Southern Idaho
Twin Falls, Idaho

Denise J. DeDeaux, AAS, BS, MBA*
Fayetteville Technical Community College
Fayetteville, North Carolina

Anita Denson, BS, CMA
National College of Business and Technology
Danville, Kentucky

Susan D. Dooley, CMT*
Seminole Community College
Sorrento, Florida

Vickie Findley, MPA, RHIA
Fairmont State College
Fairmont, West Virginia

Kathie Folsom, MS, BSN, RN
Skagit Valley College—Whidbley Island Campus
Oak Harbor, Washington

Joyce Foster
State Fair Community College
Sedalia, Missouri

Elaine Garcia, RHIT
Spokane Community College
Spokane, Washington

Suzanne B. Garrett, MSA, RHIA
Central Florida Community College
Ocala, Florida

Cheryl Gates, RN, MSN, PHN
Cerro Coso Community College
Ridgecrest, California

Barbara E. Geary, RN, MA
North Seattle Community College
Seattle, Washington

Paige Gebhardt, RMT
Sussex County Community College
Newton, New Jersey

Laura Ristrom Goodman, MSSW
Pima Medical Institute
Tucson, Arizona

Patricia Goshorn, MA, RN, CMA-AC
Cosumnes River College
Sacramento, California

Debra Griffin, RN, BSN
Tidewater Community College
Virginia Beach, Virginia

Dawn Guzicki, RN
Detroit Business Institute—Downriver
Riverview, Michigan

Paula Hagstrom, MM, RHIA
Ferris State University
Big Rapids, Michigan

Dotty Hall, RN, MSN, CST
Ivy Tech Community College
Lafayette, Indiana

Karen Hardney, MSEd, RT
Chicago State University
Chicago, Illinois

Marie Hattabaugh, RT(R)(M)
Pensacola Junior College
Pensacola, Florida

Barbara L. Henry, RN, BSN
Gateway Technical College
Racine, Wisconsin

Forrest Heredia
Pima Medical Institute
Tucson, Arizona

Cathy Hess, RHIA
Texas State University
San Marcos, Texas

Dori L. Hess, MS, LMT, BS
Stark State College of Technology
Canton, Ohio

Jan C. Hess, MA
Metropolitan Community College
Omaha, Nebraska

Denise M. Hightower, RHIA
Cape Fear Community College
Wilmington, North Carolina

Beulah A. Hofmann, RN, MSN, CMA
Ivy Tech Community College
Greencastle, Indiana

Valentina Holder, MA.Ed, RHIA
Pitt Community College
Winterville, North Carolina

James E. Hudacek, MSEd*
Loraine County Community College
Amherst, Ohio

Pamela S. Huber, MS, MT(ASCP)
Erie Community College
Williamsville, New York

Bud W. Hunton, MA, RT (R) (QM)
Sinclair Community College
Dayton, Ohio

Karen Jackson, NR-CMA
Remington College
Garland, Texas

Donna Jimison RN, MSN
Cuyahoga Community College
Parma, Ohio

Tim Jones, MA
Oklahoma City Community College
Oklahoma City, Oklahoma

Kathleen Kearney, BS, MEd, EMT-P
Kent State University
Kent, Ohio

Cathy Kelley-Arney, CMA, MLTC, BSHS, AS
National College of Business and Technology
Bluefield, Virginia

Winifred Khalil, RN, MS
San Diego Mesa College
San Diego, California

Heather Kies, MHA
Goodwin College
East Hartford, Connecticut

Jan Klawitter, CMA (AAMA), CPC
San Joaquin Valley College
Bakersfield, California

Marsha Lalley, BSM, MSM
Minneapolis Community and Technical College
Minneapolis, Minnesota

Joyce Lammers, PT, MHS, PCS
University of Findlay
Findlay, Ohio

Carol A. Lehman, ART
Hocking College
Nelsonville, Ohio

Sandra Lehrke, MS, RN
Anoka Technical Community College
Anoka, Minnesota

Randall M. Levin, FACEP
Sanford Brown College
Milwaukee, Wisconsin

Maria Teresa Lopez-Hill, MS
Laredo Community College
Laredo, Texas
Bow Valley College
Calgary, Alberta
Collin County Community College
McKinney, Texas

Michelle Lovings, BA
Missouri College
Brentwood, Missouri

Carol Loyd, MSN, RN
University of Arkansas Community College
Morrilton, Arkansas

Patricia McLane, RHIA, MA
Henry Ford Community College
Dearborn, Michigan

Michael C. McMinn, MA, RRT
Mott Community College
Flint, Michigan

Aimee Michaelis
Pima Medical Institute
Denver, Colorado

Michelle G. Miller, M, CMA, COMT
Lakeland Community College
Kirtland, Ohio

Ann Minks, FAAMT
Lake Washington Technical College
Kirkland, Washington

Suzanne Moe, RN
Northwest Technical College
Bemidji, Minnesota

Barbara S. Moffet, PhD, RN
Southeastern Louisiana University
Hammond, Louisiana

Debby Montone, BS, RN, CCS-P, RCVT
Eastwick College/Ho Ho Kus Schools
Ramsey, New Jersey

Karen Myers, CPC
Pierce College Puyallup
Puyallup, Washington

Gloria Newton, MA-ED
Shasta College
Redding, California

Erin Nixon, RN
Bakersfield College
Bakersfield, California

Alice M. Noblin, MBA, RHIA, CCS, LHRM
University of Central Florida
Orlando, Florida

Wendy Oguz, AS, BA
National College
Indianapolis, Indiana

Evie O'Nan, RMA
National College
Florence, Kentucky

Kerry Openshaw, PhD
Bemidji State University
Bemidji, Minnesotta

Mirella G. Pardee, MSN, RN
University of Toledo
Toledo, Ohio

Sherry Pearsall, MSN
Bryant & Stratton College
Liverpool, New York

Tina Peer, MS, RN
The College of Southern Idaho
Twin Falls, Idaho

Tammie C. Petersen, RNC-OB, BSN
Austin Community College
Austin, Texas

Susan Prion, EdD, RN
University of San Francisco
San Francisco, California

Mary Rahr, MS, RN, CMA
Northeast Wisconsin Technical College
Madison, Wisconsin

Edilberto A. Raynes, MD
Tennessee State University
Nashville, Tennessee

Deward Reece, DC
Sanford Brown College
Milwaukee, Wisconsin

Joy Renfro, EdD, RHIA, CMA, CCS-P, CPC
Eastern Kentucky University
Richmond, Kentucky

Sheila G. Rockoff, EdD, MSN, BSN, AS, RN
Santa Ana College
Santa Ana, California

Mary Sayles, RN, MSN
Sierra College—Nevada County Campus
Rocklin, California

Jody E. Scheller, MS, RHIA
Schoolcraft College
Garden City, Michigan

Patricia Schrull, MSN, MBA, MEd, RN
Lorain County Community College
Elyria, Ohio

Theresa R. Schuldt, MEd, HT/HTL (ASCP)
Rose State College
Midwest City, Oklahoma

Jan Sesser, BS, RMA (AMT), CMA
High Tech Institute
Phoenix, Arizona

Julie A. Shellenbarger, MBA, RHIA
University of Northwestern Ohio
Lima, Ohio

Donna Sue Shellman, MA, CPC
Gaston College
Dallas, North Carolina

Karin Sherrill, BSN
Mesa Community College
Gilbert, Arizona

Erin Sitterley
North Seattle Community College
Seattle, Washington

Tim J. Skaife, RT(R), MA
National Park Community College
Hot Springs, Arizona

Lynn G. Slack, CMA
ICM School of Business and Medical Careers
Pittsburgh, Pennsylvania

Ellie Smith, RN, MSN
Cuesta College
San Luis Obispo, California

Sherman K. Sowby, PhD, CHES
California State University—Fresno
Fresno, California

Darla K. Sparacino, MEd, RHIA
Arkansas Tech University
Russelville, Arkansas

Carolyn Stariha, BS, RHIA
Houston Community College—Coleman Campus
Houston, Texas

Kathy Stau, CPhT
Medix School
Smyrna, Georgia

Twila Sterling-Guillory, RN, MSN
McNeese State University
Lake Charles, Louisiana

Deb Stockberger, MSN, RN
North Iowa Community College
Mason City, Iowa

Paula L. Stoltz, CMT-F
Medical Transcription Education Center
Fairlawn, Ohio

Diane Swift
State Fair Community College
Sedalia, Missouri

J. David Taylor, PhD, PT, CSCS
University of Central Arkansas
Conway, Arkansas

Sylvia Taylor, CMA, CPCA
Cleveland State Community College
Cleveland, Tennessee

Jean Ternus, RN, MS
Kansas City Community College
Kansas City, Kansas

Cindy B. Thompson, BSRT, MA*
Alamance Community College
Graham, North Carolina

Lenette Thompson, CST
Piedmont Technical College
Greenwood, South Carolina

Margaret A. Tiemann, RN, BS
St. Charles Community College
Cottleville, Missouri

Mary Jane Tremethick, PhD, RN, CHES
Northern Michigan University
Marquette, Michigan

Valeria D. Truitt, BS, MAEd
Craven Community College
New Bern, North Carolina

Christine Tufts-Maher, MS, RHIA
Seminole Community College
Altamonte Springs, Florida

Pam Ventgen, CMA (AAMA), CCS-P, CPC, CPC-I
University of Alaska Anchorage
Anchorage, Alaska

Patricia Von Knorring
Tacoma Community College
Gig Harbor, Washington

Mary Warren-Oliver, BA
Gibbs College
Vienna, Virginia

Kristen Waterstram-Rich, MS, CNMT
Rochester Institute of Technology
Rochester, New York

Kim Webb, RN, MN
Northern Oklahoma College
Tonkawa, Oklahoma

Richard Weidman, RHIA, CCS-P
Tacoma Community College
Tacoma, Washington

Bonnie Welniak, RN, MSN
Monroe County Community College
Monroe, Michigan

Connie Werner, MS, RHIA
York College of Pennsylvania
York, Pennsylvania

Victoria Lee Wetle, RN, EdD
Chemeketa Community College
Salem, Oregon

David J. White, MA, MLIS
Baylor University
Waco, Texas

Jay W. Wilborn, MEd, MT(ASCP)
National Park Community College
Hot Springs, Arkansas

Tammy L. Wilder, RN, MSN, CMSRN
Ivy Tech Community College
Evansville, Indiana

Scott Zimmer, MS
Metropolitan Community College
Omaha, Nebraska

Focus Group Participants

Kim Anthony Aaronson, BS, DC
Harry S. Truman College
Chicago, Illinois
Harold Washington College
Chicago, Illinois

Kendra J. Allen, LPN
Ohio Institute of Health Careers
Columbus, Ohio

Delena Kay Austin, BTIS, CMA
Macomb Community College
Clinton Township, Michigan

Molly Baxter
Baker College—Port Huron
Port Huron, Michigan

Joan Berry, RN, MSN, CNS
Lansing Community College
Lansing, Michigan

Kenneth Bretl, MA, RRT
College of DuPage
Glen Ellyn, Illinois

Carole Bretscher
Southwestern College
Bellbrook, Ohio

Adrienne L. Carter, MEd, NRMA
Riverside Community College
Moreno Valley, California

Mary Dudash-White, MA, RHIA, CCS
Sinclair Community College
Dayton, Ohio

Cathy Flite, MEd, RHIA
Temple University
Philadelphia, Pennsylvania

Sherry Gamble, RN, CNS, MSN, CNOR
University of Akron
Akron, Ohio

Mary Garcia, BA, AD, RN
Northwestern Business College
Northeastern Illinois University
Truman College
Chicago, Illinois

Joyce Garozzo, MS, RHIA, CCS
Community College of Philadelphia
Philadelphia, Pennsylvania

Patsy Gehring, PhD, RN, CS
Lakeland Community College
Kirkland, Ohio

Michelle Heller, CMA, RMA
Ohio Institute of Health Careers
Columbus, Ohio

Janet Hossli
Northwestern Business College
Chicago, Illinois

Trudi James-Parks, RT, BS,
Lorain County Community College
Elyria, Ohio

Sherry L. Jones, RN, ASN
Western School of Health and Business
Community College of Allegheny County
Pittsburgh, Pennsylvania

Esther H. Kim
Chicago State University
Chicago, Illinois

Richelle S. Laipply, PhD, CMA
University of Akron
Akron, Ohio

Andrea M. Lane, CMA-C, BAS RN, MS
Brookdale Community College
Lincroft, New Jersey

Mary Lou Liebal, BS, RTR, MA
Cuyahoga Community College
Cleveland, Ohio

Stacey Long, BS
Miami Jacobs Career College
Dayton, Ohio

Anne Loochtan, MEd
Columbus State Community College
Cincinnati, Ohio

Anne M. Lunde, BS, CMT
Waubonsee Community College
Sugar Grove, Illinois

Janice Manning, MA, PCP
Baker College
Jackson, Michigan

Sandy Marks, RN, MS(HCA)
Cerritos College
Norwalk, California

Kathleen Masters, MS, RN
Monroe County Community College
Monroe, Michigan

Mary Morgan, MS, CNMT
Columbus State Community College
Columbus, Ohio

Andrew Muniz, OT, BBA, MBA
Baker College
Auburn Hills, Michigan

Michael Murphy, AAS, CMA, CLP
Berdan Institute
Union, New Jersey

Stephen Nardozzi, BA
SUNY- Westchester Community College
Valhalla, New York

Ruth Ann O'Brien, MHA, RRT
Miami Jacobs Career College
Dayton, Ohio

Donna Schnepp, MHA, RHIA
Moraine Valley Community College
Palos Hills, Illinois

Ann M. Smith, MS
Joliet Junior College
Joliet, Illinois

Mark Velderrain
Cerritos College
Norwalk, California

Barbara Wiggins, MT(ASCP)
Delaware Technical & Community College
Georgetown, Delaware

Gail S. Williams, Ph.D., MT(ASCP)SBB, CLS(NCA)
Northern Illinois University
DeKalb, Illinois

Karen Wright, RHIA, MHA
Hocking College
Nelsonville, Ohio

Student Advisors

Tobi Burch
Community College of Philadelphia
Philadelphia, Pennsylvania

Calvin Byrd
Temple University
Philadelphia, Pennsylvania

Kimberly Clark
Community College of Philadelphia
Philadelphia, Pennsylvania

Susan DiMaria
Brookdale Community College
Lincroft, New Jersey

Avelina Elam
Thomas Jefferson University
Philadelphia, Pennsylvania

Michael Flores
Berdan Institute
Union, New Jersey

Frederick Herbert
Temple University
Philadelphia, Pennsylvania

Brenda Merlino
Thomas Jefferson University
Philadelphia, Pennsylvania

Megan Milos
Ocean County College
Toms River, New Jersey

Payam Mohadjeri
Temple University
Philadelphia, Pennsylvania

Monica Narang
Westchester Community College
Valhalla, New York

About the Author

Susan M. Turley, MA (Educ), BSN, RN, RHIT, CMT, is an adjunct professor in the School of Health Professions, Wellness, and Physical Education at Anne Arundel Community College in Arnold, Maryland, where she has taught courses in medical terminology, disease processes, and medical transcription. In the past, she was instrumental in gaining initial accreditation for the college's medical assisting program and also taught courses in pharmacology and medical office procedures. She is also currently the director of curriculum development and accreditation for the International Institute of Original Medicine in Maryland.

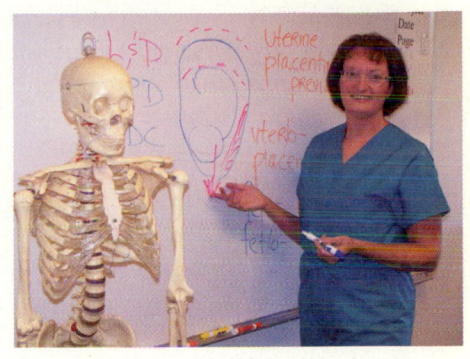

As a healthcare professional, Susan has worked in a variety of healthcare settings over the past 30 years: acute care, long-term care, physicians' offices, and managed care. She has held positions as an intensive care nurse, plasmapheresis nurse, infection control officer, medical transcriptionist, medical grant writer, manager of the Medic Alert national difficult airway database, medical record coder, director of education, and director of quality management and corporate compliance.

Susan is the author of *Understanding Pharmacology for Health Professionals, 4th edition* (Pearson, 2010), *Medical Language STAT!* with James F. Allen, Jr., RN, BSN, MBA/HCM, JD (Pearson, 2009), and of more than 40 articles published in medical transcription and health information management journals. She is a codeveloper of *The SUM Program for Medical Transcription Training* and reference books for Health Professions Institute. With a physician coauthor, she has written two nationally funded grants and a chapter in a physician's anesthesiology textbook.

She has been a guest speaker at national seminars for accreditation of utilization management programs, medical transcription teacher training, and health information management certification exam review.

Susan holds a Master of Arts degree in adult education from Norwich University in Vermont, a Bachelor of Science degree in nursing from the Pennsylvania State University, state licensure as an RN, as well as national certification in medical transcription from the Association for Healthcare Documentation Integrity (AHDI) and national certification in health information management from the American Health Information Management Association (AHIMA).

About the Illustrator

The illustrations throughout this book were carefully coordinated through a close collaborative effort between the author and artist. Every figure was custom developed specifically for this book, and refined to be precise, unique, and fresh. From a pedagogical point of view, it was important that all of the art be consistent throughout, rather than presenting a conglomeration of styles and levels of detail.

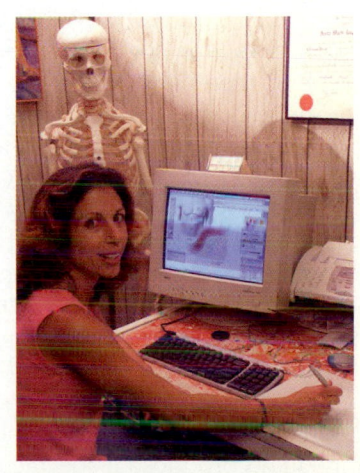

Anita Impagliazzo is a medical illustrator and designer in Charlottesville, Virginia. A graduate of the University of Virginia, she went on to complete the Biomedical Illustration Graduate Program at the University of Texas Southwestern Medical Center at Dallas and spent several years specializing in illustrating for medical malpractice litigation. She is currently self-employed, creating artwork for researchers and physicians at the University of Virginia Health System, science and surgical textbooks, medical journals, the courtroom, and presentations. She is a member of the Association of Medical Illustrators and has received several awards in its annual juried salons. She never tires of using medical language to learn new things about the human body: how it works, how it fails, how it is fixed, and how the fixing fails.

Acknowledgments

My utmost thanks go to Mark Cohen, Pearson Health Science Editor in Chief and my editor for **Medical Language**, 2nd edition. We have worked together on various projects since 1997, and his responsiveness, creative insights, and professionalism make him a delight to work with. His vision of this book was one with mine, but he also envisioned the next level of excellence and continually moved the book toward that goal. His support and enthusiasm have been constant and invaluable as he expertly managed a complexity of details and guided this book from idea to reality.

My gratitude and thanks go to Anita Impagliazzo, my medical illustrator. She embraced much more than her original role and quickly became a creative collaborator and advisor for both editions. She is a wonderfully talented medical illustrator whose efforts made this book medically accurate, artistically unique, and without equal. My thanks, too, to the many models who appear in the real-life photographs throughout the book.

My sincere thanks go to Cathy Wein, my development editor. She coordinated communication, manuscript copyediting review, and deadlines for everyone involved. She embraced both editions, and they would never have been completed without her expert, professional, all-encompassing, and timely editorial assistance and personal support.

My special thanks go to Pearson design directors Mary Siener and Maria Guglielmo. Their inspired work created a strikingly beautiful textbook.

Special thanks to Melissa Kerian, Managing Development Editor at Pearson, who has been involved in so many details—small and large. She directed the entire editorial development and quality management program for each of the ancillary materials that accompany this textbook. Instructors who appreciate complete, high-quality supplemental materials have her to thank for her tireless, precise, and impassioned work.

Special thanks go to Nicole Ragonese, Assistant Editor at Pearson, who coordinated a complex review program for the second edition, including an in-depth accuracy evaluation.

Thanks to Pearson Professional & Careers President and CEO Tim Bozik, Division Presidents Robin Baliszewski and Leah Jewell, and Vice President/Publisher Julie Alexander. Their understanding of and support for my vision allowed the entire team to put forth maximum effort toward a landmark second edition.

My thanks goes to Katrin Beacom, my marketing manager, for embracing the concept of developing a customer-driven textbook. She was committed to listening to the needs of the market and then consulting with me to help me shape the textbook around those needs.

My thanks go to the talented team at Laserwords, led by Kate Boilard, Project Manager, who oversaw the extensive editing, layout, and indexing of the second edition. In light of the complexity of the book, I especially appreciated her professionalism, flexibility, creative insights, and can-do approach.

Thanks to Patrick Walsh and Christina Zingone, who managed the complete production of the second edition. They were masters at handling the complex and ever-evolving details of this huge project while maintaining a close watch over budgets and schedules.

My thanks go to the Pearson media team lead by Amy Peltier that designed and produced a spectacular array of learning applications to support my textbook.

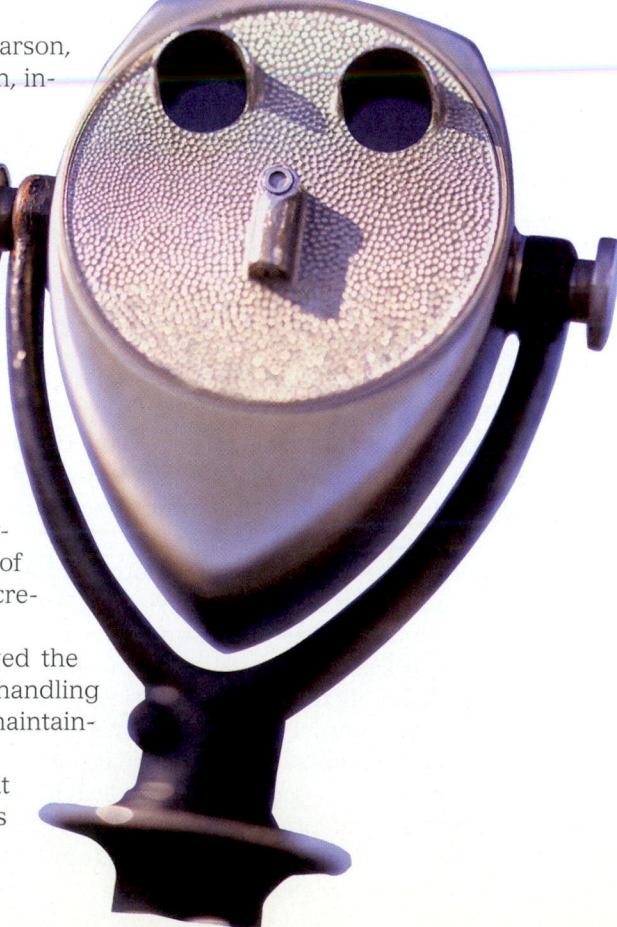

Thanks to Meg and Glenn Turner and their team at Burrston House, who got the first edition started with an extensive market development program that included focus groups, reviews, and detailed analyses that helped me to truly understand our customers' needs.

My thanks go to Sally Pitman of Health Professions Institute for granting permission for using authentic medical dictation from *The SUM Program for Medical Transcription Training* as exercises.

Thanks to the many classes of students who motivated me to continually research and present medical language clearly and thoroughly. It was their warm response to my teaching methods and materials that encouraged me to keep improving.

My thanks go to the many teachers and practitioners who have overwhelmingly validated my efforts to write about medical language with a uniquely interesting, lively, and fresh approach. Each and every person listed on pages xviii–xxii played an important role in the development of this textbook, and I hope they share my sense of pride in this second edition.

CONTENTS

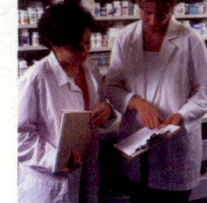
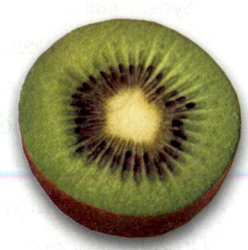
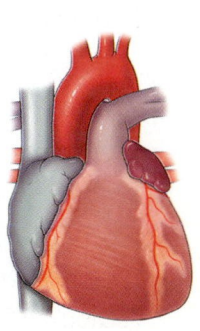

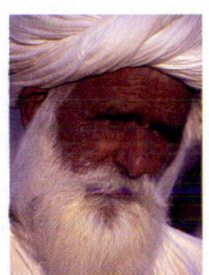
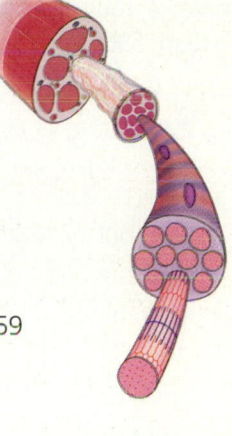
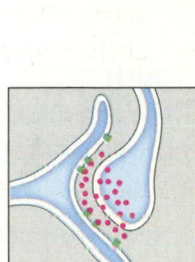
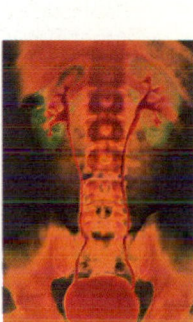

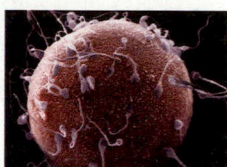

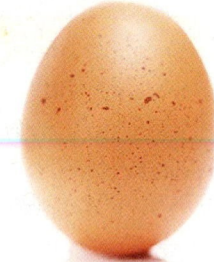

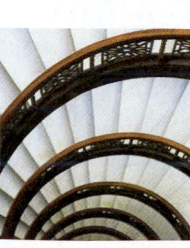

PART III   OTHER MEDICAL SPECIALTIES 848

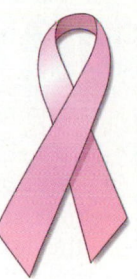

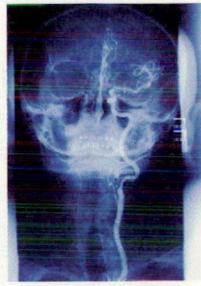

Did You Know?

Two bonus chapters are available online. Go to www.myhealthprofessionskit.com, select Medical Terminology and follow the log-in instructions for this book. Once you're inside the website, find bonus chapters on Dentistry and Dietetics inside the Medical Bag.

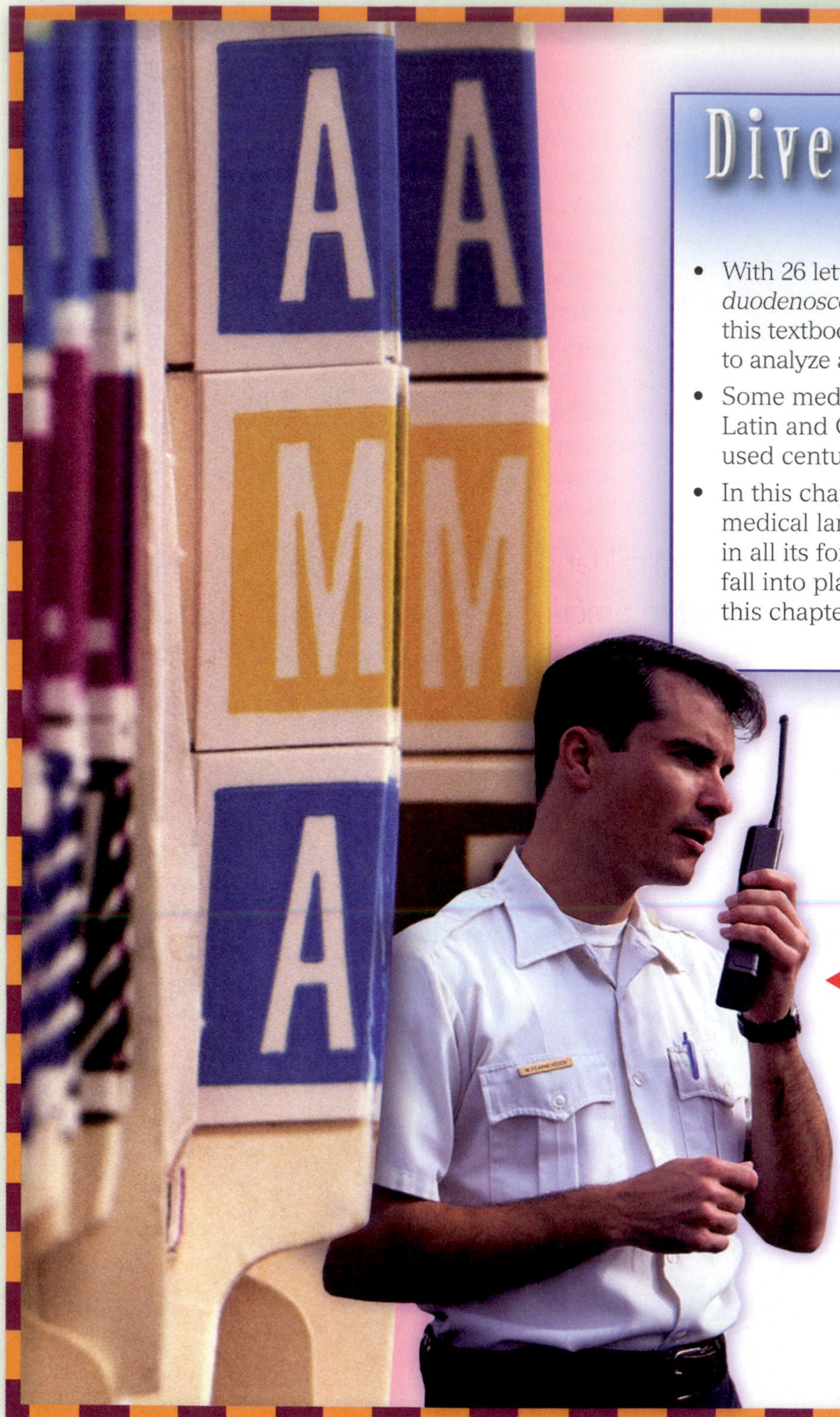

Dive In!

- With 26 letters, *esophagogastro-duodenoscopy* is the longest word in this textbook, but soon you'll be able to analyze and understand it.
- Some medical words are actual Latin and Greek words that were used centuries ago.
- In this chapter you'll explore medical language communication in all its forms. The pieces will all fall into place when you master this chapter!

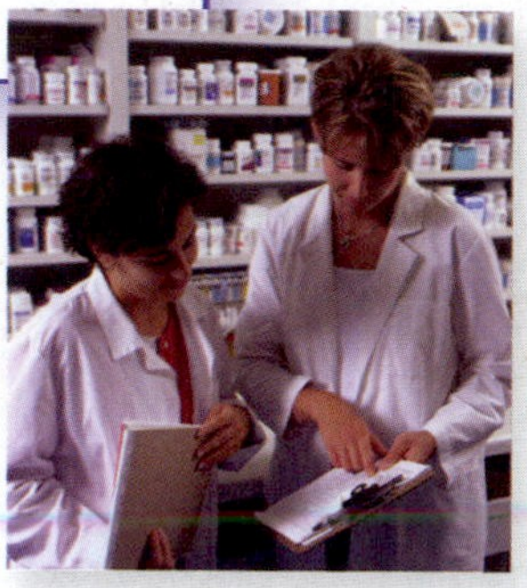

◀ Medical language is the key to a successful career in health care. If you want to "walk the walk," then you have to "talk the talk" of medical language.

Medicine Through HISTORY

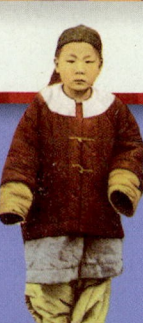

475 B.C.

The Chinese write a textbook on acupuncture and the treatment of disease

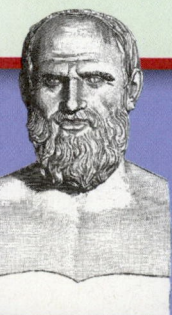

377 B.C.

Hippocrates is born, a Greek physician and the father of modern medicine

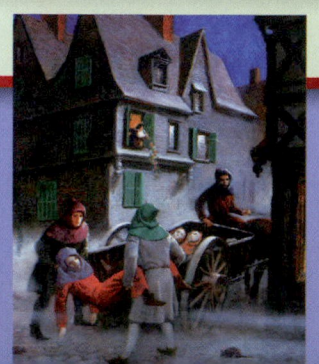

1347

The Black Death plague ravages Europe, killing one third of the population. It is transmitted by fleas carried by black rats

1

The Structure of Medical Language

Medical language is the framework on which the practice of medicine is built. Healthcare professionals use medical language every day to communicate with each other.

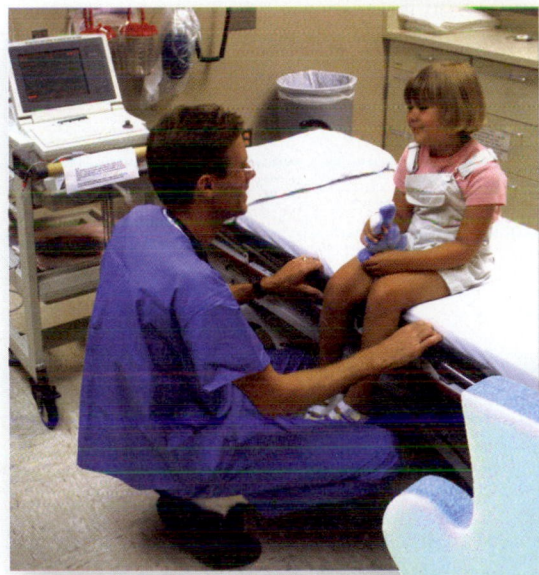

▶ Medical words are like puzzles, and their word parts are like the pieces. If you put the pieces together correctly, you can understand the meaning of the medical word.

1500

The Chinese invent the toothbrush

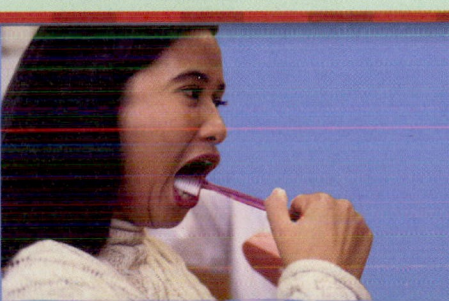

1529

French physician Ambroïse Paré devises amputation to save lives and also creates the first artificial leg. He is shown here working with wounded soldiers on the battlefield

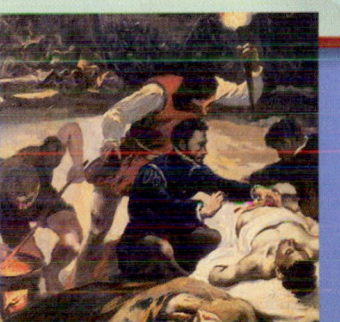

Measure Your Progress: Learning Objectives

After you study this chapter, you should be able to

1. Identify the five skills of medical language communication.

2. Describe the origins of medical language.

3. Recognize common Latin and Greek singular nouns and form their plurals.

4. Describe characteristics of combining forms, suffixes, and prefixes.

5. Give the medical meaning of common word parts.

6. Build medical words from word parts and divide medical words into word parts.

7. Spell and pronounce common medical words.

8. Describe the format and contents of common medical documents.

9. Dive deeper into the structure of medical language by reviewing the activities at the end of this chapter and online at Medical Terminology Interactive.

Welcome to Medical Language

You are about to begin the study of medical language. This will involve time and effort on your part. But what can you expect in return? What benefits come from learning medical language? To find out, read Scenario 1 (that follows) and contrast it with Scenario 2.

Scenario 1

Imagine that you just made an important decision that will affect the rest of your life: You decided to move to a foreign country. You are excited and anxious to get going! When you arrive, you are thrilled to be in this new, exotic environment. It is fascinating to you! There are so many new sights and sounds. You want to embrace this new culture and become part of it, but your first attempts at interacting are awkward because you do not know the language. You can't seem to make anyone understand you. All around you, people are engaged in interesting activities and important conversations, but you can't join in because you can't understand them. You feel confused and helpless. Your future in this country now seems uncertain, and you wonder if you will ever be anything more than just a spectator here. What went wrong?

Scenario 2

Imagine that you just made an important decision that will affect the rest of your life: You decided to pursue a career in the healthcare field. You are excited and anxious to get going! When you walk into a physician's office, clinic, or hospital, you are thrilled to be in this new, fast-paced, exotic environment. It is fascinating to you! There are so many new sights and sounds. You want to embrace the medical culture and become part of it. Your first attempts at interacting with other healthcare professionals are successful because you know medical language. Immediately, you are immersed in interesting medical activities and important conversations, and you understand what is going on. You feel excited and empowered! Your future in the healthcare field is certain because you took the time to study medical language.

Healthcare professionals know that there is no substitute for a thorough, working knowledge of medical language (see Figure 1-1 ■). Medical language is the language of the healthcare profession, and medical words are the tools of the trade! Learning medical language is your key to a successful career in the healthcare field.

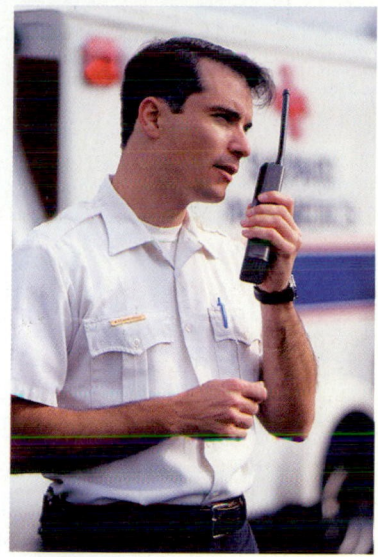

Figure 1-1 ■ Medical language.

This paramedic is using medical language to communicate with healthcare professionals in the emergency department and describe the condition of a patient in the ambulance. How important do you think it is for this paramedic to have a thorough, working knowledge of medical language?

Medical Language and Communication

Communication in any language consists of five language skills. These same skills apply to **medical language.** You need to master all five skills in order to communicate on the job with other healthcare professionals (see Figure 1-2 ■).

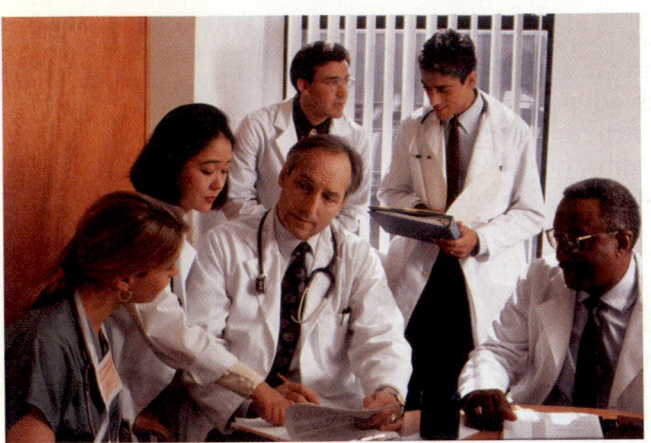

Figure 1-2 ■ Medical language communication.
These healthcare professionals are using all five medical language skills in order to communicate successfully.

1. **Reading**
2. **Listening**
   These skills involve receiving medical language. This is similar to the input coming into a computer.
   - You read medical words. Each chapter in this book contains many medical words.
   - You read actual medical reports in the Chapter Review Exercises.
   - You listen to your course instructor speak medical language.
   - You listen to exercises with actual physicians speaking medical language excerpts from medical reports.
3. **Thinking, analyzing, and understanding**
   This skill involves processing medical language. This is similar to the processing function of a computer.
   - You analyze medical words by dividing them into word parts.
   - You recall the medical meaning of word parts.
   - You build medical words from word parts.
   - You complete exercises to test your understanding of medical language.
   - You read actual medical reports and answer critical thinking questions.
   - You correlate common English words with their medical equivalents.
4. **Writing (or typing) and spelling**
5. **Speaking and pronouncing**
   These skills involve relaying medical language. This is similar to output coming from a computer.
   - You write or type a medical word and spell it correctly.
   - You spell the plural and adjective forms of medical words.
   - You identify misspelled medical words in a paragraph.
   - You speak medical words, using the "see-and-say" pronunciation guides to practice pronouncing them correctly.
   - You read a medical word and identify the primary accented syllable.
   - You read the "see-and-say" pronunciation, identify the medical word, and then spell the word correctly.

These skills are critical in the communication of medical language. This book *Medical Language* helps you develop all five skills by giving you many opportunities to practice until you have mastered all of them.

Let's begin the study of medical language by looking at how medical language began.

The Beginning of Medical Language

Etymology is the study of word origins. In medical language, many words have come from other languages, particularly from Latin and Greek. Why? Because in ancient times both the Romans and the Greeks advanced the study and practice of medicine. They named anatomical structures, diseases, and treatments in their own languages, and these Latin and Greek words remain a part of medical language today. You'll be surprised to see how many of these words are familiar to you.

WORD BUILDING

etymology (ET-ih-MAWL-oh-jee)
etym/o- *word origin*
-logy *the study of*

Word Alert

Some medical words are identical to Latin and Greek words from centuries ago.

Medical Word	Language of Origin
nucleus	Latin *nucleus*
pelvis	Latin *pelvis*
sinus	Latin *sinus*
paranoia	Greek *paranoia*
thorax	Greek *thorax*

Some medical words are similar (but not identical) to Latin and Greek words.

Medical Word	Language of Origin
artery	Latin *arteria*
muscle	Latin *musculus*
vein	Latin *vena*
phobia	Greek *phobos*
sperm	Greek *sperma*

Some medical words are similar to words from older versions of the English, Dutch, and French languages.

Medical Word	Language of Origin
bladder	English *blaedre*
heart	English *heorte*
drug	Dutch *droog*
physician	French *physicien*

This It's Greek to Me feature appears in each chapter. It lists many of the combining forms, their language of origin, and the medical words in which they were used in that chapter.

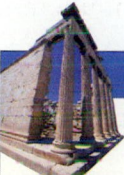

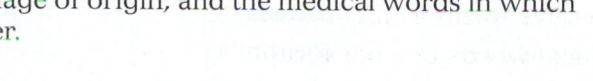

It's Greek to Me!

Did you notice that some words have two different combining forms? Combining forms from both Greek and Latin languages remain a part of medical language today.

Medical Word Singular and Plural Nouns

The Latin and Greek languages are the main sources of medical words. These languages had rules that told how to form plural nouns and how to pronounce singular and plural nouns; those rules still apply today. *Note:* When a Latin or Greek word is used in a chapter, there will be a note there to remind you of those rules. Here are some common Latin and Greek singular and plural nouns and their pronunciations.

Latin Singular and Plural Nouns and Pronunciations

When a Latin singular noun ends in *–a*, form the plural by changing *–a* to *–ae*.

Singular	Pronunciation	Plural	Pronunciation
areola	(ah-REE-oh-lah)	areolae	(ah-REE-oh-lee)
bursa	(BER-sah)	bursae	(BER-see)
conjunctiva	(CON-junk-TY-vah)	conjunctivae	(CON-junk-TY-vee)
patella	(pah-TEL-ah)	patellae	(pah-TEL-ee)
petechia	(peh-TEE-kee-ah)	petechiae	(peh-TEE-kee-ee)
ruga	(ROO-gah)	rugae	(ROO-gee)
scapula	(SKAP-yoo-lah)	scapulae	(SKAP-yoo-lee)
sclera	(SKLEER-ah)	sclerae	(SKLEER-ee)
vena	(VEE-nah)	venae	(VEE-nee)
vertebra	(VER-teh-brah)	vertebrae	(VER-teh-bree)

When a Latin singular noun ends in *–us,* form the plural by changing *–us* to *–i.*
(*Note:* Exceptions to this rule are the Latin words *fetus, virus,* and *sinus,* whose plural forms are the English-type plurals of *fetuses, viruses,* and *sinuses.*)

alveolus	(al-VEE-oh-lus)	alveoli	(al-VEE-oh-lie)
bronchus	(BRONG-kus)	bronchi	(BRONG-kigh)
calculus	(KAL-kyoo-lus)	calculi	(KAL-kyoo-lie)
decubitus	(dee-KYOO-bih-tus)	decubiti	(dee-KYOO-bih-tie)
glomerulus	(gloh-MAIR-yoo-lus)	glomeruli	(gloh-MAIR-yoo-lie)
gyrus	(JY-rus)	gyri	(JY-rye)
nucleus	(NOO-klee-us)	nuclei	(NOO-klee-eye)
sulcus	(SUL-kus)	sulci	(SUL-sigh)
thrombus	(THRAWM-bus)	thrombi	(THRAWM-by)
villus	(VIL-us)	villi	(VIL-eye)

When a Latin singular noun ends in *–um,* form the plural by changing *–um* to *–a.*

atrium	(AA-tree-um)	atria	(AA-tree-ah)
bacterium	(bak-TEER-ee-um)	bacteria	(bak-TEER-ee-ah)
diverticulum	(DY-ver-TIK-yoo-lum)	diverticula	(DY-ver-TIK-yoo-lah)
haustrum	(HAW-strum)	haustra	(HAW-strah)
hilum	(HY-lum)	hila	(HY-lah)
labium	(LAY-bee-um)	labia	(LAY-bee-ah)
ovum	(OH-vum)	ova	(OH-vah)

Singular	Pronunciation	Plural	Pronunciation
When a Latin singular noun ends in *–is,* form the plural by changing *–is* to *–es.*			
diagnosis	(DY-ag-NOH-sis)	diagnoses	(DY-ag-NOH-seez)
testis	(TES-tis)	testes	(TES-teez)
When a Latin singular noun ends in *–ex,* form the plural by changing *–ex* to *–ices.*			
apex	(AA-peks)	apices	(AA-pih-seez)
cortex	(KOR-teks)	cortices	(KOR-tih-seez)
index	(IN-deks)	indices	(IN-dih-seez)
When a Latin singular noun ends in *–ix,* form the plural by changing *–ix* to *–ices.*			
calix	(KAY-liks)	calices	(KAL-ih-seez)
helix	(HEE-liks)	helices	(HEE-lih-seez)

Greek Singular and Plural Nouns and Pronunciations

Singular	Pronunciation	Plural	Pronunciation
When a Greek singular noun ends in *–is,* form the plural by changing *–is* to *–ides.*			
epididymis	(EP-ih-DID-ih-mis)	epididymides	(EP-ih-dih-DIM-ih-deez)
iris	(EYE-ris)	irides	(IHR-ih-deez)
When a Greek singular noun ends in *–nx,* form the plural by changing *–nx* to *–nges.*			
phalanx	(FAY-langks)	phalanges	(fah-LAN-jeez)
When a Greek singular noun ends in *–oma,* form the plural by changing *–oma* to *–omata.*			
carcinoma	(KAR-sih-NOH-mah)	carcinomata	(KAR-sih-NOH-mah-tah)
fibroma	(fy-BROH-mah)	fibromata	(FY-broh-MAH-tah)
leiomyoma	(LIE-oh-my-OH-mah)	leiomyomata	(LIE-oh-my-OH-mah-tah)
When a Greek singular noun ends in *–on,* form the plural by changing *–on* to *–a.*			
ganglion	(GANG-glee-on)	ganglia	(GANG-glee-ah)
mitochondrion	(MY-toh-CON-dree-on)	mitochondria	(MY-toh-CON-dree-ah)

Medical Words and Word Parts

Medical language contains medical words, and medical words contain word parts. Word parts are the puzzle pieces that, when fit together, build a medical word.

There are three different kinds of word parts: combining form, suffix, and prefix.

Word Part	*Meaning*
combining form	the foundation of the word
suffix	the word ending
prefix	an optional word beginning

Did You Know?

When you learn something new, it is always best to learn it the right way the very first time! That is why the spelling (and punctuation) of combining forms, suffixes, and prefixes used in this book are based on those used in medical dictionaries that are the recognized authorities on medical language origin and use.

Combining Forms

Characteristics of a Combining Form

Combining forms have the following characteristics.

- A combining form is a word part that is the foundation of a word.
- A combining form gives the word its main medical meaning.
- A combining form has a **root** (with medical meaning), a forward slash (to separate the root from the combining vowel), a combining vowel (usually an *o,* but occasionally an *a, i,* or *y*), and a final hyphen (see Figure 1-3 ■).
- Most medical words contain a combining form. (*Note:* Some medical words, such as *blood, health, heart, or nurse* are from early versions of the English or French languages and do not contain any word parts.)
- Sometimes a medical word contains two or more combining forms, one right after the other.

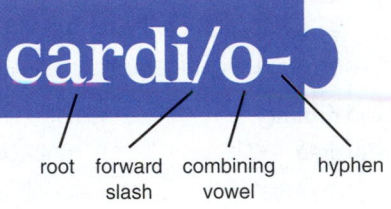

root forward   combining   hyphen
      slash   vowel

Figure 1-3 ■ Combining form.

A combining form contains a root, forward slash, combining vowel, and hyphen. The hyphen shows that the combining form is a word part, not a complete word. The combining form *cardi/o-* means *heart.*

Word Alert

Learning medical language requires some memorization of combining forms and their medical meanings. Why is this necessary? Because knowing the meaning of the combining form allows you to look at a medical word and already have an idea about its definition. Knowing the meaning of one word part allows you to apply it to the many medical words where it appears. The alternative is having to use a medical dictionary to look up the definition of each new medical word you encounter!

Here are some tips on how to manage your time and the amount of memorization you need to do as you study medical language.

Tip #1: Some combining forms are nearly identical to their medical meanings. When you see combining forms like these, you already know their medical meanings.

Combining Form	Medical Meaning
abdomin/o-	abdomen
append/o-	appendix
arteri/o-	artery
intestin/o	intestine
laryng/o-	larynx (voice box)
muscul/o-	muscle
thyroid/o-	thyroid gland
tonsill/o-	tonsil
ven/o-	vein

Tip #2: Some combining forms bring to mind a word you already know. That helps you to remember the medical meaning of combining forms like these.

Combining Form	Related Word	Medical Meaning
arthr/o-	arthritis	joint
cardi/o-	cardiac	heart
derm/o-	dermatologist	skin
gastr/o-	gastric	stomach
mamm/o-	mammogram	breast
nas/o-	nasal	nose
psych/o-	psychiatrist	mind

Tip #3: Other combining forms are very different from their medical meanings. Combining forms like these and their medical meanings need to be memorized.

Combining Form	Medical Meaning
cholecyst/o-	gallbladder
cost/o-	rib
enter/o-	intestine
hepat/o-	liver
hyster/o-	uterus
lapar/o-	abdomen

Word Alert

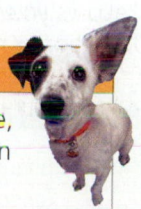

Two combining forms can have the same medical meaning. For example, the combining forms *enter/o-* and *intestin/o-* both mean *intestine*. When this occurs in a chapter, there will be a note to remind you.

Suffixes

Characteristics of a Suffix

Suffixes have the following characteristics.

- A suffix is a word part that is at the end of a word.
- A suffix modifies or clarifies the medical meaning of the combining form.
- A suffix is a single letter or group of letters that begins with a hyphen (see Figure 1-4 ▪).
- Most medical words contain a suffix (see *Note* with *Combining Forms*).

Here are some common suffixes. Take a moment to review them and learn their meanings so that you will be ready to use them in medical words.

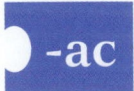

Figure 1-4 ▪ **Suffix.**
A suffix begins with a hyphen to show that it is a word part, not a complete word. The suffix -ac means *pertaining to*.

Suffixes for Adjective Forms

Suffix	Meaning	Medical Word Example	Definition
-ac	pertaining to	cardiac (KAR-dee-ak) (*cardi/o-* means *heart*)	pertaining to the heart
-al	pertaining to	intestinal (in-TES-tih-nal) (*intestin/o-* means *intestine*)	pertaining to the intestine
-ar	pertaining to	muscular (MUS-kyoo-lar) (*muscul/o-* means *muscle*)	pertaining to the muscle
-ary	pertaining to	urinary (YOO-rih-NAIR-ee) (*urin/o-* means *urine; urinary tract*)	pertaining to the urine
-ic	pertaining to	pelvic (PEL-vik) (*pelv/o-* means *pelvis*)	pertaining to the pelvis
-ine	pertaining to	uterine (YOO-ter-in) (*uter/o-* means *uterus*)	pertaining to the uterus
-ive	pertaining to	digestive (dy-JES-tiv) (*digest/o-* means *break down food; digest*)	pertaining to digestion
-ous	pertaining to	venous (VEE-nus) (*ven/o-* means *vein*)	pertaining to a vein

Suffixes for Processes

Suffix	Meaning	Medical Word Example	Definition
-ation	a process; being or having	urination (YOO-rih-NAY-shun) (*urin/o-* means *urine; urinary system*)	a process of (making) urine
-ion	action; condition	digestion (dy-JES-chun) (*digest/o-* means *break down foods; digest*)	action of breaking down food
-lysis	process of breaking down or destroying	hemolysis (hee-MAWL-ih-sis) (*hem/o-* means *blood*)	process of breaking down or destroying blood

Suffixes for Diseases and Conditions

Suffix	Meaning	Medical Word Example	Definition
-ia	condition; state; thing	pneumonia (noo-MOH-nee-ah) (*pneumon/o-* means *lung; air*)	condition of the lung
-ism	process; disease from a specific cause	hypothyroidism (HY-poh-THY-roid-izm) (*thyroid/o-* means *thyroid gland*)	disease from the specific cause of deficient thyroid (hormone)

Suffix	Meaning	Medical Word Example	Definition
-itis	inflammation of; infection of	tonsillitis (TAWN-sih-LY-tis) (*tonsill/o*- means *tonsil*)	infection of the tonsil
-megaly	enlargement	cardiomegaly (KAR-dee-oh-MEG-ah-lee) (*cardi/o*- means *heart*)	enlargement of the heart
-oma	tumor; mass	neuroma (nyoo-ROH-mah) (*neur/o*- means *nerve*)	tumor on a nerve
-osis	condition; abnormal condition; process	psychosis (sy-KOH-sis) (*psych/o*- means *mind*)	abnormal condition of the mind
-pathy	disease; suffering	arthropathy (ar-TRAWP-ah-thee) (*arthr/o*- means *joint*)	disease of the joint

Suffixes for Diagnostic, Medical, and Surgical Procedures

Suffix	Meaning	Medical Word Example	Definition
-ectomy	surgical excision	appendectomy (AP-pen-DEK-toh-mee) (*append/o*- means *appendix*)	surgical excision of the appendix
-gram	a record or picture	mammogram (MAM-oh-gram) (*mamm/o*- means *breast*)	a record or picture of the breast
-graphy	process of recording	mammography (mah-MAWG-rah-fee) (*mamm/o*- means *breast*)	process of recording the breast
-metry	process of measuring	spirometry (spih-RAWM-eh-tree) (*spir/o*- means *breathe*)	process of measuring the breathing
-scope	instrument used to examine	colonoscope (koh-LAWN-oh-skop) (*colon/o*- means *colon*)	instrument used to examine the colon
-scopy	process of using an instrument to examine	gastroscopy (gas-TRAWS-koh-pee) (*gastr/o*- means *stomach*)	process of using an instrument to examine the stomach
-stomy	surgically created opening	colostomy (koh-LAWS-toh-mee) (*col/o*- means *colon*)	surgically created opening in the colon
-therapy	treatment	psychotherapy (SY-koh-THAIR-ah-pee) (*psych/o*- means *mind*)	treatment of the mind
-tomy	process of cutting or making an incision	laparotomy (LAP-ah-RAW-toh-mee) (*lapar/o*- means *abdomen*)	process of making an incision in the abdomen

Suffixes for Medical Specialties

Suffix	Meaning	Medical Word Example	Definition
-iatry	medical treatment	psychiatry (sy-KY-ah-tree) (*psych/o*- means *mind*)	medical treatment for the mind
-ist	one who specializes in	therapist (THAIR-ah-pist) (*therap/o*- means *therapy*)	one who specializes in therapy
-logy	the study of	cardiology (KAR-dee-AWL-oh-jee) (*cardi/o*- means *heart*)	the study of the heart

Prefixes

Characteristics of a Prefix

Prefixes have the following characteristics.

- A prefix is a word part that is at the beginning of a word. A prefix is an optional word part, and not every word contains a prefix.
- A prefix modifies or clarifies the medical meaning of the combining form.
- A prefix is a single letter or group of letters that ends with a hyphen (see Figure 1-5 ■).
- Occasionally, a medical word has two prefixes, one right after the other.

Here are some common prefixes. Take a moment to review them and learn their meanings so that you will be ready to use them in medical words.

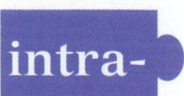

Figure 1-5 ■ **Prefix.**
A prefix ends with a hyphen to show that it is a word part, not a complete word. The prefix *intra-* means *within*.

Prefixes for Location or Direction

Prefix	Meaning	Medical Word Example	Definition
endo-	innermost; within	endotracheal (EN-doh-TRAY-kee-al) (*trache/o-* means *trachea*)	pertaining to within the trachea
epi-	upon; above	epidermal (EP-ih-DER-mal) (*derm/o-* means *skin*)	pertaining to upon the skin
inter-	between	intercostal (IN-ter-KAWS-tal) (*cost/o-* means *rib*)	pertaining to between the ribs
intra-	within	intravenous (IN-trah-VEE-nus) (*ven/o-* means *vein*)	pertaining to within a vein
peri-	around	pericardial (PAIR-ih-KAR-dee-al) (*cardi/o-* means *heart*)	pertaining to around the heart
post-	after; behind	postnasal (post-NAY-zal) (*nas/o-* means *nose*)	pertaining to behind the nose
pre-	before; in front of	premenstrual (pree-MEN-stroo-al) (*menstru/o-* means *monthly discharge of blood*)	pertaining to before menstruation
sub-	below; underneath; less than	subcutaneous (SUB-kyoo-TAY-nee-us) (*cutane/o-* means *skin*)	pertaining to underneath the skin
trans-	across; through	transvaginal (trans-VAJ-in-nal) (*vagin/o-* means *vagina*)	pertaining to through the vagina

Prefixes for Amount, Number, or Speed

Prefix	Meaning	Medical Word Example	Definition
bi-	two	bilateral (bi-LAT-er-al) (*later/o-* means *side*)	pertaining to two sides
brady-	slow	bradycardia (BRAD-ee-KAR-dee-ah) (*card/i-* means *heart*)	condition of a slow heart
hemi-	one half	hemiplegia (HEM-ee-PLEE-jee-ah) (*pleg/o-* means *paralysis*)	condition of one half (of the body) with paralysis
hyper-	above; more than normal	hypertension (HY-per-TEN-shun) (*tens/o-* means *pressure*)	condition of more than normal pressure
hypo-	below; deficient	hypothyroidism (HY-poh-THY-royd-izm) (*thyroid/o-* means *thyroid gland*)	disease from a specific cause of deficient thyroid gland (hormone)
mono-	one; single	mononucleosis (MAWN-oh-noo-klee-OH-sis) (*nucle/o-* means *nucleus*)	abnormal condition of (white blood cells that each have) one (large) nucleus
poly-	many; much	polyneuritis (PAWL-ee-nyoo-RY-tis) (*neur/o-* means *nerve*)	inflammation of many nerves
quadri-	four	quadriplegia (KWAH-drih-PLEE-jee-ah) (*pleg/o-* means *paralysis*)	condition of four (limbs) with paralysis
tachy-	fast	tachycardia (TAK-ih-KAR-dee-ah) (*card/i-* means *heart*)	condition of a fast heart
tri-	three	trigeminal (try-JEM-ih-nal) (*gemin/o-* means *set or group*)	pertaining to three (nerve branches in a) group

Prefixes for Degree or Quality

Prefix	Meaning	Medical Word Example	Definition
a-	away from; without	aspermia (aa-SPER-mee-ah) (*sperm/o-* means *sperm*)	condition (of being) without sperm
an-	without; not	anesthesia (AN-es-THEE-zee-ah) (*esthes/o-* means *sensation; feeling*)	condition (of being) without sensation
anti-	against	antibiotic (AN-tee-by-AWT-ik) (*bi/o-* means *living organisms*	pertaining to against living organisms (such as bacteria)
de-	reversal of; without	dementia (dee-MEN-shee-ah) (*ment/o-* means *mind*)	condition (of being) without a mind
dys-	painful; difficult; abnormal	dysphagia (dis-FAY-jee-ah) (*phag/o-* means *eating; swallowing*)	condition of painful or difficult eating and swallowing
eu-	normal; good	euthyroidism (yoo-THY-royd-izm) (*thyroid/o-* means *thyroid gland*)	process of normal thyroid gland (function)
mal-	bad; inadequate	malnutrition (MAL-noo-TRISH-un) (*nutri/o-* means *nourishment*)	being or having inadequate nourishment
re-	again and again	respiration (RES-pih-RAY-shun) (*spir/o-* means *breathe*)	a process of again and again breathing

Analyze and Define Medical Words

The third skill of medical language involves thinking, analyzing, and understanding. When you analyze something, you break it into smaller pieces that are easier to understand. To analyze a medical word, break it into its word parts. Then you combine the meanings of the word parts to give you the definition of the medical word. Here are the steps for analyzing and defining a medical word.

Medical Word with a Combining Form and Suffix
Follow these steps to analyze and define a medical word that has a combining form and a suffix.

Medical word example: **cardiology.**

Step 1. Divide the medical word into its combining form and suffix.
    (Note: At this point in your study, you will not be able to look at a medical word and know that it contains a combining form and a suffix. However, as you memorize various word parts and their meanings, you will be able to do this.)

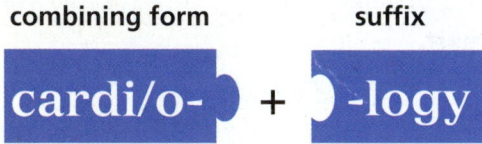

Step 2. Define each word part.

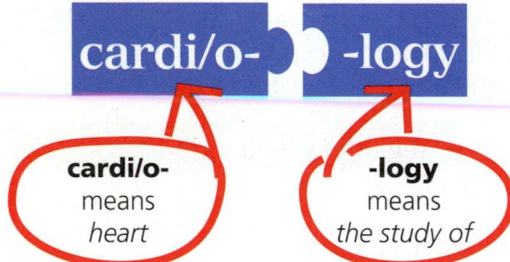

Step 3. Put the word part meanings in this order: the meaning of the suffix first, followed by the meaning of the combining form.

    suffix   **combining form**
    the study of   *heart*

Step 4. Add small connecting words, if needed, to make a correct and complete definition of the medical word.

Cardiology: The study of (the) heart (and related structures).

Medical Word with a Combining Form, Suffix, and Prefix
Follow these steps to analyze and define a medical word that has a combining form, suffix, and prefix.

Medical word example: **pericardial.**

Step 1. Divide the medical word into its prefix, combining form, and suffix.

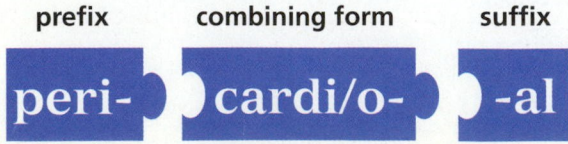

Step 2. Define each word part.

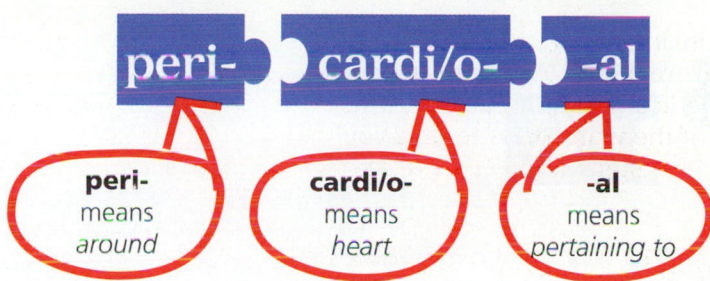

Step 3. Put the word part meanings in this order: the meaning of the suffix first, followed by the meaning of the prefix, followed by the meaning of the combining form.

suffix	prefix	combining form
pertaining to	around	heart

Step 4. Add small connecting words, if needed, to make a correct and complete definition of the medical word.

Pericardial: Pertaining to around the heart.

Build Medical Words

Medical words are like puzzles, and their word parts are the pieces of the puzzle. To build a medical word, begin with its definition. Select word parts that match that definition, and then put the word part puzzle pieces together in the correct way. Here are the steps for building a medical word.

Suffix that Begins with a Consonant Follow these steps to build a medical word when the suffix begins with a consonant.

Medical word definition: **The study of the heart.**

Step 1. Select the suffix and combining form whose meanings match the definition of the medical word.

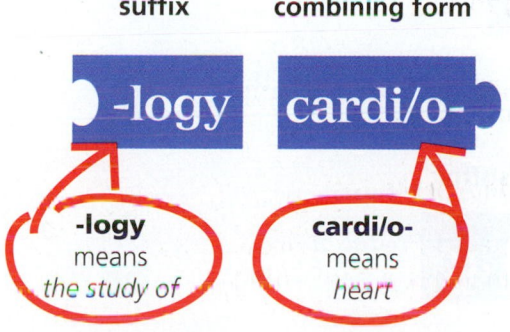

Step 2. Change the order of the word parts to put the suffix last.

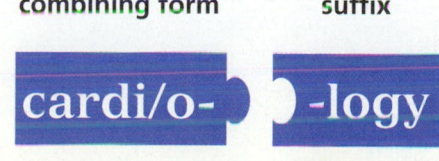

Step 3. Delete the forward slash and hyphen from the combining form. Delete the hyphen from the suffix.

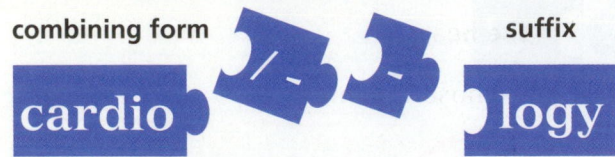

Step 4. Join the two word parts.

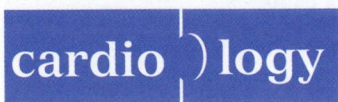

Suffix that Begins with a Vowel
Follow these steps to build a medical word when the suffix begins with a vowel.

Medical word definition: **Pertaining to the heart.**

Step 1. Select the suffix and combining form whose meanings match the definition of the medical word.

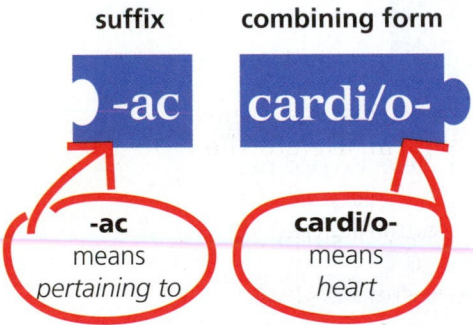

Step 2. Change the order of the word parts to put the suffix last.

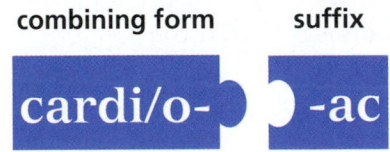

Step 3. Delete the forward slash, combining vowel, and hyphen from the combining form. Delete the hyphen from the suffix.

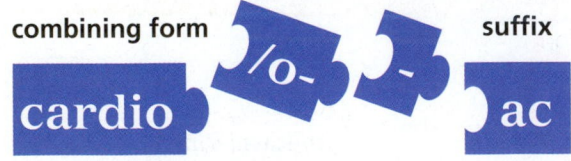

Step 4. Join the two word parts.

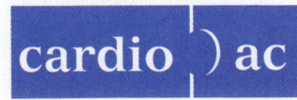

Contains a Prefix   Follow these steps to build a medical word that contains a prefix.

Medical word definition: **Pertaining to within the heart.**

Step 1. Select the suffix, prefix, and combining form whose meanings match the definition of the medical word.

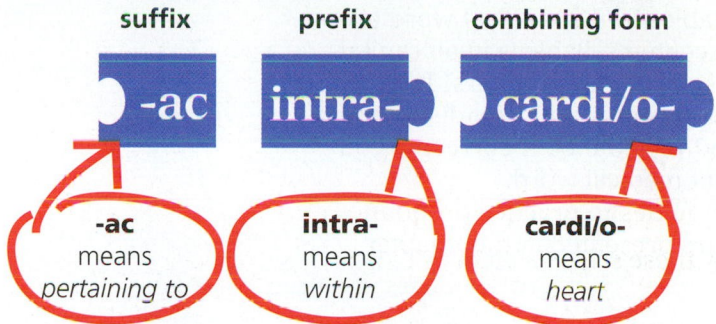

Step 2. Change the order of the word parts to put the suffix last.

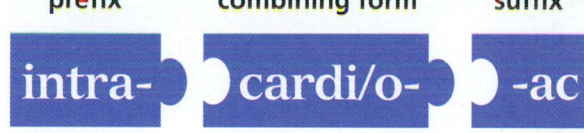

Step 3. Delete the hyphen from the prefix. Delete the forward slash, combining vowel, and hyphen from the combining form. Delete the hyphen from the suffix.

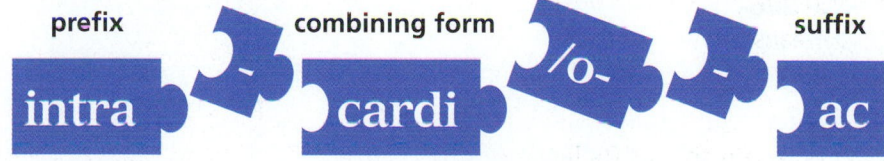

Step 4. Join the three word parts.

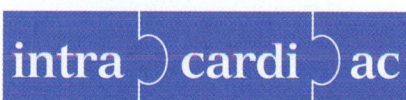

Word Alert

Some medical words contain two or more combining forms.

Example:

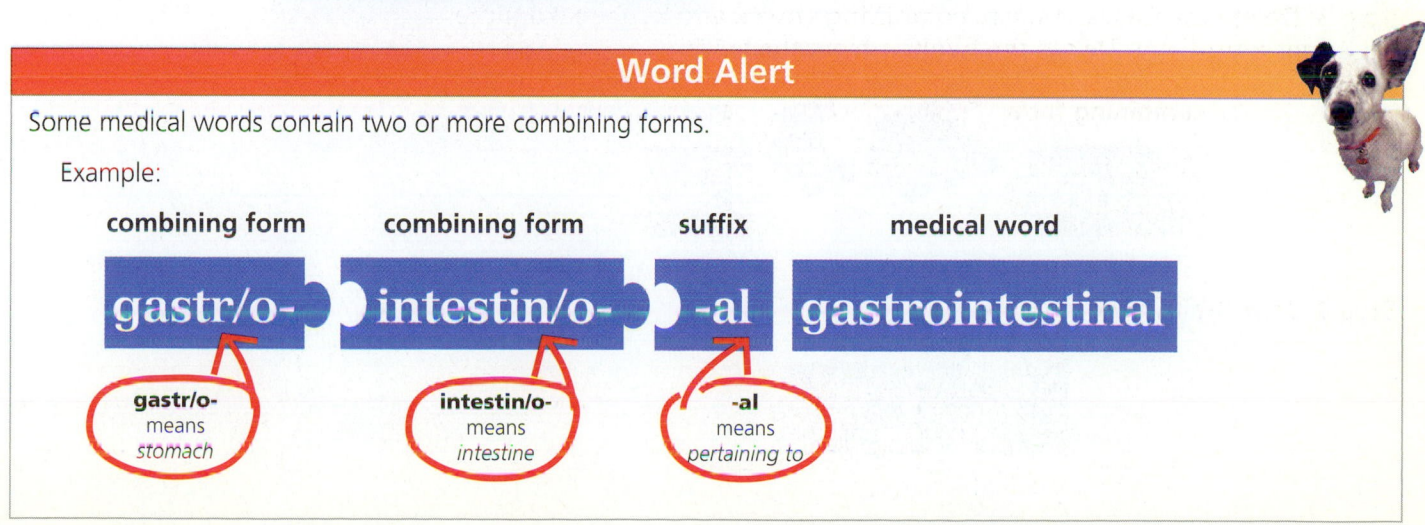

Pronounce Medical Words

Knowing the definition of a medical word is important, but being able to pronounce the word correctly is equally important. One of the five medical language skills is pronunciation. In each chapter, as you read a medical word (in bold), there is an accompanying "see and say" pronunciation, so you can immediately pronounce the word you are learning. These guides are straightforward and easy to use. The syllables in the medical word are separated by hyphens. The primary (main) accented syllable is in all capital letters. The secondary accented syllable is in smaller capital letters. Just say each syllable by following the "see-and-say" pronunciation guide. When you read a medical word and then speak and pronounce it correctly, you are forming an accurate word memory for that medical word.

Now use the "see-and-say" pronunciation guides to practice pronouncing common medical words, many of which are presented in this chapter.

Pronouncing Medical Words   Look at each medical word and its pronunciation guide. Practice pronouncing the word several times.

Medical Word	Medical Word Pronunciation
1. abdominal	(ab-DAWM-ih-nal)
2. appendectomy	(AP-pen-DEK-toh-mee)
3. arthritis	(ar-THRY-tis)
4. cardiac	(KAR-dee-ak)
5. cardiology	(KAR-dee-AWL-oh-jee)
6. digestion	(dy-JES-chun)
7. gastric	(GAS-trik)
8. intestinal	(in-TES-tih-nal)
9. intravenous	(IN-trah-VEE-nus)
10. laryngitis	(LAIR-in-JY-tis)
11. mammography	(mah-MAWG-rah-fee)
12. muscular	(MUS-kyoo-lar)
13. pneumonia	(noo-MOH-nee-ah)
14. psychiatry	(sy-KY-ah-tree)
15. therapist	(THAIR-ah-pist)
16. tonsillectomy	(TAWN-sih-LEK-toh-mee)
17. urinary	(YOO-rih-NAIR-ee)

Vocabulary Review

Here are the word parts presented in this chapter. (They are also used in other chapters as well.) Take time to review them and learn their meanings so that you will be ready to use them in medical words.

Combining Forms

Combining Form	Medical Meaning	Combining Form	Medical Meaning
abdomin/o-	abdomen	mamm/o-	breast
append/o-	appendix	menstru/o-	monthly discharge of blood
arteri/o-	artery	ment/o-	mind
arthr/o-	joint	muscul/o-	muscle
bi/o-	life; living organisms	nas/o-	nose
card/i-	heart	neur/o-	nerve
cardi/o-	heart	nucle/o-	nucleus
cholecyst/o-	gallbladder	nutri/o-	nourishment
col/o-	colon	pelv/o-	pelvis
colon/o-	colon	phag/o-	eating; swallowing
cost/o-	rib	pleg/o-	paralysis
cutane/o-	skin	pneumon/o-	lung; air
derm/o-	skin	psych/o-	mind
digest/o-	break down food; digest	sperm/o-	sperm
enter/o-	intestine	spir/o-	breathe
esthes/o-	sensation; feeling	tens/o-	pressure
gastr/o-	stomach	therap/o-	therapy
gemin/o-	set or group	thyroid/o-	thyroid gland
hem/o-	blood	tonsill/o-	tonsil
hepat/o-	liver	trache/o-	trachea
hyster/o-	uterus (womb)	urin/o-	urine; urinary system
intestin/o-	intestine	uter/o-	uterus (womb)
lapar/o-	abdomen	vagin/o-	vagina
laryng/o-	larynx (voice box)	ven/o-	vein
later/o-	side		

Suffixes

Suffix	Medical Meaning	Suffix	Medical Meaning
-ac	pertaining to	-ine	pertaining to
-al	pertaining to	-ion	action; condition
-ar	pertaining to	-ism	process; disease from a specific cause
-ary	pertaining to	-ist	one who specializes in
-ation	a process; being or having	-itis	inflammation of; infection of
-ectomy	surgical excision	-ive	pertaining to
-gram	a record or picture	-logy	the study of
-graphy	process of recording	-lysis	process or breaking down or destroying
-ia	condition; state; thing	-megaly	enlargement
-iatry	medical treatment	-metry	process of measuring
-ic	pertaining to	-oma	tumor; mass

Suffix	Medical Meaning	Suffix	Medical Meaning
-osis	condition; abnormal condition; process	-scopy	process of using an instrument to examine
-ous	pertaining to	-stomy	surgically created opening
-pathy	disease; suffering	-therapy	treatment
-scope	instrument used to examine	-tomy	process of cutting or making an incision

Prefixes

Prefix	Medical Meaning	Prefix	Medical Meaning
a-	away from; without	intra-	within
an-	without; not	mal-	bad; inadequate
anti-	against	mono-	one; single
bi-	two	peri-	around
brady-	slow	poly-	many; much
de-	reversal of; without	post-	after; behind
dys-	painful; difficult; abnormal	pre-	before; in front of
endo-	innermost; within	quadri-	four
epi-	upon; above	re-	again and again
eu-	normal; good	sub-	below; underneath; less than
hemi-	one half	tachy-	fast
hyper-	above; more than normal	trans-	across; through
hypo-	below; deficient	tri-	three
inter-	between		

The Medical Record

Many of the medical language skills discussed at the beginning of the chapter are used when dealing with medical documents. Let's briefly look at some of the more common types of medical documents.

The **medical record** is where healthcare professionals document all care provided to a patient. In the past, the medical record was mainly used to document diseases, treatments, surgeries, etc. Now, the medical record reflects an emphasis on keeping the patient in good health and preventing disease. Most physicians' office medical records include a checklist that documents preventive care given to the patient (immunizations, routine physical exams, etc.), as well as things the patient should do (limit sun exposure and apply sunscreen, have smoke detectors in the home, use seat belts, do monthly self-examination of the breasts or testicles, secure firearms kept in the home, etc.).

The paper medical record has been the traditional form of medical record. Its disadvantages are that only one healthcare professional can access it at a time, it can become lost or damaged, and it can take hours or even days to retrieve a patient's past medical records that are stored off-site. This delay can compromise the delivery of quality care.

Recently, however, more and more offices, hospitals, and other healthcare facilities are converting some or all of their paper medical records to **computerized patient records (CPRs)** (see Figure 1-6 ■). In these facilities, several healthcare professionals can access the same record at the same time, the record cannot be lost or damaged (because there is always a back-up electronic copy), it takes only seconds to retrieve a patient's past medical records (because the record is stored in a computer that is on-site or can be accessed electronically in a remote location).

WORD BUILDING

medical (MED-ih-kal)
  medic/o- *physician; medicine*
  -al *pertaining to*

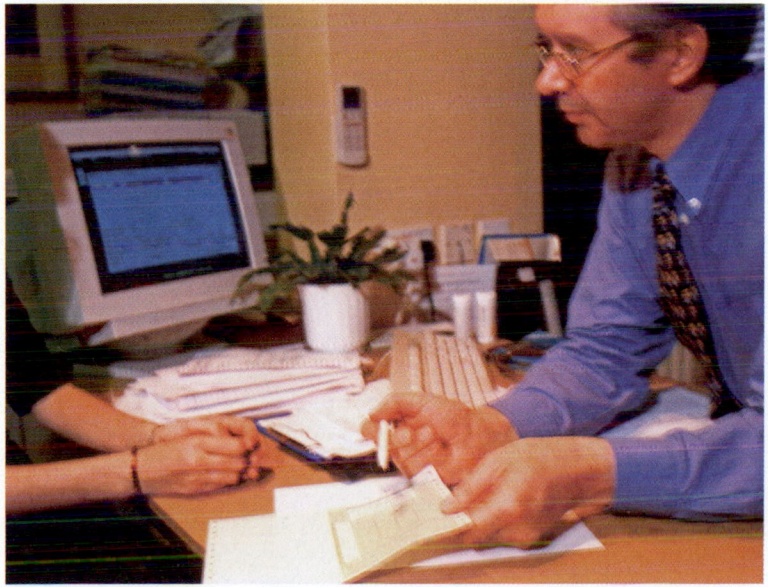

Figure 1-6 ■ Computerized patient record (CPR).
The computerized patient record can provide immediate access to a patient's current and previous medical records from within one facility or between related facilities. The computerized patient record has not yet entirely replaced the paper record.

In the future, it is hoped that an all-encompassing **electronic medical record (EMR), electronic patient record (EPR),** or **electronic health record (EHR)** will provide seamless, immediate, and simultaneous access for several healthcare professionals to all parts of a patient's record regardless of where those parts were created or stored. The federal government set a goal to have the electronic medical record and electronic prescribing of drugs (e-prescribing) done everywhere in health care.

Types of Documents in the Medical Record

The medical record is a medicolegal record. This means that it not only contains medical documents but that those are also legal documents that can be used in a court of law.

The medical record varies in format and content from one facility to the next. Short narrative notes and checklists are used in many physicians' offices and clinics. These notes usually contain a brief history of the present illness, pertinent past medical or surgical history, a physical examination, a diagnosis, treatments given, and a follow-up plan.

Hospitals use more extensive documentation than physicians' offices. Common documents for a hospitalized patient include the Admission History and Physical Examination (H&P), Operative Report, and Discharge Summary (DS). These documents include standard headings, as described below.

Standard Headings in Hospital Admission and Discharge Documents

- Chief Complaint (CC)
- History of Present Illness (HPI)
- Past Medical (and Surgical) History (PMH)
- Social History (SH) and Family History (FH)
- Review of Systems (ROS)
- Physical Examination (PE)
- Laboratory and X-Ray Data
- Diagnosis (Dx)
- Disposition

Before patients can be treated at any type of healthcare facility, they must sign a **consent to treatment** form that gives physicians and other healthcare professionals the right to treat them. Treatment without consent is against the law and could constitute battery (touching another person without his or her consent or causing harm). For a patient who is a minor, the parent or legal guardian signs the consent to treatment form. In an emergency situation, implied consent allows care to be provided until the patient is awake and able to consent or until a legally appropriate person is able to consent for the patient. Prior to a surgery, the physician describes the purpose of the surgery and informs the patient of alternatives, risks, and possible outcomes or complications. Then the patient signs a consent to surgery form.

A patient must also sign a form that allows the facility to contact the insurance company to obtain payment for any health care that is provided. Under the federal regulations of **HIPAA (the Health Insurance Portability and Accountability Act of 1996),** all healthcare settings must provide patients with a statement verifying that their medical record information is secure and is released only to authorized healthcare providers, insurance companies, or healthcare quality monitoring organizations.

In addition, physicians write orders and progress notes, nurses write nurses' notes, and other departments contribute to these notes or use preprinted forms to record information in the medical record.

Abbreviations

Abbreviations are commonly used in medical language and understanding their meanings is a part of learning medical language. Each chapter in this book includes a list of commonly used abbreviations.

CC	chief complaint	**H&P**	history and physical (examination)
CPR	computerized patient record	**HIPAA**	Health Insurance Portability and Accountability Act (pronounced "HIP-ah")
DS	discharge summary		
Dx	diagnosis	**HPI**	history of present illness
EHR	electronic health record	**PE**	physical examination
EMR	electronic medical record	**PMH**	past medical history
EPR	electronic patient record	**ROS**	review of systems
FH	family history	**SH**	social history

Word Alert

ABBREVIATIONS

Abbreviations are commonly used in all types of medical documents; however, they can mean different things to different people and their meanings can be misinterpreted. Always verify the meaning of an abbreviation.

CC means *chief complaint,* but it also means *cubic centimeter* (a measure of volume).

CPR means *computerized patient record,* but it also means *cardiopulmonary resuscitation.*

H&P means *history and physical (examination),* but the sound-alike abbreviation *HNP* stands for *herniated nucleus pulposus.*

Did You Know?

Each healthcare facility develops its own list of acceptable abbreviations (that can be used in documents produced in that facility) and a list of unacceptable or "do not use" abbreviations. In addition to that, the Joint Commission on Accreditation of Healthcare Organizations (JCAHO) has a list of abbreviations that should not be used because they cause errors. JCAHO's National Safety Goal states that these abbreviations must appear on a facility's "Do Not Use" list. The JCAHO list is a short list because it is the minimum required for a facility to be accredited. Some of these "do not use" abbreviations are included in this book because they are still in common use by some healthcare providers, but they are marked with an asterisk (*) and a reminder note. Other "do not use" abbreviations compiled by the Institute for Safe Medication Practices (ISMP) are also marked (■). Finally, some abbreviations (such as the abbreviation *SOB,* meaning *shortness of breath*) have an alternate undesirable meaning. Even though many hospitals have removed some or all of these abbreviations from their official list of abbreviations, they still continue to be used and are noted when they are included in a chapter.

CAREER FOCUS

Meet Erica, a paramedic

"I was always interested in health care. EMTs give basic life support. They can do things such as backboarding a patient, splinting, giving oxygen, taking vital signs, and transporting patients to the hospital. Paramedics give advanced life support. We can start intravenous lines, give medications. We can defibrillate, give electrocardiotherapy. It's hard to describe a typical day, because no day is like any other. We give care to patients with chest pain, shortness of breath, diabetes, seizures, and trauma (obviously auto accidents, but also industrial accidents) and transport them to the hospital. I use medical terminology when I'm writing my run reports. Those reports are medical and legal documents. They can be looked at by lawyers in the future. I always want my reports to look professional and be medically correct."

Paramedics are allied health professionals who respond to emergency calls from the community, treat patients in ambulances, and transport them to the emergency department of the hospital. The paramedic provides medical care in a setting that is apart from a hospital or physician's office.

paramedic (PAIR-ah-MED-ik)
Paramedic contains the prefix *para-* (apart from) and *medic* (a shortened form of *medical*). A paramedic works apart from the medical personnel in healthcare facilities.

PEARSON myhealthprofessionskit To see Erica's complete video profile, visit Medical Terminology Interactive at www.myhealthprofessionskit.com. Select this book, log in, and go to the 1st floor of Pearson General Hospital. Enter the Laboratory, and click on the computer screen.

CHAPTER REVIEW EXERCISES

Test your knowledge of the chapter by completing these review questions. Use the Answer Key at the end of the book to check your answers.

Welcome to Medical Language

Matching Exercise

Match each word part to its description. The word parts may be used more than once.

1. combining form
2. suffix
3. prefix

_____ Begins with a hyphen

_____ Contains the main meaning of a medical word

_____ Ends with a combining vowel

_____ Always positioned at the end of a medical word

_____ If present, it is always at the beginning of a medical word

_____ When there is no prefix, this is the first part of a medical word

True or False Exercise

Indicate whether each statement is true or false by writing T or F on the line.

1. _____ The three word parts in medical language are spelling, reading, and Greek.
2. _____ Every medical word contains a prefix.
3. _____ The suffix is the foundation of a medical word.
4. _____ You can form the plural of a Latin singular noun that ends in –a by changing the -a to -ae.
5. _____ A root and a combining vowel together form a medical word.
6. _____ The suffixes -ac and -al both mean *pertaining to*.
7. _____ All medical words originally come from Latin words.
8. _____ You can increase your chances of success in a healthcare career by learning medical language.

Fill in the Blank Exercise

1. Name the three word parts that are used to build medical words.
   a. _____
   b. _____
   c. _____

2. Name the five medical language skills needed for successful communication.
   a. _____   d. _____
   b. _____   e. _____
   c. _____

3. Write the two combining forms that have a medical meaning of
   a. skin _____   _____
   b. intestine _____   _____
   c. mind _____   _____

4. Write the prefix that has the *opposite* medical meaning of
   a. hypo- _____
   b. epi- _____
   c. pre- _____

Latin and Greek Singular and Plural Nouns Exercise

Write the plural form of these Latin or Greek singular nouns. Be sure to check your spelling. The first one has been done for you.

Latin Singular	Latin Plural	Latin Singular	Latin Plural
1. vertebra	*vertebrae*	9. bacterium	_____
2. bursa	_____	10. hilum	_____
3. petechia	_____	11. diverticulum	_____
4. ruga	_____	12. labium	_____
5. bronchus	_____	13. ovum	_____
6. alveolus	_____	14. testis	_____
7. thrombus	_____	15. diagnosis	_____
8. nucleus	_____		

Greek Singular	Greek Plural	Greek Singular	Greek Plural
16. iris	_____	20. leiomyoma	_____
17. epididymis	_____	21. ganglion	_____
18. phalanx	_____	22. mitochondrion	_____
19. carcinoma	_____		

Building Medical Words

Word Parts Exercise

Before you build medical words, review these word parts. Next to each word part, indicate what type it is, and then write its medical meaning. Be sure to check your spelling. The first one has been done for you.

Prefix = P   Combining Form = CF   Suffix = S

Word Part	Type	Medical Meaning	Word Part	Type	Medical Meaning
1. a-	P	away from; without	18. cholecyst/o-	____	_____
2. abdomin/o-	____	_____	19. col/o-	____	_____
3. -ac	____	_____	20. colon/o-	____	_____
4. -al	____	_____	21. cost/o-	____	_____
5. an-	____	_____	22. cutane/o-	____	_____
6. anti-	____	_____	23. de-	____	_____
7. append/o-	____	_____	24. derm/o-	____	_____
8. -ar	____	_____	25. digest/o-	____	_____
9. arteri/o-	____	_____	26. dys-	____	_____
10. arthr/o-	____	_____	27. -ectomy	____	_____
11. -ary	____	_____	28. endo-	____	_____
12. -ation	____	_____	29. enter/o-	____	_____
13. bi-	____	_____	30. epi-	____	_____
14. bi/o-	____	_____	31. esthes/o-	____	_____
15. brady-	____	_____	32. eu-	____	_____
16. card/i-	____	_____	33. gastr/o-	____	_____
17. cardi/o-	____	_____	34. gemin/o-	____	_____

Word Part	Type	Medical Meaning		Word Part	Type	Medical Meaning
35. -gram	_____	_____		71. nutri/o-	_____	_____
36. -graphy	_____	_____		72. -oma	_____	_____
37. hemi-	_____	_____		73. -osis	_____	_____
38. hem/o-	_____	_____		74. -ous	_____	_____
39. hepat/o-	_____	_____		75. -pathy	_____	_____
40. hyper-	_____	_____		76. pelv/o-	_____	_____
41. hypo-	_____	_____		77. peri-	_____	_____
42. hyster/o-	_____	_____		78. phag/o-	_____	_____
43. -ia	_____	_____		79. pleg/o-	_____	_____
44. -iatry	_____	_____		80. pneumon/o-	_____	_____
45. -ic	_____	_____		81. poly-	_____	_____
46. -ine	_____	_____		82. post-	_____	_____
47. inter-	_____	_____		83. pre-	_____	_____
48. intestin/o-	_____	_____		84. psych/o-	_____	_____
49. intra-	_____	_____		85. quadri-	_____	_____
50. -ion	_____	_____		86. re-	_____	_____
51. -ism	_____	_____		87. -scope	_____	_____
52. -ist	_____	_____		88. -scopy	_____	_____
53. -itis	_____	_____		89. sperm/o-	_____	_____
54. -ive	_____	_____		90. spir/o-	_____	_____
55. lapar/o-	_____	_____		91. -stomy	_____	_____
56. laryng/o-	_____	_____		92. sub-	_____	_____
57. later/o-	_____	_____		93. tachy-	_____	_____
58. -logy	_____	_____		94. tens/o-	_____	_____
59. -lysis	_____	_____		95. therap/o-	_____	_____
60. mal-	_____	_____		96. -therapy	_____	_____
61. mamm/o-	_____	_____		97. thyroid/o-	_____	_____
62. -megaly	_____	_____		98. -tomy	_____	_____
63. menstru/o-	_____	_____		99. tonsill/o-	_____	_____
64. ment/o-	_____	_____		100. trache/o-	_____	_____
65. -metry	_____	_____		101. trans-	_____	_____
66. mono-	_____	_____		102. tri-	_____	_____
67. muscul/o-	_____	_____		103. urin/o-	_____	_____
68. nas/o-	_____	_____		104. uter/o-	_____	_____
69. neur/o-	_____	_____		105. vagin/o-	_____	_____
70. nucle/o-	_____	_____		106. ven/o-	_____	_____

Meaning of a Word Part Exercise

Read the meaning of the word part. Write the word part on the line. Be sure to include a hyphen or forward slash, if needed. Then write a medical word from this chapter that includes that word part. Be sure to check your spelling. The first one has been done for you.

Word Part Meaning	Word Part	Medical Word Example
1. many; much	poly-	polyneuritis
2. joint		
3. the study of		
4. surgical excision		
5. slow		
6. tonsil		
7. muscle		
8. vein		
9. disease from a specific cause		
10. lung; air		
11. inflammation of; infection of		
12. below; underneath; less than		
13. enlargement		
14. disease; suffering		
15. stomach		
16. sensation; feeling		
17. process of using an instrument to examine		

Analyze and Define Medical Words Exercise

Read the sentence. Look at the medical word in bold. Divide it into its word parts. Write the suffix and its meaning on the lines. Write the prefix and its meaning on the lines. (Note: Not every medical word contains a prefix). Write the combining form and its meaning on the lines. Join the suffix, prefix (if present), and combining form meanings together (adding small connecting words as necessary) to make the definition of the medical word and write that on the line. The first one has been done for you.

1. Patients with **cardiac** disease can have an abnormal heart rhythm.

cardiac Suffix _-ac_   Combining Form _cardi/o_

(KAR-dee-ak) Meaning _pertaining to_   Meaning _heart_

Medical Word Definition _pertaining to the heart_

2. Hepatitis and cancer are **hepatic** diseases that affect the liver.

hepatic Suffix _____   Combining Form _____

(heh-PAT-ik) Meaning _____   Meaning _____

Medical Word Definition _____

3. When you have **laryngitis,** you often lose your voice.

laryngitis Suffix _____   Combining Form _____

(LAIR-in-JY-tis) Meaning _____   Meaning _____

Medical Word Definition _____

4. A patient with chronically infected tonsils may need to have a **tonsillectomy.**

tonsillectomy Suffix _____   Combining Form _____

(TAWN-sil-LEK-toh-mee) Meaning _____   Meaning _____

Medical Word Definition _____

5. Patients with diseases such as multiple sclerosis and Parkinson's disease are treated in a **neurology** clinic (see Figure 1-7 ■).

neurology   Suffix _____   Combining Form _____

(nyoo-RAWL-oh-jee)   Meaning _____   Meaning _____

                       Medical Word Definition _____

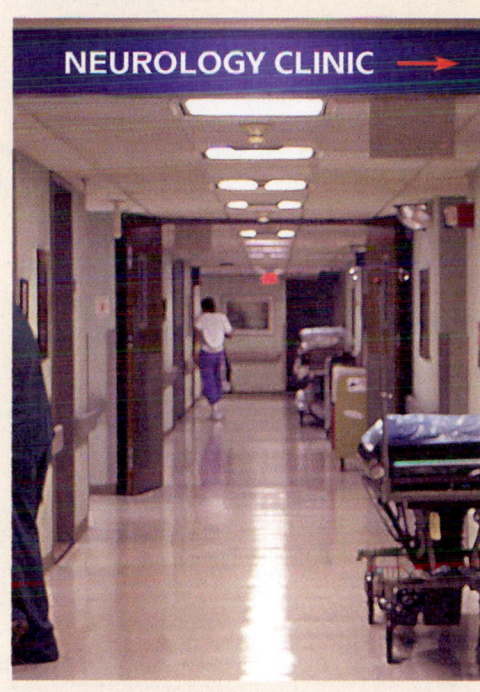

Figure 1-7 ■ Neurology clinic.
There are many types of clinics. Clinics are located in a hospital or in a separate healthcare facility.

6. Knowledge of **psychology** helps healthcare professionals understand patients and their behaviors.

psychology   Suffix _____   Combining Form _____

(sy-KAWL-oh-jee)   Meaning _____   Meaning _____

                       Medical Word Definition _____

7. **Pneumonia,** an infection in the lungs, causes hazy, white areas on a chest x-ray.

pneumonia   Suffix _____   Combining Form _____

(noo-MOH-nee-ah)   Meaning _____   Meaning _____

                       Medical Word Definition _____

8. In older adults, **arthritis** in the hip and knee joints can make walking very painful.

arthritis   Suffix _____   Combining Form _____

(ar-THRY-tis)   Meaning _____   Meaning _____

                       Medical Word Definition _____

9. A patient with constant stomach pain may need to have a **gastroscopy** to look for ulcers or bleeding.

gastroscopy   Suffix _____   Combining Form _____

(gas-TRAWS-koh-pee)   Meaning _____   Meaning _____

                       Medical Word Definition _____

10. **Polyneuropathy** is a disease condition that affects many nerves.

polyneuropathy   Suffix _____   Prefix _____   Combining Form _____

(PAWL-ee-nyoo-RAWP-ah-thee) Meaning _____   Meaning _____   Meaning _____

                       Medical Word Definition _____

11. Drugs are used to numb the skin and produce **anesthesia** prior to a procedure.

anesthesia   Suffix _____   Prefix _____   Combining Form _____

(AN-es-THEE-see-ia)   Meaning _____   Meaning _____   Meaning _____

                          Medical Word Definition _____

12. Diabetic patients give themselves insulin injections under the skin into the fatty **subcutaneous** tissue.

subcutaneous   Suffix _____   Prefix _____   Combining Form _____

(SUB-kyoo-TAY-nee-us)   Meaning _____   Meaning _____   Meaning _____

                          Medical Word Definition _____

13. **Tachycardia** is a medical condition in which the heart has an abnormally fast rate.

tachycardia   Suffix _____   Prefix _____   Combining Form _____

(TAK-ih-KAR-dee-ah)   Meaning _____   Meaning _____   Meaning _____

                          Medical Word Definition _____

14. Patients who are unable to eat are given fluids through an **intravenous** line into a vein.

intravenous   Suffix _____   Prefix _____   Combining Form _____

(IN-trah-VEE-nus)   Meaning _____   Meaning _____   Meaning _____

                          Medical Word Definition _____

15. An **intranasal** gauze pad is placed in the nostril to control bleeding from the nose.

intranasal   Suffix _____   Prefix _____   Combining Form _____

(IN-trah-NAY-zal)   Meaning _____   Meaning _____   Meaning _____

                          Medical Word Definition _____

16. An **endotracheal** tube is inserted through the mouth and into the trachea to help a patient breathe (see Figure 1-8 ■).

endotracheal   Suffix _____   Prefix _____   Combining Form _____

(EN-doh-TRAY-kee-al)   Meaning _____   Meaning _____   Meaning _____

                          Medical Word Definition _____

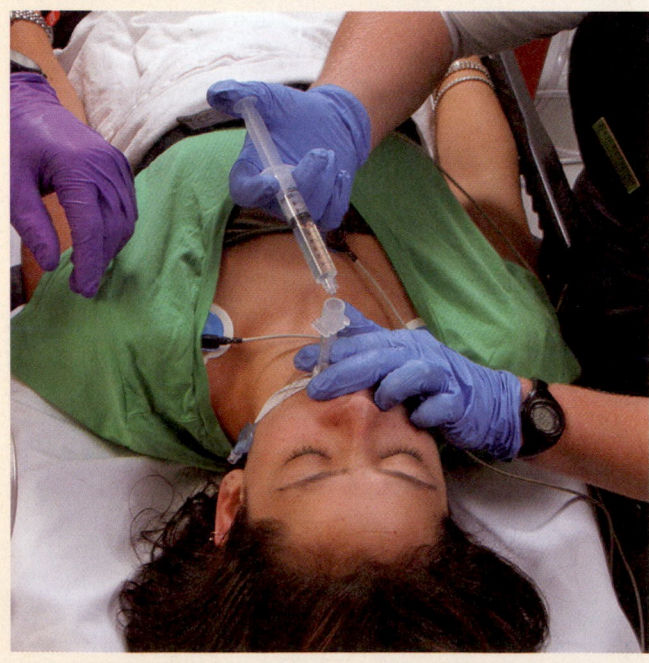

Figure 1-8 ■ Endotracheal tube.
An endotracheal tube is connected to a ventilator that breathes for a patient, but it can also be used to give a solution of a drug in an emergency situation.

Combining Form and Suffix Exercise

Practice building medical words by joining these combining forms and suffixes. Write the medical word on the line. Be sure to check your spelling. The first one has been done for you.

Combining Form	Suffix that Begins with a Vowel	Medical Word
1. cardi/o-	-ac	cardiac
2. digest/o-	-ive	_____
3. intestin/o-	-al	_____
4. append/o-	-ectomy	_____
5. neur/o-	-oma	_____
6. pneumon/o-	-ia	_____
7. therap/o-	-ist	_____
8. tonsill/o-	-itis	_____
9. urin/o-	-ary	_____
10. urin/o-	-ation	_____

Combining Form	Suffix that Begins with a Consonant	Medical Word
11. arthr/o-	-pathy	_____
12. cardi/o-	-logy	_____
13. cardi/o-	-megaly	_____
14. colon/o-	-scope	_____
15. hem/o-	-lysis	_____

Prefix Exercise

Read the definition of the medical word. Look at the medical word or partial word that is given (it already contains a combining form and a suffix). Select the correct prefix from the Prefix List and write it on the blank line. Then build the medical word and write it on the blank line. Be sure to check your spelling. The first one has been done for you.

PREFIX LIST		
an- (without; not)	hyper- (above; more than normal)	post- (after; behind)
dys- (painful; difficult; abnormal)	intra- (within)	tachy- (fast)
epi- (upon; above)	poly- (many; much)	

Definition of the Medical Word	Prefix	Word or Partial Word	Build the Medical Word
1. Disease from a specific cause of **more than normal** thyroid gland (hormone)	hyper-	thyroidism	hyperthyroidism
2. Condition of **much** urine	_____	uria	_____
3. Pertaining to **above** the stomach	_____	gastric	_____
4. Condition of (being) **without** urine	_____	uria	_____
5. Pertaining to **within** a muscle	_____	muscular	_____
6. Condition of a **fast** heart (rate)	_____	cardia	_____
7. Pertaining to **behind** the nose	_____	nasal	_____
8. Condition of **painful** urine	_____	uria	_____

Matching Exercise

Match each word or word part to its description.

1. arthr/o-   _____ Medical word definition is *pertaining to within the trachea*

2. brady-   _____ Combining form meaning *blood*

3. laryngitis   _____ Medical word definition is *pertaining to the heart*

4. endotracheal   _____ Combining form meaning *skin*

5. lapar/o-   _____ Combining form meaning *abdomen*

6. cutane/o-   _____ Suffix meaning *inflammation of; infection of*

7. -ectomy   _____ Prefix meaning *slow*

8. hem/o-   _____ Medical word definition is *pertaining to within a vein*

9. -itis   _____ Combining form meaning *joint*

10. intravenous   _____ Medical word definition is *enlargement of the heart*

11. cardiomegaly   _____ Medical word definition is *inflammation or infection of the voice box*

12. cardiac   _____ Suffix meaning *surgical excision*

Word Analysis Exercise

These are the two longest words you will study in this textbook. See if you can break apart each word into its word parts, define the word parts, and then define the entire medical word. Some of the word parts will be familiar to you. For those that are not, use Appendix A at the back of this book to look up the meanings.

1. esophagogastroduodenoscopy

Suffix _____   Suffix Meaning _____

Combining Form _____   Combining Form Meaning _____

Combining Form _____   Combining Form Meaning _____

Combining Form _____   Combining Form Meaning _____

Medical Word Definition _____

2. otorhinolaryngology

Suffix _____   Suffix Meaning _____

Combining Form _____   Combining Form Meaning _____

Combining Form _____   Combining Form Meaning _____

Combining Form _____   Combining Form Meaning _____

Medical Word Definition _____

The Medical Record

True or False Exercise

Indicate whether each statement is true or false by writing T or F on the line.

1. _____ The medical record is where healthcare professionals document care provided to a patient.

2. _____ The medical record of today is mainly used to document diseases, treatments, and surgeries.

3. _____ The medical record is a medicolegal document.

4. _____ By law, the format of a medical record must be the same in all healthcare facilities.

5. _____ A consent to treat form signed by the patient allows the healthcare facility to contact HIPAA for payment for any medical care provided.

Critical Thinking Questions

1. Describe three advantages of the newer computerized patient record.

   a. _____

   b. _____

   c. _____

2. Name five things that might be included on a preventive care checklist in a patient's medical record.

   a. _____

   b. _____

   c. _____

   d. _____

   e. _____

3. Give the three names used for a future, all-encompassing medical record that will provide immediate access to all parts of a patient's record.

   a. _____

   b. _____

   c. _____

Abbreviations

Abbreviation Exercise

Write the definition for each abbreviation on the line provided.

1. CPR _____

2. DS _____

3. CC _____

4. H&P _____

5. Dx _____

6. ROS _____

Applied Skills

Circle Exercise

Circle the correct word from the choices given.

1. Daniel Frist broke his left middle (**phalanges, phalanx**) while playing baseball.

2. Baby Phong Nyugen's mother took him to the doctor when she noticed that his left (**testes, testis**) was not present in the scrotum.

3. On the x-ray, Leona Calvin's spine showed several (**vertebra, vertebrae**) that were misaligned.

4. Dr. James Gibbons treated Al Smith's (**gastric, gastroscopy**) ulcer by prescribing medication.

5. The physical examination at the walk-in clinic revealed that Jose Rodriguez had (**tonsillectomy, tonsillitis**).

6. The laboratory identified several (**bacteria, bacterium**) that were present in the patient's wound.

7. Alan Witherspoon underwent a (**cardiac, cardiomegaly**) stress test to evaluate his heart.

8. Alicyn Smart experienced severe abdominal pain, and the emergency department physician scheduled her to have this surgery: (**appendectomy, appendicitis**).

9. Dr. Matthew Cohen decided to specialize in treating the (**tonsillectomy, urinary**) system.

10. When Briana Wright began feeling depressed, she made an appointment with a (**psychotherapy, psychiatrist**).

Spelling Exercise

Look at each medical word and detect the spelling error. Then write the correct spelling of the medical word on the line provided. The first one has been done for you.

Misspelled Medical Word	Correct Spelling	Misspelled Medical Word	Correct Spelling
1. cardeac	<u>cardiac</u>	6. sychiatry	_____
2. appendektomee	_____	7. takicardia	_____
3. subcutayneous	_____	8. tonsilitis	_____
4. larinjitis	_____	9. urinashun	_____
5. mamografee	_____	10. venus	_____

Hearing Medical Words Exercise

You hear someone speaking the medical words given below. Read each pronunciation and then write the medical word it represents. Be sure to check your spelling. The first one has been done for you.

1. KAR-dee-ac	<u>cardiac</u>	6. nyoo-RAWL-oh-jee	_____
2. AP-pen-DEK-toh-mee	_____	7. TAWN-sih-LY-tis	_____
3. YOO-rih-NAY-shun	_____	8. YOO-ter-in	_____
4. SY-koh-THAIR-ah-tree	_____	9. SUB-kyoo-TAY-nee-us	_____
5. IN-trah-VEE-nus	_____	10. noo-MOH-nee-ah	_____

Pronunciation Exercise

Read the medical word that is given. Then review the syllables in its pronunciation. Circle the primary (main) accented syllable. The first one has been done for you.

1. cardiac (kar-dee-ak)
2. urinary (yoo-rih-nair-ee)
3. endotracheal (en-doh-tray-kee-al)
4. muscular (mus-kyoo-lar)
5. psychology (sy-kawl-oh-jee)
6. hepatic (heh-pat-ik)
7. cardiomegaly (kar-dee-oh-meg-ah-lee)
8. mammography (mah-mawg-rah-fee)
9. psychosis (sy-koh-sis)
10. laparotomy (lap-ah-raw-toh-mee)

Multimedia Preview

Immerse yourself in a variety of activities inside Medical Terminology Interactive. Getting there is simple:

1. Click on www.myhealthprofessionskit.com.
2. Select "Medical Terminology" from the choice of disciplines.
3. First-time users must create an account using the scratch-off code on the inside front cover of this book.
4. Find this book and log in using your username and password.
5. Click on Medical Terminology Interactive.
6. Take the elevator to the 1st Floor to begin your virtual exploration of this chapter!

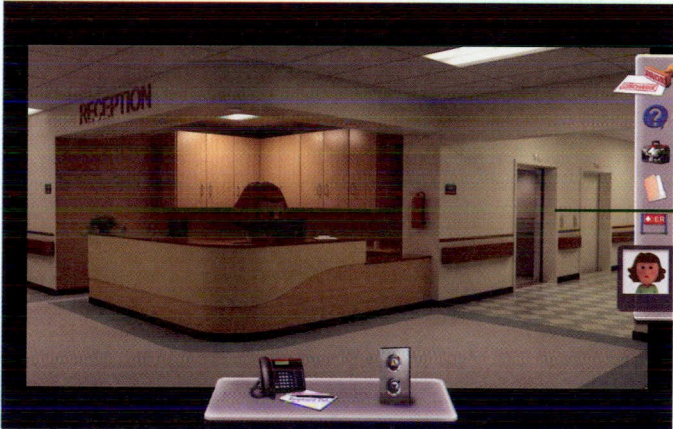 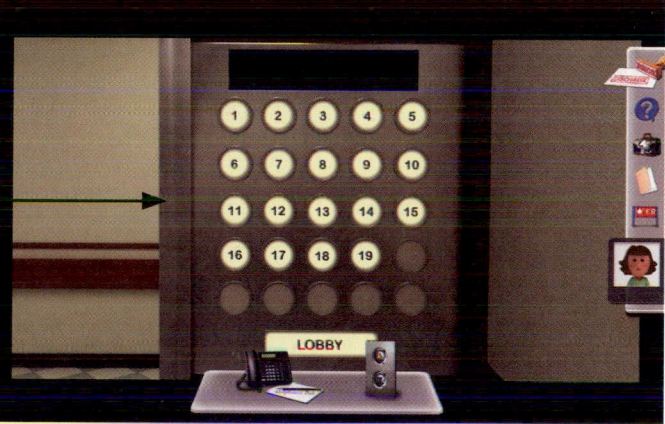

Beat the Clock   Challenge the clock by testing your medical terminology smarts against time. Click here for a game of knowledge, spelling, and speed. Can you correctly answer 20 questions before the final tick?

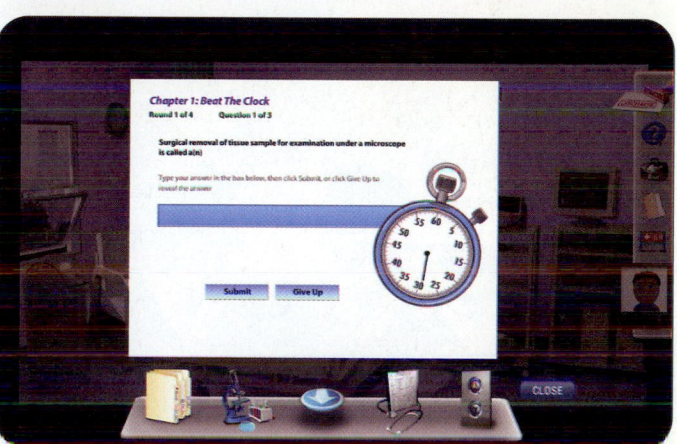

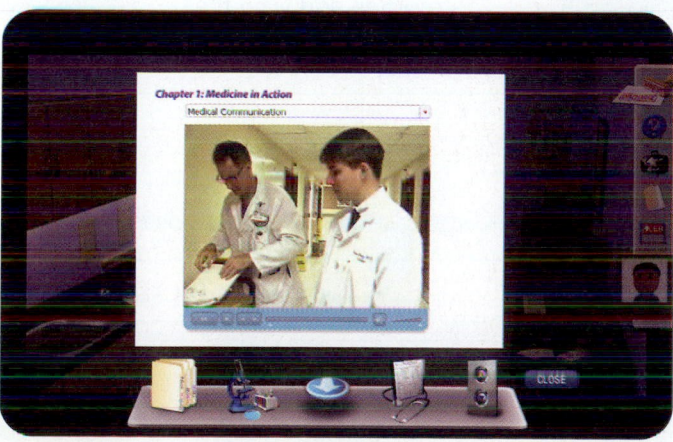

Medicine in Action   These videos breathe life into the concepts presented in the pages of this book. The videos give you a better understanding of the material by allowing you to see it in action.

PEARSON
myhealthprofessionskit

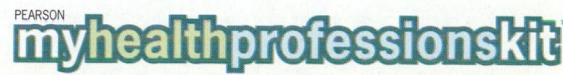

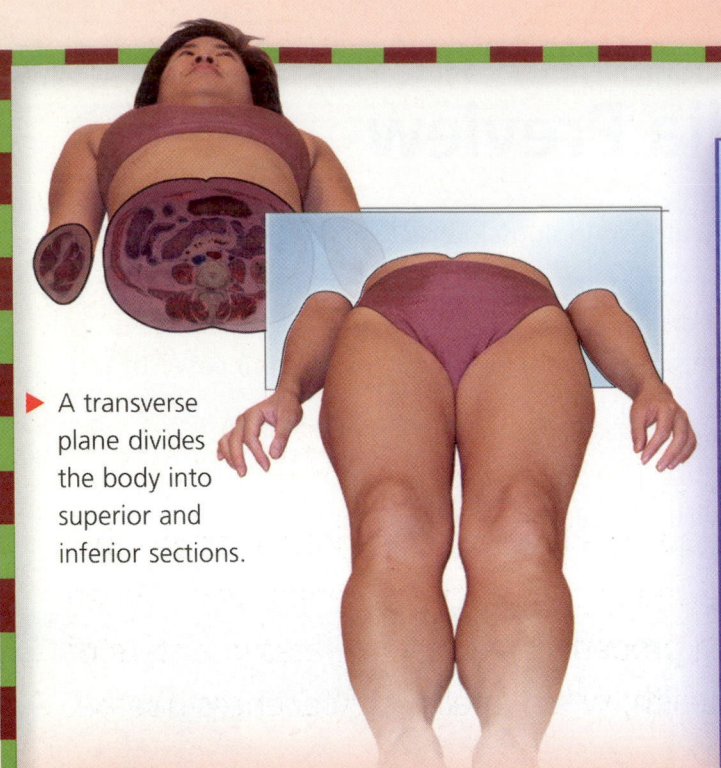

A transverse plane divides the body into superior and inferior sections.

Dive In!

- Attention! Stand up! Arms at your sides and palms forward. Look straight ahead. Now you are in anatomical position.
- The first human dissection was performed about 2,500 years ago in Greece.
- In this chapter you'll explore body positions, cavities, systems, and medical specialties. Then you'll be in a position to master the language of the body as a whole!

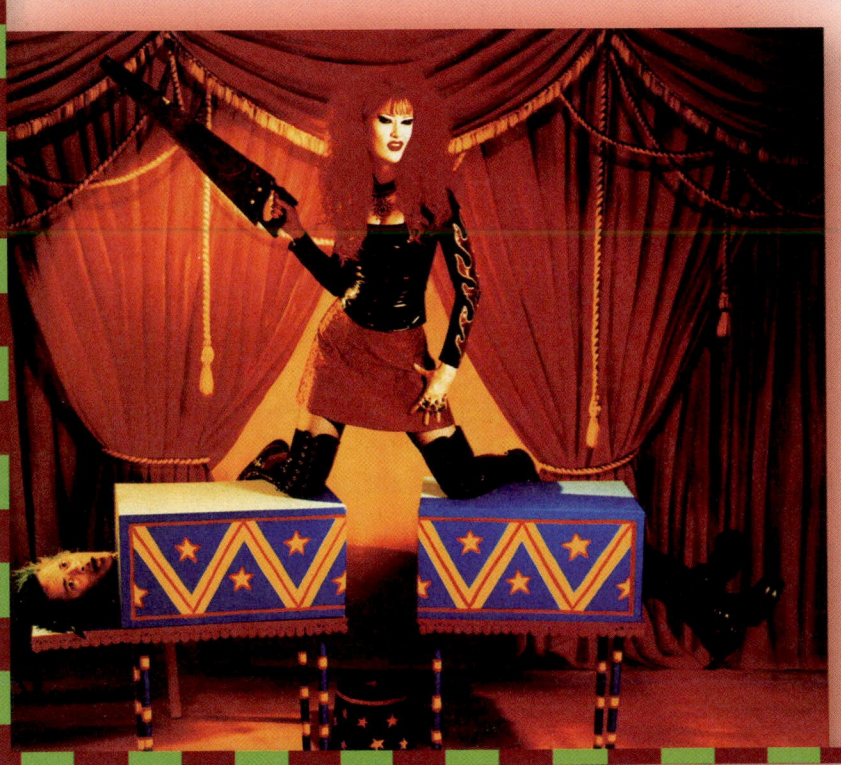

The magic of advanced medical imaging techniques allows healthcare professionals to divide and view the body in various ways.

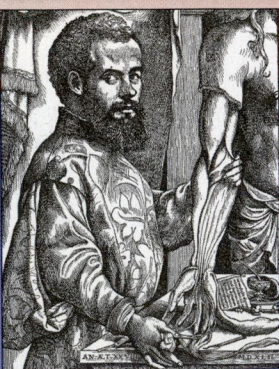

1543

The first complete anatomy textbook is written and illustrated by Andreas Vesalius of Brussels, Belgium

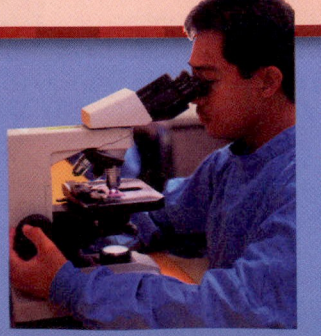

1609

Galileo invents a microscope that includes a magnifying lens and focusing mechanism

The Body in Health and Disease

2

The human body is a marvelous, intricate creation that can be organized and studied in different ways. When functioning properly, the body operates in a state of health; when it fails, it experiences disease.

▶ A diet that includes a variety of nutritious foods helps to maintain the body in health and aids in the prevention of disease.

◀ A hospital is just one of the many different settings where health care takes place.

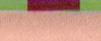

1616

William Harvey, an English physician, describes the circulation of the blood throughout the body

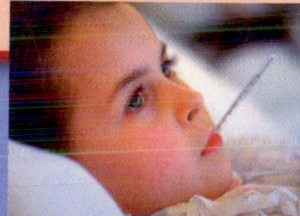

German physicist Gabriel Fahrenheit invents the mercury thermometer

1714

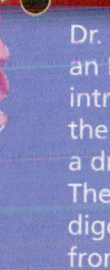

1741

Dr. William Withering, an English physician, introduces the use of the foxglove plant as a drug for the heart. The modern drug digoxin is derived from it

Measure Your Progress: Learning Objectives

After you study this chapter, you should be able to

1. Describe approaches used to organize information about the human body.

2. Identify body directions, body cavities, body systems, and medical specialties.

3. Describe various categories of diseases.

4. Describe techniques used to perform a physical examination.

5. Describe categories of healthcare professionals and settings in which health care is provided.

6. Give the medical meaning of word parts related to the body, health, and disease.

7. Build medical words about the body, health, and disease from word parts and divide and define words.

8. Spell and pronounce medical words about the body, health, and disease.

9. Dive deeper into the body, health, and disease by reviewing the activities at the end of this chapter and online at Medical Terminology Interactive.

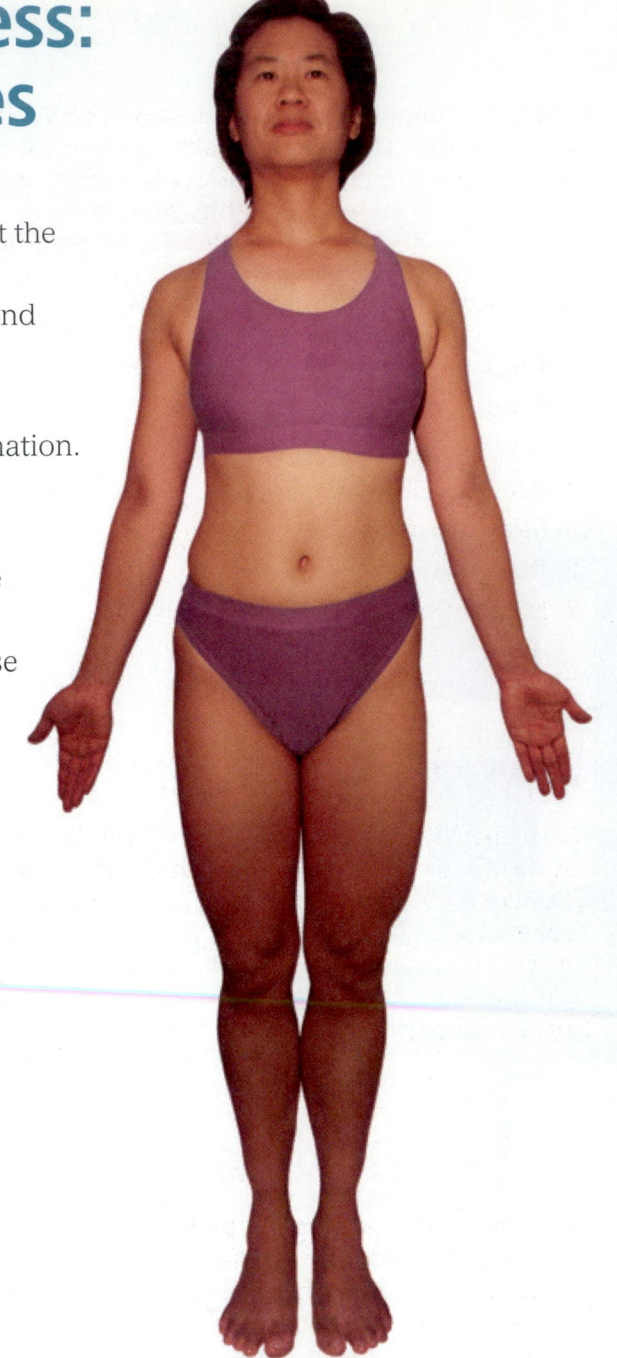

Figure 2-1 ■ Human body in anatomical position.

Anatomical position is a standard position in which the body is standing erect, the head is up with the eyes looking forward, the arms are by the sides with the palms facing forward, and the legs are straight with the toes pointing forward.

The Body in Health

WORD BUILDING

When the human body's countless parts function correctly, the body is in a state of **health.** The World Health Organization defines health as a state of complete physical, mental, and social well-being (and not just the absence of disease or infirmity).The healthy human body can be studied in several different ways. Each way approaches the body from a specific point of view and provides unique information by dividing or organizing the body in a logical way. These ways include the following

1. Body planes and body directions
2. Body cavities
3. Quadrants and regions
4. Anatomy and physiology
5. Microscopic to macroscopic
6. Body systems
7. Medical specialties.

Body Planes and Body Directions

When the human body is in the **anatomical position** (see Figure 2-1 ■), it can be studied by dividing it with planes. A **plane** is an imaginary flat surface (like a plate of glass) that divides the body into two parts. There are three main body planes: the coronal or frontal plane, the sagittal plane, and the transverse plane. These planes divide the body into front and back, right and left, and top and bottom sections respectively. Body directions represent movement away from or toward these planes.

The Coronal Plane and Body Directions

The **coronal plane** or **frontal plane** is a vertical plane that divides the body into front and back sections (see Figure 2-2 ■). The coronal plane is named for the coronal suture in the cranium (see Figure 2-3 ■).

The front of the body is the **anterior** or **ventral** section. The back of the body is the **posterior** or **dorsal** section. Lying face down is being in the **prone** position. Lying on the back is being in the **dorsal** or **dorsal supine** position.

Moving toward the front of the body is moving in an anterior direction, or anteriorly. Moving toward the back of the body is moving in a posterior direction, or posteriorly (see Figure 2-4 ■). The directions anterior and posterior can be combined as anteroposterior or posteroanterior. An **anteroposterior (AP)** direction involves moving from outside the body through the anterior section and then through the posterior section. A **posteroanterior (PA)** direction involves moving from outside the body through the posterior section and then through the anterior section (see Figure 2-5 ■).

health (HELTH)

anatomical (AN-ah-TAWM-ih-kal)
 ana- *apart from; excessive*
 tom/o- *cut; slice; layer*
 -ical *pertaining to*

plane (PLAYN)

coronal (kor-OH-nal)
 coron/o- *structure that encircles like a crown*
 -al *pertaining to*

frontal (FRUN-tal)
 front/o- *front*
 -al *pertaining to*

anterior (an-TEER-ee-or)
 anter/o- *before; front part*
 -ior *pertaining to*

ventral (VEN-tral)
 ventr/o- *front; abdomen*
 -al *pertaining to*

posterior (pohs-TEER-ee-or)
 poster/o- *back part*
 -ior *pertaining to*

dorsal (DOR-sal)
 dors/o- *back; dorsum*
 -al *pertaining to*

prone (PROHN)

supine (soo-PINE) (SOO-pine)

anteroposterior
(AN-ter-oh-pohs-TEER-ee-or)
 anter/o- *before; front part*
 poster/o- *back part*
 -ior *pertaining to*

posteroanterior
(POHS-ter-oh-an-TEER-ee-or)
 poster/o- *back part*
 anter/o- *before; front part*
 -ior *pertaining to*

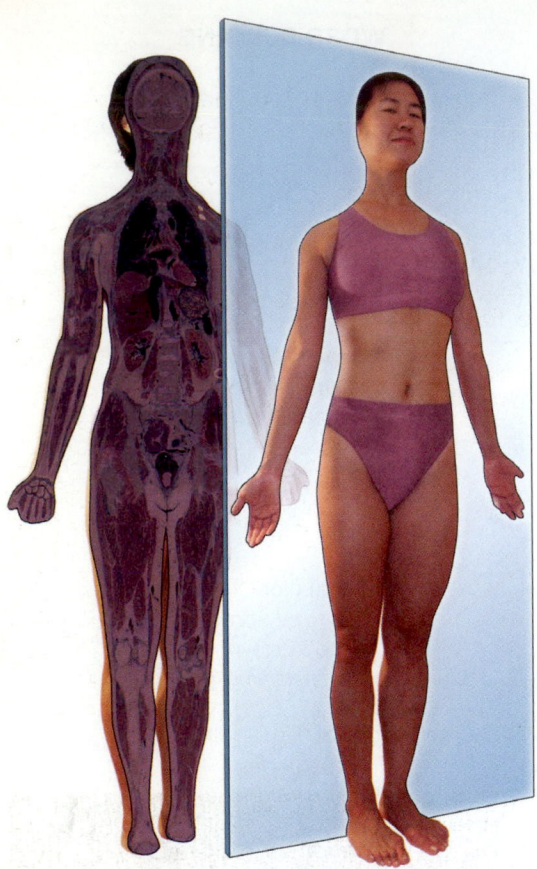

Figure 2-2 ■ Coronal plane.
The coronal or frontal plane divides the body into anterior (front) and posterior (back) sections.

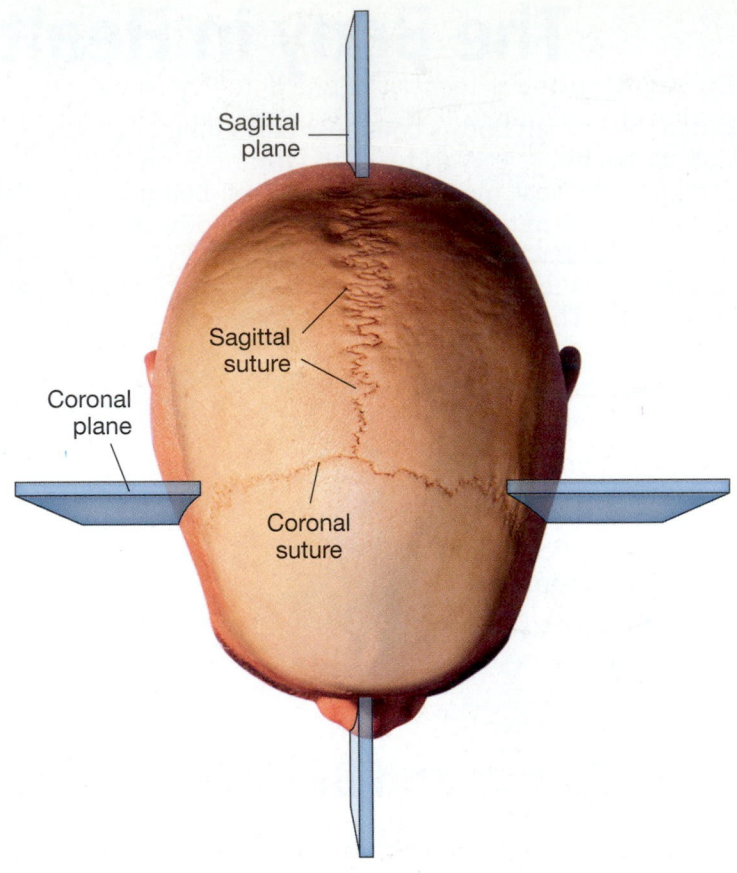

Figure 2-3 ■ Coronal and sagittal sutures of the cranium.
The coronal and sagittal planes are named for the coronal and sagittal sutures that join together the bones of the cranium. Each plane is oriented in the same direction as the suture for which it is named.

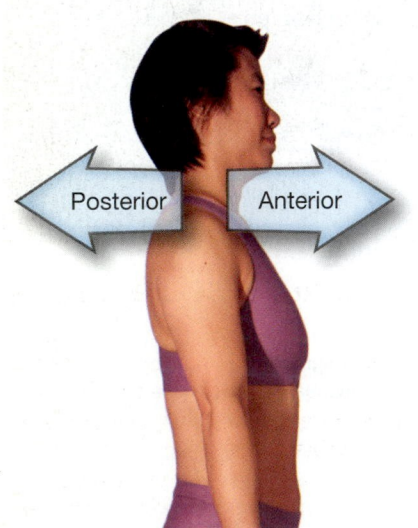

Figure 2-4 ■ Anterior and posterior directions.
Moving in an anterior direction is moving toward the front of the body. Moving in a posterior direction is moving toward the back of the body. Anterior and posterior are opposite directions.

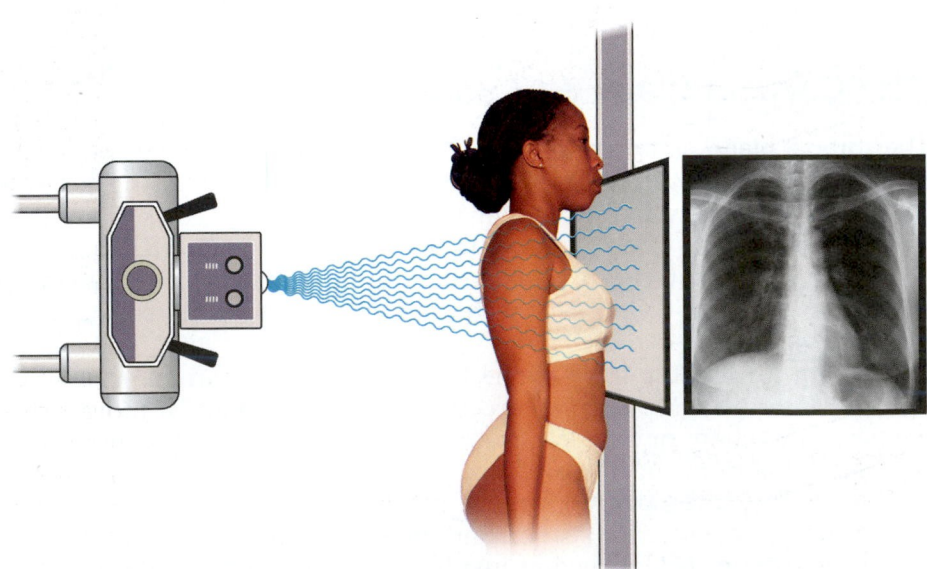

Figure 2-5 ■ Posteroanterior direction.
Anteroposterior and *posteroanterior* are commonly used in radiology to indicate the path of the x-ray beam. For a posteroanterior (PA) chest x-ray, the x-ray beam enters the posterior chest, goes through the anterior chest, and enters the x-ray plate to produce an image.

The Sagittal Plane and Body Directions

The **sagittal plane** is a vertical plane that divides the body into right and left sections (see Figure 2-6 ■). The sagittal plane is named for the sagittal suture in the cranium (see Figure 2-3). If this plane divides the body at the midline into equal right and left sections, it is a midsagittal plane (see Figure 2-7 ■).

Moving from either side of the body toward the midline is moving in a **medial** direction, or medially. Moving from the midline toward either side of the body is moving in a **lateral** direction, or laterally (see Figure 2-8 ■).

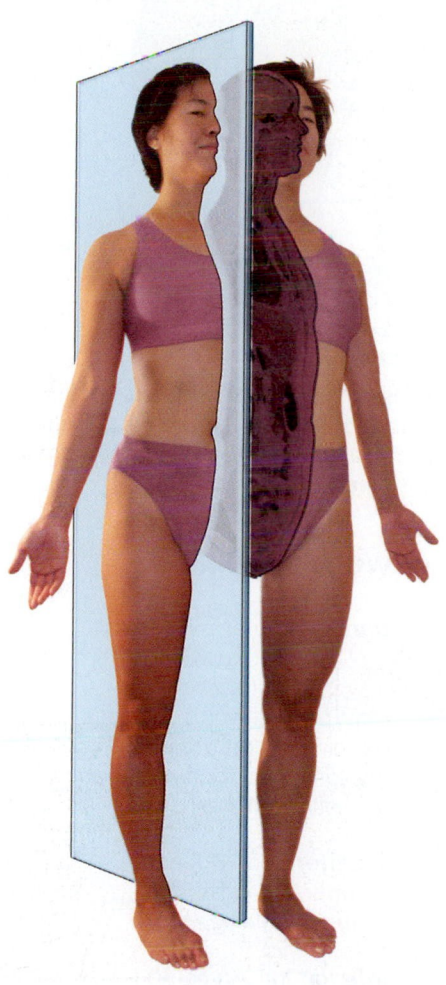

Figure 2-6 ■ Sagittal plane.
The sagittal plane divides the body into right and left sections.

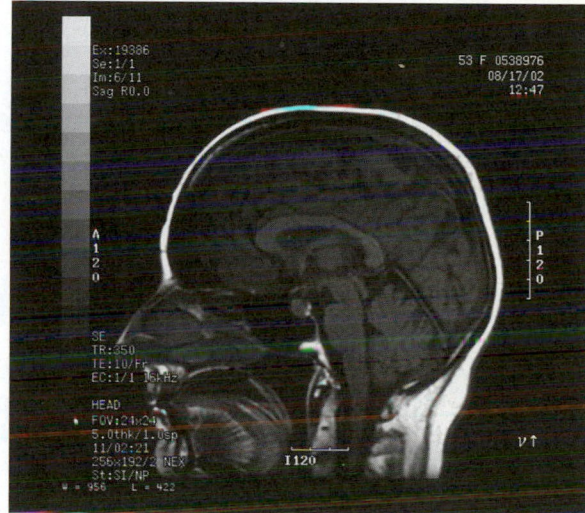

Figure 2-7 ■ **Midsagittal image of the head on an MRI scan.**

A magnetic resonance imaging (MRI) scan uses a magnetic field to create many individual images of the body in "slices." This image was taken along the midsagittal plane. The prefix *mid-* means *middle*. Other images taken during this scan would show "slices" along many parasagittal planes on either side of the midline. The prefix *para-* means *beside; apart from.*

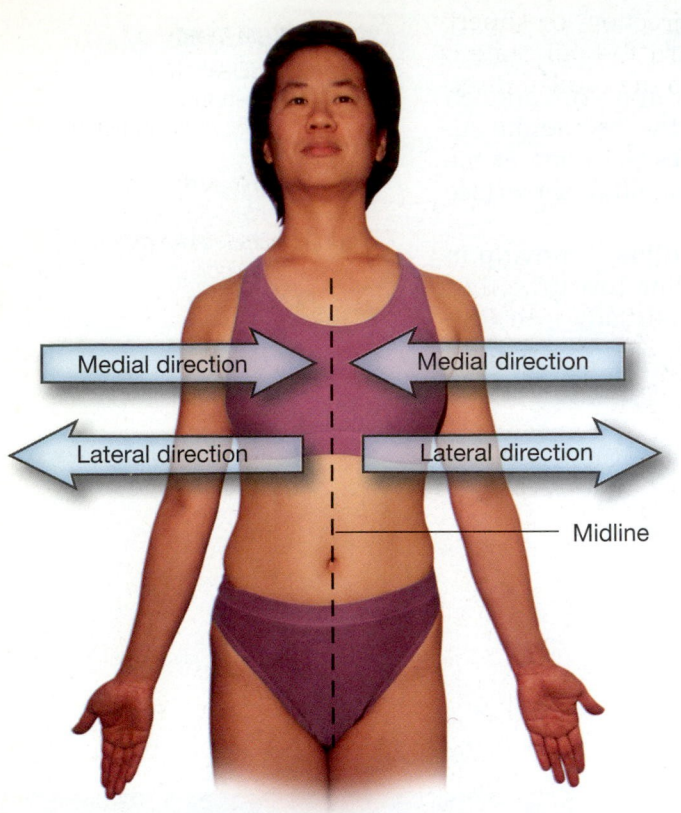

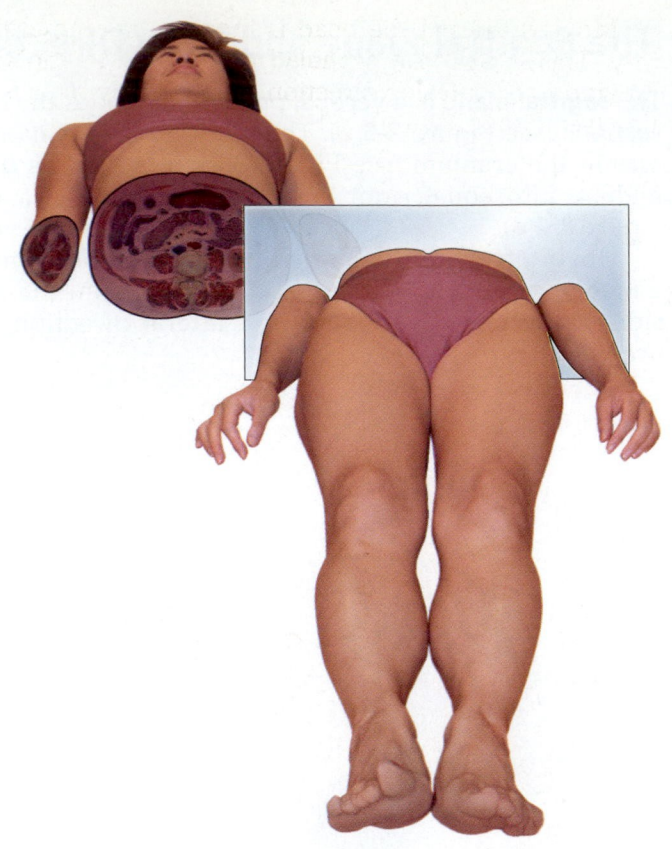

Figure 2-8 ■ **Medial and lateral directions.**
Moving in a medial direction is moving toward the midline of the body. Moving in a lateral direction is moving away from the midline of the body. Medial and lateral are opposite directions.

Figure 2-9 ■ **Transverse plane.**
The transverse plane divides the body into superior (top) and inferior (bottom) sections.

The Transverse Plane and Body Directions

The **transverse plane** is a horizontal plane that divides the body into top and bottom sections (see Figure 2-9 ■). The upper half of the body is the **superior** section, and the lower half is the **inferior** section. Some anatomical structures have superior and inferior parts (see Figure 2-10 ■).

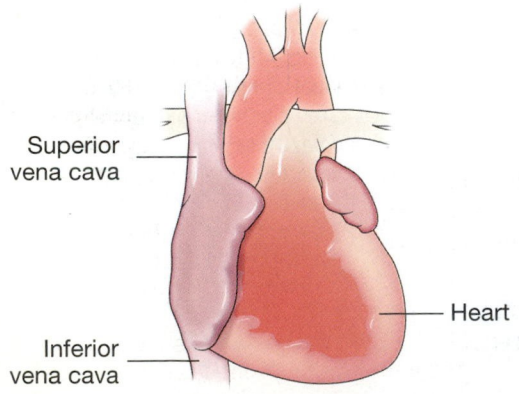

Figure 2-10 ■ **Superior and inferior parts.**
The superior vena cava is a large vein that is above the heart. It carries blood from the head and brings it to the heart. The inferior vena cava is a large vein below the heart. It carries blood from the lower body and brings it to the heart.

WORD BUILDING

transverse (trans-VERS)
 trans- *across; through*
 -verse *to travel; to turn*
Most medical words contain a combining form. *Transverse* contains the combining form *vers/o-* and the one-letter suffix *-e.*

superior (soo-PEER-ee-or)
 super/o- *above*
 -ior *pertaining to*

inferior (in-FEER-ee-or)
 infer/o- *below*
 -ior *pertaining to*

Moving toward the head is moving in a superior direction, or superiorly. This is also the **cephalad** direction. Moving toward the tail bone is moving in an inferior direction, or inferiorly. This is also the **caudad** direction (see Figure 2-11 ■).

WORD BUILDING

cephalad (SEF-ah-lad)
  cephal/o- *head*
  -ad *toward; in the direction of*

caudad (KAW-dad)
  caud/o- *tail (tail bone)*
  -ad *toward; in the direction of*

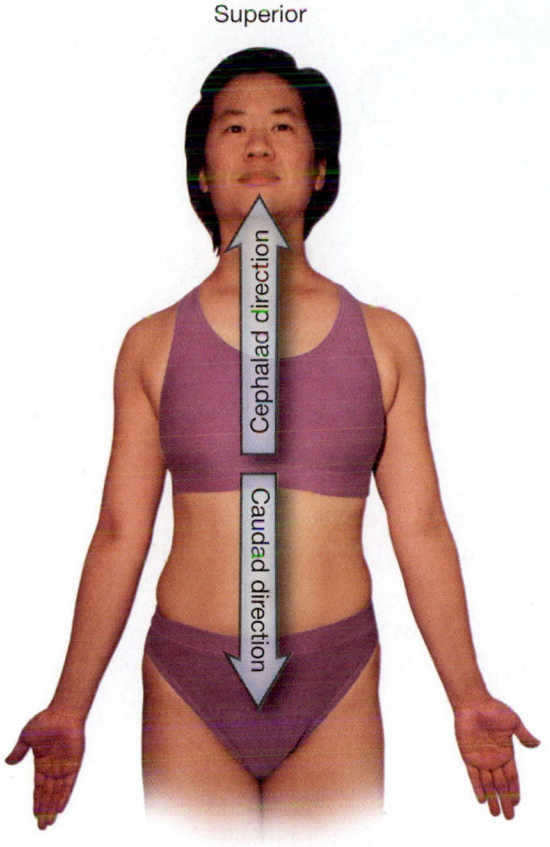

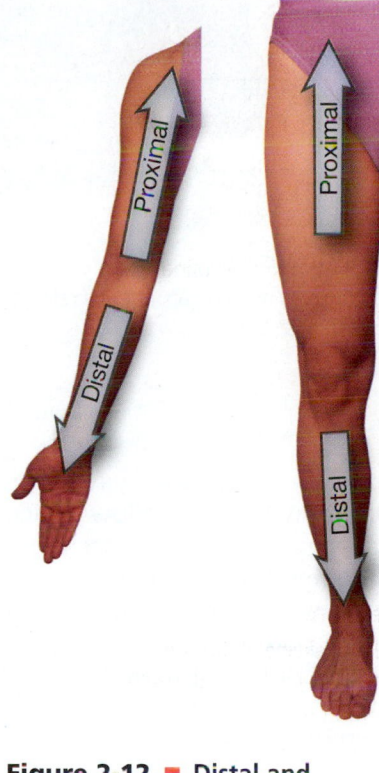

Figure 2-12 ■ Distal and proximal directions.

Moving in a distal direction is moving from where the limb is attached to the body toward the fingers or toes (at the end of the limb). Moving in a proximal direction is moving from the fingers or toes toward where the limb is attached to the body. Distal and proximal are opposite directions.

Figure 2-11 ■ Cephalad and caudad directions.

Moving in a cephalad direction is moving toward the head. Moving in a caudad direction is moving toward the tail bone. Cephalad and caudad are opposite directions.

Other Body Directions and Positions

Moving from the trunk of the body toward the end of a limb (arm or leg) is moving in a **distal** direction, or distally. Moving from the end of a limb toward the trunk of the body is moving in a **proximal** direction, or proximally (see Figure 2-12 ■).

Structures on the surface of the body are superficial or **external** structures. Structures below the surface and inside the body are deep or **internal** structures (see Figure 2-13 ■).

distal (DIS-tal)
  dist/o- *away from the center or point of origin*
  -al *pertaining to*

proximal (PRAWK-sih-mal)
  proxim/o- *near the center or point of origin*
  -al *pertaining to*

external (eks-TER-nal)
  extern/o- *outside*
  -al *pertaining to*

internal (in-TER-nal)
  intern/o- *inside*
  -al *pertaining to*

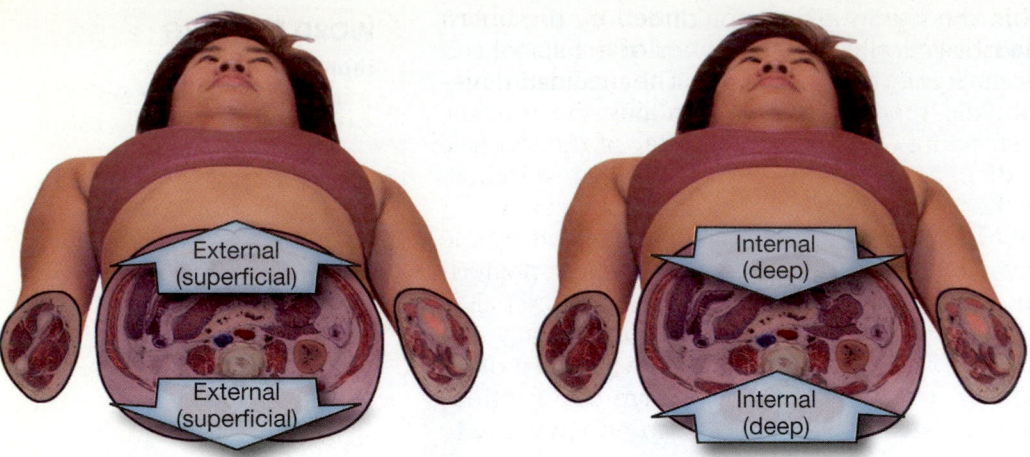

External (superficial)

External (superficial)

Internal (deep)

Internal (deep)

Figure 2-13 ■ External and internal positions.

External refers to the superficial or outer part of the body or an organ. *Internal* refers to deep inside the body or an organ. Internal and external are opposite positions.

Body Cavities

The human body can be studied according to its body cavities and their internal organs (see Figure 2-14 ■). A **cavity** is a hollow space. It is surrounded by bones or muscles that support and protect the organs and structures within the cavity. There are five body cavities.

The **cranial cavity** is within the bony cranium. The cranial cavity contains the brain, cranial nerves, and other structures.

The **spinal cavity** or spinal canal is a continuation of the cranial cavity as it travels down the midline of the back. The spinal cavity is within the bones of the spinal column. The spinal cavity contains the spinal cord, spinal nerves, and other structures.

WORD BUILDING
cavity (KAV-ih-tee)
cav/o- *hollow space*
-ity *state; condition*
cranial (KRAY-nee-al)
crani/o- *cranium (skull)*
-al *pertaining to*
spinal (SPY-nal)
spin/o- *spine; backbone*
-al *pertaining to*

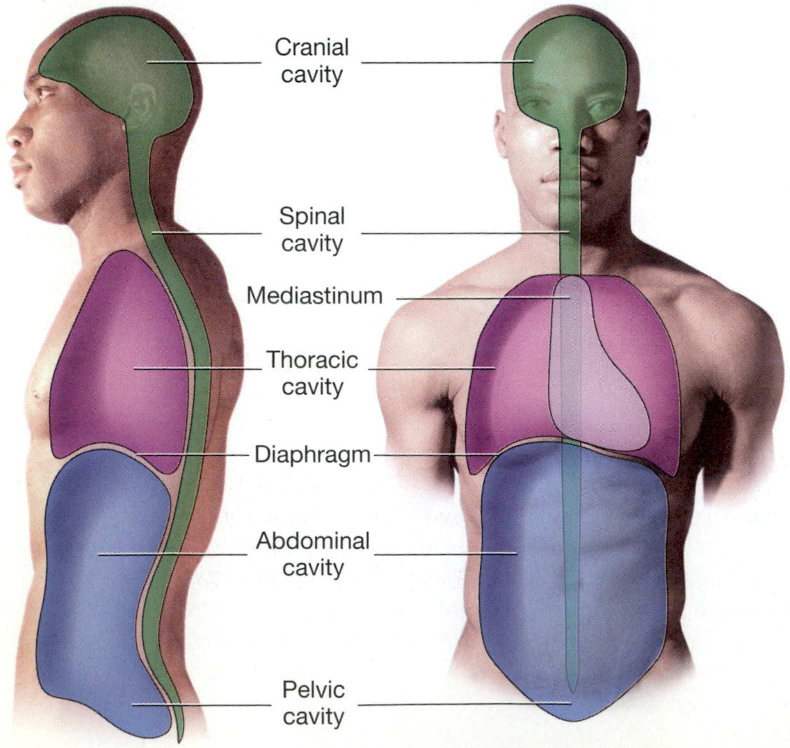

Cranial cavity

Spinal cavity

Mediastinum

Thoracic cavity

Diaphragm

Abdominal cavity

Pelvic cavity

Figure 2-14 ■ Body cavities.

The cranial and spinal cavities are continuous with each other. The thoracic cavity is separated from the abdominal cavity by the diaphragm. The abdominal cavity is continuous with the pelvic cavity and is often referred to as the abdominopelvic cavity.

The **thoracic cavity** is within the chest and is surrounded by the breast bone (sternum) anteriorly, the ribs laterally, and the bones of the spinal column posteriorly. The thoracic cavity contains the lungs. The mediastinum—a smaller, central area within the thoracic cavity—contains the trachea, esophagus, heart, and other structures. The inferior border of the thoracic cavity is the large, muscular diaphragm that functions during respiration. The diaphragm separates the thoracic cavity from the abdominal cavity.

The **abdominal cavity** is within the abdomen. It is surrounded by the abdominal muscles anteriorly and the bones of the spinal column posteriorly. The **pelvic cavity** is a continuation of the abdominal cavity. The pelvic cavity is surrounded by the pelvic (hip) bones anteriorly and laterally and the bones of the spinal column posteriorly. These two cavities are often referred to as the **abdominopelvic cavity** because they form one continuous cavity that has no dividing structure in it. The abdominopelvic cavity contains many of the organs of the gastrointestinal, reproductive, and urinary systems. These internal organs in the abdominopelvic cavity are known as the **viscera.**

Quadrants and Regions

The human body can be studied according to its quadrants and regions. The anterior surface of the abdominopelvic area can be divided into four quadrants or nine regions, either of which is helpful as a reference during a physical examination of the internal organs.

The four **quadrants** include the left upper quadrant (LUQ), right upper quadrant (RUQ), left lower quadrant (LLQ), and right lower quadrant (RLQ) (see Figure 2-15 ■).

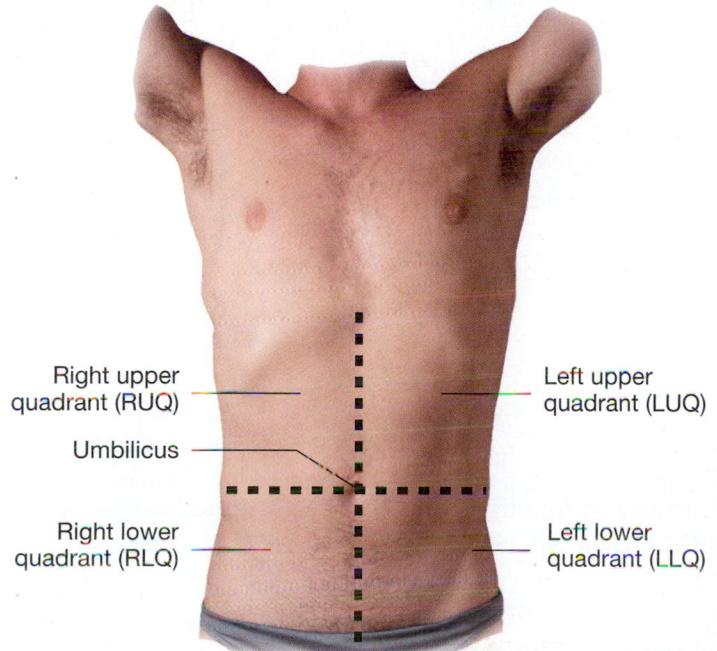

Right upper quadrant (RUQ)

Umbilicus

Right lower quadrant (RLQ)

Left upper quadrant (LUQ)

Left lower quadrant (LLQ)

Figure 2-15 ■ Quadrants of the abdominopelvic area.
Four quadrants are formed when a horizontal line and a vertical line cross at the umbilicus (navel). Remember, when you are facing the patient (as in this illustration), your right side corresponds to the patient's left side.

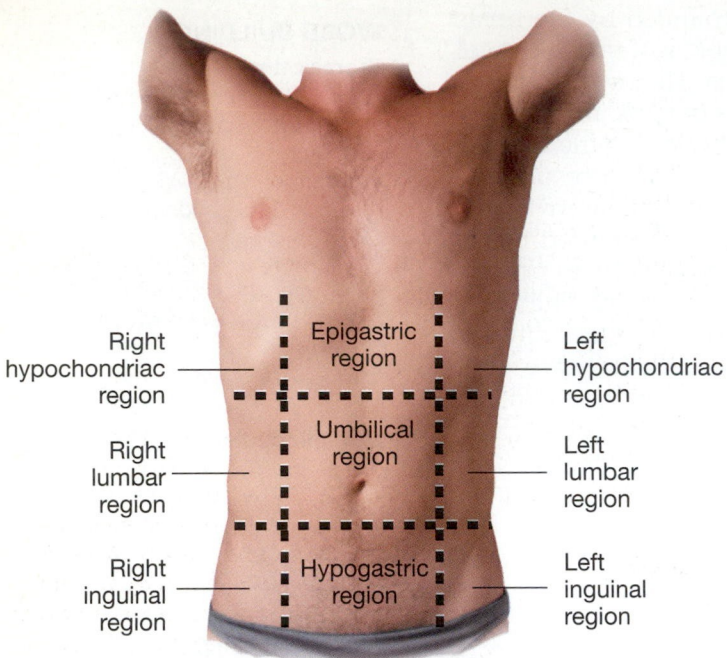

Right hypochondriac region

Epigastric region

Left hypochondriac region

Right lumbar region

Umbilical region

Left lumbar region

Right inguinal region

Hypogastric region

Left inguinal region

Figure 2-16 ■ Regions of the abdominopelvic area.
Nine regions are formed when two horizontal lines and two vertical lines form a square around the umbilicus.

The nine regions include the right and left **hypochondriac** regions, the **epigastric** region, the right and left **lumbar** regions, the **umbilical** region, the right and left **inguinal** or **iliac** regions, and the **hypogastric** region (see Figure 2-16 ■).

Did You Know?

The Greeks considered the hypochondriac regions to be the seat of melancholy (sad feelings) because they contained the liver and spleen, and it was thought that these organs released humors that caused different moods. This is the basis for the word *hypochondriac*, a person who is anxious and talks excessively about real or imagined illnesses. Many of the symptoms of these illnesses occur in the abdominal and pelvic areas of the body which are "below the cartilage (of the ribs)."

Anatomy and Physiology

The human body can be studied according to its structures and functions. **Anatomy** is the study of the structures of the human body. **Physiology** is the study of the functions of those structures.

Clinical Connections

The anatomy of the human body was first studied by physicians who secretly carried away and dissected the unclaimed dead bodies of criminals.

WORD BUILDING

hypochondriac
(HY-poh-CON-dree-ak)
  hypo- *below; deficient*
  chondr/o- *cartilage*
  -iac *pertaining to*
Add words to make a complete definition of *hypochondriac: pertaining to below the cartilage (of the ribs).*

epigastric (EP-ih-GAS-trik)
  epi- *upon; above*
  gastr/o- *stomach*
  -ic *pertaining to*

lumbar (LUM-bar)
  lumb/o- *lower back; area between the ribs and pelvis*
  -ar *pertaining to*

umbilical (um-BIL-ih-kal)
  umbilic/o- *umbilicus; navel*
  -al *pertaining to*

inguinal (ING-gwih-nal)
  inguin/o- *groin*
  -al *pertaining to*

iliac (IL-ee-ak)
  ili/o- *ilium (hip bone)*
  -ac *pertaining to*

hypogastric (HY-poh-GAS-trik)
  hypo- *below; deficient*
  gastr/o- *stomach*
  -ic *pertaining to*

anatomy (ah-NA-toh-mee)
  ana- *apart from; excessive*
  -tomy *process of cutting or making an incision*
The ending *-tomy* contains the combining form *tom/o-* and the one-letter suffix *-y.*

physiology (FIZ-ee-AWL-oh-jee)
  physi/o- *physical function*
  -logy *the study of*

Microscopic to Macroscopic

The human body can be studied according to its smallest parts and how they combine to make larger and more complex structures and systems.

A **cell** is the smallest independently functioning structure in the body that can reproduce itself by division. (The structures and functions of a cell are discussed in "Oncology," Chapter 18.) Most cells and cellular structures are **microscopic** in size, that is, they can be seen only through a **microscope** (see Figure 2-17 ■). (*Note:* Some cells—a female ovum, for example—are large enough to be seen with the naked eye.) Cells combine to form **tissues,** and tissues combine to form **organs.** (The different kinds of tissues and organs are discussed in specific chapters.) Tissues and organs are **macroscopic,** that is, they can be seen with the naked eye. Organs combine to form a body system. The human body contains several different body systems, as discussed in the next section.

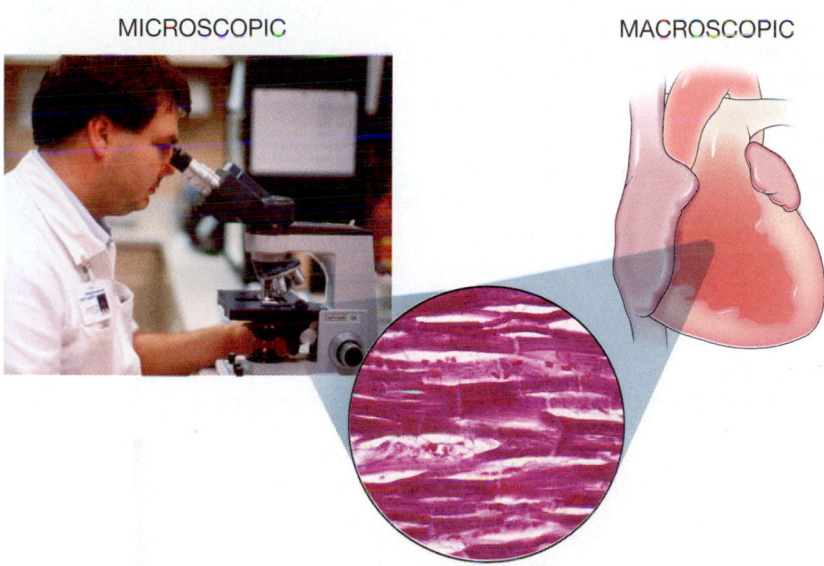
MICROSCOPIC   MACROSCOPIC

Figure 2-17 ■ Using a microscope to study the human body.

A microscope enhances our ability to understand the human body because it allows us to see anatomical structures not visible to the naked eye. With its magnification, we can see cells and even tiny structures within the cells.

Body Systems

The human body can be studied according to its various structures and how they function together as a **body system.** The following is a list of those body systems.

- Gastrointestinal (GI) system
- Respiratory system
- Cardiovascular (CV) system
- Blood
- Lymphatic system
- Integumentary system
- Skeletal system
- Muscular system
- Nervous system
- Urinary system
- Male genital and reproductive system
- Female genital and reproductive system
- Endocrine system
- Eyes
- Ears, nose, and throat (ENT) system

WORD BUILDING

cell (SEL)

microscopic (MY-kroh-SKAWP-ik)
  micr/o- *one millionth; small*
  scop/o- *examine with an instrument*
  -ic *pertaining to*

microscope (MY-kroh-skohp)
  micr/o- *one millionth; small*
  -scope *instrument used to examine*
A microscope is *an instrument used to examine small (things). Note:* To define this word correctly, you must follow the standard rule to start with the definition of the suffix followed by the definition of the combining form. If not, you will get the incorrect definition of *small instrument used to examine (things).*

tissue (TISH-yoo)

organ (OR-gan)

macroscopic (MAK-roh-SKAWP-ik)
  macr/o- *large*
  scop/o- *examine with an instrument*
  -ic *pertaining to*

system (SIS-tem)

Medical Specialties

The human body can be studied according to the **medical specialties** that make up the practice of medicine. Each medical specialty includes the anatomy (structures), physiology (functions), diseases and conditions, laboratory and diagnostic procedures, medical and surgical procedures, and drugs for that body system. Medical specialties (not body systems) are used to name departments in the hospital and other facilities where medicine is practiced (example: the Cardiology Department).

Medical Specialty and Body System	Structures	Functions	Word Building

Gastroenterology Gastrointestinal System (Chapter 3)
 	
 Gastroenterology is the study of the stomach and intestines (and related structures). A gastroenterologist is a physician who specializes in gastroenterology.
	• mouth (teeth and tongue)
	• salivary glands
	• pharynx (throat)
	• esophagus
	• stomach
	• small intestine
	• large intestine
	• liver
	• gallbladder
	• pancreas
		• taste (receive sensory information)
		• digest food (mechanically and chemically)
		• absorb nutrients into the blood
		• excrete undigested wastes
			gastroenterology (GAS-troh-EN-ter-AWL-oh-jee)
			  gastr/o- *stomach*
			  enter/o- *intestine*
			  -logy *the study of*
			
			 gastrointestinal (GAS-troh-in-TES-tih-nal)
			  gastr/o- *stomach*
			  intestin/o- *intestine*
			  -al *pertaining to*

Pulmonology Respiratory System (Chapter 4)
 	
 Pulmonology is the study of the lungs (and related structures). A pulmonologist is a physician who specializes in pulmonology.
	• nose
	• pharynx (throat)
	• larynx (voice box)
	• trachea
	• bronchi
	• bronchioles
	• alveoli (in the lungs)
		• inhale oxygen
		• exhale carbon dioxide
		• exchange gases in the alveoli
			pulmonology (PUL-moh-NAWL-oh-jee)
			  pulmon/o- *lung*
			  -logy *the study of*
			
			 respiratory (RES-pih-rah-TOR-ee) (reh-SPYR-ah-tor-ee)
			  re- *again and again; backward; unable to*
			  spir/o- *breathe*
			  -atory *pertaining to*

Medical Specialty and Body System	Structures	Functions	Word Building

Cardiology
Cardiovascular System (Chapter 5)
 	
Cardiology is the study of the heart (and related structures). A cardiologist is a physician who specializes in cardiology.
	• heart
	• arteries
	• veins
	• capillaries
		• circulate blood throughout the body	**cardiology**
			(KAR-dee-AWL-oh-jee)
			    cardi/o- *heart*
			    -logy *the study of*
			
			cardiovascular
			(KAR-dee-oh-VAS-kyoo-lar)
			    cardi/o- *heart*
			    vascul/o- *blood vessel*
			    -ar *pertaining to*

Hematology
Blood (Chapter 6)
 	
Hematology is the study of the blood. A hematologist is a physician who specializes in hematology.
	• blood (blood cells and plasma)	• transport oxygen and nutrients to the cells
		• transport carbon dioxide to the lungs and wastes to the kidneys
			hematology
			(HEE-mah-TAWL-oh-jee)
			    hemat/o- *blood*
			    -logy *the study of*
			
			blood (BLUD)

Immunology
Blood, Lymphatic System (Chapter 6)
 	
Immunology is the study of the immune response. An immunologist is a physician who specializes in immunology.
	• lymphatic vessels, lymph nodes, and lymph fluid
	• spleen
	• thymus
	• white blood cells
		• recognize and destroy disease-causing organisms and abnormal cells	**immunology**
			(IM-myoo-NAWL-oh-jee)
			    immun/o- *immune response*
			    -logy *the study of*
			
			lymphatic (lim-FAT-ik)
			    lymph/o- *lymph; lymphatic system*
			    -atic *pertaining to*

Dermatology
Integumentary System (Chapter 7)
 	
Dermatology is the study of the skin (and related structures). A dermatologist is a physician who specializes in dermatology.
	• skin
	• hair
	• nails
	• sweat glands
	• oil glands
		• pain, touch, temperature (receive sensory information)
		• protect internal organs
		• regulate body temperature by sweating
			dermatology
			(DER-mah-TAWL-oh-jee)
			    dermat/o- *skin*
			    -logy *the study of*
			
			integumentary
			(in-TEG-yoo-MEN-tair-ee)
			    integument/o- *skin*
			    -ary *pertaining to*

Medical Specialty and Body System	Structures	Functions	Word Building

Orthopedics
Skeletal System
(Chapter 8)
 	
Orthopedics is the knowledge and practice of producing straightness of the bones and muscles in a child or other person. An orthopedist is a physician who specializes in orthopedics.
	• bones
	• cartilage
	• ligaments
	• joints
		• support the body	**orthopedics** (OR-thoh-PEE-diks)
			  orth/o- *straight*
			  ped/o- *child*
			  -ics *knowledge; practice*
			Add words to make a complete definition of *orthopedics: knowledge and practice (of producing) straight(ness of the bones and muscles in a) child (or other person).*
			
			skeletal (SKEL-eh-tal)
			  skelet/o- *skeleton*
			  -al *pertaining to*

Orthopedics
Muscular System
(Chapter 9)
	• muscles
	• tendons
		• produce movement of the body	**muscular** (MUS-kyoo-lar)
			  muscul/o- *muscle*
			  -ar *pertaining to*

Neurology
Nervous System
(Chapter 10)
 	
Neurology is the study of the nerves (and related structures). A neurologist is a physician who specializes in neurology.
	• brain
	• cranial nerves
	• spinal cord
	• spinal nerves
	• cerebrospinal fluid
	• neurons
		• receive, relay, and interpret sensory information (vision, hearing, smell, taste, pain, touch, temperature, body position, balance)
		• coordinate movement
		• store and interpret memory and emotion
			neurology (nyoo-RAWL-oh-jee)
			  neur/o- *nerve*
			  -logy *the study of*
			nervous (NER-vus)
			  nerv/o- *nerve*
			  -ous *pertaining to*

Medical Specialty and Body System	Structures	Functions	Word Building
Urology Urinary System (Chapter 11) Urology is the study of the urine and the urinary system. A urologist is a physician who specializes in urology.	• kidneys • ureters • bladder • urethra • nephrons	• excrete urine and waste products	**urology** (yoo-RAWL-oh-jee) **ur/o-** *urine; urinary system* **-logy** *the study of* **urinary** (YOO-rih-NAIR-ee) **urin/o-** *urine; urinary system* **-ary** *pertaining to*
Male Reproductive Medicine Male Genital and Reproductive System (Chapter 12) Reproductive medicine studies the structures that produce children. A reproductive specialist is a physician who specializes in reproductive medicine.	• scrotum • testes • epididymides • vas deferens • seminal vesicles • prostate gland • urethra • penis	• secrete male hormones • produce sperm • deliver sperm to the female reproductive system	**reproductive** (REE-proh-DUK-tiv) **re-** *again and again; backward; unable to* **product/o-** *produce* **-ive** *pertaining to* Select the correct prefix meaning to get the definition of *reproductive: pertaining to again and again produc(ing children).* **genital** (JEN-ih-tal) **genit/o-** *genitalia* **-al** *pertaining to*
Gynecology (GYN) and Obstetrics (OB) Female Genital and Reproductive System (Chapter 13) Gynecology is the study of females. A gynecologist is a physician who specializes in gynecology. Obstetrics is the knowledge and practice of treating women during pregnancy and childbirth. An obstetrician is a physician who specializes in obstetrics.	• breasts • ovaries • uterine tubes • uterus • vagina • external genitalia	• secrete female hormones • produce ova • menstruation • accept sperm from the male • pregnancy • milk production after childbirth	**gynecology** (GY-neh-KAWL-oh-jee) **gynec/o-** *female; woman* **-logy** *the study of* **obstetrics** (awb-STET-riks) **obstetr/o-** *pregnancy and childbirth* **-ics** *knowledge; practice* Add words to make a complete definition of *obstetrics: knowledge and practice (of treating women during) pregnancy and childbirth.* **genital** (JEN-ih-tal) **genit/o-** *genitalia* **-al** *pertaining to*

Medical Specialty and Body System	Structures	Functions	Word Building

Endocrinology Endocrine System (Chapter 14)
 	
Endocrinology is the study of an organ or gland within the body that secretes hormones. An endocrinologist is a physician who specializes in endocrinology.
	• pituitary gland
	• pineal gland
	• thyroid gland
	• parathyroid glands
	• thymus
	• pancreas
	• adrenal glands
	• ovaries
	• testes
		• secrete hormones into the blood
		• direct the activities of other body organs
			endocrinology (EN-doh-krih-NAWL-oh-jee)
			  endo- *innermost; within*
			  crin/o- *secrete*
			  -logy *the study of*
			Add words to make a complete definition of *endocrinology: the study of (an organ or gland) within (the body that) secretes (hormones).*
			
			endocrine (EN-doh-krin) (EN-doh-krine)
			  endo- *innermost; within*
			  -crine *thing that secretes*
			This medical word does contain a combining form. The ending *-crine* contains the combining form *crin/o-* and the one-letter suffix *-e*.

Ophthalmology Eyes (Chapter 15)
 	
Ophthalmology is the study of the eye (and other structures). An ophthalmologist is a physician who specializes in ophthalmology.
	• eyes	• vision (receive sensory information)	**ophthalmology** (OFF-thal-MAWL-oh-jee)
			  ophthalm/o- *eye*
			  -logy *the study of*

Otolaryngology Ears, Nose, and Throat (ENT) System (Chapter 16)
 	
Otolaryngology is the study of the ears, nose, pharynx (throat), and (larynx, and related structures). An otolaryngologist is a physician who specializes in otolaryngology.
	• ears
	• nose
	• sinuses
	• pharynx (throat)
	• larynx (voice box)
		• hearing (receive sensory information)
		• balance (receive sensory information)
		• smell (receive sensory information)
		• speech
			otolaryngology (OH-toh-LAIR-ing-GAWL-oh-jee)
			  ot/o- *ear*
			  laryng/o- *larynx (voice box)*
			  -logy *the study of*

Other Medical Specialties

These medical specialties are not directly related to body systems.

Medical Specialty	Chapter	Description	Word Building
Psychiatry	17	Psychiatry is the medical treatment of the mind. A psychiatrist is a physician who specializes in psychiatry.	**psychiatry** (sy-KY-ah-tree) **psych/o-** *mind* **-iatry** *medical treatment*
Oncology	18	Oncology is the study of a (cancerous) tumor or mass. An oncologist is a physician who specializes in oncology.	**oncology** (ong-KAWL-oh-jee) **onc/o-** *tumor; mass* **-logy** *the study of*
Radiology and Nuclear Medicine	19	Radiology is the study and use of x-rays, sound waves, and other forms of radiation and energy to diagnose diseases and conditions. A radiologist is a physician who specializes in radiology.	**radiology** (RAY-dee-AWL-oh-jee) **radi/o-** *radius (forearm bone); x-rays; radiation* **-logy** *the study of* Select the correct combining form meaning to get the definition of *radiology: the study of x-rays.* **nuclear** (NOO-klee-ar) **nucle/o-** *nucleus (of an atom)* **-ar** *pertaining to* **medicine** (MED-ih-sin) **medic/o-** *physician; medicine* **-ine** *thing pertaining to*
Dentistry	*	Dentistry is a process related to the specialty of the teeth. A dentist is a doctor of dentistry who specializes in the teeth.	**dentistry** (DEN-tis-tree) **dent/o-** *tooth* **-istry** *process related to the specialty of*
Dietetics	*	Dietetics is the knowledge and practice of foods and diet. A dietician is a healthcare professional who specializes in dietetics.	**dietetics** (DY-eh-TET-iks) **dietet/o-** *foods; diet* **-ics** *knowledge; practice*
Pharmacology	**	Pharmacology is the study of medicines and drugs. A pharmacist is a doctor of pharmacy who specializes in medicines and drugs.	**pharmacology** (FAR-mah-KAWL-oh-jee) **pharmac/o-** *medicine; drug* **-logy** *the study of*
Neonatology	**	Neonatology is the study of new babies at birth. A neonatologist is a physician who specializes in neonatology.	**neonatology** (NEE-oh-nay-TAWL-oh-jee) **ne/o-** *new* **nat/o-** *birth* **-logy** *the study of*
Pediatrics	**	Pediatrics is the knowledge and practice of children and their medical treatment. A pediatrician is a physician who specializes in pediatrics.	**pediatrics** (PEE-dee-AT-riks) **ped/o-** *child* **iatr/o-** *physician; medical treatment* **-ics** *knowledge; practice*
Geriatrics	**	Geriatrics is the knowledge and practice of persons of old age and their medical treatment. A gerontologist is a physician who specializes in geriatrics.	**geriatrics** (JAIR-ee-AT-riks) **ger/o-** *old age* **iatr/o-** *physician; medical treatment* **-ics** *knowledge; practice*

*For more information about Dentistry and Dietetics visit the eChapter on the website that accompanies this book.
**These medical specialties are mentioned in feature boxes throughout the book.

Vocabulary Review

The Body in Health

Word or Phrase	Description	Combining Forms
abdominal cavity	Cavity that is surrounded by the diaphragm superiorly, the abdominal wall anteriorly, and the spinal column posteriorly	**abdomin/o-** *abdomen*
abdominopelvic cavity	Continuous cavity formed by the abdominal and pelvic cavities	**abdomin/o-** *abdomen* **pelv/o-** *pelvis (hip bone; renal pelvis)*
anatomical position	Standard position of the body for the purpose of study. The body is erect, head up, hands by the side with palms facing forward, and the legs are straight with toes pointing forward.	**tom/o-** *cut; slice; layer*
anatomy	The study of the structure of the human body and its parts	**tom/o-** *cut; slice; layer*
anterior	Pertaining to the front of the body, an organ, or a structure	**anter/o-** *before; front part*
anteroposterior	Moving through the anterior section and then the posterior section of the body	**anter/o-** *before; front part* **poster/o-** *back part*
blood	Includes blood cells and plasma. It transports oxygen and nutrients to the cells, carbon dioxide to the lungs, and wastes to the kidneys.	**hemat/o-** *blood*
body system	A way to study the body according to its structures and how they function	
cardiology	Medical specialty that deals with the cardiovascular system	**cardi/o-** *heart*
cardiovascular system	Body system that includes the heart, arteries, veins, and capillaries. It circulates the blood throughout the body.	**cardi/o-** *heart* **vascul/o-** *blood vessel*
caudad	Toward the tail bone	**caud/o-** *tail (tail bone)*
cavity	Hollow space surrounded by bones or muscles and containing organs and other structures	**cav/o-** *hollow space*
cell	Smallest independently functioning structure in the body that can reproduce itself by division	
cephalad	Toward the head	**cephal/o-** *head*
coronal plane	Plane that divides the body into front and back sections, anterior and posterior. It is also known as the **frontal plane.**	**coron/o-** *structure that encircles like a crown* **front/o-** *front*
cranial cavity	Cavity in the head that is surrounded by the bony cranium and contains the brain, cranial nerves, and other structures	**crani/o-** *cranium (skull)*
dentistry	Medical specialty that deals with the teeth and gums	**dent/o-** *tooth*
dermatology	Medical specialty that deals with the integumentary system	**dermat/o-** *skin*
dietetics	Medical specialty that deals with nutrition, nutrients, foods, and diet	**dietet/o-** *foods; diet*
distal	Away from the point of origin of an arm or leg	**dist/o-** *away from the center or point of origin*
dorsal	Pertaining to the posterior of the body, particularly the back. Lying on the back is being in the dorsal or **dorsal supine** position.	**dors/o-** *back; dorsum*

Word or Phrase	Description	Combining Forms
endocrine system	Body system that includes the pituitary gland, pineal gland, thyroid gland, parathyroid glands, thymus, pancreas, adrenal glands, ovaries, and testes. It produces and secretes hormones into the blood that direct other body organs.	**crin/o-** *secrete*
endocrinology	Medical specialty that deals with the endocrine system	**crin/o-** *secrete*
epigastric region	Region on the surface of the abdominopelvic area. It is superior to the umbilical region and between the right and left hypochondriac regions.	**gastr/o-** *stomach*
external	Pertaining to the outer, superficial surface of the body, an organ, or other structure	**extern/o-** *outside*
gastroenterology	Medical specialty that deals with the gastrointestinal system	**gastr/o-** *stomach* **enter/o-** *intestine*
gastrointestinal system	Body system that includes the mouth, teeth, tongue, salivary glands, pharynx (throat), esophagus, stomach, small intestine, large intestine, liver, gallbladder, and pancreas. It digests food, absorbs nutrients into the blood, and excretes undigested wastes. It receives sensory information for the sense of taste.	**gastr/o-** *stomach* **intestin/o-** *intestine*
genital	Pertaining to the male or female genitalia	**genit/o-** *genitalia*
geriatrics	Medical specialty that deals with older adults	**ger/o-** *old age* **iatr/o-** *physician; medical treatment*
gynecology	Medical specialty that deals with the female genital system	**gynec/o-** *female; woman*
health	State of complete physical, mental, and social well-being	
hematology	Medical specialty that deals with the blood	**hemat/o-** *blood*
hypochondriac regions	Left and right regions on the surface of the abdominopelvic area. They are inferior to the ribs.	**chondr/o-** *cartilage*
hypogastric region	Region on the surface of the abdominopelvic area. It is inferior to the umbilical region and between the right and left inguinal regions.	**gastr/o-** *stomach*
immunology	Medical specialty that deals with the lymphatic system and the immune response	**immun/o-** *immune response*
inferior	Pertaining to the lower part of the body, an organ, or a structure	**infer/o-** *below*
inguinal regions	Left and right regions on the surface of the abdominopelvic area. They are inferior to the lumbar regions. They are also known as the **iliac regions.**	**inguin/o-** *groin* **ili/o-** *ilium (hip bone)*
integumentary system	Body system that includes the skin, hair, nails, sweat glands, and oil glands. It receives sensory information for the sensations of pain, touch, and temperature. It protects the internal organs from infection and trauma. It regulates the body temperature by sweating.	**integument/o-** *skin*
internal	Within the body or an organ	**intern/o-** *inside*
lateral	Pertaining to the side of the body, an organ, or a structure	**later/o-** *side*
lumbar regions	Left and right regions on the surface of the abdominopelvic area. They are on either side of the umbilical region.	**lumb/o-** *lower back; area between the ribs and pelvis*
lymphatic system	Body system that includes the lymphatic vessels, lymph nodes, lymph fluid, spleen, thymus, and white blood cells. It recognizes and destroys disease-causing organisms and abnormal cells.	**lymph/o-** *lymph; lymphatic system*

Word or Phrase	Description	Combining Forms
macroscopic	Pertaining to structures that can be seen with the naked eye	**macr/o-** *large* **scop/o-** *examine with an instrument*
medial	Pertaining to the middle of the body, an organ, or a structure	**medi/o-** *middle*
medical specialty	Basis of the practice of medicine. Each medical specialty includes the structures, functions, and diseases for a body system plus related laboratory and diagnostic procedures, medical and surgical procedures, and drugs.	**medic/o-** *physician; medicine*
microscope	Instrument used to examine very small structures	**micr/o-** *one millionth; small*
microscopic	Pertaining to structures that cannot be seen with the naked eye	**micr/o-** *one millionth; small* **scop/o-** *examine with an instrument*
muscular system	Body system that includes the muscles and tendons. It produces body movement.	**muscul/o-** *muscle*
neonatology	Medical specialty that deals with newborns	**ne/o-** *new* **nat/o-** *birth*
nervous system	Body system that includes the brain, cranial nerves, spinal cord, spinal nerves, cerebrospinal fluid, and neurons. It receives, relays, and interprets sensory information from the body for the senses of vision, hearing, smell, and taste and for the sensations of pain, touch, temperature, and body position. It co-ordinates body movement and stores and interprets memory and emotion.	**nerv/o-** *nerve*
neurology	Medical specialty that deals with the nervous system	**neur/o-** *nerve*
obstetrics	Medical specialty that deals with the female reproductive system during pregnancy and childbirth	**obstetr/o-** *pregnancy and childbirth*
oncology	Medical specialty that deals with cancer	**onc/o-** *tumor; mass*
ophthalmology	Medical specialty that deals with the eyes. The eyes receive sensory information for the sense of vision.	**ophthalm/o-** *eye*
organ	Body structure formed of tissues	
orthopedics	Medical specialty that deals with the skeletal system and muscular system	**orth/o-** *straight* **ped/o-** *child*
otolaryngology	Medical specialty that deals with the ears, nose, and throat. The ears receive sensory information for the sense of hearing and the sensation of balance. The nose receives sensory information for the sense of smell. The pharynx (throat) and the larynx (voice box) help produce speech.	**ot/o-** *ear* **laryng/o-** *larynx (voice box)*
pediatrics	Medical specialty that deals with infants and children	**ped/o-** *child* **iatr/o-** *physician; medical treatment*
pelvic cavity	Cavity that is continuous with and inferior to the abdominal cavity. It is surrounded by the pelvic bones and the spinal column.	**pelv/o-** *pelvis (hip bone; renal pelvis)*
pharmacology	The study of drugs used as medicines	**pharmac/o-** *medicine; drug*
physiology	The study of the function of the human body	**physi/o-** *physical function*
plane	An imaginary flat surface that divides the body into sections. There are three planes: the coronal plane (frontal plane), sagittal plane, and transverse plane.	
posterior	Pertaining to the back of the body, an organ, or a structure	**poster/o-** *back part*
posteroanterior	Moving through the posterior section and then the anterior section of the body	**poster/o-** *back part* **anter/o-** *before; front part*

Word or Phrase	Description	Combining Forms
prone	Position of lying on the anterior surface of the body	
proximal	Toward or near the point of origin of an arm or leg	**proxim/o-** *near the center or point of origin*
psychiatry	Medical specialty that deals with the mind	**psych/o-** *mind*
pulmonology	Medical specialty that deals with the respiratory system	**pulmon/o-** *lung*
quadrant	The four equal reference squares on the surface of the abdominopelvic area: the left upper quadrant (LUQ), right upper quadrant (RUQ), left lower quadrant (LLQ), and right lower quadrant (RLQ)	
radiology and nuclear medicine	Medical specialty that deals with the use of x-rays, sound waves, and other forms of radiation and energy to create images and diagnose disease	**radi/o-** *radius (forearm bone); x-rays; radiation* **nucle/o-** *nucleus (of an atom)*
reproductive medicine	Medical specialty that deals with the reproductive system	**product/o-** *produce*
reproductive system	Body system that, in the female, includes the breasts, ovaries, uterine tubes, uterus, vagina, and external genitalia. It secretes hormones, produces ova, and regulates menstruation, pregnancy, and milk production from the breasts. In the male, it includes the scrotum, testes, epididymides, vas deferens, seminal vesicles, prostate gland, and penis. It secretes hormones and produces sperm.	**product/o-** *produce*
respiratory system	Body system that includes the nose, pharynx (throat), larynx (voice box), trachea, bronchi, bronchioles, and alveoli (in the lungs). It inhales oxygen, exhales carbon dioxide, and exchanges gases in the alveoli.	**spir/o-** *breathe*
sagittal plane	Plane that divides the body into right and left sections	**sagitt/o-** *going from front to back*
skeletal system	Body system that includes the bones, cartilage, ligaments, and joints. It supports the body.	**skelet/o-** *skeleton*
spinal cavity	Cavity that is within the bones of the spinal column and contains the spinal cord, spinal nerves, and spinal fluid	**spin/o-** *spine; backbone*
superior	Pertaining to the upper part of the body, an organ, or a structure	**super/o-** *above*
thoracic cavity	Cavity that is surrounded by the breast bone (sternum), ribs, and spinal column. The diaphragm is the inferior border of the cavity. The thoracic cavity contains the lungs and the mediastinum (and the structures within it).	**thorac/o-** *thorax (chest)*
tissue	Body structure formed of cells	
transverse plane	Plane that divides the body into top and bottom sections, superior and inferior	**vers/o-** *to travel; to turn*
umbilical region	Center region on the surface of the abdominopelvic area. It is located around the umbilicus.	**umbilic/o-** *umbilicus; navel*
urinary system	Body system that includes the kidneys, ureters, bladder, urethra, and nephrons. It excretes urine and waste products.	**urin/o-** *urine; urinary system*
urology	Medical specialty that deals with the urinary system	**ur/o-** *urine; urinary system*
ventral	Pertaining to the anterior of the body, particularly the abdomen	**ventr/o-** *front; abdomen*
viscera	All of the internal organs in a body cavity	**viscer/o-** *large internal organs*

Labeling Exercise

A. *Match each direction to its arrow and write it in the numbered box. Be sure to check your spelling. Use the Answer Key at the end of the book to check your answers.*

anterior (ventral)	distal	lateral	medial	posterior (dorsal)	proximal

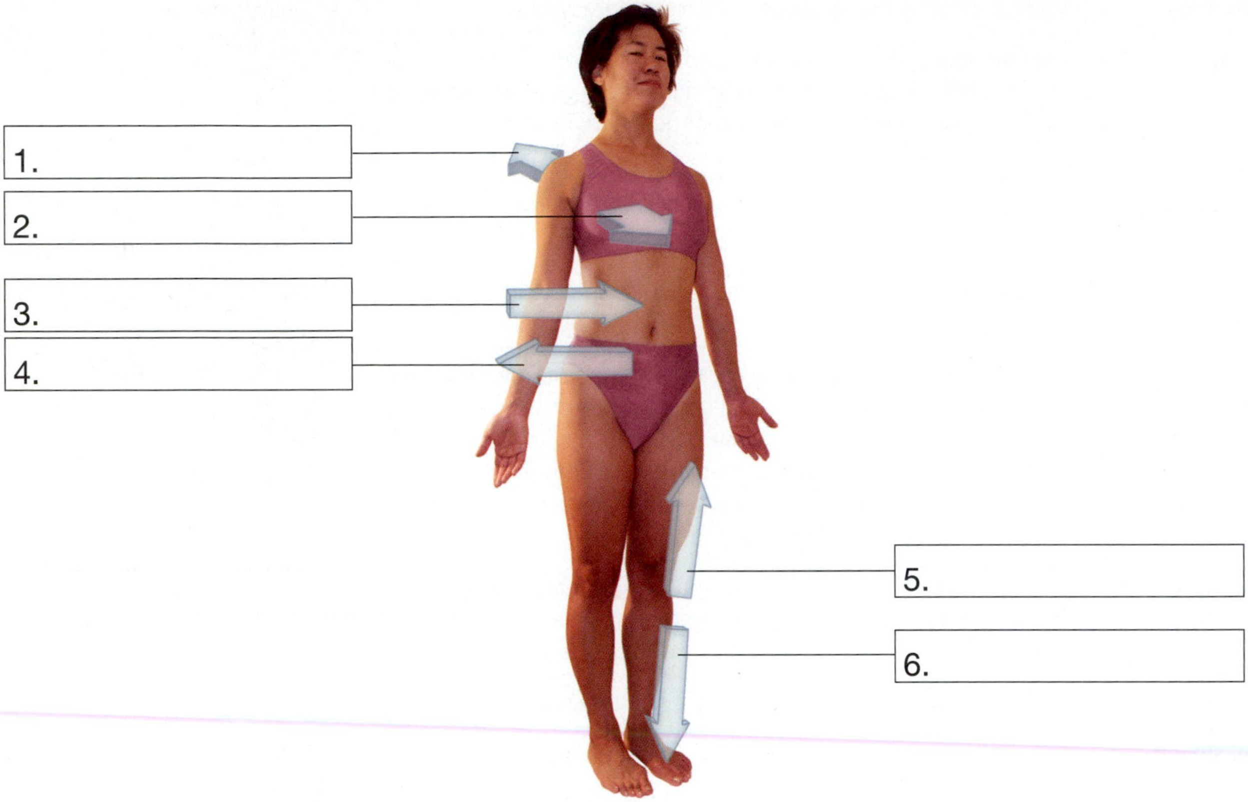

1. _____

2. _____

3. _____

4. _____

5. _____

6. _____

B. *Match each anatomy word or phrase to its structure and write it in the numbered box.*

abdominal cavity	cranial cavity	diaphragm	pelvic cavity	spinal cavity	thoracic cavity

1. _____

2. _____

3. _____

4. _____

5. _____

6. _____

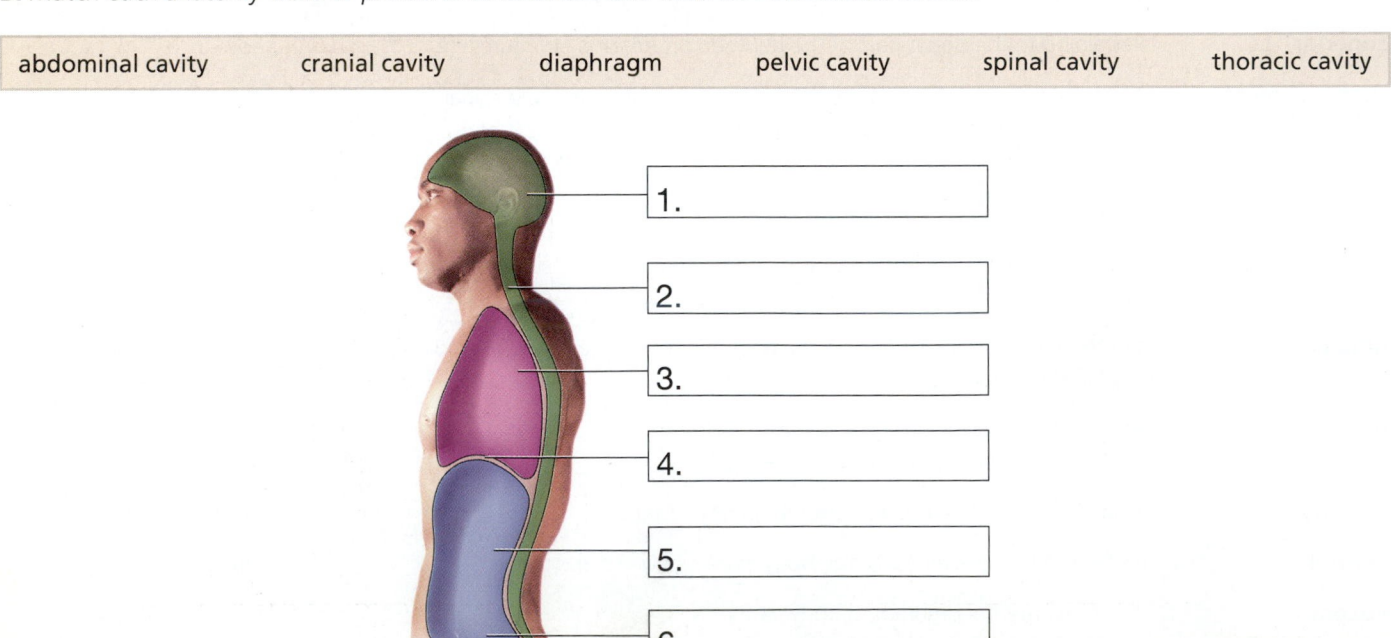

C. *Write the name of each body system and its related medical specialty on the lines under each illustration.*

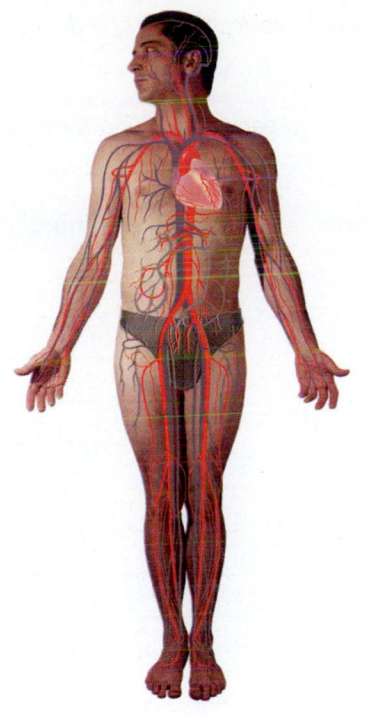

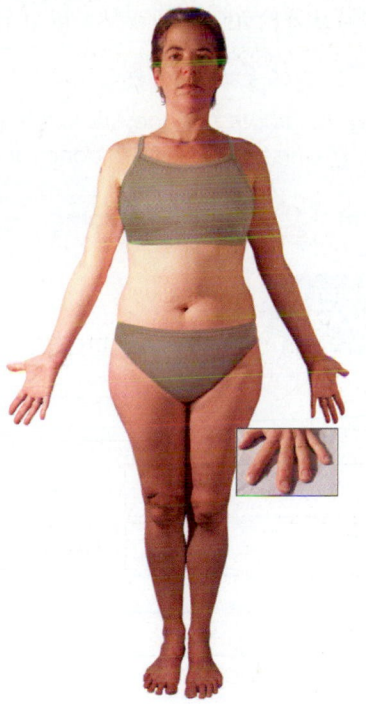

1. _____

2. _____

3. _____

4. _____

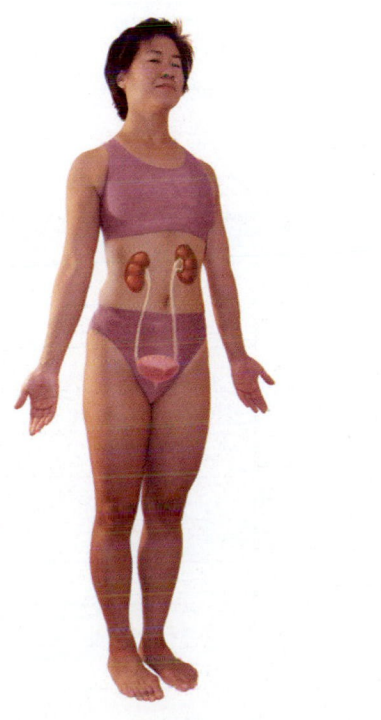

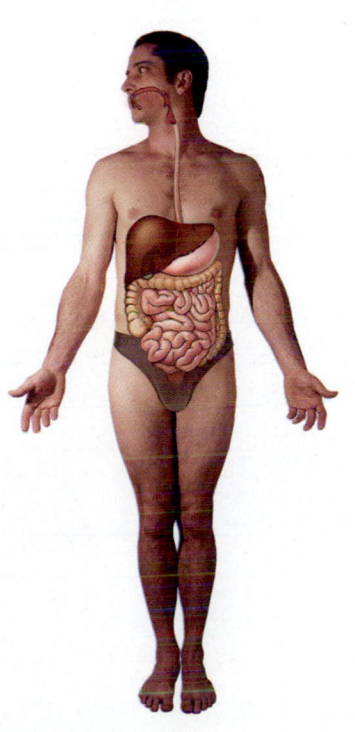

5. _____

6. _____

7. _____

8. _____

Building Medical Words

Use the Answer Key at the end of the book to check your answers.

Combining Forms Exercise

Before you build words about the body in health, review these combining forms. Next to each combining form, write its medical meaning. The first one has been done for you.

Combining Form	Medical Meaning	Combining Form	Medical Meaning
1. **dors/o-**	back; dorsum	34. lumb/o-	
2. abdomin/o-		35. lymph/o-	
3. anter/o-		36. macr/o-	
4. cardi/o-		37. medic/o-	
5. caud/o-		38. medi/o-	
6. cav/o-		39. micr/o-	
7. cephal/o-		40. muscul/o-	
8. chondr/o-		41. nat/o-	
9. coron/o-		42. ne/o-	
10. crani/o-		43. nerv/o-	
11. crin/o-		44. neur/o-	
12. dent/o-		45. nucle/o-	
13. dermat/o-		46. obstetr/o-	
14. dietet/o-		47. onc/o-	
15. dist/o-		48. ophthalm/o-	
16. enter/o-		49. orth/o-	
17. extern/o-		50. ot/o-	
18. front/o-		51. ped/o-	
19. gastr/o-		52. pelv/o-	
20. genit/o-		53. pharmac/o-	
21. ger/o-		54. physi/o-	
22. gynec/o-		55. poster/o-	
23. hemat/o-		56. product/o-	
24. iatr/o-		57. proxim/o-	
25. ili/o-		58. psych/o-	
26. immun/o-		59. pulmon/o-	
27. infer/o-		60. radi/o-	
28. inguin/o-		61. sagitt/o-	
29. integument/o-		62. scop/o-	
30. intern/o-		63. skelet/o-	
31. intestin/o-		64. spin/o-	
32. laryng/o-		65. spir/o-	
33. later/o-		66. super/o-	

Combining Form	Medical Meaning	Combining Form	Medical Meaning
67. thorac/o-	_____	72. vascul/o-	_____
68. tom/o-	_____	73. ventr/o-	_____
69. umbilic/o-	_____	74. vers/o-	_____
70. urin/o-	_____	75. viscer/o-	_____
71. ur/o-	_____		

Combining Form and Suffix Exercise

Read the definition of the medical word. Look at the combining form that is given. Select the correct suffix from the Suffix List and write it on the blank line. Then build the medical word and write it on the line. (Remember: You may need to remove the combining vowel. Always remove the hyphens and slash.) Be sure to check your spelling. The first one has been done for you.

SUFFIX LIST			
-ad (toward; in the direction of)	-ary (pertaining to)	-ics (knowledge; practice)	-ity (state; condition)
-al (pertaining to)	-atic (pertaining to)	-ior (pertaining to)	-logy (the study of)
-ar (pertaining to)	-iatry (medical treatment)	-istry (process related to the specialty of)	-ous (pertaining to)
	-ic (pertaining to)		

Definition of the Medical Word	Combining Form	Suffix	Build the Medical Word

1. Pertaining to the abdomen

abdomin/o-   **-al**   abdominal

(You think *pertaining to* (-al) + *the abdomen* (abdomin/o-). You change the order of the word parts to put the suffix last. You write *abdominal*.)

Definition of the Medical Word	Combining Form	Suffix	Build the Medical Word
2. The study of the physical function (of the body)	physi/o-	_____	_____
3. Pertaining to the lower back	lumb/o-	_____	_____
4. In the direction of the head	cephal/o-	_____	_____
5. Pertaining to away from the point of origin	dist/o-	_____	_____
6. Pertaining to the chest	thorac/o-	_____	_____
7. Pertaining to the skull	crani/o-	_____	_____
8. Pertaining to the back part	poster/o-	_____	_____
9. The study of the skin	dermat/o-	_____	_____
10. Pertaining to the lymph (system)	lymph/o-	_____	_____
11. Pertaining to the side	later/o-	_____	_____
12. Pertaining to inside	intern/o-	_____	_____
13. The study of the heart	cardi/o-	_____	_____
14. The knowledge and practice of pregnancy and childbirth	obstetr/o-	_____	_____
15. The study of the urine and the urinary system	ur/o-	_____	_____
16. The study of the lungs	pulmon/o-	_____	_____
17. The study of the eye	ophthalm/o-	_____	_____
18. Pertaining to the skin	integument/o-	_____	_____
19. The study of females	gynec/o-	_____	_____
20. Medical treatment of the mind	psych/o-	_____	_____

Definition of the Medical Word	Combining Form	Suffix	Build the Medical Word
21. Pertaining to the nerves	nerv/o-	_____	_____
22. Pertaining to the urine (and its system)	urin/o-	_____	_____
23. The study of (cancerous) tumors	onc/o-	_____	_____
24. Pertaining to the front part	anter/o	_____	_____
25. Pertaining to the groin	inguin/o-	_____	_____
26. State of (having) a hollow space	cav/o-	_____	_____
27. The study of the blood	hemat/o-	_____	_____
28. Process related to the specialty of the teeth	dent/o-	_____	_____
29. The study of the nerves	neur/o-	_____	_____
30. Pertaining to the muscles	muscul/o-	_____	_____
31. Pertaining to the middle	medi/o-	_____	_____
32. Pertaining to (being) above	super/o-	_____	_____
33. The study of the heart	cardi/o-	_____	_____
34. The study of medicines and drugs	pharmac/o-	_____	_____
35. Knowledge and practice of foods and diet	dietet/o-	_____	_____
36. The study of x-rays	radi/o-	_____	_____
37. Pertaining to the large internal organs	viscer/o-	_____	_____

Prefix Exercise

Read the definition of the medical word. Look at the medical word or partial word that is given (it already contains a combining form and a suffix). Select the correct prefix from the Prefix List and write it on the blank line. Then build the medical word and write it on the line. Be sure to check your spelling. The first one has been done for you.

PREFIX LIST			
ana- (apart from; excessive)	epi- (upon; above)	mid- (middle)	re- (again and again; backward; unable to)
endo- (innermost; within)	hypo- (below; deficient)		

Definition of the Medical Word	Prefix	Word or Partial Word	Build the Medical Word
1. Thing that secretes (hormones) within (the body)	**endo-**	**-crine**	_endocrine_
2. Pertaining to apart from (the body by making) a cut, slice, or layer	_____	tomical	_____
3. Pertaining to in the middle (of the body with a plane) going front to back	_____	sagittal	_____
4. Pertaining to (a region) below the cartilage (of the ribs)	_____	chondriac	_____
5. Pertaining to again and again breathing	_____	spiratory	_____
6. Pertaining to (a region) above the stomach	_____	gastric	_____
7. Pertaining to again and again producing	_____	productive	_____

The Body in Disease

WORD BUILDING

preventive (pree-VEN-tiv)
prevent/o- *prevent*
-ive *pertaining to*

medicine (MED-ih-sin)
medic/o- *physician; medicine*
-ine *pertaining to*

disease (dih-ZEEZ)

etiology (EE-tee-AWL-oh-jee)
eti/o- *cause of disease*
-logy *the study of*

Preventive medicine is the healthcare specialty that focuses on keeping a person healthy and preventing disease. But despite the best efforts of modern medicine, the human body does not always remain in a state of health. Much of medical language deals with diseases and conditions and how they are diagnosed and treated. **Disease** is any change in the normal structure or function of the body. This change might be slight and short lived or severe and life threatening. The **etiology** is the cause or origin of a disease. In most cases, the cause of a disease is known or can be discovered through laboratory and diagnostic procedures. In some cases, however, the exact cause of a disease is never completely understood.

Disease Categories

Diseases can be divided into different categories based on their etiology (cause or origin).

Disease Type	Etiology	Word Building
congenital	Caused by an abnormality in the fetus as it develops or caused by an abnormal process that occurs during gestation or birth Examples: Cleft lip and palate, cerebral palsy	**congenital** (con-JEN-ih-tal) **congenit/o-** *present at birth* **-al** *pertaining to*
degenerative	Caused by the progressive destruction of cells due to disease or the aging process Examples: Multiple sclerosis, loss of hearing, arthritis	**degenerative** (dee-JEN-er-ah-tiv) **de-** *reversal of; without* **gener/o-** *production; creation* **-ative** *pertaining to*
environmental	Caused by exposure to external substances Examples: Smoke, allergies to pollen, skin cancer from the sun	**environmental** (en-VY-rawn-MEN-tal)
hereditary	Caused by an inherited or spontaneous mutation in the genetic material of a cell Examples: Cystic fibrosis, Down syndrome, sickle cell disease	**hereditary** (heh-RED-ih-TAIR-ee) **heredit/o-** *genetic inheritance* **-ary** *pertaining to*
iatrogenic	Caused by medicine or treatment that was given to the patient Examples: Wrong drug given to a patient, surgery performed on the wrong leg, an incompatible blood type given as a blood transfusion	**iatrogenic** (eye-AT-roh-JEN-ik) **iatr/o-** *physician; medical treatment* **gen/o-** *arising from; produced by* **-ic** *pertaining to*
idiopathic	Having no identifiable or confirmed cause Example: Sudden infant death syndrome (SIDS)	**idiopathic** (ID-ee-oh-PATH-ik) **idi/o-** *unknown; individual* **path/o-** *disease; suffering* **-ic** *pertaining to*

Disease Type	Etiology	Word Building

infectious	Caused by a **pathogen** (a disease-causing microorganism such as a bacterium, virus, fungus, etc.). A **communicable** disease is an infectious disease that is transmitted by direct or indirect contact with an infected person, animal, or insect.
	Examples: Gonorrhea (a sexually transmitted disease), rabies from an animal bite, tuberculosis from being in close proximity to a person with tuberculosis
		infectious (in-FEK-shus)
		  infect/o- *disease within*
		  -ious *pertaining to*
		Add words to make a complete definition of *infectious: pertaining to disease(-causing organisms) within (the body)*.
		
		pathogen (PATH-oh-jen)
		  path/o- *disease; suffering*
		  -gen *that which produces*
		
		communicable (koh-MYOON-ih-kah-bl)
		  communic/o- *impart; transmit*
		  -able *able to be*

neoplastic	Caused by the new growth of either a benign (not cancerous) or a malignant (cancerous) tumor
	Examples: Benign cyst, cancerous tumor of the skin
		neoplastic (NEE-oh-PLAS-tik)
		  ne/o- *new*
		  plast/o- *growth; formation*
		  -ic *pertaining to*

nosocomial	Caused by exposure to a disease while in the hospital environment
	Example: Surgical wound infection
		nosocomial (NOS-oh-KOH-mee-al)
		  nosocomi/o- *hospital*
		  -al *pertaining to*

nutritional	Caused by a lack of nutritious food, insufficient amounts of food, or an inability to utilize the nutrients in food
	Examples: Malnutrition, pernicious anemia caused by a lack of intrinsic factor in the stomach
		nutritional (noo-TRISH-un-al)
		  nutri/o- *nourishment*
		  -tion *a process; being or having*
		  -al *pertaining to*

Onset, Course, and Outcome of Disease

Onset of a Disease

The beginning or onset of disease is often noticed because of symptoms and/or signs. A **symptom** is any deviation from health that is experienced or felt by the patient. When a symptom can be seen or detected by others, it is known as a **sign.** An elevated temperature, coughing, tremors, paleness, vomiting, or a lump that can be seen or felt would all be signs of disease. **Symptomatology** is the clinical picture of all of the patient's symptoms and signs. A **syndrome** is a set of symptoms and signs associated with and characteristic of one particular disease. Patients who are **asymptomatic** (showing no symptoms or signs) can still have a disease, but one that can only be detected by laboratory and diagnostic procedures.

To fully understand the patient's symptoms and signs, the physician takes a history and performs a physical examination. For the history of the present illness, the physician asks the patient in detail about the location, onset, duration, and severity of the symptoms. The physician also asks about the patient's past medical history, past surgical history, family history, social history, and history of allergies to drugs. Then the physician performs a physical examination to look for signs of disease. The physician

WORD BUILDING

symptom (SIMP-tom)

symptomatology (SIMP-toh-mah-TAWL-oh-jee)
  symptomat/o- *collection of symptoms*
  -logy *the study of*

syndrome (SIN-drohm)
  syn- *together*
  -drome *a running*
Most medical words contain a combining form. The ending *-drome* contains the combining form *drom/o-* and the one-letter suffix *-e.*

asymptomatic (AA-simp-toh-MAT-ik)
  a- *away from; without*
  symptomat/o- *collection of symptoms*
  -ic *pertaining to*

uses the following techniques (as needed) during the physical examination: **inspection**, **palpation**, **auscultation**, and **percussion** (see Figures 2-18 ■ through 2-21 ■).

WORD BUILDING

inspection (in-SPEK-shun)
 inspect/o- *looking at*
 -ion *action; condition*

palpation (pal-PAY-shun)
 palpat/o- *touching; feeling*
 -ion *action; condition*

auscultation (aws-kul-TAY-shun)
 auscult/o- *listening*
 -ation *a process; being or having*

percussion (per-KUH-shun)
 percuss/o- *tapping*
 -ion *action; condition*

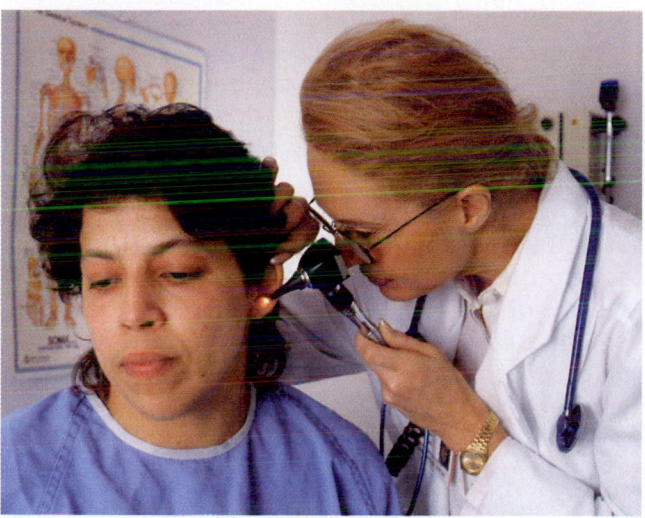

Figure 2-18 ■ Inspection.
Inspection is using the eyes or an instrument to examine the external surfaces or the internal cavities of the body. This physician is using her eyes and a lighted instrument (an otoscope) to examine the patient's internal ear canal.

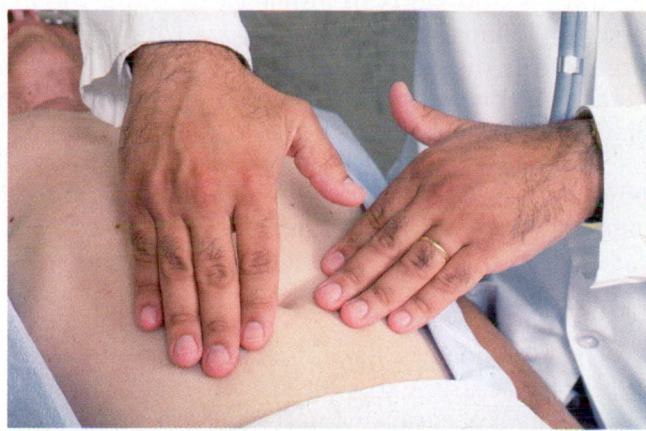

Figure 2-19 ■ Palpation.
Palpation is using the fingers to feel masses or enlarged organs or to detect tenderness or pain. This physician is palpating the patient's abdomen.

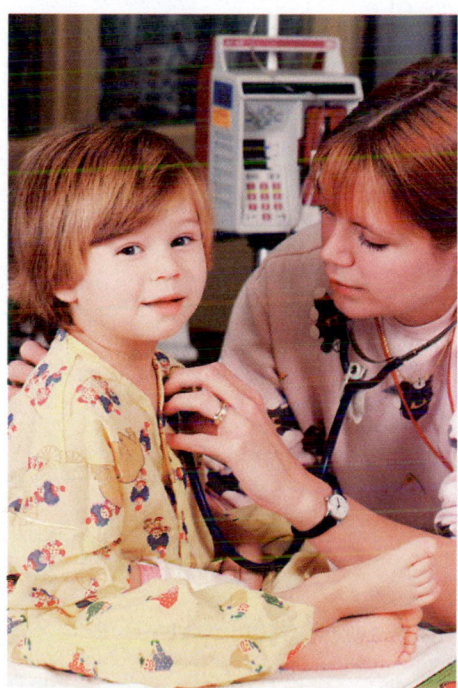

Figure 2-20 ■ Auscultation.
Auscultation is using a stethoscope to listen to the sounds of the heart, lungs, or intestines. This nurse is using a stethoscope to listen to this child's lungs and breath sounds.

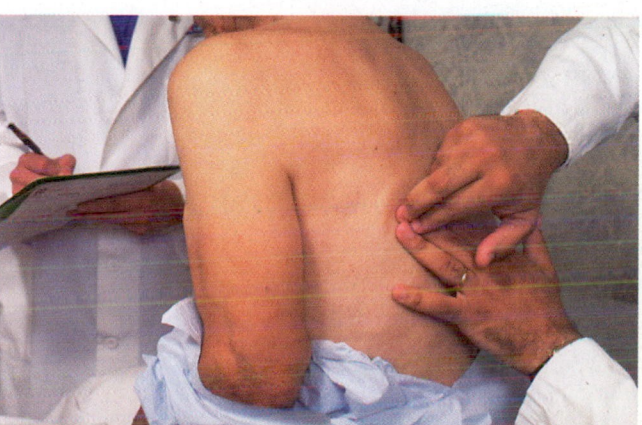

Figure 2-21 ■ Percussion.
Percussion is using the finger of one hand to tap on the finger of the other hand that is spread over a body cavity. After a few taps, the hand is moved to another location. This physician is using percussion over the thoracic cavity and left lung and listening to the sound that is produced.

Based on the patient's history and the results of the physical examination, the physician makes a **diagnosis** and identifies the nature and cause of the disease or condition. If it is not possible to make a diagnosis, the physician makes a tentative or working diagnosis and orders further diagnostic procedures or refers the patient to a specialist for a more detailed evaluation.

Course and Outcome of a Disease

The course of a disease includes all events from the onset of the disease until its final outcome. During the course of a disease, the symptoms and signs may be **acute** (sudden in nature and severe in intensity), **subacute** (less severe in intensity), or **chronic** (continuing for 3 months or more). An **exacerbation** is a sudden worsening in the severity of the symptoms or signs. A **remission** is a temporary improvement in the symptoms and signs of a disease without the underlying disease being cured. A relapse or recurrence is a return of the original symptoms and signs of the disease. A **sequela** is an abnormal condition or complication that arises because of the original disease and remains after the original disease has resolved.

The course and outcome of a disease can be affected by treatment: the physician prescribes drugs or orders therapy for the patient. If the treatment is **therapeutic,** the symptoms or signs of the disease disappear. A disease that is **refractory** (resistant) to treatment is one that does not respond to treatment. Certain diseases that cannot be treated with drugs or therapy may require **surgery.**

The **prognosis** is the predicted outcome of a disease. The natures of many diseases are so well known that the physician can predict with a great deal of accuracy what the patient's prognosis will be. The course of a disease ends in one of the following outcomes. **Recuperation** or recovery is a return to a normal state of health. When recuperation is not complete, residual chronic disease or disability remains. A **disability** is a permanent loss of the ability to perform certain activities or to function in a given way. A **terminal illness** is one from which the patient cannot recover, and which eventually results in death.

WORD BUILDING

diagnosis (DY-ag-NOH-sis)
  dia- *complete; completely through*
  gnos/o- *knowledge*
  -osis *condition; abnormal condition; process*
Diagnosis is a Greek noun. Form the plural by changing *-is* to *–es.*

acute (ah-KYOOT)

subacute (SUB-ah-KYOOT)

chronic (KRAW-nik)
  chron/o- *time*
  -ic *pertaining to*

exacerbation (eg-ZAS-er-BAY-shun)
  exacerb/o- *increase; provoke*
  -ation *a process; being or having*

remission (ree-MISH-un)
  remiss/o- *send back*
  -ion *action; condition*

sequela (see-KWEL-ah)
Sequela is a Latin singular noun. Form the plural by changing *-a* to *-ae.*

therapeutic (THAIR-ah-PYOO-tik)
  therapeut/o- *therapy; treatment*
  -ic *pertaining to*

refractory (ree-FRAK-tor-ee)
  re- *again and again; backward; unable to*
  fract/o- *break up*
  -ory *having the function of*
Add words to make a complete definition of *refractory: having the function of (being) unable to break up (treat or cure a disease).*

surgery (SER-jer-ee)
  surg/o- *operative procedure*
  -ery *process of*

prognosis (prawg-NOH-sis)
  pro- *before*
  gnos/o- *knowledge*
  -osis *condition; abnormal condition; process*

recuperation (ree-KOO-per-AA-shun)
  recuper/o- *recover*
  -ation *a process; being or having*

disability (DIS-ah-BIL-ah-tee)

terminal (TER-mih-nal)
  termin/o- *end; boundary*
  -al *pertaining to*

Healthcare Professionals and Healthcare Settings

Healthcare Professionals

Physicians

A **physician** or **doctor** leads the members of the healthcare team and directs their activities. The physician examines the patient, orders tests (if necessary), diagnoses diseases, and treats diseases by prescribing medicines or therapy. Physicians who graduate from medical school receive a Doctor of Medicine (M.D.) degree. Physicians who graduate from a school of osteopathy receive a Doctor of Osteopathy or Osteopathic Medicine (D.O.) degree. After medical school, physicians complete residency training and select a specialized area for their medical practice (examples: family practice, pediatrics, psychiatry, etc.). **Surgeons** are physicians who complete additional training in surgical techniques.

Primary care physicians (PCPs) are physicians who specialize in family practice or pediatrics. They see the majority of patients on a day-to-day basis. A physician who is on the medical staff of a hospital and admits a patient to the hospital is known as the **attending physician.**

Other doctors graduate from schools that focus their training on just one part of the body or one aspect of medicine. Chiropractors have a Doctor of Chiropracty or Chiropractic Medicine (D.C.) degree and only treat the alignment of the bones, muscles, and nerves. Optometrists have a Doctor of Optometry (O.D.) degree and only treat the eyes. Podiatrists have a Doctor of Podiatric Medicine (D.P.M.) degree and only treat the feet. Dentists have a Doctor of Dental Surgery (D.D.S.) degree and only treat the teeth. Pharmacists have a Doctor of Pharmacy (Pharm. D.) degree. They fill prescriptions for medicines as well as consult with physicians and patients.

Physician Extenders

Physician extenders are healthcare professionals who perform some of the duties of a physician. They examine, diagnose, and treat patients and some of them can prescribe medicines. They work under the supervision of a physician (M.D. or D.O.).

Physician extenders include physician's assistants (PAs), nurse practitioners (NPs), certified nurse midwives (CNMs), and certified registered nurse anesthetists (CRNAs).

Allied Health Professionals

Nurses, such as a registered nurse (RN), licensed practical nurse (LPN), or licensed vocational nurse (LVN), are allied health professionals who examine patients, make nursing diagnoses, and administer treatments or medicines ordered by the physician. Nurses give hands-on care and focus on the physical and emotional needs of the patient and the family.

Other allied health professionals include **technologists, technicians,** and **therapists,** as well as dietitians, medical assistants, phlebotomists, dental hygienists, and audiologists.

Healthcare Settings

Health care is provided in many different settings, depending on the healthcare needs of the patient and which setting can most cost effectively meet those needs.

Hospital

A **hospital** is a healthcare facility that is the traditional setting for providing care for patients who are acutely ill and require medical or surgical care for longer than 24 hours. Each hospital stay begins with admission and ends with discharge from the hospital. The attending physician must write an order in the patient's medical record to admit or **discharge** the patient. The attending physician also monitors the patient's care and orders diagnostic tests, treatments, therapies, medicines, and surgeries, as needed. A patient in the hospital is an **inpatient.**

A hospital is divided into floors or nursing units that provide care for specific types of patients. There are also specialty care units such as the intensive care unit (ICU). **Ancillary** departments in the hospital provide additional types of services and include the radiology department, physical therapy (PT) department, dietary department, emergency department (ED) or emergency room (ER), clinical laboratory, and pharmacy. Nonmedical departments provide other services such as health information management (medical records), finances and billing, housekeeping, etc.

hospital (HAWS-pih-tal)

discharge (DIS-charj)

inpatient (IN-pay-shent)

ancillary (AN-sih-LAIR-ee)
ancill/o- *servant; accessory*
-ary *pertaining to*

Physician's Office

The physician's office is one of the most frequently used healthcare settings. A single physician (or group of physicians in a group practice) maintains an office where patients are seen, diagnosed, treated, and counseled. Some offices have their own laboratory and x-ray equipment for performing diagnostic tests. Seriously ill patients who cannot be quickly diagnosed or adequately treated in the office are sent to a hospital.

Clinic

A **clinic** provides healthcare services similar to that of a physician's office but for just one type of patient or one type of disease. For example, a well-baby clinic provides care to newborn infants, and a methadone clinic treats former drug addicts. Outpatient clinics are located in a hospital or in their own separate facility. Their patients are known as **outpatients** because they are not admitted to the clinic and do not stay overnight.

clinic (KLIN-ik)

outpatient (OUT-pay-shent)

Ambulatory Surgery Center

An **ambulatory surgery center (ASC)** is a facility where minor surgery is performed and the patient does not stay overnight.

ambulatory (AM-byoo-lah-TOR-ee)
ambulat/o- *walking*
-ory *having the function of*

Long-Term Care Facility

A **long-term care facility,** previously known as a nursing home, is primarily a residential facility for older adults or those with disabilities who are unable to care for themselves. Long-term care facilities provide 24-hour nursing care. Persons in long-term care facilities are referred to as **residents** rather than patients, because the facility is considered their home or residence. **Skilled nursing facilities (SNFs)** are long-term care facilities with a special nursing unit that provides a higher level of medical and nursing care that is needed for patients who have recently been discharged from the hospital. Many long-term care facilities also provide **rehabilitation** services to prepare a patient to live independently at home.

Home Health Agency

A **home health agency** provides a range of healthcare services to persons (**clients**) in their homes. These services are particularly useful for those who are unable to come to a physician's office or clinic and do not want to live in a long-term care facility (see Figure 2-22 ■).

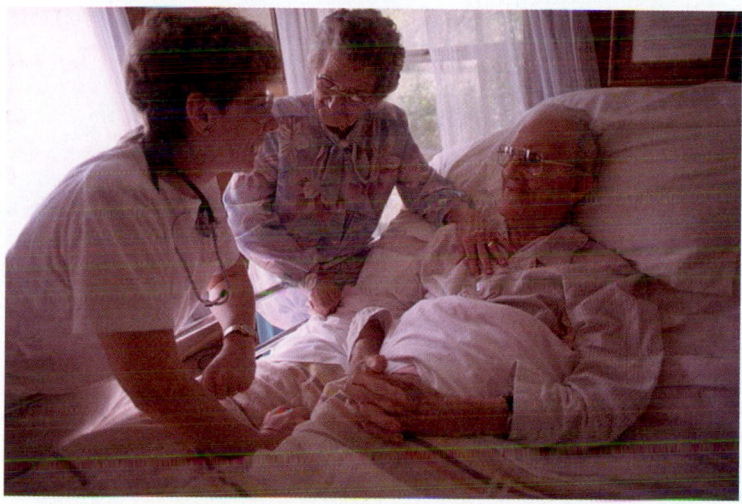

Figure 2-22 ■ Home Health Nurse.

This home health nurse is making one of her routinely scheduled visits to an elderly client in his home. She will assess his physical status, emotional needs, and medications. She will also offer emotional support to other family members. She supervises the home health aide who sees the client several times a week to help him with his physical care.

Hospice

A **hospice** is an inpatient facility for patients who are dying from a terminal illness, and their physicians have certified that they have less than 6 months to live. Hospice services include **palliative** care (supportive medical and nursing care to keep the patient comfortable), counseling, and emotional support for the patient and family. Hospice care can also be provided in the patient's home.

Across the Life Span

Most people think of the healthcare settings of a long-term care facility and hospice as only pertaining to older adults. In fact, some chronically ill or severely handicapped children and young adults are cared for in long-term care facilities. All ages of patients who are terminally ill can receive hospice care in a hospice facility or at home.

WORD BUILDING

rehabilitation
(REE-hah-BIL-ih-TAY-shun)
  re- *again and again; backward; unable to*
  habilitat/o- *give ability*
  -ion *action; condition*

hospice (HAWS-pis)

palliative (PAL-ee-ah-tiv)
  palliat/o- *reduce the severity of*
  -ive *pertaining to*

Vocabulary Review

The Body in Disease

Word or Phrase	Description	Combining Forms
acute	Symptoms and signs that occur suddenly and are severe in nature	
allied health professionals	Healthcare professionals who support the work of physicians and perform specific services ordered by the physician. Allied health professionals include nurses, technologists, technicians, therapists, and others.	
ambulatory surgery center (ASC)	Facility where minor surgical procedures are performed. The person is an **outpatient** who arrives in time for the surgery and does not stay overnight.	**ambulat/o-** *walking* **surg/o-** *operative procedure*
ancillary department	Department that provides services to support the medical and surgical care given in a hospital. Examples: Radiology department, physical therapy department, dietary department, emergency department, clinical laboratory, and pharmacy.	**ancill/o-** *servant; accessory*
asymptomatic	Showing no symptoms or signs of disease	**symptomat/o-** *collection of symptoms*
attending physician	Physician on the medical staff of a hospital who admits patients, directs their care, and discharges them	**physic/o-** *body*
auscultation	Using a stethoscope to listen to the heart, lungs, or intestines	**auscult/o-** *listening*
chronic	Symptoms or signs that continue for 3 months or longer	**chron/o-** *time*
clinic	An ambulatory facility that provides healthcare services, often for just one type of patient or one type of disease. Example: Well-baby clinic for newborns, cleft lip/palate clinic, diabetes clinic. Clinic patients are known as **outpatients** and the facility is an outpatient clinic.	
congenital	Disease caused by an abnormality in fetal development or an abnormal process that occurs during gestation or birth. Examples: Cleft lip, cerebral palsy.	**congenit/o-** *present at birth*
degenerative	Disease caused by progressive destruction of cells due to disease or the aging process. Examples: Multiple sclerosis, hearing loss, arthritis.	**gener/o-** *production; creation*
diagnosis	A determination based on knowledge about the cause of the patient's symptoms and signs	**gnos/o-** *knowledge*
disability	Permanent inability to perform certain activities or function in a given way	
discharge	Release by the hospital of a patient who no longer needs hospital-level care. The patient can be discharged to home or transferred to another healthcare facility. (*Note:* Discharge also refers to a fluid or semisolid substance produced by a disease process or condition.)	
disease	Any change in the normal structure or function of the body	
environmental	Disease caused by exposure to substances in the environment. Examples: Smoke, pollen, sun rays, etc.	
etiology	The cause or origin of a disease	**eti/o-** *cause of disease*
exacerbation	Sudden worsening in the severity of symptoms or signs	**exacerb/o-** *increase; provoke*

Word or Phrase	Description	Combining Forms
hereditary	Disease caused by an inherited or spontaneous mutation in the genetic material of a cell. Examples: Cystic fibrosis, Down syndrome, sickle cell disease.	**heredit/o-** *genetic inheritance*
home health agency	Agency that provides nursing and non-nursing services to patients in their homes. These patients are known as **clients.**	
hospice	Facility for patients who have a terminal illness and require **palliative** supportive care, counseling, and emotional support for themselves and their families. Hospice care can also be provided in the patient's home.	**palliat/o-** *reduce the severity of*
hospital	Healthcare facility that provides care for acutely ill medical and surgical patients for longer than 24 hours. The person being treated is an **inpatient.** The patient is admitted, occupies a bed in the hospital, and is discharged.	
iatrogenic	Disease caused by medicine or treatment given to the patient. Examples: Wrong drug or blood given to a patient; surgery on the wrong part.	**iatr/o-** *physician; medical treatment* **gen/o-** *arising from; produced by*
idiopathic	Disease having no identifiable or confirmed cause. Example: Sudden infant death syndrome.	**idi/o-** *unknown; individual* **path/o-** *disease; suffering*
infectious	Disease caused by a pathogen. A **communicable** disease is an infectious disease that is transmitted by direct or indirect contact with an infected person, animal, or insect. Examples: Gonorrhea, rabies, tuberculosis.	**infect/o-** *disease within* **communic/o-** *impart; transmit*
inpatient	A patient in a hospital	
inspection	Using the eyes or an instrument to examine the body	**inspect/o-** *looking at*
long-term care facility	Residential facility for persons who are unable to take care of themselves. A long-term care facility, also known as a nursing home, provides 24-hour nursing care and rehabilitation services. Persons in this facility are known as **residents.**	**habilitat/o-** *give ability*
neoplastic	Disease caused by the growth of a benign (not cancerous) tumor or mass or by a malignant (cancerous) tumor or mass	**ne/o-** *new* **plast/o-** *growth; formation*
nosocomial	Disease caused by exposure to an infection while the patient is in the hospital. Example: Surgical wound infection.	**nosocomi/o-** *hospital*
nurse	Allied health professional who examines patients, makes nursing diagnoses, and gives medicines and treatment ordered by a physician	
nutritional disease	Disease caused by lack of nutritious food, too little food, or an inability to utilize the food that is eaten. Example: Malnutrition.	**nutri/o-** *nourishment*
palliative care	Supportive medical and nursing care that keeps the patient comfortable but does not cure the disease	**palliat/o-** *reduce the severity of*
palpation	Using the fingers to press on a body part to detect a mass, an enlarged organ, tenderness, or pain	**palpat/o-** *touching; feeling*
pathogen	Disease-causing microorganism, such as a bacterium, virus, fungus, etc.	**path/o-** *disease; suffering*
percussion	Tapping one finger on another finger of a hand that is spread across the chest or abdomen to listen for differences in sound in a body cavity	**percuss/o-** *tapping*
physician	Healthcare professional who directs the activities of the healthcare team. The physician orders tests and diagnoses and treats patients. Other healthcare professionals who graduate from schools that focus their training on just one part of the body or one aspect of medicine are known as **doctors.** A primary care physician (PCP) is a general practitioner who specializes in family practice or pediatrics.	**physic/o-** *body*

Word or Phrase	Description	Combining Forms
physician extender	Healthcare professionals who perform some of the duties of a physician and work under the supervision of a physician (M.D. or D.O.). They examine, diagnose, and treat patients. Some can prescribe medicines. Physician extenders include physician's assistants, nurse practitioners, certified nurse midwives, and certified registered nurse anesthetists.	
physician's office	Ambulatory facility where a physician (or a group of physicians in a group practice) maintains an office. The patients are outpatients and are seen for a short period of time to diagnose and prescribe treatment for diseases that do not require hospitalization.	
preventive medicine	Keeps a person in a state of health and prevents the occurrence of disease	**prevent/o-** *prevent* **medic/o-** *physician; medicine*
prognosis	Predicted course and outcome of a disease	**gnos/o-** *knowledge*
recuperation	Return to a normal state of health	**recuper/o-** *recover*
refractory	Pertaining to a disease that does not respond well to treatment	**fract/o-** *break up*
remission	Temporary improvement in the symptoms and signs of a disease without the underlying disease being cured	**remiss/o-** *send back*
sequela	Abnormal condition or complication that is caused by the original disease and remains after the original disease has resolved	
skilled nursing facility (SNF)	Long-term care facility with a special nursing unit that can admit patients directly from the hospital and provide a higher level of medical and nursing care. Persons in this facility are known as **residents.**	
symptom	A deviation from health that is only experienced and felt by the patient	
symptomatology	The clinical picture of all the patient's symptoms and signs	**symptomat/o-** *collection of symptoms*
syndrome	Set of symptoms and signs associated with one particular disease	
subacute	Symptoms and signs that are less severe in intensity than acute symptoms	
surgeon	Physician or doctor who performs surgery	**surg/o-** *operative procedure*
surgery	A treatment that involves invading the patient's body, often by cutting	**surg/o-** *operative procedure*
technician	Allied health professional who has technical skill in a particular field of medicine	**techn/o-** *technical skill*
technologist	Allied health professional who specializes in a technical area of a field of medicine and performs technical tests	**techn/o-** *technical skill* **log/o-** *word; the study of*
terminal illness	A disease from which there is no hope of recovery and one that will eventually result in the patient's death	**termin/o-** *end; boundary*
therapeutic	Pertaining to an action (from therapy or medicines) that results in improvement in the symptoms or signs of a disease	**therapeut/o-** *therapy; treatment*
therapist	Allied health professional who performs therapy on patients to treat a specific disease or condition	**therap/o-** *treatment*

Building Medical Words

Use the Answer Key at the end of the book to check your answers.

Combining Forms Exercise

Before you build words about the body in disease, review these combining forms. Next to each combining form, write its medical meaning. The first one has been done for you.

Combining Form	Medical Meaning	Combining Form	Medical Meaning
1. **termin/o-**	end; boundary	20. log/o-	
2. ambulat/o-		21. medic/o-	
3. ancill/o-		22. ne/o-	
4. auscult/o-		23. nosocomi/o-	
5. chron/o-		24. nutri/o-	
6. communic/o-		25. palliat/o-	
7. congenit/o-		26. palpat/o-	
8. eti/o-		27. path/o-	
9. exacerb/o-		28. percuss/o-	
10. fract/o-		29. physic/o-	
11. gener/o-		30. plast/o-	
12. gen/o-		31. prevent/o-	
13. gnos/o-		32. recuper/o-	
14. habilitat/o-		33. remiss/o-	
15. heredit/o-		34. surg/o-	
16. iatr/o-		35. symptomat/o-	
17. idi/o-		36. techn/o-	
18. infect/o-		37. therapeut/o-	
19. inspect/o-		38. therap/o-	

Combining Form and Suffix Exercise

Read the definition of the medical word. Look at the combining form that is given. Select the correct suffix from the Suffix List and write it on the blank line. Then build the medical word and write it on the line. (Remember: You may need to remove the combining vowel. Always remove the hyphens and slash.) Be sure to check your spelling. The first one has been done for you.

SUFFIX LIST

-al (pertaining to)	-eon (one who performs)	-ician (a skilled professional or expert)	-ist (one who specializes in)
-ary (pertaining to)	-ery (process of)		-ive (pertaining to)
-ation (a process; being or having)	-gen (that which produces)	-ion (action; condition)	-logy (the study of)
	-ic (pertaining to)	-ious (pertaining to)	

Definition of the Medical Word	Combining Form	Suffix	Build the Medical Word
1. Action of looking at (the body)	inspect/o-	-ion	inspection

(You think *action* (-ion) + *looking at* (inspect/o-). You change the order of the word parts to put the suffix last. You write *inspection*.)

2. Pertaining to the end (of life)	termin/o-	_____	_____
3. One who specializes in treatment	therap/o-	_____	_____
4. One who performs operative procedures	surg/o-	_____	_____
5. Pertaining to reducing the severity of	palliat/o-	_____	_____
6. Skilled professional or expert (with) technical skill	techn/o-	_____	_____
7. Pertaining to genetic inheritance	heredit/o-	_____	_____
8. That which produces disease or suffering	path/o-	_____	_____
9. The study of the collection of symptoms	symptomat/o-	_____	_____
10. Action of touching or feeling	palpat/o-	_____	_____
11. A process of listening	auscult/o-	_____	_____
12. Pertaining to disease(-causing organisms) within (the body)	infect/o-	_____	_____
13. Pertaining to therapy or treatment	therapeut/o-	_____	_____
14. Process of an operative procedure	surg/o-	_____	_____
15. Action of tapping	percuss/o-	_____	_____
16. Pertaining to (continuing over) time	chron/o-	_____	_____
17. Pertaining to (being) present at birth	congenit/o-	_____	_____
18. The study of the cause of disease	eti/o-	_____	_____

Prefix Exercise

Read the definition of the medical word. Look at the medical word or partial word that is given (it already contains a combining form and a suffix). Select the correct prefix from the Prefix List and write it on the blank line. Then build the medical word and write it on the line. Be sure to check your spelling. The first one has been done for you.

PREFIX LIST

a- (away from; without)	dia- (complete; completely through)	re- (again and again; backward; unable to)
de- (reversal of; without)	pro- (before)	

Definition of the Medical Word	Prefix	Word or Partial Word	Build the Medical Word
1. Condition of complete knowledge	dia-	gnosis	diagnosis
2. Pertaining to the reversal of the creation (of tissues)	_____	generative	_____
3. Pertaining to without symptoms	_____	symptomatic	_____
4. Condition of before knowledge (foreknowledge about the course of a disease)	_____	gnosis	_____
5. Pertaining to (being) unable to break up	_____	fractory	_____

Abbreviations

A&P	anatomy and physiology		**LPN**	licensed practical nurse
AP	anteroposterior		**LUQ**	left upper quadrant
ASC	ambulatory surgery center		**LVN**	licensed vocational nurse
CNM	certified nurse midwife		**M.D.**	Doctor of Medicine
CRNA	certified registered nurse anesthetist		**NP**	nurse practitioner
CV	cardiovascular		**OB**	obstetrics
D.C.	Doctor of Chiropracty (or Chiropractic Medicine)		**OB/GYN**	obstetrics and gynecology
D.D.S.	Doctor of Dental Surgery		**O.D.**	Doctor of Optometry
D.O.	Doctor of Osteopathy (or Osteopathic Medicine)		**PA**	physician's assistant
D.P.M.	Doctor of Podiatric Medicine			posteroanterior
Dr.	doctor		**PCP**	primary care physician
Dx	diagnosis		**PE**	physical examination
ED	emergency department		**Pharm. D.**	Doctor of Pharmacy
ENT	ears, nose, and throat		**PT**	physical therapy
ER	emergency room		**RLQ**	right lower quadrant
GI	gastrointestinal		**RN**	registered nurse
GYN	gynecology		**R/O**	rule out
H&P	history and physical (examination)		**RUQ**	right upper quadrant
Hx	history		**SNF**	skilled nursing facility (pronounced "sniff")
ICU	intensive care unit		**Sx**	symptoms
LLQ	left lower quadrant		**Tx**	treatment

Word Alert

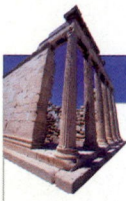

ABBREVIATIONS

Abbreviations are commonly used in all types of medical documents; however, they can mean different things to different people and their meanings can be misinterpreted. Always verify the meaning of an abbreviation.

PA means *physician's assistant,* but it also means *posteroanterior.*

PCP means *primary care physician,* but it also means *phencyclidine* (the street drug known as "angel dust").

It's Greek to Me!

Some words are related to two different combining forms. Why? In ancient times, the Greeks and the Romans independently advanced the study and practice of medicine, naming things in their own languages. Combining forms from both Greek and Latin languages remain a part of medical language today.

Word	Greek	Latin	Medical Word Examples
intestine	enter/o-	intestin/o-	gastroenterology, gastrointestinal
nerve	neur/o	nerv/o-	neurology, nervous system
skin	dermat/o-	integument/o-	dermatology, integumentary system

CAREER FOCUS

Meet April, a health information manager

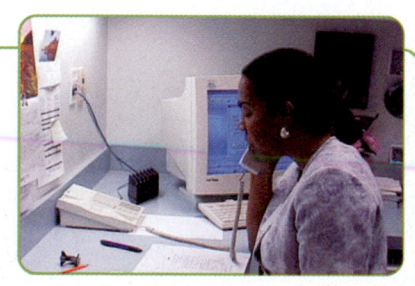

"My title is Applications Manager for the Health Information Management Department. We were previously known as the Medical Records Department. Within the department, I've moved to managing software and how we use the software to gather information. For anything that is done to the patient, there would be documentation, and all of it comes to this department to be stored. We end up interacting with every single clinical department. Since we hold the information, we also help to disseminate it. You get to know a whole lot about medicine without actually being the person who takes care of a patient. You definitely have to have a strong background in medical terminology in order to be really effective in this kind of setting. You're looking at patients' records and trying to make sure that things are correct, and a misunderstood word can change the meaning. Not only for transcription, but for coding, for analysis of the record—there's almost no area here that it's not important. The tasks that we perform really help make health care run smoothly for the patients and for the people who are delivering the care."

Health information management professionals work in physician group practices, clinics, hospitals, nursing homes, and for transcription and coding companies.

CHAPTER REVIEW EXERCISES

Test your knowledge of the chapter by completing these review exercises. Use the Answer Key at the end of the book to check your answers.

The Body in Health and Disease

Matching Exercise

Match each word to its description.

1. anatomy
2. cephalad
3. cranial
4. sagittal
5. muscular
6. physiology
7. psychiatry
8. superficial
9. ventral

_____ Medical specialty that diagnoses and treats mental illness

_____ Body system that supports the body and produces motion

_____ The study of the structures of the human body

_____ The front of the body

_____ Plane that divides the body into right and left sections

_____ Moving toward the head from a lower area of the body

_____ The study of the functions of the human body

_____ Structures that are on the surface of the body

_____ Body cavity that contains the brain

Circle Exercise

Circle the correct word or phrase from the choices given.

1. Hematology is the study of the (**blood, brain, muscles**).
2. Which of the following is related to a body cavity? (**endocrine, thoracic, ventral**)
3. The microscopic approach to the human body helps us gain knowledge about (**body systems, cavities, cells**).
4. The medical specialty of (**gastroenterology, immunology, obstetrics**) studies the stomach, intestines, and other structures.
5. The (**anatomical, anatomy, plane**) position is a standard position of the body for study purposes.
6. If you move your arm and point to something ahead of you, you have moved it in a/an (**anterior, lateral, superficial**) direction.
7. The (**cranial, pelvic, thoracic**) cavity contains the lungs.
8. The (**endocrine, reproductive, respiratory**) system provides oxygen to the body and rids the body of carbon dioxide.
9. The tips of the fingers are (**anterior, distal, proximal**) to the elbow.

True or False Exercise

Indicate whether each statement is true or false by writing T or F on the line.

1. _____ The lymphatic system contains the lymph nodes.
2. _____ Things on the macroscopic level cannot be seen with the naked eye.
3. _____ The coronal plane is also known as the transverse plane.
4. _____ When you lie on your back, you are in the dorsal supine position.
5. _____ The abdominopelvic cavity contains the heart and the lungs.
6. _____ The integumentary system consists of the skin and related structures.

7. _____ The medical specialty of orthopedics includes the skeletal system and the muscular system.

8. _____ Dermatology and the integumentary system both pertain to the skin.

9. _____ Something in a lateral position is located toward the side.

10. _____ Going from your waist toward your head would be moving in a caudad direction.

Healthcare Professionals and Healthcare Settings

Circle Exercise

Circle the correct word or phrase from the choices given.

1. The (**clinic, hospital, physician's office**) is one of the most frequently used healthcare settings.

2. The cause of a disease is the (**etiology, sequela, syndrome**).

3. A disease that does not respond well to treatment is said to be (**acute, refractory, therapeutic**).

4. A/an (**exacerbation, remission, sequela**) is a temporary improvement in the symptoms and signs of a disease.

5. A disease that is inherited from one's parents is (**congenital, hereditary, nutritional**).

Fill in the Blank Exercise

Fill in the blank with the correct word from the word list.

auscultation	clinic	idiopathic	palpation	subacute	symptomatology	syndrome

1. _____ symptoms are slightly less severe than acute symptoms.

2. _____ is performed by pressing the fingers on the abdomen.

3. _____ is using a stethoscope to listen to the heart sounds.

4. A/an _____ is a set of symptoms and signs associated with one particular disease.

5. A/an _____ disease has no known cause.

6. _____ is all of the patient's symptoms and signs.

7. A healthcare facility that sees just one type of outpatient is called a/an _____.

True or False Exercise

Indicate whether each statement is true or false by writing T or F on the line.

1. _____ Doctors and therapists form the core of the healthcare team.

2. _____ A hospital stay begins with the physician's order to admit the patient.

3. _____ Lung disease caused by smoking would be an example of an environmental exposure that caused disease.

4. _____ The predicted outcome of a disease is known as the diagnosis.

5. _____ A pathogen is a microorganism that produces disease in the body.

6. _____ A nurse orders therapy for a patient.

7. _____ A Doctor of Chiropractic treats only the eyes.

8. _____ A dietitian is an example of a technologist.

Building Medical Words

Matching Exercise

Match each word part to its definition.

1. cardi/o-
2. cephal/o-
3. dietet/o-
4. enter/o-
5. extern/o-
6. hemat/o-
7. integument/o-
8. -logy
9. medi/o-
10. onc/o-
11. ot/o-
12. pulmon/o-
13. radi/o-
14. super/o-
15. thorac/o-
16. tom/o-
17. ventr/o-

_____ x-rays; radiation
_____ lung
_____ skin
_____ middle
_____ blood
_____ intestine
_____ cut; slice; layer
_____ tumor; mass
_____ front; abdomen
_____ head
_____ thorax (chest)
_____ ear
_____ above
_____ heart
_____ outside
_____ the study of
_____ foods; diet

Word Parts Exercise

Read the definition of the medical word. Select the correct suffix and combining form from the Word Parts List. Then build the medical word and write it on the line. Be sure to check your spelling. The first one has been done for you.

SUFFIX LIST	COMBINING FORM LIST	
-al (pertaining to)	anter/o- (before; front part)	ne/o- (new)
-ation (a process; being or having)	auscult/o- (listening)	neur/o- (nerve)
-gen (that which produces)	cardi/o- (heart)	path/o- (disease; suffering)
-ic (pertaining to)	congenit/o- (present at birth)	plast/o- (growth; formation)
-ics (knowledge; practice)	dermat/o- (skin)	super/o- (above)
-ior (pertaining to)	dietet/o- (foods; diet)	symptomat/o- (collection of
-logy (the study of)	interno- (inside)	symptoms)
-scope (instrument used to examine)	micr/o- (one millionth; small)	thorac/o- (thorax; chest)

Definition of the Medical Word

1. The study of the nerves
2. Pertaining to the front part
3. Instrument used to examine small (things)
4. Pertaining to a new growth or formation
5. The study of the heart
6. That which produces disease

Build the Medical Word

1. *neurology* _____
2. _____
3. _____
4. _____
5. _____
6. _____

Definition of the Medical Word

Build the Medical Word

7. Pertaining to above _____

8. Pertaining to (the body cavity in) the chest _____

9. Pertaining to (being) present at birth _____

10. Pertaining to inside _____

11. The study of the skin _____

12. A process of listening _____

13. Pertaining to (having) symptoms _____

14. Knowledge and practice of foods and diet _____

Dividing Medical Words

Separate these words into their component parts (prefix, combining form, suffix). Note: Some words do not contain all three word parts. The first one has been done for you.

Medical Word	Prefix	Combining Form	Suffix	Medical Word	Prefix	Combining Form	Suffix
1. anatomical	ana-	tom/o-	-ical	7. ophthalmology	_____	_____	_____
2. nosocomial	_____	_____	_____	8. asymptomatic	_____	_____	_____
3. cephalad	_____	_____	_____	9. posterior	_____	_____	_____
4. endocrinology	_____	_____	_____	10. reproductive	_____	_____	_____
5. gynecology	_____	_____	_____	11. thoracic	_____	_____	_____
6. degenerative	_____	_____	_____	12. urinary	_____	_____	_____

Abbreviations

Matching Exercise

Match each abbreviation to its description.

1. M.D. _____ Minor outpatient surgery is performed here

2. NP _____ Physician extender who delivers babies

3. SNF _____ Doctor who treats the feet

4. ASC _____ Female genital system

5. CNM _____ Physician who graduated from a medical school

6. D.P.M. _____ Registered nurse

7. GI _____ Acts as a physician extender

8. RN _____ Patients here are known as residents

9. D.D.S. _____ Ancillary department within a hospital

10. ED _____ Doctor who treats the teeth

11. GYN _____ Has to do with the stomach and intestines

Applied Skills

Fill in the Blank Exercise

Complete each sentence with the correct medical specialty. Be sure to check your spelling. The first one has been done for you.

1. Diseases of the female genital system are studied in the medical specialty of <u>gynecology</u>.

2. Mrs. Claire English is four months pregnant. She is under the care of a physician who specializes in _____.

3. Bobby McCollum seems to constantly have a runny nose, a sore throat, and repeated ear infections. His regular physician may refer him to a specialist in the field of _____ for possible surgery on his ears.

4. _____ is the medical specialty that helps patients who have diseases of the nervous system.

5. County road worker Jeremy Walker accidentally touched poison ivy while clearing some brush. He has severe itching and redness on the skin of his hands and arms. He has an appointment this afternoon in the _____ clinic.

6. Alfred Dunley has a chronic lung condition and is seen annually for pulmonary function tests that are performed in the _____ Department of Allegheny General Hospital.

7. Sarah Gibbs was born 4 weeks prematurely, but is going home today after being cared for by the nurses and doctors who specialize in _____.

8. When Chris Sutton fell down the steps, she went to the emergency room and a physician from the medical specialty of _____ read her x-rays and found she had fractured her little toe.

9. The team physician for the Baltimore Ravens football team is a specialist in the field of _____, because team members have so many bone and muscle injuries during the season.

Proofreading and Spelling Exercise

Read the following paragraph. Identify each misspelled word and write the correct spelling of it on the line.

Beginning with the body in anetomical position is a good way to study the human body. Traveling posteriorily from the breast bone to the spine takes you through the tharacic cavty that holds the heart, the main organ of the kardiovascular system. The study of the eye is known as ophthamology, while the study of the ears, nose, and throat is otolarngology. The study of the lungs, which are in the thoracic cavity, is known as pulmonawlogy. However, most students like gyenecology the best because of its interesting anatomy and fisiology.

1. _____   6. _____
2. _____   7. _____
3. _____   8. _____
4. _____   9. _____
5. _____   10. _____

English and Medical Word Equivalents Exercise

For each English word, write its equivalent medical word. Be sure to check your spelling. The first one has been done for you.

English Word	Medical Word	English Word	Medical Word
1. front	<u>anterior</u> or <u>ventral</u>	6. lying on the stomach	_____
2. back	_____ or _____	7. upper half	_____
3. side	_____	8. lower half	_____
4. midline	_____	9. going toward the head	_____
5. lying on the back	_____	10. going toward the tail bone	_____

Hearing Medical Words Exercise

You hear someone speaking the medical words given below. Read each pronunciation and then write the medical word it represents. Be sure to check your spelling. The first one has been done for you.

1. dih-ZEEZ   *disease*
2. AM-byoo-lah-TOR-ee   _____
3. KAR-dee-oh-VAS-kyoo-lar   _____
4. dee-JEN-er-ah-tiv   _____
5. EP-ih-GAS-trik   _____
6. eg-ZAS-er-BAY-shun   _____
7. heh-RED-ih-TAIR-ee   _____

8. HAWS-pis   _____
9. in-TEG-yoo-MEN-tair-ee   _____
10. NEE-oh-PLAS-tik   _____
11. PAL-ee-ah-tiv   _____
12. PEE-dee-AT-riks   _____
13. prawg-NOH-sis   _____
14. THAIR-ah-PYOO-tik   _____

Pronunciation Exercise

Read the medical word that is given. Then review the syllables in the pronunciation. Circle the primary (main) accented syllable. The first one has been done for you.

1. anterior (an-teer-ee-or)
2. anatomical (an-ah-tawm-ih-kal)
3. auscultation (aws-kul-tay-shun)
4. congenital (con-jen-ih-tal)
5. endocrinology (en-doh-krih-nawl-oh-jee)

6. geriatrics (jair-ee-at-riks)
7. idiopathic (id-ee-oh-path-ik)
8. prognosis (prawg-noh-sis)
9. superficial (soo-per-fish-al)
10. technologist (tek-nawl-oh-jist)

Multimedia Preview

Immerse yourself in a variety of activities inside Medical Terminology Interactive. Getting there is simple:

1. Click on www.myhealthprofessionskit.com.
2. Select "Medical Terminology" from the choice of disciplines.
3. First-time users must create an account using the scratch-off code on the inside front cover of this book.
4. Find this book and log in using your username and password.
5. Click on Medical Terminology Interactive.
6. Take the elevator to the 2nd Floor to begin your virtual exploration of this chapter!

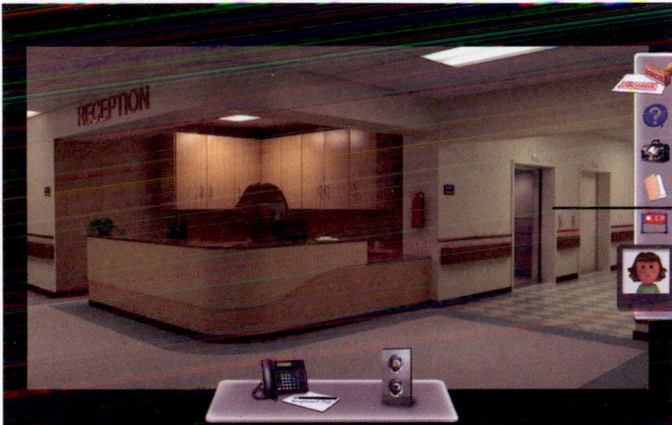 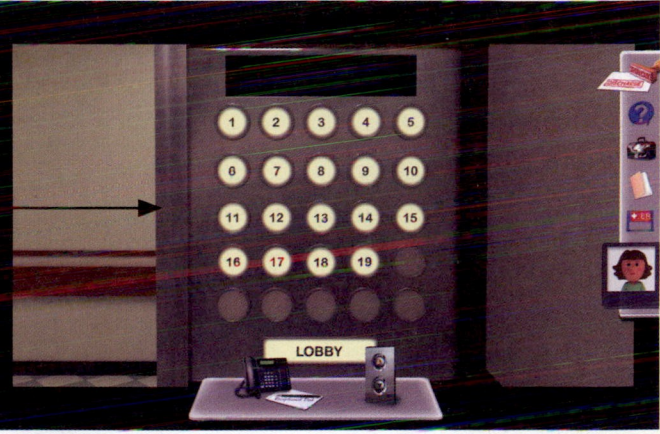

■ **Crossword**   Here's where learning and fun intersect! Simply use the clues to complete the puzzle grid. Whether you're a crossword wizard or only a novice, this activity will reinforce your understanding of key terms and concepts.

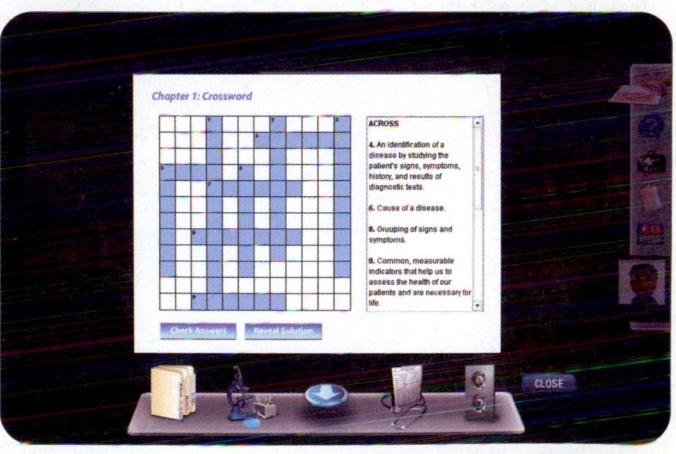

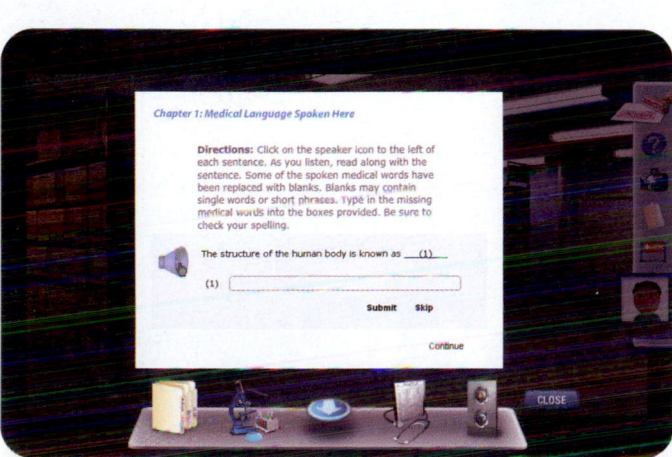

■ **Medical Language Spoken Here**   Click here to immerse yourself in the world of real physician dictation. Listen carefully to these actual medical reports. Can you correctly spell the missing medical words?

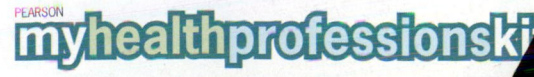

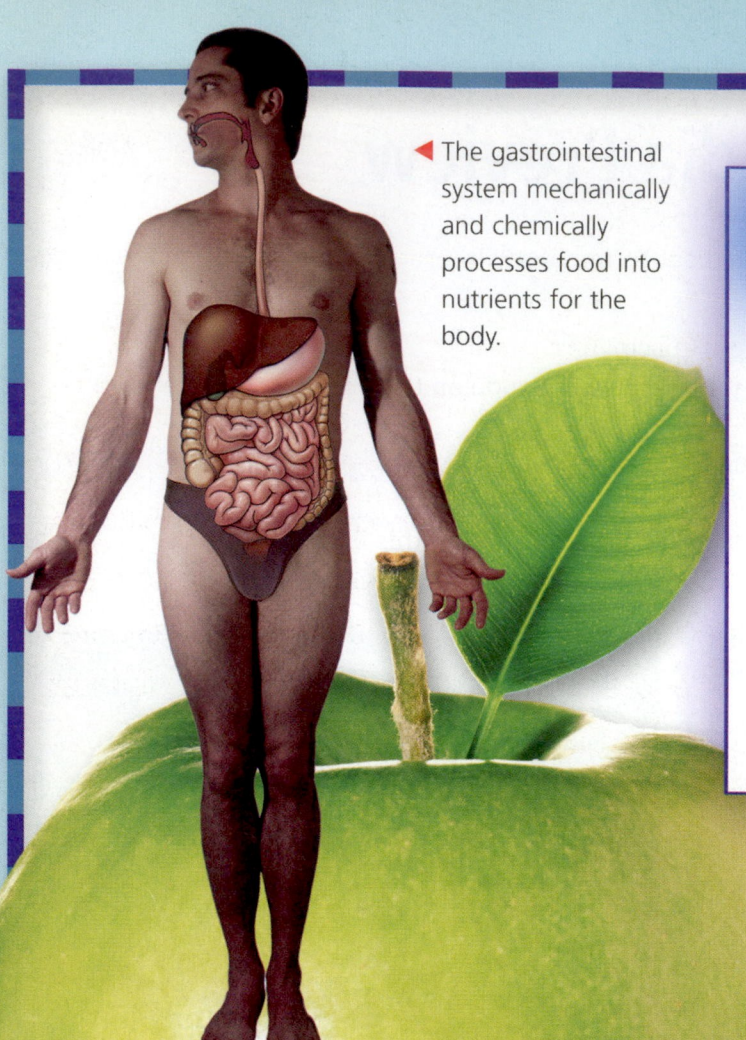

◄ The gastrointestinal system mechanically and chemically processes food into nutrients for the body.

Dive In!

- The small intestine is 21 feet long and the large intestine adds another 5 feet.
- The average person eats 11 pounds per year of spaghetti sauce and ketchup.
- The first nasogastric tube (a feeding tube through the nose to the stomach) was made from eel skin.
- In this chapter you'll explore the gastrointestinal system. Satisfy your hunger for the medical language of gastroenterology!

◄ Taking a bite of an apple and chewing it is the process known as *mastication.* Swallowing is known as *deglutition.*

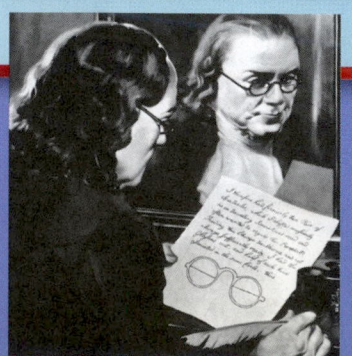

1747

Scottish surgeon James Lind discovers that a substance in citrus fruits (vitamin C) keeps sailors from developing scurvy

1760

Benjamin Franklin invents bifocal glasses

3

Gastroenterology

Gastrointestinal System

Gastroenterology (GAS-troh-EN-ter-AWL-oh-jee) is the medical specialty that studies the anatomy and physiology of the gastrointestinal system and uses diagnostic tests, medical and surgical procedures, and drugs to treat gastrointestinal diseases.

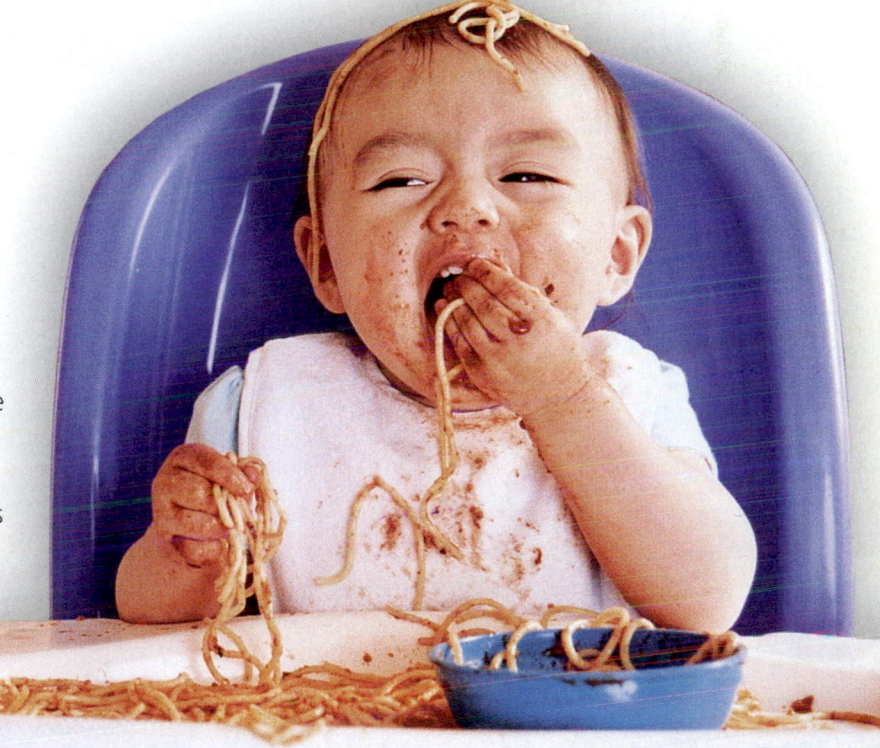

▶ The sense of taste can detect sweet, salty, sour, bitter, umami (the savory taste of amino acids), fatty acids, and the sensation of metals and water.

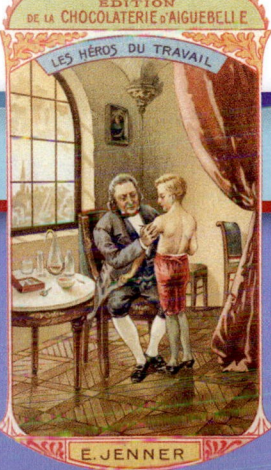

1796

Edward Jenner, an English physician, devises the first vaccination by injecting material from cowpox sores to prevent smallpox

1798

John Dalton, an English physicist, describes color blindness

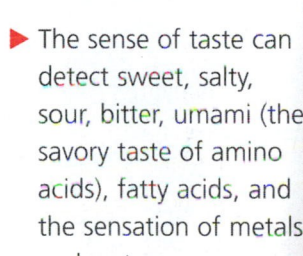

1806

The painkilling drug morphine is isolated from the opium poppy

Measure Your Progress: Learning Objectives

After you study this chapter, you should be able to

1. Identify the structures of the gastrointestinal system.

2. Describe the process of digestion.

3. Describe common gastrointestinal diseases and conditions, laboratory and diagnostic procedures, medical and surgical procedures, and drug categories.

4. Give the medical meaning of word parts related to the gastrointestinal system.

5. Build gastrointestinal words from word parts and divide and define gastrointestinal words.

6. Spell and pronounce gastrointestinal words.

7. Analyze the medical content and meaning of a gastroenterology report.

8. Dive deeper into gastroenterology by reviewing the activities at the end of this chapter and online at Medical Terminology Interactive.

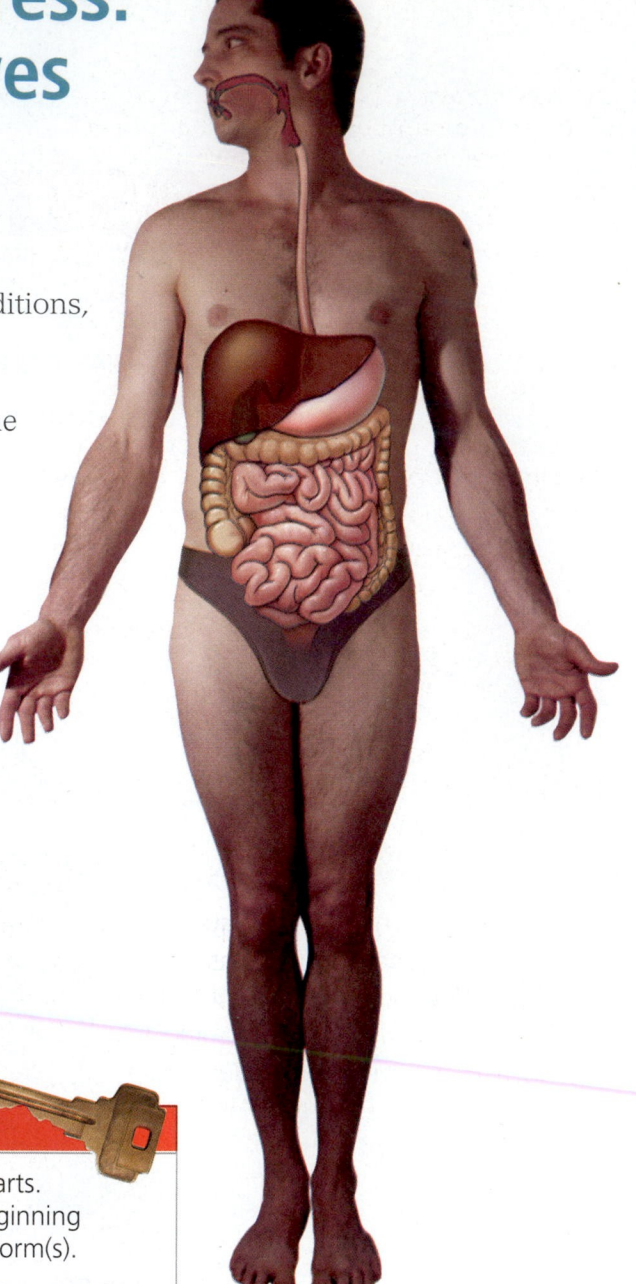

Figure 3-1 ■ **Gastrointestinal system.**

The gastrointestinal system consists of organs and glands connected in a pathway. Food enters the body, is digested, and undigested wastes are eliminated from the body.

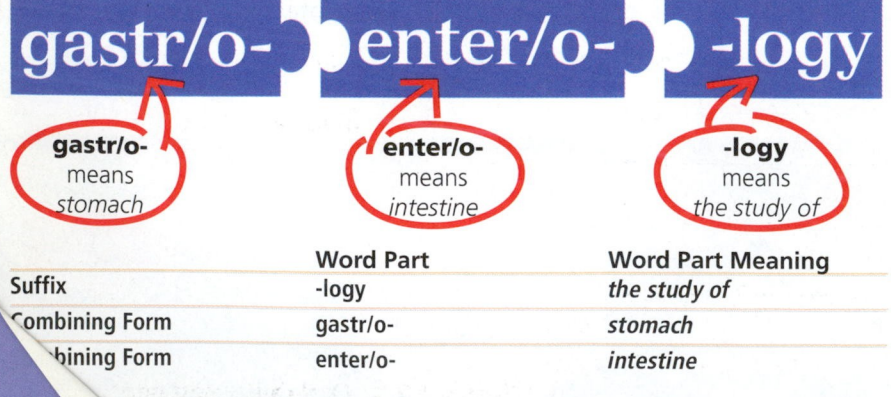

Medical Language Key

To unlock the definition of a medical word, break it into word parts. Define each word part. Put the word part meanings in order, beginning with the suffix, then the prefix (if present), then the combining form(s).

gastr/o- enter/o- -logy

gastr/o-
means
stomach

enter/o-
means
intestine

-logy
means
the study of

	Word Part	Word Part Meaning
Suffix	-logy	*the study of*
Combining Form	gastr/o-	*stomach*
Combining Form	enter/o-	*intestine*

Gastroenterology: *The study of the stomach and intestines (and related structures).*

Anatomy and Physiology

The **gastrointestinal (GI) system** is an elongated body system that begins at the mouth, continues through the thoracic cavity, and fills much of the abdominopelvic cavity (see Figure 3-1 ■). The upper gastrointestinal system includes the structures from the mouth through the stomach. The lower gastrointestinal system includes the structures from the small intestine through the anus. The purpose of the gastrointestinal system is to digest food, absorb nutrients, and remove undigested material (waste) from the body.

WORD BUILDING

gastrointestinal
(GAS-troh-in-TES-tih-nal)
  gastr/o- *stomach*
  intestin/o- *intestine*
  -al *pertaining to*

system (SIS-tem)

Word Alert

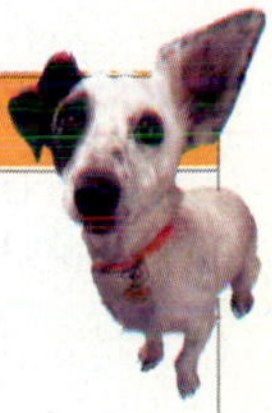

The gastrointestinal system is also known as the **gastrointestinal tract,** the **digestive system** or digestive tract, and the **alimentary canal.** Each name highlights a different characteristic of this body system.

1. Tract: a continuing pathway
2. Digestive: describes the purpose of the system
3. Alimentary: refers to food and nourishment
4. Canal: a tubular channel

digestive (dy-JES-tiv)
  digest/o- *break down food; digest*
  -ive *pertaining to*

alimentary (AL-ih-MEN-tair-ee)
  aliment/o- *food; nourishment*
  -ary *pertaining to*

Anatomy of the Gastrointestinal System

Oral Cavity and Pharynx

The gastrointestinal system begins in the mouth or **oral cavity** (see Figure 3-2 ■). It contains the teeth, gums, **tongue,** hard **palate,** and soft palate with its fleshy, hanging **uvula.** The oral cavity is lined with **mucosa,** a mucous

oral (OR-al)
  or/o- *mouth*
  -al *pertaining to*
Oral is the adjective form for *mouth.* The combining form *stomat/o-* also means *mouth.*

tongue (TUNG)
  lingu/o- *tongue*
  -al *pertaining to*
The combining form *gloss/o-* also means *tongue.*

palate (PAL-at)

uvula (YOO-vyoo-lah)

mucosa (myoo-KOH-sah)

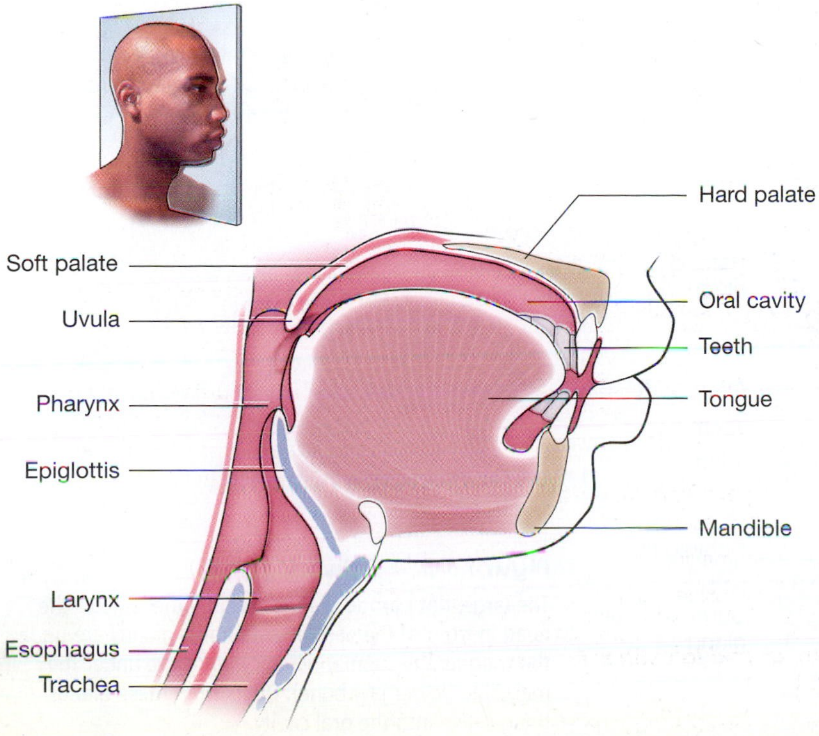

Soft palate
Uvula
Pharynx
Epiglottis
Larynx
Esophagus
Trachea

Hard palate
Oral cavity
Teeth
Tongue
Mandible

Figure 3-2 ■ **Oral cavity and pharynx.**
The oral cavity contains the teeth, gums, tongue, and palate. Food passes from the oral cavity into the pharynx (throat) and then into the esophagus.

membrane that produces thin mucus. The sense of taste is also associated with the gastrointestinal system. Receptors on the tongue perceive taste and send this information to the **gustatory cortex** in the brain.

The sight, smell, and taste of food cause the salivary glands to release saliva into the mouth. **Saliva** is a lubricant that moistens food as it is chewed and swallowed. Saliva also contains the enzyme amylase that begins the process of digestion. There are three pairs of **salivary glands:** the **parotid glands, sublingual glands,** and **submandibular glands** (see Figure 3-3 ■).

The teeth tear, chew, and grind food during the process of **mastication.** The tongue moves food toward the teeth and mixes food with saliva. Swallowing or **deglutition** moves food into the throat or pharynx. The **pharynx** is a passageway for food as well as for inhaled and exhaled air. When food is swallowed, the larynx moves upward to close against the epiglottis, so that food in the pharynx does not enter the larynx, trachea, and lungs. If the entrance to the larynx is not closed when food is in the back of the pharynx pressing on the uvula, this initiates the gag reflex.

Across the Life Span

Pediatrics. The first food for many babies is colostrum from the mother's breast. Colostrum is rich in nutrients and contains maternal antibodies. For the first few days of life, the newborn's intestinal tract is permeable and allows these antibodies to be absorbed from the intestine into the blood, where they provide passive immunity to common diseases.

Geriatrics. Older adults often complain that food does not seem as flavorful as when they were younger. The aging process causes a very real decline in the ability to smell and taste food as the number of receptors in the nose and on the tongue decreases.

WORD BUILDING

gustatory (GUS-tah-TOR-ee)
  gustat/o- *the sense of taste*
  -ory *having the function of*

saliva (sah-LY-vah)

salivary (SAL-ih-VAIR-ee)
  saliv/o- *saliva*
  -ary *pertaining to*
The combining form *sial/o-* also means *salivary gland* or *saliva.*

parotid (pah-RAWT-id)
  par- *beside*
  ot/o- *ear*
  -id *resembling; source or origin*

sublingual (sub-LING-gwal)
  sub- *below; underneath; less than*
  lingu/o- *tongue*
  -al *pertaining to*

submandibular
(SUB-man-DIB-yoo-lar)
  sub- *below; underneath; less than*
  mandibul/o- *mandible (lower jaw)*
  -ar *pertaining to*

mastication (MAS-tih-KAY-shun)
  mastic/o- *chewing*
  -ation *a process; being or having*

deglutition (DEE-gloo-TISH-un)
  degluti/o- *swallowing*
  -tion *a process; being or having*

pharynx (FAIR-ingks)

pharyngeal (fah-RIN-jee-al)
  pharyng/o- *pharynx (throat)*
  -eal *pertaining to*

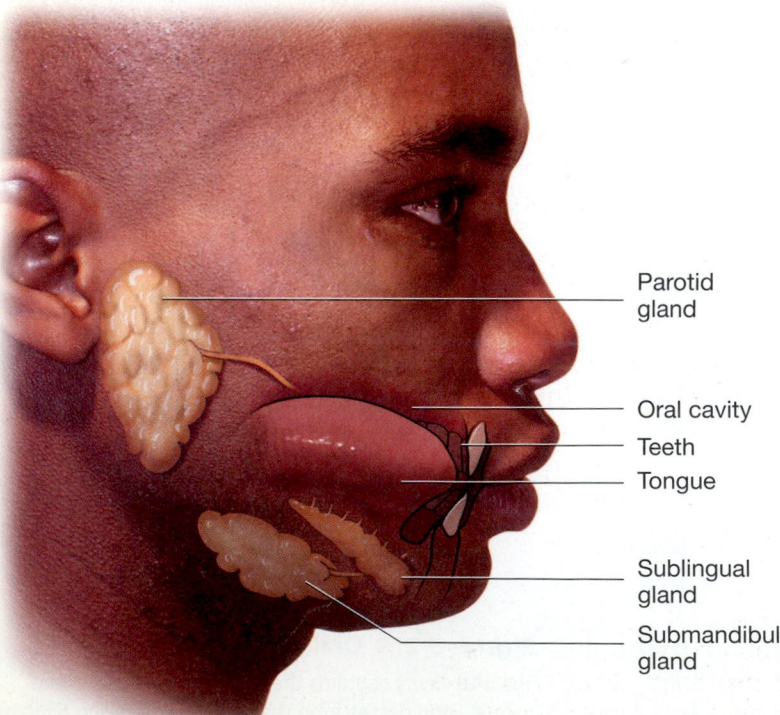

Parotid gland

Oral cavity

Teeth

Tongue

Sublingual gland

Submandibular gland

Figure 3-3 ■ Salivary glands.

The large, flat parotid glands are on either side of the head in front of the ear. The sublingual glands are under the tongue. The submandibular glands are under the mandible (lower jaw bone). Ducts from these glands bring saliva into the oral cavity.

Esophagus

The **esophagus** is a flexible, muscular tube that connects the pharynx to the stomach. It is lined with mucosa that produces mucus. With coordinated contractions of its wall—a process known as **peristalsis**—the esophagus moves food toward the stomach.

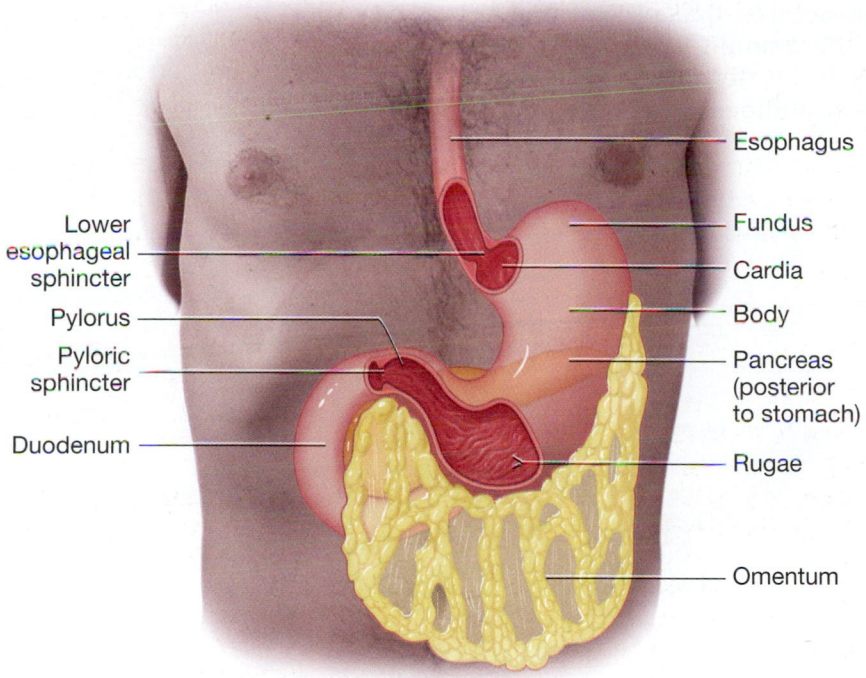

Labels on figure:
Esophagus
Lower esophageal sphincter
Pylorus
Pyloric sphincter
Duodenum
Fundus
Cardia
Body
Pancreas (posterior to stomach)
Rugae
Omentum

Figure 3-4 ■ **Stomach.**

The stomach has four regions. The cardia is the small area where the esophagus joins the stomach. The fundus is the rounded top of the stomach. The body is the large, curved part of the stomach. The pylorus is the narrowed canal at the end.

Stomach

The **stomach** (see Figure 3-4 ■) is a large, elongated sac in the upper abdominal cavity. It receives food from the esophagus. The stomach is divided into four regions: the **cardia, fundus, body,** and **pylorus** (see Figure 3-4). The gastric mucosa is arranged in thick, deep folds or **rugae** that expand as the stomach fills with food. The stomach produces hydrochloric acid, pepsinogen, and gastrin to aid in the digestion of food. The mucosa produces mucus that protects the lining of the stomach from the hydrochloric acid.

Two sphincters (muscular rings) keep food in the stomach. The **lower esophageal sphincter (LES)** is located at the distal end of the esophagus. The **pyloric sphincter** is located at the distal end of the stomach. **Chyme** is a semisolid mixture of partially digested food, saliva, digestive enzymes, and fluids in the stomach. An hour or so after eating, the pyloric sphincter opens and waves of peristalsis propel the chyme into the small intestine.

Small Intestine

The **small intestine** or **small bowel** is a long, hollow tube that receives chyme from the stomach. The small intestine produces three digestive enzymes: lactase, maltase, and sucrase. The small intestine consists of three parts: the duodenum, jejunum, and ileum (see Figure 3-5 ■). The

WORD BUILDING

esophagus (eh-SAWF-ah-gus)

esophageal (eh-SAWF-ah-JEE-al)
  esophag/o- *esophagus*
  -eal *pertaining to*

peristalsis (PAIR-ih-STAL-sis)
  peri- *around*
  stal/o- *contraction*
  -sis *process; condition; abnormal condition*

gastric (GAS-trik)
  gastr/o- *stomach*
  -ic *pertaining to*
Gastric is the adjective form for stomach.

cardia (KAR-dee-ah)

fundus (FUN-dus)

pylorus (py-LOR-us)

pyloric (py-LOR-ik)
  pylor/o- *pylorus*
  -ic *pertaining to*

rugae (ROO-gee)
The singular form *ruga* is seldom used.

sphincter (SFINGK-ter)

chyme (KIME)

intestine (in-TES-tin)

intestinal (in-TES-tih-nal)
  intestin/o- *intestine*
  -al *pertaining to*
The combining form *enter/o-* also means *intestine*.

duodenum is a 10-inch, C-shaped segment that begins at the stomach and ends at the jejunum. Digestive enzymes from the gallbladder and pancreas flow through ducts into the duodenum. The **jejunum,** the second part of the small intestine, is an 8-foot segment that repeatedly twists and turns in the abdominal cavity. Digestion continues in the jejunum. Peristalsis slowly moves the chyme along for several hours until it reaches the ileum, the final part of the small intestine. The **ileum** is a 12-foot segment where absorption of nutrients is completed. The ileum contains **villi,** thousands of small, thin structures that project into the **lumen** (central, open area) and increase the amount of surface area to maximize the absorption of food nutrients and water through the intestinal wall and into the blood. The remaining undigested material (waste) and water move into the large intestine.

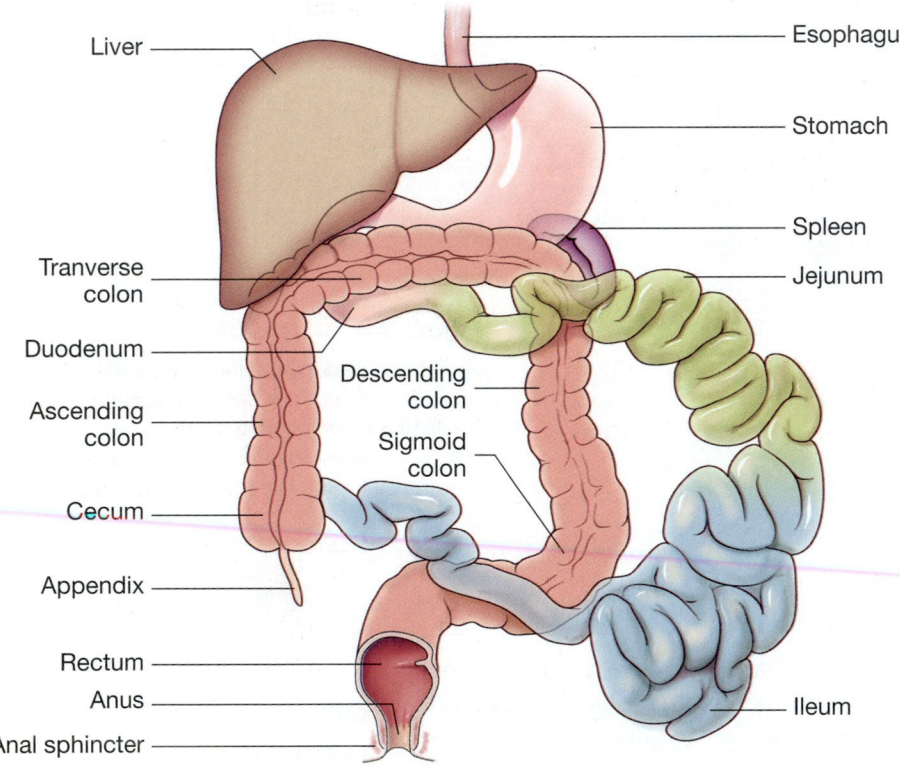

Figure 3-5 ■ Small and large intestines.
The small intestine consists of the duodenum, jejunum, and ileum. The large intestine consists of the cecum (and appendix), colon, rectum, and anus. The colon can be divided into the ascending colon, transverse colon, descending colon, and sigmoid colon. The bends (flexures) in the colon are landmarks that are mentioned in x-ray reports. The bend near the liver is the hepatic flexure. The bend near the spleen is the splenic flexure.

Large Intestine

The **large intestine** or **large bowel** is a larger, hollow tube that receives undigested material and some water from the small intestine. The large intestine consists of the cecum, colon, rectum, and anus (see Figure 3-5). The **cecum** is a short sac. Hanging from its external wall is the **appendix,** a thin tube that is closed at its distal end.

The walls of the large intestine contain **haustra** (puckered pouches) that can greatly expand as needed. Waves of peristalsis slowly move undigested material through the large intestine as water is absorbed through the intestinal wall and into the blood.

The **colon** is the longest part of the large intestine. It travels through all four quadrants of the abdomen as the **ascending colon, transverse colon, descending colon,** and **sigmoid colon** (see Figure 3-5). As the ascending colon nears the liver, it bends in a right angle at the hepatic flexure. As the transverse colon nears the spleen, it bends in a right angle at the splenic flexure. The sigmoid colon bends toward the midline in an S-shaped curve that joins the rectum. The **rectum** is a short, straight segment that connects to the outside of the body. The **anus,** the external opening of the rectum, is located between the buttocks. The anal sphincter is a muscular ring whose opening and closing is under conscious, voluntary control.

Did You Know?

The appendix or vermiform appendix can be up to 8 inches in length. *Vermiform* is a Latin word meaning *wormlike.* The appendix plays no role in digestion. It is part of the lymphatic system and the immune response (discussed in "Hematology and Immunology," Chapter 6).

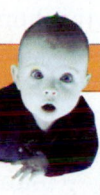

Clinical Connections

Immunology (Chapter 6). Some parts of the gastrointestinal system are also part of the body's immune response. Saliva contains antibodies that destroy microorganisms in the food we eat. Small areas on the walls of the intestines (Peyer's patches) and in the appendix contain white blood cells that destroy microorganisms. However, ingested microorganisms can still cause gastrointestinal illness.

Abdomen and Abdominopelvic Cavity

The anterior **abdominal wall** can be divided into four quadrants or nine regions (discussed in "The Body in Health and Disease," Chapter 2).

The **abdominopelvic cavity** contains the largest organs (viscera) of the gastrointestinal system. The **peritoneum** is a double-layer serous membrane. One layer lines the walls of the abdominopelvic cavity. The other layer surrounds each of the organs. The peritoneum secretes **peritoneal fluid,** a watery fluid that fills the spaces between the organs and allows them to slide past each other during the movements of digestion.

The peritoneum extends into the center of the abdominopelvic cavity as the **omentum** (see Figure 3-4). The omentum supports the stomach and hangs down as a fatty apron to cover and protect the small intestine. The peritoneum also extends as the **mesentery,** a thick, fan-shaped sheet that supports the jejunum and ileum.

The blood supply to the stomach, small intestine, liver, gallbladder, and pancreas comes from the **celiac trunk** of the abdominal aorta, the largest artery in the body.

Accessory Organs of Digestion

The liver, gallbladder, and pancreas are accessory organs of digestion. They contribute to, but are not physically involved in, the process of digestion.

WORD BUILDING

colon (KOH-lon)

colonic (koh-LAWN-ik)
  colon/o- *colon*
  -ic *pertaining to*
The combining form *col/o-* also means *colon.*

sigmoid (SIG-moyd)
The combining form *sigmoid/o-* means *sigmoid colon.*

rectum (REK-tum)

rectal (REK-tal)
  rect/o- *rectum*
  -al *pertaining to*
The combining form *proct/o-* also means *rectum.*

anus (AA-nus)

anal (AA-nal)
  an/o- *anus*
  -al *pertaining to*

abdominal (ab-DAWM-ih-nal)
  abdomin/o- *abdomen*
  -al *pertaining to*
The combining forms *celi/o-* and *lapar/o-* also mean *abdomen.*

abdominopelvic
(ab-DAWM-ih-noh-PEL-vik)
  abdomin/o- *abdomen*
  pelv/o- *pelvis (hip bone; renal pelvis)*
  -ic *pertaining to*

peritoneum (PAIR-ih-toh-NEE-um)

peritoneal (PAIR-ih-toh-NEE-al)
  peritone/o- *peritoneum*
  -al *pertaining to*
The combining form *periton/o-* also means *peritoneum.*

omentum (oh-MEN-tum)

mesentery (MEZ-en-TAIR-ee)

mesenteric (MEZ-en-TAIR-ik)
  meso- *middle*
  enter/o- *intestine*
  -ic *pertaining to*
Delete the *o-* on *meso-* before building the word.

celiac (SEE-lee-ak)
  celi/o- *abdomen*
  -ac *pertaining to*

The **liver,** a large, dark red-brown organ, is located in the upper abdomen (see Figure 3-6 ■). Liver cells **(hepatocytes)** continuously produce **bile,** a yellow-green, bitter-tasting, thick fluid. Bile is a combination of bile acids, mucus, fluid, and two pigments: the yellow pigment **bilirubin** and the green pigment **biliverdin.** Bile produced by the liver flows through the common hepatic duct and into the common bile duct to the duodenum. When the duct is full, bile flows into the cystic duct and gallbladder. All of the **bile ducts** collectively are known as the **biliary tree.**

The **gallbladder** is a teardrop-shaped, dark green sac posterior to the liver (see Figure 3-6). It concentrates and stores bile from the liver. The presence of fatty chyme in the duodenum causes the gallbladder to contract, sending bile into the common bile duct and then into the duodenum to digest fats.

The **pancreas** is a yellow, somewhat lumpy gland shaped like an elongated triangle (see Figure 3-6). It is located posterior to the stomach. The presence of food in the duodenum causes the pancreas to secrete digestive enzymes (amylase, lipase, and others) through the pancreatic duct and into the duodenum. The pancreas also functions as an organ of the endocrine system (discussed in "Endocrinology," Chapter 14).

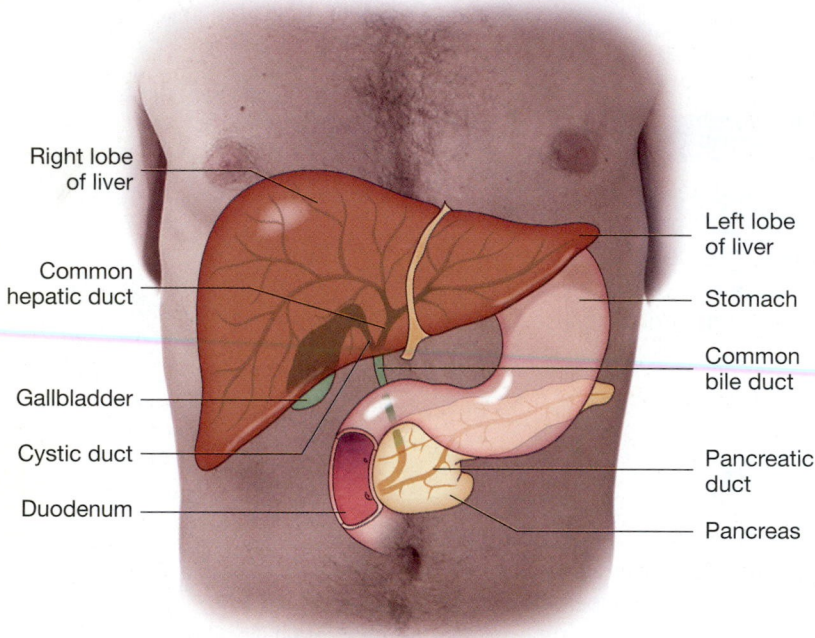

Right lobe of liver
Left lobe of liver
Common hepatic duct
Stomach
Common bile duct
Gallbladder
Cystic duct
Pancreatic duct
Duodenum
Pancreas

Figure 3-6 ■ **Biliary tree.**
Bile flows through hepatic ducts in the liver that merge to form the common hepatic duct. It joins the cystic duct from the gallbladder to form the common bile duct. Because of their appearance, these ducts are known as the biliary tree. The pancreatic duct joins the common bile duct just before it enters the duodenum.

Physiology of Digestion

The process of **digestion** begins in the oral cavity (see Figure 3-7 ■). There are two parts to digestion: mechanical and chemical.

Mechanical digestion uses mastication (tearing, crushing, and grinding of food in the mouth), deglutition (swallowing), and peristalsis (mixing and moving a bolus of food through the esophagus, and mixing and moving chyme and undigested material through the stomach and intestines). Mechanical digestion also involves breaking apart fats in the duodenum. Fatty chyme stimulates the duodenum to secrete the hormone **cholecystokinin,** which stimulates the gallbladder to contract and release bile. Bile breaks apart large globules of fat during the process of **emulsification.**

Chemical digestion uses **enzymes** and acid to break down foods. The enzyme amylase in saliva begins to break down carbohydrate foods in the mouth. The stomach secretes the following substances that continue the process of chemical digestion.

- **Hydrochloric acid (HCl).** This strong acid breaks down food fibers, converts pepsinogen to the digestive enzyme pepsin, and kills microorganisms in food.

- **Pepsinogen.** This inactive substance is converted by hydrochloric acid to **pepsin,** a digestive enzyme that breaks down protein foods into large protein molecules.

- **Gastrin.** This hormone stimulates the release of more hydrochloric acid and pepsinogen.

WORD BUILDING

cholecystokinin
(KOH-lee-SIS-toh-KY-nin)
  cholecyst/o- *gallbladder*
  kin/o- *movement*
  -in *a substance*

emulsification
(ee-MUL-sih-fih-KAY-shun)
  emulsific/o- *droplets of fat suspended in a liquid*
  -ation *a process; being or having*

enzyme (EN-zime)

hydrochloric acid
(HY-droh-KLOR-ik AS-id)
  hydr/o- *water; fluid*
  chlor/o- *chloride*
  -ic *pertaining to*

pepsinogen (pep-SIN-oh-jen)
  pepsin/o- *pepsin*
  -gen *that which produces*

pepsin (PEP-sin)
  peps/o- *digestion*
  -in *a substance*

gastrin (GAS-trin)
  gastr/o- *stomach*
  -in *a substance*

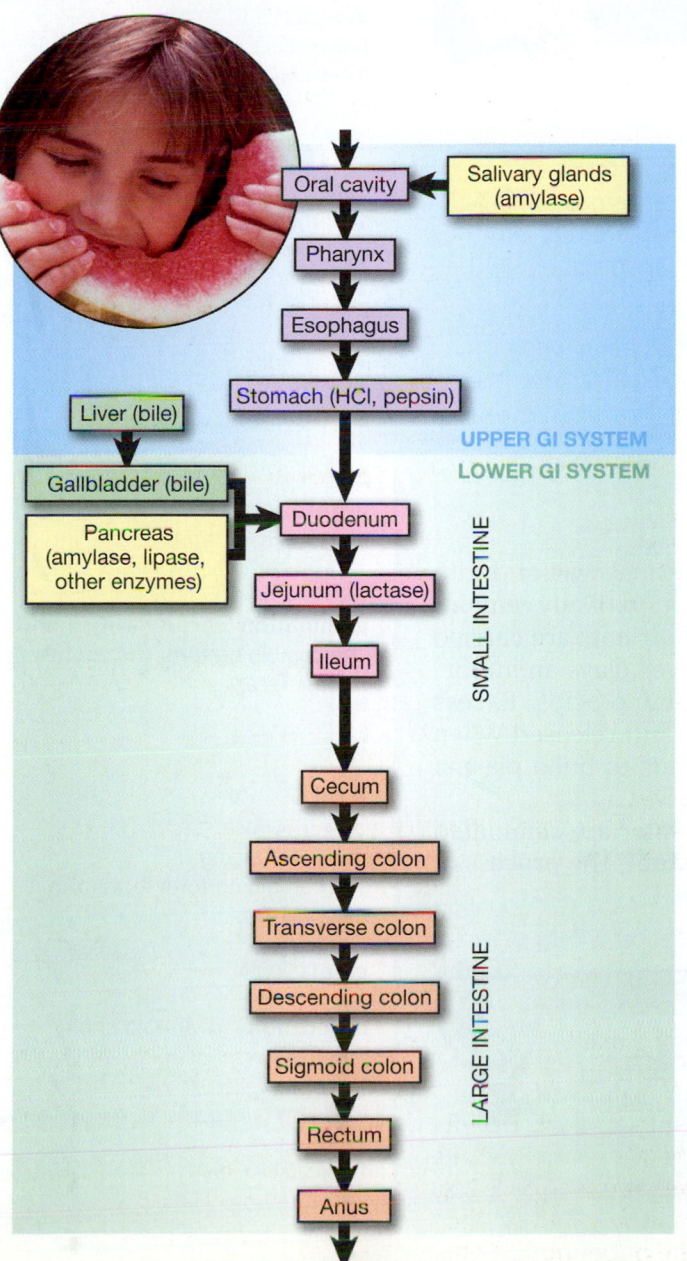

Figure 3-7 ■ Gastrointestinal system.
Everyone enjoys eating! The gastrointestinal system helps you taste and enjoy the food you eat and then uses mechanical and chemical means to break down that food into nutrients that nourish your body.

Chemical digestion continues in the small intestine as cholecystokinin from the duodenum also stimulates the pancreas to secrete its digestive enzymes into the duodenum.

- **Amylase** continues the digestion of carbohydrates that was begun by amylase in the saliva. It breaks down carbohydrates and starches into sugars and food fibers.
- **Lipase** breaks down small fat globules into fatty acids.
- Other enzymes break down large protein molecules into peptide chains and then break down peptide chains into amino acids.

The villi of the small intestine produce digestive enzymes such as **lactase** to break down sugars. The simple sugar glucose is the only source of energy that body cells can use.

Clinical Connections

Hematology (Chapter 6). The stomach plays an indirect role in the production of red blood cells. It secretes intrinsic factor that allows vitamin B_{12} (a building block of red blood cells) to be absorbed from the intestine into the blood. When the stomach does not produce enough intrinsic factor or when part of the stomach is removed (gastrectomy) because of a cancerous tumor, vitamin B_{12} is not absorbed; the red blood cells that are formed are very large, fragile, and die prematurely. This disease is called pernicious anemia.

Dietetics. Individuals whose small intestine does not produce enough of the digestive enzyme lactase experience gas and bloating when they drink milk or eat dairy products. This is caused by undigested lactose (the sugar in milk).

Absorption of nutrients and water through the intestinal wall and into the blood takes place in the small intestine, while absorption of any remaining water takes place in the large intestine. Absorbed nutrients are carried in the blood of a large vein that goes to the liver. The liver plays an important role in regulating nutrients such as glucose and amino acids. Excess glucose in the blood is stored in the liver as glycogen and released when the blood glucose level is low. The liver uses amino acids to build plasma proteins and clotting factors for the blood.

Elimination occurs when undigested materials and water are eliminated from the body in a solid waste form known as **feces** or **stool.** The process of elimination is a bowel movement or **defecation.**

A Closer Look

The large intestine is inhabited by millions of beneficial bacteria that produce vitamin K to supplement what is in the diet. These bacteria also change the yellow-green pigment in bile to the characteristic brown color of feces. Bacteria in the large intestine feed on undigested materials and produce intestinal gas or **flatus.**

WORD BUILDING

amylase (AM-il-ace)
  amyl/o- *carbohydrate; starch*
  -ase *enzyme*

lipase (LIP-ace)
  lip/o- *lipid (fat)*
  -ase *enzyme*

lactase (LAK-tace)
  lact/o- *milk*
  -ase *enzyme*

absorption (ab-SORP-shun)
  absorpt/o- *absorb; take in*
  -ion *action; condition*

elimination (ee-LIM-ih-NAY-shun)
The combining form *chez/o-* means *to pass feces.*

feces (FEE-seez)

fecal (FEE-kal)
  fec/o- *feces; stool*
  -al *pertaining to*
The combining form *fec/a-* also means *feces.*

stool (STOOL)

defecation (DEF-eh-KAY-shun)
  de- *reversal of; without*
  fec/o- *feces; stool*
  -ation *a process; being or having*

flatus (FLAY-tus)

Vocabulary Review

Anatomy and Physiology

Word or Phrase	Description	Combining Forms
alimentary canal	Alternate name for the gastrointestinal system	aliment/o- *food; nourishment*
digestive system	Alternate name for the gastrointestinal system. It is also known as the **digestive tract.**	digest/o- *break down food; digest*
gastrointestinal system	Body system that includes the salivary glands, oral cavity (teeth, gums, palate, and tongue), pharynx, esophagus, stomach, small and large intestines, and the accesssory organs of the liver, gallbladder, and pancreas. Its function is to digest food, absorb nutrients into the blood, and remove undigested material from the body. It is also known as the **gastrointestinal tract,** digestive tract or system, and alimentary canal.	gastr/o- *stomach* intestin/o- *intestine*

Oral Cavity and Pharynx

Word or Phrase	Description	Combining Forms
deglutition	Process of swallowing food	degluti/o- *swallowing*
gustatory cortex	Area of the brain that receives and interprets tastes from the tongue	gustat/o- *the sense of taste*
mastication	Process of chewing. This is part of the process of mechanical digestion.	mastic/o- *chewing*
mucosa	Mucous membrane that lines the gastrointestinal system and produces mucus	
oral cavity	Mouth. Hollow area that contains the hard palate, soft palate, uvula, tongue, gums, and teeth	or/o- *mouth* stomat/o- *mouth*
palate	The hard bone and posterior soft tissues that form the roof of the mouth	
pharynx	Throat. The passageway for both food and inhaled and exhaled air	pharyng/o- *pharynx (throat)*
salivary glands	Three pairs of glands (**parotid, submandibular,** and **sublingual**) that secrete saliva into the mouth. Saliva is a watery substance that contains the digestive enzyme amylase.	saliv/o- *saliva* sial/o- *saliva* ot/o- *ear* mandibul/o- *mandible (lower jaw)* lingu/o- *tongue*
tongue	Large muscle that fills the oral cavity and assists with eating and talking. It contains receptors for the sense of taste.	lingu/o- *tongue* gloss/o- *tongue*
uvula	Fleshy hanging part of the soft palate. It plays a role in speech and, during swallowing, it initiates the gag reflex to prevent food from entering the pharynx before the epiglottis closes over the larynx.	

Esophagus and Stomach

Word or Phrase	Description	Combining Forms
cardia	Small area where the esophagus enters the stomach	
chyme	Partially digested food, saliva, and digestive enzymes in the stomach and small intestine	
esophagus	Flexible, muscular tube that moves food from the pharynx to the stomach	esophag/o- *esophagus*

Word or Phrase	Description	Combining Forms
fundus	Rounded, most superior part of the stomach	
lower esophageal sphincter (LES)	Muscular ring at the distal end of the esophagus. It keeps food in the stomach from going back into the esophagus.	esophag/o- esophagus
peristalsis	Contractions of smooth muscle that propel a bolus of food, and then chyme, waste products, and water through the gastrointestinal tract	stal/o- contraction
pyloric sphincter	Muscular ring that keeps chyme in the stomach or opens to let chyme into the duodenum	pylor/o- pylorus
pylorus	Narrowing area of the stomach just before it joins the duodenum. It contains the pyloric sphincter.	pylor/o- pylorus
rugae	Deep folds in the gastric mucosa that expand to accommodate food	
stomach	Organ of digestion between the esophagus and the small intestine. Areas of the stomach: cardia, fundus, body, and pylorus. The stomach secretes hydrochloric acid, pepsinogen, and gastrin. The stomach secretes intrinsic factor needed to absorb vitamin B_{12}.	gastr/o- stomach

Small and Large Intestines

Word or Phrase	Description	Combining Forms
anus	External opening of the rectum. The external anal sphincter is under voluntary control.	an/o- anus
appendix	Long, thin pouch on the exterior wall of the cecum. It does not play a role in digestion. It contains lymphatic tissue and is active in the body's immune response.	appendic/o- appendix append/o- appendix
cecum	Short, pouch-like first part of the large intestine. The appendix is attached to the cecum's external wall.	cec/o- cecum
colon	Longest part of the large intestine. It consists of the **ascending colon, transverse colon, descending colon,** and S-shaped **sigmoid colon.**	col/o- colon colon/o- colon sigmoid/o- sigmoid colon
duodenum	First part of the small intestine. It secretes the hormone cholecystokinin. Digestion takes place there, as well as some absorption of nutrients and water.	duoden/o- duodenum
haustra	Pouches in the wall of the large intestine that expand to accommodate the bulk of undigested materials	
ileum	Third part of the small intestine. It connects to the cecum of the large intestine. Some digestion takes place there. There is absorption of nutrients and water through the wall of the ileum and into the blood.	ile/o- ileum
jejunum	Second part of the small intestine. Digestion takes place there, as well as some absorption of nutrients and water through the intestinal wall and into the blood.	jejun/o- jejunum
large intestine	Organ of absorption between the small intestine and the anus. The large intestine includes the cecum, colon, rectum, and anus. It is also known as the **large bowel.**	intestin/o- intestine

Word or Phrase	Description	Combining Forms
lumen	Open channel inside a tubular structure such as the esophagus, small intestine, and large intestine	
rectum	Final part of the large intestine. It is a short, straight segment that lies between the sigmoid colon and the anus.	**rect/o-** rectum **proct/o-** rectum
small intestine	Organ of digestion between the stomach and the large intestine. The duodenum, jejunum, and ileum are the three parts of the small intestine. It is also known as the **small bowel.**	**intestin/o-** intestine **enter/o-** intestine
villi	Microscopic projections of the mucosa in the small intestine. They produce digestive enzymes such as lactase to break down sugars. They have a very large combined surface area to maximize the absorption of nutrients into the blood.	

Abdomen, Liver, Gallbladder, and Pancreas

Word or Phrase	Description	Combining Forms
abdominopelvic cavity	Continuous cavity within the **abdomen** and pelvis that contains the largest organs (viscera) of the gastrointestinal system	**abdomin/o-** abdomen **celi/o-** abdomen **lapar/o-** abdomen **pelv/o-** pelvis (hip bone; renal pelvis)
bile	Bitter fluid produced by the liver and stored in the gallbladder. It is released into the duodenum to digest the fat in foods. It contains the green pigment biliverdin and the yellow pigment bilirubin.	**bili/o-** bile; gall **chol/e-** bile; gall
bile ducts	Bile produced by the liver flows through the hepatic ducts to the common hepatic duct. Then it goes into the common bile duct to the duodenum. When that duct is full, bile goes into the cystic duct and gallbladder. All of these ducts form the **biliary tree,** a treelike structure.	**bili/o-** bile; gall **cholangi/o-** bile duct **choledoch/o-** common bile duct
celiac trunk	Part of the abdominal aorta where arteries branch off to take blood to the stomach, small intestine, liver, gallbladder, and pancreas	**celi/o-** abdomen
gallbladder	Small, dark green sac posterior to the liver that stores and concentrates bile. When stimulated by cholecystokinin from the duodenum, it contracts and releases bile into the common bile duct to the duodenum.	**cholecyst/o-** gallbladder
liver	Largest solid organ in the body. It contains **hepatocytes** that produce bile.	**hepat/o-** liver
mesentery	Thick sheet of peritoneum that supports the jejunum and ileum	**enter/o-** intestine
omentum	Broad, fatty apron of peritoneum. It supports the stomach and protects the small intestine.	
pancreas	Triangular organ located posterior to the stomach. It secretes digestive enzymes (amylase, lipase, and other enzymes) into the duodenum.	**pancreat/o-** pancreas
peritoneum	Double-layer serous membrane that lines the abdominopelvic cavity and surrounds each gastrointestinal organ. It secretes peritoneal fluid to fill the spaces between the organs.	**peritone/o-** peritoneum **periton/o-** peritoneum

Digestion

Word or Phrase	Description	Combining Forms
absorption	Process by which digested nutrients move through villi of the small intestine and into the blood	**absorpt/o-** *absorb; take in*
amylase	Digestive enzyme in saliva that begins digestion of carbohydrates in the mouth. It is also secreted by the pancreas to finish the digestion of carbohydrates in the small intestine.	**amyl/o-** *carbohydrate; starch*
cholecystokinin	Hormone secreted by the duodenum when it receives fatty chyme from the stomach. Cholecystokinin stimulates the gallbladder to release bile and the pancreas to release its digestive enzymes.	**cholecyst/o-** *gallbladder* **kin/o-** *movement*
defecation	Process by which undigested materials and water are removed from the body as a bowel movement	**fec/o-** *feces; stool*
digestion	Process of mechanically and chemically breaking down food into nutrients that can be used by the body	**digest/o-** *break down food; digest*
elimination	Process in which undigested materials and water are eliminated from the body	**chez/o-** *to pass feces*
emulsification	Process in which bile breaks down large fat droplets into smaller droplets	**emulsific/o-** *droplets of fat suspended in a liquid*
enzymes	Proteins that speed up chemical reactions in the body. During chemical digestion, enzymes break the chemical bonds in large food molecules. Enzymes are produced by the salivary glands, stomach, small intestine, and pancreas. An enzyme name usually ends in *-ase*.	
feces	Formed, solid waste composed of undigested material, bacteria, and water that is eliminated from the body. It is also known as **stool.**	**fec/a-** *feces; stool* **fec/o-** *feces; stool*
flatus	Gas produced by bacteria that inhabit the large intestine	
gastrin	Hormone produced by the stomach. It stimulates the release of hydrochloric acid and pepsinogen in the stomach.	**gastr/o-** *stomach*
hydrochloric acid	Strong acid produced by the stomach. It breaks down food, kills microorganisms in food, and converts pepsinogen to pepsin.	**chlor/o-** *chloride* **hydr/o-** *water; fluid*
lactase	Digestive enzyme from villi in the small intestine. It breaks down lactose, the sugar in milk.	**lact/o-** *milk*
lipase	Digestive enzyme secreted by the pancreas. It breaks down fat globules in the duodenum into fatty acids.	**lip/o-** *lipid (fat)*
pepsin	Digestive enzyme in the stomach that breaks down protein foods into large protein molecules.	**peps/o-** *digestion*
pepsinogen	Inactive substance produced by the stomach that is converted by hydrochloric acid to the digestive enzyme pepsin.	**pepsin/o-** *pepsin*

Labeling Exercise

Match each anatomy word or phrase to its structure and write it in the numbered box for each figure. Be sure to check your spelling. Use the Answer Key at the end of the book to check your answers.

esophagus	parotid gland	sublingual gland	teeth
oral cavity	pharynx	submandibular gland	tongue

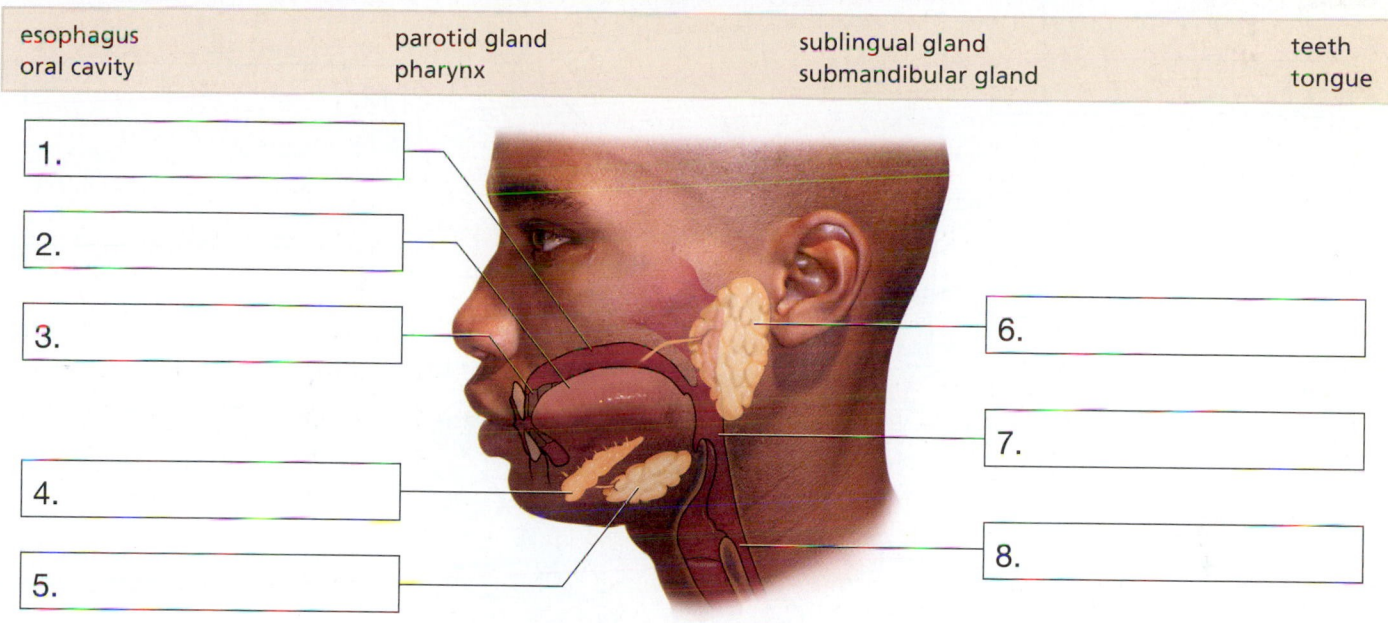

1.

2.

3.

4.

5.

6.

7.

8.

body of stomach	esophagus	omentum	pylorus
cardia	fundus	pancreas	rugae
duodenum	lower esophageal sphincter	pyloric sphincter	

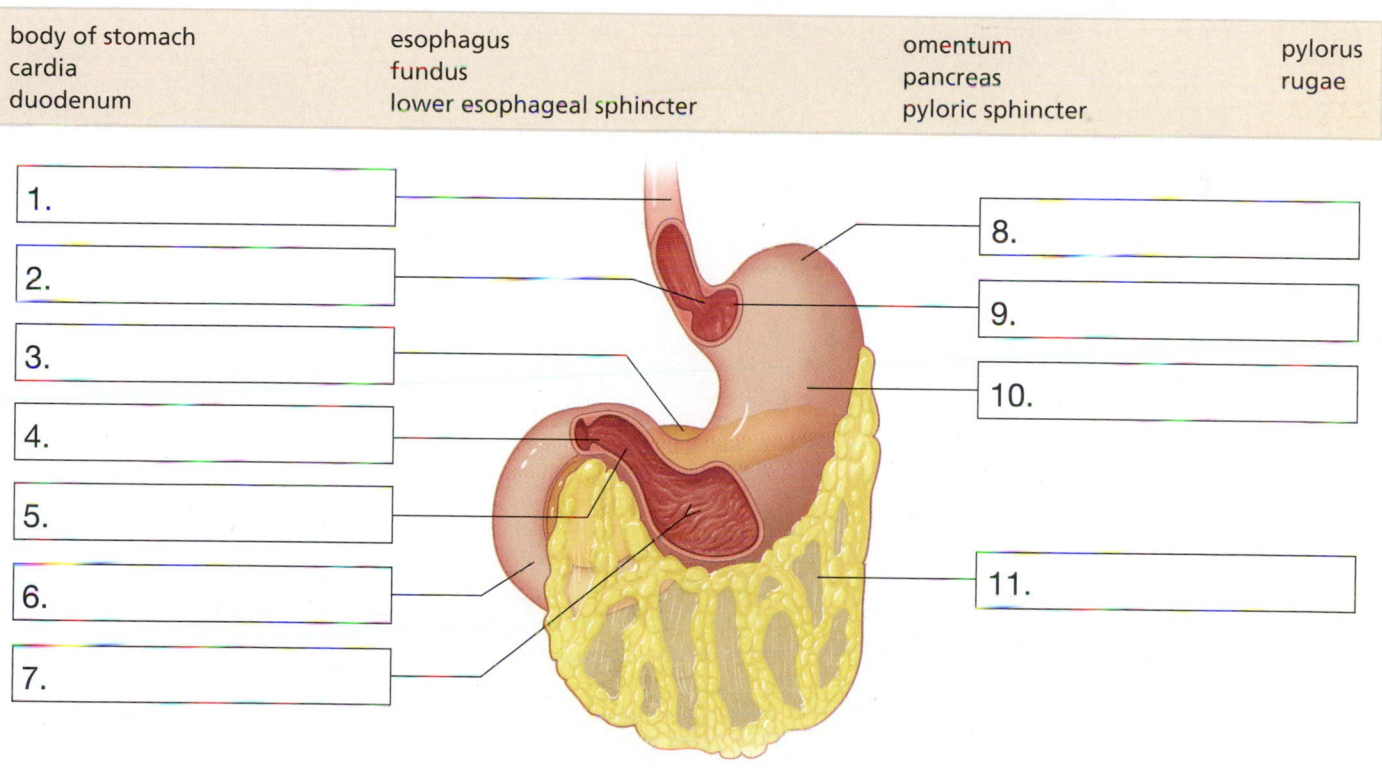

1.

2.

3.

4.

5.

6.

7.

8.

9.

10.

11.

anus
appendix
ascending colon
cecum

descending colon
duodenum
gallbladder
ileum

jejunum
liver
pancreas
rectum

sigmoid colon
sphincter, anal
stomach
transverse colon

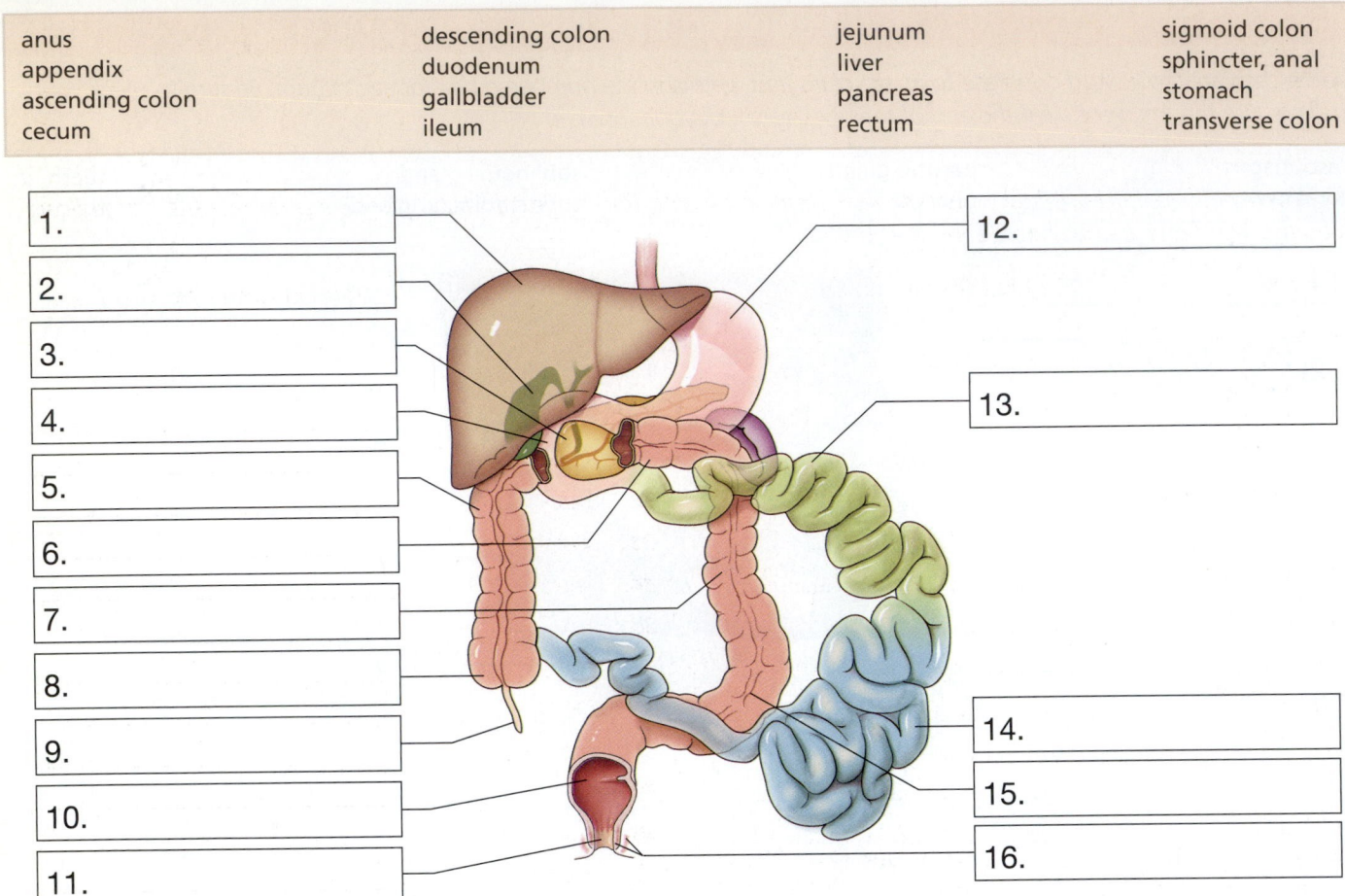

1.

2.

3.

4.

5.

6.

7.

8.

9.

10.

11.

12.

13.

14.

15.

16.

Building Medical Words

Use the Answer Key at the end of the book to check your answers.

Combining Forms Exercise

Before you build gastrointestinal words, review these combining forms. Next to each combining form, write its medical meaning. The first one has been done for you.

Combining Form	Medical Meaning	Combining Form	Medical Meaning
1. hydr/o-	water; fluid	30. gustat/o-	
2. abdomin/o-		31. hepat/o-	
3. absorpt/o-		32. ile/o-	
4. aliment/o-		33. intestin/o-	
5. amyl/o-		34. jejun/o-	
6. an/o-		35. kin/o-	
7. appendic/o-		36. lact/o-	
8. append/o-		37. lapar/o-	
9. bili/o-		38. lingu/o-	
10. cec/o-		39. lip/o-	
11. celi/o-		40. mandibul/o-	
12. chez/o-		41. mastic/o-	
13. chlor/o-		42. or/o-	
14. cholangi/o-		43. ot/o-	
15. chol/e-		44. pancreat/o-	
16. cholecyst/o-		45. pelv/o-	
17. choledoch/o-		46. peps/o-	
18. col/o-		47. pepsin/o-	
19. colon/o-		48. peritone/o-	
20. degluti/o-		49. periton/o-	
21. digest/o-		50. pharyng/o-	
22. duoden/o-		51. proct/o-	
23. emulsific/o-		52. pylor/o-	
24. enter/o-		53. rect/o-	
25. esophag/o-		54. saliv/o-	
26. fec/a-		55. sial/o-	
27. fec/o-		56. sigmoid/o-	
28. gastr/o-		57. stal/o-	
29. gloss/o-		58. stomat/o-	

Combining Form and Suffix Exercise

Read the definition of the medical word. Look at the combining form that is given. Select the correct suffix from the Suffix List and write it on the blank line. Then build the medical word and write it on the line. (Remember: You may need to remove the combining vowel. Always remove the hyphens and slash.) Be sure to check your spelling. The first one has been done for you.

SUFFIX LIST			
-ac (pertaining to)	-ation (a process; being or having)	-gen (that which produces)	-ion (action; condition)
-al (pertaining to)	-cyte (cell)	-ic (pertaining to)	-ive (pertaining to)
-ary (pertaining to)	-eal (pertaining to)	-in (a substance)	-ory (having the function of)
-ase (enzyme)			

Definition of the Medical Word	Combining Form	Suffix	Build the Medical Word
1. Pertaining to the intestine	intestin/o-	-al	intestinal

(You think *pertaining to* (-al) + *the intestine* (intestin/o-). You change the order of the word parts to put the suffix last. You write *intestinal*.)

2. Pertaining to the stomach	gastr/o-	_____	_____
3. Liver cell	hepat/o-	_____	_____
4. Pertaining to the mouth	or/o-	_____	_____
5. Pertaining to (a gland that makes) saliva	saliv/o-	_____	_____
6. Action that breaks down or digests food	digest/o-	_____	_____
7. Process of chewing	mastic/o-	_____	_____
8. Pertaining to the rectum	rect/o-	_____	_____
9. Enzyme (that digests) fat	lip/o-	_____	_____
10. Pertaining to the appendix	appendic/o-	_____	_____
11. Pertaining to food and nourishment	aliment/o-	_____	_____
12. Pertaining to the colon	colon/o-	_____	_____
13. Pertaining to digestion	digest/o-	_____	_____
14. Pertaining to the esophagus	esophag/o-	_____	_____
15. That which produces pepsin	pepsin/o-	_____	_____
16. Pertaining to the pancreas	pancreat/o-	_____	_____
17. Pertaining to bile	bil/i-	_____	_____
18. Pertaining to the duodenum	duoden/o-	_____	_____
19. Having the function of the sense of taste	gustat/o-	_____	_____
20. Pertaining to the throat	pharyng/o-	_____	_____
21. A substance (produced by the) stomach	gastr/o-	_____	_____
22. Pertaining to the pylorus	pylor/o-	_____	_____
23. Pertaining to the jejunum	jejun/o-	_____	_____
24. Pertaining to the abdomen	celi/o-	_____	_____
25. Pertaining to feces	fec/o-	_____	_____
26. Action (in which something is) absorbed	absorpt/o-	_____	_____
27. Enzyme (that digests) milk	lact/o-	_____	_____
28. A process of having fat droplets suspended in a liquid	emulsific/o-	_____	_____
29. Pertaining to the peritoneum	peritone/o-	_____	_____

Prefix Exercise

Read the definition of the medical word. Look at the medical word or partial word that is given (it already contains a combining form and a suffix). Select the correct prefix from the Prefix List and write it on the blank line. Then build the medical word and write it on the line. Be sure to check your spelling. The first one has been done for you.

PREFIX LIST

de- (reversal of; without)	meso- (middle)	peri- (around)	sub- (below; underneath; less than)

Definition of the Medical Word	Prefix	Word or Partial Word	Build the Medical Word
1. Pertaining to (the salivary gland that is) underneath the mandible	sub-	mandibular	submandibular
2. Process around (the intestine of) contraction	_____	stalsis	_____
3. Pertaining to the middle of the intestine *Hint: Delete the o on the prefix before building this word.*	_____	enteric	_____
4. A process (of being) without stool	_____	fecation	_____
5. Pertaining to (being) underneath the tongue	_____	lingual	_____

Multiple Combining Forms and Suffix Exercise

Read the definition of the medical word. Select the correct suffix and combining forms. Then build the medical word and write it on the line. Be sure to check your spelling. The first one has been done for you.

SUFFIX LIST	COMBINING FORM LIST		
-al (pertaining to) -ic (pertaining to) -in (a substance) -logy (the study of)	abdomin/o- (abdomen) chlor/o- (chloride) cholecyst/o- (gallbladder)	enter/o- (intestine) gastr/o- (stomach) hydr/o- (water; fluid)	intestin/o- (intestine) kin/o- (movement) pelv/o- (pelvis)

Definition of the Medical Word	Combining Form	Combining Form	Suffix	Build the Medical Word
1. Pertaining to (an acid made of) water and chloride (You think *pertaining to* (-ic) + *water* (hydr/o-) + *chloride* (chlor/o-). You change the order of the word parts to put the suffix last. You write *hydrochloric*.)	hydr/o-	chlor/o-	-ic	hydrochloric
2. Pertaining to the stomach and intestine	_____	_____	_____	_____
3. Pertaining to the abdomen and pelvis	_____	_____	_____	_____
4. The study of the stomach and intestines	_____	_____	_____	_____
5. A substance (that causes the) gallbladder to move (and contract)	_____	_____	_____	_____

Diseases and Conditions

Eating

Word or Phrase	Description	Word Building
anorexia	Decreased appetite because of disease or the gastrointestinal side effects of a drug. The patient is said to be **anorexic.** Treatment: Correct the underlying cause.	**anorexia** (AN-oh-REK-see-ah) **an-** *without; not* **orex/o-** *appetite* **-ia** *condition; state; thing* **anorexic** (AN-oh-REK-sik)

Clinical Connections

Psychiatry (Chapter 17). Anorexia nervosa is a psychiatric disorder in which patients have an obsessive desire to be thin. They decrease their food intake to the point of starvation, not because they have no appetite, but because they see themselves as being fat.

Word or Phrase	Description	Word Building
dysphagia	Difficult or painful eating or swallowing. A stroke can make it difficult to coordinate the muscles for eating and swallowing. An oral infection or poorly fitted dentures can cause painful eating. Treatment: Soft foods and thickened liquids. Antibiotic drugs for an oral bacterial infection.	**dysphagia** (dis-FAY-jee-ah) **dys-** *painful; difficult; abnormal* **phag/o-** *eating; swallowing* **-ia** *condition; state; thing*
polyphagia	Excessive overeating due to an overactive thyroid gland, diabetes mellitus, or a psychiatric illness. Treatment: Correct the underlying cause.	**polyphagia** (PAWL-ee-FAY-jee-ah) **poly-** *many; much* **phag/o-** *eating; swallowing* **-ia** *condition; state; thing*

Mouth and Lips

Word or Phrase	Description	Word Building
cheilitis	Inflammation and cracking of the lips and corners of the mouth due to infection, allergies, or nutritional deficiency. Treatment: Correct the underlying cause.	**cheilitis** (ky-LY-tis) **cheil/o-** *lip* **-itis** *inflammation of; infection of*
sialolithiasis	A stone (**sialolith**) that forms in the salivary gland and becomes lodged in the duct, blocking the flow of saliva. The salivary gland, mouth, and face become swollen. When the salivary gland contracts, the duct spasms, causing pain. Treatment: Surgical removal of the stone.	**sialolithiasis** (sy-AL-oh-lih-THY-ah-sis) **sial/o-** *saliva; salivary gland* **lith/o-** *stone* **-iasis** *state of; process of* **sialolith** (sy-AL-oh-lith) **sial/o-** *saliva; salivary gland* **-lith** *stone*

Word or Phrase	Description	Word Building

stomatitis	Inflammation of the oral mucosa. Stomatitis can be caused by poorly fitting dentures or infection. **Aphthous stomatitis** consists of small ulcers (canker sores) of the oral mucosa. Its cause is unknown. **Glossitis** is an inflammation that involves only the tongue (see Figure 3-8 ■). Treatment: Correct the underlying cause.	**stomatitis** (STOH-mah-TY-tis)
		  stomat/o- *mouth*
		  -itis *inflammation of; infection of*
		aphthous (AF-thus)
		  aphth/o- *ulcer*
		  -ous *pertaining to*
		glossitis (glaw-SY-tis)
		  gloss/o- *tongue*
		  -itis *inflammation of; infection of*

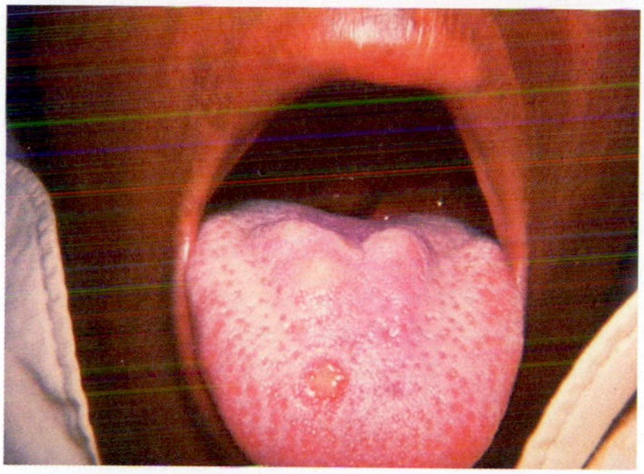

Figure 3-8 ■ Glossitis.
This inflammation of the tongue was caused by a viral infection. Other causes of glossitis include bacterial infection, food allergy, abrasive or spicy foods, or a vitamin B deficiency.

Esophagus and Stomach

Word or Phrase	Description	Word Building

dyspepsia	**Indigestion** or epigastric pain that may be accompanied by gas or nausea. It can be caused by excess stomach acid or reflux of stomach acid into the esophagus, overeating, spicy foods, or stress. Treatment: Antacid drugs. Avoid things that cause it.	**dyspepsia** (dis-PEP-see-ah)
		  dys- *painful; difficult; abnormal*
		  peps/o- *digestion*
		  -ia *condition; state; thing*

esophageal varices	Swollen, protruding veins in the mucosa of the lower esophagus or stomach (see Figure 3-9 ■). When liver disease causes blood to back up in the large vein from the intestines to the liver, the blood is forced to take an alternate route through the gastroesophageal veins, but eventually these veins become engorged. Esophageal and gastric varices are easily irritated by passing food. They can hemorrhage suddenly, causing death. Treatment: Correct the underlying liver disease. Surgery: A drug is injected into the varix to harden it and block the blood flow.	**varix** (VAIR-iks) **varices** (VAIR-ih-seez) *Varix* is a Latin singular noun. Form the plural by changing *-ix* to *-ices*.

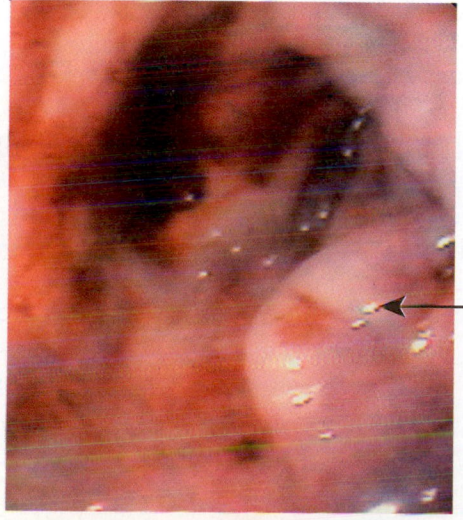

Figure 3-9 ■ Esophageal varix.
A varix is a dilated, swollen vein in the mucosa. This esophageal varix was seen through an endoscope passed through the mouth and into the esophagus. There are dark areas of old blood from previous bleeding.

Word or Phrase	Description	Word Building

gastritis	Acute or chronic inflammation of the stomach due to spicy foods, excess acid production, or a bacterial infection. Treatment: Antacid drugs, antibiotic drugs for a bacterial infection.	**gastritis** (gas-TRY-tis)
		  gastr/o- *stomach*
		  -itis *inflammation of; infection of*

gastroenteritis	Acute inflammation or infection of the stomach and intestines due to a virus (flu) or bacterium (contaminated food). There is abdominal pain, nausea, vomiting, and diarrhea. Treatment: Antiemetic drugs (to prevent vomiting), antidiarrheal drugs, antibiotic drugs for a bacterial infection.	**gastroenteritis**
		(GAS-troh-EN-ter-EYE-tis)
		  gastr/o- *stomach*
		  enter/o- *intestine*
		  -itis *inflammation of; infection of*

gastroesophageal reflux disease (GERD)	Chronic inflammation and irritation due to **reflux** of stomach acid back into the esophagus. This occurs because the lower esophageal sphincter does not close tightly. There is a sore throat, belching, and **esophagitis** with chronic inflammation. This can lead to esophageal ulcers or cancer of the esophagus. Treatment: Eat small, frequent meals, not large meals. Elevate the head of the bed while sleeping. Avoid alcohol and foods that stimulate acid secretion. Treatment: Antacid drugs to neutralize acid, drugs that decrease the production of acid.	**gastroesophageal**
		(GAS-troh-ee-SAWF-ah-JEE-al)
		  gastr/o- *stomach*
		  esophag/o- *esophagus*
		  -eal *pertaining to*
		reflux (REE-fluks)
		esophagitis (ee-SAWF-ah-JY-tis)
		  esophag/o- *esophagus*
		  -itis *inflammation of; infection of*

heartburn	Temporary inflammation of the esophagus due to reflux of stomach acid. It is also known as **pyrosis.** Treatment: Antacid drugs.	**pyrosis** (py-ROH-sis)
		  pyr/o- *fire; burning*
		  -osis *condition; abnormal condition; process*

hematemesis	Vomiting of blood (emesis) because of bleeding in the stomach or esophagus. This can be due to an esophageal or gastric ulcer or esophageal varices. Coffee-grounds emesis contains old, dark blood that has been partially digested by the stomach. Treatment: Correct the underlying cause.	**hematemesis**
		(HEE-mah-TEM-eh-sis)
		  hemat/o- *blood*
		  -emesis *vomiting*

nausea and vomiting (N&V)	Nausea is an unpleasant, queasy feeling in the stomach that precedes the urge to vomit. The patient is said to be nauseated. It is caused by inflammation or infection of the stomach or by motion sickness. Vomiting or **emesis** is the expelling of food from the stomach through the mouth. It is triggered when impulses from the stomach or inner ear stimulate the vomiting center in the brain.
	
	    Vomit or **vomitus** is the expelled food or chyme. Projectile vomiting is vomitus expelled with force and projected a distance from the patient. Retching (dry heaves) is continual vomiting when there is no longer anything in the stomach. **Regurgitation** is the reflux of small amounts of food and acid back into the mouth, but without vomiting. Treatment: Antiemetic drugs.
		nausea (NAW-see-ah) (NAW-zha)
		emesis (EM-eh-sis)
		vomitus (VAWM-ih-tus)
		regurgitation
		(ree-GER-jih-TAY-shun)
		  regurgitat/o- *flow backward*
		  -ion *action; condition*

Clinical Connections

Obstetrics (Chapter 13). Hyperemesis gravidarum is excessive vomiting during the first months of pregnancy. It is thought to be due to changes in hormone levels that occur during pregnancy.

hyperemesis (HY-per-EM-eh-sis)
  hyper- *above; more than normal*
  -emesis *condition of vomiting*

gravidarum (GRAV-ih-DAIR-um)
Gravidarum means of pregnancy.

Word or Phrase	Description	Word Building
peptic ulcer disease (PUD)	Chronic irritation, burning pain, and erosion of the mucosa to form an ulcer. An esophageal ulcer, a gastric ulcer in the stomach, and a duodenal ulcer are all peptic ulcers. Gastric ulcers are most commonly caused by the bacterium *Helicobacter pylori* (see Figure 3-10 ■). Ulcers can also be caused by excessive hydrochloric acid, stress, and by drugs (such as aspirin) that irritate the mucosa. Treatment: Antibiotic drugs to treat *H. pylori* infection. Drugs to decrease acid production. Antacid drugs. Avoid spicy foods, smoking, alcohol, caffeine, and aspirin-containing drugs.	**peptic** (PEP-tik) **pept/o-** *digestion* **-ic** *pertaining to* **ulcer** (UL-ser)

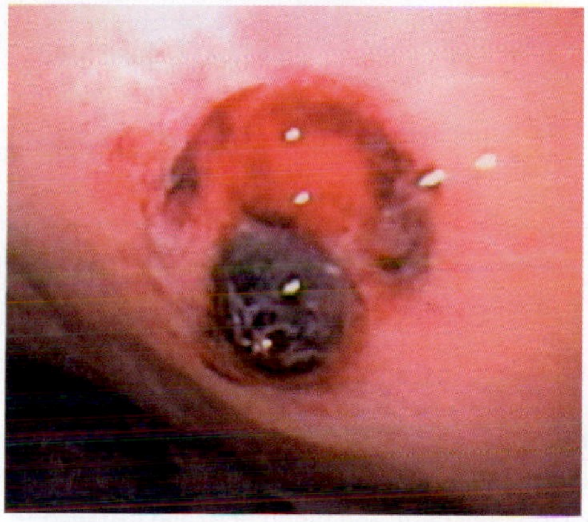

Figure 3-10 ■ Gastric ulcer.
This gastric mucosa is raw and irritated with a large central ulcer crater. The dark blood clot indicates a recent episode of bleeding from the ulcer.

Word or Phrase	Description	Word Building
stomach cancer	**Cancerous** tumor of the stomach that usually begins in glands in the gastric mucosa. It is also known as gastric **adenocarcinoma.** It can develop due to chronic irritation from a *Helicobacter pylori* infection. Treatment: Surgery to remove the cancerous tumor and part of the stomach (gastrectomy).	**cancerous** (KAN-ser-us) **cancer/o-** *cancer* **-ous** *pertaining to* **adenocarcinoma** (AD-eh-noh-KAR-sih-NOH-mah) **aden/o-** *gland* **carcin/o-** *cancer* **-oma** *tumor; mass*

Duodenum, Jejunum, Ileum

Word or Phrase	Description	Word Building
ileus	Abnormal absence of peristalsis in the small and large intestines. Obstipation, a tumor, adhesions, or a hernia can cause a mechanical obstruction. A severe infection in the intestine or abdominopelvic cavity, trauma, shock, or drugs can cause a paralytic ileus. **Postoperative ileus** occurs after the intestines are manipulated during abdominal surgery and peristalsis is slow to return. Treatment: Intravenous fluids for temporary nutritional support. Surgery (bowel resection and anastomosis) may be needed.	**ileus** (IL-ee-us) **postoperative** (post-AWP-er-ah-tiv) **post-** *after; behind* **operat/o-** *perform a procedure; surgery* **-ive** *pertaining to*

Word or Phrase	Description	Word Building
intussusception	Telescoping of one segment of intestine inside the lumen of the next segment (see Figure 3-11a ■). There is vomiting and abdominal pain. The cause is unknown. Treatment: Surgery (bowel resection and anastomosis).	**intussusception** (IN-tus-suh-SEP-shun) **intussuscep/o-** *to receive within* **-tion** *a process; being or having*

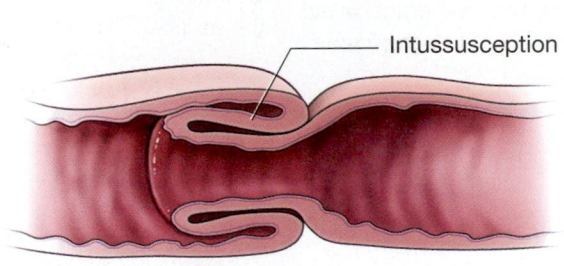
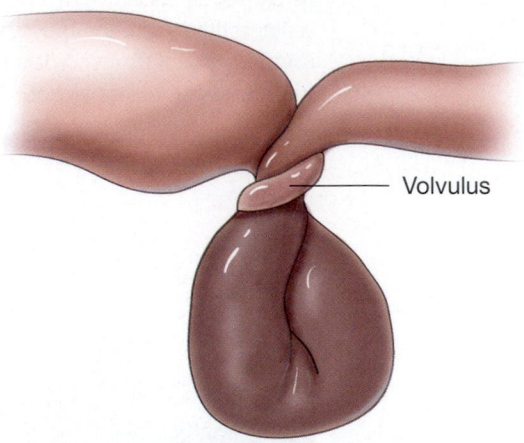

(a)   **(b)**

Figure 3-11 ■ Intussusception and volvulus of the intestine.

(a) In an intussusception, the intestine folds back on itself in the same way that one part of a telescope slides into the other. (b) In a volvulus, the intestine becomes twisted. Both of these conditions stop peristalsis and blood flow and can lead to tissue death.

volvulus	Twisting of the intestine around itself because of a structural abnormality of the mesentery (see Figure 3-11b). There is vomiting and abdominal pain. If the blood vessels are also twisted, blood flow is stopped and the tissues die. It is also known as **malrotation** of the intestines. Treatment: Surgery (bowel resection and anastomosis).	**volvulus** (VAWL-vyoo-lus) **malrotation** (MAL-roh-TAY-shun) **mal-** *bad; inadequate* **rotat/o-** *rotate* **-ion** *action; condition*

Cecum and Colon

appendicitis	Inflammation and infection of the appendix. Undigested material becomes trapped in the lumen of the appendix. There is steadily increasing abdominal pain that finally localizes to the right lower quadrant. If the physician presses on that area and then quickly removes the hand and releases the pressure, the patient complains of severe rebound pain. An inflamed appendix can rupture (burst), spilling infection into the abdominopelvic cavity and causing peritonitis. Treatment: Surgery to remove the appendix (appendectomy).	**appendicitis** (ah-PEN-dih-SY-tis) **appendic/o-** *appendix* **-itis** *inflammation of; infection of*
colic	Common disorder in babies. There is crampy abdominal pain soon after eating. It can be caused by overfeeding, feeding too quickly, inadequate burping, or food allergies to milk. Treatment: Correct the underlying cause.	**colic** (KAWL-ik) **col/o-** *colon* **-ic** *pertaining to*
colon cancer	Cancerous tumor of the colon. It occurs when colonic polyps or ulcerative colitis become cancerous. It is also linked to a high-fat diet. There can be blood in the feces. It is also known as **colorectal adenocarcinoma.** Treatment: Preventive surgery to remove polyps before they become cancerous. Surgery to remove the cancer and the affected intestine (bowel resection) and reroute the colon to a new opening in the abdominal wall (colostomy).	**colorectal** (KOH-loh-REK-tal) **col/o-** *colon* **rect/o-** *rectum* **-al** *pertaining to* **adenocarcinoma** (AD-eh-noh-KAR-sih-NOH-mah) **aden/o-** *gland* **carcin/o-** *cancer* **-oma** *tumor; mass*

Word or Phrase	Description	Word Building
diverticulum	Weakness in the wall of the colon where the mucosa forms a pouch or tube. Diverticula can be caused by eating a low-fiber diet that forms small, compact feces. Then, increased intra-abdominal pressure and straining to pass those feces eventually creates diverticula. **Diverticulosis** or diverticular disease is the condition of multiple diverticula (see Figure 3-12 ■). If feces become trapped inside a diverticulum, this causes inflammation, infection, abdominal pain, and fever, a condition known as **diverticulitis** (see Figure 3-13 ■). Prevention: High-fiber diet. Treatment: Antibiotic drugs to treat diverticulitis. Surgery (bowel resection and anastomosis) to remove the affected segment of intestine.	**diverticulum** (DY-ver-TIK-yoo-lum) **diverticula** (DY-ver-TIK-yoo-lah) *Diverticulum* is a Latin singular noun. Form the plural by changing *-um* to *-a*. **diverticulosis** (DY-ver-TIK-yoo-LOH-sis) **diverticul/o-** *diverticulum* **-osis** *condition; abnormal condition; process* **diverticulitis** (DY-ver-TIK-yoo-LY-tis) **diverticul/o-** *diverticulum* **-itis** *inflammation of; infection of*

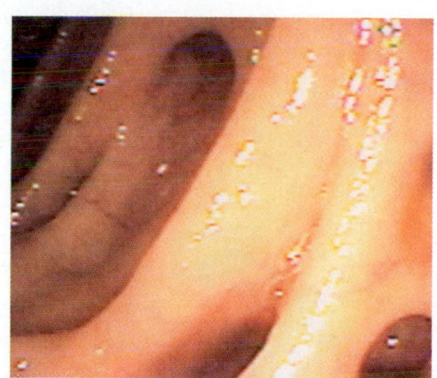

Figure 3-12 ■ Diverticula.
These openings in the wall of the colon lead to diverticular sacs where feces can become trapped.

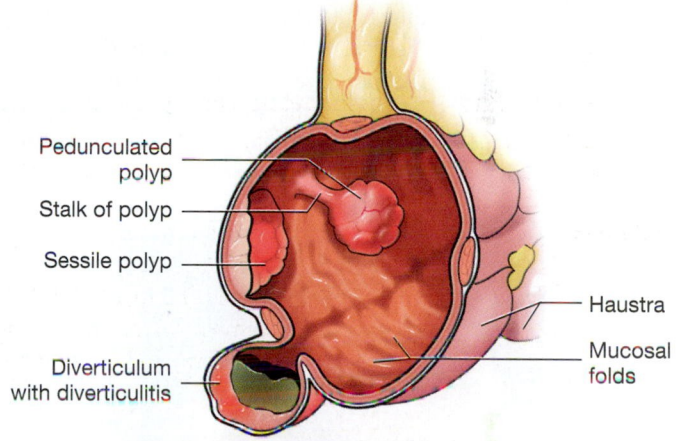

Pedunculated polyp
Stalk of polyp
Sessile polyp
Diverticulum with diverticulitis
Haustra
Mucosal folds

Figure 3-13 ■ Diverticulitis and polyposis.
This diverticulum has become infected from trapped feces. These polyps are irritated by the passage of feces and can become cancerous.

Clinical Connections

Dietetics. Diverticular disease was unknown until the early 1900s, when refined flour began to replace whole wheat flour. Diverticular disease is common in countries where people eat a low-fiber diet, but is uncommon in third-world countries where there is a high-fiber diet. Fiber creates bulk and holds water to keep the feces soft.

Word or Phrase	Description	Word Building
dysentery	Bacterial infection caused by an unusual strain of *E. coli*, a common bacterium in the large intestine. There is watery diarrhea mixed with blood and mucus. Treatment: Antibiotic drugs.	**dysentery** (DIS-en-TAIR-ee) **dys-** *painful; difficult; abnormal* **-entery** *condition of the intestine* The ending *-entery* contains the combining form *enter/o-* and the one-letter suffix *-y*.

Word or Phrase	Description	Word Building

gluten enteropathy	A food allergy and toxic reaction to the gluten found in certain grains (wheat, barley, rye, oats). The small intestine is damaged by the allergic response. It is also known as **celiac disease.** Treatment: Avoid eating foods and food products that contain gluten.	**gluten** (GLOO-ten)
		
		enteropathy (EN-ter-AWP-ah-thee)
		   enter/o- *intestine*
		   -pathy *disease; suffering*
		
		celiac (SEE-lee-ak)
		   celi/o- *abdomen*
		   -ac *pertaining to*

inflammatory bowel disease (IBD)	Chronic inflammation of various parts of the small and large intestines. There is diarrhea, bloody feces, abdominal cramps, and fever. The cause is not known. There are two types of inflammatory bowel disease: (1) **Crohn's disease** or **regional enteritis** affects the ileum and colon (see Figure 3-14 ■). There are areas of normal mucosa ("skip areas") and then inflammation. There are ulcers and thickening of the intestinal wall that can cause a partial obstruction in the intestine. (2) **Ulcerative colitis** affects the colon and rectum and causes inflammation and ulcers. Treatment: Corticosteroid drugs to decrease inflammation. Surgery (bowel resection) to remove the affected area and reroute the intestine to a new opening in the abdominal wall (ileostomy, colostomy).	**Crohn** (KROHN)
		
		enteritis (EN-ter-EYE-tis)
		   enter/o- *intestine*
		   -itis *inflammation of; infection of*
		
		ulcerative (UL-sir-ah-tiv)
		   ulcerat/o- *ulcer*
		   -ive *pertaining to*
		
		colitis (koh-LY-tis)
		   col/o- *colon*
		   -itis *inflammation of; infection of*

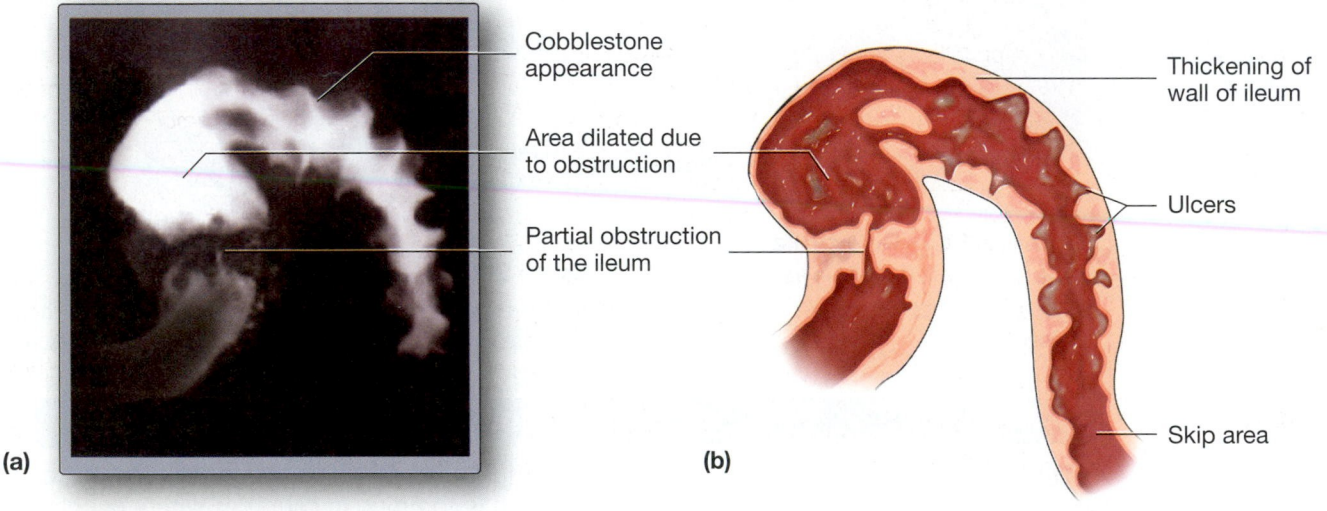

Cobblestone appearance

Area dilated due to obstruction

Partial obstruction of the ileum

Thickening of wall of ileum

Ulcers

Skip area

(a)

(b)

Figure 3-14 ■ Crohn's disease.
(a) This x-ray shows the characteristic cobblestone appearance of Crohn's disease. (b) It is due to thickening of the intestinal wall and ulcers. There is also a partial obstruction.

irritable bowel syndrome (IBS)	Disorder of the function of the colon, although the mucosa of the colon never shows any visible signs of inflammation. A syndrome consists of interrelated symptoms and signs. There is cramping, abdominal pain, diarrhea, bloating alternating with constipation, and excessive mucus. The cause is not known but may be related to lactose intolerance and emotional stress. It is also known as **spastic colon** or **mucous colitis.** Treatment: Antidiarrheal, antispasmodic, and antianxiety drugs. High-fiber diet and laxative drugs to prevent constipation.	**spastic** (SPAS-tik)
		   spast/o- *spasm*
		   -ic *pertaining to*
		
		colitis (koh-LY-tis)
		   col/o- *colon*
		   -itis *inflammation of; infection of*

Word or Phrase	Description	Word Building

polyp	Small, fleshy, benign or precancerous growth in the mucosa of the colon. A **pedunculated polyp** has a thin stalk that supports an irregular, ball-shaped top (see Figure 3-13). A **sessile polyp** is a mound with a broad base (see Figure 3-15 ■). **Benign familial polyposis** is an inherited condition in which family members have multiple colon polyps. Although all polyps initially are benign, they can become cancerous. Treatment: Surgery to remove the polyps (polypectomy).
	
	Figure 3-15 ■ Colonic polyps.
	This patient has multiple sessile polyps protruding through the many haustra (folds) in the wall of the colon.
		polyp (PAW-lip)
		
		pedunculated
		(peh-DUNG-kyoo-lay-ted)
		
		sessile (SES-il)
		
		benign (bee-NINE)
		
		polyposis (PAWL-ee-POH-sis)
		  polyp/o- *polyp*
		  -osis *condition; abnormal condition; process*

Rectum and Anus

Word or Phrase	Description	Word Building

hemorrhoids	Swollen, protruding veins in the rectum (internal hemorrhoids) or on the skin around the anus (external hemorrhoids). They are caused by increased intra-abdominal pressure from straining during a bowel movement. This dilates the veins with blood until they permanently protrude. They are also known as **piles.** A hemorrhoid is irritated as feces go by it, and its surface bleeds easily. Treatment: Topical corticosteroid drugs to decrease itching and irritation. Surgery to remove the hemorrhoids (hemorrhoidectomy).	**hemorrhoid** (HEM-oh-royd)
		  hemorrh/o- *a flowing of blood*
		  -oid *resembling*

proctitis	Inflammation of the rectum due to radiation therapy or ulcers or infection of the rectum	**proctitis** (prawk-TY-tis)
		  proct/o- *rectum*
		  -itis *inflammation of; infection of*

rectocele	Protruding wall of the rectum pushes on the adjacent vaginal wall, causing it to collapse inward and block the vaginal canal. Treatment: Surgery to repair the defect.	**rectocele** (REK-toh-seel)
		  rect/o- *rectum*
		  -cele *hernia*

Defecation and Feces

Word or Phrase	Description	Word Building

constipation	Failure to have regular, soft bowel movements. This can be due to decreased peristalsis, lack of dietary fiber, inadequate water intake, or the side effect of a drug. **Obstipation** is severe, unrelieved constipation that can lead to a mechanical obstruction of the bowel. The patient is said to be obstipated. A **fecalith** is hardened feces that becomes a stonelike mass. This can form in the appendix or in a diverticulum. It can be seen when an abdominal x-ray is done. Treatment: Laxative drugs, a high-fiber diet, increased water intake, enemas.	**constipation** (CON-stih-PAY-shun)
		  constip/o- *compacted feces*
		  -ation *a process; being or having*
		
		obstipation (AWB-stih-PAY-shun)
		  obstip/o- *severe constipation*
		  -ation *a process; being or having*
		
		fecalith (FEE-kah-lith)
		  fec/a- *feces; stool*
		  -lith *stone*

Word or Phrase	Description	Word Building
diarrhea	Abnormally frequent, loose, and sometimes watery feces. It is caused by an infection (bacteria, viruses), irritable bowel syndrome, ulcerative colitis, lactose intolerance, or the side effect of a drug. There is increased peristalsis, and the feces move through the large intestine before the water can be absorbed. Treatment: Antidiarrheal drugs, lactase supplements. Antibiotic drugs to treat bacterial infections.	**diarrhea** (DY-ah-REE-ah) **dia-** *complete; completely through* **-rrhea** *flow; discharge* The ending *-rrhea* contains the combining form *rrhe/o-* and the one-letter suffix *-a*.
flatulence	Presence of excessive amounts of flatus (gas) in the stomach or intestines. It can be caused by milk (lactose intolerance), indigestion, or incomplete digestion of carbohydrates such as beans. Treatment: Lactase supplements, antigas drugs.	**flatulence** (FLAT-yoo-lens) **flatul/o-** *flatus (gas)* **-ence** *state of*
hematochezia	Blood in the feces. The source of bleeding can be an ulcer, cancer, Crohn's disease, polyp, diverticulum, or hemorrhoid. Bright red blood indicates active bleeding in the lower gastrointestinal system. **Melena** is a dark, tar-like feces that contains digested blood from bleeding in the esophagus or stomach. Treatment: Correct the underlying cause of bleeding.	**hematochezia** (hee-MAH-toh-KEE-zee-ah) **hemat/o-** *blood* **chez/o-** *to pass feces* **-ia** *condition; state; thing* **melena** (meh-LEE-nah)
incontinence	Inability to voluntarily control bowel movements. A patient with paralysis of the lower extremities lacks sensation and motor control of the external anal sphincter and is incontinent. Patients with dementia are unaware of a bowel movement. Treatment: None.	**incontinence** (in-CON-tih-nens) **in-** *in; within, not* **contin/o-** *hold together* **-ence** *state of* Select the correct prefix meaning to get the definition of *incontinence: a state of not holding together (feces).*
steatorrhea	Greasy, frothy, foul-smelling feces that contain undigested fats. There is not enough of the enzyme lipase because of pancreatic disease or cystic fibrosis. Treatment: Correct the underlying cause.	**steatorrhea** (stee-AT-oh-REE-ah) **steat/o-** *fat* **-rrhea** *flow; discharge*

Across the Life Span

Pediatrics. Feces forms in the intestine while the fetus is in the uterus. Swallowed amniotic fluid and sloughed-off fetal skin cells mix with mucus and bile to form **meconium,** a thick, sticky, green-to-black waste that is passed after birth. In the newborn nursery, the nurse checks to see that the anus and rectum are **patent** (open). Occasionally, a newborn will have an **imperforate anus.** This is a congenital (present at birth) abnormality in which there is no anal opening. Treatment: Immediate surgery to open the anus and connect the rectum to the outside of the body.

Geriatrics. Constipation is a common complaint in older adults. A diet of refined foods with low fiber, lack of water intake, and inactivity contribute to the formation of small, hard feces. Narcotic drugs used to treat chronic pain cause constipation and can actually cause a bowel obstruction in older adults. Some older patients are incontinent of feces (unable to voluntarily control their bowel movements). This can be due to a decrease in the size of the rectum because of a rectocele, impairment of anal sphincter function because of nerve damage, or mental impairment and dementia in which the patient is unaware that a bowel movement is occurring.

meconium (meh-KOH-nee-um)

patent (PAY-tent)

imperforate anus
(im-PER-for-ate)
im- *not*
perfor/o- *to have an opening*
-ate *composed of; pertaining to*

Abdominal Wall and Abdominal Cavity

Word or Phrase	Description	Word Building
adhesions	Fibrous bands that form after abdominal surgery. They bind the intestines to each other or to other organs. They can bind so tightly that peristalsis and intestinal function are affected. Treatment: Surgery to cut the fibrous adhesions (lysis of adhesions).	**adhesion** (ad-HEE-zhun) **adhes/o-** *to stick to* **-ion** *action; condition*
hernia	Weakness in the muscle of the diaphragm or abdominal wall. The intestine bulges through the defect. There is swelling and pain. There is an inherited tendency to hernias, but hernias can also be caused by pregnancy, obesity, or heavy lifting. Treatment: Surgery to correct the hernia (herniorrhaphy). 1. Hernias are named according to how easily the intestines can move back into their normal position. A sliding or reducible hernia moves back and forth between the hernia sac and the abdominopelvic cavity (see Figure 3-16a ■). In an **incarcerated (irreducible) hernia**, the intestine swells in the hernia sac and becomes trapped. The intestine can no longer be pushed back into the abdomen. A **strangulated hernia** is an incarcerated hernia whose blood supply has been cut off (see Figure 3-16b). This leads to tissue death (necrosis). 2. Hernias are named according to their location. With a **hiatal hernia**, the stomach bulges through the normal opening in the diaphragm for the esophagus. A **ventral hernia** is anywhere on the anterior abdominal wall (except at the umbilicus). An **umbilical hernia** is at the umbilicus (navel). An **omphalocele** is an umbilical hernia that is present at birth and is only covered with peritoneum, without any fat or abdominal skin (see Figure 3-16c). An **inguinal hernia** is in the groin. In a male patient with an inguinal hernia, the intestine slides through the inguinal canal and into the scrotum. An **incisional hernia** is along the suture line of a prior abdominal surgical incision.	**hernia** (HER-nee-ah) **incarcerated** (in-KAR-seh-ray-ted) **incarcer/o-** *to imprison* **-ated** *pertaining to a condition; composed of* **hiatal** (hy-AA-tal) **hiat/o-** *gap; opening* **-al** *pertaining to* **ventral** (VEN-tral) **ventr/o-** *front; abdomen* **-al** *pertaining to* **umbilical** (um-BIL-ih-kal) **umbilic/o-** *umbilicus; navel* **-al** *pertaining to* **omphalocele** (OM-fal-oh-seel) **omphal/o-** *umbilicus; navel* **-cele** *hernia* **inguinal** (ING-gwih-nal) **inguin/o-** *groin* **-al** *pertaining to* **incisional** (in-SIH-shun-al) **incis/o-** *to cut into* **-ion** *action; condition* **-al** *pertaining to*

SLIDING HERNIA
Loop of intestine in
hernia sac

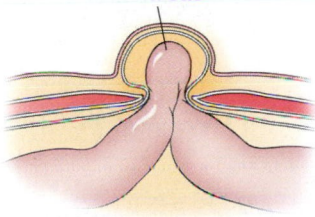

(a)

STRANGULATED HERNIA
Entrapped, necrotic
loop of intestine

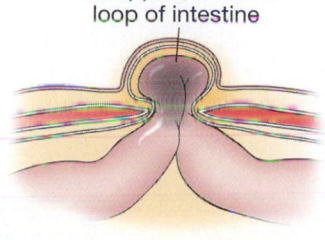

(b)

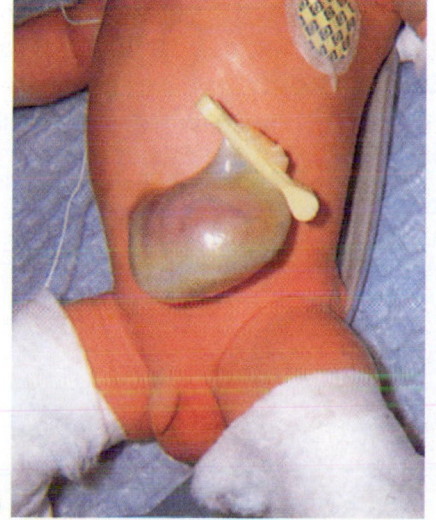

(c)

Figure 3-16 ■ Hernia.

(a) In a sliding hernia, the intestine moves in and out of the hernia sac. (b) In a strangulated hernia, the intestine is trapped in the hernia sac and becomes necrotic. (c) This baby was born with an omphalocele, a hernia at the umbilicus. The hernia sac is only a layer of peritoneum, and the intestine inside is visible. This baby will have immediate surgery to repair the hernia.

Word or Phrase	Description	Word Building
peritonitis	Inflammation and infection of the peritoneum (see Figure 3-17 ■). It occurs when an ulcer, diverticulum, or cancerous tumor eats through the wall of the stomach or intestines or when an inflamed appendix ruptures. Drainage and bacteria spill into the abdominopelvic cavity. Treatment: Surgery (exploratory laparotomy) to clean out the abdominal cavity. Correct the underlying cause. Antibiotic drugs for bacterial infection. **Figure 3-17 ■ Peritonitis.** This patient developed peritonitis when a duodendal ulcer perforated the intestinal wall and spilled green bile and chyme into the abdominal cavity. The areas of white are large numbers of white blood cells (pus) that are fighting this infection.	peritonitis (PAIR-ih-toh-NY-tis) **periton/o-** *peritoneum* **-itis** *inflammation of; infection of*

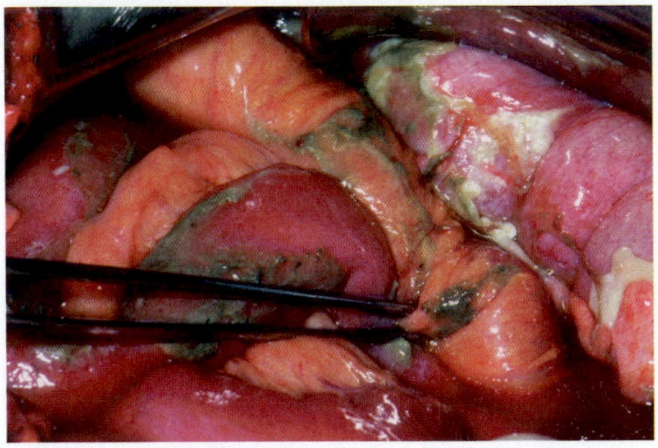

Liver

ascites	Accumulation of **ascitic** fluid in the abdominopelvic cavity. Liver disease and congestive heart failure cause a backup of blood. This increases the blood pressure in the veins of the abdomen. This pressure pushes fluid out of the blood and into the abdominopelvic cavity. Treatment: Removal of ascitic fluid from the abdomen using a needle (abdominocentesis). Surgery: Permanent drainage of excess fluid via an implanted tube (shunt).	ascites (ah-SY-teez) ascitic (ah-SIT-ik) **ascit/o-** *ascites* **-ic** *pertaining to*

Word Alert

SOUND-ALIKE WORDS

acidic   (adjective)   Pertaining to an acid, having a low pH
Example: Hydrochloric acid creates an acidic (low pH) environment in the stomach.

ascitic   (adjective)   Pertaining to ascites
Example: Ascitic fluid accumulates and causes the abdominal wall to bulge outward.

Word or Phrase	Description	Word Building
cirrhosis	Chronic, progressive inflammation and finally irreversible degeneration of the liver, with nodules and scarring (see Figure 3-18 ■). The cirrhotic liver is enlarged, and its function is severely impaired. There is nausea and vomiting, weakness, and jaundice. Cirrhosis is caused by alcoholism, viral hepatitis, or chronic obstruction of the bile ducts. Severe cirrhosis can progress to liver failure. Treatment: Correct the underlying cause. 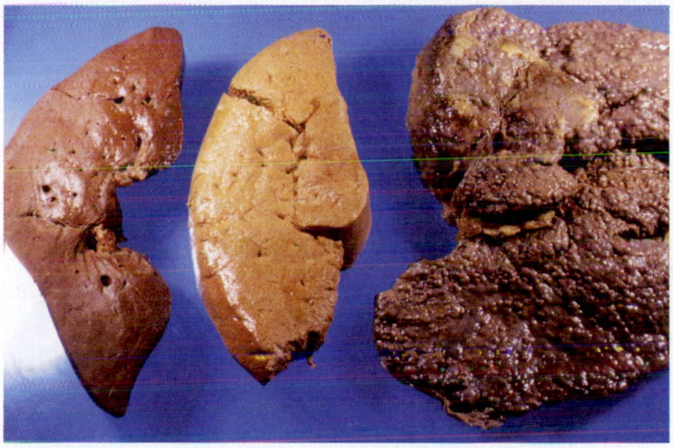 **Figure 3-18 ■ Fatty liver disease and cirrhosis of the liver.** The liver on the left is normal. The liver in the center shows fatty liver disease, which is common in alcoholics because the sugar in alcohol is converted to triglycerides (fats) and stored in the liver. Diabetes mellitus and lipid (fat) disorders also cause this yellow, fatty appearance. The liver on the right shows cirrhosis. It is deformed with nodules and scar tissue that affect liver function.	**cirrhosis** (sih-ROH-sis) **cirrh/o-** *yellow* **-osis** *condition; abnormal condition; process*
hepatitis	Inflammation and infection of the liver from the hepatitis virus. There is weakness, anorexia, nausea, fever, dark urine, and jaundice. It is also known as **viral hepatitis**. <div align="right">*(continued)*</div>	**hepatitis** (HEP-ah-TY-tis) **hepat/o-** *liver* **-itis** *inflammation of; infection of* **viral** (VY-ral) **vir/o-** *virus* **-al** *pertaining to*

Word or Phrase	Description	Word Building

hepatitis
(continued)

A Closer Look

Hepatitis is the most common chronic liver disease. There are five types of hepatitis.

- **Hepatitis A** is an acute but short-lived infection and most persons recover completely. There is no chronic form. It is caused by exposure to water or food that is contaminated with feces from a person who is infected with the hepatitis A virus (HAV). It is also known as **infectious hepatitis.** Treatment: Vaccination to prevent hepatitis A.

- **Hepatitis B** is an acute infection, but many persons recover completely. When it is chronic, there may be no symptoms for 20 years. During that time, however, the infected person is a carrier and can infect others. Hepatitis B is caused by exposure to the blood of a person who is already infected with the hepatitis B virus (HBV) (see Figure 3-19 ■). It is also spread during sexual activity by contact with saliva and vaginal secretions. An infected mother can pass hepatitis B to her fetus before birth or when breastfeeding. It is also known as **serum hepatitis.** Treatment: Vaccination. Healthcare workers are vaccinated because of their constant exposure to blood and body fluids.

- **Hepatitis C** begins as an acute infection that continues as a chronic infection. It is caused by exposure to contaminated needles or to the blood of a person who is already infected with the hepatitis C virus (HCV). Hepatitis C is not readily transmitted by sexual activity or from a mother to her fetus. Chronic hepatitis C is the main cause of chronic liver disease, cirrhosis, and liver cancer. Treatment: Antiviral drugs.

- **Hepatitis D** is a secondary infection caused by a mutated (changed) hepatitis virus. It only develops in patients who already have hepatitis B. It is also known as **delta hepatitis.**

- **Hepatitis E** is similar to hepatitis A, but rarely occurs in the United States.

infectious (in-FEK-shus)
   infect/o- *disease within*
   -ous *pertaining to*

serum (SEER-um)
Serum is the fluid portion of the blood (without the cells and clotting factors).

delta (DEL-tah)

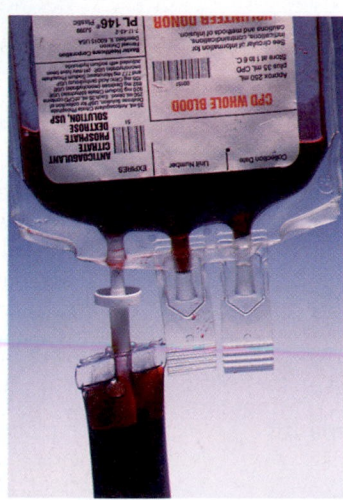

Figure 3-19 ■ Blood transfusion.
Receiving infected blood during a blood transfusion, coming in contact with blood-contaminated instruments, or the sharing of needles by drug addicts can result in hepatitis B or hepatitis C.

| **hepatomegaly** | Enlargement of the liver due to cirrhosis, hepatitis, or cancer (see Figures 3-18 and 3-21). The enlarged liver can be felt on palpation of the abdomen. The degree of enlargement is measured as the number of fingerbreadths from the edge of the right rib cage to the inferior edge of the liver. **Hepatosplenomegaly** is enlargement of both the liver and the spleen. Treatment: Correct the underlying cause. | **hepatomegaly** (HEP-ah-toh-MEG-ah-lee)
   hepat/o- *liver*
   -megaly *enlargement*

hepatosplenomegaly (HEP-ah-toh-SPLEN-oh-MEG-ah-lee)
   hepat/o- *liver*
   splen/o- *spleen*
   -megaly *enlargement* |

Word or Phrase	Description	Word Building

jaundice	Yellowish discoloration of the skin and whites of the eyes (the sclerae) (see Figure 3-20 ■). There is an increased level of unconjugated bilirubin in the blood. This bilirubin enters the tissues, giving them a yellow color. Jaundice occurs:
	
	1. If the liver is too diseased to conjugate bilirubin.
	2. If the liver is too immature to conjugate bilirubin. This occurs in premature newborns.
	3. If there is too much unconjugated bilirubin in the blood because of the destruction of large numbers of red blood cells.
	4. If a gallstone is obstructing the flow of bile in the bile ducts (**obstructive jaundice**).
	
	Treatment: Correct the underlying disease.
		jaundice (JAWN-dis)
		  jaund/o- *yellow*
		  -ice *state; quality*
		
		obstructive (awb-STRUK-tiv)
		  obstruct/o- *blocked by a barrier*
		  -ive *pertaining to*

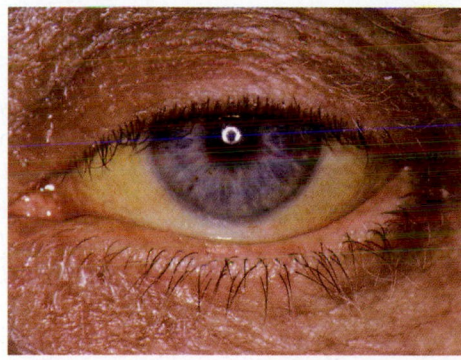

Figure 3-20 ■ Jaundice.

Jaundice can be seen as a yellow discoloration of the whites of the eyes (sclerae). The skin is also yellow, but skin pigmentation masks this to some extent.

A Closer Look

Bilirubin is produced when old red blood cells are broken down by the spleen. This is unconjugated (unjoined) bilirubin. The liver joins this bilirubin to another substance to make conjugated (joined) bilirubin, which is used to make bile. When the liver is damaged, the amount of unconjugated bilirubin in the blood increases. When gallstones obstruct the flow of bile, conjugated bilirubin leaves the bile and moves into the blood.

Word or Phrase	Description	Word Building

liver cancer	Cancerous tumor of the liver (see Figure 3-21 ■). This is usually a secondary cancer that began in another place and spread (metastasized) to the liver. It is also known as a **hepatoma** or **hepatocellular carcinoma.** Treatment: Surgery to remove the tumor; chemotherapy.	**hepatoma** (HEP-ah-TOH-mah)
		  hepat/o- *liver*
		  -oma *tumor; mass*
		
		hepatocellular
		(HEP-ah-toh-SEL-yoo-lar)
		  hepat/o- *liver*
		  cellul/o- *cell*
		  -ar *pertaining to*
		
		carcinoma (KAR-sih-NOH-mah)
		  carcin/o- *cancer*
		  -oma *tumor; mass*

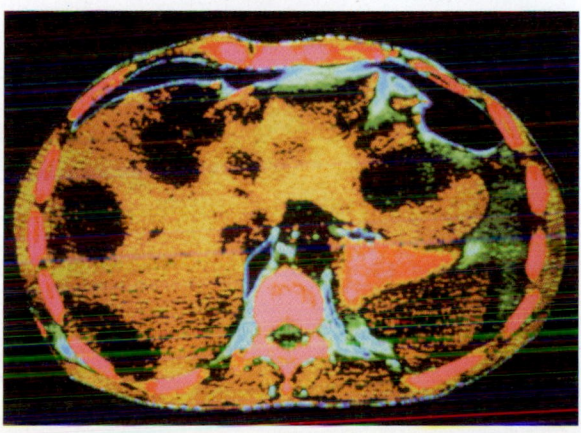

Figure 3-21 ■ Liver cancer.

This colorized computed tomography (CT) scan of the abdomen shows an enlarged (yellow) liver with several large, dark areas where cancer has spread.

Gallbladder and Bile Ducts

Word or Phrase	Description	Word Building
cholangitis	Acute or chronic inflammation of the bile ducts because of cirrhosis or gallstones. Treatment: Correct the underlying disease.	**cholangitis** (KOH-lan-JY-tis) **cholangi/o-** *bile duct* **-itis** *inflammation of; infection of* Delete the duplicate *i* when building the word.
cholecystitis	Acute or chronic inflammation of the gallbladder. Acute cholecystitis occurs when a gallstone blocks the cystic duct of the gallbladder. When the gallbladder contracts, the duct spasms, causing severe pain (**biliary colic**). Chronic cholecystitis occurs when a gallstone partially blocks the cystic duct, causing backup of bile and thickening of the gallbladder wall. Treatment: Avoid fatty foods that cause the gallbladder to contract. Drugs to dissolve the gallstone. Surgery to remove the gallbladder (cholecystectomy).	**cholecystitis** (KOH-lee-sis-TY-tis) **cholecyst/o-** *gallbladder* **-itis** *inflammation of; infection of*
cholelithiasis	One or more gallstones in the gallbladder (see Figure 3-22 ■). When the bile is too concentrated, it forms a thick sediment (sludge) that gradually becomes gallstones. Cholelithiasis causes mild symptoms or can cause severe biliary colic when the gallbladder contracts or when a gallstone becomes lodged in a bile duct. **Choledocholithiasis** is a gallstone that is stuck in the common bile duct (see Figure 3-23 ■). Treatment: Avoid fatty foods that cause the gallbladder to contract. Drugs to dissolve the gallstone. Surgery to remove the gallbladder (cholecystectomy) or to remove a gallstone from the common bile duct (choledocholithotomy).	**cholelithiasis** (KOH-lee-lih-THY-ah-sis) **chol/e-** *bile; gall* **lith/o-** *stone* **-iasis** *state of; process of* **choledocholithiasis** (koh-LED-oh-koh-lith-EYE-ah-sis) **choledoch/o-** *common bile duct* **lith/o-** *stone* **-iasis** *state of; process of*

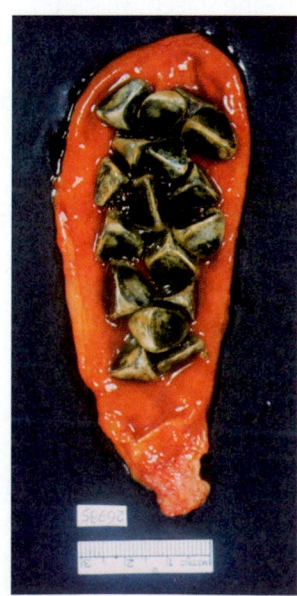

Figure 3-22 ■ **Cholelithiasis.**

This patient's gallbladder was removed during surgery. When it was opened by the pathologist, it contained numerous small and large gallstones.

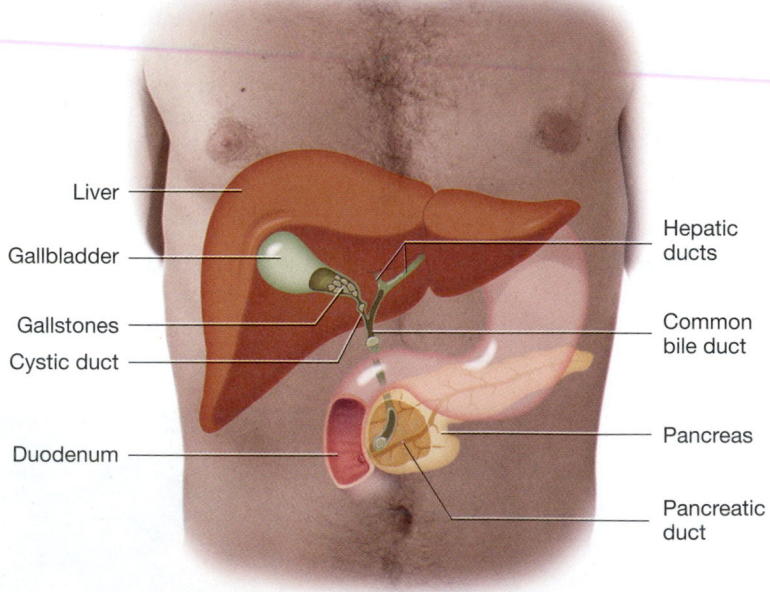

Figure 3-23 ■ **Gallstones in the biliary and pancreatic ducts.**

A gallstone in the cystic duct causes bile to back up into the gallbladder. A gallstone in the proximal common bile duct causes bile to back up into the gallbladder and liver. A gallstone in the distal common bile duct keeps pancreatic digestive enzymes from entering the duodenum.

Pancreas

Word or Phrase	Description	Word Building
pancreatic cancer	Cancerous tumor (**adenocarcinoma**) of the pancreas. Most patients are in the advanced stage when they are diagnosed and so survival is usually less than one year. Treatment: Chemotherapy; surgery to remove the tumor.	**adenocarcinoma** (AD-eh-noh-KAR-sih-NOH-mah) **aden/o-** *gland* **carcin/o-** *cancer* **-oma** *tumor; mass*
pancreatitis	Inflammation or infection of the pancreas. There is abdominal pain, nausea, and vomiting. Inflammation occurs when a gallstone blocks the lower common bile duct and pancreatic enzymes back up into the pancreas. Inflammation of the pancreas can also be due to chronic alcoholism. Infection in the pancreas is caused by bacteria or viruses. Treatment: Stop drinking alcohol. Antibiotic drugs to treat a bacterial infection. Surgery to remove a gallstone (choledocholithotomy).	**pancreatitis** (PAN-kree-ah-TY-tis) **pancreat/o-** *pancreas* **-itis** *inflammation of; infection of*

Laboratory and Diagnostic Procedures

Blood Tests

Word or Phrase	Description	Word Building
albumin	Test for albumin, the major protein molecule in the blood. Because albumin is produced by the liver, liver disease results in a low albumin level. The albumin level is also low in patients with malnutrition from poor protein intake.	albumin (al-BYOO-min)
alkaline phosphatase (ALP)	Test for the enzyme alkaline phosphatase that is found in both liver cells and bone cells. An elevated blood level is due to liver disease or bone disease.	alkaline phosphatase (AL-kah-lin FAWS-fah-tays)
ALT and AST	Test for the enzymes alanine transaminase (ALT) and aspartate transaminase (AST), which are mainly found in the liver. Elevated blood levels occur when damaged liver cells release these enzymes. Formerly known as **SGPT** and **SGOT.**	
bilirubin	Test for unconjugated, conjugated, and total bilirubin levels. These levels are abnormal when there is liver disease or gallstones. Conjugated bilirubin is also known as **direct bilirubin** because it reacts directly with the reagent used to perform the lab test. Unconjugated bilirubin or **indirect bilirubin** only reacts when another substance is added to the reagent.	bilirubin (BIL-ih-ROO-bin) **bili/o-** *bile; gall* **rub/o-** *red* **-in** *a substance*
GGT	Test for the enzyme gamma-glutamyl transpeptidase (GGT or GGTP), which is mainly found in the liver. An elevated blood level occurs when damaged liver cells release this enzyme into the blood.	
liver function tests (LFTs)	Panel of individual blood tests performed at the same time to give a comprehensive picture of liver function. It includes albumin, bilirubin, ALT, AST, and GGT, as well as prothrombin time (to evaluate blood clotting factors produced by the liver).	

Gastric and Feces Specimen Tests

Word or Phrase	Description	Word Building
CLO test	Rapid screening test to detect the presence of the bacterium *Helicobacter pylori*. A biopsy of the patient's gastric mucosa is placed in urea. If *H. pylori* bacteria are present, they metabolize the urea to ammonia, and ammonia changes the color of the test pad.	CLO (kloh) *CLO* stands for *Campylobacter-like organism* (because *H. pylori* used to be categorized with the genus Campylobacter).
culture and sensitivity (C&S)	Diagnostic test of a culture that determines which bacterium is causing an intestinal infection and a sensitivity test to determine which antibiotic drugs it is sensitive to. The patient's feces are swabbed onto a culture dish that contains a nutrient medium for growing bacteria. After the bacterium grows, it can be identified by the appearance of the colonies. Then disks of antibiotic drugs are placed in the culture dish. If the bacteria are resistant to that antibiotic drug, there will only be a small zone of inhibition (no growth) around it. If the bacteria are sensitive to that antibiotic drug, there will be a medium or large zone of inhibition around that disk.	sensitivity (SEN-sih-TIV-ih-tee) **sensitiv/o-** *affected by; sensitive to* **-ity** *state; condition*

Word or Phrase	Description	Word Building
fecal occult blood test	Diagnostic test for occult (hidden) blood in the feces. The feces are mixed with the chemical reagent guaiac. This is also known as a **stool guaiac test.** If blood is present, the guaiac will turn a blue color (guaiac-positive). Hemoccult and Coloscreen cards can be purchased by consumers for home testing. The results of these tests are heme positive or heme negative because they detect the heme molecule of hemoglobin from the blood.	**occult** (oh-KULT) **guaiac** (GWY-ak)
gastric analysis	Diagnostic test to determine the amount of hydrochloric acid in the stomach. A nasogastric (NG) tube is inserted, and gastric fluid is collected. Then a drug is given to stimulate acid production, and another sample is collected.	**gastric** (GAS-trik) **gastr/o-** *stomach* **-ic** *pertaining to*
ova and parasites (O&P)	Diagnostic test to determine if there is a parasitic infection in the gastrointestinal tract. Ova are the eggs of parasitic worms. They can be seen in the feces or by examining a sample under a microscope.	**ovum** (OH-vum) **ova** (OH-va) *Ovum* is a Latin singular noun. Form the plural by changing *-um* to *-a.* **parasite** (PAIR-ah-site)

Radiologic Procedures

barium enema (BE)	Procedure that uses liquid radiopaque contrast medium (barium) instilled into the rectum and colon (see Figure 3-24 ■). Barium outlines and coats the walls, and an x-ray is then taken. This test is used to identify polyps, diverticula, ulcerative colitis, and colon cancer.	**barium** (BAIR-ee-um) **enema** (EN-eh-mah)

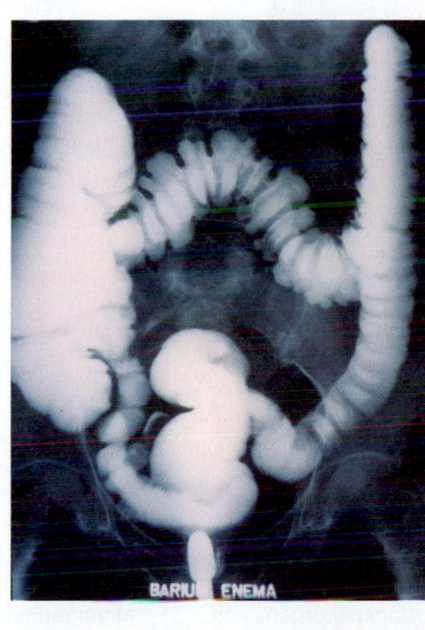

Figure 3-24 ■ Barium enema.
Barium contrast medium inserted through the rectum fills the rectum, sigmoid colon, descending colon, transverse colon, and ascending colon on this x-ray.

Word or Phrase	Description	Word Building

cholangiography	Procedure that uses a contrast dye to outline the bile ducts. Then an x-ray is taken to show stones in the gallbladder and bile ducts or thickening of the gallbladder wall. The x-ray image is a **cholangiogram.**
	
	For an **intravenous cholangiography (IVC),** the contrast dye is injected intravenously, travels through the blood to the liver, and is excreted with bile into the gallbladder.
	
	For a **percutaneous transhepatic cholangiography (PTC),** a needle is passed through the abdominal wall, and the contrast dye is injected into the liver.
	
	For an **endoscopic retrograde cholangiopancreatography (ERCP),** the contrast dye is injected going backward (in the opposite direction of the flow of bile and enzymes) to visualize the common bile duct and pancreatic duct (see Figure 3-25 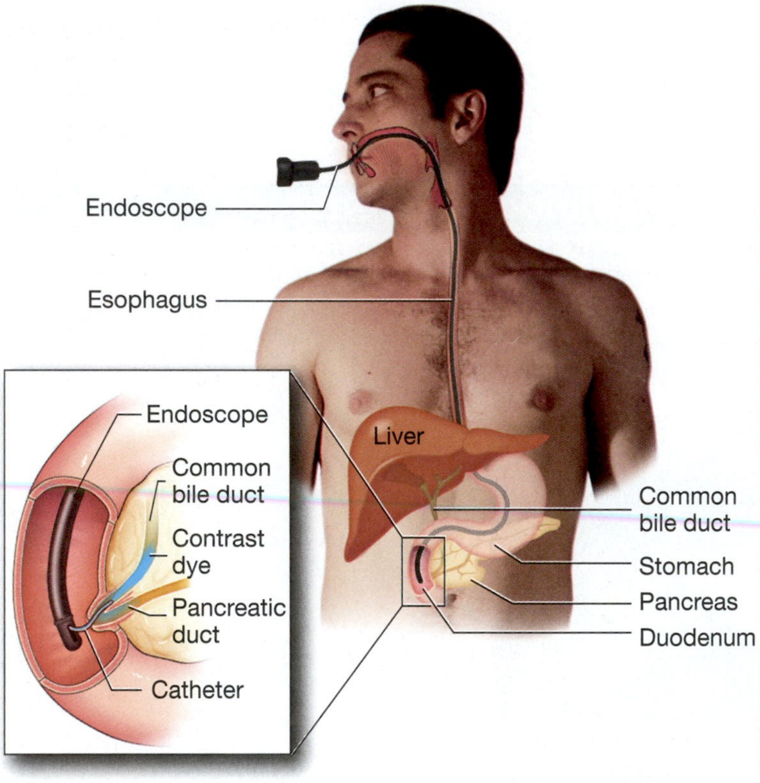 ■).
	
	Figure 3-25 ■ Endoscopic retrograde cholangiopancreatography.
	
	In this procedure, an endoscope is passed through the mouth and into the duodenum. A catheter is passed through the endoscope, and contrast dye is injected to visualize the common bile duct and pancreatic duct.
		cholangiography
		(koh-LAN-jee-AWG-rah-fee)
		  cholangi/o- *bile duct*
		  -graphy *process of recording*
		
		cholangiogram
		(koh-LAN-jee-oh-gram)
		  cholangi/o- *bile duct*
		  -gram *a record or picture*
		
		intravenous (IN-trah-VEE-nus)
		  intra- *within*
		  ven/o- *vein*
		  -ous *pertaining to*
		
		percutaneous (PER-kyoo-TAY-nee-us)
		  per- *through; throughout*
		  cutane/o- *skin*
		  -ous *pertaining to*
		
		transhepatic (TRANS-heh-PAT-ik)
		  trans- *across; through*
		  hepat/o- *liver*
		  -ic *pertaining to*
		
		endoscopic (EN-doh-SKAW-pik)
		  endo- *innermost; within*
		  scop/o- *examine with an instrument*
		  -ic *pertaining to*
		
		retrograde (RET-roh-grayd)
		  retro- *behind; backward*
		  -grade *pertaining to going*
		
		cholangiopancreatography
		(koh-LAN-jee-oh-PAN-kree-ah-TAWG-rah-fee)
		  cholangi/o- *bile duct*
		  pancreat/o- *pancreas*
		  -graphy *process of recording*

computerized axial tomography (CAT, CT scan)	Procedure that uses x-rays to create images of abdominal organs and structures in many thin, successive "slices"	**tomography** (toh-MAWG-rah-fee)
		  tom/o- *cut; slice; layer*
		  -graphy *process of recording*

flat plate of the abdomen	An x-ray without contrast dye. The patient lies flat, in the supine position, on the x-ray table for this procedure.	

Word or Phrase	Description	Word Building
gallbladder ultrasound	Procedure that uses ultra high-frequency sound waves to create images of the gallbladder. It is used to identify gallstones and thickening of the gallbladder wall. The image is a **gallbladder sonogram.**	**ultrasound** (UL-trah-sound) **sonogram** (SAWN-oh-gram) **son/o-** *sound* **-gram** *a record or picture*
magnetic resonance imaging (MRI scan)	Procedure that uses a strong magnetic field to align protons in the atoms of the patient's body. The protons emit signals to form images of abdominal organs and structures as thin, successive "slices."	**magnetic** (mag-NET-ik) **magnet/o-** *magnet* **-ic** *pertaining to*
oral cholecysto-graphy (OCG)	Procedure that uses tablets of radiopaque contrast dye taken orally. The tablets dissolve in the intestine. The contrast dye is absorbed into the blood, travels to the liver, and is excreted with bile into the gallbladder. An x-ray is taken to identify stones in the gallbladder and biliary ducts or thickening of the gallbladder wall. The x-ray image is a **cholecystogram.**	**cholecystography** (KOH-lee-sis-TAWG-rah-fee) **cholecyst/o-** *gallbladder* **-graphy** *process of recording* **cholecystogram** (KOH-lee-SIS-toh-gram) **cholecyst/o-** *gallbladder* **-gram** *a record or picture*
upper gastro-intestinal series (UGI)	Procedure that uses a liquid radiopaque contrast medium (barium) that is swallowed (a barium meal). Barium coats and outlines the walls of the esophagus, stomach, and duodenum. It is also known as a **barium swallow.** Fluoroscopy (a continuously moving x-ray image on a screen) is used to follow the barium through the small intestine. This is a **small bowel follow-through.** Individual x-rays are taken at specific times throughout the procedure (see Figure 19-4). This test identifies ulcers, tumors, or obstruction in the esophagus, stomach, and small intestine.	

Medical and Surgical Procedures

Medical Procedures

Word or Phrase	Description	Word Building
insertion of nasogastric tube (NG tube)	Procedure to insert a long, flexible **nasogastric tube** through the nostril into the stomach. It is used to drain secretions from the stomach or give feedings to the patient on a temporary basis (see Figure 3-26 ■).	**nasogastric** (NAY-zoh-GAS-trik) **nas/o-** *nose* **gastr/o-** *stomach* **-ic** *pertaining to*

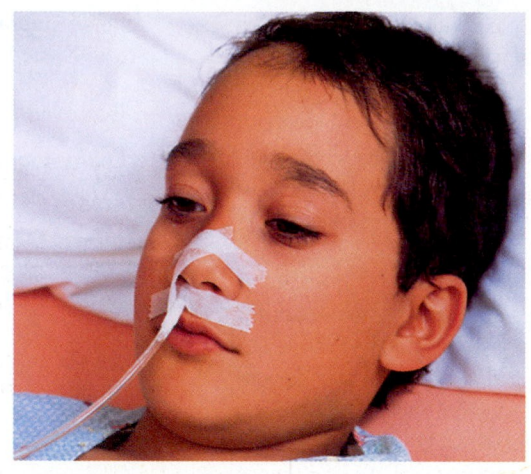

Did You Know?

The first nasogastric tube, developed in the late 1700s, was constructed from eel skin. It was used for several weeks to feed a patient who could not eat.

Figure 3-26 ■ **Nasogastric tube.**
This patient has a nasogastric (NG) tube. It was inserted into one nostril and, as he swallowed, it was advanced through the esophagus and into the stomach. Only liquid feedings or liquid drugs can be given through an NG tube.

Surgical Procedures

Word or Phrase	Description	Word Building
abdominocentesis	Procedure to remove fluid from the abdomen using a needle and a vacuum container. It is done to relieve abdominal pressure from fluid produced by ascites. It is also done to see if there are cancer cells in the peritoneal fluid or to see if there is blood in the peritoneal fluid after abdominal trauma.	**abdominocentesis** (ab-DAWM-ih-noh-sen-TEE-sis) **abdomin/o-** *abdomen* **-centesis** *procedure to puncture*
appendectomy	Procedure to remove the appendix because of appendicitis	**appendectomy** (AP-pen-DEK-toh-mee) **append/o-** *small structure hanging from a larger structure; appendix* **-ectomy** *surgical excision*
biopsy	Procedure to remove a small piece of tissue from an ulcer, polyp, mass, or tumor to look for abnormal or cancerous cells	**biopsy** (BY-awp-see) **bi/o-** *life; living organisms; living tissue* **-opsy** *process of viewing*
bowel resection and anastomosis	Procedure to remove a section of diseased intestine and rejoin the intestine. An end-to-end anastomosis joins the two cut ends together. An end-to-side anastomosis joins one end to the side of another segment.	**resection** (ree-SEK-shun) **resect/o-** *to cut out; remove* **-ion** *action; condition* **anastomosis** (ah-NAS-toh-MOH-sis) **anastom/o-** *create an opening between two structures* **-osis** *condition; abnormal condition; process*

Word or Phrase	Description	Word Building
cholecystectomy	Procedure to remove the gallbladder. This is done as a minimally invasive **laparoscopic cholecystectomy** that uses a **laparoscope** (see Figure 3-27 ■). 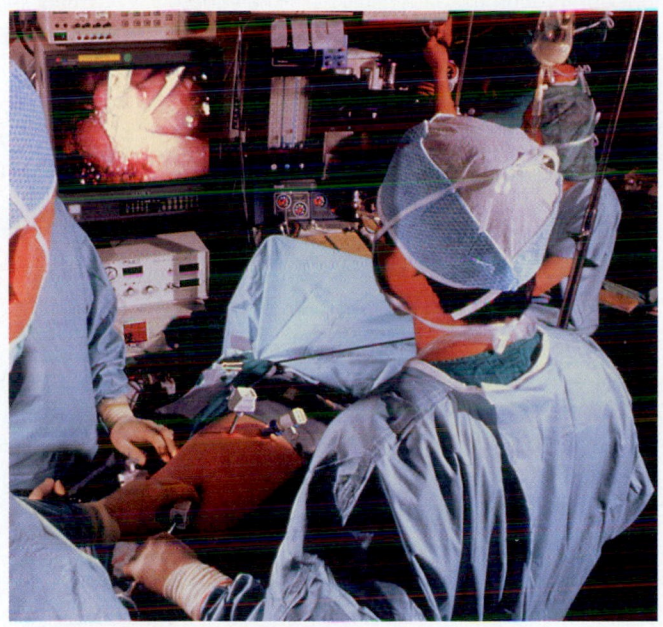 **Figure 3-27 ■ Laparoscopic cholecystectomy.** Carbon dioxide gas is used to inflate the abdominal cavity and separate the organs. A laparoscope is inserted through one of several small incisions; it is used to visualize the gallbladder (on the computer screen), while other instruments grasp and remove the gallbladder.	**cholecystectomy** (KOH-lee-sis-TEK-toh-mee) **cholecyst/o-** *gallbladder* **-ectomy** *surgical excision* **laparoscopic** (LAP-ah-roh-SKAWP-ik) **lapar/o-** *abdomen* **scop/o-** *examine with an instrument* **-ic** *pertaining to* **laparoscope** (LAP-ah-roh-skohp) **lapar/o-** *abdomen* **-scope** *instrument used to examine*

Did You Know?

At one time, a cholecystectomy to remove the gallbladder required a 5- to 7-inch abdominal incision, followed by a painful 6-week recovery. The first minimally invasive surgical procedure ever performed was done in 1989 to remove a gallbladder. Minimally invasive surgery is done with instruments inserted through several tiny incisions at various places on the abdominal wall.

Word or Phrase	Description	Word Building
choledocholitho-tomy	Procedure to make an incision in the common bile duct to remove a gallstone	**choledocholithotomy** (koh-LED-oh-koh-lih-THAW-toh-mee) **choledoch/o-** *common bile duct* **lith/o-** *stone* **-tomy** *process of cutting or making an incision*

Word or Phrase	Description	Word Building
colostomy	Procedure to remove the diseased part of the colon and create a new opening in the abdominal wall where feces can leave the body (see Figure 3-28 ■). The colon is brought out through the abdominal wall. The edges of the colon are rolled to make a mouth (**stoma**) and sutured to the abdominal wall. The patient wears a plastic disposable pouch that adheres to the abdominal wall to collect feces. If part of the ileum and colon are removed and a stoma created, the procedure is known as an **ileostomy**.	**colostomy** (koh-LAWS-toh-mee) **col/o-** *colon* **-stomy** *surgically created opening* **stoma** (STOH-mah) **ileostomy** (IL-ee-AWS-toh-mee) **ile/o-** *ileum* **-stomy** *surgically created opening*

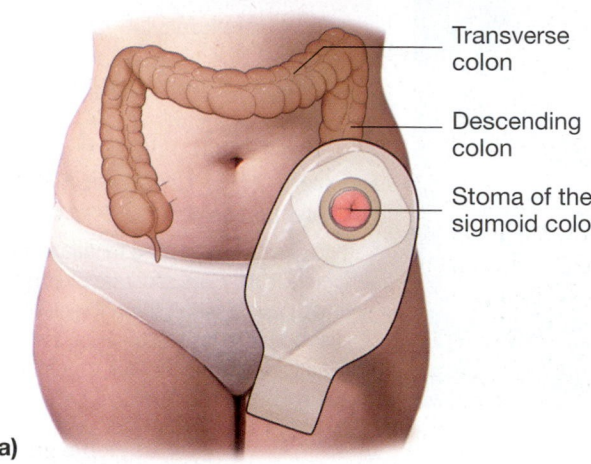

Transverse colon

Descending colon

Stoma of the sigmoid colon

(a)

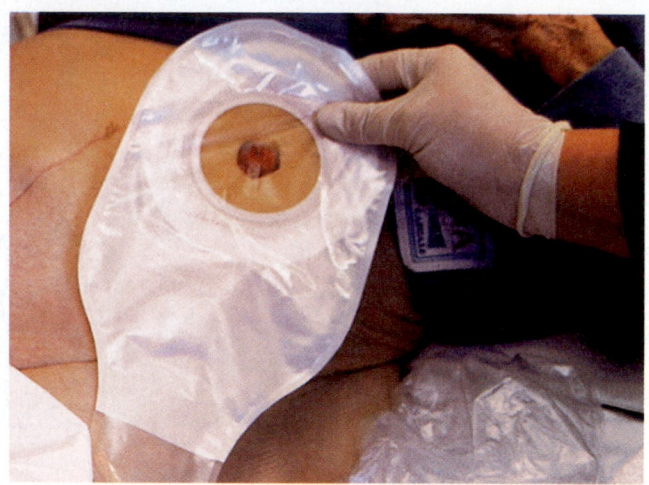

(b)

Figure 3-28 ■ Colostomy and stoma.

(a) A colostomy is done in the transverse, descending, or sigmoid colon. Here the red mucosa of the colon is rolled back on itself to create a stoma, which is sutured to the abdominal wall. (b) The patient wears a plastic disposable bag that adheres to the skin to collect feces.

Word Alert

SOUND-ALIKE WORDS

stoma (noun) A surgically created opening like a mouth

Example: The colostomy patient wears a disposable pouch around the stoma on his abdominal wall.

stomatitis (noun) Inflammation of the oral mucosa of the mouth

Example: The patient was losing weight because of a painful stomatitis that prevented him from chewing his food.

Word or Phrase	Description	Word Building
endoscopy	Procedure that uses an **endoscope** (a flexible, fiberoptic scope with a magnifying lens and a light source) to internally examine the gastrointestinal tract. An endoscopic procedure can be coupled with another procedure such as a biopsy or removal of a polyp.	**endoscopy** (en-DAWS-koh-pee) **endo-** *innermost; within* **-scopy** *process of using an instrument to examine* **endoscope** (EN-doh-skohp) **endo-** *innermost; within* **-scope** *instrument used to examine*

A Closer Look

These procedures use an endoscope inserted through the nose or mouth.

- **esophagoscopy:** visualization and examination of the esophagus
- **gastroscopy:** visualization and examination of the stomach (after the endoscope first passes through the esophagus)
- **esophagogastroduodenoscopy (EGD):** visualization and examination of the esophagus first, followed by the stomach, and then the duodenum

The ileum, cecum, and ascending colon cannot be visualized with endoscopy. Instead, the patient swallows a capsule that contains a small camera. It uses wireless technology to transmit pictures until it is excreted from the body.

These procedures use an endoscope inserted through the rectum.

- **sigmoidoscopy:** visualization and examination of the rectum and sigmoid colon using a sigmoidoscope
- **colonoscopy:** visualization and examination of the entire colon after the colonoscope is passed through the rectum (see Figure 3-29 ■)

esophagoscopy
(ee-SAWF-ah-GAWS-koh-pee)
esophag/o- *esophagus*
-scopy *process of using an instrument to examine*

gastroscopy (gas-TRAWS-koh-pee)
gastr/o- *stomach*
-scopy *process of using an instrument to examine*

esophagogastroduodenoscopy
(ee-SAWF-ah-goh-GAS-troh-DOO-oh-den-AWS-koh-pee)
esophag/o- *esophagus*
gastr/o- *stomach*
duoden/o- *duodenum*
-scopy *process of using an instrument to examine*

sigmoidoscopy
(SIG-moy-DAWS-koh-pee)
sigmoid/o- *sigmoid colon*
-scopy *process of using an instrument to examine*

colonoscopy (KOH-lon-AWS-koh-pee)
colon/o- *colon*
-scopy *process of using an instrument to examine*

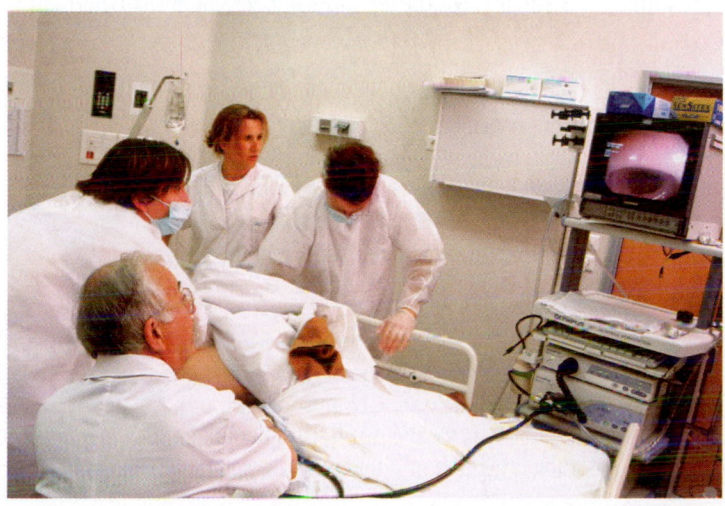

Figure 3-29 ■ Colonoscopy.
A colonoscope with a camera is passed through the anus to examine the rectum and colon. The images are transmitted to a computer screen for viewing and also recorded for the patient's medical record.

Word or Phrase	Description	Word Building
exploratory laparotomy	Procedure that uses an abdominal incision to open the abdominopelvic cavity widely so that it can be explored	**laparotomy** (LAP-ah-RAW-toh-mee) **lapar/o-** *abdomen* **-tomy** *process of cutting or making an incision*

Word or Phrase	Description	Word Building
gastrectomy	Procedure to remove all or part of the stomach because of a cancerous or benign tumor	**gastrectomy** (gas-TREK-toh-mee) **gastr/o-** *stomach* **-ectomy** *surgical excision*
gastroplasty	Procedure to treat severe obesity. Staples are used to make a small stomach pouch. A gastroplasty can be combined with a gastric bypass in which the stapled stomach pouch is anastomosed (connected) to the cut end of the jejunum. This bypasses the duodenum, where most fats are absorbed. It is also known as **gastric stapling** or **gastric bypass.**	**gastroplasty** (GAS-troh-PLAS-tee) **gastr/o-** *stomach* **-plasty** *process of reshaping by surgery*
gastrostomy	Procedure to create a temporary or permanent opening from the abdominal wall into the stomach to insert a gastrostomy feeding tube. For a **percutaneous endoscopic gastrostomy (PEG),** a PEG tube is inserted through the abdominal wall. Then under visual guidance from an endoscope that was previously passed through the mouth into the stomach, a catheter inside the PEG tube is positioned in the stomach (see Figure 3-30 ■). **Figure 3-30 ■ PEG tube.** This permanent feeding tube is inserted during a percutaneous endoscopic gastrostomy.	**gastrostomy** (gas-TRAWS-toh-mee) **gastr/o-** *stomach* **-stomy** *surgically created opening* **percutaneous** (PER-kyoo-TAY-nee-us) **per-** *through; throughout* **cutane/o-** *skin* **-ous** *pertaining to* **endoscopic** (EN-doh-SKAW-pik) **endo-** *innermost; within* **scop/o-** *examine with an instrument* **-ic** *pertaining to*
hemorrhoid-ectomy	Procedure to remove hemorrhoids from the rectum or around the anus	**hemorrhoidectomy** (HEM-oh-roy-DEK-toh-mee) **hemorrhoid/o-** *hemorrhoid* **-ectomy** *surgical excision*
herniorrhaphy	Procedure that uses sutures to close a defect in the muscle wall where there is a hernia	**herniorrhaphy** (HER-nee-OR-ah-fee) **herni/o-** *hernia* **-rrhaphy** *procedure of suturing*
jejunostomy	Procedure to create a temporary or permanent opening from the abdominal wall into the jejunum through which to insert a jejunostomy feeding tube. For a **percutaneous endoscopic jejunostomy (PEJ),** a PEJ tube is inserted through the abdominal wall. Then under visual guidance from an endoscope that was previously passed through the mouth, the PEJ tube is positioned in the jejunum.	**jejunostomy** (JEH-joo-NAWS-toh-mee) **jejun/o-** *jejunum* **-stomy** *surgically created opening*
liver transplantation	Procedure to remove a severely damaged liver from a patient with end-stage liver disease and insert a new liver from a donor. The patient (the recipient) is matched by blood type and tissue type to the donor. Liver transplant patients must take immunosuppressant drugs for the rest of their lives to keep their bodies from rejecting the foreign tissue that is their new liver.	**transplantation** (TRANS-plan-TAY-shun) **transplant/o-** *move something to another place* **-ation** *a process; being or having*
polypectomy	Surgical excision of polyps from the colon using forceps	**polypectomy** (PAWL-ih-PEK-toh-mee) **polyp/o-** *polyp* **-ectomy** *surgical excision*

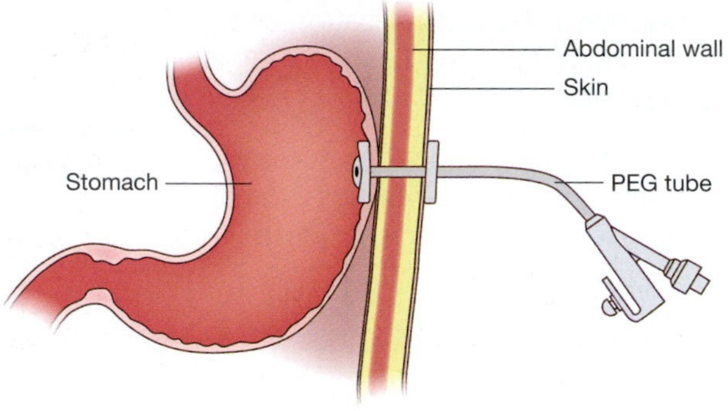

Drug Categories

These categories of drugs are used to treat gastrointestinal diseases and conditions. The most common generic and trade name drugs in each category are listed.

Category	Indication	Examples	Word Building
antacid drugs	Treat heartburn and peptic ulcer disease by neutralizing acid in the stomach	Maalox, Mylanta, Tums	**antacid** (ant-AS-id) *Antacid* is a combination of *anti-* (against) and the word *acid*. The *i* in *anti-* is deleted.
antibiotic drugs	Treat gastrointestinal infections caused by bacteria, including *Helicobacter pylori*. Antibiotic drugs are not effective against viral gastrointestinal infections.	amoxicillin (Amoxil), ciprofloxacin (Cipro), doxycycline (Vibramycin), Helidac (bismuth, metronidazole, tetracycline)	**antibiotic** (AN-tee-by-AWT-ik) (AN-tih-by-AWT-ik) **anti-** *against* **bi/o-** *life; living organisms; living tissue* **-tic** *pertaining to*
antidiarrheal drugs	Treat diarrhea. They slow peristalsis and this increases water absorption from the feces.	loperamide (Imodium), Lomotil (atropine, diphenoxylate)	**antidiarrheal** (AN-tee-DY-ah-REE-al) **anti-** *against* **dia-** *complete; completely through* **-rrhe/o-** *flow; discharge* **-al** *pertaining to*
antiemetic drugs	Treat nausea and vomiting and motion sickness	dimenhydrinate (Dramamine), meclizine (Antivert), prochlorperazine (Compazine)	**antiemetic** (AN-tee-eh-MET-ik) **anti-** *against* **emet/o-** *to vomit* **-ic** *pertaining to*
H₂ blocker drugs	Treat peptic ulcers by blocking H_2 (histamine 2) receptors in the stomach that trigger the release of hydrochloric acid	cimetidine (Tagamet), famotidine (Pepcid), ranitidine (Zantac)	
laxative drugs	Treat constipation by softening the stool, adding dietary fiber, or directly stimulating the intestinal mucosa	bisacodyl (Dulcolax), docusate (Colace, Surfak), psyllium (Fiberall, Metamucil)	**laxative** (LAK-sah-tiv)
proton pump inhibitor drugs	Treat heartburn, peptic ulcers, and gastroesophageal reflux disease (GERD) by blocking the final step in the production of hydrochloric acid	esomeprazole (Nexium), omeprazole (Prilosec)	

Did You Know?

A **suppository** is a bullet-shaped capsule that contains a drug. It is inserted into the rectum, where it melts and releases the drug.

suppository (soo-PAWZ-ih-TOR-ee)
supposit/o- *placed beneath*
-ory *having the function of*

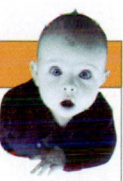

Abbreviations

ABD	abdomen		**LFTs**	liver function tests
a.c.	before meals (Latin, *ante cibum*)		**LLQ**	left lower quadrant
ALP	alkaline phosphatase		**LUQ**	left upper quadrant
ALT	alanine aminotransferase		**N&V**	nausea and vomiting
AST	aspartate aminotransferase		**NG**	nasogastric
BE	barium enema		**NPO (n.p.o.)**	nothing by mouth (Latin, *nil per os*)
BM	bowel movement			
BRBPR	bright red blood per rectum		**OCG**	oral cholecystography
BS	bowel sounds		**O&P**	ova and parasites
CBD	common bile duct		**p.c.**	after meals (Latin, *post cibum*)
EGD	esophagogastroduodenoscopy		**PEG**	percutaneous endoscopic gastrostomy
ERCP	endoscopic retrograde cholangiopancreatography		**PEJ**	percutaneous endoscopic jejunostomy
GERD	gastroesophageal reflux disease		**PO (p.o.)**	by mouth (Latin, *per os*)
GI	gastrointestinal		**PTC**	percutaneous transhepatic cholangiography
HAV	hepatitis A virus		**PUD**	peptic ulcer disease
HBV	hepatitis B virus		**RLQ**	right lower quadrant
HCl	hydrochloric acid		**RUQ**	right upper quadrant
HCV	hepatitis C virus		**SGOT**	serum glutamic-oxaloacetic transaminase (older name for AST)
IBD	inflammatory bowel disease			
IBS	irritable bowel syndrome		**SGPT**	serum glutamic-pyruvic transaminase (older name for ALT)
IVC	intravenous cholangiography			
LES	lower esophageal sphincter		**UGI**	upper gastrointestinal (series)

Word Alert

ABBREVIATIONS

Abbreviations are commonly used in all types of medical documents; however, they can mean different things to different people and their meanings can be misinterpreted. Always verify the meaning of an abbreviation.

BS means *bowel sounds*, but it also means *breath sounds*.

PUD means *peptic ulcer disease*, but when handwritten the *U* can look like a *V*; *PVD* means *peripheral vascular disease*.

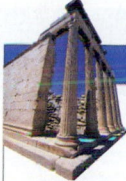

It's Greek to Me!

Did you notice that some words have two different combining forms? Combining forms from both Greek and Latin languages remain a part of medical language today.

Word	Greek	Latin	Medical Word Examples
abdomen	celi/o-	abdomin/o-	celiac trunk, celiac disease, abdominal
	lapar/o-	ventr/o-	laparoscopy, laparotomy, ventral
bile duct	cholangi/o-	bili/o-	cholangitis, cholangiography, biliary
	choledoch/o-		choledocholithiasis, choledocholithotomy
digest	peps/o-	digest/o-	pepsin, pepsinogen, digestive, digestion
	pept/o-		peptic
fats	steat/o-	lip/o-	steatorrhea, lipase
intestine	enter/o-	intestin/o-	enteropathy, gastroenteritis, gastroenterologist, gastroenterology, intestinal, gastrointestinal
mouth	stomat/o-	or/o-	stomatitis, oral
pass feces	chez/o-	fec/a-, fec/o-	hematochezia, fecalith, defecation
rectum	proct/o-	rect/o-	proctitis, rectal
saliva	sial/o-	saliv/o-	sialolith, sialolithiasis, salivary
tongue	gloss/o-	lingu/o-	glossitis, sublingual
umbilicus, navel	omphal/o-	umbilic/o-	omphalocele, umbilical

CAREER FOCUS

Meet Patricia, a medical assistant

"The best part of my job as a medical assistant is dealing with the patients. I love coming to work and doing it every day. It's just very fulfilling to me. I love helping people. I love talking to them. I love learning about their families, and that's what you find in this kind of practice. This is a huge clinic. It has internal medicine, pediatrics, OB/GYN, and plastic surgery. We have a specialty department with ears, nose, and throat doctors. We have optometry; we have physical therapy. I work with patients. I bring them in, I weigh them, take their blood pressure, find out what their problem is, write down their problem, and go to the physician and tell why the patient is here. I definitely think medical assistants are the first line of defense for the doctor. I bring everything to the doctor. We work as a team. We have a great rapport together and with our patients."

Medical assistants are allied health professionals who perform and document a variety of clinical and laboratory procedures and assist the physician during medical procedures in the office or clinic.

Gastroenterologists are physicians who practice in the medical specialty of gastroenterology. They diagnose and treat patients with diseases of the gastrointestinal system. Physicians can take additional training and become board certified in the subspecialty of pediatric gastroenterology. Cancerous tumors of the gastrointestinal system are treated medically by an **oncologist** or surgically by a general **surgeon.**

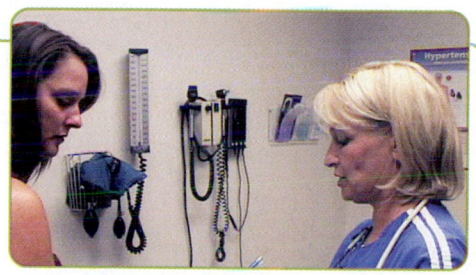

gastroenterologist
(GAS-troh-EN-ter-AWL-oh-jist)
  gastr/o- stomach
  enter/o- intestine
  log/o- word; the study of
  -ist one who specializes in

oncologist (ong-KAWL-oh-jist)
  onc/o- tumor; mass
  log/o- word; the study of
  -ist one who specializes in

surgeon (SER-jun)
  surg/o- operative procedure
  -eon one who performs

CHAPTER REVIEW EXERCISES

Test your knowledge of the chapter by completing these review exercises. Use the Answer Key at the end of the book to check your answers.

Anatomy and Physiology

Matching Exercise

Match each word or phrase to its description.

1. cholecystokinin
2. chyme
3. deglutition
4. enzyme
5. haustra
6. jejunum
7. lipase
8. lumen
9. mastication
10. meconium
11. omentum
12. parotid gland
13. rectum

_____ Enzyme that breaks apart fats

_____ The act of chewing

_____ One of the three salivary glands

_____ Hormone from the duodenum that stimulates the gallbladder to contract

_____ Fatty sheet of peritoneum that supports the stomach

_____ Last part of the large intestine

_____ First feces of newborn infants

_____ Second part of the small intestine

_____ Substance that breaks the chemical bonds between molecules of food

_____ Pouches in the mucosa of the large intestine

_____ The act of swallowing

_____ Open channel inside the intestines

_____ Partially digested food and digestive enzymes in the stomach

Circle Exercise

Circle the correct word from the choices given.

1. The first part of the small intestine is the (**cecum, colon, duodenum**).
2. The process of having a bowel movement is known as (**defecation, emulsification, mastication**).
3. The part of the stomach that is closest to the esophagus is the (**body, cardia, pylorus**).
4. What structure secretes a digestive enzyme? (**esophagus, pharynx, salivary gland**)
5. The digestive enzyme (**amylase, hydrochloric acid, lipase**) is *not* secreted by the pancreas.
6. The S-shaped segment of colon is the (**jejunum, sigmoid, transverse**).
7. Emulsification of fat globules in food is done by (**bile, flatus, lactase**).

True or False Exercise

Indicate whether each statement is true or false by writing T *or* F *on the line.*

1. _____ The stomach is superior to the small intestine.
2. _____ The salivary glands and pancreas both secrete amylase.
3. _____ The structure that comes after the duodenum is the ileum.
4. _____ The colon is the longest part of the large intestine.
5. _____ The appendix is considered to be part of the gastrointestinal system and the endocrine system.

6. _____ Mucosa lines the gastrointestinal tract.

7. _____ You can find villi in the large intestine.

8. _____ Deglutition is waves of contractions that propel food through the GI tract.

9. _____ The omentum carries food nutrients from the intestines to the liver.

10. _____ The parotid gland is one of the salivary glands.

Sequencing Exercise

Beginning with food entering the mouth, write each structure of the gastrointestinal system in the order in which food moves through it.

Structure	Correct Order
anus	1. _____
cecum	2. _____
colon	3. _____
duodenum	4. _____
esophagus	5. _____
ileum	6. _____
jejunum	7. _____
oral cavity	8. _____
pharynx	9. _____
rectum	10. _____
stomach	11. _____

Diseases and Conditions

Matching Exercise

Match each word or phrase to its description.

1. hematochezia   _____ Chronic liver disease with nodular liver

2. choledocholithiasis   _____ Dark, tar-like feces that contain old blood

3. incontinence   _____ Gallstones in the common bile duct

4. hematemesis   _____ Inflammation of the lips

5. obstipation   _____ Enlargement of the liver and spleen

6. cheilitis   _____ Fatty feces and malabsorption of dietary fat

7. hepatosplenomegaly   _____ A type of stomach cancer

8. steatorrhea   _____ Blood in the feces

9. melena   _____ Excessive vomiting of pregnancy

10. varices   _____ Severe constipation

11. hyperemesis gravidarum _____ Inability to control bowel movements

12. adenocarcinoma   _____ Vomiting blood

13. cirrhosis   _____ Swollen veins in the esophagus

True or False Exercise

Indicate whether each statement is true or false by writing T or F on the line.

1. _____ Indigestion is known by the medical name *dyspepsia*.

2. _____ A hiatal hernia occurs in the groin.

3. _____ A peptic ulcer is an ulcer in the esophagus, stomach, or duodenum.

4. _____ An ileus is an abnormal fibrous band that forms between two organs following abdominal surgery.

5. _____ A ruptured appendix can cause diverticulosis.

6. _____ Hepatoma is another name for liver cancer.

7. _____ Pancreatitis can occur when a gallstone blocks the common bile duct near the duodenum.

Laboratory, Radiology, Surgery, and Drugs

Fill in the Blank Exercise

Fill in the blank with the correct word from the word list.

albumin	cholangiography	nasogastric tube	sonogram
antiemetic	herniorrhaphy	ova and parasites	stoma
barium swallow	laxative		

1. Surgically created opening like a mouth _____

2. A medicine used to treat vomiting _____

3. Major protein molecule in the blood _____

4. Eggs and worms in the GI tract _____

5. Radiologic procedure that uses contrast dye to show the bile ducts _____

6. An ultrasound is also known as a _____

7. Another name for an upper GI series _____

8. Provides a temporary way to feed a patient _____

9. Procedure that sutures a weak area in the abdominal wall that protrudes outward _____

10. A drug used to treat constipation _____

Circle Exercise

Circle the correct word from the choices given.

1. The words *donor* and *recipient* are associated with this operative procedure: (**gastroplasty, liver transplantation, polypectomy**)

2. A gallbladder ultrasound is also known as a/an (**amylase test, ERCP, sonogram**).

3. Surgical removal of the gallbladder is known as a (**cholecystectomy, colectomy, colostomy**).

4. All of these are types of feeding tubes *except* (**colostomy, gastrostromy, jejunostomy**).

5. Gastroplasty is a popular surgery to treat (**colon polyps, heartburn, obesity**).

6. ALT is the newer name for the lab test (**albumin, CBD, SGPT**).

7. *Helicobacter pylori* causes what test to be positive? (**CLO, colonoscopy, gastric analysis**)

8. A/an (**anastomosis, endoscopy, laparotomy**) uses a long abdominal incision to explore the abdominal cavity.

9. The surgical procedure done to treat stomach cancer is a (**gastrectomy, gastroplasty, gastroscopy**).

Building Medical Words

Review the Combining Forms Exercise, Combining Form and Suffix Exercise, Prefix Exercise, and Multiple Combining Forms and Suffix Exercise that you already completed in the anatomy section on pages 103–105.

Combining Forms Exercise

Before you build gastrointestinal words, review these additional combining forms. Next to each combining form, write its medical meaning. The first one has been done for you.

Combining Form	Medical Meaning	Combining Form	Medical Meaning
1. anastom/o-	create an opening between two structures	16. log/o-	
2. cheil/o-		17. obstip/o-	
3. cirrh/o-		18. obstruct/o-	
4. constip/o-		19. omphal/o-	
5. contin/o-		20. orex/o-	
6. diverticul/o-		21. pept/o-	
7. emet/o-		22. perfor/o-	
8. hemat/o-		23. phag/o-	
9. hemorrhoid/o-		24. polyp/o-	
10. herni/o-		25. pyr/o-	
11. hiat/o-		26. regurgitat/o-	
12. inguin/o-		27. rotat/o-	
13. intussuscep/o-		28. splen/o-	
14. jaund/o-		29. steat/o-	
15. lith/o-		30. umbilic/o-	

Related Combining Forms Exercise

Write the combining forms on the line provided. (Hint: See the It's Greek to Me feature box.)

1. Two combining forms that mean *fats*. _____
2. Two combining forms that mean *intestine*. _____
3. Two combining forms that mean *tongue*. _____
4. Four combining forms that mean *abdomen*. _____
5. Three combining forms that mean *bile duct*. _____

Dividing Medical Words

Separate these words into their component parts (prefix, combining form, suffix). Note: Some words do not contain all three word parts. The first one has been done for you.

Medical Word	Prefix	Combining Form	Suffix	Medical Word	Prefix	Combining Form	Suffix
1. anorexia	an-	orex/o-	-ia	5. hematemesis			
2. appendectomy				6. hepatomegaly			
3. mesenteric				7. herniorrhaphy			
4. dysphagia				8. sublingual			

Combining Form and Suffix Exercise

Read the definition of the medical word. Select the correct suffix from the Suffix List. Select the correct combining form from the Combining Form List. Build the medical word and write it on the line. Be sure to check your spelling. The first one has been done for you.

SUFFIX LIST	COMBINING FORM LIST	
-ation (a process; being or having)	anastom/o- (create an opening between two structures)	gastr/o- (stomach)
-cele (hernia)		gloss/o- (tongue)
-ectomy (surgical excision)	appendic/o- (appendix)	hemat/o- (blood)
-emesis (condition of vomiting)	append/o- (appendix)	hemorrhoid/o- (hemorrhoid)
-gram (a record or picture)	cholangi/o- (bile duct)	hepat/o- (liver)
-itis (inflammation of; infection of)	cholecyst/o- (gallbladder)	herni/o- (hernia)
-lith (stone)	cirrh/o- (yellow)	lapar/o- (abdomen)
-megaly (enlargement)	col/o- (colon)	polyp/o- (polyp)
-oma (tumor; mass)	constip/o- (compacted feces)	rect/o- (rectum)
-osis (condition; abnormal condition; process)	diverticul/o- (diverticulum)	sial/o- (saliva; salivary gland)
-pathy (disease; suffering)	enter/o- (intestine)	sigmoid/o- (sigmoid colon)
-rrhaphy (procedure of suturing)		
-scope (instrument used to examine)		
-scopy (process of using an instrument to examine)		
-stomy (surgically created opening)		
-tomy (process of cutting or making an incision)		

Definition of the Medical Word

1. Being or having compacted feces
2. Inflammation or infection of the stomach
3. Condition of vomiting of blood
4. Enlargement of the liver
5. Inflammation or infection of the appendix
6. Disease of the intestine
7. Surgical excision of the gallbladder
8. Abnormal condition (of having) diverticula
9. Process of cutting or making an incision into the abdomen
10. Inflammation or infection of the liver
11. Surgical excision of a polyp
12. Tumor of the liver
13. Surgical excision of the appendix
14. Procedure of suturing a hernia
15. Process of using an instrument to examine the sigmoid colon
16. Inflammation or infection of the gallbladder
17. Create an opening between two structures (such as the intestine)
18. Inflammation or infection of the tongue
19. Surgically created opening in the colon
20. Instrument used to examine (the inside of) the abdomen

Build the Medical Word

1. constipation

Definition of the Medical Word

21. Surgical excision of hemorrhoids
22. Hernia in the rectum
23. Stone in a salivary gland
24. Abnormal condition (of the liver that causes the skin to be) yellow
25. A record or (x-ray) picture of the bile ducts

Build the Medical Word

_____

_____

_____

_____

_____

Prefix Exercise

Read the definition of the medical word. Look at the medical word or partial word that is given (it already contains a combining form and a suffix.) Select the correct prefix from the Prefix List and write it on the blank line. Then build the medical word and write it on the line. Be sure to check your spelling. The first one has been done for you.

PREFIX LIST

an- (without; not)	in- (in; within; not)	sub- (below; underneath; less than)
anti- (against)	mal- (bad; inadequate)	trans- (across; through)
dys- (painful; difficult; abnormal)	poly- (many; much)	
im- (not)		

Definition of the Medical Word	Prefix	Word or Partial Word	Build the Medical Word
1. Condition of not digesting	in-	digestion	indigestion
2. Condition of (being) without an appetite	_____	orexia	_____
3. Condition of painful or abnormal digestion	_____	pepsia	_____
4. Condition of bad rotation (of the intestine)	_____	rotation	_____
5. Pertaining to underneath the tongue	_____	lingual	_____
6. Condition of much eating	_____	phagia	_____
7. Pertaining to (a drug that is) against vomiting	_____	emetic	_____
8. Condition of painful or difficult eating or swallowing	_____	phagia	_____
9. Pertaining to not having an opening (at the anus)	_____	perforate	_____
10. State of not (being able to) hold together (feces in the rectum)	_____	continence	_____

Multiple Combining Forms and Suffix Exercise

Read the definition of the medical word. Select the correct suffix and combining forms. Then build the medical word and write it on the line. Be sure to check your spelling. The first one has been done for you.

SUFFIX LIST	COMBINING FORM LIST	
-al (pertaining to)	bili/o- (bile; gall)	hepat/o- (liver)
-ia (condition; state; thing)	chez/o- (to pass feces)	lapar/o- (abdomen)
-ic (pertaining to)	col/o- (colon)	lith/o- (stone)
-in (a substance)	choledoch/o- (common bile duct)	log/o- (word; the study of)
-ist (one who specializes in)	duoden/o- (duodenum)	nas/o- (nose)
-itis (inflammation of; infection of)	enter/o- (intestine)	rect/o- (rectum)
-megaly (enlargement)	esophag/o- (esophagus)	rub/o- (red)
-scopy (process of using an instrument to examine)	gastr/o- (stomach)	scop/o- (examine with an instrument)
-tomy (process of cutting or making an incision)	hemat/o- (blood)	splen/o- (spleen)

Definition of the Medical Word

Build the Medical Word

1. A substance (composed of) bile and (taken from blood cells that are) red   <u>bilirubin</u>

2. Process of using an instrument to examine the esophagus, stomach, and duodenum   _____

3. Inflammation or infection of the stomach and intestine   _____

4. Enlargement of the liver and spleen   _____

5. Pertaining to (a tube that goes through) the nose (to) the stomach   _____

6. Condition of blood (when you) pass feces   _____

7. Pertaining to the colon and rectum   _____

8. One who specializes in stomach and intestines the study of   _____

9. Process of cutting or making an incision into the common bile duct (to remove) a stone   _____

10. Process of using an instrument to examine (inside) the abdomen   _____

Abbreviations

Matching Exercise

Match each abbreviation to its description.

1. ALT   _____ Also known as a barium swallow

2. C&S   _____ SGPT was its former name

3. CBD   _____ A duct that bile flows through

4. CLO test   _____ Screening test for *Helicobacter pylori*

5. GERD   _____ Feeding tube from nose to stomach

6. LFTs   _____ Stomach acid irritates the esophagus

7. N&V   _____ Blood tests for hepatic function

8. NG   _____ Tells which antibiotic drug a bacterium is sensitive to

9. NPO   _____ Feeding tube surgically inserted in the stomach

10. O&P   _____ Upset stomach and emesis

11. PEG   _____ One of four abdominal quadrants

12. RUQ   _____ Nothing by mouth

13. UGI   _____ Test for worms and eggs of parasites in the feces

Applied Skills

Adjective Spelling Exercise

Read the noun and write the adjective form. Be sure to check your spelling. The first one has been done for you.

Noun	Adjective Form		Noun	Adjective Form
1. abdomen	abdominal	9. cecum		
2. mouth		10. appendix		
3. pharynx		11. colon		
4. esophagus		12. rectum		
5. stomach		13. anus		
6. pylorus		14. peritoneum		
7. duodenum		15. liver		
8. jejunum		16. pancreas		

Proofreading and Spelling Exercise

Read the following paragraph. Identify each misspelled medical word and write the correct spelling of it on the line provided.

Gastrointerology is the study of the digestive organs. Food moves into the pharinxy from the mouth and then down the esophogus. You won't develop diverticulee or hemorroids if you eat a high-fiber diet, but cholelithasis could still be a problem. If the lumin of your bowel is filled with polips, then you may need to have surgery. A rectoseel can affect the vagina in women. If you do not eat enough protein, the albumen level in your blood will be low.

1. _____   6. _____
2. _____   7. _____
3. _____   8. _____
4. _____   9. _____
5. _____   10. _____

English and Medical Word Equivalents Exercise

For each English word, write its equivalent medical word. Be sure to check your spelling. The first one has been done for you.

English Word	Medical Word		English Word	Medical Word
1. belly	abdomen	8. indigestion		
2. belly button		9. mouth		
3. bowel, gut		10. piles		
4. bowel movement		11. swallowing		
5. chewing		12. throat		
6. gas		13. throwing up		
7. heartburn				

You Write the Medical Report

You are a healthcare professional interviewing a patient. Listen to the patient's statements and then enter them in the patient's medical record using medical words and phrases. Be sure to check your spelling. The first one has been done for you.

1. The patient says, "I can't explain it. I just don't seem to have any appetite at all for the past few weeks, and that's not like me at all."

   You write: The patient is complaining of _____*anorexia*_____ that has been present for the past few weeks.

2. The patient says, "I had cancer of the colon in 2008 and they took out my colon and made this new opening in my abdomen."

   You write: The patient had cancer of the colon in 2008 and a _____ was performed.

3. The patient says, "Oh that bug was going around and I caught it from my kids—you know that intestinal virus with nausea, vomiting, and diarrhea. I had it for 4 days."

   You write: The patient developed viral _____ with symptoms of nausea, vomiting, and diarrhea for 4 days.

4. The patient says, "I strain most times when I try to pass a stool, but it never gets really bad."

   You write: The patient reports that she has frequent episodes of _____, but denies having any _____.

5. The patient says, "I don't want to but I know I am supposed to have one of those procedures where they use an instrument to look into your bowel, so I guess it's time to go."

   You write: The patient is apprehensive about having a _____ performed, but is agreeable to my referring her for this procedure.

6. The patient says, "I went to see that doctor at the hospital who specializes in treating the GI system, and he said I have an ulcer."

   You write: The patient was seen by a _____ at the hospital who diagnosed her as having an ulcer.

7. The patient says, "This is an emergency. I have an old ulcer in my esophagus, but today I just started vomiting up blood. I know I am an alcoholic, and my liver has disease and my abdomen is all swollen up with fluid, too."

   You write: The patient has a history of an _____ ulcer and today had an episode of _____. He has a past history of alcoholism with a diagnosis of _____, and now has an enlarged abdomen with _____.

8. The patient says, "I have an acidy, irritated stomach with gas when I eat spicy foods."

   You write: The patient complains of _____ with _____ after eating spicy foods.

9. The patient says, "You know I have had these stones in my gallbladder that keep giving me trouble, so is it time for me to have them taken out?"

   You write: The patient has frequent bouts of _____ and is now considering the surgical option of having a _____ done.

10. The patient says, "You know that past stroke I had. Well, I still have difficulty eating from that. I also lost weight and now my dentures don't fit right and they hurt when I eat."

    You write: The patient is complaining of _____ due to impairment from a past stroke and also weight loss that resulted in poorly fitting dentures that cause pain.

Medical Report Exercise

This exercise contains two related reports: a hospital Admission History and Physical Examination and a Pathology Report. Read both reports and answer the questions.

ADMISSION HISTORY AND PHYSICAL EXAMINATION

PATIENT NAME: MARTINEZ, Javier

HOSPITAL NUMBER: 138-524-7193

DATE OF ADMISSION: NOVEMBER 19, 20xx

HISTORY OF PRESENT ILLNESS
This is a 20-year-old Hispanic male who experienced severe abdominal pain beginning on the morning of admission. He was awakened at 6:00 A.M. by sharp pains in the stomach. Drinking a glass of milk, which usually helps this type of pain, was not effective. He also took his customary antacid, but with no relief. He went to college and ate lunch there and then developed nausea and vomiting. An hour later, he developed watery diarrhea with approximately 3–4 bowel movements over the next few hours. He denies any history of ulcerative colitis or Crohn's disease. By this evening, his pain was so severe that he came to the emergency room to be seen.

PHYSICAL EXAMINATION
Temperature 100.2, pulse 84, respiratory rate 30, blood pressure 132/88. He is alert and oriented, lying uncomfortably in bed. Abdominal examination: Abdomen is soft. There is rebound tenderness in the RLQ.

LABORATORY DATA
Labs drawn in the emergency room showed an elevated white blood cell count of 14.6. Bilirubin and amylase were within normal limits. Urinalysis was unremarkable.

IMPRESSION
Acute appendicitis.

DISCUSSION
A detailed discussion was carried out with the patient and his parents. The dangers of waiting and observing his condition were discussed as well as the indications, possible risks, complications, and alternatives to an appendectomy. They agree with the plan to perform an appendectomy, and the patient will be taken to the operating room shortly.

James R. Rodgers, M.D.

James R. Rodgers, M.D.

JRR/bjg
D: 11/19/xx
T: 11/19/xx

PATHOLOGY REPORT

PATIENT NAME: MARTINEZ, Javier

HOSPITAL NUMBER: 138-524-7193

DATE OF REPORT: NOVEMBER 19, 20xx

SPECIMEN: Appendix

GROSS EXAMINATION
The specimen identified as "appendix" is an inflamed, vermiform appendix with an attached piece of the mesoappendix. The appendix measures 6.5 cm in length and up to 1.3 cm in diameter. There is a yellow-gray exudate noted inside with marked hemorrhage of the mucosa. There is no evidence of tumor or fecalith.

PATHOLOGICAL DIAGNOSIS
Acute appendicitis.

Leona T. Parkins, M.D.

Leona T. Parkins, M.D.

LTP:rrg
D: 11/19/xx
T: 11/19/xx

Word Analysis Questions

1. The patient had sharp pains in his stomach. If you wanted to use the adjective form of *stomach,* you would say, "He had sharp _____ pains."

2. Divide *appendicitis* into its two word parts and define each word part.

Word Part	Definition
_____	_____
_____	_____

3. Divide *fecalith* into its two word parts and define each word part.

Word Part	Definition
_____	_____
_____	_____

4. Where is the RLQ? _____

5. What is the abbreviation for *nausea and vomiting*? _____

Fact Finding Questions

1. What is the name of the category of drug that neutralizes acid in the stomach?

   _____

2. What is another medical name for *vomiting*?

   _____

3. Ulcerative colitis and Crohn's disease both affect which part of the gastrointestinal system?

   _____

4. What does *vermiform* mean?

_____

5. What is the medical word that means *surgical excision of the appendix*?

_____

6. According to the pathology report on the specimen removed during surgery, what was the patient's diagnosis?

_____

Critical Thinking Questions

1. The patient has taken milk and an antacid in the past for his stomach pains. This suggests he has a previous history of what disease condition? Circle the correct answer.

   pyrosis   **colon cancer**   **hemorrhoids**

2. Acute symptoms of nausea and vomiting with diarrhea might lead you to think that the patient has what disease? Circle the correct answer.

   jaundice   **hematochezia**   **gastroenteritis**

3. An elevated white blood cell count is associated with an infection. Where was the site of this patient's infection?

   _____

4. The danger in waiting and observing the patient's condition was that he could develop a ruptured appendix that would lead to what condition? Circle the correct answer.

   peritonitis   **gastritis**   **cholecystitis**

5. The patient had a finding of "rebound tenderness" on the physical examination. Describe what the physician did to check for rebound tenderness.

   _____

6. The patient's bilirubin was within normal limits. This tells you that he is not having any problems with which of these organs?

   stomach   **liver**   **pancreas**

7. The patient's amylase was within normal limits. This tells you that he is not having any problems with which of these organs?

   pancreas   **colon**   **esophagus**

On the Job Challenge Exercise

On the job, you will encounter new medical words. Practice your medical dictionary skills by looking up the medical words in bold and writing their definitions on the lines provided.

OFFICE CHART NOTE

This is a 68-year-old white female with episodic abdominal pain, some headaches, heartburn symptoms, **aerophagia** and **eructation**, obstipation, and **tenesmus**. The patient presented with a 3-day history of **singultus**, unrelieved by any medications. Her physical examination revealed **borborygmus** and a slightly tender abdomen, but no evidence of rebound.

---

1. aerophagia _____

2. eructation _____

3. tenesmus _____

4. singultus _____

5. borborygmus _____

Hearing Medical Words Exercise

You hear someone speaking the medical words given below. Read each pronunciation and then write the medical word it represents. Be sure to check your spelling. The first one has been done for you.

1. AN-oh-REK-see-ah   <u>anorexia</u>

2. ah-SY-teez   _____

3. KOH-lee-sis-TY-tis   _____

4. sih-ROH-sis   _____

5. koh-LAWS-toh-mee   _____

6. GAS-troh-EN-ter-EYE-tis   _____

7. HER-nee-OR-ah-fee   _____

8. LAP-ah-RAW-toh-mee   _____

9. NAY-zoh-GAS-trik   _____

10. SIG-moy-DAWS-koh-pee   _____

Pronunciation Exercise

Read the medical word that is given. Then review the syllables in the pronunciation. Circle the primary (main) accented syllable. The first one has been done for you.

1. gastric (gas-trik)

2. appendicitis (ah-pen-dih-sy-tis)

3. cholecystectomy (koh-lee-sis-tek-toh-mee)

4. dysphagia (dis-fay-jee-ah)

5. gastroenterologist (gas-troh-en-ter-awl-oh-jist)

6. gastrointestinal (gas-troh-in-tes-tih-nal)

7. hepatic (heh-pat-ik)

8. hepatitis (hep-ah-ty-tis)

9. hepatosplenomegaly (hep-ah-toh-splen-oh-meg-ah-lee)

10. peristalsis (pair-ih-stal-sis)

Multimedia Preview

Immerse yourself in a variety of activities inside Medical Terminology Interactive. Getting there is simple:

1. Click on www.myhealthprofessionskit.com.
2. Select "Medical Terminology" from the choice of disciplines.
3. First-time users must create an account using the scratch-off code on the inside front cover of this book.
4. Find this book and log in using your username and password.
5. Click on Medical Terminology Interactive.
6. Take the elevator to the 3rd Floor to begin your virtual exploration of this chapter!

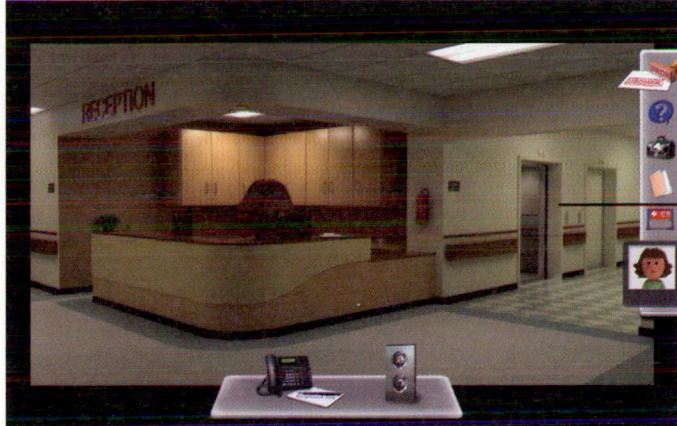 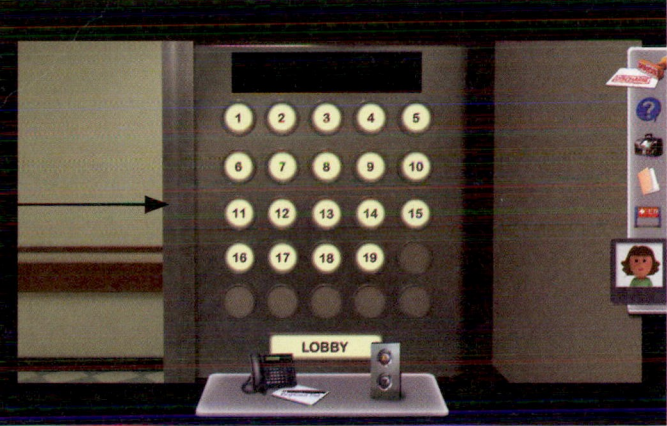

■ **Racing Pulse**   Don't miss a beat! Your challenge is to answer quiz show questions to top the computer. With each correct answer you earn a spin of the dial which tells you how many pulses to advance. First around the body is a winner.

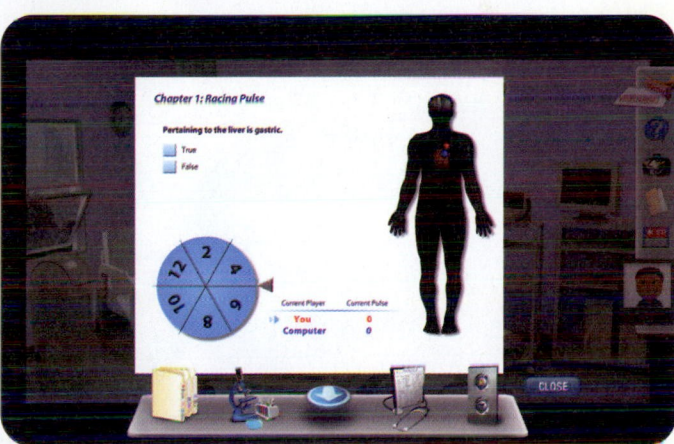

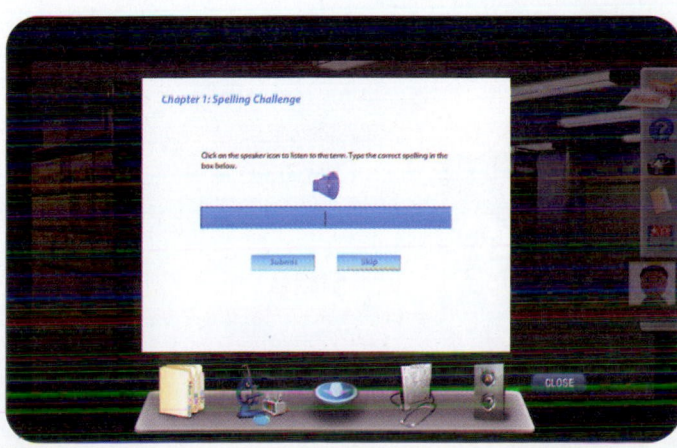

■ **Spelling Challenge**   Would you be the winner in a medical terminology spelling bee? Test your skills, listen to a pronounced medical word and then attempt to spell it correctly.

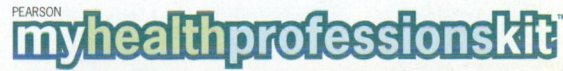
PEARSON
myhealthprofessionskit™

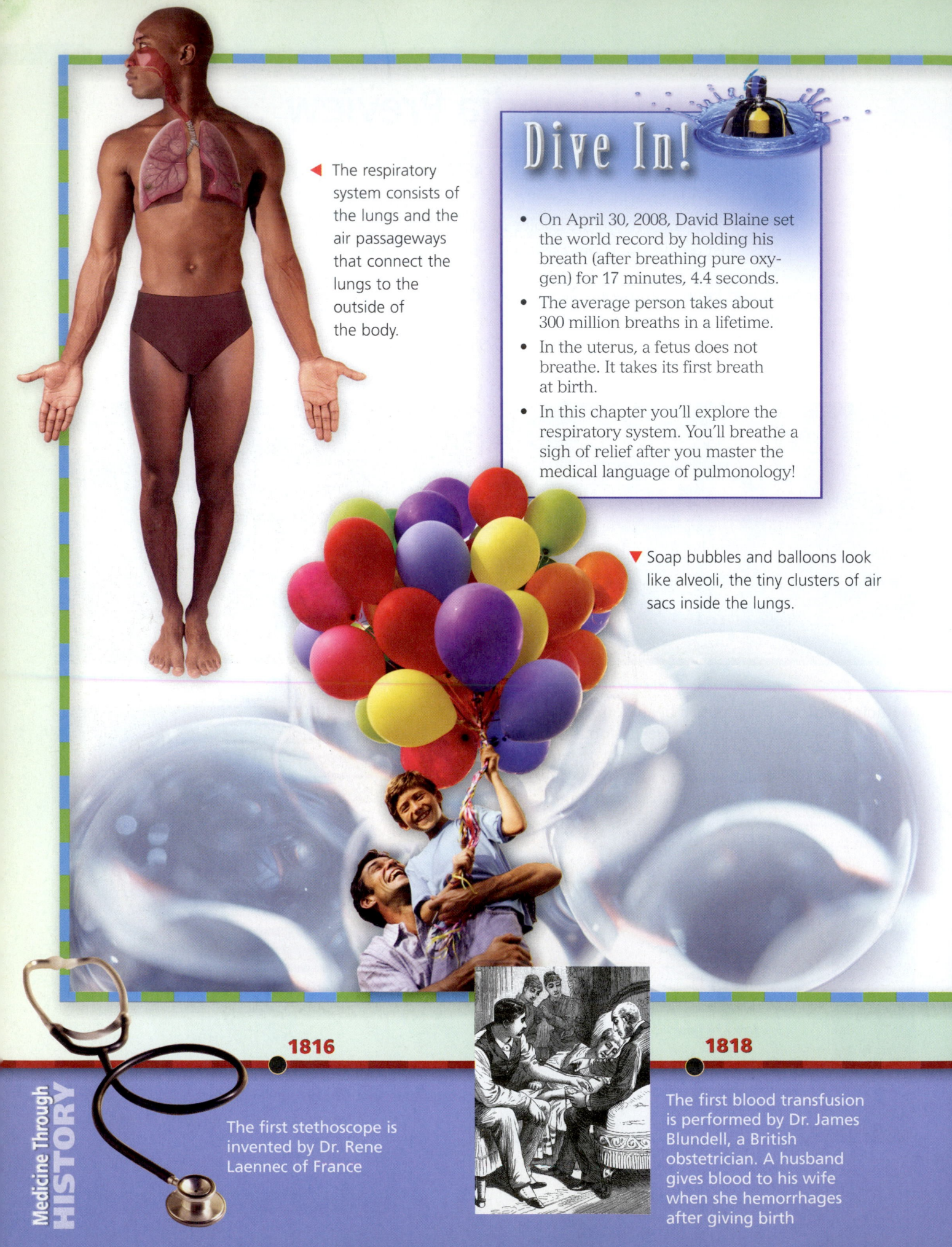

◀ The respiratory system consists of the lungs and the air passageways that connect the lungs to the outside of the body.

Dive In!

- On April 30, 2008, David Blaine set the world record by holding his breath (after breathing pure oxygen) for 17 minutes, 4.4 seconds.

- The average person takes about 300 million breaths in a lifetime.

- In the uterus, a fetus does not breathe. It takes its first breath at birth.

- In this chapter you'll explore the respiratory system. You'll breathe a sigh of relief after you master the medical language of pulmonology!

▼ Soap bubbles and balloons look like alveoli, the tiny clusters of air sacs inside the lungs.

Medicine Through HISTORY

1816

The first stethoscope is invented by Dr. Rene Laennec of France

1818

The first blood transfusion is performed by Dr. James Blundell, a British obstetrician. A husband gives blood to his wife when she hemorrhages after giving birth

Pulmonology

Respiratory System

Pulmonology (PUL-moh-NAWL-oh-jee) is the medical specialty that studies the anatomy and physiology of the respiratory system and uses diagnostic tests, medical and surgical procedures, and drugs to treat respiratory diseases.

▶ Blowing up a balloon may look simple, but there's a lot happening in those little lungs.

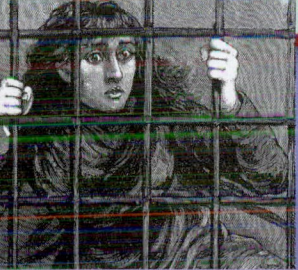

1841

Dorthea Dix advocates for the mentally ill and better conditions in mental hospitals

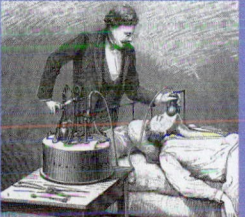

1846

Dr. William Morton uses ether gas to perform the first surgery under general anesthesia

1847

The American Medical Association (AMA) is founded

Measure Your Progress: Learning Objectives

After you study this chapter, you should be able to

1. Identify the structures of the respiratory system.

2. Describe the process of respiration.

3. Describe common respiratory diseases and conditions, laboratory and diagnostic procedures, medical and surgical procedures, and drug categories.

4. Give the medical meaning of word parts related to the respiratory system.

5. Build respiratory words from word parts and divide and define respiratory words.

6. Spell and pronounce respiratory words.

7. Analyze the medical content and meaning of a pulmonology report.

8. Dive deeper into pulmonology by reviewing the activities at the end of this chapter and online at Medical Terminology Interactive.

Figure 4-1 ■ **Respiratory system.**

The respiratory system consists of two main organs—the lungs—and other structures connected to the lungs. These form a pathway through which air flows into and out of the body.

Medical Language Key

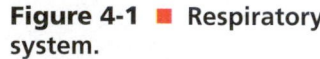

To unlock the definition of a medical word, break it into word parts. Define each word part. Put the word part meanings in order, beginning with the suffix, then the prefix (if present), then the combining form(s).

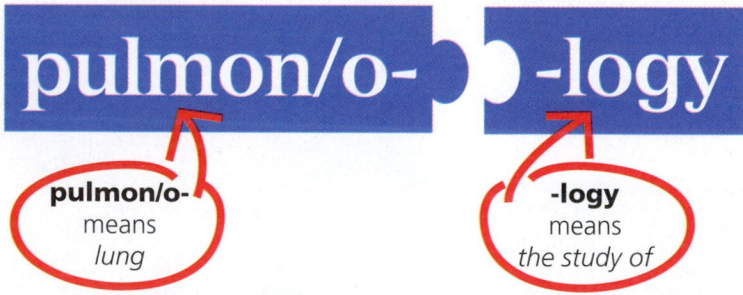

pulmon/o-
means
lung

-logy
means
the study of

	Word Part	Word Part Meaning
Suffix	-logy	*the study of*
Combining Form	pulmon/o-	*lung*

Pulmonology: *The study of the lungs (and related structures).*

Anatomy and Physiology

The **respiratory system** consists of the right and left lungs and the air passageways that connect the lungs to the outside of the body (see Figure 4-1 ■). The upper respiratory system in the head and neck includes the nose, nasal cavity, and pharynx (throat). The upper respiratory system shares these structures with the ears, nose, and throat system (discussed in "Otolaryngology," Chapter 16). The lower respiratory system includes the larynx (voice box) and trachea (windpipe) in the neck and the bronchi, bronchioles, and alveoli in the lungs. The lungs fill much of the thoracic cavity. The purpose of the respiratory system is to bring oxygen into the body and expel the waste product carbon dioxide.

WORD BUILDING

respiratory (RES-pih-rah-TOR-ee) (reh-SPYR-ah-TOR-ee)
  re- *again and again; backward; unable to*
  spir/o- *breathe; a coil*
  -atory *pertaining to*
Select the correct prefix meaning to get the definition of *respiratory*: *pertaining to again and again breathing.*

nasal (NAY-zal)
  nas/o- *nose*
  -al *pertaining to*
Nasal is the adjective form for *nose*.

Word Alert

The respiratory system is also known as the **respiratory tract.** A tract is a pathway. The adjective **cardiopulmonary** reflects the connection between the heart and the respiratory system. Without the heart, oxygen brought into the lungs would never reach the rest of the body, and carbon dioxide produced by the cells in the body would never reach the lungs to be exhaled.

cardiopulmonary (KAR-dee-oh-PUL-moh-NAIR-ee)
  cardi/o- *heart*
  pulmon/o- *lung*
  -ary *pertaining to*

Anatomy of the Respiratory System

Nose and Nasal Cavity

The nose contains the **nasal cavity,** which is divided in the center by the **nasal septum.** On each side of the cavity are three long, bony projections: the superior, middle, and inferior **turbinates** or **nasal conchae** (see Figure 4-2 ■). These jut into the nasal cavity and slow down inhaled air so that it can be warmed and moistened. The nasal cavity is lined with **mucosa,** a **mucous membrane** that humidifies the air and produces **mucus.** Mucus and hairs in the nose trap inhaled particles of dust, pollen, smoke, and bacteria and keep them from entering the lungs. The sinuses in the bones

septum (SEP-tum)

septal (SEP-tal)
  sept/o- *septum (dividing wall)*
  -al *pertaining to*

turbinate (TER-bih-nayt)
  turbin/o- *scroll-like structure; turbinate*
  -ate *composed of; pertaining to*

concha (CON-kah)

conchae (CON-kee)
Form the plural by changing *–a* to *–ae*.

mucosa (myoo-KOH-sah)

mucosal (myoo-KOH-sal)
  mucos/o- *mucous membrane*
  -al *pertaining to*

mucous (MYOO-kus)
  muc/o- *mucus*
  -ous *pertaining to*

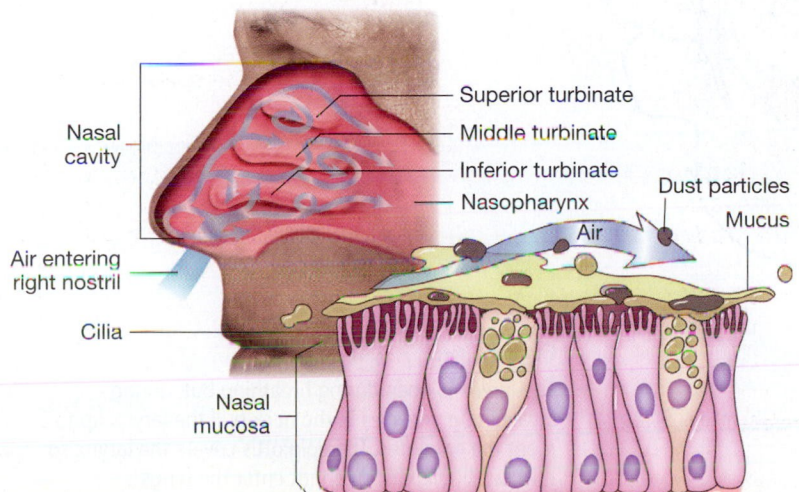

Figure 4-2 ■ Nasal cavity.

Air entering the nasal cavity swirls around the turbinates, allowing the mucosa to warm and moisten it before it goes to the lungs. This helps the body maintain its core temperature and keeps the tissues of the lungs from becoming dehydrated. The mucosa also produces mucus to trap inhaled particles and bacteria before they enter the lungs.

around the nose and elsewhere in the skull are discussed in "Otolaryngology," Chapter 16.

Pharynx

Posteriorly, the nasal cavity merges with the throat or **pharynx.** The **nasopharynx** is the area of the throat that is posterior to the nasal cavity, the **oropharynx** is the area of the throat that is posterior to the oral cavity, and the **laryngopharynx** is posterior to the larynx. The mucous membranes of the pharynx also warm and moisten inhaled air and trap particles. The pharynx is a common passageway for both air and food.

Larynx

At its inferior end, the pharynx divides into two parts: the larynx that leads to the trachea and the esophagus that leads to the stomach (see Figure 4-3 ■). The **larynx** or voice box remains open during respiration and speech, allowing air to pass in and out through the vocal cords. During swallowing, muscles in the neck pull the larynx up to meet the **epiglottis,** a lidlike structure. It seals off the entrance to the larynx so that swallowed food moves across the epiglottis and into the esophagus, not into the trachea.

WORD BUILDING
pharynx (FAIR-ingks)

pharyngeal (fah-RIN-jee-al)
   pharyng/o- *pharynx (throat)*
   -eal *pertaining to*

nasopharynx (NAY-soh-FAIR-ingks)
   nas/o- *nose*
   -pharynx *pharynx (throat)*

oropharynx (OR-oh-FAIR-ingks)
   or/o- *mouth*
   -pharynx *pharynx (throat)*

laryngopharynx
 (lah-RING-goh-FAIR-ingks)
   laryng/o- *larynx (voice box)*
   -pharynx *pharynx (throat)*

larynx (LAIR-ingks)

laryngeal (lah-RIN-jee-al)
   laryng/o- *larynx (voice box)*
   -eal *pertaining to*

epiglottis (EP-ih-GLAWT-is)

epiglottic (EP-ih-GLAWT-ik)
   epi- *upon; above*
   glott/o- *glottis (of the larynx)*
   -ic *pertaining to*

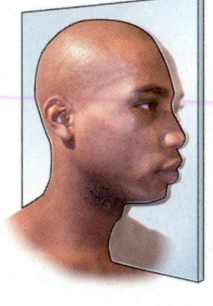

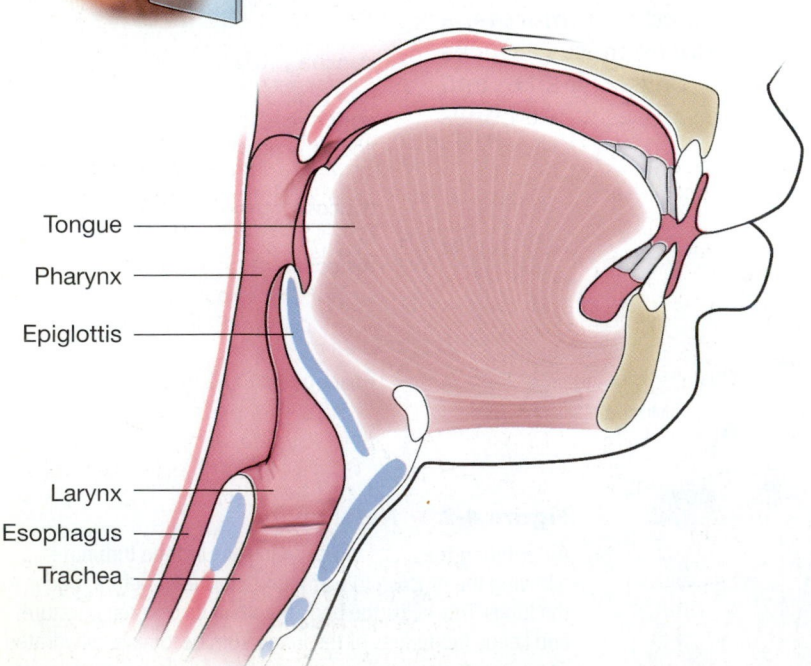

Tongue
Pharynx
Epiglottis
Larynx
Esophagus
Trachea

Figure 4-3 ■ **Larynx.**

The larynx is open during breathing but, during swallowing, muscles in the neck pull the larynx up to meet the epiglottis. The epiglottis covers the larynx so that swallowed food cannot enter the lungs.

Trachea

Below the vocal cords, the larynx merges into the trachea. The **trachea** or windpipe is about 1 inch in diameter and 4 inches in length. It is a passageway for inhaled and exhaled air (see Figure 4-4 ■). A column of C-shaped rings of cartilage provide support to the trachea. On the posterior surface where there is no cartilage, the trachea is flexible and can flatten to make room when a large amount of swallowed food passes through the esophagus.

Bronchi

The inferior end of the trachea splits to become the right and left primary **bronchi** (see Figure 4-4). The primary bronchi contain cartilage rings for support. Each primary bronchus enters a lung and branches into smaller **bronchioles.** The smallest bronchioles (with a diameter of 1 mm or less) have smooth muscle around them, but no cartilage. The **lumen** is the central opening in the bronchi and bronchioles through which air passes. **Bronchopulmonary** refers to the bronchi and the lungs.

The trachea, bronchi, and bronchioles look like the trunk and branches of an upside-down tree and are called the **bronchial tree.** The bronchial tree is lined with **cilia,** small hairs that flow in coordinated waves to move mucus and trapped particles toward the throat where they are expelled by coughing or are swallowed.

Did You Know?

Smoking immobilizes and eventually destroys the cilia. Without cilia, smoke particles easily enter the lung and are deposited there permanently. The normally pink lung tissue becomes gray in color with speckles of black.

WORD BUILDING

trachea (TRAY-kee-ah)

tracheal (TRAY-kee-al)
  trache/o- *trachea (windpipe)*
  -al *pertaining to*

bronchus (BRONG-kus)

bronchi (BRONG-kigh)
Form the plural by changing the *-us* to *-i*.

bronchial (BRONG-kee-al)
  bronchi/o- *bronchus*
  -al *pertaining to*
The combining form *bronch/o-* also means *bronchus*.

bronchiole (BRONG-kee-ohl)
  bronchi/o- *bronchus*
  -ole *small thing*

bronchiolar (BRONG-kee-OH-lar)
  bronchiol/o- *bronchiole*
  -ar *pertaining to*

lumen (LOO-men)

bronchopulmonary
(BRONG-koh-PUL-moh-NAIR-ee)
  bronch/o- *bronchus*
  pulmon/o- *lung*
  -ary *pertaining to*

cilia (SIL-ee-ah)
Cilium is a Latin singular noun. Form the plural by changing *-um* to *-a*. Because there are so many cilia, the singular form *cilium* is seldom used.

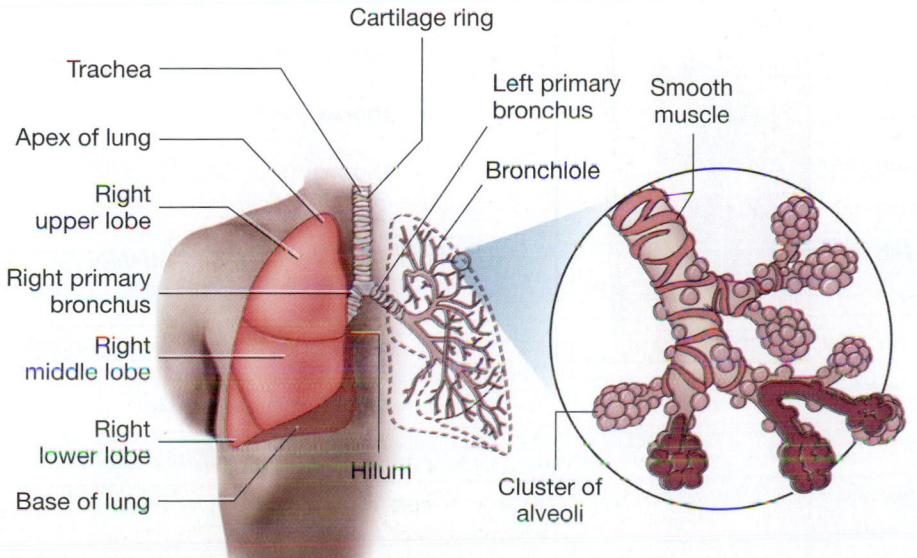

Trachea
Cartilage ring
Apex of lung
Left primary bronchus
Smooth muscle
Right upper lobe
Bronchiole
Right primary bronchus
Right middle lobe
Right lower lobe
Hilum
Base of lung
Cluster of alveoli

Figure 4-4 ■ **Trachea, lung, bronchi, bronchioles, and alveoli.**

The larger right lung has three lobes. The trachea divides into the right and left primary bronchi. A bronchus enters the lung at the hilum and then divides into bronchioles. Alveoli are clusters of microscopic air sacs at the end of each bronchiole where oxygen and carbon dioxide are exchanged.

Lungs

The **lungs** are spongy, air-filled structures. Each lung contains **lobes,** large divisions whose dividing lines are visible on the outer surface of the lung (see Figure 4-4). The right lung, which is larger, has three lobes: the right upper lobe (RUL), the right middle lobe (RML), and the right lower lobe (RLL). The left lung has two lobes: the left upper lobe (LUL) and the left lower lobe (LLL). The rounded top of each lung is the **apex.** The base of each lung lies along the diaphragm (see Figure 4-4). A bronchus enters the lung at the **hilum** (an indentation on the medial surface of the lung). The pulmonary arteries and pulmonary veins for each of the lobes also enter and exit there.

Inside the lung, the bronchus branches into bronchioles, which branch into alveoli. An **alveolus** is a hollow sphere of cells that expands and contracts with each breath (see Figure 4-4). Oxygen and carbon dioxide are exchanged between the alveolus and a nearby small blood vessel (capillary). The alveolus secretes **surfactant,** a protein-fat compound that reduces surface tension and keeps the walls of the alveolus from collapsing with each exhalation. Collectively, the alveoli are the pulmonary **parenchyma,** the functional part of the lung, as opposed to the connective tissue framework around them.

Thoracic Cavity

The **thorax** is a bony cage that consists of the sternum (breast bone) anteriorly, the ribs laterally, and the spinal column posteriorly. The thorax surrounds and protects the **thoracic cavity.** The lungs take up most of the space on either side of the thoracic cavity. Between the lungs lies the **mediastinum,** an irregularly shaped area that contains the trachea (and the heart and esophagus). The **diaphragm,** a sheet of skeletal muscle, lies along the inferior border of the thoracic cavity (see Figure 4-5 ■). The diaphragm is active during breathing.

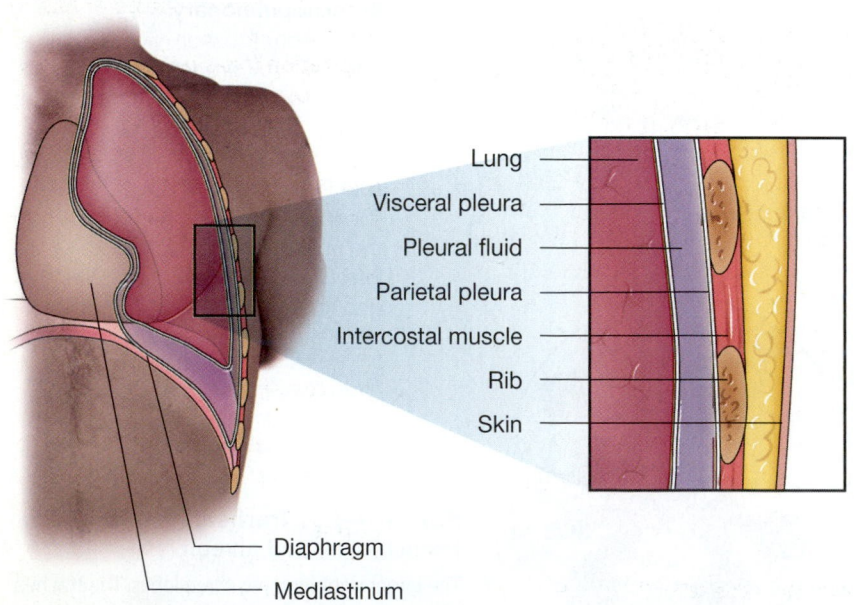

Lung
Visceral pleura
Pleural fluid
Parietal pleura
Intercostal muscle
Rib
Skin

Diaphragm
Mediastinum

Figure 4-5 ■ Diaphragm and pleura.
The diaphragm is the inferior border of the thoracic cavity. The pleura folds back on itself to make two layers. The visceral pleura covers the surface of the lungs. The parietal pleura lines the thoracic cavity. The pleural space between the two layers is filled with pleural fluid.

WORD BUILDING

pulmonary (PUL-moh-NAIR-ee)
  pulmon/o- *lung*
  -ary *pertaining to*
Pulmonary is the adjective form for *lung.* The combining forms *pneum/o-* and *pneumon/o-* also mean *lung.*

lobe (LOHB)

apex (AA-peks)

apices (AA-pih-sees)
Apex is a Latin singular noun. Form the plural by changing *-ex* to *-ices.*

hilum (HY-lum)

hila (HY-lah)
Hilum is a Latin singular noun. Form the plural by changing *-um* to *-a.*

hilar (HY-lar)
  hil/o- *hilum (indentation in an organ)*
  -ar *pertaining to*

alveolus (al-VEE-oh-lus)

alveoli (al-VEE-oh-lie)
Alveolus is a Latin singular noun. Form the plural by changing *-us* to *-i.*

alveolar (al-VEE-oh-lar)
  alveol/o- *alveolus (air sac)*
  -ar *pertaining to*

surfactant (ser-FAK-tant)
Surfactant is a combination of the words *surface* and *active* plus the suffix *-ant* (pertaining to).

parenchyma (pah-RENG-kih-mah)

thorax (THOR-aks)

thoracic (thoh-RAS-ik)
  thorac/o- *thorax (chest)*
  -ic *pertaining to*
The combining forms *steth/o-* and *pector/o-* also mean *chest.*

mediastinum (MEE-dee-as-TY-num)

diaphragm (DY-ah-fram)

diaphragmatic (DY-ah-frag-MAT-ik)
  diaphragmat/o- *diaphragm*
  -ic *pertaining to*

Each lung is located within a **pleural cavity** that is surrounded by **pleura,** a double-layered serous membrane (see Figure 4-5). The **visceral pleura** is the layer next to the lung surface, while the **parietal pleura** is the layer next to the wall of the thorax. The pleura secretes pleural fluid into the **pleural space,** the narrow space between its two layers. **Pleural fluid** is a slippery, watery fluid that allows the two layers to slide smoothly past each other as the lungs expand and contract during respiration.

Physiology of Respiration

Respiration consists of breathing in and breathing out. Breathing in is **inhalation** or **inspiration.** Breathing out is **exhalation** or **expiration.**

Breathing is normally an involuntary process that occurs without any conscious effort. **Respiratory control centers** in the brain regulate the depth and rate of respiration. Receptors in large arteries in the chest and neck send these centers information about the blood level of oxygen, and receptors in the brain send information about the blood level of carbon dioxide. Based on this information, the respiratory control centers control the rate of respiration by sending nerve impulses to the **phrenic nerve,** causing the diaphragm to contract. You can voluntarily control your respirations (when you hold your breath), but eventually involuntary control takes over, forcing you to breathe.

During inhalation, the diaphragm contracts and moves downward as the **intercostal muscles** between the ribs pull the ribs up and out. This enlarges the thoracic cavity and creates negative internal pressure that causes air to flow into the lungs. During exhalation, the diaphragm and intercostal muscles relax, the thoracic cavity returns to its previous size, and air flows slowly out of the nose. A different set of intercostal muscles contracts to pull the ribs down and in to expel air during forceful exhalation (see Figure 4-6 ■). Having a normal depth and rate of respiration is known as **eupnea.**

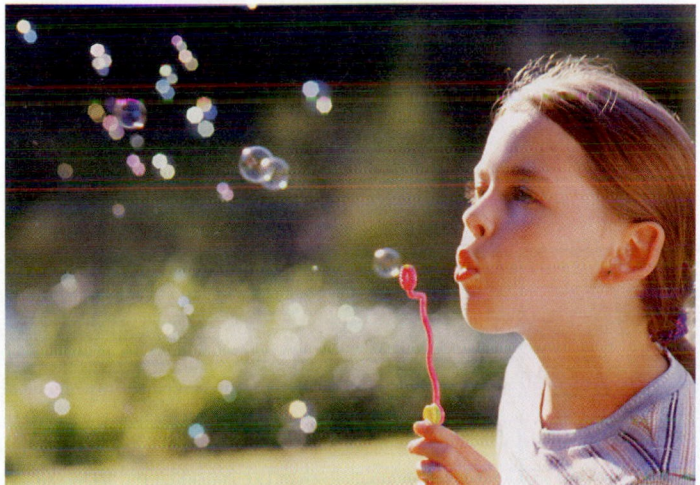

Figure 4-6 ■ Exhalation.
When you want to forcefully exhale air, your brain tells one set of the intercostal muscles between the ribs as well as the abdominal muscles to contract. This quickly decreases the size of the thoracic cavity and expels a large volume of air in just a few seconds—perfect for blowing bubbles, blowing up a balloon, or whistling.

Respiration involves five separate processes.

1. **Ventilation.** Movement of air in and out of the lungs.
2. **External respiration.** Movement of **oxygen** from the alveoli into the blood and the movement of **carbon dioxide** from the blood into the alveoli (see Figure 4-7 ■).
3. **Gas transport.** Transport of oxygen and carbon dioxide in the blood. Oxygen molecules in the blood bind with the hemoglobin in red blood cells to form **oxyhemoglobin. Oxygenated** blood travels from the lungs to the heart, where it is pumped throughout the body to reach every cell. Carbon dioxide also binds with hemoglobin in the red blood cells.
4. **Internal respiration.** Movement of oxygen from the blood into the cells and movement of carbon dioxide from the cells into the blood. Internal respiration is the exchange of these gases at the cellular level.
5. **Cellular respiration.** Oxygen is used by the cell to produce energy in the process of **metabolism.** Carbon dioxide is a gaseous waste product of metabolism.

The respiratory system is solely responsible for the first process. The respiratory system and cardiovascular system share responsibility for the second process. The rest of the processes are done by the cardiovascular system and/or the individual cell.

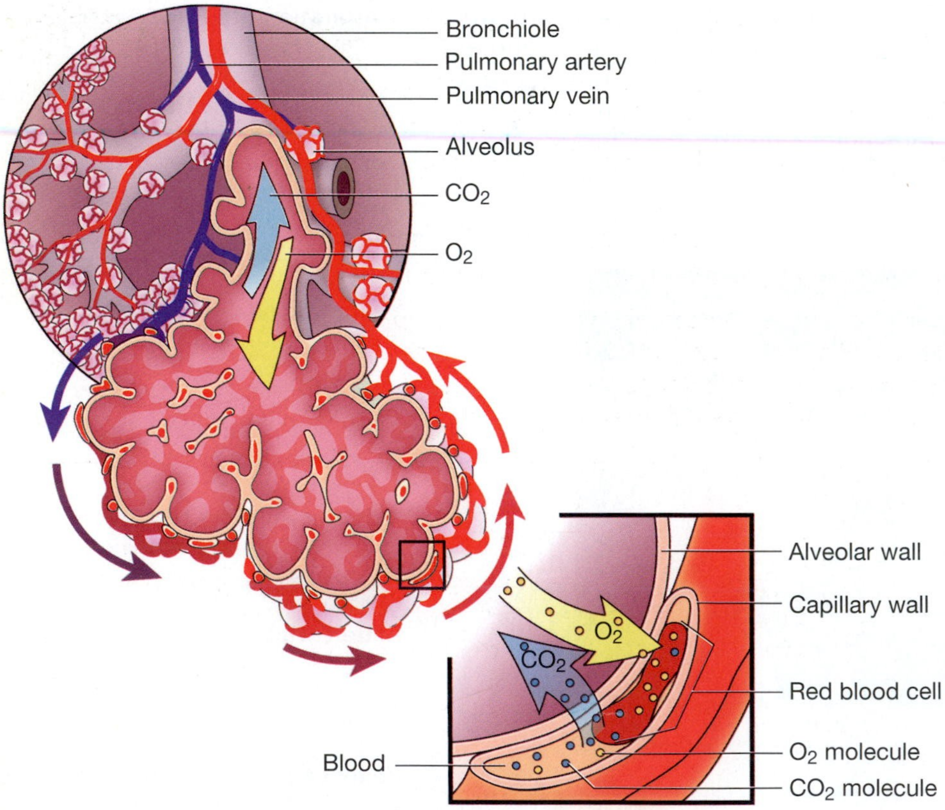

Figure 4-7 ■ Gas exchange.

Oxygen moves from the alveolus into the blood, binds to hemoglobin in a red blood cell, and is carried to the cells of the body. Carbon dioxide comes from each cell as a waste product of metabolism. It dissolves in the blood or binds to hemoglobin and is carried to the lungs where it is exhaled by the lung.

WORD BUILDING

ventilation (VEN-tih-LAY-shun)
   ventil/o- *movement of air*
   -ation *a process; being or having*

oxygen (AWK-seh-jen)
The combining forms *ox/i-, ox/o-,* and *ox/y-* mean *oxygen.*

carbon dioxide
(KAR-bun dy-AWK-side)
The combining form *capn/o-* means *carbon dioxide.*

oxyhemoglobin
(AWK-see-HEE-moh-GLOH-bin)
   ox/y- *oxygen; quick*
   hem/o- *blood*
   glob/o- *shaped like a globe; comprehensive*
   -in *a substance*

oxygenated (AWK-see-jen-AA-ted)
   ox/y- *oxygen; quick*
   gen/o- *arising from; produced by*
   -ated *pertaining to a condition; composed of*

cellular (SEL-yoo-lar)
   cellul/o- *cell*
   -ar *pertaining to*

metabolism (meh-TAB-oh-lizm)
   metabol/o- *change; transformation*
   -ism *process; disease from a specific cause*

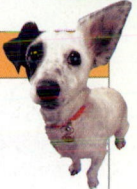

Word Alert

SOUND-ALIKE WORDS

breath   (noun)   the air that flows in and out of the lungs
(BRETH)   *Example: The breath of a diabetic patient can have a fruity odor to it.*

breathe   (verb)   the action of inhaling and exhaling
(BREETH)   *Example: If you ask an asthmatic patient to breathe deeply, you might hear a wheezing sound.*

mucosa   (noun)   a Latin word that means *mucous membrane*
(myoo-KOH-sah)   *Example: If a patient needs more oxygen, the oral mucosa might have a bluish color to it.*

mucous   (adjective)   pertaining to a membrane (the mucosa) that secretes mucus
(MYOO-kus)   *Example: Allergies make the mucous membranes of the nose swollen and inflamed.*

mucus   (noun)   a secretion from a mucous membrane
(MYOO-kus)   *Example: A chronic smoker coughs often and produces a significant amount of mucus.*

Across the Life Span

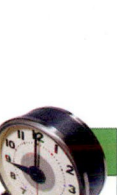

Pediatrics. In the uterus, the fetus does not breathe, and its lungs are collapsed. Instead, it receives oxygen from the mother's lungs via the placenta and umbilical cord. The lungs of the fetus do not function until the very first breath after birth. At that time, they must expand fully and stay expanded (which is helped by the presence of surfactant).

The normal respiratory rate for a newborn infant is 30–60 breaths per minute. The normal respiratory rate for an adult is 12–20 breaths per minute. One inhalation and one exhalation are counted as one respiration.

Geriatrics. As a person ages, some alveoli deteriorate. Because the body does not repair or replace alveoli, the total number of alveoli in the lungs continues to decline with age, and the remaining alveoli are less elastic. The thorax becomes stiff and less able to expand on inhalation. In addition, a lifetime of exposure to air pollution, chemical fumes, and smoke causes damage to the lungs. All of these changes decrease the pulmonary function in older adults.

Vocabulary Review

Anatomy and Physiology

Word or Phrase	Description	Combining Forms
cardiopulmonary	Pertaining to the heart and lungs	**cardi/o-** *heart* **pulmon/o-** *lung*
respiratory system	Body system that brings oxygen into the body and expels carbon dioxide. The upper respiratory system includes the nose, nasal cavity, and pharynx (throat). The lower respiratory system includes the larynx (voice box), trachea (windpipe) in the neck and the bronchi, bronchioles, and alveoli (in the lungs). It is also known as the **respiratory tract.**	**spir/o-** *breathe; a coil*

Upper Respiratory System

mucosa	**Mucous membrane** that lines the entire respiratory system. It warms and humidifies incoming air. It produces **mucus** to trap foreign particles.	**mucos/o-** *mucous membrane* **muc/o-** *mucus*
nasal cavity	Hollow area inside the nose	**nas/o-** *nose*
pharynx	The throat. A shared passageway for both air and food. The **nasopharynx** is posterior to the nasal cavity, the **oropharynx** is posterior to the oral cavity, and the **laryngopharynx** is posterior to the larynx.	**pharyng/o-** *pharynx (throat)* **nas/o-** *nose* **or/o-** *mouth* **laryng/o-** *larynx (voice box)*
septum	Wall of cartilage and bone that divides the nasal cavity into right and left sides	**sept/o-** *septum (dividing wall)*
turbinates	Three long, bony projections (superior, middle, and inferior) on either side of the nasal cavity. They break up and slow down inhaled air. They are also known as the **nasal conchae.**	**turbin/o-** *scroll-like structure; turbinate*

Lower Respiratory System

alveolus	Hollow sphere of cells in the lungs where oxygen and carbon dioxide are exchanged	**alveol/o-** *alveolus (air sac)*
apex	Rounded top of each lung	
bronchiole	Small tubular air passageway that branches off from a bronchus and then branches into several alveoli. Its wall contains smooth muscle.	**bronchiol/o-** *bronchiole*
bronchus	Tubular air passageway that forms an inverted Y below the trachea. Each primary bronchus enters a lung and branches into bronchioles. The **bronchial tree** includes the trachea, bronchi, and bronchioles. **Bronchopulmonary** refers to the bronchi and the lungs.	**bronchi/o-** *bronchus* **bronch/o-** *bronchus* **pulmon/o-** *lung*
cilia	Small hairs that flow in waves to move foreign particles away from the lungs and toward the nose and the throat where they can be expelled	
epiglottis	Lidlike structure that seals off the larynx, so that swallowed food goes into the esophagus, not into the trachea	**glott/o-** *glottis (of the larynx)*

Word or Phrase	Description	Combining Forms
hilum	Indentation on the medial side of a lung where the bronchus, pulmonary arteries, and nerves enter the lung and the pulmonary veins exit	**hil/o-** hilum (indentation in an organ)
larynx	Structure that contains the vocal cords and is a passageway for inhaled and exhaled air. It is also known as the **voice box.**	**laryng/o-** larynx (voice box)
lobe	Large division of a lung, visible on the outer surface	**lob/o-** lobe of an organ
lumen	Central opening through which air flows inside the trachea, a bronchus, or a bronchiole	
lung	Organ of respiration that contains alveoli	**pneum/o-** lung; air **pneumon/o-** lung; air **pulmon/o-** lung
parenchyma	Functional part of the lung (i.e., the alveoli) as opposed to the connective tissue framework	
surfactant	Protein–fat compound that reduces surface tension and keeps the walls of the alveolus from collapsing with each exhalation	
trachea	Vertical tube with C-shaped rings of cartilage in it. It is an air passageway between the larynx and the bronchi.	**trache/o-** trachea (windpipe)

Thoracic Cavity

diaphragm	Muscular sheet that divides the thoracic cavity from the abdominal cavity	**diaphragmat/o-** diaphragm
intercostal muscles	Two sets of muscles between the ribs that contract to pull the ribs up and out during inhalation or down and in during forceful exhalation	**cost/o-** rib
mediastinum	Smaller cavity within the thoracic cavity. It contains the trachea (and other structures such as the heart).	
phrenic nerve	Nerve that, when stimulated, causes the diaphragm to contract and move inferiorly to expand the thoracic cavity during inspiration	**phren/o-** diaphragm; mind
pleura	Double-layered serous membrane. The **visceral pleura** is next to the lung surface. The **parietal pleura** is next to the wall of the thorax. The pleura secretes **pleural fluid** into the **pleural space** (the space between the two layers of pleura).	**pleur/o-** pleura (lung membrane) **viscer/o-** large internal organs **pariet/o-** wall of a cavity
pleural cavity	Hollow space that contains each lung	**pleur/o-** pleura (lung membrane)
thoracic cavity	Hollow space that is filled with the lungs and structures in the mediastinum	**thorac/o-** thorax (chest)
thorax	Bony cage of the sternum and ribs and the spinal column posteriorly that surrounds and protects the lungs and other organs in the thoracic cavity	**thorac/o-** thorax (chest) **pector/o-** chest **steth/o-** chest

Respiration

Word or Phrase	Description	Combining Forms
carbon dioxide	Exhaled gas that is a waste product of cellular metabolism. It is carried in the blood and by the hemoglobin in red blood cells.	**capn/o-** *carbon dioxide*
eupnea	Normal rate and rhythm of breathing	**pne/o-** *breathing*
exhalation	Breathing out. It is also known as **expiration.**	**hal/o-** *breathe* **spir/o-** *breathe; a coil*
inhalation	Breathing in. It is also known as **inspiration.**	**hal/o-** *breathe* **spir/o-** *breathe; a coil*
metabolism	Process of using oxygen to produce energy for cells. Metabolism produces carbon dioxide and other waste products.	**metabol/o-** *change; transformation*
oxygen	Inhaled gas that is used by each cell to produce energy in the process of metabolism. Oxygen is carried in the blood and by the hemoglobin in red blood cells. Blood that contains a high level of oxygen is **oxygenated.**	**ox/y-** *oxygen; quick* **ox/i-** *oxygen* **ox/o-** *oxygen* **gen/o-** *arising from; produced by*
oxyhemoglobin	Compound formed when oxygen combines with the hemoglobin in red blood cells	**ox/y-** *oxygen; quick* **hem/o-** *blood* **glob/o-** *shaped like a globe; comprehensive*
respiration	Consists of five processes: **ventilation** (movement of air in and out of the lungs), **external respiration** (exchange of oxygen and carbon dioxide between the alveoli and the blood), **gas transport** through the blood, **internal respiration** (exchange of oxygen and carbon dioxide between the blood and the cells), and **cellular respiration** (use of oxygen to produce energy in the cell and the production of carbon dioxide as a waste product of metabolism).	**spir/o-** *breathe; a coil* **ventil/o-** *movement of air* **cellul/o-** *cell*
respiratory control centers	Centers in the brain that regulate the depth and rate of respiration	**spir/o-** *breathe; a coil*

Labeling Exercise

Match each anatomy word or phrase to its structure and write it in the numbered box for each figure. Be sure to check your spelling. Use the Answer Key at the end of the book to check your answers.

apex of lung	cluster of alveoli	lower lobe of lung	rib
bronchioles	diaphragm	nasal cavity	sternum
bronchus	larynx	pharynx	trachea

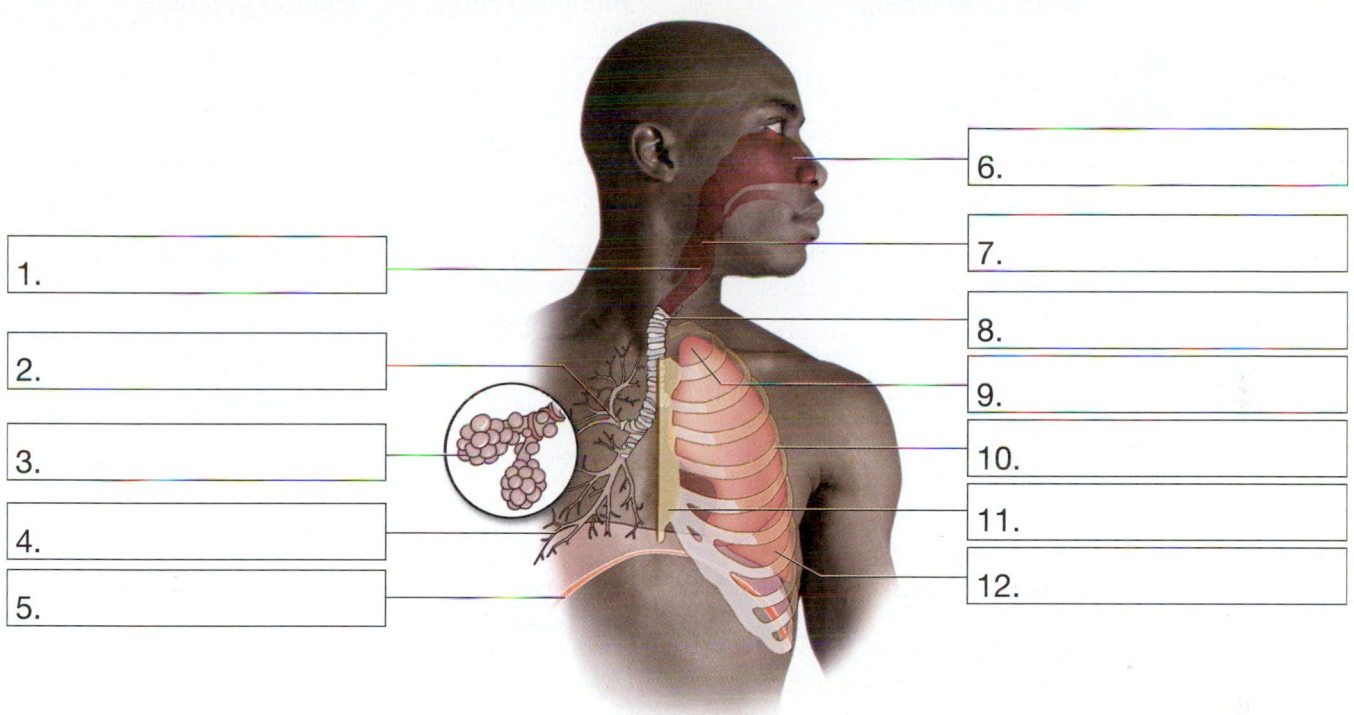

1.

2.

3.

4.

5.

6.

7.

8.

9.

10.

11.

12.

bronchiole	capillary wall	carbon dioxide	cluster of alveoli	oxygen	red blood cell

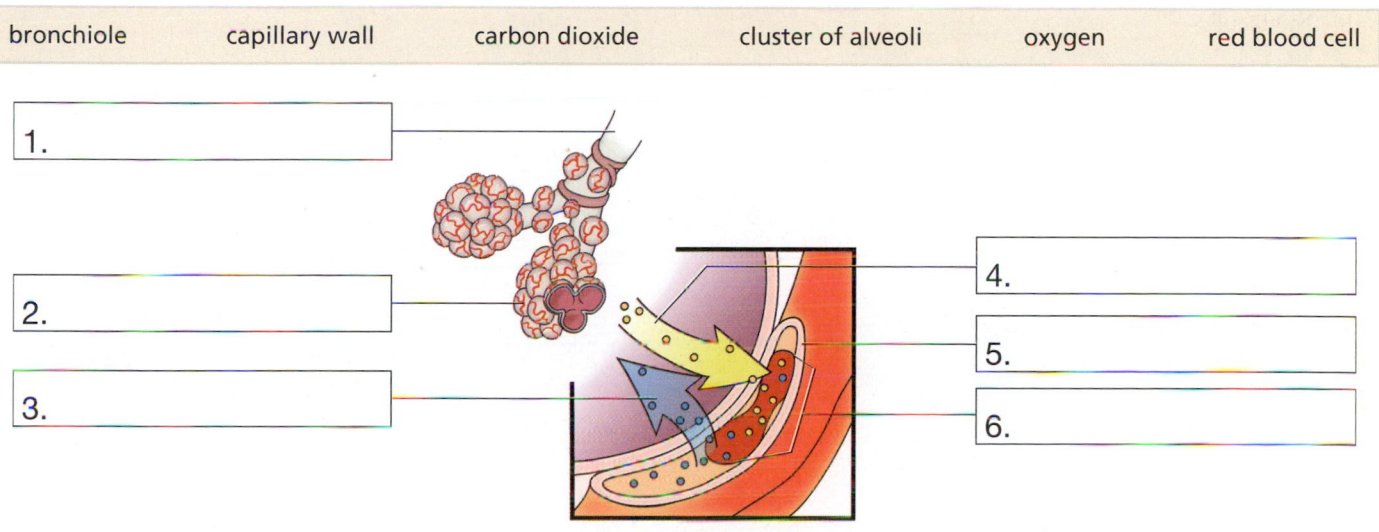

1.

2.

3.

4.

5.

6.

Building Medical Words

Use the Answer Key at the end of the book to check your answers.

Combining Forms Exercise

Before you build respiratory words, review these combining forms. Next to each combining form, write its medical meaning. The first one has been done for you.

Combining Form	Medical Meaning		Combining Form	Medical Meaning
1. **alveol/o-**	alveolus (air sac)	22.	or/o-	
2. bronchi/o-		23.	ox/i-	
3. bronchiol/o-		24.	ox/o-	
4. bronch/o-		25.	ox/y-	
5. capn/o-		26.	pariet/o-	
6. cardi/o-		27.	pector/o-	
7. cellul/o-		28.	pharyng/o-	
8. cost/o-		29.	phren/o-	
9. diaphragmat/o-		30.	pleur/o-	
10. gen/o-		31.	pne/o-	
11. glob/o-		32.	pneum/o-	
12. glott/o-		33.	pneumon/o-	
13. hal/o-		34.	pulmon/o-	
14. hem/o-		35.	sept/o-	
15. hil/o-		36.	spir/o-	
16. laryng/o-		37.	steth/o-	
17. lob/o-		38.	thorac/o-	
18. metabol/o-		39.	trache/o-	
19. muc/o-		40.	turbin/o-	
20. mucos/o-		41.	ventil/o-	
21. nas/o-		42.	viscer/o-	

Combining Form and Suffix Exercise

Read the definition of the medical word. Look at the combining form that is given. Select the correct suffix from the Suffix List and write it on the blank line. Then build the medical word and write it on the line. (Remember: You may need to remove the combining vowel. Always remove the hyphens and slash.) Be sure to check your spelling. The first one has been done for you.

SUFFIX LIST

-al (pertaining to)	-ation (a process; being or having)	-ism (process; disease from a specific cause)
-ar (pertaining to)	-eal (pertaining to)	-logy (the study of)
-ary (pertaining to)	-ic (pertaining to)	-ole (small thing)

	Definition of the Medical Word	Combining Form	Suffix	Build the Medical Word
1.	Pertaining to the alveolus	alveol/o- ⟩ ⟨ -ar		_alveolar_

(You think *pertaining to* (-ar) + *the alveolus* (alveol/o-). You change the order of the word parts to put the suffix last. You write *alveolar*.)

2.	Pertaining to the nose	nas/o-	_____	_____
3.	Pertaining to the trachea	trache/o-	_____	_____
4.	Pertaining to the lungs	pulmon/o-	_____	_____
5.	Pertaining to (the nerve for) the diaphragm	phren/o-	_____	_____
6.	Small thing (that comes from a) bronchus	bronchi/o-	_____	_____
7.	Pertaining to the chest	thorac/o-	_____	_____
8.	Pertaining to a lobe of the lung	lob/o-	_____	_____
9.	The study of the lung (and related structures)	pulmon/o-	_____	_____
10.	A process of movement of air	ventil/o-	_____	_____
11.	Process of change or transformation (that happens within a cell)	metabol/o-	_____	_____
12.	Pertaining to the bronchus	bronchi/o-	_____	_____
13.	Pertaining to the bronchiole	bronchiol/o-	_____	_____
14.	Pertaining to the larynx	laryng/o-	_____	_____
15.	Pertaining to the mucosa	mucos/o-	_____	_____
16.	Pertaining to the diaphragm	diaphragmat/o-	_____	_____
17.	Pertaining to the pharynx	pharyng/o-	_____	_____

Prefix Exercise

Read the definition of the medical word. Look at the medical word or partial word that is given (it already contains a combining form and suffix). Select the correct prefix from the Prefix List and write it on the blank line. Then build the medical word and write it on the line. Be sure to check your spelling. The first one has been done for you.

PREFIX LIST

epi- (upon; above)   in- (in; without; not)   re- (again and again; backward; unable to)
ex- (out; away from)   inter- (between)

	Definition of the Medical Word	Prefix	Word or Partial Word	Build the Medical Word
1.	Process of (taking) in a breath	**in-**	**spiration**	*inspiration*
2.	Pertaining to between the ribs	_____	costal	_____
3.	Process of again and again breathing	_____	spiration	_____
4.	Pertaining to above the glottis	_____	glottic	_____
5.	Process of (letting) out a breath	_____	halation	_____
6.	Pertaining to again and again breathing	_____	spiratory	_____

Multiple Combining Forms and Suffix Exercise

Read the definition of the medical word. Select the correct suffix and combining forms. Then build the medical word and write it on the line. Be sure to check your spelling. The first one has been done for you.

SUFFIX LIST	COMBINING FORM LIST	
-ary (pertaining to)	bronch/o- (bronchus)	hem/o- (blood)
-ated (pertaining to a condition; composed of)	cardi/o- (heart)	ox/y- (oxygen; quick)
	gen/o- (arising from; produced by)	pulmon/o- (lung)
-in (a substance)	glob/o- (shaped like a globe; comprehensive)	

	Definition of the Medical Word	Combining Form	Combining Form	Suffix	Build the Medical Word
1.	Pertaining to the heart and lungs	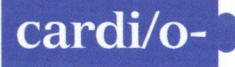 **cardi/o-**	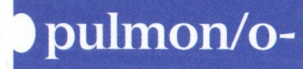 **pulmon/o-**	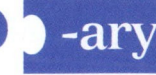 **-ary**	*cardiopulmonary*

(You think *pertaining to* (-ary) + *the heart* (cardi/o-) + *lungs* (pulmon/o-). You change the order of the word parts to put the suffix last. You write *cardiopulmonary*.)

2.	Pertaining to a condition (in which there is) oxygen arising from (the blood)	_____	_____	_____	_____
3.	Pertaining to the bronchi and lungs	_____	_____	_____	_____
4.	A substance (that carries) oxygen (in the) blood (and is) shaped like a globe	_____	_____	_____	_____

Diseases and Conditions

Note: Diseases and conditions of the nose and pharynx are discussed in "Otolaryngology," Chapter 16.

Nose and Pharynx

Word or Phrase	Description	Word Building
upper respiratory infection (URI)	Bacterial or viral infection of the nose and/or throat. It is also known as the common cold or a head cold (see Figure 4-8 ■). Treatment: Antibiotic drugs for bacterial infections.	**infection** (in-FEK-shun) **infect/o-** *disease within* **-ion** *action; condition*

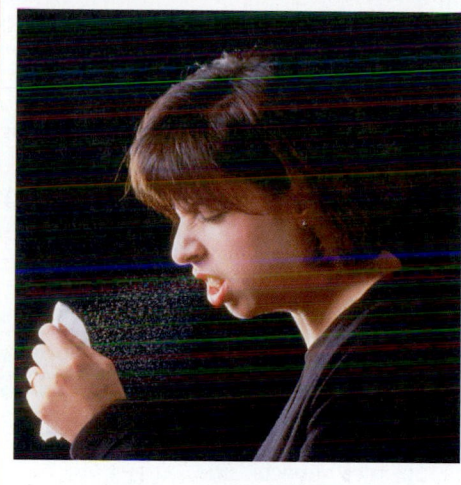

Figure 4-8 ■ Upper respiratory infection.
The common cold is an upper respiratory infection caused by a bacterium or virus. It spreads easily to others on unwashed hands or by droplets of mucus and saliva that are expelled into the air during sneezing and coughing.

Trachea, Bronchi, and Bronchioles

asthma	Hyperreactivity of the bronchi and bronchioles with **bronchospasm** (contraction of the smooth muscle). Inflammation and swelling severely narrow the lumens. Attacks are triggered by exposure to allergens, dust, mold, smoke, inhaled chemicals, exercise, cold air, or emotional stress. It is also known as **reactive airway disease.** There is severe shortness of breath, mucus production, coughing, audible wheezing, and difficulty exhaling. Patients with asthma are said to be **asthmatic. Status asthmaticus** is a prolonged, extremely severe, life-threatening asthma attack. Treatment: Avoid things that trigger asthma attacks. Corticosteroid drugs, bronchodilator drugs, and leukotriene receptor blocker drugs to prevent attacks. Inhaled bronchodilator drugs during attacks. Oxygen and epinephrine (Adrenalin) for severe attacks.	**asthma** (AZ-mah) **bronchospasm** (BRONG-koh-spazm) **bronch/o-** *bronchus* **-spasm** *sudden, involuntary muscle contraction* **asthmatic** (az-MAT-ik) **asthm/o-** *asthma* **-atic** *pertaining to* **status asthmaticus** (STAT-us az-MAT-ih-kus)

Clinical Connections

Public Health. Asthma is prevalent in poor inner-city children. Researchers found that exposure to cockroaches appears to be a strong asthma trigger. Extermination of live cockroaches does not eliminate the problem because cockroach droppings and carcasses remain behind the walls of apartment buildings.

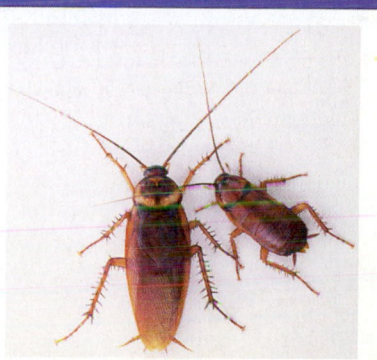

Word or Phrase	Description	Word Building
bronchitis	Acute or chronic inflammation or infection of the bronchi. Inflammation is due to pollution or smoking, and this causes a constant cough, mucus production (**sputum**), and wheezing. Chronic bronchitis is part of chronic obstructive pulmonary disease (COPD). Bronchitis with infection is due to bacteria or viruses. There is coughing, mucus production, wheezing, and a fever. Treatment: Bronchodilator drugs and corticosteroid drugs for inflammation. Antibiotic drugs for a bacterial infection.	**bronchitis** (brong-KY-tis) **bronch/o-** *bronchus* **-itis** *inflammation of; infection of* **sputum** (SPYOO-tum)

Did You Know?

Pack-years are a standardized way to express as a single number the amount and duration of cigarette smoking. Pack-years equal the number of packs smoked per day multiplied by the number of years of smoking.

Word or Phrase	Description	Word Building
bronchiectasis	Chronic, permanent enlargement and loss of elasticity of the bronchioles. Chronic inflammation destroys the smooth muscle, and the bronchioles become overdilated. There is a large amount of mucus with coughing. It is often seen in patients with cystic fibrosis. Treatment: Bronchodilator drugs. Oxygen therapy.	**bronchiectasis** (BRONG-kee-EK-tah-sis) **bronchi/o-** *bronchus* **-ectasis** *condition of dilation*

Lungs

Word or Phrase	Description	Word Building
abnormal breath sounds	Normal inspiration sounds like a soft wind rushing through a tunnel. Abnormal breath sounds include a pleural friction rub, rales, rhonchi, stridor, or wheezes.	

A Closer Look

Pleural friction rub: Creaking, grating, or rubbing sound when the two layers of inflamed pleura rub against each other during inspiration.

Rales: Irregular crackling or bubbling sounds during inspiration. Wet rales are caused by fluid or infection in the alveoli. Dry rales are caused by chronic irritation or fibrosis.

rales (RAWLZ)

Rhonchi: Humming, whistling, or snoring sounds during inspiration or expiration. They are caused by swelling, mucus, or a foreign body that partially obstructs the bronchi.

rhonchi (RONG-kigh)

Stridor: High-pitched, harsh, crowing sound due to edema or obstruction in the trachea or larynx.

stridor (STRY-dor)

Wheezes: High-pitched whistling or squeaking sounds during inspiration or expiration. They are caused by extreme narrowing of the lumen due to bronchospasm from asthma.

wheezes (WHEE-zes)

Word or Phrase	Description	Word Building
adult respiratory distress syndrome (ARDS)	A severe infection, extensive burns, or injury to the lungs (aspiration of vomit or inhalation of chemical fumes) damage the alveoli (see Figure 4-9 ■). The alveoli are edematous (filled with fluid) and do not make surfactant; they collapse with each breath. Treatment: Oxygen therapy. Use of a respirator. Surfactant drug through an endotracheal tube. Treat the underlying cause.	

Poor blood flow

Air flow

Capillary

Fluid in alveoli

Edema of alveolar wall

Poor oxygenation of blood

Blood and fluid leak from capillary wall

Blood clot

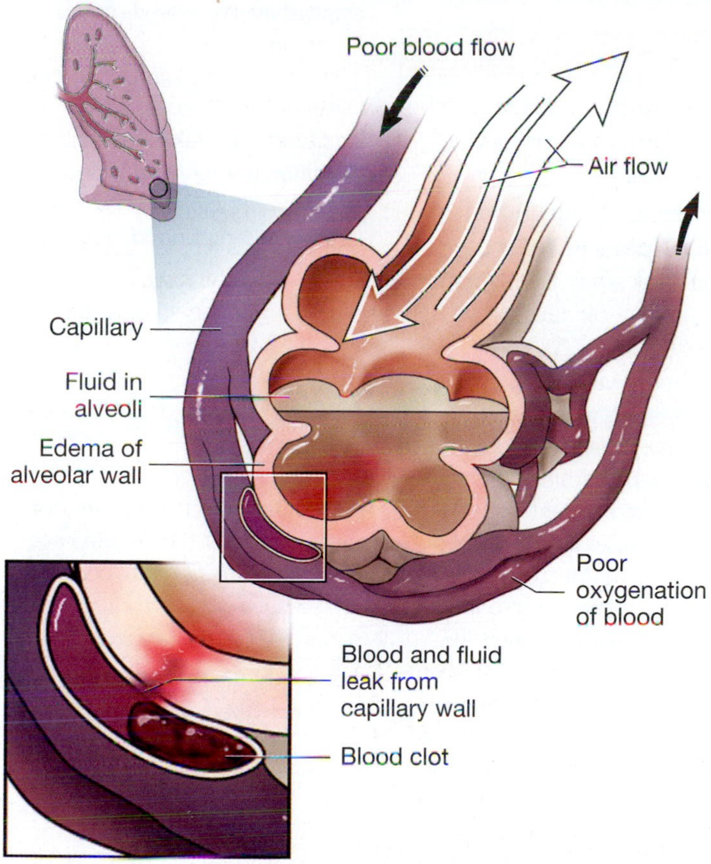

Figure 4-9 ■ Adult respiratory distress syndrome.
The wall of each alveolus is edematous and filled with fluid. There is poor blood flow in the capillary around the alveolus with some blood clots. The capillary walls leak fluid and blood into the alveolus. Capillary blood coming back to the heart (and going to the rest of the body) does not contain enough oxygen.

A Closer Look

Infant **respiratory distress syndrome (RDS)** develops in premature infants who produce too little surfactant because their lungs are not fully mature. There is nasal flaring (the nostrils flare with each breath to draw in more air), grunting (the larynx closes against the epiglottis to maintain pressure in the lungs and keep the alveoli from collapsing), and retractions. Sternal **retractions** bend the flexible breast bone inward. Intercostal retractions pull in the soft tissue and muscles between the ribs. It is also known as **hyaline membrane disease (HMD).**

retraction (re-TRAK-shun)
  re- *again and again; backward; unable to*
  tract/o- *pulling*
  -ion *action; condition*
Select the correct prefix meaning to get the definition of *retraction*: *action of backward pulling.*

atelectasis	Incomplete expansion or collapse of part or all of a lung due to mucus, tumor, trauma, or a foreign body that blocks the bronchus. The lung is said to be **atelectatic.** It is also known as **collapsed lung.** This can develop postoperatively in patients who have shallow breathing and no cough reflex. It appears on a chest x-ray as a hazy, white patch. Treatment: Treat the underlying cause. A chest tube can be inserted to reinflate the lung.	**atelectasis** (AT-eh-LEK-tah-sis) **atel/o-** *incomplete* **-ectasis** *condition of dilation* **atelectatic** (AT-eh-lek-TAT-ik)

Word or Phrase	Description	Word Building

chronic obstructive pulmonary disease (COPD)	Combination of chronic bronchitis and **emphysema** caused by chronic exposure to pollution or smoking. In emphysema, the alveoli become hyperinflated and often rupture, creating large air pockets in the lungs. Air can be inhaled but not exhaled. There is severe coughing, shortness of breath (dyspnea), **sputum** production, fatigue, and sometimes cyanosis. The chronic overexpansion of the lungs deforms the thorax (barrel chest). Treatment: Bronchodilator drugs and corticosteroid drugs. Oxygen therapy.	**chronic** (KRAW-nik)
		  chron/o- *time*
		  -ic *pertaining to*
		
		obstructive (awb-STRUK-tiv)
		  obstruct/o- *blocked by a barrier*
		  -ive *pertaining to*
		
		emphysema (EM-fih-SEE-mah)
		  em- *in*
		  phys/o- *inflate; distend; grow*
		  -ema *condition*
		Add words to make a complete definition of *emphysema*: *condition in (which the lungs are excessively) inflated and distended.*

Did You Know?

In healthy persons, an increased level of carbon dioxide stimulates breathing. Patients with COPD have a constantly increased level of carbon dioxide, so they depend on a decreased level of oxygen (hypoxic drive) to stimulate them to take a breath. Oxygen therapy for COPD patients must be carefully controlled so that it does not take away the hypoxic drive.

Word or Phrase	Description	Word Building

cystic fibrosis (CF)	Inherited, eventually fatal disease caused by a recessive gene. Cystic fibrosis affects all the exocrine cells (those that secrete mucus, digestive enzymes, or sweat), but the respiratory system is particularly affected. Mucus is abnormally viscous (thick), and it blocks the alveoli, causing dyspnea. Constant coughing causes bronchiectasis. There are frequent bacterial infections in the lungs. The chronic lack of oxygen causes cyanosis and clubbing, a deformity of the fingertips (see Figure 4-10 ■). Mucus blocks pancreatic ducts and the secretion of pancreatic enzymes, and so fat is not digested properly. The patient has diarrhea and is undernourished. The pancreas develops cysts that become fibrous, hence the name cystic fibrosis. The sweat glands are overactive; the patient perspires excessively, losing large amounts of sodium. A sweat test shows increased amounts of sodium and chloride in the sweat. Treatment: Daily postural drainage and chest percussion (see Figure 4-11 ■) to remove mucus. Bronchodilator drugs and corticosteroid drugs, digestive enzymes, and a high-salt diet.	**cystic** (SIS-tik)
		  cyst/o- *bladder; fluid-filled sac; semisolid cyst*
		  -ic *pertaining to*
		Select the correct combining form meaning to get the definition of *cystic* (in *cystic fibrosis*): *pertaining to semisolid cysts (which are in the pancreas, not the lungs).*
		
		fibrosis (fy-BROH-sis)
		  fibr/o- *fiber*
		  -osis *condition; abnormal condition; process*

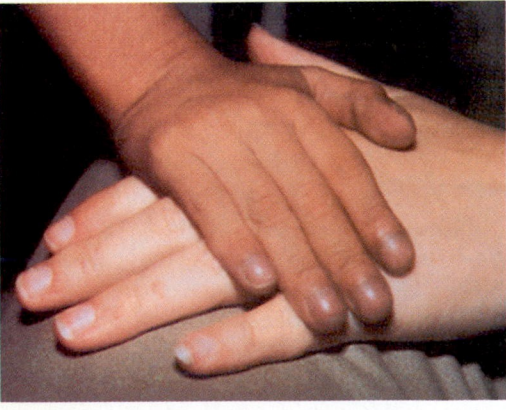

Figure 4-10 ■ Cystic fibrosis.
The hand of a child with cystic fibrosis compared to a normal adult hand (beneath). Cyanosis and clubbing of the fingertips are common in cystic fibrosis. A low level of oxygen causes blood in the arteries to be bluish rather than bright red, and the skin color is cyanotic. The chronic lack of oxygen causes the fingertips and fingernails to grow abnormally.

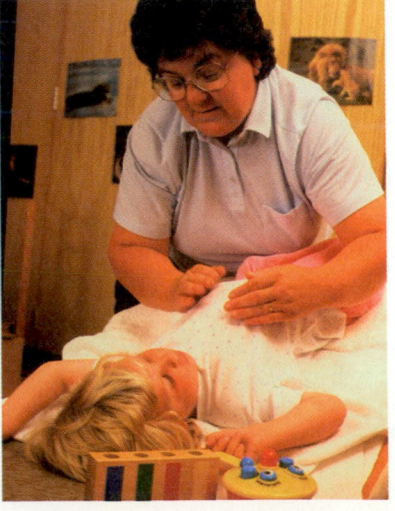

Figure 4-11 ■ Postural drainage and percussion.

This child with cystic fibrosis is lying on a downward incline to promote mucus drainage. The respiratory therapist is using cupped hands to do chest percussion to shake loose the thick mucus in her lungs.

Word or Phrase	Description	Word Building
empyema	Localized collection of **purulent** material (pus) in the thoracic cavity from an infection in the lungs. It is also known as **pyothorax.** Treatment: Antibiotic drugs or surgery to drain the pus.	**empyema** (EM-py-EE-mah) **em-** *in* **py/o-** *pus* **-ema** *condition* Add words to make a complete definition of *empyema*: *Condition in (the lungs of) pus.* **purulent** (PYOOR-yoo-lent) **purul/o-** *pus* **-ent** *pertaining to* **pyothorax** (PY-oh-THOR-aks) **py/o-** *pus* **-thorax** *thorax (chest)*

Word Alert

SOUND-ALIKE WORDS

emphysema   (noun)   Chronic, irreversibly damaged alveoli that are enlarged and trap air in the lungs.
Example: Emphysema caused this patient to have a barrel chest.

empyema   (noun)   Localized collection of pus in the thoracic cavity.
Example: She will be started immediately on intravenous antibiotic drugs for her empyema.

Word or Phrase	Description	Word Building
influenza	Acute viral infection of the upper and lower respiratory system. There is fever, severe muscle aches, and a cough. It is also known as the flu. It occurs most often in the fall and winter months. Influenza plus a secondary bacterial infection can cause pneumonia and death in older adults. Prevention: An annual flu shot. Treatment: Rest, analgesic drugs, and fluids. Antibiotic drugs for a secondary bacterial infection.	**influenza** (IN-floo-EN-zah)

Clinical Connections

Pharmacology. There have been influenza epidemics in the past that killed thousands of people. Today, the most deadly strain of influenza is swine flu (H1N1 strain). (*Note:* For a discussion of flu shots, see the Clinical Connections feature box on page 186.) The use of aspirin to relieve the symptoms of the flu can cause **Reye's syndrome.** The reason for this is not known. There is a very high level of ammonia in the blood and brain, with vomiting, seizures, and liver failure; it is sometimes fatal. Prevention: Use of acetaminophen (Tylenol) instead of aspirin to treat the symptoms of any viral infection.

Reye (RYE)

syndrome (SIN-drohm)
syn- *together*
-drome *a running*
The ending *-drome* contains the combining form *drom/o-* and the one-letter suffix *–e.*

Word or Phrase	Description	Word Building
Legionnaire's disease	Severe, sometimes fatal, bacterial infection. There are flu-like symptoms, body aches, and fever, followed by severe pneumonia with liver and kidney degeneration. Treatment: Antibiotic drug that is effective against this bacterium.	**Legionnaire** (LEE-jen-AIR)

Did You Know?

Legionnaire's disease was first identified in 1976 when many people at an American Legion convention in Philadelphia became sick. Physicians and epidemiologists from the Centers for Disease Control and Prevention (CDCP) were called in to investigate this unknown disease. It was caused by an air conditioning system contaminated by a bacterium that is attracted to the lungs. The bacterium was named *Legionella pneumophilia.*	**Legionella** (LEE-jeh-NEL-ah) **pneumophilia** (NOO-moh-FIL-ee-ah) **pneum/o-** *lung; air* **phil/o-** *attraction to; fondness for* **-ia** *condition; state; thing*

Word or Phrase	Description	Word Building
lung cancer	Cancerous tumor of the lungs that is more common in smokers (see Figure 4-12 ■) than nonsmokers. Lung cancer destroys normal tissue as it spreads (see Figure 4-13 ■). The different types of lung cancer are named for the characteristics of the original **malignant** cell or tissue: squamous cell **carcinoma, adenocarcinoma,** large cell carcinoma, small cell carcinoma, and oat cell carcinoma. Treatment: Surgery, chemotherapy, or radiation therapy.	**cancer** (KAN-ser) **malignant** (mah-LIG-nant) **malign/o-** *intentionally causing harm; cancer* **-ant** *pertaining to* **carcinoma** (KAR-sih-NOH-mah) **carcin/o-** *cancer* **-oma** *tumor; mass* **adenocarcinoma** (AD-eh-noh-KAR-sih-NOH-mah) **aden/o-** *gland* **carcin/o-** *cancer* **-oma** *tumor; mass*

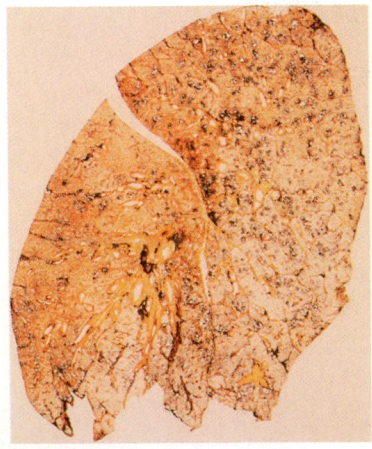

Figure 4-12 ■ Tar deposits in the lung.

This section of lung tissue shows hundreds of large and small deposits of black tar from years of smoking. Cigarette tar also contains carcinogens that can cause cancer.

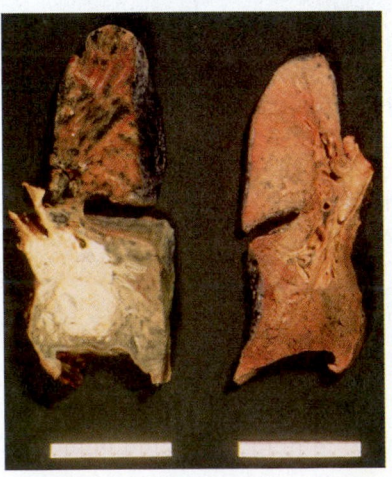

Figure 4-13 ■ Lung cancer.

These are two autopsy specimens of lungs. The normal lung on the right has some small darkened areas due to air pollution or smoking. The lung on the left shows a large, white cancerous tumor in the base of the lung, as well as darkened areas throughout due to heavy smoking.

Word or Phrase	Description	Word Building
occupational lung diseases	Constant exposure to inhaled particles causes pulmonary fibrosis, and the alveoli lose their elasticity. **Anthracosis** (coal miner's lung or black lung disease) is caused by coal dust. **Asbestosis** is caused by asbestos fibers. **Pneumoconiosis** is a general word for any occupational lung disease caused by chronically inhaling some type of dust or particle. Treatment: Wear a filtering mask to prevent inhalation. Bronchodilator drugs and corticosteroid drugs.	**anthracosis** (AN-thrah-KOH-sis) **anthrac/o-** *coal* **-osis** *condition; abnormal condition; process* Add words to make a complete definition of *anthracosis*: *abnormal condition (of the lungs from inhaling) coal (dust).*
	<div align="center">**Clinical Connections**</div> **Public Health.** Sick building syndrome consists of symptoms such as headache; eye, nose, or throat irritation; cough; dizziness; difficulty concentrating; and fatigue. These are not related to any specific illness, and the symptoms subside or disappear shortly after a person leaves that building. Sick building syndrome is caused by inadequate ventilation coupled with indoor pollutants released by carpeting, adhesives, paint that contains volatile organic compounds (VOCs), copy machines, cleaning agents, etc.	**asbestosis** (AS-bes-TOH-sis) **asbest/o-** *asbestos* **-osis** *condition; abnormal condition; process* **pneumoconiosis** (NOO-moh-KOH-nee-OH-sis) **pneum/o-** *lung; air* **coni/o-** *dust* **-osis** *condition; abnormal condition; process*
pneumonia	Infection of some or all of the lobes of the lungs (see Figure 4-14 ■). Fluid, microorganisms, and white blood cells fill the alveoli and air passages. There is difficulty breathing, with coughing and mucus production. Inflammation of the pleura causes pain on inspiration. Pneumonia is named according to its cause or its location in the lungs. Treatment: Antibiotic drugs for bacterial pneumonia. Oxygen therapy and mechanical ventilation, if needed.	**pneumonia** (noo-MOH-nee-ah) **pneumon/o-** *lung; air* **-ia** *condition; state; thing*

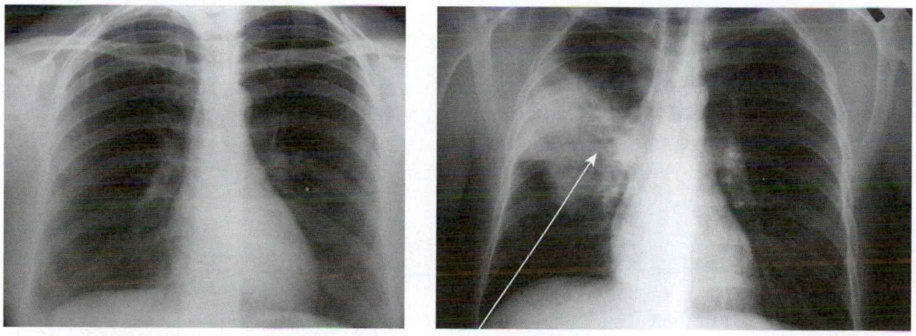

Figure 4-14 ■ Pneumonia.
Compare the normal chest x-ray on the left with the chest x-ray on the right that shows a patchy gray-white area of pneumonia in the right upper and right middle lobes. Remember, when you look at the x-ray, the patient's right lung corresponds to your left side.

Word or Phrase	Description	Word Building
aspiration pneumonia	Caused by foreign matter (chemicals, vomit, etc.) that is inhaled into the lungs	**aspiration** (AS-pih-RAY-shun) **aspir/o-** *to breathe in; to suck in* **-ation** *a process; being or having*

Word or Phrase	Description	Word Building
bacterial pneumonia	Pneumonia caused by bacteria	**bacterial** (bak-TEER-ee-al) **bacteri/o-** *bacterium* **-al** *pertaining to*
broncho-pneumonia	Affects the bronchi, bronchioles, and alveoli in the lung	**bronchopneumonia** (BRONG-koh-noo-MOH-nee-ah) **bronch/o-** *bronchus* **pneumon/o-** *lung; air* **-ia** *condition; state; thing*
double pneumonia	Involves both lungs	
lobar pneumonia	Affects part or all of one lobe of the lung. **Panlobar** pneumonia affects all of the lobes in one lung.	**lobar** (LOH-bar) **lob/o-** *lobe of an organ* **-ar** *pertaining to* **panlobar** (pan-LOH-bar) **pan-** *all* **lob/o-** *lobe of an organ* **-ar** *pertaining to*
pneumococcal pneumonia	Acute pneumonia caused by the bacterium *Streptococcus pneumoniae*. Prevention: Pneumococcal vaccine.	**pneumococcal** (NOO-moh-KAW-kal) **pneum/o-** *lung; air* **cocc/o-** *spherical bacterium* **-al** *pertaining to*
***Pneumocystis jiroveci* pneumonia**	Severe pneumonia caused by the fungus *Pneumocystis jiroveci*. Most people are infected with this microorganism in childhood. It causes a mild infection, and then lies dormant in small cysts. In patients with AIDS, it emerges from the cysts and causes disease. It is known as an **opportunistic infection** because it waits for an opportunity to cause disease. *Note:* In the past, this disease was known as *Pneumocystis carinii* pneumonia (PCP). Treatment: Antifungal and antiprotozoal drugs.	***Pneumocystis jiroveci*** (NOO-moh-SIS-tis YEE-roh-VET-zee) **opportunistic** (AWP-or-too-NIS-tik) **opportun/o-** *well timed; taking advantage of an opportunity* **-istic** *pertaining to*
viral pneumonia	Pneumonia caused by a virus	**viral** (VY-ral) **vir/o-** *virus* **-al** *pertaining to*
walking pneumonia	Mild form of pneumonia caused by the bacterium *Mycoplasma pneumoniae*. The patient does not feel well but can continue daily activities.	
pulmonary edema	Fluid (edema) collects in the alveoli. This is a result of backup of blood in the pulmonary circulation because of failure of the left side of the heart to adequately pump blood. There is dyspnea and orthopnea. Treatment: Correct the underlying heart failure. Oxygen therapy.	**edema** (eh-DEE-mah)

Word or Phrase	Description	Word Building
pulmonary embolism	Blockage of a pulmonary artery or one of its branches by an **embolus** (see Figure 4-15 ■). A patient on prolonged bedrest or one with an injury to the leg can develop a blood clot in the leg (deep vein thrombosis), or a fractured bone can release a fat globule. The embolus (blood clot or fat globule) travels in the circulatory system to a pulmonary artery where it is trapped and blocks the blood flow. There is decreased oxygenation of the blood and dyspnea. A large pulmonary embolus can be fatal. Treatment: Oxygen therapy, thrombolytic drugs (to dissolve a blood clot), and anticoagulant drugs (to prevent more blood clots from forming).	**embolism** (EM-boh-lizm) **embol/o-** embolus (occluding plug) **-ism** process; disease from a specific cause **embolus** (EM-boh-lus)

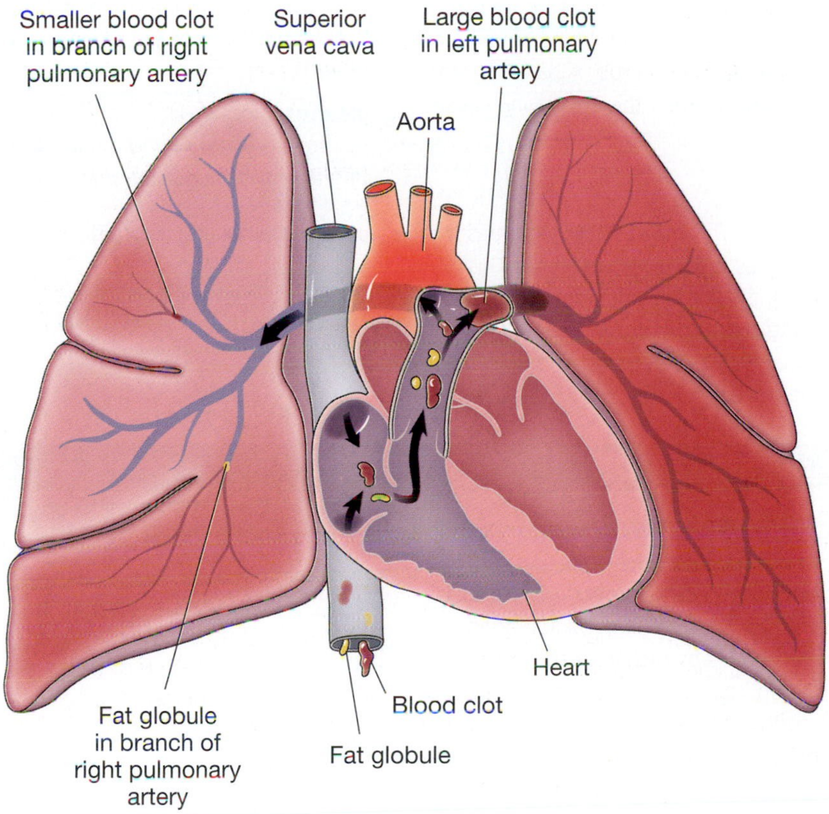

Smaller blood clot in branch of right pulmonary artery — Superior vena cava — Large blood clot in left pulmonary artery — Aorta — Heart — Blood clot — Fat globule — Fat globule in branch of right pulmonary artery

Figure 4-15 ■ Pulmonary embolus.
An embolus (blood clot or fat globule) in a pulmonary artery blocks the flow of blood to the lung. The blood never reaches the alveoli to pick up oxygen. This lowers the overall oxygen content of the blood in the body. The alveoli collapse in that area of the lung.

Word or Phrase	Description	Word Building
severe acute respiratory syndrome (SARS)	Acute viral respiratory illness that can be fatal. There is fever, dyspnea, and cough, together with a history of travel in an airplane or close contact with another SARS patient. Chest x-ray shows pneumonia or adult respiratory distress syndrome. Treatment: Oxygen therapy and ventilator support. Antibiotic drugs are not effective against a viral illness.	
tuberculosis (TB)	Lung infection caused by the bacterium *Mycobacterium tuberculosis* and spread by airborne droplets and coughing. If the patient's immune system is strong, the bacteria remain dormant and cause no symptoms. Otherwise, the bacteria multiply, producing **tubercles** (soft nodules of necrosis) in the lungs. There is fever, cough, weight loss, night sweats, and hemoptysis (coughing up blood). When this bacterium is stained in the laboratory, it holds an acid stain, and so it is known as an acid-fast bacillus (AFB). Treatment: The waxy, external coating around this bacterium makes it resistant to regular antibiotic drugs. Several antitubercular drugs are used in combination for 9 months to treat tuberculosis.	**tuberculosis** (too-BER-kyoo-LOH-sis) **tubercul/o-** nodule; tuberculosis **-osis** condition; abnormal condition; process **tubercle** (TOO-ber-kl) **tuber/o-** nodule **-cle** small thing

Pleura and Thorax

Word or Phrase	Description	Word Building
hemothorax	Presence of blood in the thoracic cavity, usually from trauma. Treatment: Thoracentesis or insertion of a chest tube to remove blood and fluid.	**hemothorax** (HEE-moh-THOR-aks) **hem/o-** *blood* **-thorax** *thorax (chest)*
pleural effusion	Accumulation of fluid in the pleural space due to inflammation or infection of the pleura and lungs. Treatment: Antibiotic drugs or thoracentesis to remove the fluid.	**effusion** (ee-FYOO-zhun) **effus/o-** *a pouring out* **-ion** *action; condition*
pleurisy	Inflammation or infection of the pleura due to pneumonia, trauma, or tumor. It is also known as **pleuritis.** The inflamed layers of pleura rub against each other, causing pain on inspiration. The rubbing sound heard through the stethoscope is a pleural friction rub. A patient with pleurisy is said to be pleuritic. Treatment: Correct the underlying cause.	**pleurisy** (PLOOR-ih-see) **pleur/o-** *pleura (lung membrane)* **-isy** *condition of inflammation or infection* **pleuritis** (ploo-RY-tis) **pleur/o-** *pleura (lung membrane)* **-itis** *inflammation of; infection of*
pneumothorax	Large volume of air in the pleural space. This increasingly separates the two layers of the pleura and compresses or collapses the lung. This is caused by a penetrating injury, or a spontaneous pneumothorax can occur when alveoli rupture from lung disease. *Note:* Air within the lung is normal; air within the pleural space is not. Treatment: Thoracentesis or insertion of a chest tube to remove the air.	**pneumothorax** (NOO-moh-THOR-aks) **pneum/o-** *lung; air* **-thorax** *thorax (chest)*

Respiration

apnea	Brief or prolonged absence of spontaneous respirations due to respiratory failure or respiratory arrest. In premature infants, the immature central nervous system fails to maintain a consistent respiratory rate, and there are long pauses between periods of regular breathing. Middle-aged, obese patients who snore excessively have **obstructive sleep apnea.** They stop breathing as many as 30 times an hour during the night because of obstruction of the airway (by the soft palate or obesity of the neck), and then take a gasping breath that often awakens them. This causes sleep deprivation, fatigue, and difficulty concentrating during the day. Patients having an episode of apnea are said to be **apneic.** Treatment: Home apnea monitors for infants. A continuous positive airway pressure (CPAP) apparatus on the nose to give positive pressure to keep the airway open.	**apnea** (AP-nee-ah) **a-** *away from; without* **-pnea** *breathing* **obstructive** (awb-STRUK-tiv) **obstruct/o-** *blocked by a barrier* **-ive** *pertaining to* **apneic** (AP-nee-ik) **a-** *away from; without* **pne/o-** *breathing* **-ic** *pertaining to*
bradypnea	Abnormally slow rate of breathing (less than 10 breaths per minute). This can be caused by a chemical imbalance in the blood or by neurologic damage that affects the respiratory centers of the brain. Treatment: Correct the underlying cause.	**bradypnea** (BRAD-ip-NEE-ah) **brady-** *slow* **-pnea** *breathing*
cough	Protective mechanism to forcefully expel accidentally inhaled food, irritating particles (smoke, dust), or internally produced mucus. A cough may be nonproductive or productive of sputum. **Expectoration** is coughing up sputum from the lungs. **Hemoptysis** is coughing up blood-tinged sputum. Treatment: Expectorant drugs for a productive cough, antitussive drugs for a nonproductive cough. Correct the underlying cause.	**expectoration** (ek-SPEK-toh-RAY-shun) **ex-** *out; away from* **pector/o-** *chest* **-ation** *a process; being or having* Add words to make a complete definition of *expectoration: a process (of expelling sputum) out (of the) chest.* **hemoptysis** (hee-MAWP-tih-sis) **hem/o-** *blood* **-ptysis** *abnormal condition of coughing up*

Word or Phrase	Description	Word Building

dyspnea	Difficult, labored, or painful respirations due to lung disease. It is also known as **shortness of breath (SOB). Dyspnea on exertion (DOE)** occurs after brief activity in patients with severe chronic obstructive pulmonary disease (COPD). **Paroxysmal nocturnal dyspnea (PND)** is shortness of breath that occurs at night (nocturnal) because fluid builds up in the lungs while the patient is lying down. Patients are said to be **dyspneic.** Treatment: Sleeping propped up on pillows or in a chair. Oxygen therapy. Correct the underlying cause.	**dyspnea** (DISP-nee-ah)
		  dys- *painful; difficult; abnormal*
		  -pnea *breathing*
		
		paroxysmal (PAIR-awk-SIZ-mal)
		  paroxysm/o- *sudden, sharp attack*
		  -al *pertaining to*
		
		dyspneic (DISP-nee-ik)
		  dys- *painful; difficult; abnormal*
		  pne/o- *breathing*
		  -ic *pertaining to*

orthopnea	The need to be propped in an upright or semi-upright position in order to breathe and sleep comfortably. Dyspnea and congestion occur if the patient lies down. The patient is said to be orthopneic. The severity of the orthopnea is expressed as the number of pillows that are needed (i.e., two-pillow orthopnea). Treatment: Oxygen therapy. Correct the underlying cause.	**orthopnea** (or-THAWP-nee-ah)
		  orth/o- *straight*
		  -pnea *breathing*
		Add words to make a complete definition of *orthopnea: breathing (that is only comfortable in a) straight (up position).*

tachypnea	Abnormally rapid rate of breathing (greater than 20 breaths per minute in adults), that is caused by lung disease. The patient is said to be **tachypneic.** Treatment: Oxygen therapy. Correct the underlying cause.	**tachypnea** (TAK-ip-NEE-ah)
		  tachy- *fast*
		  -pnea *breathing*
		
		tachypneic (TAK-ip-NEE-ik)
		  tachy- *fast*
		  pne/o- *breathing*
		  -ic *pertaining to*

Oxygen and Carbon Dioxide Levels

anoxia	Complete lack of oxygen in the arterial blood and body tissues. It is caused by a lack of oxygen in the inhaled air or by an obstruction that prevents oxygen from reaching the lungs. The patient is said to be **anoxic.** Treatment: Oxygen therapy. Correct the underlying cause.	**anoxia** (an-AWK-see-ah)
		  an- *without; not*
		  ox/o- *oxygen*
		  -ia *condition; state; thing*
		
		anoxic (an-AWK-sik)

asphyxia	An abnormally high level of carbon dioxide and an abnormally low level of oxygen. Asphyxia can occur in a fetus during the birth process or at any age if a person chokes, drowns, or suffocates. Treatment: Cardiopulmonary resuscitation.	**asphyxia** (as-FIK-see-ah)

Clinical Connections

Obstetrics. Birth **asphyxia** occurs when the fetus in the uterus does not get enough oxygen through the umbilical cord and placenta before or during birth. This can be caused by premature separation of the placenta from the uterine wall, an umbilical cord that is wrapped tightly around the neck, or an umbilical cord that is compressed by the weight of the fetus during delivery.

Sudden infant death syndrome (SIDS). is an acute event in which an apparently healthy infant under 1 year of age suddenly dies. The cause is unknown; it may be due to respiratory arrest from vomiting and aspirating stomach contents, from asphyxiation from soft bedding blocking the nose, from sleep apnea, or from an imbalance of neurotransmitters in the brain. Parents are cautioned to position babies on their backs (or their sides) to sleep.

Word or Phrase	Description	Word Building
cyanosis	Bluish-gray discoloration of the skin because of a very low level of oxygen and a very high level of carbon dioxide in the blood and tissues. It can be seen around the mouth (**circumoral cyanosis**) or in the nailbeds (see Figure 4-10). The patient is said to be **cyanotic.** Treatment: Oxygen therapy. Correct the underlying cause.	**cyanosis** (SY-ah-NOH-sis) **cyan/o-** blue **-osis** condition; abnormal condition; process **circumoral** (SIR-kum-OR-al) **circum-** around **or/o-** mouth **-al** pertaining to **cyanotic** (SY-ah-NAWT-ik) **cyan/o-** blue **-tic** pertaining to

Clinical Connections

Forensic Science. When a person drowns or suffocates, there is a high level of carbon dioxide (CO_2) in the blood, and the skin shows cyanosis. However, when a person dies in a fire or from inhaling the fumes from car exhaust or a faulty space heater, there is a high level of carbon monoxide (CO) in the blood. Carbon monoxide binds to the same site on the hemoglobin molecule as oxygen does, and the hemoglobin is unable to carry any oxygen. Carbon monoxide poisoning causes a characteristic cherry red skin color.

Public Health. One new car in 1960 generated as much air pollution as 20 new cars today. According to the Foundation for Clean Air Progress, air pollution in the United States has decreased dramatically since 1970. The Air Quality Index is a numeral scale that rates the quality of the air daily. An AQI of 0–50 is good, over 100 is unhealthy for sensitive people, and over 300 is hazardous for everyone. California was the first of 23 states to ban smoking in public places such as restaurants and bars, because even secondhand smoke is a carcinogen according to the Environmental Protection Agency. In children, exposure to it is linked to asthma, respiratory infections, and middle ear infections.

Word or Phrase	Description	Word Building
hypercapnia	Very high level of carbon dioxide (CO_2) in the arterial blood. Treatment: Oxygen therapy. Correct the underlying cause.	**hypercapnia** (HY-per-KAP-nee-ah) **hyper-** above; more than normal **capn/o-** carbon dioxide **-ia** condition; state; thing
hypoxemia	Very low level of oxygen in the arterial blood. **Hypoxia** is a very low level of oxygen in the cells. The patient is said to be **hypoxic.** Treatment: Oxygen therapy. Correct the underlying cause.	**hypoxemia** (HY-pawk-SEE-mee-ah) **hypo-** below; deficient **ox/o-** oxygen **-emia** condition of the blood; substance in the blood **hypoxia** (hy-PAWK-see-ah) **hypo-** below; deficient **ox/o-** oxygen **-ia** condition; state; thing **hypoxic** (hy-PAWK-sik)

Laboratory and Diagnostic Procedures

Word or Phrase	Description	Word Building
arterial blood gases (ABG)	Blood test to measure the partial pressure (P) of the gases oxygen (PO_2) and carbon dioxide (PCO_2) in arterial blood. The pH, how acidic or alkaline the blood is, is also measured. The higher the level of carbon dioxide, the more acidic the blood and the lower the pH.	**arterial** (ar-TEER-ee-al) **arteri/o-** *artery* **-al** *pertaining to*
carboxyhemo-globin	Blood test to measure the level of carbon monoxide in the blood of patients exposed to fires or fumes in unventilated spaces. Carbon monoxide is carried by hemoglobin as carboxyhemoglobin. A blood level above 50% is fatal.	**carboxyhemoglobin** (kar-BAWK-see-HEE-moh-gloh-bin) **carbox/y-** *carbon monoxide* **hem/o-** *blood* **glob/o-** *shaped like a globe; comprehensive* **-in** *a substance*
oximetry	Diagnostic procedure in which an **oximeter,** a small, noninvasive clip device, is placed on the patient's index finger or earlobe to measure the degree of oxygen saturation of the blood (see Figure 4-16 ■). It emits light waves that penetrate the skin and are absorbed or reflected by saturated hemoglobin (that is bound to oxygen) versus unsaturated hemoglobin. The oximeter calculates and displays a number for the oxygen saturation of the blood. It does not measure the CO_2 level. Some oximeters also measure the pulse rate; they are known as pulse oximeters.	**oximetry** (awk-SIM-eh-tree) **ox/i-** *oxygen* **-metry** *process of measuring* **oximeter** (awk-SIM-eh-ter) **ox/i-** *oxygen* **-meter** *instrument used to measure*

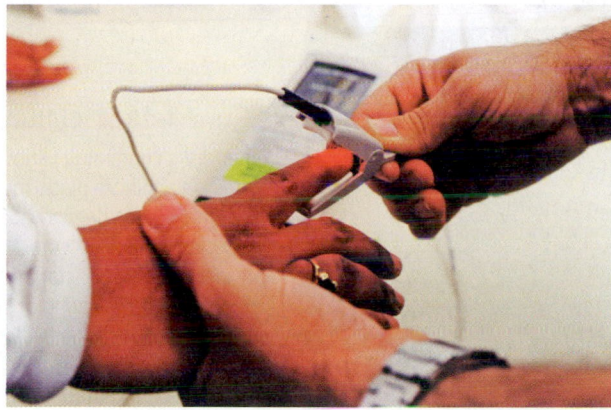

Figure 4-16 ■ Oximeter.

This device is used in ambulances and in hospitals (at the patient's bedside) to provide a quick and accurate readout of the degree of oxygen saturation of the patient's blood.

Word or Phrase	Description	Word Building
pulmonary function test (PFT)	Diagnostic procedure to measure the capacity of the lungs and the volume of air during inhalation and exhalation (see Figure 4-17 ■). The FVC (forced vital capacity) measures the amount of air that can be forcefully exhaled from the lungs after the deepest inhalation. The FEV$_1$ (forced expiratory volume in 1 second) measures the volume of air that can be forcefully exhaled during the first second of measuring the FVC. **Spirometry** measures the FEV$_1$ and FVC and produces a tracing on a graph.	**spirometry** (spih-RAWM-eh-tree) **spir/o-** *breathe; a coil* **-metry** *process of measuring*

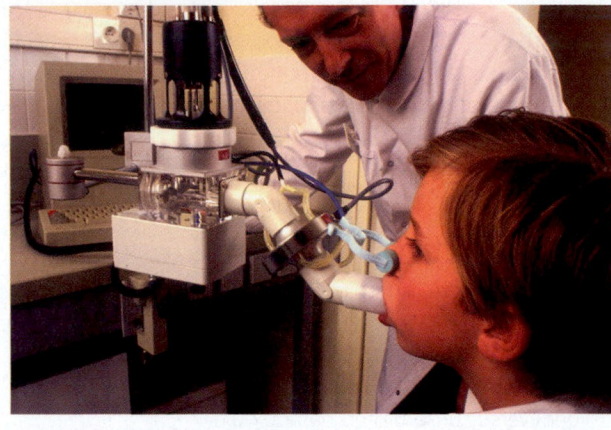

Figure 4-17 ■ Pulmonary function test.
This child who has asthma is having a pulmonary function test. The blue clip on his nose ensures that air only flows in and out of his mouth so that the volume of air in his lungs can be accurately measured.

Word or Phrase	Description	Word Building
sputum culture and sensitivity (C&S)	Diagnostic test to identify which bacterium is causing a pulmonary infection and to determine its sensitivity to various antibiotic drugs (see Figure 4-18 ■).	**sensitivity** (SEN-sih-TIV-ih-tee) **sensitiv/o-** *affected by; sensitive to* **-ity** *state; condition*

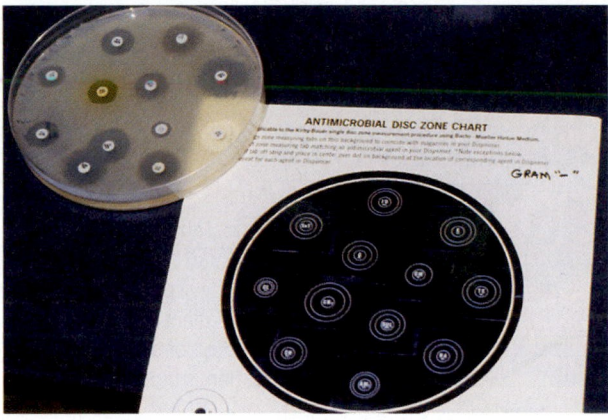

Figure 4-18 ■ Culture and sensitivity.
Paper disks containing various antibiotic drugs are placed on a culture plate. The plate contains a growth medium that has been swabbed with a specimen from the patient (mucus, pleural fluid, etc.). If the bacteria in the specimen are resistant to that antibiotic drug, there will only be a small zone of inhibition (no growth) around that disk. If the bacteria are sensitive to that antibiotic drug, there will be a medium or large zone of inhibition around that disk, and the physician may prescribe that drug to treat the patient's infection.

Word or Phrase	Description	Word Building
tuberculosis tests	Tests to determine if a patient has been exposed to tuberculosis. The **tine test** is a screening test that uses a four-pronged device (similar to the tines on a fork) to puncture the skin and introduce PPD (purified protein derivative), part of the bacterium *Mycobacterium tuberculosis*. The **Mantoux test** is a diagnostic test that uses an intradermal injection of PPD. A raised skin reaction after 48 to 72 hours indicates a prior exposure to tuberculosis with antibodies to the tuberculosis bacterium. A positive Mantoux test is followed up with a chest x-ray to confirm whether or not the patient has active tuberculosis. A sputum specimen can be smeared on a glass slide, stained, and examined under the microscope to look for the acid-fast bacilli of *Mycobacterium tuberculosis*.	**Mantoux** (man-TOO)

Radiology and Nuclear Medicine Procedures

Word or Phrase	Description	Word Building
chest radiography	Radiologic procedure that uses x-rays to create an image of the lungs. It is also known as a **chest x-ray (CXR).** In an AP (anteroposterior) chest x-ray, the x-rays enter the patient's body through the anterior chest and then enter the x-ray plate. In a PA (posteroanterior) chest x-ray, the x-rays enter through the patient's back (see Figure 2-5). In a lateral chest x-ray, the x-rays enter through the patient's side. PA and lateral chest x-rays are often done during the same examination.	**radiography** (RAY-dee-AWG-rah-fee) **radi/o-** radius (forearm bone); x-rays; radiation **-graphy** process of recording
CT scan and MRI scan	Radiologic procedures that scan a narrow slice of tissue and create an image. This process is known as **tomography.** A computer then assembles all of the "slices" into a three-dimensional image. A CT scan (which uses x-rays) and an MRI scan (which uses a magnetic field) are better at showing soft tissue structures than is radiography.	**tomography** (toh-MAWG-rah-fee) **tom/o-** cut; slice; layer **-graphy** process of recording
lung scan	Nuclear medicine procedure that uses inhaled radioactive gas to show air flow (ventilation) in the lungs. Areas of decreased uptake ("cold spots") indicate pneumonia, atelectasis, or pleural effusion. A radioactive solution is given intravenously for the perfusion part of the scan. Areas of decreased uptake indicate poor blood flow to that part of the lung (and possible pulmonary embolus). It is also known as a **ventilation-perfusion (V/Q) scan.**	**ventilation** (VEN-tih-LAY-shun) **ventil/o-** movement of air **-ation** a process; being or having **perfusion** (per-FYOO-zhun) **per-** through; throughout **fus/o-** pouring **-ion** action; condition

Medical and Surgical Procedures

Medical Procedures

Word or Phrase	Description	Word Building
auscultation and percussion	Procedure that uses a **stethoscope** to listen to breath sounds (see Figures 2-20 and 4-21). Percussion uses the finger of one hand to tap over the finger of the other hand that is spread across the patient's back over a lobe of the lung. After a few taps, the hand is moved over another lobe. The sound tells the physician if the lung is clear or if there is fluid or a tumor present (see Figure 2-21).	**auscultation** (AWS-kul-TAY-shun) **auscult/o-** *listening* **-ation** *a process; being or having* **percussion** (per-KUSH-un) **percuss/o-** *tapping* **-ion** *action; condition* **stethoscope** (STETH-oh-skohp) **steth/o-** *chest* **-scope** *instrument used to examine*
cardiopulmonary resuscitation (CPR)	Procedure to ventilate the lungs and artificially circulate the blood if the patient has stopped breathing and the heart has stopped beating. Mouth-to-mouth resuscitation involves forcing air into the victim's lungs; chest compressions pump blood through the heart.	**cardiopulmonary** (KAR-dee-oh-PUL-moh-NAIR-ee) **cardi/o-** *heart* **pulmon/o-** *lung* **-ary** *pertaining to* **resuscitation** (ree-SUS-ih-TAY-shun) **resuscit/o-** *revive; raise up again* **-ation** *a process; being or having*

Clinical Connections

Public Health. Many persons with chronic health problems wear a Medic Alert emblem bracelet or necklace. The back of the emblem describes their disease or condition so that this information is available in an emergency even if they are unconscious.

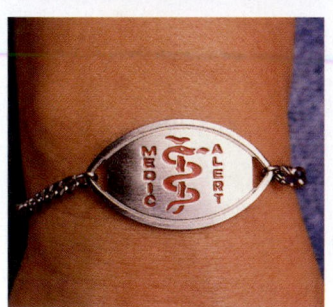

Word or Phrase	Description	Word Building
endotracheal intubation	Procedure in which an endotracheal tube (ETT) is inserted. A lighted **laryngoscope** helps visualize the vocal cords. The tube goes from outside the mouth, between the vocal cords of the larynx, and into the trachea. This establishes an airway for a patient who is not breathing or needs a ventilator (see Figure 4-19 ■). This procedure is performed by paramedics in the field, by physicians in the emergency department, or by anesthesiologists in the operating room prior to surgical procedures. Alternatively, a **nasotracheal tube** that goes from outside the nose, between the vocal cords, and into the trachea can be used. 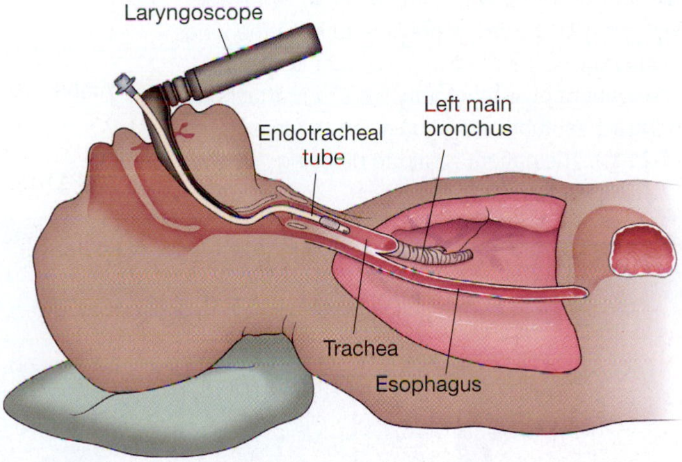 Laryngoscope Endotracheal tube Left main bronchus Trachea Esophagus **Figure 4-19 ■ Endotracheal intubation.** A laryngoscope is used to visualize the vocal cords prior to insertion of an endotracheal tube. The endotracheal tube is positioned in the trachea, just above the bronchi. A small balloon at the tip of the tube is inflated to hold the tube in place, and the external part of the tube is taped to the patient's cheek.	**endotracheal** (EN-doh-TRAY-kee-al) **endo-** innermost; within **trache/o-** trachea (windpipe) **-al** pertaining to **intubation** (IN-too-BAY-shun) **in-** in; within; not **tub/o-** tube **-ation** a process; being or having **laryngoscope** (lah-RING-goh-skohp) **laryng/o-** larynx (voice box) **-scope** instrument used to examine **nasotracheal** (NAY-soh-TRAY-kee-al) **nas/o-** nose **trache/o-** trachea (windpipe) **-al** pertaining to
Heimlich maneuver	Procedure to assist a choking victim with an airway obstruction. The rescuer stands behind the victim and places a fist on the victim's abdominal wall just below the diaphragm and, with both hands, gives a sudden push inward and upward. This generates a burst of air that pushes the obstruction into the mouth where it can be expelled.	**Heimlich** (HYM-lik)
incentive spirometer	Medical device to encourage patients to breathe deeply to prevent atelectasis. A **spirometer** is a portable plastic device with a mouthpiece and balls that move as the patient inhales forcefully.	**spirometer** (spih-RAWM-eh-ter) **spir/o-** breathe; a coil **-meter** instrument used to measure

Word or Phrase	Description	Word Building
oxygen therapy	Procedure to provide additional oxygen to patients with pulmonary disease. Room air is 21% oxygen. A patient can need amounts of oxygen ranging from 22% to 100%. Oxygen is delivered to the patient via a **nasal cannula** (see Figure 4-20 ■) or a face mask. An infant can receive oxygen through a rigid plastic hood placed over the head or in an oxygen tent. Oxygen is drying, and so patients who need a high flow of oxygen or prolonged oxygen therapy receive humidified oxygen (bubbled through water). A patient who requires respiratory assistance as well as oxygen is placed on a **ventilator (respirator),** a mechanical device that breathes for the patient or assists with some breaths. Ventilators can provide up to 100% oxygen, as well as pressure to keep the lungs from collapsing. An **Ambu bag** is a hand-held device that is used to manually breathe for the patient on a temporary basis. It is attached to a face mask or to an endotracheal tube and is squeezed to force air into the lungs (see Figure 4-21 ■). The patient is said to be being "bagged."	**cannula** (KAN-yoo-lah) **ventilator** (VEN-tih-LAY-tor) **ventil/o-** *movement of air* **-ator** *person or thing that produces or does* **respirator** (RES-pih-RAY-tor) **re-** *again and again; backward; unable to* **spir/o-** *breathe; a coil* **-ator** *person or thing that produces or does* **Ambu** (AM-boo)

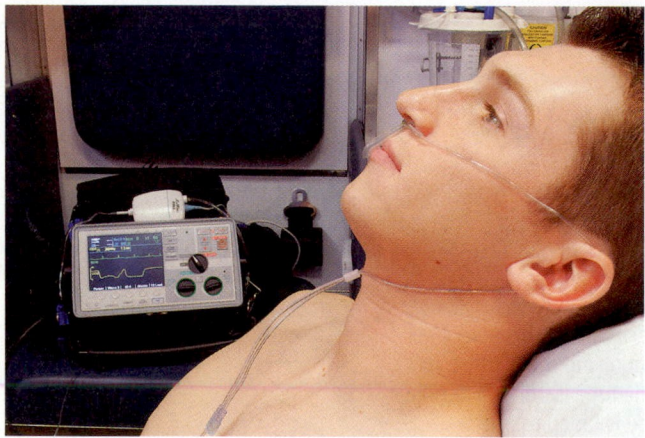

Figure 4-20 ■ Nasal cannula.

This patient is receiving oxygen therapy through a nasal cannula, a plastic tube with two short, flexible prongs that rest just inside the nostrils. A nasal cannula can provide an oxygen concentration up to 45%.

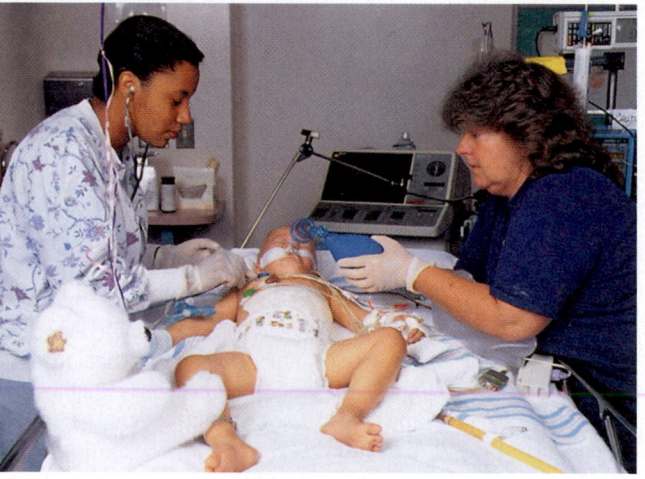

Figure 4-21 ■ Endotracheal tube and Ambu bag.

This infant in the pediatric intensive care unit has an endotracheal tube to assist with breathing. The nurse on the left is using a stethoscope to auscultate the breath sounds in the infant's right lung. The other nurse is squeezing a blue Ambu bag to breathe for the infant until the endotracheal tube is reconnected to the ventilator. The left chest is bandaged where a chest tube was inserted, and the yellow drainage tube for the chest tube is at the bottom right. The infant's pink skin color shows that the level of oxygen in the blood is adequate because of treatment with the ventilator and oxygen.

Word or Phrase	Description	Word Building
vital signs	Procedure during a physical examination in which the temperature, pulse, respirations (TPR), and blood pressure (BP) are measured. The respirations are measured for 1 minute by counting each rise and fall of the thorax as one breath. An assessment of pain is often done as well as the fifth vital sign.	

Surgical Procedures

Word or Phrase	Description	Word Building
bronchoscopy	Procedure that uses a lighted **bronchoscope** inserted through the mouth and larynx to examine the trachea and bronchi. Attachments on the bronchoscope can remove foreign bodies, suction thick mucus, or perform a biopsy.	**bronchoscopy** (brong-KAWS-koh-pee) **bronch/o-** *bronchus* **-scopy** *process of using an instrument to examine* **bronchoscope** (BRONG-koh-skohp) **bronch/o-** *bronchus* **-scope** *instrument used to examine*
chest tube insertion	Procedure that inserts a plastic tube between the ribs and into the thoracic cavity to remove accumulated air or blood due to trauma or infection. The tube is connected to a container (to measure the drainage) and to a suction device. A chest tube is used to treat pneumothorax, pyothorax, or hemothorax.	
lung resection	Procedure to remove part or all of a lung. A wedge resection removes a small wedge-shaped piece of lung tissue. A segmental resection removes a large piece or a segment of a lobe. A **lobectomy** removes an entire lobe (see Figure 4-22 ■). A **pneumonectomy** removes an entire lung. A lung resection is done as a biopsy procedure or to treat severe emphysema or lung cancer.	**resection** (ree-SEK-shun) **resect/o-** *to cut out; remove* **-ion** *action; condition* **lobectomy** (loh-BEK-toh-mee) **lob/o-** *lobe of an organ* **-ectomy** *surgical excision* **pneumonectomy** (NOO-moh-NEK-toh-mee) **pneumon/o-** *lung; air* **-ectomy** *surgical excision*

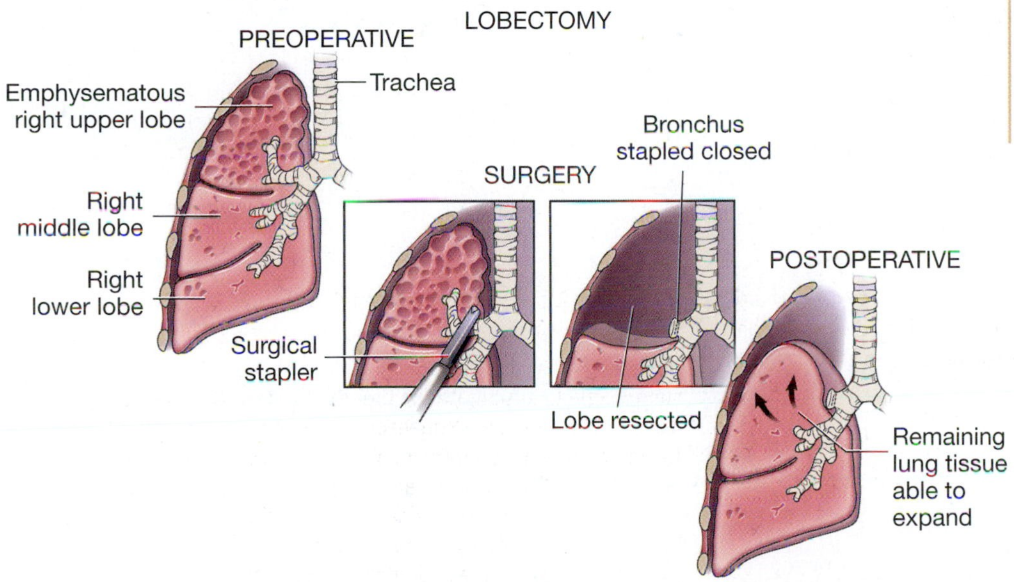

Figure 4-22 ■ Lobectomy.
A surgical stapler is used to staple and seal spongy lung tissue and the bronchus. Then the emphysematous right upper lobe is removed (resected). The remaining lung tissue has more room to normally expand with each breath.

Word or Phrase	Description	Word Building
thoracentesis	Procedure that uses a needle and a vacuum container to remove pleural fluid from the pleural space. It is used to treat a pleural effusion or obtain fluid for the diagnosis of lung cancer. It is also known as a **thoracocentesis.**	**thoracentesis** (THOR-ah-sen-TEE-sis) **thorac/o-** *thorax (chest)* **-centesis** *procedure to puncture* Note: The duplicated c is deleted.
thoracotomy	Incision into the thoracic cavity. This is the first step of a surgical procedure involving the thoracic cavity and lungs.	**thoracotomy** (THOR-ah-KAW-toh-mee) **thorac/o-** *thorax (chest)* **-tomy** *process of cutting or making an incision*

Word or Phrase	Description	Word Building
tracheostomy	This procedure begins with an incision into the trachea (**tracheotomy**) to create an opening. A tracheostomy tube is then inserted to keep the opening from closing (see Figure 4-23 ■). A tracheostomy provides temporary or permanent access to the lungs in patients who need respiratory support, usually with a ventilator. The patient is said to have a "trach." 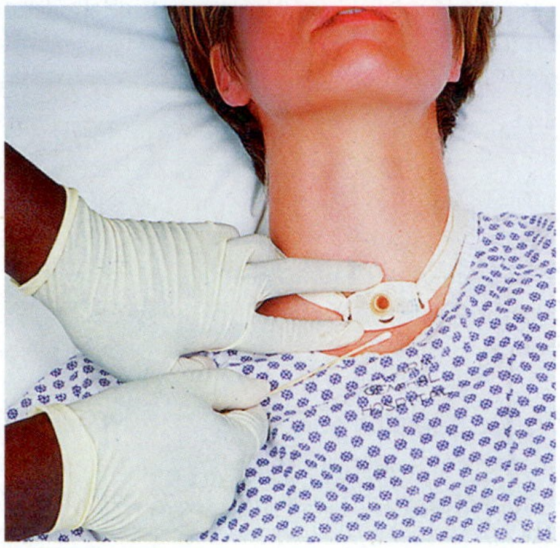	**tracheostomy** (TRAY-kee-AWS-toh-mee) **trache/o-** *trachea (windpipe)* **-stomy** *surgically created opening* **tracheotomy** (TRAY-kee-AW-toh-mee) **trache/o-** *trachea (windpipe)* **-tomy** *process of cutting or making an incision*

Figure 4-23 ■ Tracheostomy.

This patient has a permanent tracheostomy. The tracheostomy tube has a wide flange around it with slots where cotton tape can be inserted and tied around the patient's neck to secure the tube in the trachea.

Drug Categories

These categories of drugs are used to treat respiratory diseases and conditions. The most common generic and trade name drugs in each category are listed.

Category	Indication	Examples	Word Building
antibiotic drugs	Treat respiratory infections caused by bacteria. Antibiotic drugs are not effective against viral respiratory infections.	ampicillin (Principen), amoxicillin (Amoxil), ciprofloxacin (Cipro), ceftriaxone (Rocephin)	**antibiotic** (AN-tee-by-AWT-ik) (AN-tih-by-AWT-ik) **anti-** *against* **bi/o-** *life; living organisms; living tissue* **-tic** *pertaining to*
antitubercular drugs	Treat tuberculosis. Several of these drugs must be used together in combination to be effective.	isoniazid (INH), ethambutol (Myambutol), rifampin (Rifadin)	**antitubercular** (AN-tee-too-BER-kyoo-lar) **anti-** *against* **tubercul/o-** *nodule; tuberculosis* **-ar** *pertaining to*
antitussive drugs	Suppress the cough center in the brain. They are used to treat chronic bronchitis and nonproductive coughs. Some of these contain a narcotic drug.	dextromethorphan (Robitussin), hydrocodone (Hycodan)	**antitussive** (AN-tee-TUS-iv) **anti-** *against* **tuss/o-** *cough* **-ive** *pertaining to*
antiviral drugs	Prevent and treat influenza virus infection in at-risk patients with asthma or lung disease.	oseltamivir (Tamiflu)	**antiviral** (AN-tee-VY-ral) **anti-** *against* **vir/o-** *virus* **-al** *pertaining to*
bronchodilator drugs	Dilate constricted airways by relaxing the smooth muscles that surround the bronchioles. They are used to treat asthma, COPD, emphysema, and cystic fibrosis. They are given orally or inhaled through a metered-dose inhaler (MDI) (see Figure 4-24 ■).	albuterol (Proventil), salmeterol (Serevent), theophylline (Bronkodyl)	**bronchodilator** (BRONG-koh-DY-lay-tor) **bronch/o-** *bronchus* **dilat/o-** *dilate; widen* **-or** *person or thing that produces or does*

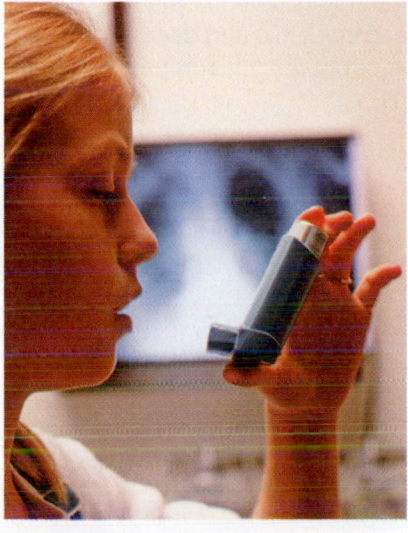

Figure 4-24 ■ Metered-dose inhaler.

A metered-dose inhaler (MDI) automatically delivers a premeasured dose of a bronchodilator drug or corticosteroid drug into the lungs as the patient inhales through the mouth. The dose is prescribed as the number of metered sprays or puffs.

Category	Indication	Examples	Word Building
corticosteroid drugs	Block the immune system from causing inflammation in the lung. They are used to treat asthma and COPD. They are given by a metered-dose inhaler, orally, or intravenously.	fluticasone (Flovent), mometasone (Asmanex), prednisolone (Orapred), prednisone (Deltasone), triamcinolone (Azmacort)	**corticosteroid** (KOR-tih-koh-STAIR-oyd) **cortic/o-** *cortex (outer region)* **-steroid** *steroid* Corticosteroids are hormones secreted by the cortex (outer region) of the adrenal glands; they have a powerful, anti-inflammatory effect. Corticosteroid drugs have this same effect.
expectorant drugs	Reduce the thickness of sputum so that it can be coughed up. They are used to treat productive coughs.	guaifenesin (Mucinex)	**expectorant** (ek-SPEK-toh-rant) **ex-** *out; away from* **pector/o-** *chest* **-ant** *pertaining to*
leukotriene receptor blocker drugs	Block leukotriene, which causes inflammation and edema. They are used to treat asthma.	montelukast (Singulair)	**leukotriene** (LOO-koh-TRY-een)
mast cell stabilizer drugs	Stabilize mast cells and prevent them from releasing histamine that causes bronchospasm during an allergic reaction. They are used to treat asthma.	cromolyn (Intal)	

Clinical Connections

Public Health. Flu shots are given to prevent influenza. Each February, the Centers for Disease Control and Prevention (CDCP) selects those strains of influenza that are most prevalent in Asia and other parts of the world to include in the flu vaccine that will be offered in the United States the following fall before the start of flu season. Flu viruses mutate constantly, and so the influenza vaccine must be reformulated every year. Persons who get flu shots can still get the flu from other strains of influenza not included in the flu vaccine. The concern about a possible widespread epidemic and deaths from swine flu (H1N1 strain) has resulted in a massive public vaccination program to prevent infection from this specific strain of virus.

Abbreviations

ABG	arterial blood gases	**MDI**	metered-dose inhaler
AFB	acid-fast bacillus	**O₂**	oxygen
A&P	auscultation and percussion	**PA**	posteroanterior (view on chest x-ray)
AP	anteroposterior (view on chest x-ray)	**PCO₂**	partial pressure of carbon dioxide (also pCO_2)
ARDS	adult respiratory distress syndrome; acute respiratory distress syndrome	**PCP***	*Pneumocystis carinii* pneumonia
		PFT	pulmonary function test
BS	breath sounds	**PND**	paroxysmal noctural dyspnea
C&S	culture and sensitivity	**PO₂**	partial pressure of oxygen (also pO_2)
CF	cystic fibrosis	**PPD**	protein purified derivative (TB test); packs per day (of cigarettes)
CO	carbon monoxide		
CO₂	carbon dioxide	**RA**	room air (no supplemental oxygen)
COPD	chronic obstructive pulmonary disease	**RDS**	respiratory distress syndrome
CPAP	continuous positive airway pressure	**RLL**	right lower lobe (of the lung)
CPR	cardiopulmonary resuscitation	**RML**	right middle lobe (of the lung)
CXR	chest x-ray	**RRT**	registered respiratory therapist
DOE	dyspnea on exertion	**RUL**	right upper lobe (of the lung)
ETT	endotracheal tube	**SARS**	severe acute respiratory syndrome
FEV₁	forced expiratory volume (in one second)	**SIDS**	sudden infant death syndrome
FiO₂	fraction (percentage) of inspired oxygen	**SOB****	shortness of breath
FVC	forced vital capacity	**TB**	tuberculosis
HMD	hyaline membrane disease	**TPR**	temperature, pulse, and respiration
LLL	left lower lobe (of the lung)	**URI**	upper respiratory infection
LUL	left upper lobe (of the lung)	**V/Q**	ventilation-perfusion (scan)

*This abbreviation is still used, but it is incorrect, as the name of this organism is now *Pneumocystis jiroveci*.

**This abbreviation is still in use, but many hospitals have removed it from their official list of abbreviations because it also has an undesirable meaning that is unrelated to the respiratory system.

Word Alert

ABBREVIATIONS

Abbreviations are commonly used in all types of medical documents; however, they can mean different things to different people and their meanings can be misinterpreted. Always verify the meaning of an abbreviation.

A&P means *auscultation and percussion*, but it also means *anatomy and physiology*.

BS means *breath sounds*, but it also means *bowel sounds*.

C&S means *culture and sensitivity*, but it can also be confused with the sound-alike abbreviation *CNS* (central nervous system).

PND means *paroxysmal nocturnal dyspnea*, but it also means *postnasal drip*.

PPD means *purified protein derivative* (TB test), but it also means *packs per day (of cigarettes smoked)*.

RA means *room air*, but it also means *rheumatoid arthritis* or *right atrium* (of the heart).

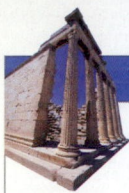

It's Greek to Me!

Did you notice that some words have two different combining forms? Combining forms from both Greek and Latin languages remain a part of medical language today.

Word	Greek	Latin	Medical Word Examples
breathe, breathing	spir/o- pne/o-	hal/o-	respiration, inspiration, inhalation, exhalation eupnea, bradypnea, tachypnea
chest	thorac/o pector/o-	steth/o-	thoracic, stethoscope expectorant
lung	pneum/o- pneumon/o-	pulmon/o-	pneumococcus, pneumoconiosis, pulmonary pneumonia, pneumonectomy
pus	py/o-	purul/o-	pyothorax, empyema, purulent

CAREER FOCUS

Meet Susan, a respiratory therapist in a hospital

"I love my job. I've been doing it for 36 years. I probably could retire, but I choose not to. We treat neonates to geriatric patients. We treat asthma, COPD, and pulmonary fibrosis patients and give information to the patients' families. We also manage oxygen therapy, nebulizer therapy, and medication therapy. We do pulmonary function technology and blood gases. I feel that being a respiratory therapist allows me to feel respected and appreciated, not only by the medical staff, but by the patients because you are giving patient care. You are dealing with the patient directly, as well as the physician. You feel good at the end of the day when you leave."

Respiratory therapists are allied health professionals who perform pulmonary function tests and administer respiratory therapy with various types of equipment that provide oxygen or respiratory assistance to a patient.

　　Pulmonologists are physicians who practice in the medical specialty of pulmonology. They diagnose and treat patients with respiratory problems. Physicians can take additional training and become board certified in the subspecialty of pediatric pulmonology. Cancerous tumors of the lungs are treated medically by an oncologist or surgically by a thoracic or **cardiothoracic** surgeon.

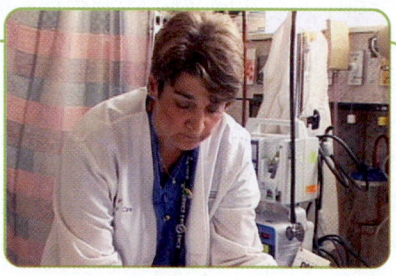

therapist (THAIR-ah-pist)
　therap/o- *treatment*
　-ist *one who specializes in*

pulmonologist
(PUL-moh-NAWL-oh-jist)
　pulmon/o- *lung*
　log/o- *word; the study of*
　-ist *one who specializes in*

cardiothoracic
(KAR-dee-oh-thoh-RAS-ik)
　cardi/o- *heart*
　thorac/o- *thorax (chest)*
　-ic *pertaining to*

PEARSON myhealthprofessionskit™ To see Susan's complete video profile, visit Medical Terminology Interactive at www.myhealthprofessionskit.com. Select this book, log in, and go to 4th floor of Pearson General Hospital. Enter the Laboratory, and click on the computer screen.

CHAPTER REVIEW EXERCISES

Test your knowledge of the chapter by completing these review exercises. Use the Answer Key at the end of the book to check your answers.

Anatomy and Physiology

Matching Exercise

Match each word or phrase to its description.

1. apex
2. turbinates
3. cilia
4. trachea
5. bronchus
6. bronchiole
7. alveoli
8. pleura
9. diaphragm
10. thorax
11. phrenic nerve

_____ Small passageway that ends in several alveoli

_____ Impulse from this structure causes the diaphragm to contract

_____ Projections of bone in the nasal cavity that break up inhaled air

_____ Small hairs in the mucosa that move in waves

_____ Connecting passageway between the trachea and the bronchioles

_____ Air sacs that are the functional units of the lung

_____ Double-layered membrane around the lungs and thoracic cavity

_____ Muscular wall that moves on inhalation

_____ Topmost part of a lung

_____ Bony cage surrounding the lungs

_____ Connecting passageway between the larynx and the bronchi

Circle Exercise

Circle the correct word from the choices given.

1. A large division of a lung that is visible on its surface is known as the (**alveolus, apex, lobe**).

2. The (**bronchioles, lungs, pleura**) have smooth muscle around them that can contract.

3. The bronchus, pulmonary arteries, and pulmonary veins enter and exit the lung at the (**alveolus, base, hilum**).

4. The functional part of the lung that is made up of the alveoli is known collectively as the (**bronchioles, mediastinum, parenchyma**).

5. Swallowed food does not go into the trachea or lungs because of the (**epiglottis, pharynx, turbinates**).

6. (**Carbon dioxide, Oxygen, Surfactant**) keeps the alveoli from collapsing with each breath.

7. The (**diaphragm, phrenic nerve, thorax**) carries an impulse from the respiratory centers of the brain to initiate inspiration.

True or False Exercise

Indicate whether each statement is true or false by writing T or F on the line.

1. _____ Inhalation is another word for inspiration.

2. _____ The upper respiratory system includes the nose, throat, and lungs.

3. _____ Oxygen is carried in the blood in the form of oxyhemoglobin in a red blood cell.

4. _____ The pharynx is an air passageway that connects the nasal cavity and the bronchi.

5. _____ The alveoli are divided into lobes.

6. _____ The visceral pleura is a serous membrane on the surface of the lung.

7. _____ A normal depth and rate of respirations is known as eupnea.

8. _____ Oxygenated blood contains low levels of oxygen.

Diseases and Conditions

Matching Exercise

Match each word or phrase to its description.

1. apnea
2. asthma
3. hemothorax
4. pleurisy
5. pneumoconiosis
6. pulmonary embolus
7. retractions
8. Reye's syndrome

_____ Caused by trauma; treated with a chest tube

_____ Blood clot or fat globule in a pulmonary artery

_____ Creates a pleural friction rub

_____ Premature babies often have this lapse in breathing

_____ Caused by allergies, exercise, cold air, or stress

_____ Sternal and intercostal are two types

_____ Caused by taking aspirin during a viral illness

_____ Occupational lung disease

True or False Exercise

Indicate whether each statement is true or false by writing T or F on the line.

1. _____ Bronchospasm occurs during an asthma attack.

2. _____ Patients who have orthopnea use pillows to prop themselves up to sleep.

3. _____ Hemoptysis means blood in the thoracic cavity.

4. _____ Asthma is also known as reactive airway disease.

5. _____ The two components of COPD are chronic bronchitis and emphysema.

6. _____ Lobar pneumonia is caused by aspirating food while eating.

7. _____ Tuberculosis is spread by air-borne droplets from an infected person coughing.

8. _____ Purulent sputum contains pus.

9. _____ Double pneumonia is twice as serious as regular pneumonia.

Fill in the Blank Exercise

Fill in the blank with the correct word from the word list.

bronchopneumonia	Legionnaire's disease	status asthmaticus	tuberculosis
carcinoma	pulmonary edema	tachypnea	wheezing
cystic fibrosis			

1. Infection that affects the bronchi, bronchioles, and adjacent lung tissue _____

2. Extremely severe, sustained attack of wheezing and difficulty exhaling _____

3. High-pitched whistling or squeaking breath sound _____

4. Eventually fatal, inherited disease of the mucus glands _____

5. Abnormally rapid breathing _____

6. First identified in 1976 _____

7. Malignant tumor of the lung _____

8. Fluid in the lungs from heart failure _____

9. The bacterium that causes this disease has a waxy, resistant coating _____

Laboratory, Radiology, Surgery, and Drugs

Matching Exercise

Match each word or phrase to its description.

1. bronchoscopy
2. carboxyhemoglobin
3. chest tube
4. culture and sensitivity
5. intubation
6. radiography
7. resuscitation
8. spirometer
9. thoracotomy

_____ Taking a chest x-ray

_____ Carries carbon monoxide in the blood

_____ Encourages patients to breathe deeply

_____ Using a scope to look at the bronchi

_____ Used to treat a pneumothorax

_____ Procedure to ventilate the lungs and circulate the blood

_____ Diagnoses a bacterial infection and which antibiotic drug to use

_____ Incision into the chest

_____ Uses an endotracheal tube

Circle Exercise

Circle the correct word from the choices given.

1. A pneumonectomy involves surgical removal of the (**alveoli, lung, trachea**).

2. Oxygen therapy is administered by using a/an (**ABG, nasal cannula, tracheotomy**).

3. (**Carboxyhemoglobin, CXR, Pulmonary function test**) measures the amount of carbon monoxide in the blood.

4. Expectorant drugs are used to treat (**apnea, productive coughs, pneumothorax**).

Dividing Medical Words

Separate these words into their component parts (prefix, combining form, suffix). Note: Some words do not contain all three word parts. The first one has been done for you.

Medical Word	Prefix	Combining Form	Suffix	Medical Word	Prefix	Combining Form	Suffix
1. inhalation	in	hal/o-	-ation	5. circumoral	_____	_____	_____
2. pharyngeal	_____	_____		6. bronchiectasis	_____	_____	_____
3. respiratory	_____	_____	_____	7. panlobar	_____	_____	_____
4. hemoptysis	_____	_____	_____	8. pneumothorax	_____	_____	_____

Building Medical Words

Review the Combining Forms Exercise, Combining Form and Suffix Exercise, Prefix Exercise, and Multiple Combining Forms and Suffix Exercise that you already completed in the anatomy section on pages 162–164.

Combining Forms Exercise

Before you build respiratory words, review these additional combining forms. Next to each combining form, write its medical meaning. The first one has been done for you.

Combining Form	Medical Meaning	Combining Form	Medical Meaning
1. aden/o-	gland	13. embol/o-	
2. anthrac/o-		14. log/o-	
3. aspir/o-		15. obstruct/o-	
4. asthm/o-		16. percuss/o-	
5. atel/o-		17. purul/o-	
6. auscult/o-		18. py/o-	
7. carbox/y-		19. resect/o-	
8. carcin/o-		20. resuscit/o-	
9. cocc/o-		21. therap/o-	
10. coni/o-		22. tubercul/o-	
11. cyan/o-		23. tuber/o-	
12. dilat/o-		24. tuss/o-	

Multiple Combining Forms and Suffix Exercise

Read the definition of the medical word. Select the correct suffix and combining forms. Then build the medical word and write it on the line. Be sure to check your spelling. The first one has been done for you.

SUFFIX LIST	COMBINING FORM LIST	
-al (pertaining to)	aden/o- (gland)	glob/o- (shaped like a globe; comprehensive)
-ia (condition; state; thing)	bronch/o- (bronchus)	hem/o- (blood)
-ic (pertaining to)	carbox/y- (carbon monoxide)	log/o- (word; the study of)
-in (a substance)	carcin/o- (cancer)	pneum/o- (lung; air)
-ist (one who specializes in)	cardi/o- (heart)	pneumon/o- (lung; air)
-oma (tumor; mass)	cocc/o- (spherical bacterium)	pulmon/o- (lung)
-or (person or thing that produces or does)	dilat/o- (dilate; widen)	thorac/o- (thorax; chest)

Definition of the Medical Word

1. Pertaining to the heart and thorax
2. Tumor of a gland that is a cancer
3. Thing (a drug) that produces or does (something to make the) bronchus widen
4. Condition of (inflammation or infection) of the bronchi and lung
5. Pertaining to (an infection in the) lung (that is caused by a) spherical bacterium
6. A substance (that carries) carbon monoxide (in the) blood (and is) shaped like a globe
7. One who specializes in the lung (and) the study of (it)

Build the Medical Word

1. cardiothoracic
2.
3.
4.
5.
6.
7.

Combining Form and Suffix Exercise

Read the definition of the medical word. Select the correct suffix from the Suffix List. Select the correct combining form from the Combining Form List. Build the medical word and write it on the line. Be sure to check your spelling. The first one has been done for you.

SUFFIX LIST	COMBINING FORM LIST
-atic (pertaining to)	anthrac/o- (coal)
-ation (a process; being or having)	asthm/o- (asthma)
-ator (person or thing that produces or does)	auscult/o- (listening)
-centesis (procedure to puncture)	bronchi/o- (bronchus)
-ectasis (condition of dilation)	bronch/o- (bronchus)
-ectomy (surgical excision)	cyan/o- (blue)
-ia (condition; state; thing)	hem/o- (blood)
-ist (one who specializes in)	laryng/o- (larynx; voice box)
-isy (condition of inflammation or infection)	lob/o- (lobe of an organ)
-itis (inflammation of; infection of)	orth/o- (straight)
-meter (instrument used to measure)	ox/i- (oxygen)
-metry (process of measuring)	pleur/o- (pleura; lung membrane)
-osis (condition; abnormal condition; process)	pneum/o- (lung; air)
-pnea (breathing)	pneumon/o- (lung; air)
-ptysis (abnormal condition of coughing up)	py/o- (pus)
-scope (instrument used to examine)	resuscit/o- (revive; raise up again)
-scopy (process of using an instrument to examine)	spir/o- (breathe; a coil)
-spasm (sudden, involuntary muscle contraction)	steth/o- (chest)
-stomy (surgically created opening)	therap/o- (treatment)
-thorax (thorax; chest)	thorac/o- (thorax; chest)
-tomy (process of cutting or making an incision)	trache/o- (trachea; windpipe)
	ventil/o- (movement of air)

Definition of the Medical Word

Build the Medical Word

1. Pertaining to asthma — asthmatic

2. Inflammation of or infection of the bronchus

3. Thorax (that contains) pus

4. A process of listening (to the lung sounds)

5. Abnormal condition (of the skin being) blue

6. Surgically created opening into the trachea

7. Abnormal condition of coughing up blood

8. Surgical excision of a lung

9. Instrument used to examine (listen to) the chest

10. Sudden, involuntary muscle contraction (around the) bronchus

11. Condition of dilation of the bronchus

12. Instrument used to measure the oxygen (content of the blood)

13. Person or thing that produces movement of air

14. Instrument used to examine the larynx

15. Condition of inflammation or infection of the pleura

16. Condition (of infection) in the lung

17. Abnormal condition (of having) coal (dust in the lungs)

18. Process of cutting or making an incision (into the) thorax

Definition of the Medical Word

Build the Medical Word

19. Process of using an instrument to examine the bronchus _____

20. Surgical excision of a lobe (of the lung) _____

21. One who specializes in treatment _____

22. (Abnormal condition of) the thorax (having) air (in it) _____

23. Thorax (that contains) blood _____

24. Instrument used to measure (the volume that the patient) breathes _____

25. A process to revive or raise up again (a patient) _____

26. Process of measuring oxygen (in the blood) _____

27. Procedure to puncture the thorax (with a needle) _____

28. Breathing (in a) straight (up position) _____

Related Combining Forms Exercise

Write the combining forms on the line provided. (Hint: See the It's Greek to Me feature box.)

1. Three combining forms that mean *breathe, breathing*. _____

2. Three combining forms that mean *chest*. _____

3. Three combining forms that mean *lung*. _____

Prefix Exercise

Read the definition of the medical word. Look at the medical word or partial word that is given (it already contains a combining form and suffix). Select the correct prefix from the Prefix List and write it on the blank line. Then build the medical word and write it on the line. Be sure to check your spelling. The first one has been done for you.

PREFIX LIST			
an- (without; not)	em- (in)	hyper- (above; more than normal)	pan- (all)
anti- (against)	endo- (innermost; within)	in- (in; within; not)	tachy- (fast)
dys- (painful; difficult; abnormal)	ex- (out; away from)		

Definition of the Medical Word	**Prefix**	**Word or Partial Word**	**Build the Medical Word**
1. A process of within (the trachea putting) a tube	in-	tubation	intubation
2. Pertaining to difficult breathing	_____	pneic	_____
3. Pertaining to (being in) all lobes (of the lung)	_____	lobar	_____
4. Condition of more than normal carbon dioxide	_____	capnia	_____
5. Pertaining to (a drug that is) against cough(ing)	_____	tussive	_____
6. Pertaining to fast breathing	_____	pneic	_____
7. Condition (of being) without oxygen	_____	oxia	_____
8. Condition in (the lung of) pus	_____	pyemia	_____
9. Pertaining to within the trachea	_____	tracheal	_____
10. Pertaining to (a drug that takes sputum) out (of the) chest	_____	pectorant	_____

Abbreviations

Matching Exercise

Match each abbreviation to its description.

1.	SOB	_____ Inhaler device used to give a bronchodilator drug
2.	FVC	_____ Forced vital capacity
3.	PFT	_____ Disease that includes bronchitis and emphysema
4.	TB	_____ Resuscitation
5.	COPD	_____ Synonym for *dyspnea*
6.	CXR	_____ Tuberculosis
7.	MDI	_____ Radiology test of the chest
8.	CPR	_____ Includes FVC and FEV_1

Applied Skills

Plural Noun and Adjective Spelling Exercise

Read the noun and write its plural form and/or adjective form. Be sure to check your spelling. The first one has been done for you.

Singular Noun	Plural Noun	Adjective	Singular Noun	Plural Noun	Adjective
1. nose		nasal	10. hilum	_____	_____
2. alveolus	_____	_____	11. larynx		_____
3. anoxia		_____	12. lung	_____	_____
4. apex	_____		13. mucosa		_____
5. apnea		_____	14. pharynx		_____
6. asthma		_____	15. pleura		_____
7. bronchus	_____	_____	16. tachypnea		_____
8. cyanosis		_____	17. thorax		_____
9. diaphragm		_____	18. trachea		_____

English and Medical Word Equivalents Exercise

For each English word, write its equivalent medical word. Be sure to check your spelling. The first one has been done for you.

English Word	Medical Word	English Word	Medical Word
1. throat	pharynx	6. flu	_____
2. black lung disease	_____	7. shortness of breath	_____
3. chest	_____	8. common cold	_____
4. collapsed lung	_____	9. voice box	_____
5. crib death	_____	10. windpipe	_____

Medical Report Exercise

This exercise contains a report of an admission to an acute care hospital. Read the report and answer the questions.

ADMISSION HISTORY AND PHYSICAL EXAMINATION

PATIENT NAME: OTT, George
HOSPITAL NUMBER: 208-333-7943
DATE OF ADMISSION: November 19, 20xx

HISTORY OF PRESENT ILLNESS
This 65-year-old Caucasian male was evaluated by me in the emergency department on the above date, complaining of progressive shortness of breath, coughing, fever, and fatigue.

PAST HISTORY
The patient was a coal miner for 25 years before he retired on disability with black lung disease at age 55. He currently smokes 2 packs of cigarettes per day and has done so for the past 22 years. Past surgical history of an appendectomy in the remote past. Chest x-ray done recently showed a suspicious lesion in the LLL; a bronchoscopy was performed and a biopsy was done, but the biopsy results were negative for malignancy.

PHYSICAL EXAMINATION
VITAL SIGNS: Pulse 110, respiratory rate 42 per minute, temperature 100.6, blood pressure 156/96.
GENERAL: The patient appears older than his stated age and quite tired at this time.
HEENT: Negative, except for slight cyanosis of the lips. The neck is supple and free of any masses.
CHEST: There is an increased anteroposterior diameter to the chest. There are no intercostal retractions during inspiration. There are diffuse expiratory wheezes, but no rales or rhonchi.
HEART: Normal heart sounds without murmur, gallop, or rub.
ABDOMEN: Soft and nontender.
EXTREMITIES: Normal with full range of motion noted. There was no clubbing of the fingers noted.

LABORATORY DATA
Complete blood count showed an elevated white blood cell count of 17,600 with 80 segs, 4 bands, and 2 lymphs. Oximeter showed 70% saturation. Sputum was sent for C&S. Chest x-ray: Patchy infiltrates from the apex to the midlung on the right with some consolidative changes involving the entire right lower lobe. There is no pleural fluid noted. There is a density seen in the left lower lobe posterolaterally, which extends to the pleural surface. It is most probably focal scarring or atelectasis from old inflammation.

IMPRESSION
1. Right-sided pneumonia.
2. Chronic obstructive pulmonary disease, secondary to anthracosis and smoking.

Christina S. Jencks, M.D.
Christina S. Jencks, M.D.

CSJ: lcc
D: 11/19/xx
T: 11/19/xx

Word Analysis Questions

1. This patient has dyspnea. What phrase in the History of Present Illness says the same thing? _____ What is the medical abbreviation for this phrase? _____

2. If you wanted to use the adjective form of *dyspnea*, you would say, "The patient is _____."

3. Divide *bronchoscopy* into its two word parts and define each word part.

Word Part	Definition
_____	_____
_____	_____

4. Divide *cyanosis* into its two word parts and define each word part.

Word Part	Definition
_____	_____
_____	_____

5. What do these abbreviations stand for?

   a. C&S _____

   b. COPD _____

   c. LLL _____

Fact Finding Questions

1. What is the medical word for *black lung disease*?

   _____

2. What respiratory surgery did the patient have in the past?

   _____

3. What other surgery did the patient have?

   _____

4. Circle all of the abnormalities that were seen on the patient's CXR.

   intercostal muscles   **consolidative changes**   **density in LLL**   **patchy infiltrates**

   atelectasis   **cyanosis**   **oximeter**   **pleural fluid**

Critical Thinking Questions

1. Of the four medical complaints the patient had when he came to the emergency department, which one was directly related to an infection?

   _____

2. What is the descriptive name that laypersons give for the medical condition of increased anteroposterior diameter of the chest that is seen in patients with chronic obstructive pulmonary disease?

   _____

3. What method of examination would the physician use to hear the patient's expiratory wheezes? (Circle one)

   auscultation   **percussion**   **postural drainage**   **oximeter**

4. The patient has an elevated white blood cell count of 17,600, which indicates an infection. This is due to which of the two diagnoses listed in the Impression section?

   _____

5. Calculate the number of pack-years for this patient's history of smoking.

   _____

On the Job Challenge Exercise

On the job, you will encounter new medical words. Practice your medical dictionary skills by looking up the phrases **cystic fibrosis** *and* **respiratory distress syndrome.** *Did you find the complete definition under the first, second, or third word of the phrase? Which way of word searching is more effective? Write a word searching rule to help you remember how to look up these phrases.*

1. cystic fibrosis

   Complete definition is under: **cystic** **fibrosis** (Circle one)

2. respiratory distress syndrome

   Complete definition is under: **respiratory** **distress** **syndrome** (Circle one)

3. Wordsearching rule: _____

Hearing Medical Words Exercise

You hear someone speaking the medical words given below. Read each pronunciation and then write the medical word it represents. Be sure to check your spelling. The first one has been done for you.

1. an-AWK-see-ah _anoxia_
2. az-MAT-ik _____
3. AWS-kul-TAY-shun _____
4. brong-KAWS-koh-pee _____
5. EM-fih-SEE-mah _____

6. hee-MAWP-tih-sis _____
7. lah-RIN-jee-al _____
8. loh-BEK-toh-mee _____
9. NOO-moh-THOR-aks _____
10. TRAY-kee-AWS-toh-mee _____

Pronunciation Exercise

Read the medical word. Then review the syllables in the pronunciation. Circle the primary (main) accented syllable. The first one has been done for you.

1. bronchitis (brong-ky-tis)
2. bronchopulmonary (brong-koh-pul-moh-nair-ee)
3. cyanosis (sy-ah-noh-sis)
4. pneumonia (noo-moh-nee-ah)

5. respiration (res-pih-ray-shun)
6. thoracic (thoh-ras-ik)
7. tracheal (tray-kee-al)
8. tracheostomy (tray-kee-aws-toh-mee)

Multimedia Preview

Immerse yourself in a variety of activities inside Medical Terminology Interactive. Getting there is simple:

1. Click on www.myhealthprofessionskit.com.
2. Select "Medical Terminology" from the choice of disciplines.
3. First-time users must create an account using the scratch-off code on the inside front cover of this book.
4. Find this book and log in using your username and password.
5. Click on Medical Terminology Interactive.
6. Take the elevator to the 4th Floor to begin your virtual exploration of this chapter!

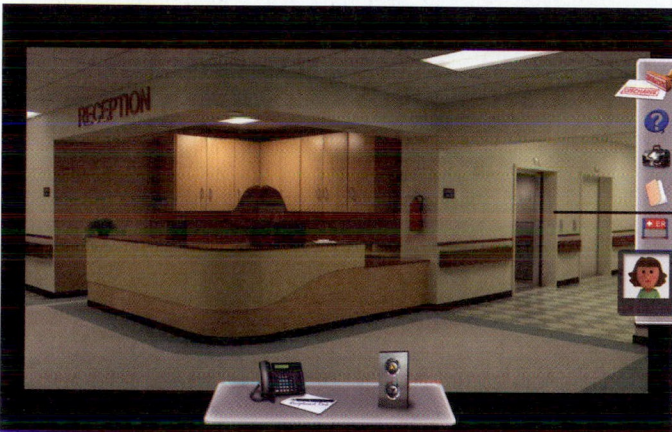 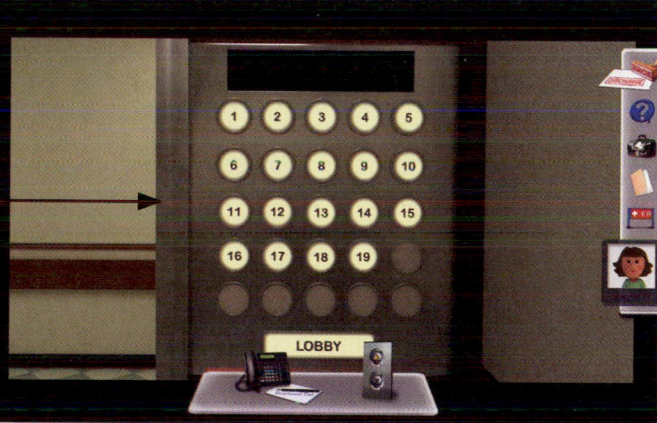

■ Popping Words   Popping pills won't help you study, but popping words might do the trick. Test your knowledge by launching the term pill into the correct container. Ready, aim, fire!

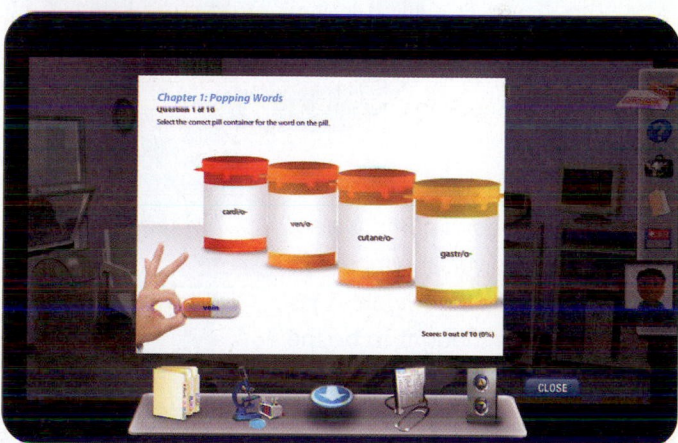

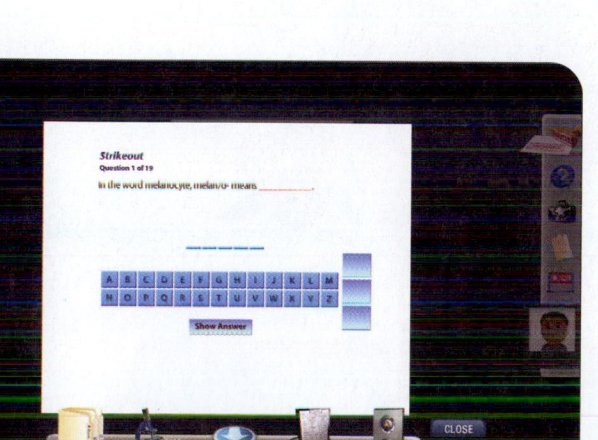

■ Strikeout   Click on the alphabet tiles to fill in the empty squares in the word or phrase to complete the sentence. This game quizzes your vocabulary and spelling. But choose your letters carefully because three strikes and you're out!

PEARSON
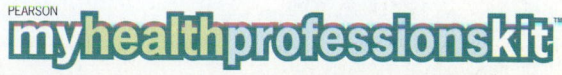
myhealthprofessionskit™

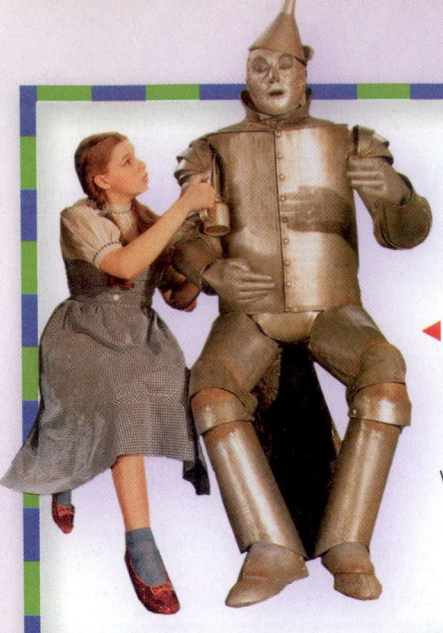

◀ Everyone needs a heart. Just ask the Tin Man from the classic story The Wizard of Oz.

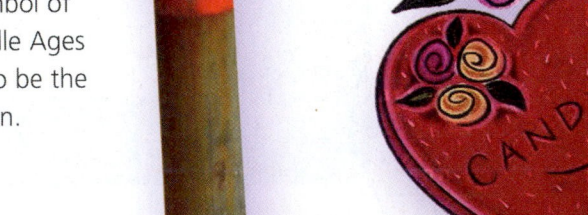

▶ The body's pump is also the universal symbol of love. In the Middle Ages it was thought to be the center of emotion.

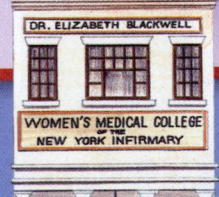

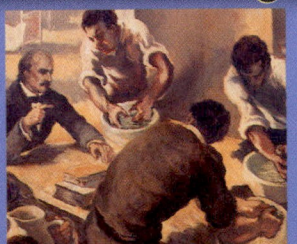

1847

Handwashing is found to prevent the spread of disease, as discovered by Ignaz Semmelweis, a Hungarian physician

Brian Warling/International Museum of Surgical Science, Chicago, IL

1849

Elizabeth Blackwell becomes the first woman physician

1849

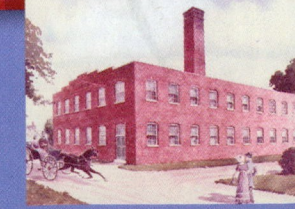

Pfizer pharmaceutical compan[y] is founded in Brooklyn, NY

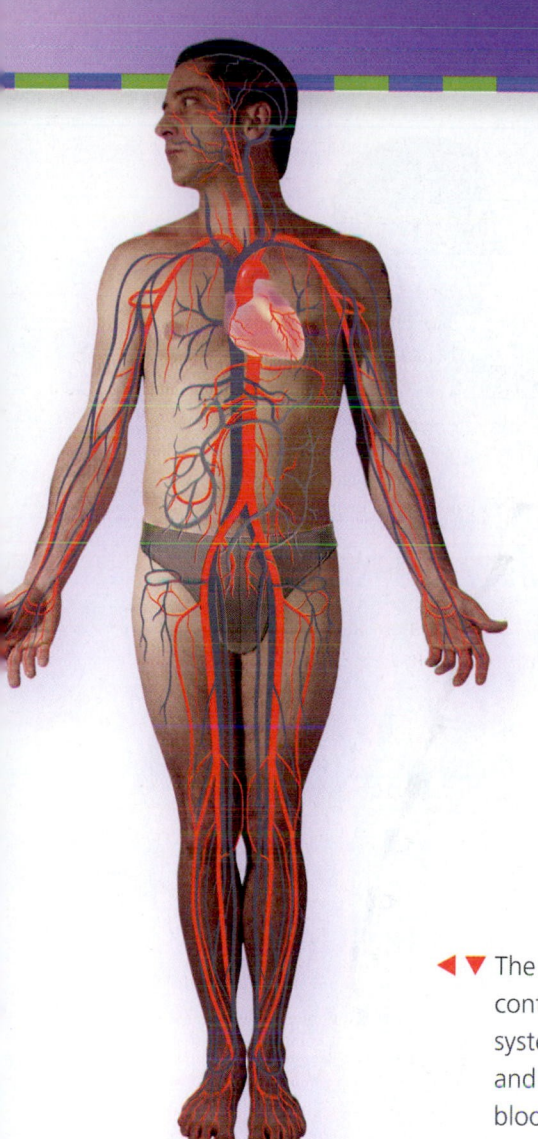

5
Cardiology
Cardiovascular System

Cardiology (KAR-dee-AWL-oh-jee) is the medical specialty that studies the anatomy and physiology of the cardiovascular system and uses diagnostic tests, medical and surgical procedures, and drugs to treat cardiovascular diseases.

◀▼ The cardiovascular system is a continuous, circular body system—containing the heart and blood vessels—that moves blood throughout the body to transport oxygen, nutrients, and waste products.

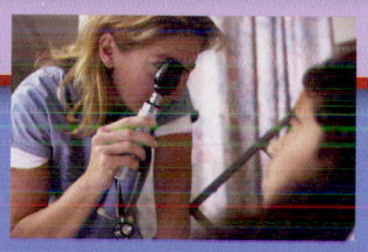

1851

The ophthalmoscope, an instrument used to view the inside of the eye, is invented by Hermann von Helmholtz, a German physiologist

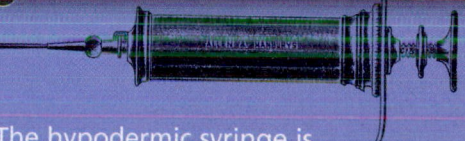

1853

The hypodermic syringe is invented by Dr. Alexander Wood of Scotland

Measure Your Progress: Learning Objectives

After you study this chapter, you should be able to

1. Identify the structures of the cardiovascular system.
2. Describe the process of circulation.
3. Describe common cardiovascular diseases and conditions, laboratory and diagnostic procedures, medical and surgical procedures, and drug categories.
4. Give the medical meaning of word parts related to the cardiovascular system.
5. Build cardiovascular words from word parts and divide and define cardiovascular words.
6. Spell and pronounce cardiovascular words.
7. Analyze the medical content and meaning of a cardiology report.
8. Dive deeper into cardiology by reviewing the activities at the end of this chapter and online at Medical Terminology Interactive.

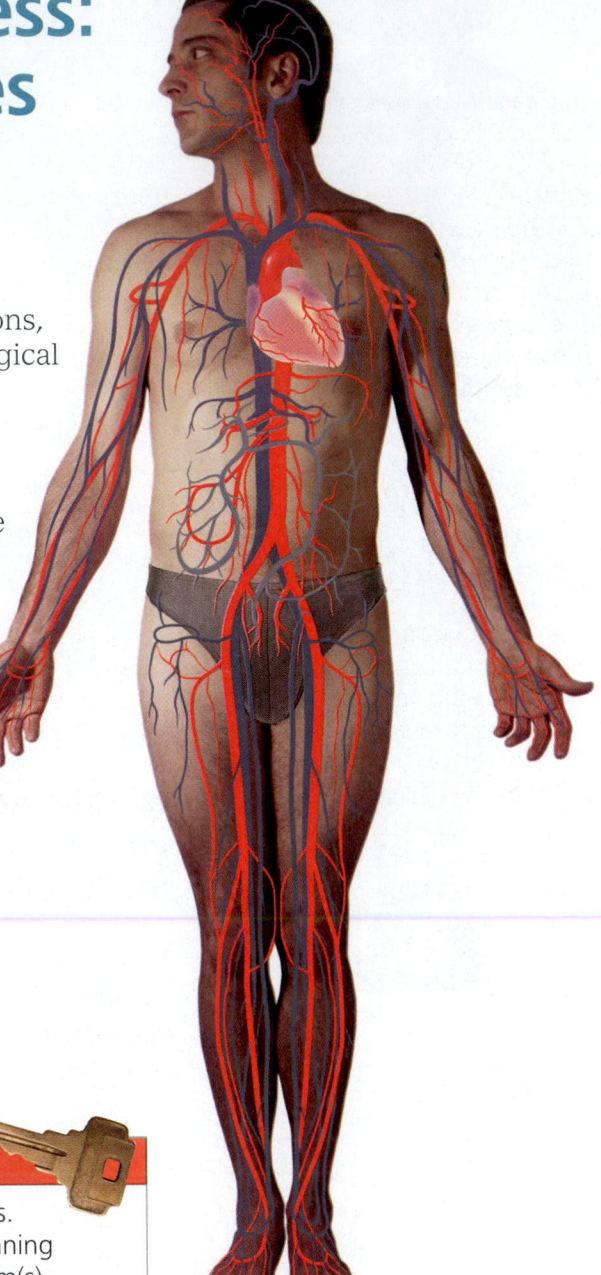

Figure 5-1 ■ **Cardiovascular system.**

The cardiovascular system consists of the heart and blood vessels connected in a common pathway that carries blood to and from all parts of the body.

Medical Language Key

To unlock the definition of a medical word, break it into word parts. Define each word part. Put the word part meanings in order, beginning with the suffix, then the prefix (if present), then the combining form(s).

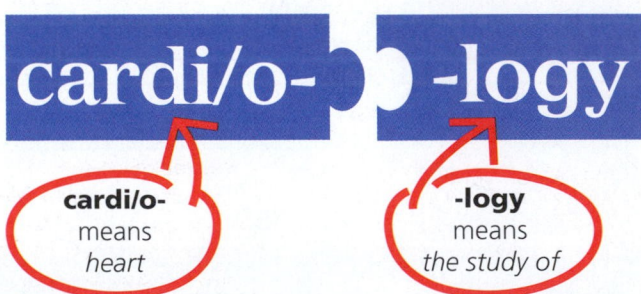

cardi/o-
means
heart

-logy
means
the study of

	Word Part	Word Part Meaning
Suffix	-logy	*the study of*
Combining Form	cardi/o-	*heart*

Cardiology: *The study of the heart (and related structures).*

Anatomy and Physiology

The **cardiovascular system** is a continuous, circular body system that includes the heart and the **vascular** structures (blood vessels such as arteries, capillaries, and veins) (see Figure 5-1 ■). It is also known as the **circulatory system.** To study the cardiovascular system, you can begin with the heart or you can begin with the capillaries, the tiniest blood vessels in the farthest parts of the body. Either way you will pass through every part of the cardiovascular system and arrive back at your starting point. The purpose of the cardiovascular system is to move (circulate) the blood to every part of the body as it transports oxygen, carbon dioxide, nutrients, and wastes. The blood itself is discussed in "Hematology and Immunology," Chapter 6.

Anatomy of the Cardiovascular System

Heart

The **heart** is perhaps the best-known organ in the body and certainly one of the most important. It is a muscular organ that contracts at least once every second to pump blood throughout the body. It also has an extensive electrical system that initiates and coordinates its contractions.

Heart Chambers   The heart contains four chambers, two on the top and two on the bottom (see Figures 5-2 ■ and 5-3 ■). Each small upper chamber is an **atrium.** Each large lower chamber is a **ventricle.** The **septum,** a central wall, divides the heart into right and left sides. The inferior tip of the heart is the **apex.**

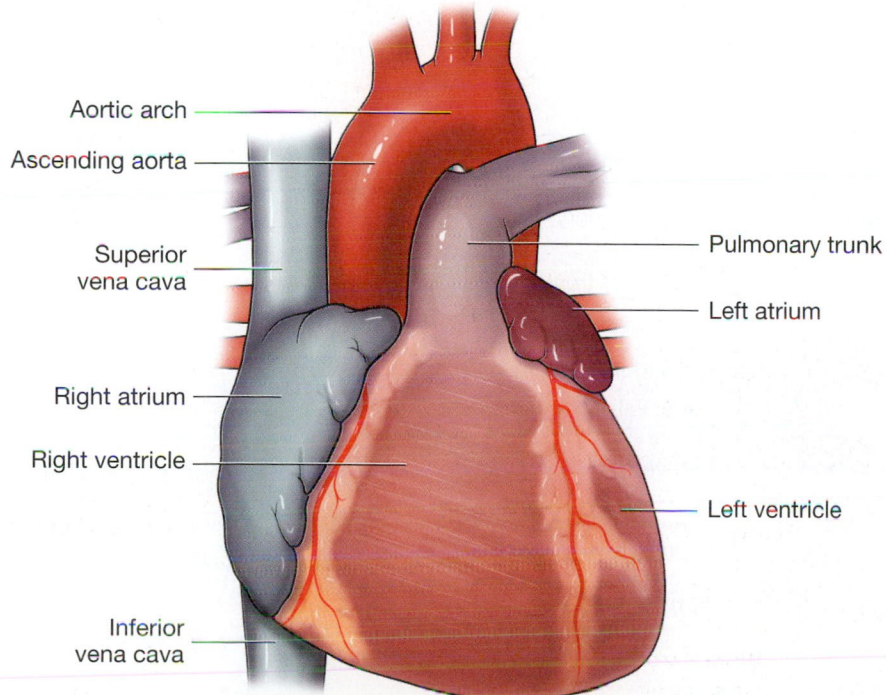

Aortic arch
Ascending aorta
Superior vena cava
Right atrium
Right ventricle
Inferior vena cava

Pulmonary trunk
Left atrium
Left ventricle

Figure 5-2 ■ Surface of the heart.
The boundaries of the internal chambers of the heart can be seen on the surface of the heart as elevated mounds and grooves that are filled with fat, blood vessels, and nerves.

Heart Valves   Four **valves** control the flow of blood through the heart. They are the tricuspid valve, pulmonary valve, mitral valve, and aortic valve (see Figure 5-3).

The **tricuspid valve** is between the right atrium and right ventricle. It has three triangular cusps (leaflets). It opens as the right atrium contracts to allow blood to flow from the right atrium into the right ventricle. Then it closes to prevent blood from flowing back into the right atrium.

The **pulmonary valve** is between the right ventricle and the pulmonary trunk. It opens as the right ventricle contracts to allow blood to flow into the pulmonary trunk and pulmonary arteries. Then it closes to prevent blood from flowing back into the right ventricle.

The **mitral valve** is between the left atrium and left ventricle. It has two cusps and is also known as the **bicuspid valve.** It opens as the left atrium contracts to allow blood to flow from the left atrium into the left ventricle. Then it closes to prevent blood from flowing back into the left atrium.

The **aortic valve** is between the left ventricle and the aorta (see Figure 5-4 ■). It opens as the left ventricle contracts to allow blood to flow from the left ventricle into the aorta. Then it closes to prevent blood from flowing back into the left ventricle.

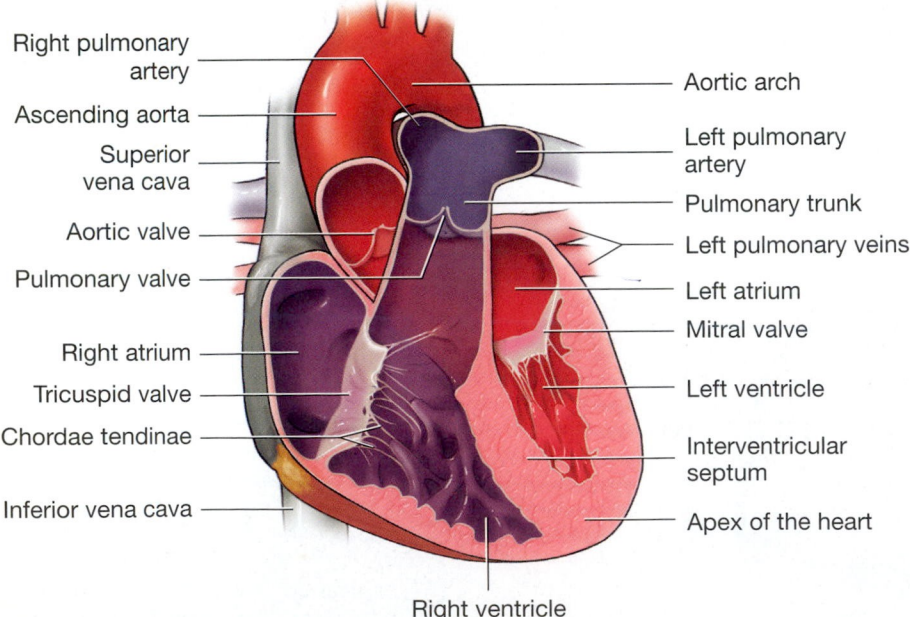

Right pulmonary artery
Ascending aorta
Superior vena cava
Aortic valve
Pulmonary valve
Right atrium
Tricuspid valve
Chordae tendinae
Inferior vena cava
Right ventricle

Aortic arch
Left pulmonary artery
Pulmonary trunk
Left pulmonary veins
Left atrium
Mitral valve
Left ventricle
Interventricular septum
Apex of the heart

Figure 5-3 ■ Chambers and valves of the heart.
The heart has four chambers: right atrium, right ventricle, left atrium, and left ventricle. The heart has four valves: tricuspid valve, pulmonary valve, mitral valve, and aortic valve.

Leaflets open   Leaflets closed

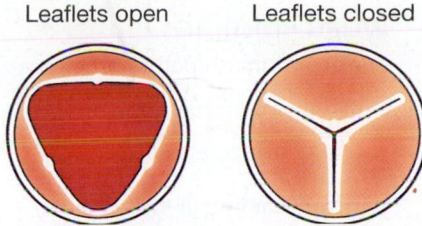

Figure 5-4 ■ Aortic valve.
With the three valve leaflets open, blood flows freely through the valve. When the valve leaflets close, their edges seal tightly against one another, preventing the backflow of blood.

The tricuspid and mitral valves have **chordae tendineae,** ropelike connective tissues attached to their valve leaflets (see Figure 5-3). The other end of the chordae tendineae is anchored to small muscles on the wall of the ventricles. When the ventricles contract, these small muscles also contract and pull on the chordae tendineae. This stabilizes the valve leaflets and keeps them firmly sealed together to keep blood from flowing back into the atria, even during the strong force of a ventricular contraction.

The sounds of the valves closing are commonly known as "lubb-dupp" (a phonetic approximation of the actual sounds). The "lubb" is made as the tricuspid and mitral valves close. This first heart sound is abbreviated as S_1. The "dupp" is made as the pulmonary and aortic valves close. This second heart sound is abbreviated as S_2.

Heart Muscle   The **myocardium** is the muscular layer of the heart (see Figure 5-5 ■ and Table 5-1). The myocardium is composed of cardiac muscle. Its muscle fibers (muscle cells) respond to electrical impulses

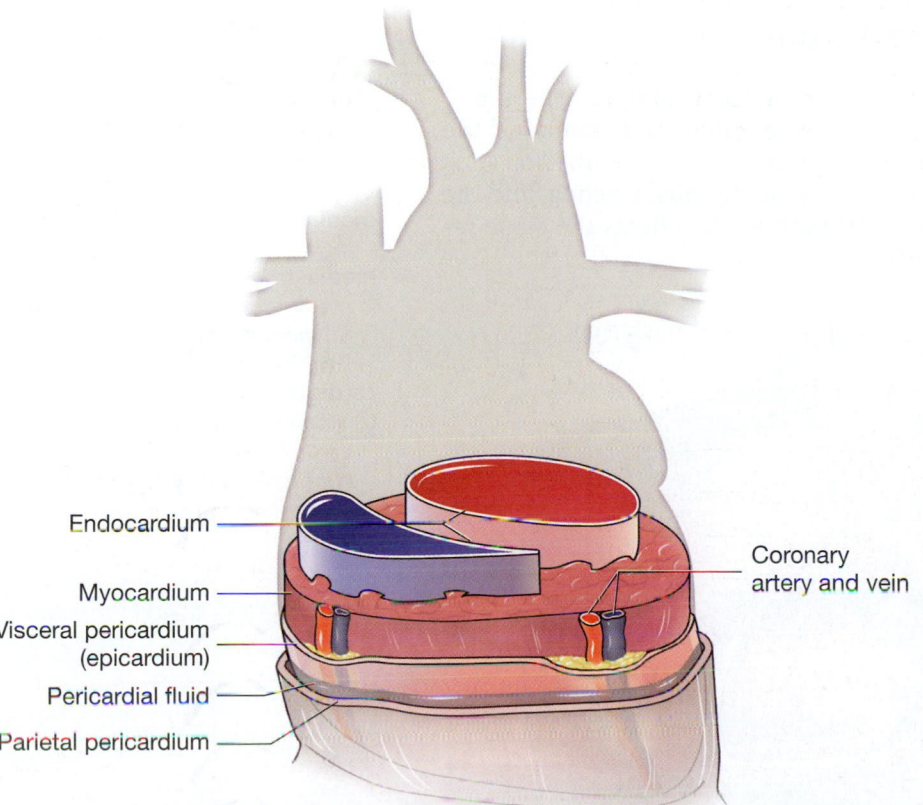

Figure 5-5 ■ Layers and membranes of the heart.
The endocardium lines the four chambers and valves inside the heart. The myocardium is the muscular layer of the heart. The pericardium is the membrane around the pericardial sac that contains pericardial fluid.

WORD BUILDING

chordae tendineae
(KOHR-dee TEN-dih-nee-ee)

myocardium (MY-oh-KAR-dee-um)
 my/o- *muscle*
 cardi/o- *heart*
 -um *a structure; period of time*

myocardial (MY-oh-KAR-dee-al)
 my/o- *muscle*
 cardi/o- *heart*
 -al *pertaining to*

Table 5-1   Layers and Membranes of the Heart

endocardium	Innermost layer of cells that lines the atria, ventricles, and heart valves. (*Note:* This layer also extends into the blood vessels where it is known as the endothelium or intima.)
myocardium	Muscular layer of the heart
pericardium	Outermost layer. This membrane surrounds the heart as the **pericardial sac** and secretes pericardial fluid. The pericardial sac is U-shaped, and the heart is within the U. The part of the membrane that is next to the surface of the heart is the **visceral pericardium** or **epicardium** because it is upon the heart. The part that is the outer wall of the pericardial sac is the **parietal pericardium. Pericardial fluid** is a watery, slippery fluid that allows the two membranes to slide past each other as the heart contracts and relaxes.

generated by a node within the right atrium. This process is discussed in a later section.

The myocardium contracts in a coordinated way to pump blood. First the myocardium around the two atria contracts, forcing blood into the two ventricles. Then the myocardium around the two ventricles contracts. The blood in the right ventricle goes into the pulmonary trunk and the pulmonary arteries (that go to the lungs). The blood in the left ventricle goes into the aorta (that goes to the entire body). The myocardium is thickest on the left side of the heart because it is the left ventricle that must work the hardest to pump blood to the entire body.

Thoracic Cavity and Mediastinum

The **thoracic cavity** contains the lungs and the **mediastinum,** an irregularly shaped central area between the lungs. The mediastinum contains the heart and parts of the **great vessels** (aorta, superior vena cava, inferior vena cava, pulmonary arteries and veins), as well as the thymus, trachea, and the esophagus (see Figure 5-6 ■). The word **cardiothoracic** reflects the close relationship between the heart and the thoracic cavity.

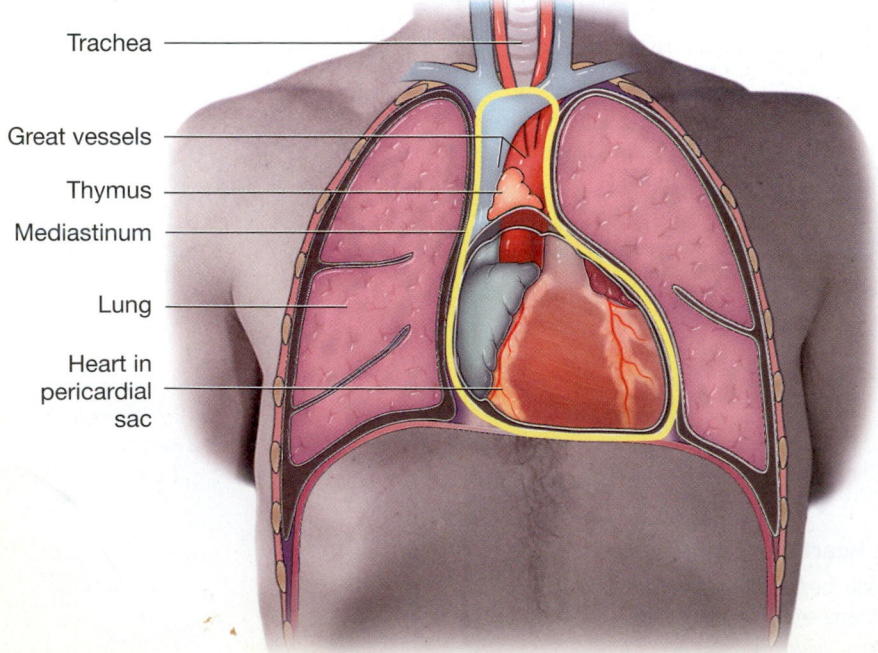

Trachea

Great vessels

Thymus

Mediastinum

Lung

Heart in pericardial sac

Figure 5-6 ■ Mediastinum.

The connective tissue of the mediastinum holds the heart and pericardial sac, great vessels, trachea, esophagus, and thymus in place within the thoracic cavity.

Blood Vessels

The blood vessels are vascular channels through which blood circulates in the body. **Vasculature** refers to the blood vessels associated with a particular organ. Blood vessels have a central opening or **lumen** through which the blood flows. Blood vessels are lined with **endothelium,** a smooth inner layer that promotes the flow of blood. This layer is also known as the **intima.**

There are three kinds of blood vessels: arteries, capillaries, and veins. Each performs a different function in the circulatory system.

Arteries   **Arteries** are large blood vessels that branch into smaller arteries known as **arterioles.** All arteries share some important characteristics and functions.

1. All arteries carry blood away from the heart to the body or to the lungs.

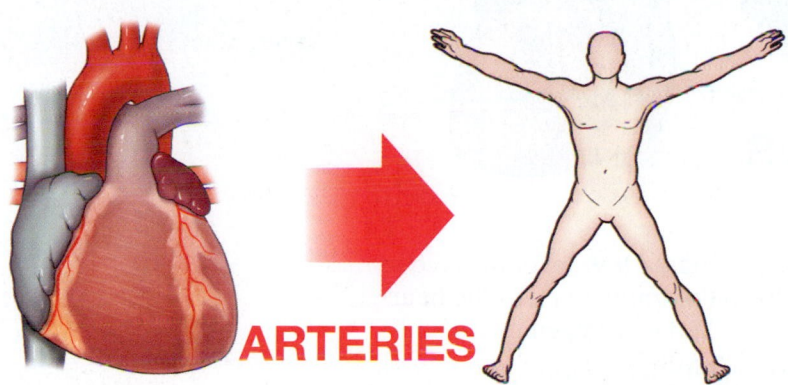

ARTERIES

2. All arteries carry bright red blood that has a high level of oxygen. The exception is the pulmonary arteries from the heart to the lungs. They carry dark red-purple blood that has a low level of oxygen. This blood has come from the body and is going to the lungs to pick up oxygen.

3. Most arteries lie deep beneath the skin. A few, however, lie near the surface. Their walls bulge outward each time the heart contracts, and this can be felt as a **pulse** (see Figure 5-27).

4. All arteries have smooth muscle in their walls. When the smooth muscle contracts (**vasoconstriction**), the lumen of the artery decreases in size, and the pressure of the blood in the artery increases (see Figure 5-7 ■). When the smooth muscle relaxes (**vasodilation**), the lumen of the artery increases in size, and the pressure of the blood in the artery decreases.

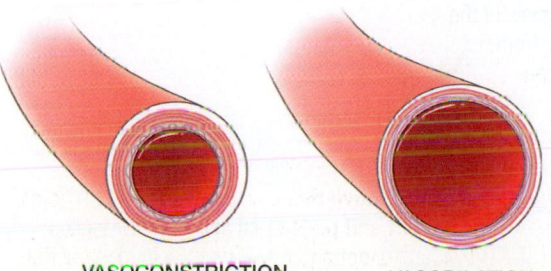

VASOCONSTRICTION   **VASODILATION**

Figure 5-7 ■ Vasoconstriction and vasodilation.

Vasoconstriction and vasodilation of the arteries are important ways in which the body regulates the blood pressure.

WORD BUILDING

vasculature (VAS-kyoo-lah-chur)
  vascul/o- *blood vessel*
  -ature *system composed of*

lumen (LOO.men)

endothelium (EN-doh-THEE-lee-um)
  endo- *innermost; within*
  theli/o- *cellular layer*
  -um *a structure; period of time*

intima (IN-tih-mah)

artery (AR-ter-ee)

arterial (ar-TEER-ee-al)
  arteri/o- *artery*
  -al *pertaining to*
The combining form *arter/o-* also means *artery.*

arteriole (ar-TEER-ee-ohl)
  arteri/o- *artery*
  -ole *small thing*

arteriolar (ar-TEER-ee-OH-lar)
  arteriol/o- *arteriole*
  -ar *pertaining to*

pulse (PULS)

vasoconstriction
(VAY-soh-con-STRIK-shun)
  vas/o- *blood vessel; vas deferens*
  constrict/o- *drawn together; narrowed*
  -ion *action; condition*

vasodilation (VAY-soh-dy-LAY-shun)
  vas/o- *blood vessel; vas deferens*
  dilat/o- *dilate; widen*
  -ion *action; condition*

Capillaries   **Capillaries** are the smallest blood vessels in the body. The lumen of a capillary is so small that blood cells must pass through in single file. Capillaries connect arterioles and venules, as an arteriole branches into a network of capillaries that reaches each cell in the body and then re-combines into a venule.

Veins   Capillaries combine to form small veins known as **venules,** which then combine to form a large **vein.** All veins share some important characteristics and functions.

1. All veins carry blood back to the heart from the body or from the lungs.

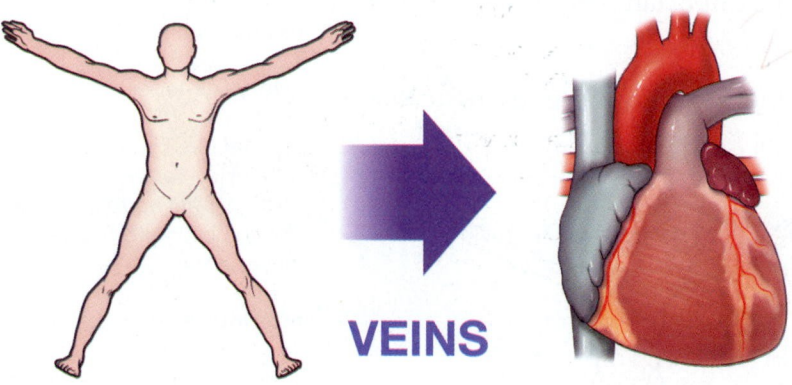

2. All veins carry dark red-purple blood that has a low level of oxygen. The exception is the pulmonary veins from the lungs back to the heart. They carry bright red blood that has just picked up oxygen in the lungs.

3. The largest veins have valves that keep the blood flowing in one direction—back toward the heart (see Figure 5-8 ▪).

4. Many veins are near the surface of the body and can be seen just under the skin as bluish, sometimes bulging lines.

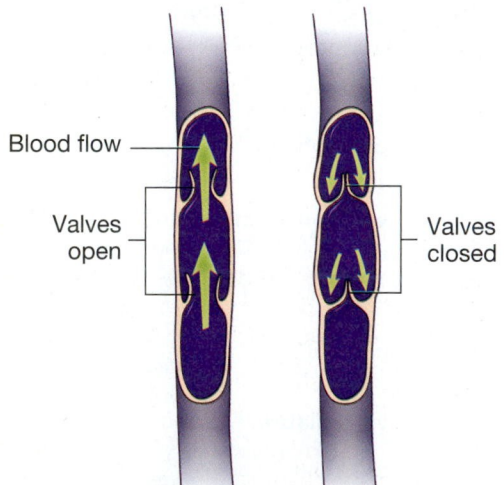

Figure 5-8 ▪ **Valves in a vein.**
As the large muscles in an arm or leg contract, they compress the vein and this moves blood through the vein. Valves in the vein then close to prevent gravity from pulling the blood back to its original location.

Blood Vessel Names and Locations

The names of most arteries and veins come from the names of nearby anatomic structures, such as bones or muscles. Capillaries are not named.

WORD BUILDING

capillary (KAP-ih-LAIR-ee)
   capill/o- *hairlike structure; capillary*
   -ary *pertaining to*

venule (VEN-yool)
   ven/o- *vein*
   -ule *small thing*

vein (VAYN)

venous (VEE-nus)
   ven/o- *vein*
   -ous *pertaining to*
The combining form *phleb/o-* also means *vein.*

Left common
carotid artery

Brachiocephalic
trunk

Left subclavian
artery

Aortic arch

Superior
vena cava

Left pulmonary
arteries

Right pulmonary
arteries

Ascending aorta

Pulmonary trunk

Left atrium

Right pulmonary
veins

Left pulmonary
veins

Right atrium

Left coronary
artery

Right coronary
artery

Left ventricle

Right ventricle

Inferior
vena cava

Figure 5-9 ■ **Arteries and veins around the heart.**
The aorta is the largest artery in the body. The coronary arteries to the heart receive oxygenated blood directly from the aorta. The aortic arch contains the first three major branches of arteries. The superior vena cava and inferior vena cava are the largest veins in the body.

Ascending Aorta and Arterial Branches

The **aorta** is the largest artery in the body (see Figures 5-9 ■ and 5-10 ■). It receives oxygenated blood from the left ventricle of the heart. The **ascending aorta** travels from the heart in a superior direction. The **coronary arteries** branch off directly from the ascending aorta. Before oxygenated blood goes to any other part of the body, it goes to the heart muscle via the coronary arteries. This is because of the importance of the heart in maintaining life.

aorta (aa-OR-tah)

coronary (KOR-oh-NAIR-ee)
 coron/o- *structure that encircles like a crown*
 -ary *pertaining to*

Did You Know?

Even though the chambers of the heart are filled with blood, the myocardium cannot use this blood. It must get its oxygen from the blood that flows through the coronary arteries.

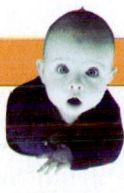

aortic (aa-OR-tik)
 aort/o- *aorta*
 -ic *pertaining to*

carotid (kah-ROT-id)
 carot/o- *stupor; sleep*
 -id *resembling; source or origin*

The ascending aorta then becomes the **aortic arch,** an inverted, U-shaped segment. Three major arteries branch off from the aortic arch (see Figure 5-9): the brachiocephalic trunk (that branches into the right common carotid artery and right subclavian artery), the left common carotid artery, and the left subclavian artery. The **carotid arteries** bring oxygenated blood to the neck, face, head, and brain (see Figure 5-10). The **subclavian arteries** bring oxygenated blood to the shoulders. Each subclavian artery goes

subclavian (sub-KLAY-vee-an)
 sub- *below; underneath; less than*
 clav/o- *clavicle (collar bone)*
 -ian *pertaining to*

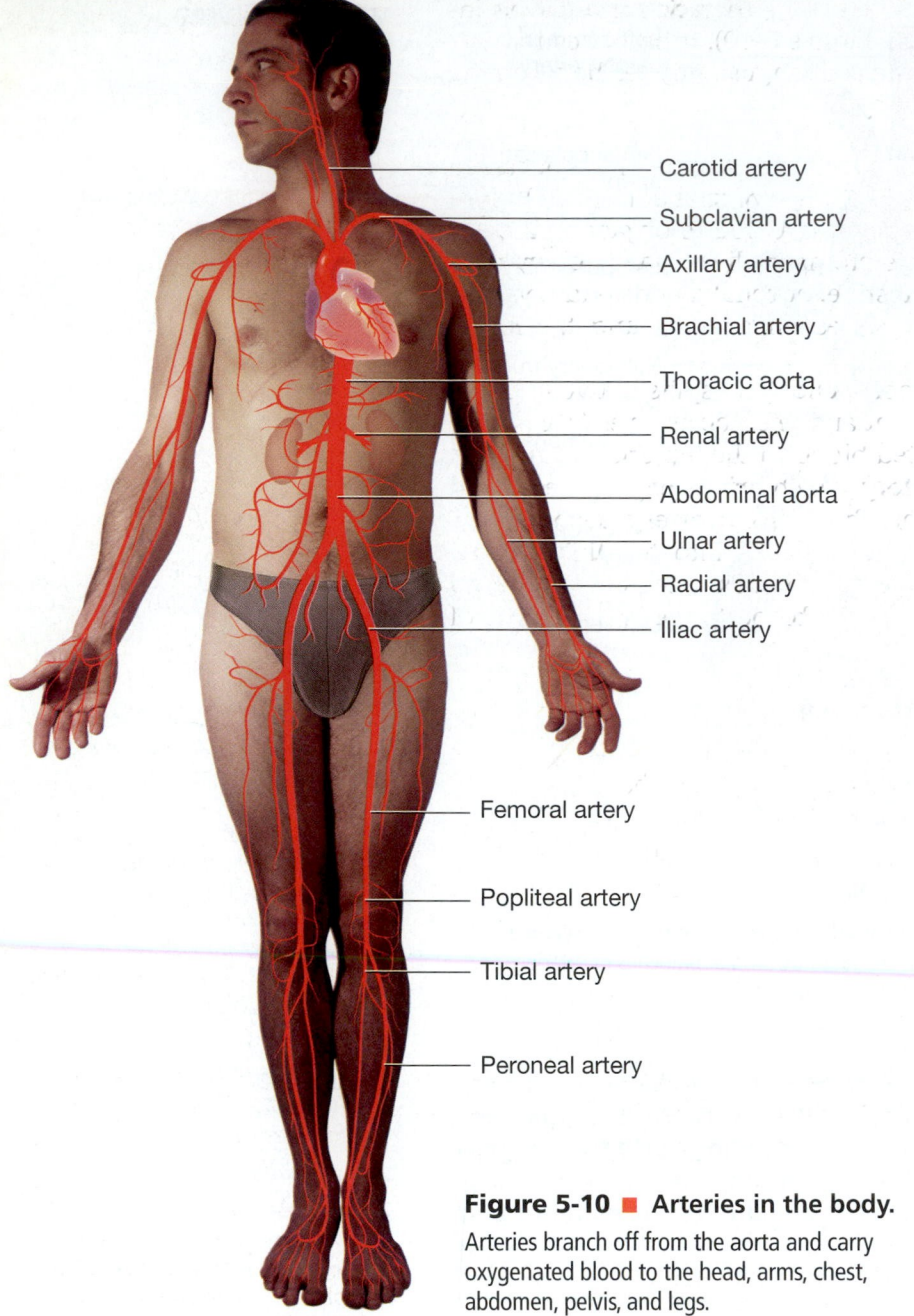

Figure 5-10 ■ **Arteries in the body.**
Arteries branch off from the aorta and carry oxygenated blood to the head, arms, chest, abdomen, pelvis, and legs.

Carotid artery
Subclavian artery
Axillary artery
Brachial artery
Thoracic aorta
Renal artery
Abdominal aorta
Ulnar artery
Radial artery
Iliac artery
Femoral artery
Popliteal artery
Tibial artery
Peroneal artery

underneath the clavicle (collar bone) and then continues as the **axillary artery** (in the area of the armpit). The axillary artery divides into the **brachial artery,** which brings oxygenated blood to the upper arm, and then into the **radial artery** and **ulnar artery,** which bring oxygenated blood to the lower arm.

Did You Know?

The brachial artery takes its name from the biceps brachii muscle of the upper arm. The radial and ulnar arteries take their names from the radius (the bone on the thumb side of the lower arm) and the ulna (the bone on the little finger side of the lower arm).

WORD BUILDING

axillary (AK-zih-LAIR-ee)
axill/o- *axilla (armpit)*
-ary *pertaining to*

brachial (BRAY-kee-al)
brachi/o- *arm*
-al *pertaining to*

radial (RAY-dee-al)
radi/o- *radius (forearm bone); x-rays; radiation*
-al *pertaining to*
Select the correct combining form meaning to get the definition of *radial: pertaining to the radius (forearm bone).*

ulnar (UL-nar)
uln/o- *ulna (forearm bone)*
-ar *pertaining to*

Thoracic Aorta and Arterial Branches

The **thoracic aorta** travels inferiorly through the thoracic cavity (see Figure 5-10). It branches into arteries that bring oxygenated blood to the esophagus, muscles between the ribs, diaphragm, upper spinal cord, and back.

Abdominal Aorta and Arterial Branches

As the thoracic aorta goes through the diaphragm, it becomes the **abdominal aorta** (see Figure 5-10). The abdominal aorta brings oxygenated blood to organs in the abdominopelvic cavity. These include the stomach, liver, gallbladder, pancreas, spleen, small intestine, large intestine, adrenal glands, kidneys (the **renal arteries**), ovaries (in a woman), testes (in a man), and the lower spinal cord.

In the pelvic cavity, the abdominal aorta ends and splits in two (a bifurcation) to form the inverted Y of the right and left iliac arteries (see Figure 5-10). The **iliac arteries** bring oxygenated blood to the hip and groin. Each iliac artery continues as the **femoral artery,** which brings oxygenated blood to the upper leg. Near the knee joint, the femoral artery becomes the **popliteal artery.** The popliteal artery then divides into the **tibial artery,** which brings oxygenated blood to the front and back of the lower leg, and the **peroneal artery,** which brings oxygenated blood to the little toe side of the lower leg.

Did You Know?

The femoral artery takes its name from the femur (the bone in the upper leg). The popliteal artery takes its name from the popliteus, a small muscle at the back of the knee. The tibial and peroneal arteries take their names from the tibia (the main bone in the lower leg) and the fibula (the narrow bone on the little toe side of the lower leg). *Peroneal* is the adjective form for *fibula*.

Pulmonary Arteries

The **pulmonary arteries** originate from the pulmonary trunk, which comes from the right ventricle of the heart, not from the aorta (see Figure 5-9).

Venae Cavae

The two major veins of the body are the superior vena cava and inferior vena cava (see Figure 5-9). The **superior vena cava** carries blood from the head, neck, arms, and chest to the right atrium. The **inferior vena cava** carries blood from the rest of the body (except the lungs) to the right atrium. The **pulmonary veins** carry blood from the lungs to the left atrium of the heart. Other major veins include the **jugular vein** (that carries blood from the head to the superior vena cava), the **portal vein** (that carries blood from the intestines to the liver), and the **saphenous vein** and **femoral vein** (that carry blood from the leg to the groin).

Did You Know?

The jugular vein takes its name from a Latin word that means *neck*. The portal vein takes its name from the porta hepatis, the Latin phrase for the portal or site where the vein enters the liver. (*Hepatis* is a Latin word meaning *of the liver*.) The saphenous vein takes its name from a Latin word that means *clearly visible*, as this vein often can be seen through the skin of the posterior lower leg.

WORD BUILDING

thoracic (thoh-RAS-ik)
   thorac/o- *thorax (chest)*
   -ic *pertaining to*

abdominal (ab-DAWM-ih-nal)
   abdomin/o- *abdomen*
   -al *pertaining to*

renal (REE-nal)
   ren/o- *kidney*
   -al *pertaining to*

iliac (IL-ee-ak)
   ili/o- *ilium (hip bone)*
   -ac *pertaining to*

femoral (FEM-oh-ral)
   femor/o- *femur (thigh bone)*
   -al *pertaining to*

popliteal
(pop-LIT-ee-al) (pop-lih-TEE-al)
   poplite/o- *back of the knee*
   -al *pertaining to*

tibial (TIB-ee-al)
   tibi/o- *tibia (shin bone)*
   -al *pertaining to*

peroneal (PAIR-oh-NEE-al)
   perone/o- *fibula (lower leg bone)*
   -al *pertaining to*

pulmonary (PUL-moh-NAIR-ee)
   pulmon/o- *lung*
   -ary *pertaining to*

vena cava (VEE-nah KAY-vah)
Vena is a Latin singular noun. Form the plural by changing *-a* to *-ae*. Example: The superior and inferior venae cavae.

jugular (JUG-yoo-lar)
   jugul/o- *jugular (throat)*
   -ar *pertaining to*

portal (POR-tal)
   port/o- *point of entry*
   -al *pertaining to*

saphenous (sah-FEE-nus)
   saphen/o- *clearly visible*
   -ous *pertaining to*

Circulation

Circulation of the blood occurs through two different pathways (see Figure 5-11 ■): the systemic circulation and the pulmonary circulation.

1. **Systemic circulation.** Arteries, arterioles, capillaries, venules and veins everywhere in the body, except in the lungs.
2. **Pulmonary circulation.** Arteries, arterioles, capillaries, venules, and veins going to, within, and coming from the lungs. The word **cardiopulmonary** reflects the close connection between the heart and the lungs.

Now let's trace the route that blood takes through the systemic and pulmonary circulations as it makes one complete trip through the whole body.

WORD BUILDING

circulation (SIR-kyoo-LAY-shun)
  circulat/o- *movement in a circular route*
  -ion *action; condition*

systemic (sis-TEM-ik)
  system/o- *the body as a whole*
  -ic *pertaining to*

cardiopulmonary
(KAR-dee-oh-PUL-moh-NAIR-ee)
  cardi/o- *heart*
  pulmon/o- *lung*
  -ary *pertaining to*

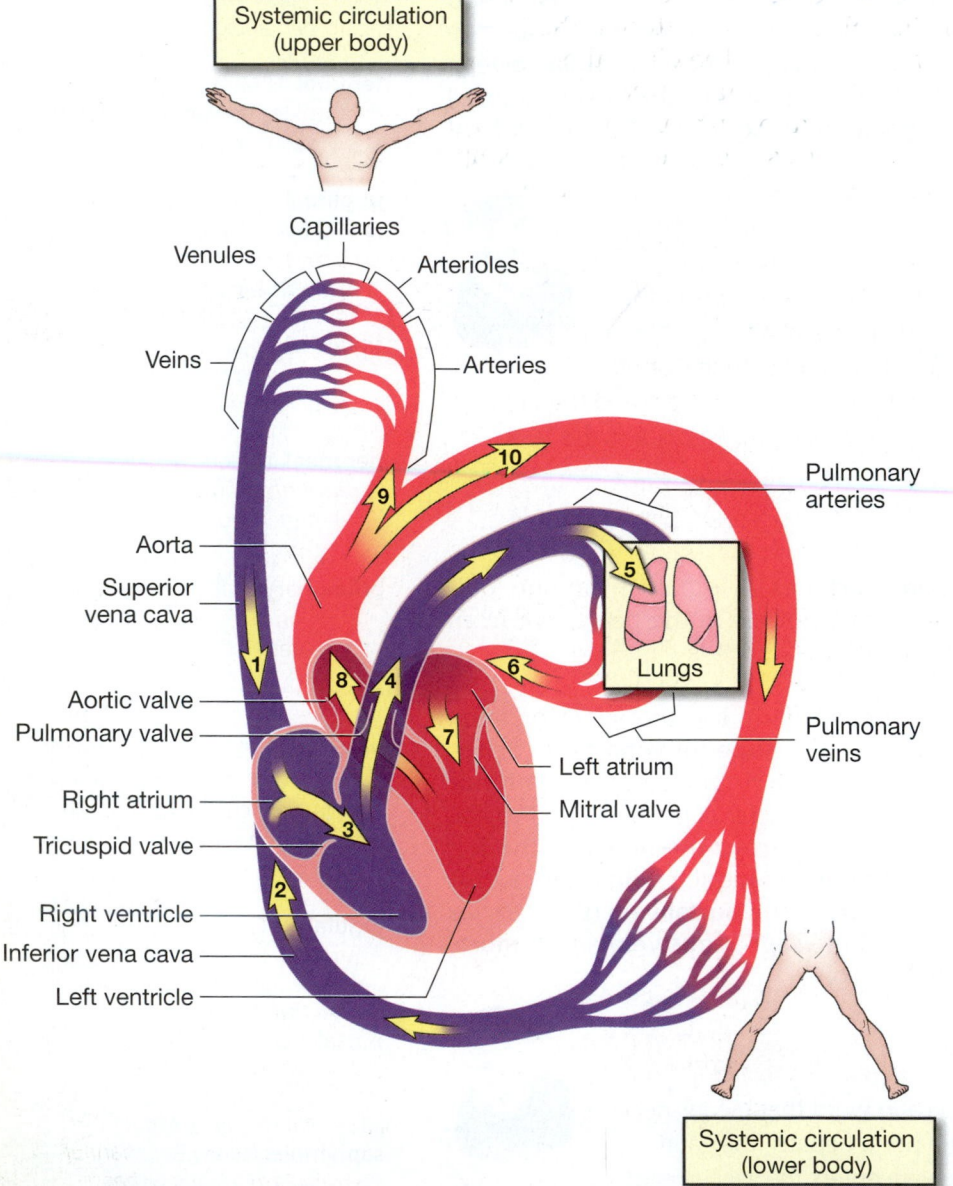

Figure 5-11 ■ **Circulation of the blood.**
Each time the heart contracts, it pumps blood from the right ventricle through the pulmonary circulation and from the left ventricle through the systemic circulation.

Systemic Circulation through the Veins   Blood coming from cells in the body is dark red–purple in color because it has a low level of oxygen. (1) Blood coming from cells in the upper body travels through capillaries, venules, and veins and the superior vena cava. (2) Blood coming from cells in the lower body travels through capillaries, venules, and veins and the inferior vena cava. (3) Then all of this blood travels through the right atrium, tricuspid valve, and right ventricle.

Pulmonary Circulation   (4) At this point, the blood enters the pulmonary circulation. The blood travels through the pulmonary valve, pulmonary trunk, and pulmonary arteries, arterioles, and capillaries in the lungs. (5) In a capillary beside an alveolus, the blood releases carbon dioxide, picks up oxygen, and becomes bright red in color. (6) The blood then travels through the pulmonary veins to the left atrium of the heart.

Systemic Circulation through the Arteries   (7) At this point, the blood is back in the systemic circulation. From the left atrium, the blood travels through the mitral valve and left ventricle. (8) The blood then travels through the aortic valve and into the aorta. The aorta, arteries, arterioles, and capillaries distribute this oxygenated blood to every part of the body. In a capillary beside a body cell, the blood releases oxygen, and picks up carbon dioxide, and becomes dark red-purple in color. This completes one trip around the circulatory system.

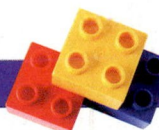

Clinical Connections

Neonatology. The fetal heart begins to beat just 4 weeks after conception. The circulation of blood in a fetus is different from that of an adult. The fetus receives oxygenated blood and nutrients from the mother through the placenta, via arteries in the umbilical cord that merge with the inferior vena cava of the fetus. The fetal heart has two unique structures that allow this oxygenated blood to bypass the (not yet functioning) lungs and go directly to the body. The **foramen ovale,** a small, oval opening in the septum between the atria, allows some of the oxygenated blood to enter the left side of the heart where it is immediately pumped out to the body. The **ductus arteriosus,** a connecting blood vessel between the pulmonary trunk and the aorta, allows the rest of the oxygenated blood to go into the right ventricle and pulmonary trunk but then diverts it to the aorta. These two unique structures in the fetal heart should close automatically within 24 hours after birth.

foramen ovale
(foh-RAY-men oh-VAH-lee)

ductus arteriosus
(DUK-tus ar-TEER-ee-OH-sus)

Did You Know?

The normal heart rate for a newborn is 110–150 beats per minute. The normal heart rate for an adult is 70–80 beats per minute. A well-trained athlete can have a resting heart rate lower than 60 beats per minute.

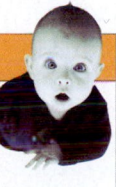

conduction (con-DUK-shun)
conduct/o- *carrying; conveying*
-ion *action; condition*

sinoatrial (SY-noh-AA-tree-al)
sin/o- *hollow cavity; channel*
atri/o- *atrium (upper heart chamber)*
-al *pertaining to*

node (NOHD)

Physiology of the Conduction System

The heart contracts and relaxes in a regular rhythm that is coordinated by the **conduction system** of the heart (see Figure 5-12 ■). The **sinoatrial node (SA node),** or pacemaker of the heart (a small area in the posterior wall of the right atrium), initiates the electrical impulse that begins each heartbeat. This impulse causes both atria to contract simultaneously. The electrical

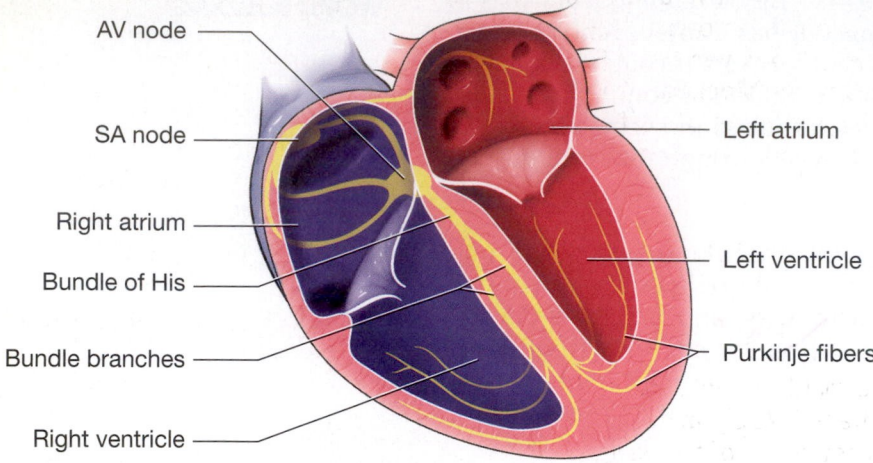

AV node
SA node
Right atrium
Bundle of His
Bundle branches
Right ventricle
Left atrium
Left ventricle
Purkinje fibers

Figure 5-12 ■ Conduction system of the heart.
The SA node (pacemaker) initiates an electrical impulse that travels through the AV node, the bundle of His, the right and left bundle branches, and then to the Purkinje fibers, causing the atria and then the ventricles to contract.

impulse then travels through the **atrioventricular node (AV node)** (a small area in the right atrium near the interatrial septum), through the **bundle of His,** and into both the right and left **bundle branches** that each end in a network of nerves (the **Purkinje fibers**). Then both ventricles contract simultaneously. A contraction is known as **systole,** and the resting period between contractions is known as **diastole.**

WORD BUILDING

atrioventricular
(AA-tree-oh-ven-TRIK-yoo-lar)
   atri/o- *atrium (upper heart chamber)*
   ventricul/o- *ventricle (lower heart chamber; chamber in the brain)*
   -ar *pertaining to*

bundle of His (HISS)

Purkinje (per-KIN-jee)

systole (SIS-toh-lee)

systolic (sis-TAWL-ik)
   systol/o- *contracting*
   -ic *pertaining to*

diastole (dy-AS-toh-lee)

diastolic (DY-ah-STAWL-ik)
   diastol/o- *dilating*
   -ic *pertaining to*

Clinical Connections

Neurology. Because the heart is such an important organ, the heart rate is influenced by the SA node, as well as by the parasympathetic and the sympathetic divisions of the nervous system. The SA node continually generates an impulse all on its own of about 80–100 beats each minute. However, the parasympathetic division (through the vagal nerve) releases the neurotransmitter acetylcholine; this slows the heart to its normal resting heart rate of 70–80 beats each minute. The sympathetic division (through the spinal cord nerves) releases the neurotransmitter norepinephrine to increase the heart rate. So, fine adjustments in the heart rate are possible from moment to moment. Sometimes, however, the heart needs to beat much faster to support increased activity during exercise (see Figure 5-13 ■) or to escape danger (the "fight or flight" response). At those times, the sympathetic division stimulates the adrenal gland to secrete the hormone **epinephrine.** It travels through the blood to the heart, overrides the normal sinus rhythm, and causes the heart to beat much faster.

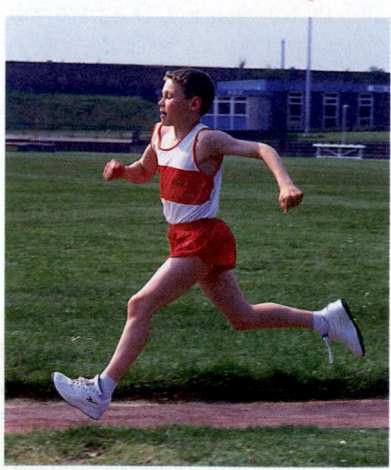

Figure 5-13 ■ Exercise increases the heart rate.

During exercise, epinephrine secreted by the adrenal glands increases the heart rate, constricts the arteries to increase the blood pressure, and dilates the bronchi to increase the flow of air into the lungs.

Besides the SA node, several other areas in the atria and ventricles can spontaneously produce electrical impulses on their own. These impulses are usually too weak to override the SA node. However, if the SA node fails to produce impulses, if the SA node impulses are blocked, or if these other areas become hyperexcited (from excessive amounts of caffeine or smoking), then these **ectopic** sites can take over, control the conduction system, and produce an abnormal heart rhythm.

WORD BUILDING

ectopic (ek-TOP-ik)
ectop/o- *outside of a place*
-ic *pertaining to*

A Closer Look

Electrical Activity of the Heart. On a molecular level, an elegant and intricate system allows the heart to contract tirelessly, approximately 100,000 times each day. To begin a contraction of the heart, an electrical impulse from the SA node changes the permeability of the membrane around a myocardial cell. Sodium ions (Na^+) outside the cell move through the cell membrane, followed (more slowly) by calcium ions (Ca^{++}). This gives the inside of the cell a more positive charge, which triggers the release of calcium ions stored inside the cell. This process is known as **depolarization** because it reverses the normal, slightly negative charge in the cell. The calcium ions cause the myocardial cell to contract. As one cell depolarizes and contracts, it triggers the next myocardial cell to do the same.

A contraction ends when potassium ions (K^+) move out of the cell, while tiny molecular pumps move sodium ions and some calcium ions out of the cell and move the rest of the calcium ions back into storage within the cell. This process is known as **repolarization.** This restores the normal, slightly negative charge of a resting myocardial cell. The myocardial cell is now ready for another impulse from the SA node.

A myocardial cell cannot respond to another electrical impulse from the SA node until the full cycle of depolarization and repolarization is complete. This period of unresponsiveness is known as the **refractory period.** The refractory period is a very, very short period of time, and so theoretically the heart could contract again almost instantly, but this would not allow enough time for the chambers of the heart to fill with blood. The optimum heart rate allows time for the heart chambers to fill with blood and to empty during a contraction.

depolarization
(dee-POH-lar-ih-ZAY-shun)
de- *reversal of; without*
polar/o- *positive or negative state*
-ization *the process of making, creating, or inserting*

repolarization
(ree-POH-lar-ih-ZAY-shun)
re- *again and again; backward; unable to*
polar/o- *positive or negative state*
-ization *process of making, creating, or inserting*

refractory (ree-FRAK-tor-ee)
re- *again and again; backward; unable to*
fract/o- *break up*
-ory *having the function of*
Select the correct prefix meaning to get the definition of *refractory:* having the function of (being) unable to break up.

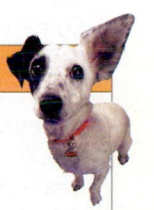

Word Alert

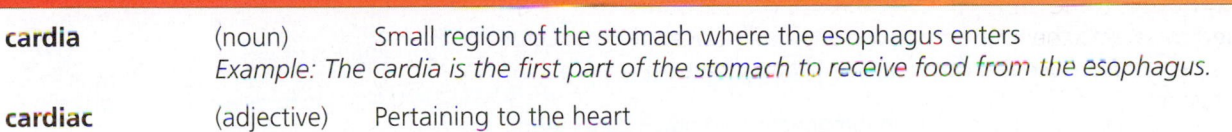

cardia	(noun)	Small region of the stomach where the esophagus enters
		Example: The cardia is the first part of the stomach to receive food from the esophagus.
cardiac	(adjective)	Pertaining to the heart
		Example: During a cardiac arrest, the heart stops beating.
cardiac valve	(noun)	Structure between two chambers of the heart (or between a heart chamber and a blood vessel) that opens and closes to regulate the flow of blood
		Example: A stethoscope allows you to hear the sound that a cardiac valve makes as it opens and closes.

Vocabulary Review

Anatomy and Physiology

Word or Phrase	Description	Combining Forms
cardiopulmonary	Pertaining to the heart and lungs.	**cardi/o-** *heart* **pulmon/o-** *lung*
cardiothoracic	Pertaining to the heart and thoracic cavity	**cardi/o-** *heart* **thorac/o-** *thorax (chest)*
cardiovascular system	Body system that includes the heart and the blood vessels (vascular structures)	**cardi/o-** *heart* **vascul/o-** *blood vessel*
circulatory system	Circular route that the blood takes as it moves through the body. **Circulation** is the process of moving the blood through the system. The circulatory system consists of the systemic circulation and the pulmonary circulation.	**circulat/o-** *movement in a circular route*
mediastinum	Irregularly shaped, central area in the **thoracic cavity** that lies between the lungs. It contains the heart, great vessels, thymus, trachea, and esophagus.	**mediastin/o-** *mediastinum* **thorac/o-** *thorax (chest)*
pulmonary circulation	The arteries, arterioles, capillaries, venules, and veins going to, within, and coming from the lungs (but not in the rest of the body)	**pulmon/o-** *lung*
systemic circulation	The arteries, arterioles, capillaries, venules, and veins everywhere in the body, except in the lungs	**system/o-** *the body as a whole*

Heart

Word or Phrase	Description	Combining Forms
aortic valve	Heart valve between the left ventricle and the aorta	**aort/o-** *aorta* **valvul/o-** *valve*
atrium	Each of the two upper chambers of the heart	**atri/o-** *atrium (upper heart chamber)*
chordae tendineae	Ropelike strands that support the tricuspid and mitral valves and keep their leaflets tightly closed when the ventricles are contracting	
ductus arteriosus	Temporary, small blood vessel in the fetal heart that connects the pulmonary trunk to the aorta. It should close within 24 hours after birth.	
endocardium	Layer of cells that lines the atria, ventricles, and valves of the heart	**cardi/o-** *heart*
foramen ovale	Temporary, oval-shaped opening in the interatrial septum of the fetal heart. It should close within 24 hours after birth.	
heart	Organ that pumps blood throughout the body. It contains four chambers, the **septum** (a center wall), and four valves. The lower tip of the heart is the **apex.** The adjective form for heart is **cardiac.**	**cardi/o-** *heart* **card/i-** *heart* **sept/o-** *septum (dividing wall)* **apic/o-** *apex (tip)*
mitral valve	Heart valve between the left atrium and the left ventricle. It is also known as the **bicuspid valve.** It has two (*bi-*) pointed **leaflets** or **cusps.**	**mitr/o-** *structure like a miter (tall hat with two points)* **valvul/o-** *valve* **cusp/o-** *projection; point*

Word or Phrase	Description	Combining Forms
myocardium	Muscular layer of the heart	**my/o-** *muscle* **cardi/o-** *heart*
pericardium	Membrane that surrounds the heart as the **pericardial sac** and is filled with **pericardial fluid.** The part of the membrane next to the heart is the **visceral pericardium** or **epicardium.** The part in the outer wall of the pericardial sac is the **parietal pericardium.**	**cardi/o-** *heart* **viscer/o-** *large internal organs* **pariet/o-** *wall of a cavity*
pulmonary valve	Heart valve between the right ventricle and the pulmonary trunk and the pulmonary arteries	**pulmon/o-** *lung* **valvul/o-** *valve*
tricuspid valve	Heart valve between the right atrium and right ventricle. It has three (*tri-*) pointed **leaflets** or **cusps.**	**cusp/o-** *projection; point* **valvul/o-** *valve*
valve	Structure that opens and closes to control the flow of blood. Heart valves include the tricuspid valve, pulmonary valve, mitral valve, and aortic valve. There are also valves in some of the large veins to prevent backflow of blood.	**valvul/o-** *valve* **valv/o-** *valve*
ventricle	Each of the two large, lower chambers of the heart	**ventricul/o-** *ventricle (lower heart chamber; chamber in the brain)*

Conduction System

Word or Phrase	Description	Combining Forms
atrioventricular (AV) node	Small area of tissue between the right atrium and right ventricle. The AV node is part of the conduction system of the heart and receives electrical impulses from the SA node.	**atri/o-** *atrium (upper heart chamber)* **ventricul/o-** *ventricle (lower heart chamber; chamber in the brain)*
bundle branches	Part of the conduction system of the heart after the bundle of His. The branches continue down the interventricular septum. At the apex of the heart, they split into the right bundle branch to the right ventricle and the left bundle branch to the left ventricle. Then, each divides into the **Purkinje fibers** that spread across the ventricles.	
bundle of His	Part of the conduction system of the heart after the AV node. It splits into the right and left bundle branches.	
conduction system	System that carries the electrical impulse that makes the heart beat. It consists of the SA node, AV node, bundle of His, bundle branches, and Purkinje fibers.	**conduct/o-** *carrying; conveying*
depolarization	To begin a contraction of the heart, an impulse from the SA node changes the permeability of the myocardial cell membrane. Positive sodium ions, then positive calcium ions, outside the cell move through the cell membrane, and more calcium ions stored in the cell are released. This reverses the normally negative charge in a resting myocardial cell and causes a contraction.	**polar/o-** *positive or negative state*
diastole	Resting period between contractions	**diastol/o-** *dilating*
ectopic site	Area within the heart that can produce its own electrical impulse but is not part of the conduction system. It sometimes overrides the impulse of the SA node and produces an abnormal heart rhythm.	**ectop/o-** *outside of a place*
refractory period	Short period of time when the myocardium is unresponsive to electrical impulses	**fract/o-** *break up*

Word or Phrase	Description	Combining Forms
repolarization	To end a contraction of the heart, positive potassium ions diffuse out of the cell, while molecular pumps move positive sodium and some calcium ions out of the cell and move the rest of the calcium ions into storage within the cell. This restores the slightly negative charge of a resting myocardial cell.	**polar/o-** *positive or negative state*
sinoatrial node	Pacemaker of the heart. Small area of tissue in the posterior wall of the right atrium. The SA node originates the electrical impulse for the entire conduction system of the heart.	**sin/o-** *hollow cavity; channel* **atri/o-** *atrium (upper heart chamber)*
systole	Contraction of the atria or the ventricles	**systol/o-** *contracting*

Blood Vessels

Word or Phrase	Description	Combining Forms
aorta	Largest artery in the body. It carries oxygenated blood from the left ventricle to the body. It includes the **ascending aorta,** the **aortic arch,** the **thoracic aorta,** and the **abdominal aorta.**	**aort/o-** *aorta* **thorac/o-** *thorax (chest)* **abdomin/o-** *abdomen*
arteriole	Smallest branch of an artery	**arteriol/o-** *arteriole*
artery	Blood vessel that carries oxygenated blood away from the heart to the body. This bright red blood has a high level of oxygen. (The exception is the pulmonary arteries that carry blood from the heart to the lungs. They carry dark red-purple blood with a low level of oxygen.)	**arteri/o-** *artery* **arter/o-** *artery*
axillary artery	Artery that carries oxygenated blood to the axilla (armpit) area	**axill/o-** *axilla (armpit)*
blood vessels	Channels through which the blood circulates throughout the body. These include arteries, arterioles, capillaries, venules, and veins. These are also known as **vascular structures.** The **lumen** is the central opening inside a blood vessel through which the blood flows.	**angi/o-** *blood vessel; lymphatic vessel* **vascul/o-** *blood vessel* **vas/o-** *blood vessel; vas deferens*
brachial artery	Artery that carries oxygenated blood to the upper arm	**brachi/o-** *arm*
capillary	Smallest blood vessel in the body. A capillary network connects the arterioles to the venules. The exchange of oxygen and carbon dioxide takes place in the capillaries.	**capill/o-** *hairlike structure; capillary*
carotid artery	Artery that carries oxygenated blood to the neck, face, head, and brain. If these arteries are compressed, the lack of blood to the brain will cause a person to become unconscious.	**carot/o-** *stupor; sleep*
coronary artery	Artery that carries oxygenated blood to the myocardium (heart muscle)	**coron/o-** *structure that encircles like a crown*
endothelium	Layer of cells that lines the wall of a blood vessel. It is also known as the **intima.**	**theli/o-** *cellular layer*
femoral artery	Artery that carries oxygenated blood to the upper leg	**femor/o-** *femur (thigh bone)*
great vessels	Collective phrase for the aorta (the largest artery), the superior and inferior venae cavae (the largest veins), and the pulmonary trunk, pulmonary arteries, and pulmonary veins	
iliac artery	Artery that carries oxygenated blood to the hip and groin area	**ili/o-** *ilium (hip bone)*
jugular vein	Vein that carries blood from the head to the superior vena cava	**jugul/o-** *jugular (throat)*

Word or Phrase	Description	Combining Forms
peroneal artery	Artery that carries oxygenated blood to the little toe side of the lower leg (along the fibula bone)	**perone/o-** *fibula (lower leg bone)*
popliteal artery	Artery that carries oxygenated blood to the back of the knee and then branches into the tibial and peroneal arteries	**poplite/o-** *back of the knee*
portal vein	Vein that carries blood from the intestines to the liver	**port/o-** *point of entry*
pulmonary artery	Artery that carries blood away from the heart to the lungs. The pulmonary artery is the only artery that carries blood that has a low level of oxygen.	**pulmon/o-** *lung*
pulmonary vein	Vein that carries oxygenated blood from the lungs to the heart. The pulmonary vein is the only vein that carries blood that has a high level of oxygen.	**pulmon/o-** *lung*
pulse	The bulging of an artery wall from blood pumped by the heart	
radial artery	Artery that carries oxygenated blood to the thumb side of the lower arm (along the radius bone)	**radi/o-** *radius (forearm bone); x-rays; radiation*
renal artery	Artery that carries oxygenated blood to the kidney	**ren/o-** *kidney*
saphenous vein	Vein that carries blood from the leg to the groin	**saphen/o-** *clearly visible*
subclavian artery	Artery that carries oxygenated blood to the shoulder. It goes underneath (sub-) the clavicle (collar bone).	**clav/o-** *clavicle (collar bone)*
tibial artery	Artery that carries oxygenated blood to the front and back of the lower leg	**tibi/o-** *tibia (shin bone)*
ulnar artery	Artery that carries oxygenated blood to the little finger side of the lower arm (along the ulna bone)	**uln/o-** *ulna (forearm bone)*
vasculature	Network of blood vessels in a particular organ	**vascul/o-** *blood vessel*
vasoconstriction	Constriction of smooth muscle in the wall of a blood vessel that causes it to become smaller in diameter	**vas/o-** *blood vessel; vas deferens* **constrict/o-** *drawn together; narrowed*
vasodilation	Relaxation of smooth muscle in the wall of a blood vessel that causes it to become larger in diameter	**vas/o-** *blood vessel; vas deferens* **dilat/o-** *dilate; widen*
vein	Blood vessel that carries blood from the body back to the heart. This blood has a low level of oxygen and a high level of carbon dioxide and waste products of cellular metabolism from the cells. The exception is the pulmonary veins that carry blood that has a high level of oxygen from the lungs back to the heart.	**ven/o-** *vein* **phleb/o-** *vein*
venae cavae	Largest veins in the body. The **superior vena cava** carries blood from the head, neck, arms, and chest back to the right atrium of the heart. The **inferior vena cava** carries blood from the abdomen, pelvis, and legs back to the right atrium.	
venule	Smallest branch of a vein	**ven/o-** *vein*

Labeling Exercise

Match each anatomy word or phrase to its structure and write it in the numbered box for each figure. Be sure to check your spelling. Use the Answer Key at the end of the book to check your answers.

aortic arch	inferior vena cava	left ventricle	right pulmonary artery
aortic valve	interventricular septum	mitral valve	right ventricle
apex of the heart	left atrium	pulmonary trunk	superior vena cava
ascending aorta	left pulmonary artery	pulmonary valve	tricuspid valve
chordae tendinae	left pulmonary veins	right atrium	

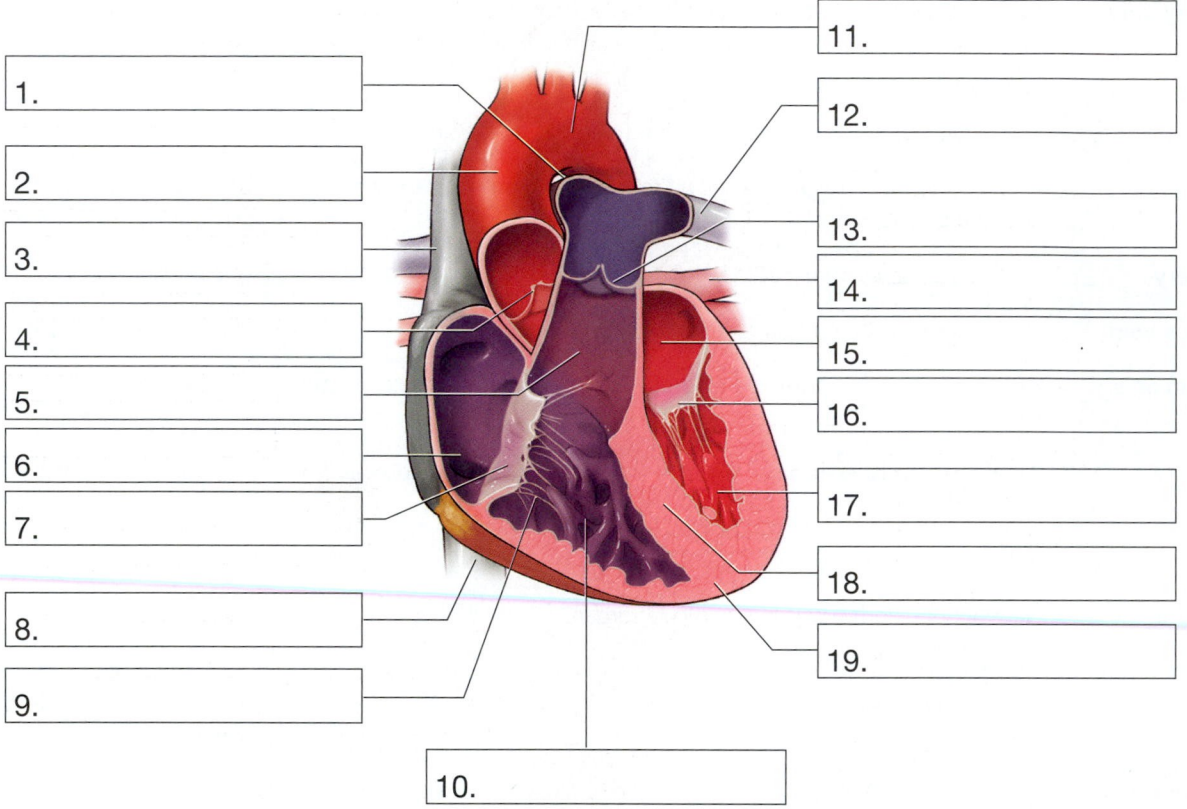

1.
2.
3.
4.
5.
6.
7.
8.
9.
10.
11.
12.
13.
14.
15.
16.
17.
18.
19.

atrioventricular node	bundle of His	left ventricle	right atrium	sinoatrial node
bundle branches	left atrium	Purkinje fibers	right ventricle	

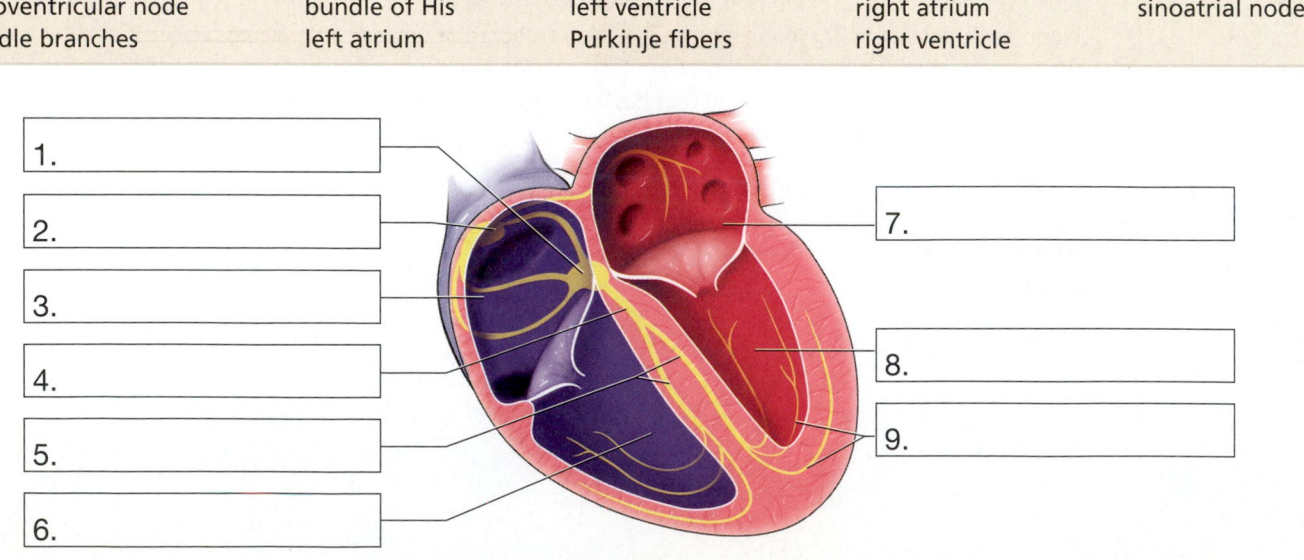

1.
2.
3.
4.
5.
6.
7.
8.
9.

abdominal aorta   carotid artery   iliac artery   radial artery   tibial artery
axillary artery   coronary artery   peroneal artery   renal artery   thoracic aorta
brachial artery   femoral artery   popliteal artery   subclavian artery   ulnar artery

1. _____

2. _____

3. _____

4. _____

5. _____

6. _____

7. _____

8. _____

9. _____

10. _____

11. _____

12. _____

13. _____

14. _____

15. _____

Building Medical Words

Use the Answer Key at the end of the book to check your answers.

Combining Forms Exercise

Before you build cardiovascular words, review these combining forms. Next to each combining form, write its medical meaning. The first one has been done for you.

Combining Form	Medical Meaning	Combining Form	Medical Meaning
1. **axill/o-**	axilla (armpit)	29. mitr/o-	
2. abdomin/o-		30. my/o-	
3. angi/o-		31. pariet/o-	
4. aort/o-		32. perone/o-	
5. apic/o-		33. phleb/o-	
6. arteri/o-		34. polar/o-	
7. arteriol/o-		35. poplite/o-	
8. arter/o-		36. port/o-	
9. atri/o-		37. pulmon/o-	
10. brachi/o-		38. radi/o-	
11. capill/o-		39. ren/o-	
12. card/i-		40. saphen/o-	
13. cardi/o-		41. sept/o-	
14. carot/o-		42. sin/o-	
15. circulat/o-		43. system/o-	
16. clav/o-		44. systol/o-	
17. conduct/o-		45. theli/o-	
18. constrict/o-		46. thorac/o-	
19. coron/o-		47. tibi/o-	
20. cusp/o-		48. uln/o-	
21. diastol/o-		49. valv/o-	
22. dilat/o-		50. valvul/o-	
23. ectop/o-		51. vascul/o-	
24. femor/o-		52. vas/o-	
25. fract/o-		53. ven/o-	
26. ili/o-		54. ventricul/o-	
27. jugul/o-		55. viscer/o-	
28. mediastin/o-			

Combining Form and Suffix Exercise

Read the definition of the medical word. Look at the combining form that is given. Select the correct suffix from the Suffix List and write it on the blank line. Then build the medical word and write it on the line. (Remember: You may need to remove the combining vowel. Always remove the hyphens and slash.) Be sure to check your spelling. The first one has been done for you.

SUFFIX LIST

-ac (pertaining to)	-ary (pertaining to)	-ion (action; condition)	-ous (pertaining to)
-al (pertaining to)	-ature (system composed of)	-ole (small thing)	-ule (small thing)
-ar (pertaining to)	-ic (pertaining to)	-ory (having the function of)	

	Definition of the Medical Word	Combining Form	Suffix	Build the Medical Word
1.	Pertaining to the thorax (chest)	**thorac/o-**	**-ic**	*thoracic*
	(You think *pertaining to* (-ic) + *the thorax* (thorac/o-). You change the order of the word parts to put the suffix last. You write *thoracic*.)			
2.	Pertaining to an artery	arteri/o-	_____	_____
3.	Pertaining to a valve	valvul/o-	_____	_____
4.	Action of movement in a circular route	circulat/o-	_____	_____
5.	Pertaining to the heart	cardi/o-	_____	_____
6.	Pertaining to a hairlike structure (blood vessel)	capill/o-	_____	_____
7.	Pertaining to a vein	ven/o-	_____	_____
8.	Pertaining to the body as a whole	system/o-	_____	_____
9.	Pertaining to the atrium	atri/o-	_____	_____
10.	Pertaining to the arm	brachi/o-	_____	_____
11.	Small artery	arteri/o-	_____	_____
12.	Pertaining to (a structure that is) clearly visible	saphen/o-	_____	_____
13.	Pertaining to the aorta	aort/o-	_____	_____
14.	System composed of blood vessels	vascul/o-	_____	_____
15.	Pertaining to contracting	systol/o-	_____	_____
16.	Having the function of movement in a circular route	circulat/o-	_____	_____
17.	Pertaining to the ventricle	ventricul/o-	_____	_____
18.	Small vein	ven/o-	_____	_____

Multiple Combining Forms and Suffix Exercise

Read the definition of the medical word. Look at the correct suffix that is given. Select the two correct combining forms from the Combining Form List. Then build the medical word and write it on the line. Be sure to check your spelling. The first one has been done for you.

COMBINING FORM LIST

atri/o- (atrium; upper heart chamber)	my/o- (muscle)	vas/o- (blood vessel; vas deferens)
cardi/o- (heart)	pulmon/o- (lung)	ventricul/o- (ventricle; lower heart chamber)
constrict/o- (drawn together; narrowed)	sin/o- (hollow cavity; channel)	
dilat/o- (dilate; widen)	vascul/o- (blood vessel)	

Definition of the Medical Word	Combining Form	Combining Form	Suffix	Build the Medical Word
1. Condition of blood vessels dilated	**vas/o-**	**dilat/o-**	**-ion**	*vasodilation*
(You think *condition* (-ion) + *the blood vessel* (vas/o-) + *dilated* (dilat/o-). You change the order of the word parts to put the suffix last. You write *vasodilation*.)				
2. Pertaining to the heart and lungs	_____	_____	-ary	_____
3. Pertaining to the heart and blood vessels	_____	_____	-ar	_____
4. Pertaining to the SA node	_____	_____	-al	_____
5. Condition of blood vessels narrowed	_____	_____	-ion	_____
6. Pertaining to the muscle of the heart	_____	_____	-al	_____
7. Pertaining to the atrium and ventricle	_____	_____	-ar	_____

Diseases and Conditions

Myocardium

Word or Phrase	Description	Word Building
acute coronary syndrome	Category that includes acute **ischemia** of the myocardium (because of a blood clot or atherosclerosis blocking blood flow through a coronary artery) with unstable angina pectoris. Treatment: Nitroglycerin drugs, thrombolytic drugs, oxygen therapy.	**ischemia** (is-KEE-mee-ah) **isch/o-** *keep back; block* **-emia** *condition of the blood; substance in the blood*
angina pectoris	Mild-to-severe chest pain caused by ischemia of the myocardium. Atherosclerosis blocks the flow of oxygenated blood through the coronary arteries to the myocardium. There can be a crushing, pressure-like sensation in the chest, with pain extending up into the neck or down the left arm, often accompanied by extreme sweating (diaphoresis) and a sense of doom. Angina pectoris can occur during exercise or while resting. It is a warning sign of an impending myocardial infarction. Treatment: Nitroglycerin drugs, oxygen therapy.	**angina** (AN-jih-nah) (an-JY-nah) **anginal** (AN-jih-nal) (an-JY-nal) **angin/o-** *angina* **-al** *pertaining to* **pectoris** (PEK-toh-ris) The combining form *pector/o-* means *chest*.

Did You Know?

For many years, newspaper and magazine articles described the classic symptoms of angina pectoris in order to raise public awareness and encourage those with angina to promptly seek medical help. Now it is known that those symptoms occur in men, but women most often experience angina as indigestion, nausea, anxiety, extreme fatigue, or trouble sleeping.

Word or Phrase	Description	Word Building
cardiomegaly	Enlargement of the heart, usually due to congestive heart failure. Treatment: Correct the underlying cause.	**cardiomegaly** (KAR-dee-oh-MEG-ah-lee) **cardi/o-** *heart* **-megaly** *enlargement*
cardiomyopathy	Any disease condition of the heart muscle that includes heart enlargement and heart failure. In **dilated cardiomyopathy,** the left ventricle is dilated and the myocardium is so stretched that it can no longer contract to pump blood. **Idiopathic cardiomyopathy** has an unknown cause. Treatment: Correct the underlying cause, if known.	**cardiomyopathy** (KAR-dee-oh-my-AWP-ah-thee) **cardi/o-** *heart* **my/o-** *muscle* **-pathy** *disease; suffering* **idiopathic** (ID-ee-oh-PATH-ik) **idi/o-** *unknown; individual* **path/o-** *disease; suffering* **-ic** *pertaining to*

Word or Phrase	Description	Word Building

congestive heart failure (CHF)	Inability of the heart to pump sufficient amounts of blood. It is caused by coronary artery disease or hypertension. During early CHF, the myocardium undergoes **hypertrophy** (enlargement). This temporarily improves blood flow, and the patient is in **compensated** heart failure. In the later stages of CHF, the heart can no longer enlarge. Instead, the myocardium becomes flabby and loses its ability to contract, and the patient is in **decompensated** heart failure.
	
	In right-sided congestive heart failure, the right ventricle is unable to adequately pump blood. Blood backs up in the superior vena cava, causing **jugular venous distention** (dilated jugular veins in the neck). Blood also backs up in the inferior vena cava, causing hepatomegaly (enlargement of the liver) and **peripheral edema** in the legs, ankles, and feet (see Figure 5-14 ■). When there is lung disease and the right ventricle enlarges to pump harder, this condition is known as **cor pulmonale.**
	
	In left-sided congestive heart failure, the left ventricle is unable to adequately pump blood. The blood backs up into the lungs, causing pulmonary congestion and edema that can be seen on a chest x-ray. There is also shortness of breath, cough, and an inability to sleep while lying flat. Treatment: Diuretic drugs, digitalis drugs, and antihypertensive drugs. Severe left-sided heart failure is life-threatening; it may require surgery for a heart transplant or a left ventricular assist device (LVAD).
	
	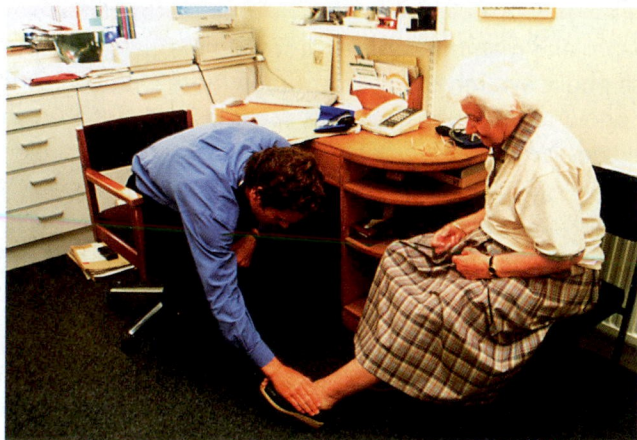
	
	Figure 5-14 ■ Peripheral edema.
	This physician knows that fluid-filled soft tissues in the feet and lower legs can be a sign of right-sided congestive heart failure. He will also examine the neck veins to look for jugular venous distention, another sign of right-sided congestive heart failure. He will also use a stethoscope to listen to the lungs to detect pulmonary edema, a sign of left-sided heart failure.
		congestive (con-JES-tiv)
		  congest/o- *accumulation of fluid*
		  -ive *pertaining to*
		
		hypertrophy (hy-PER-troh-fee)
		  hyper- *above; more than normal*
		  -trophy *process of development*
		The ending *-trophy* contains the combining form *troph/o-* and the one-letter suffix *–y.*
		
		compensated (KAWM-pen-SAY-ted)
		  compens/o- *counterbalance; compensate*
		  -ated *pertaining to a condition; composed of*
		
		decompensated
		(dee-KAWM-pen-SAY-ted)
		  de- *reversal of; without*
		  compens/o- *counterbalance; compensate*
		  -ated *pertaining to a condition; composed of*
		
		peripheral (peh-RIF-eh-ral)
		  peripher/o- *outer aspects*
		  -al *pertaining to*
		
		edema (eh-DEE-mah)
		
		cor pulmonale (KOR PUL-moh-NAL-ee)

myocardial infarction (MI)	Death of myocardial cells due to severe ischemia. The flow of oxygenated blood in a coronary artery is blocked by a blood clot or atherosclerosis. The patient may experience severe angina pectoris, may have mild symptoms similar to indigestion, or may have no symptoms at all (a silent MI). The infarcted area of myocardium has **necrosis.** If the area of necrosis is small, it will eventually be replaced by scar tissue. If the area is large, the heart muscle may be unable to contract. Treatment: Aspirin taken to prevent an MI or at the first sign of an MI. Thrombolytic drugs to dissolve a clot during an MI.	**myocardial** (MY-oh-KAR-dee-al)
		  my/o- *muscle*
		  cardi/o- *heart*
		  -al *pertaining to*
		
		infarction (in-FARK-shun)
		  infarct/o- *area of dead tissue*
		  -ion *action; condition*
		
		necrosis (neh-KROH-sis)
		  necr/o- *dead cells, tissue, or body*
		  -osis *condition; abnormal condition; process*

Heart Valves and Layers of the Heart

Word or Phrase	Description	Word Building
endocarditis	Inflammation and bacterial infection of the endocardium lining a heart valve. This occurs in patients who have a structural defect of the valve. Bacteria from an infection elsewhere in the body travel through the blood, are trapped by the structural defect, and cause infection. Acute endocarditis causes a high fever and shock, while **subacute bacterial endocarditis (SBE)** causes fever, fatigue, and aching muscles. Treatment: Antibiotic drugs.	**endocarditis** (EN-doh-kar-DY-tis) **endo-** *innermost; within* **card/i-** *heart* **-itis** *inflammation of; infection of* The combining vowel *i* of *card/i-* is deleted before it is joined to the suffix *-itis*. **subacute** (SUB-ah-KYOOT)
mitral valve prolapse (MVP)	Structural abnormality in which the leaflets of the mitral valve do not close tightly. This can be a congenital condition or can occur if the valve is damaged by infection. There is **regurgitation** as blood flows back into the left atrium with each contraction. A slight prolapse is a common condition and does not require treatment. Treatment: Valvoplasty or valve replacement surgery.	**prolapse** (PROH-laps) **regurgitation** (ree-GER-jih-TAY-shun) **regurgitat/o-** *flow backward* **-ion** *action; condition*

Clinical Connections

Neonatology. Congenital abnormalities can occur in the fetal heart as it develops:

1. **Coarctation of the aorta.** The aorta is abnormally narrow.
2. **Atrial septal defect (ASD).** There is a permanent hole in the interatrial septum.
3. **Ventricular septal defect (VSD).** There is a permanent hole in the interventricular septum.
4. **Tetralogy of Fallot.** There are four defects: a ventricular septal defect, narrowing of the pulmonary trunk, hypertrophy of the right ventricle, and abnormal position of the aorta.
5. **Transposition of the great vessels.** The aorta incorrectly originates from the right ventricle, and the pulmonary trunk incorrectly originates from the left ventricle.

The following abnormalities occur at the time of birth during the change from fetal circulation to normal newborn circulation:

1. **Patent ductus arteriosus (PDA).** The ductus arteriosus fails to close.
2. **Patent foramen ovale.** The foramen ovale fails to close.

coarctation (KOH-ark-TAY-shun)
 coarct/o- *pressed together*
 -ation *a process; being or having*

tetralogy (tet-RAL-oh-jee)
 tetr/a- *four*
 -logy *the study of*

Fallot (fah-LOW)

patent (PAY-tent)
 pat/o- *to be open*
 -ent *pertaining to*

Word or Phrase	Description	Word Building
murmur	Abnormal heart sound created by turbulence as blood leaks through a defective heart valve. Murmurs are described according to their volume (soft or loud), their sound, and when they occur. Functional murmurs are mild murmurs that are not associated with disease and are not clinically significant. Treatment: Surgery to correct the defective heart valve (valvuloplasty), if needed.	murmur (MER-mer)

Did You Know?

Heart murmurs can sound like the call of a sea gull, blowing wind, the clatter of machinery, high-pitched musical notes, or like churning, humming, or clicking.

Word or Phrase	Description	Word Building
pericarditis	Inflammation or infection of the pericardial sac with an excessive accumulation of pericardial fluid. When the fluid compresses the heart and prevents it from beating, this is **cardiac tamponade.** Treatment: Antibiotic drugs. Surgery to remove the fluid (pericardiocentesis), if necessary.	**pericarditis** (PAIR-ee-kar-DY-tis) **peri-** *around* **card/i-** *heart* **-itis** *inflammation of; infection of* **tamponade** (tam-poh-NAYD) **tampon/o-** *stop up* **-ade** *action; process*
rheumatic heart disease	Autoimmune response to a previous streptococcal infection, such as a strep throat. Rheumatic heart disease occurs most often in children and is known as rheumatic fever. The body makes antibodies to fight the bacteria, but after the infection is gone the antibodies attack the connective tissue in the body, particularly the joints and/or the heart. The joints become swollen with fluid and inflamed. The mitral and aortic valves of the heart become inflamed and damaged. **Vegetations** (irregular collections of platelets, fibrin, and bacteria) form on the valves (see Figure 5-15 ■). The valves become scarred and narrowed, a condition known as **stenosis.** Treatment: Antibiotic drug to treat the initial infection. After rheumatic heart disease has occurred, a prophylactic (preventative) antibiotic drug is given prior to any dental or surgical procedure that might release bacteria that could further damage the valves. Valve replacement surgery, if needed.	**rheumatic** (roo-MAT-ik) **rheumat/o-** *watery discharge* **-ic** *pertaining to* **vegetation** (VEJ-eh-TAY-shun) **vegetat/o-** *growth* **-ion** *action; condition* **stenosis** (steh-NOH-sis) **sten/o-** *narrowness; constriction* **-osis** *condition; abnormal condition; process*

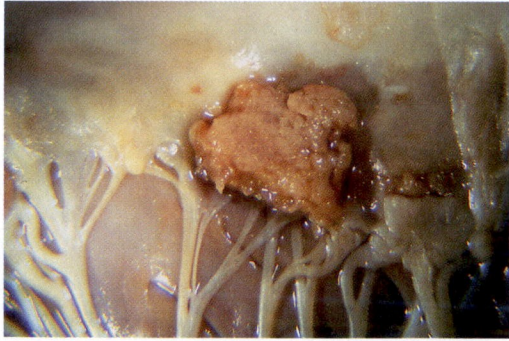

Figure 5-15 ■ Vegetation on the mitral valve.

There is an irregular, brown vegetation growing on the otherwise smooth surface of the mitral valve. The multiple ropelike structures below are the chordae tendineae attached to the valve.

Conduction System

Word or Phrase	Description	Word Building
arrhythmia	Any type of irregularity in the rate or rhythm of the heart. It is also known as **dysrhythmia.** Arrhythmias include bradycardia, fibrillation, flutter, heart block, premature contraction, sick sinus syndrome, and tachycardia. Electrocardiography is performed to diagnose the type of arrhythmia (see Figure 5-16 ■). Treatment: Antiarrhythmic drugs, cardioversion, or pacemaker, depending on the type of arrhythmia. 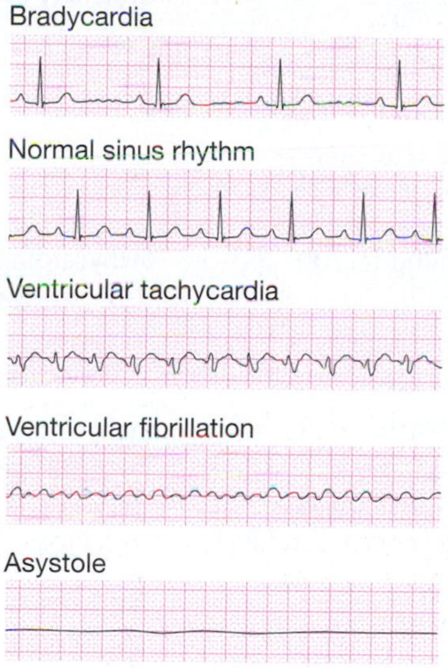 Bradycardia Normal sinus rhythm Ventricular tachycardia Ventricular fibrillation **Figure 5-16 ■ Arrhythmias on an ECG tracing.** (a) Bradycardia with a heart rate of 60 beats per minute. (b) A normal heart rate at 80 beats per minute. (c) Ventricular tachycardia at 150 beats per minute. (d) Ventricular fibrillation. (e) Asystole is not an arrythmia because there is no heart beat. Asystole	**arrhythmia** (aa-RITH-mee-ah) **a-** *away from; without* **rrhythm/o-** *rhythm* **-ia** *condition; state; thing* **dysrhythmia** (dis-RITH-mee-ah) **dys-** *painful; difficult; abnormal* **rhythm/o-** *rhythm* **-ia** *condition; state; thing* Select the correct prefix meaning to get the definition of *dysrhythmia: condition of an abnormal rhythm*
bradycardia	Arrhythmia in which the heart beats too slowly (see Figure 5-16). A patient with bradycardia is **bradycardic.** Treatment: Intravenous atropine (drug). Insertion of a pacemaker.	**bradycardia** (BRAD-ee-KAR-dee-ah) **brady-** *slow* **card/i-** *heart* **-ia** *condition; state; thing* **bradycardic** (BRAD-ee-KAR-dik) **brady-** *slow* **card/i-** *heart* **ic-** *pertaining to*
fibrillation	Arrhythmia in which there is a very fast, uncoordinated quivering of the myocardium (see Figure 5-16). It can affect the atria or ventricles. Ventricular fibrillation, a life-threatening emergency in which the heart is unable to pump blood, can progress to cardiac arrest. Treatment: Defibrillation.	**fibrillation** (FIB-rih-LAY-shun) **fibrill/o-** *muscle fiber; nerve fiber* **-ation** *a process; being or having*
flutter	Arrhythmia in which there is a very fast but regular rhythm (250 beats per minute) of the atria or ventricles. The chambers of the heart do not have time to completely fill with blood before the next contraction. Flutter can progress to fibrillation. Treatment: Antiarrhythmic drugs; cardioversion.	
heart block	Arrhythmia in which electrical impulses cannot travel normally from the SA node to the Purkinje fibers. In **first-degree heart block,** the electrical impulses reach the ventricles but are very delayed. In **second-degree heart block,** only some of the electrical impulses reach the ventricles. In **third-degree heart block** (complete heart block), no electrical impulses reach the ventricles. In **right or left bundle branch block,** the electrical impulses are unable to travel down the right or left bundle of His. Treatment: Antiarrhythmic drugs. Surgery to insert a pacemaker.	

Word or Phrase	Description	Word Building
premature contraction	Arrhythmia in which there are one or more extra contractions within a cardiac cycle. This is also known as an **extrasystole.** There are two types of premature contractions: **premature atrial contractions (PACs)** and **premature ventricular contractions (PVCs).** A repeating pattern of one normal contraction followed by one premature contraction is **bigeminy.** A repeating pattern of two normal contractions followed by one premature contraction is **trigeminy.** Two premature contractions occurring together is a **couplet.** Treatment: Antiarrhythmic drugs. Surgical insertion of a pacemaker.	**contraction** (con-TRAK-shun) **contract/o-** *pull together* **-ion** *action; condition* **extrasystole** (EKS-trah-SIS-toh-lee) **extra-** *outside of* **-systole** *contraction* **bigeminy** (by-JEM-ih-nee) **trigeminy** (try-JEM-in-nee)
sick sinus syndrome	Arrhythmia in which bradycardia alternates with tachycardia. It occurs when the sinoatrial node and an ectopic site elsewhere in the myocardium take turns being the heart's pacemaker. Treatment: Antiarrhythmic drugs. Surgery to insert a pacemaker.	
tachycardia	Arrhythmia in which there is a fast but regular rhythm (up to 200 beats/minute) (see Figure 5-16). A patient with tachycardia is **tachycardic. Sinus tachycardia** occurs because of an abnormality in the sinoatrial (SA) node. Atrial tachycardia occurs when an ectopic site somewhere in the atrium produces an electrical impulse that overrides the SA node rhythm. **Supraventricular tachycardia** occurs when an ectopic site superior to the ventricles produces an electrical impulse. **Paroxysmal tachycardia** is an episode of tachycardia that occurs suddenly and then goes away without treatment. Treatment: Antiarrhythmic drugs. Surgery to insert a pacemaker; cardioversion.	**tachycardia** (TAK-ih-KAR-dee-ah) **tachy-** *fast* **card/i-** *heart* **-ia** *condition; state; thing* **tachycardic** (TAK-ih-KAR-dik) **tachy-** *fast* **card/i-** *heart* **-ic** *pertaining to* **supraventricular** (SOO-prah-ven-TRIK-yoo-lar) **supra-** *above* **ventricul/o-** *ventricle (lower heart chamber; chamber in the brain)* **-ar** *pertaining to* **paroxysmal** (PAIR-awk-SIZ-mal)
asystole	Complete absence of a heartbeat (see Figure 5-16) This is also known as **cardiac arrest.** Treatment: Cardiopulmonary resuscitation (CPR).	**asystole** (aa-SIS-toh-lee) **a-** *away from; without* **-systole** *contraction*
palpitation	An uncomfortable sensation felt in the chest during a premature contraction of the heart. It is often described as a "thump." Treatment: None, unless it becomes an arrhythmia.	**palpitation** (PAL-pih-TAY-shun) **palpit/o-** *to throb* **-ation** *a process; being or having*

Word Alert

SOUND-ALIKE WORDS

palpation   (noun)   A process of touching and feeling.
Example: Palpation allowed the physician to identify a tumor in the abdomen.

palpitation   (noun)   Being or having (the heart) throb
Example: Her occasional palpitations concerned the patient until the physician reassured her.

Blood Vessels

Word or Phrase	Description	Word Building

aneurysm	Area of dilation and weakness in the wall of an artery (see Figure 5-17 ■). This can be congenital or where arteriosclerosis has damaged the artery. With each heartbeat, the weakened artery wall balloons outward. An aneurysm can rupture without warning. A **dissecting aneurysm** is one that enlarges by tunneling between the layers of the artery wall. Treatment: Placement of a metal clip on the neck (narrowest part) of a small **aneurysmal** dilation to occlude the blood flow. Surgical excision of a large aneurysm and replacement with a synthetic tubular graft.	**aneurysm** (AN-yoo-rizm)
		
		dissecting (dy-SEK-ting)
		   dissect/o- *to cut apart*
		   -ing *doing*
		
		aneurysmal (AN-yoo-RIZ-mal)
		   aneurysm/o- *aneurysm (dilation)*
		   -al *pertaining to*

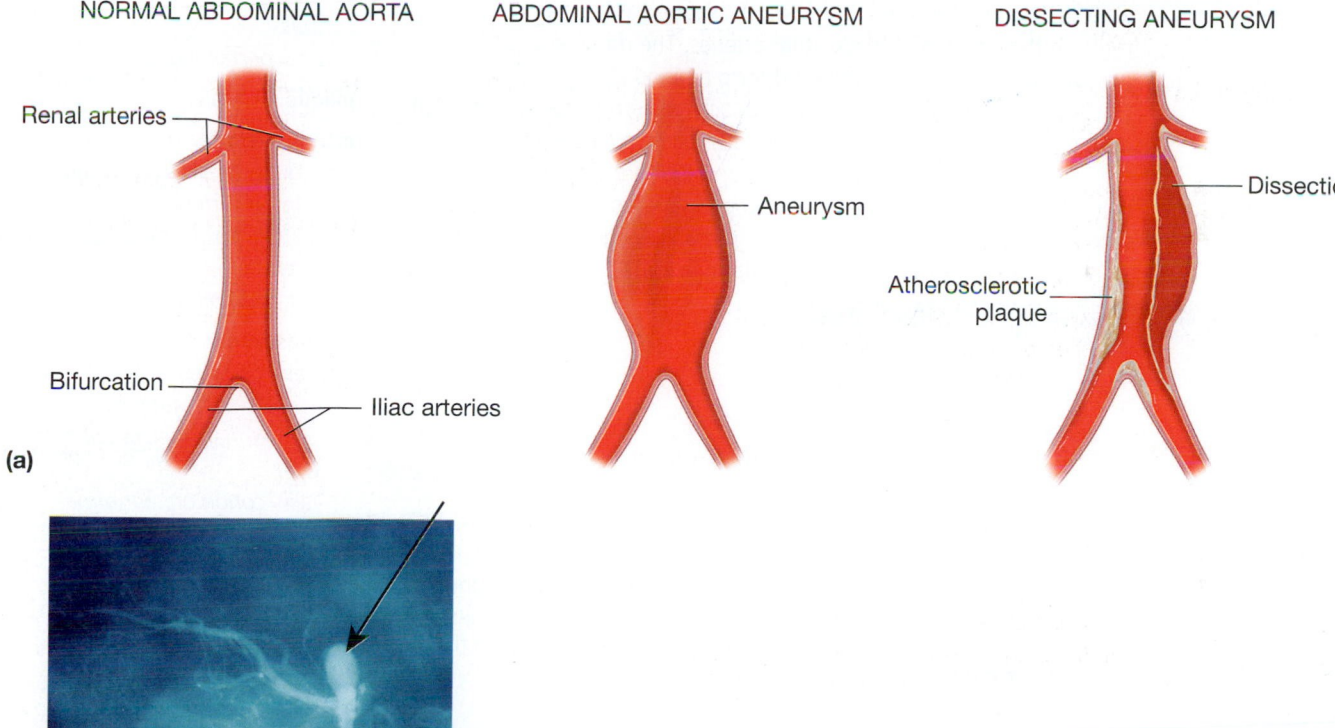

NORMAL ABDOMINAL AORTA

Renal arteries

Bifurcation

Iliac arteries

(a)

ABDOMINAL AORTIC ANEURYSM

Aneurysm

DISSECTING ANEURYSM

Dissection

Atherosclerotic plaque

(b)

Figure 5-17 ■ Aneurysm.

(a) A normal abdominal aorta, a large abdominal aortic aneurysm, and a dissecting aneurysm that has tunneled between and separated the atherosclerotic plaque from the artery wall. (b) This aneurysm is in an artery in the brain. Arteriography was performed, and the arteriogram shows contrast dye outlining the bulging aneurysm.

Word or Phrase	Description	Word Building

arteriosclerosis	Progressive degenerative changes that produce a narrowed, hardened artery. The process begins with a small tear in the endothelium that is caused by chronic hypertension. Then low-density lipoproteins (LDLs) in the blood deposit cholesterol and form an **atheroma** or **atheromatous plaque** inside the artery (see Figure 5-18 ■). Collagen fibers form underneath the plaque, so that the artery wall becomes hard and nonelastic. An artery with arteriosclerosis is said to be **arteriosclerotic.** This is also known as arteriosclerotic cardiovascular disease (ASCVD).
	
	Fatty plaque deposits enlarge more rapidly in patients who eat high-fat diets, have diabetes mellitus, or have a genetic predisposition (family history). As plaque grows on an artery wall, it makes the lumen narrower and narrower (see Figure 5-19 ■). This process is known as **atherosclerosis.** Pieces of atheromatous plaque easily break off, travel through the blood, and block other arteries. The rough edges of the plaque can trap red blood cells and form a blood clot.
	
	Severe atherosclerosis completely blocks the artery (see Figure 5-19). In the carotid arteries to the brain, this can cause a stroke. In the coronary arteries to the heart muscle, this can cause angina pectoris and a myocardial infarction. In the renal arteries to the kidney, this can cause kidney failure. Treatment: Lipid-lowering drugs. Surgery: Angioplasty or stent to press down the plaque or endarterectomy to remove the plaque.
		arteriosclerosis (ar-TEER-ee-oh-skleh-ROH-sis)
		   arteri/o- *artery*
		   scler/o- *hard; sclera (white of the eye)*
		   -osis *condition; abnormal condition; process*
		
		atheroma (ATH-eh-ROH-mah)
		   ather/o- *soft, fatty substance*
		   -oma *tumor; mass*
		
		atheromatous (ATH-eh-ROH-mah-tus)
		   atheromat/o- *fatty deposit or mass*
		   -ous *pertaining to*
		
		plaque (PLAK)
		
		arteriosclerotic (ar-TEER-ee-oh-skleh-RAW-tik)
		   arteri/o- *artery*
		   scler/o- *hard; sclera (white of the eye)*
		   -tic *pertaining to*
		
		atherosclerosis (ATH-eh-roh-skleh-ROH-sis)
		   ather/o- *soft, fatty substance*
		   scler/o- *hard; sclera (white of the eye)*
		   -osis *condition; abnormal condition; process*

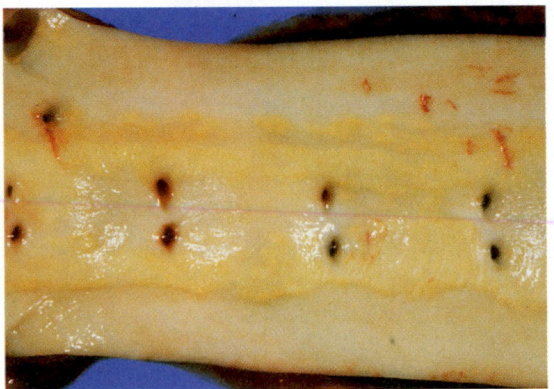

Figure 5-18 ■ Mild atheromatous plaque.

This aorta from a cadaver shows mild, slightly raised plaque along its wall. The pairs of dark areas are where right and left arteries branch off from the aorta. The plaque has not yet occluded the lumens of these arteries.

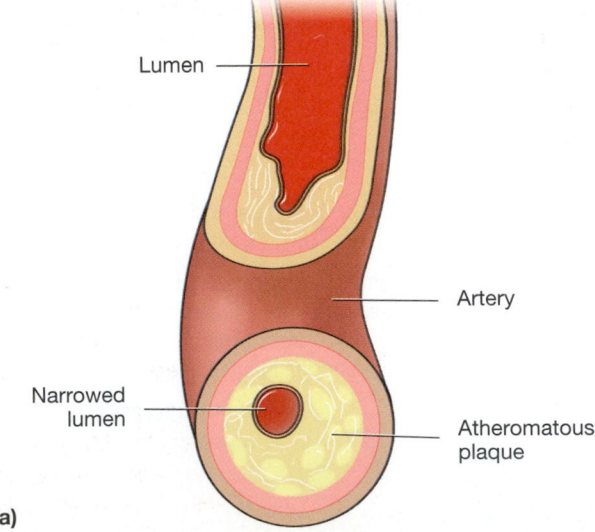

Lumen

Narrowed lumen

Artery

Atheromatous plaque

(a)

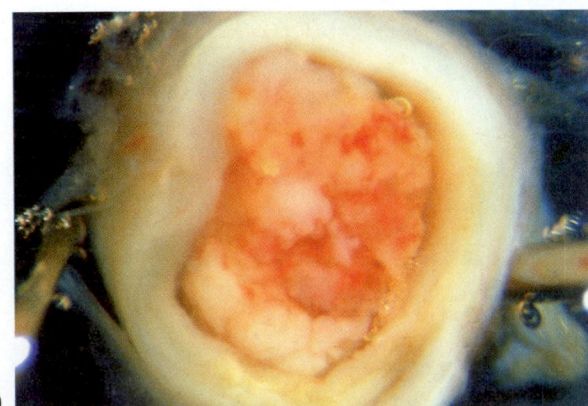

(b)

Figure 5-19 ■ Severe atherosclerotic plaque in an artery.

(a) The lumen of the artery is so small that little blood can flow through it. (b) This cut section of a coronary artery, as seen during coronary artery bypass graft surgery, is completely blocked by atheromatous plaque.

Word or Phrase	Description	Word Building
arteriosclerosis (*continued*)	**Clinical Connections**	

Dietetics. The body produces its own supply of cholesterol that is used to make bile, neurotransmitters, and sexual hormones. The diet contains additional cholesterol in foods from animal sources. An excessive amount of animal fat in the diet increases the cholesterol level in the blood. An excessive amount of sugar in the diet is converted by the body to triglycerides, and this causes an increased triglyceride level in the blood and increased storage as adipose tissue (fat).

Lipoproteins are carrier molecules produced in the liver. They transport lipids (fats such as cholesterol and triglycerides) in the blood. There are three types of lipoproteins. High-density lipoprotein (HDL) carries cholesterol to the liver where it is excreted in the bile. HDL is known by laypersons as "good cholesterol," and an increased level of HDL is beneficial. Low-density lipoprotein (LDL) carries cholesterol but deposits it on the walls of the arteries, and so it is known as "bad cholesterol." Very low-density lipoprotein (VLDL) carries triglycerides and deposits them on the walls of the arteries.

Word or Phrase	Description	Word Building
bruit	A harsh, rushing sound made by blood passing through an artery narrowed and roughened by atherosclerosis. The bruit can be heard when a stethoscope is placed over the artery.	**bruit** (BROO-ee)
coronary artery disease (CAD)	Arteriosclerosis of the coronary arteries. They are filled with atheromatous plaque, and their narrowed lumens cannot carry enough oxygenated blood to the myocardium. This results in angina pectoris. Severe atherosclerosis (or a blood clot that forms on an atherosclerotic plaque) can completely block the lumen of a coronary artery. This causes a myocardial infarction. Treatment: Lipid-lowering drugs. Surgery: Percutaneous transluminal coronary angioplasty (PTCA) or coronary artery bypass grafting (CABG).	

Clinical Connections

Public Health. There are many factors that contribute to the development of coronary artery disease. These are known as cardiac risk factors. They include demographic factors (heredity, gender, age), medical factors (hypertension, hypercholesterolemia, diabetes mellitus, obesity), and lifestyle factors (smoking, lack of exercise, poor diet, stress, alcoholism).

Word or Phrase	Description	Word Building
hyperlipidemia	Elevated levels of lipids (fats) in the blood. Lipids include cholesterol and triglycerides. **Hypercholesterolemia** is an elevated level of cholesterol in the blood. **Hypertriglyceridemia** is an elevated level of triglycerides in the blood. Normal levels are below 200 mg/dL for cholesterol and below 150 mg/dL for triglycerides. Treatment: Lipid-lowering drugs.	**hyperlipidemia** (HY-per-LIP-ih-DEE-mee-ah) **hyper-** *above; more than normal* **lipid/o-** *lipid (fat)* **-emia** *condition of the blood; substance in the blood* **hypercholesterolemia** (HY-per-koh-LES-ter-awl-EE-mee-ah) **hyper-** *above; more than normal* **cholesterol/o-** *cholesterol* **-emia** *condition of the blood; substance in the blood* **hypertriglyceridemia** (HY-per-try-GLIS-eh-ry-DEE-mee-ah) **hyper-** *above; more than normal* **triglycerid/o-** *triglyceride* **-emia** *condition of the blood; substance in the blood*

Word or Phrase	Description	Word Building
hypertension (HTN)	Elevated blood pressure. Normal blood pressure readings in an adult are less than 120/80 mm Hg. Those between 120/80 mm Hg and 140/90 mm Hg are categorized as **prehypertension.** Blood pressures above 140/90 mm Hg are categorized as hypertension, and the patient is said to be **hypertensive.** Several blood pressure readings, not just one, are needed to make a diagnosis. Essential hypertension, the most common type of hypertension, is one in which the exact cause is not known. Secondary hypertension has a known cause, such as kidney disease. Treatment: Lifestyle changes (decreased salt intake, increased exercise, weight loss) followed by antihypertensive drugs.	**hypertension** (HY-per-TEN-shun) 　**hyper-** *above; more than normal* 　**tens/o-** *pressure; tension* 　**-ion** *action; condition* **prehypertension** (pree-HY-per-TEN-shun) 　**pre-** *before; in front of* 　**hyper-** *above; more than normal* 　**tens/o-** *pressure; tension* 　**-ion** *action; condition* **hypertensive** (HY-per-TEN-siv) 　**hyper-** *above; more than normal* 　**tens/o-** *pressure; tension* 　**-ive** *pertaining to*

Did You Know?

Some people have increased blood pressure readings just because they are nervous about being in a doctor's office. This is known as white-coat hypertension. This is not a true hypertension because as soon as they leave the doctor's office, their blood pressure returns to normal.

Word or Phrase	Description	Word Building
hypotension	Blood pressure lower than 90/60 mm Hg, usually because of a loss of blood volume. A patient with hypotension is **hypotensive. Orthostatic hypotension** is the sudden, temporary, but self-correcting decrease in systolic blood pressure that occurs when the patient changes from a lying to a standing position and experiences lightheadedness. Treatment: Correct the underlying cause.	**hypotension** (HY-poh-TEN-shun) 　**hypo-** *below; deficient* 　**tens/o-** *pressure; tension* 　**-ion** *action; condition* **hypotensive** (HY-poh-TEN-siv) 　**hypo-** *below; deficient* 　**tens/o-** *pressure; tension* 　**-ive** *pertaining to* **orthostatic** (OR-thoh-STAT-ik) 　**orth/o-** *straight* 　**stat/o-** *standing still; staying in one place* 　**-ic** *pertaining to*
peripheral artery disease (PAD)	Atherosclerosis of the arteries in the legs. Blood flow (**perfusion**) to the extremities is poor, and there is ischemia of the tissues. While walking, the patient experiences pain in the calf (intermittent **claudication**). In severe PAD, the feet and toes remain cool and cyanotic and may become **necrotic** as the tissues die. Treatment: Lipid-lowering drugs. Surgery: Angioplasty.	**peripheral** (peh-RIF-eh-ral) 　**peripher/o-** *outer aspects* 　**-al** *pertaining to* **perfusion** (per-FYOO-zhun) 　**per-** *through; throughout* 　**fus/o-** *pouring* 　**-ion** *action; condition* **claudication** (KLAW-dih-KAY-shun) 　**claudicat/o-** *limping pain* 　**-ion** *action; condition* **necrotic** (neh-KRAWT-ik) 　**necr/o-** *dead cells, tissue, or body* 　**-tic** *pertaining to*
peripheral vascular disease (PVD)	Any disease of the arteries of the extremities. It includes peripheral artery disease as well as Raynaud's disease.	**peripheral** (peh-RIF-eh-ral) 　**peripher/o-** *outer aspects* 　**-al** *pertaining to*

Word or Phrase	Description	Word Building

phlebitis	Inflammation of a vein, usually accompanied by infection. The area around the vein is painful, and the skin may show a red streak that follows the course of the vein. A severe inflammation can partially occlude the vein and slow the flow of blood. **Thrombophlebitis** is phlebitis with the formation of a thrombus (blood clot). Treatment: Analgesic drugs for pain, anti-inflammatory drugs for inflammation. Antibiotic drugs. Thrombolytic drugs to dissolve a blood clot.	**phlebitis** (fleh-BY-tis)
		  phleb/o- *vein*
		  -itis *inflammation of; infection of*
		thrombophlebitis
		(THRAWM-boh-fleh-BY-tis)
		  thromb/o- *thrombus (blood clot)*
		  phleb/o- *vein*
		  -itis *inflammation of; infection of*

Raynaud's disease	Sudden, severe vasoconstriction and spasm of the arterioles in the fingers and toes, often triggered by cold or emotional upset. They become white or cyanotic and numb for minutes or hours until the attack passes. This can lead to necrosis. Treatment: Vasodilator drugs.	**Raynaud** (ray-NO)

varicose veins	Damaged or incompetent valves in a vein. They allow blood to flow backward and collect in the preceding section of vein. The vein becomes distended with blood, twisting and bulging under the surface of the skin (see Figure 5-20 ■). Varicose veins can be caused by phlebitis, injury, long periods of sitting with the legs crossed, or occupations that require constant standing. Also, during pregnancy, pressure from the enlarging uterus restricts the flow of blood in the lower extremities and can cause varicose veins. There is a family tendency to develop varicose veins. There is pain and aching; the legs feel heavy and leaden. Treatment: Destruction of the vein by injecting a sclerosing solution or foam to harden and occlude it. Laser or radiowaves to destroy the vein. These procedures redirect the blood into deeper veins.	**varicose** (VAIR-ih-kohs)
		  varic/o- *varix; varicose vein*
		  -ose *full of*

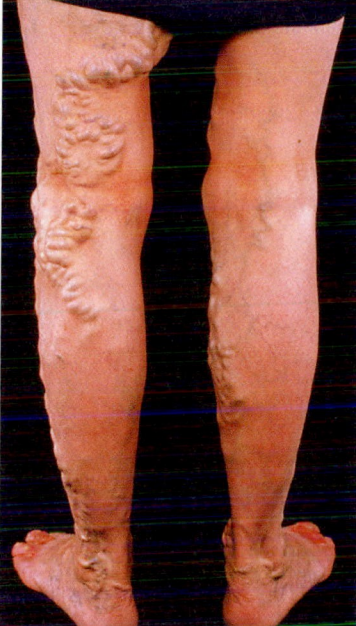

Figure 5-20 ■ Severe varicose veins in the leg.
Superficial, protruding varicose veins are unsightly and easily injured. Patients often have varicose veins treated for an improved cosmetic appearance, but this also helps decrease the chance of injury and thrombophlebitis.

Clinical Connections

Gastroenterology (Chapter 3). Varicose veins of the esophagus and stomach are esophageal and gastric varices. Varicose veins of the rectum are hemorrhoids.

Laboratory and Diagnostic Procedures

Blood Tests

Word or Phrase	Description	Word Building
cardiac enzymes	Test to measure the levels of enzymes that are released into the blood when myocardial cells die during a myocardial infarction. (These enzymes are not released during angina pectoris.) The higher the levels, the more severe the myocardial infarction and the larger the area of infarct. **Creatine kinase (CK)** is found in all muscle cells, but a specific form of it (CK-MB) is found exclusively in myocardial cells. The CK-MB level begins to rise 2–6 hours after a myocardial infarction. It is also known as **creatine phosphokinase (CPK). Lactate dehydrogenase (LDH)** is found in many different cells, including the heart. The LDH level begins to rise 12 hours after a myocardial infarction. An elevated LDH can support the CK-MB results but cannot be the only basis for a diagnosis of myocardial infarction. Cardiac enzymes are measured every few hours for several days. This test is done in conjunction with troponin.	**enzyme** (EN-zime) The suffix –ase indicates an enzyme. **creatine kinase** (KREE-ah-teen KY-nays) **creatine phosphokinase** (KREE-ah-teen FAWS-foh-KY-nays) **lactate dehydrogenase** (LAK-tayt dee-HY-droh-JEN-ase)
C-reactive protein (CRP)	Test to measure the level of inflammation in the body. Inflammation from sites other than the cardiovascular system (such as inflammation of the gums or from a chronic urinary tract infection) can produce inflammation of the walls of the blood vessels. This can lead to blood clot formation and a myocardial infarction. The high-sensitivity CRP test can detect lower blood levels of CRP and is used to predict a healthy person's risk of developing cardiovascular disease.	
homocysteine	Test included as part of a cardiac risk assessment. An elevated level increases the patient's risk of a heart attack or stroke.	**homocysteine** (HOH-moh-SIS-teen)
lipid profile	Test that provides a comprehensive picture of the levels in the blood of cholesterol and triglycerides and their lipoprotein carriers (HDL, LDL, VLDL).	**lipid** (LIP-id) **lip/o-** *lipid (fat)* **-id** *resembling; source or origin*
troponin	Test to measure the level of two proteins that are released into the blood when myocardial cells die. Troponin I and troponin T are only found in the myocardium. The troponin levels begin to rise 4–6 hours after a myocardial infarction. More importantly, they remain elevated for up to 10 days, so they can be used to diagnose a myocardial infarction many days after it occurred. Troponin levels are done in conjunction with cardiac enzyme levels.	**troponin** (troh-POH-nin)

Diagnostic Heart Procedures

cardiac catheterization	Procedure performed to study the anatomy and pressures in the heart. During a right heart catheterization, a catheter is inserted into the femoral or brachial vein and threaded to the right atrium. The catheter is used to record right heart pressures. Then a radiopaque contrast dye is injected through the catheter to outline the chambers of the heart. A right heart catheterization is used to diagnose congenital heart defects. During a left heart catheterization, a catheter is inserted into the femoral or brachial artery and threaded to the left atrium. Then radiopaque contrast dye is injected to outline the coronary arteries and show narrow or blocked areas. If a blockage of a coronary artery is present, an angioplasty can be performed at that time. This procedure is also referred to as a cardiac cath.	**catheterization** (KATH-eh-TER-ih-ZAY-shun) **catheter/o-** *catheter* **-ization** *process of making, creating, or inserting*

Word or Phrase	Description	Word Building
cardiac exercise stress test	Procedure performed to evaluate the heart's response to exercise in patients with chest pain, palpitations, or arrhythmias (see Figure 5-21 ■). The patient walks on a motorized treadmill (**treadmill exercise stress test**) or rides a stationary bicycle while an ECG is performed. The speed of the treadmill and the steepness of its incline (or the resistance of the bicycle) are gradually increased while the patient's heart rate, blood pressure, and ECG are monitored. The procedure is stopped if the patient complains of angina, palpitations, shortness of breath, or tiredness, or if the ECG pattern becomes abnormal. The patient's resting heart rate and maximum heart rate are compared to standards for other people of the same age and sex. Any abnormality in the ECG pattern is analyzed.	

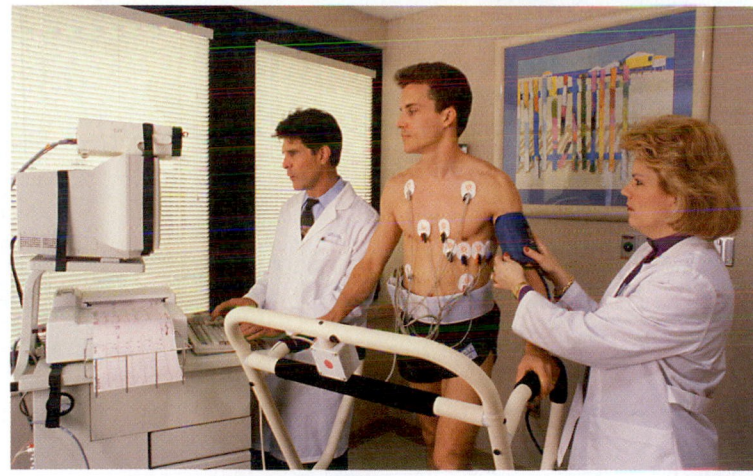

Figure 5-21 ■ Treadmill exercise stress test.

This patient is exercising on a treadmill. Electrode patches on his chest pick up the electrical impulses of the heart. The cardiologist watches the computer screen for any arrhythmias. The nurse periodically checks the patient's blood pressure.

Word or Phrase	Description	Word Building
electrocardiography (ECG, EKG)	Procedure that records the electrical activity of the heart (see Figure 5-22 ■). Electrodes (metal pieces in adhesive patches) are placed on the limbs (both arms and one leg) to send the electrical impulses of the heart to the ECG machine. These are the three limb leads (leads I–III). Electrodes placed on the chest are known as the precordial leads (V_1–V_6). A 12-lead ECG records 12 different leads that show the electrical activity between different combinations of electrodes to give an electrical picture of the heart from 12 different angles. Samples of each of these 12 tracings are mounted on a backing for an **electrocardiogram.** A longer sample of just a single lead tracing (often lead II) is known as a rhythm strip.	**electrocardiography** (ee-LEK-troh-KAR-dee-AWG-rah-fee) **electr/o-** *electricity* **cardi/o-** *heart* **-graphy** *process of recording* **electrocardiogram** (ee-LEK-troh-KAR-dee-oh-gram) **electr/o-** *electricity* **cardi/o-** *heart* **-gram** *a record or picture* *(continued)*

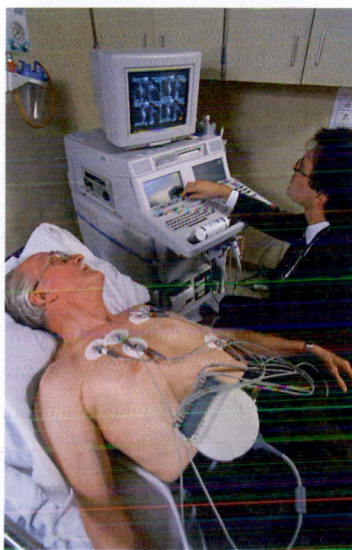

Figure 5-22 ■ Electrocardiography.

This portable ECG machine has been brought to the patient's bedside. Electrode patches attached to wire leads pick up the electrical impulses of the heart. Interpretation of an ECG includes the heart rate and rhythm and identifying abnormalities in the shape of the electrical pattern.

Word or Phrase	Description	Word Building
electrocardiography (ECG, EKG) *(continued)*		

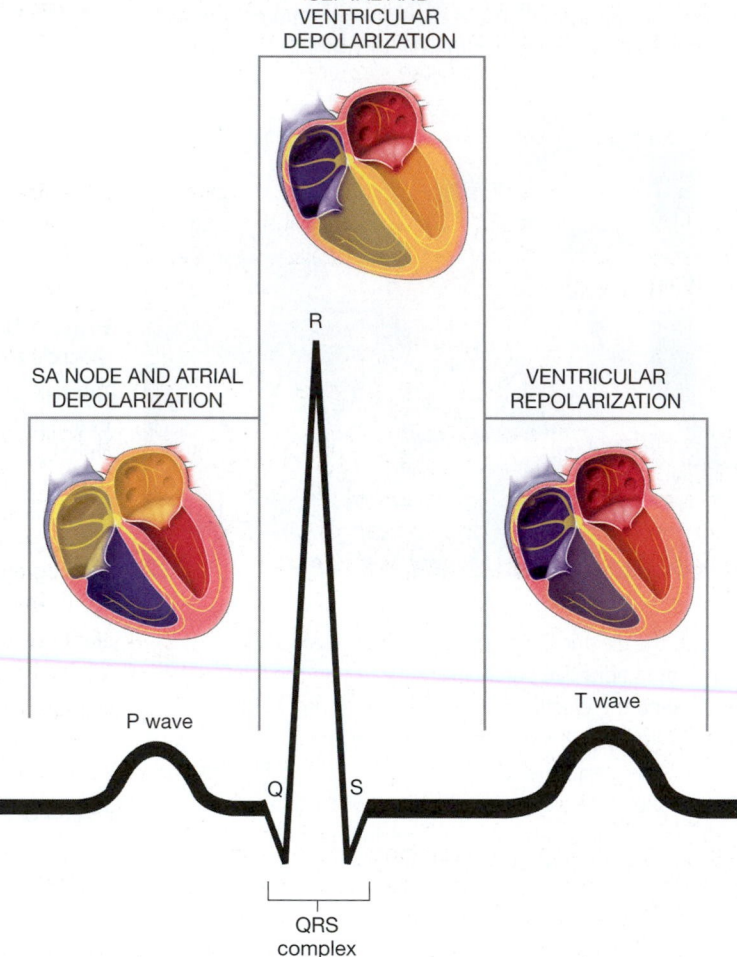

A Closer Look

ECG Interpretation. The electrical image generated by the contraction and relaxation of the heart has a characteristic pattern (see Figure 5-23 ■). The P wave corresponds to depolarization of the SA node and both atria. The QRS complex corresponds to depolarization of the septum and both ventricles. The T wave corresponds to repolarization of the ventricles. (The repolarization of the atria is hidden by the QRS complex.)

SEPTAL AND VENTRICULAR DEPOLARIZATION

R

SA NODE AND ATRIAL DEPOLARIZATION

VENTRICULAR REPOLARIZATION

P wave

Q   S

T wave

QRS complex

Figure 5-23 ■ ECG tracing.
On ECG, a normal tracing shows a P wave, QRS complex, and T wave that correspond to depolarization and repolarization changes going on in the heart.

Did You Know?

The *K* in the abbreviation *EKG* comes from the Greek word *kardia* (heart).

Word or Phrase	Description	Word Building
electrophysiologic study (EPS)	Procedure to map the heart's conduction system in a patient with an arrhythmia. While an ECG is performed, catheters are inserted into the femoral vein and subclavian vein. X-rays are used to guide the catheters to the heart. The catheters send out electrical impulses to stimulate the heart and try to induce an arrhythmia to pinpoint where the arrhythmia is originating from in the heart.	**electrophysiologic** (ee-LEK-troh-FIZ-ee-oh-LAW-jik) **electr/o-** *electricity* **physi/o-** *physical function* **log/o-** *word; the study of* **-ic** *pertaining to*

Word or Phrase	Description	Word Building
Holter monitor	Procedure during which the patient's heart rate and rhythm are continuously monitored as an outpatient for 24 hours. The patient wears electrodes attached to a small portable ECG monitor (carried in a vest or placed in a pocket). The patient also keeps a diary of activities, meals, and symptoms. A Holter monitor procedure is used to document infrequently occurring arrhythmias and to link them to activities or to symptoms such as chest pain.	**Holter** (HOL-ter)
pharmacologic stress test	Test performed in patients who cannot exercise vigorously. A vasodilator drug such as adenosine (Adenocard) or dipyridamole (Persantine) is given to cause normal coronary arteries to dilate. Occluded arteries cannot dilate, and this stresses the heart in a way that is similar to an exercise stress test and provokes angina.	**pharmacologic** (FAR-mah-koh-LAWJ-ik) **pharmac/o-** *medicine; drug* **log/o-** *word; the study of* **-ic** *pertaining to*
telemetry	Procedure to monitor a patient's heart rate and rhythm in the hospital. The patient wears electrodes connected to a device that continuously transmits an ECG tracing to a central monitoring station, usually in the coronary care unit or intensive care unit.	**telemetry** (teh-LEM-eh-tree) **tele/o-** *distance* **-metry** *process of measuring*

Radiology and Nuclear Medicine Procedures

angiography	Procedure in which radiopaque contrast dye is injected into a blood vessel to fill and outline it. In **arteriography,** it is injected into an artery to show blockage, narrowed areas, or aneurysms (see Figure 5-17). In **venography,** it is injected into a vein to show weakened valves and dilated walls. The x-ray image is an **angiogram,** or specifically an **arteriogram** or **venogram.**

In coronary angiography, a catheter is inserted into the femoral artery and threaded to the aorta. The radiopaque contrast dye is injected to outline the coronary arteries and show narrowing or blockage. The x-ray is a coronary angiogram.

In rotational angiography, multiple x-rays are taken as the x-ray machine goes around the patient. This technique is particularly helpful in documenting tortuous blood vessels in three dimensions.

Digital subtraction angiography (DSA) combines two x-ray images, one taken without radiopaque contrast dye and a second image taken after radiopaque contrast dye has been injected to outline the blood vessel. A computer compares the two images and digitally "subtracts" or removes the soft tissues, bones, and muscles, leaving just the image of the arteries. | **angiography** (AN-jee-AWG-rah-fee) **angi/o-** *blood vessel; lymphatic vessel* **-graphy** *process of recording*

arteriography (ar-TEER-ee-AWG-rah-fee) **arteri/o-** *artery* **-graphy** *process of recording*

venography (vee-NAWG-rah-fee) **ven/o-** *vein* **-graphy** *process of recording*

angiogram (AN-jee-oh-gram) **angi/o-** *blood vessel; lymphatic vessel* **-gram** *a record or picture*

arteriogram (ar-TEER-ee-oh-gram) **arteri/o-** *artery* **-gram** *a record or picture*

venogram (VEE-noh-gram) **ven/o-** *vein* **-gram** *a record or picture* |

Word or Phrase	Description	Word Building
echocardiography	Procedure that uses a transducer to produce ultra high-frequency sound waves (ultrasound) that are bounced off the heart to create an image. **Two-dimensional echocardiography** (2-D echo) creates a real-time picture of the heart and its chambers and valves as it contracts and relaxes. The image is an **echocardiogram** (see Figure 5-24 ■).	**echocardiography** (EK-oh-KAR-dee-AWG-rah-fee) **ech/o-** *echo (sound wave)* **cardi/o-** *heart* **-graphy** *process of recording* **echocardiogram** (EK-oh-KAR-dee-oh-gram) **ech/o-** *echo (sound wave)* **cardi/o-** *heart* **-gram** *a record or picture*

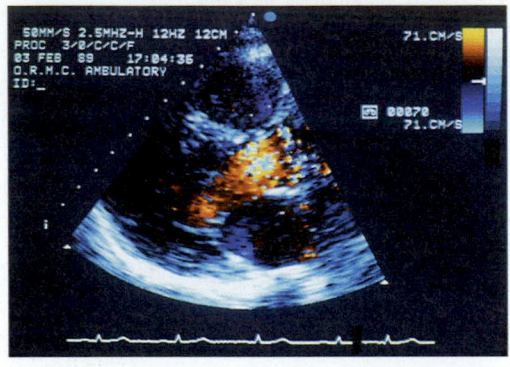

Figure 5-24 ■ Echocardiogram.

This photo was taken while a two-dimensional echocardiography produced real-time, moving images of the heart on the screen. Echocardiography uses sound waves to create images.

Transesophageal echocardiography (TEE) may be ordered when a standard echocardiogram has a poor-quality image. For a TEE, the patient swallows an endoscopic tube that contains a tiny, sound-emitting transducer. This is positioned in the esophagus directly behind, and closer to, the heart.

Color flow duplex ultrasonography combines a two-dimensional ultrasound image with another image generated by Doppler ultrasonography that color-codes images according to their velocity and direction. The image shows turbulence and variations in velocity by different degrees of brightness. This test is the "gold standard" for evaluating tortuous varicose veins.

Doppler ultrasonography images the flow of blood in a blood vessel (see Figure 5-25 ■). The reflected sound waves vary depending on how fast the blood is traveling in an artery or vein. The image can also show blockages or clots in the vessel. Doppler technology is also used in automatic blood pressure machines, in hand-held devices that give the heart rate if placed on the skin over an artery, and in fetal monitors that, when placed on the mother's abdomen, give the heart rate of the fetus.

transesophageal (TRANS-ee-SAWF-ah-JEE-al)
  trans- *across; through*
  esophag/o- *esophagus*
  -eal *pertaining to*

duplex (DOO-pleks)

ultrasonography (UL-trah-soh-NAWG-rah-fee)
  ultra- *beyond; higher*
  son/o- *sound*
  -graphy *process of recording*

Doppler (DAWP-ler)

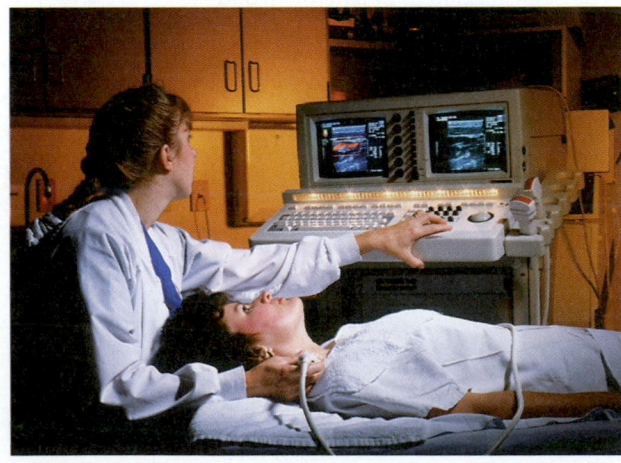

Figure 5-25 ■ Doppler ultrasonography.

This radiologic technologist has positioned an ultrasound transducer over the right carotid artery in the patient's neck. She moves the transducer to obtain the clearest image on the computer and then records this permanent image for the patient's medical record.

Word or Phrase	Description	Word Building

multiple-gated acquisition (MUGA) scan	Nuclear medicine procedure that uses the radioactive tracer technetium-99m. First, pyrophosphate is injected intravenously to allow red blood cells to bind with technetium-99m. Then technetium-99m is injected. A gamma camera records gamma rays emitted by the technetium-99m bound to red blood cells. The camera is coordinated (gated) with the patient's ECG so that images of the heart chambers (with blood—and red blood cells—in them) are taken at various times. A MUGA scan also calculates the ejection fraction (how much blood the ventricle can eject with one contraction). The ejection fraction is the most accurate indicator of overall heart function. This procedure is also known as a **radionuclide ventriculography (RNV)** or **gated blood pool scan.**	**radionuclide** (RAY-dee-oh-NOO-klide)
		  radi/o- *radius (forearm bone); x-rays; radiation*
		  nucle/o- *nucleus (of an atom)*
		  -ide *chemically modified structure*
		
		ventriculography (ven-TRIK-yoo-LAWG-rah-fee)
		  ventricul/o- *ventricle (lower heart chamber; chamber in the brain)*
		  -graphy *process of recording*

myocardial perfusion scan	Nuclear medicine procedure that combines a cardiac exercise stress test with intravenous injections of a radioactive tracer. The radioactive tracer collects in those parts of the myocardium that have the best perfusion (blood flow). A gamma camera records gamma rays emitted by the radioactive tracer and creates a two-dimensional image of the heart. Areas of decreased uptake ("cold spots") indicate poor perfusion from a blocked coronary artery. The artery must be about 70% blocked before any abnormality is evident on the image. Areas of no uptake indicate dead tissue from a previous myocardial infarction. In a **thallium stress test,** thallium-201 is the radioactive tracer, or thallium-201 and technetium-99m can be used. Technetium-99m is joined to a synthetic molecule (sestamibi). The combination of technetium-99m with sestamibi is the drug Cardiolite, so this test is also known as a **Cardiolite stress test.**	**perfusion** (per-FYOO-zhun)
		  per- *through; throughout*
		  fus/o- *pouring*
		  -ion *action; condition*
		
		thallium (THAL-ee-um)
		
		Cardiolite (KAR-dee-oh-lite)

single-photon emission computed tomography (SPECT) scan	During a myocardial perfusion scan, or a MUGA scan, the gamma camera is normally kept in a stationary position above the patient's chest. However, if the gamma camera is moved in a circle around the patient, then this becomes a SPECT scan. The computer creates many individual images or "slices" (tomography) and compiles them into a three-dimensional image of the heart.	**tomography** (toh-MAWG-rah-fee)
		  tom/o- *cut; slice; layer*
		  -graphy *process of recording*
		
		photon (FOH-tawn)
		A photon is another name for a gamma ray.

Medical and Surgical Procedures

Medical Procedures

Word or Phrase	Description	Word Building
auscultation	Procedure that uses a **stethoscope** to listen to the heart sounds. It is used to determine the heart rate or detect heart arrhythmias and murmurs.	**auscultation** (AWS-kul-TAY-shun) **auscult/o-** *listening* **-ation** *a process; being or having* **stethoscope** (STETH-oh-skohp) **steth/o-** *chest* **-scope** *instrument used to examine*
cardioversion	Procedure to treat an arrhythmia (atrial flutter, atrial fibrillation, or ventricular tachycardia) that cannot be treated with antiarrhythmic drugs. Two large, hand-held paddles are placed on either side of the patient's chest. The machine generates an electrical shock coordinated to the QRS complex of the patient's heart to restore the heart to a normal rhythm. For a patient with ventricular fibrillation, the same machine is used (it is now called a **defibrillator**) but with a much stronger electrical shock (see Figure 5-26 ■). An automatic implantable cardioverter/defibrillator (AICD) is a small device that is implanted in a patient who is at high risk for developing a serious arrhythmia. The AICD is implanted under the skin of the chest. It has leads (wires) that go to the heart, sense its rhythm, and deliver an electrical shock, if needed. An automatic external defibrillator (AED) is a portable computerized device kept on emergency response vehicles and in public places like airports. It analyzes the patient's heart rhythm and delivers an electrical shock to stimulate a heart in cardiac arrest. An AED is designed to be used by nonmedical persons.	**cardioversion** (KAR-dee-oh-VER-zhun) **cardi/o-** *heart* **vers/o-** *to travel; to turn* **-ion** *action; condition* **defibrillator** (dee-FIB-rih-LAY-tor) **de-** *reversal of; without* **fibrill/o-** *muscle fiber; nerve fiber* **-ator** *person or thing that produces or does*

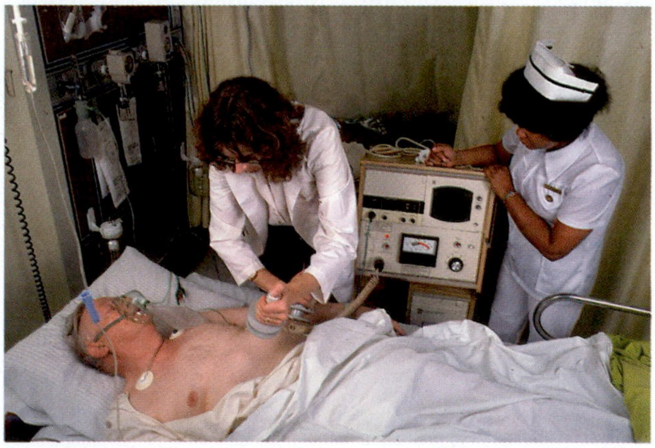

Figure 5-26 ■ Defibrillation.
This physician is about to apply defibrillator paddles to the patient's chest to convert a life-threatening ventricular fibrillation. Emergency departments, operating rooms, and intensive care units are all equipped with defibrillators that can be brought to the patient's bedside.

Word or Phrase	Description	Word Building
sclerotherapy	Procedure in which a sclerosing drug (liquid or foam) is injected into a varicose vein. The drug causes irritation and inflammation that later becomes fibrosis that occludes the vein. The blood flow is diverted to another vein, and the varicose vein is no longer distended.	**sclerotherapy** (SKLER-oh-THAIR-ah-pee) **scler/o-** *hard; sclera (white of the eye)* **-therapy** *treatment*

Word or Phrase	Description	Word Building
vital signs	Procedure during a physical examination to measure the temperature, pulse, and respirations (TPR) as well as the blood pressure (BP). Sometimes an evaluation of pain is included and it is known as the fourth vital sign. The heart rate is measured by counting the pulse. The pulse can be felt in several different parts of the body (see Figure 5-27 ■). Pulse points include the carotid pulse in the neck, apical pulse on the anterior chest, axillary pulse in the armpit, brachial pulse at the inner elbow, radial pulse at the wrist, femoral pulse in the inguinal area (groin), popliteal pulse at the back of the knee, the posterior tibial pulse at the back of the lower leg, and the dorsalis pedis pulse on the dorsum of the foot. The **radial pulse** in the wrist is the most commonly used site. In an emergency, the **carotid pulse** can be felt (see Figure 5-28 ■), particularly if the patient is in shock and little blood is flowing to the extremities. The **apical pulse** (at the apex of the heart) can be heard with a stethoscope and is also used to evaluate the heart rhythm and heart sounds. The presence of peripheral vascular disease can be determined by comparing the strength of the pulse in the right leg to the same pulse on the left.	*(continued)*

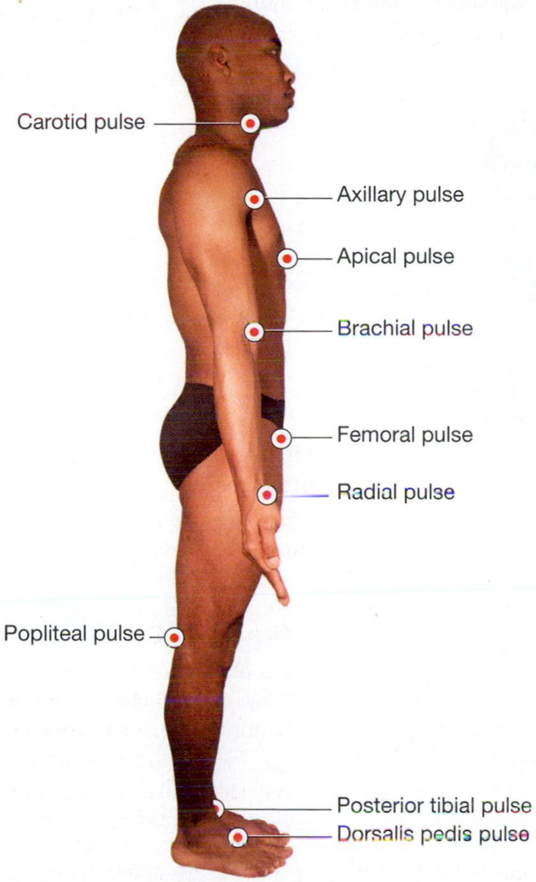

Carotid pulse

Axillary pulse

Apical pulse

Brachial pulse

Femoral pulse

Radial pulse

Popliteal pulse

Posterior tibial pulse
Dorsalis pedis pulse

Figure 5-27 ■ Pulse points.
A pulse point is where a pulse can be felt on the surface of the body. Pulse points are used to determine the heart rate and the amount of flow through the artery.

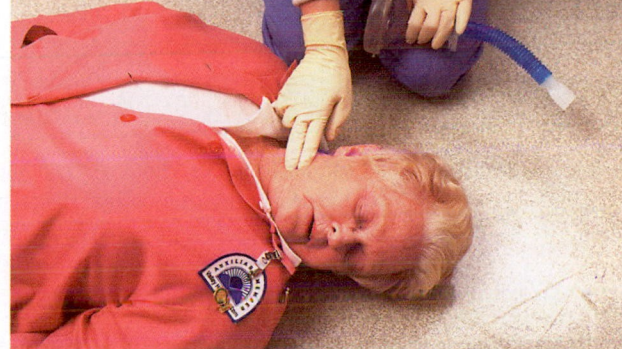

Figure 5-28 ■ Carotid pulse.
The pulse of the carotid artery can be felt easily in the neck. Emergency medical technicians use this site to quickly assess a patient's heart rate.

Word or Phrase	Description	Word Building
vital signs (*continued*)	The blood pressure is measured with a **sphygmomanometer** and a stethoscope. The sphygmomanometer consists of a thin, inflatable cuff that wraps around the arm (or leg), a hand bulb that is pumped to increase the pressure in the cuff, a regulating valve that is opened to slowly release the pressure from the cuff, and a calibrated gauge that is used to read the pressure (see Figure 5-29 ■). The stethoscope is placed at the inner elbow over the brachial pulse. As pressure increases in the cuff, it cuts off the flow of blood. The cuff pressure is decreased. When the cuff pressure is lower than the pressure in the artery, the blood spurts through and creates the first sound. This is the **systolic pressure,** the top number in a blood pressure reading. When the cuff pressure reaches the resting pressure in the artery, this is the **diastolic pressure.** A blood pressure measurement is recorded as two numbers: the systolic pressure over the diastolic pressure. Blood pressure is measured in millimeters of mercury (mm Hg). Blood pressure cuffs come in several different sizes to accommodate very thin to very large arms. There are even blood pressure cuffs for newborn and premature infants. The correct size blood pressure cuff must be used or the blood pressure reading will be either too high or too low.	**sphygmomanometer** (SFIG-moh-mah-NAWM-eh-ter) **sphygm/o-** *pulse* **man/o-** *thin; frenzy* **-meter** *instrument used to measure* Add words to make a complete definition of *sphygmomanometer: instrument used to measure (the pressure of the) pulse (by using a) thin (inflatable cuff).* **systolic** (sis-TAWL-ik) **systol/o-** *contracting* **-ic** *pertaining to* **diastolic** (DY-ah-STAWL-ik) **diastol/o-** *dilating* **-ic** *pertaining to*

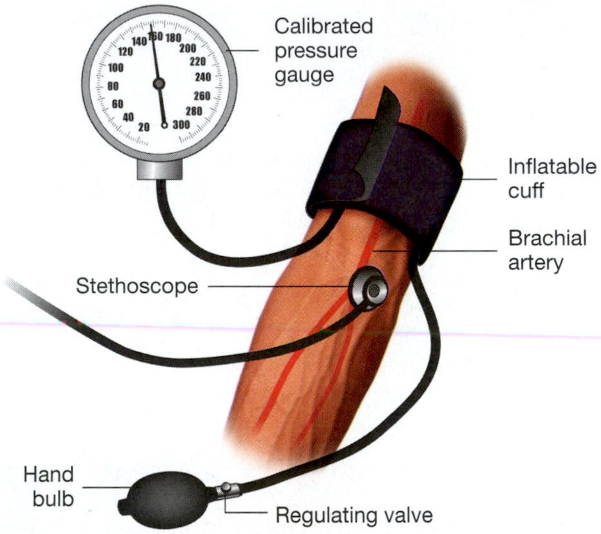

Calibrated pressure gauge

Inflatable cuff

Brachial artery

Stethoscope

Hand bulb

Regulating valve

Figure 5-29 ■ Measuring the blood pressure.

A sphygmomanometer and a stethoscope are used to measure the blood pressure.

Surgical Procedures

aneurysmectomy	Procedure to remove an aneurysm and repair the defect in the artery wall. If an aneurysm involves a large segment of artery, a flexible, tubular synthetic graft is used to replace the segment.	**aneurysmectomy** (AN-yoo-riz-MEK-toh-mee) **aneurysm/o-** *aneurysm (dilation)* **-ectomy** *surgical excision*

Word or Phrase	Description	Word Building
cardiopulmonary bypass	Technique used during open-heart surgery (see Figure 5-30 ■) in which the patient's blood is rerouted through a cannula in the femoral vein to a heart-lung machine. There, the blood is oxygenated, carbon dioxide and waste products are removed, and the blood is pumped back into the patient's body through a cannula in the femoral artery. Cardiopulmonary bypass takes over the functions of the heart and lungs during the surgery. **Figure 5-30 ■ Open heart surgery.** To perform open heart surgery, the sternum is cut in half lengthwise. Metal retractors are used to pull the two halves apart to create an operative field that allows access to the heart.	**cardiopulmonary** (KAR-dee-oh-PUL-moh-NAIR-ee) **cardi/o-** *heart* **pulmon/o-** *lung* **-ary** *pertaining to*
carotid endarterectomy	Procedure to remove plaque from an occluded carotid artery. It is used to treat carotid stenosis due to atherosclerosis.	**endarterectomy** (END-ar-ter-EK-toh-mee) **endo-** *innermost; within* **arter/o-** *artery* **-ectomy** *surgical excision* The *o* on *endo-* is deleted when the word parts are combined.
coronary artery bypass graft (CABG)	Procedure to bypass an occluded coronary artery and restore blood flow to the myocardium. A blood vessel (either the saphenous vein from the leg or the internal mammary artery from the chest) is used as the bypass graft. If the saphenous vein is used, it must be placed in a reversed position so that its valves will not obstruct the flow of blood. The suturing of one blood vessel to another is an **anastomosis.** Oxygenated blood flows through the graft, around the blockage in the coronary artery, and back into the coronary artery. The abbreviation CABG is pronounced "cabbage."	**anastomosis** (ah-NAS-toh-MOH-sis) **anastom/o-** *create an opening between two structures* **-osis** *condition; abnormal condition; process*
heart transplantation	Surgical procedure to remove a severely damaged heart from a patient with end-stage heart failure and insert a new heart from a **donor** (a patient who has recently died). The patient is matched by blood type and tissue type to the donor. Heart transplant patients must take immunosuppressant drugs for the rest of their lives to keep their bodies from rejecting the foreign tissue of their new heart. Some patients receive an artificial heart made of plastic, metal, and other synthetic materials. While awaiting a donor heart, the patient may have a left ventricular assist device (LVAD) temporarily implanted. This battery- or pneumatic-powered pump is placed in the abdomen and connected by tubes to the left ventricle and the aorta. In some patients, it becomes a permanent solution.	**transplantation** (TRANS-plan-TAY-shun) **transplant/o-** *move something to another place* **-ation** *a process; being or having* **donor** (DOH-nor)

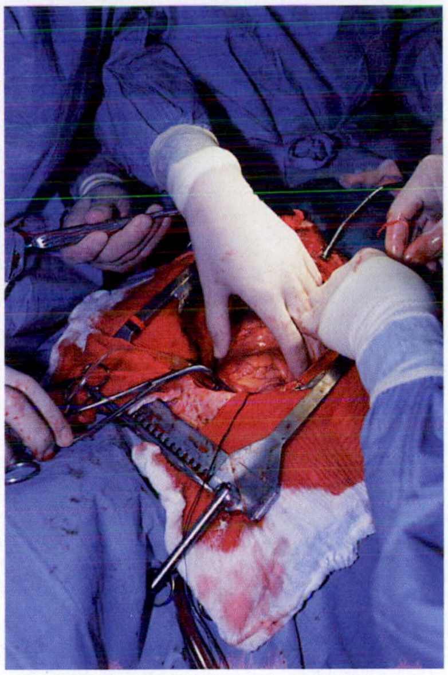

Word or Phrase	Description	Word Building
pacemaker insertion	Procedure in which an automated device is implanted to control the heart rate and rhythm (see Figure 5-31 ■). A pacemaker uses a wire positioned on the heart to coordinate the heartbeat with an electrical impulse.	

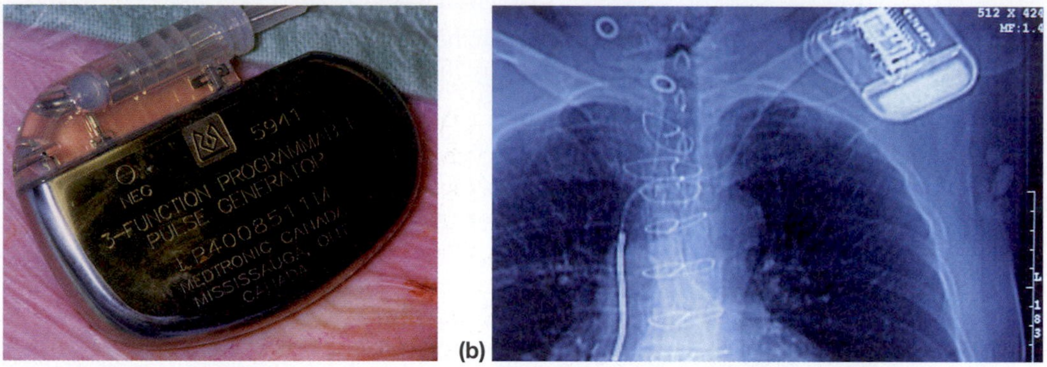

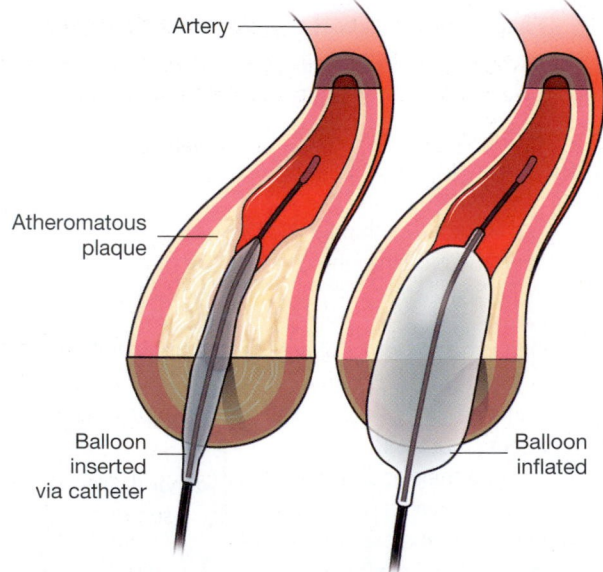

(a)

(b)

Figure 5-31 ■ Pacemaker.

(a) This pacemaker (programmable pulse generator) is placed under the skin of the anterior chest, and its wire is positioned on the heart. (b) This colorized chest x-ray shows the position of the pacemaker and the pacemaker wire on the heart.

Word or Phrase	Description	Word Building
percutaneous transluminal coronary angioplasty (PTCA)	Procedure to reconstruct an artery that is narrowed because of atherosclerosis. A catheter is inserted into the femoral artery and threaded to the site of the stenosis. During a **balloon angioplasty,** a balloon within the catheter is inflated. It compresses the atheromatous plaque and widens the lumen of the artery. Then the balloon is deflated and the catheter is removed (see Figure 5-32 ■). Alternatively, an intravascular stainless steel mesh **stent** (in a closed position) can be inserted on the catheter (see Figure 5-33 ■). The stent is expanded, the catheter is removed, and the expanded stent remains in the artery.	**percutaneous** (PER-kyoo-TAY-nee-us) **per-** *through; throughout* **cutane/o-** *skin* **-ous** *pertaining to* **transluminal** (trans-LOO-mih-nal) **trans-** *across; through* **lumin/o-** *lumen (opening)* **-al** *pertaining to* **angioplasty** (AN-jee-oh-PLAS-tee) **angi/o-** *blood vessel; lymphatic vessel* **-plasty** *process of reshaping by surgery*

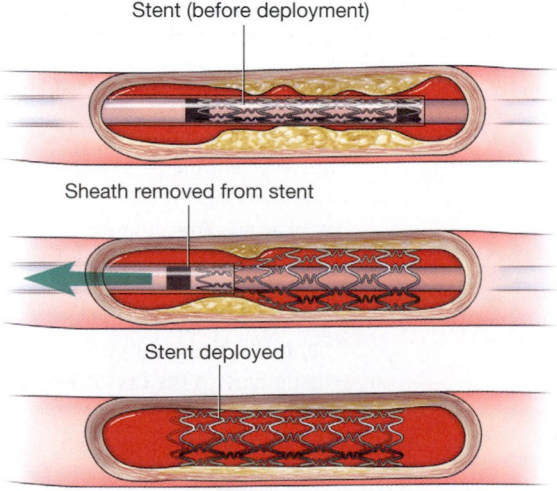

Artery

Atheromatous plaque

Balloon inserted via catheter

Balloon inflated

Stent (before deployment)

Sheath removed from stent

Stent deployed

Figure 5-32 ■ Balloon angioplasty.

The inflated balloon compresses atheromatous plaque in the artery, to open the lumen and reestablish blood flow.

Figure 5-33 ■ Stent.

A stent is expanded inside the artery to compress the atheromatous plaque and increase the blood flow. It provides continuing support to keep the lumen of the artery open over time.

Word or Phrase	Description	Word Building
pericardiocentesis	Procedure that uses a needle to puncture the pericardium and withdraw inflammatory fluid accumulated in the pericardial sac. It is used to treat pericarditis and cardiac tamponade.	**pericardiocentesis** (PAIR-ih-KAR-dee-oh-sen-TEE-sis) **peri-** *around* **cardi/o-** *heart* **-centesis** *procedure to puncture*
radiofrequency catheter ablation	Procedure to destroy ectopic areas in the heart that are emitting electrical impulses and producing arrhythmias. A catheter is inserted into the heart. Electromagnetic energy produced by a generator produces enough heat at the site to kill the cells causing the arrhythmia. It is also known as **radiofrequency ablation (RFA)**. **Radiofrequency catheter occlusion** uses heat to collapse and seal large varicose veins.	**ablation** (ah-BLAY-shun) **ablat/o-** *take away; destroy* **-ion** *action; condition* **occlusion** (oh-KLOO-zhun) **occlus/o-** *close against* **-ion** *action; condition*
valve replacement	Surgical procedure to replace a severely damaged or prolapsed heart valve (see Figure 5-34 ■). There are several types of **prosthetic** (replacement) heart valves that can be used. If the replacement heart valve comes from an animal, it is known as a **xenograft.**	**prosthetic** (praws-THET-ik) **prosthet/o-** *artificial part* **-ic** *pertaining to* **xenograft** (ZEN-oh-graft) **xen/o-** *foreign* **-graft** *tissue for implant or transplant*

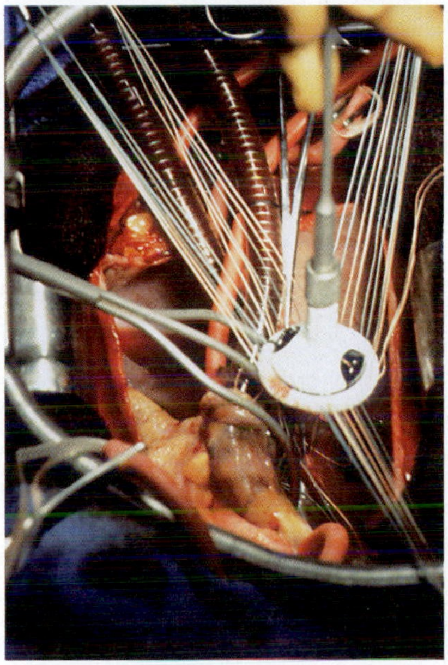

Figure 5-34 ■ Valve replacement surgery.
A white artificial valve is being implanted in the heart. Many sutures are used to attach the valve so that blood will not leak around the valve edges.

valvoplasty	Surgical procedure to reconstruct a heart valve to correct stenosis or prolapse. A **valvulotome** is used to cut the valve. This procedure is also known as a **valvuloplasty.**	**valvoplasty** (VAL-voh-PLAS-tee) **valv/o-** *valve* **-plasty** *process of reshaping by surgery* **valvulotome** (VAL-vyoo-LOH-tohm) **valvul/o-** *valve* **-tome** *instrument used to cut; area with distinct edges* **valvuloplasty** (VAL-vyoo-loh-PLAS-tee) **valvul/o-** *valve* **-plasty** *process of reshaping by surgery*

Drug Categories

These categories of drugs are used to treat cardiovascular diseases and conditions. The most common generic and trade name drugs in each category are listed.

Category	Indication	Examples	Word Building
ACE (angiotensin-converting enzyme) inhibitor drugs	Treat congestive heart failure and hypertension. Also increase the survival rate after myocardial infarction. ACE inhibitor drugs produce vasodilation and decrease the blood pressure by blocking an enzyme that converts angiotensin I to angiotensin II (a vasoconstrictor).	captopril (Capoten), lisinopril (Prinivil, Zestril), trandolapril (Mavik)	**angiotensin** (AN-jee-oh-TEN-sin) **angi/o-** *blood vessel; lymphatic vessel* **tens/o-** *pressure; tension* **-in** *a substance*
antiarrhythmic drugs	Treat arrhythmias	Intravenous atropine for brady-cardia, intravenous lidocaine (Xylocaine) for ventricular arrhythmias. See beta-blocker drugs and calcium channel blocker drugs.	**antiarrhythmic** (AN-tee-aa-RITH-mik) **anti-** *against* **a-** *away from; without* **rrhythm/o-** *rhythm* **-ic** *pertaining to*
anticoagulant drugs	Prevent a blood clot in patients with arteriosclerosis, atrial fibrillation, previous myocardial infarction, or an artificial heart valve	heparin, warfarin (Coumadin), clopidogrel (Plavix)	**anticoagulant** (AN-tee-koh-AG-yoo-lant) (AN-tih-koh-AG-yoo-lant) **anti-** *against* **coagul/o-** *clotting* **-ant** *pertaining to*
antihypertensive drugs	Treat hypertension	See ACE inhibitor drugs, beta-blocker drugs, calcium channel blocker drugs, and diuretic drugs.	**antihypertensive** (AN-tee-HY-per-TEN-siv) **anti-** *against* **hyper-** *above; more than normal* **tens/o-** *pressure; tension* **-ive** *pertaining to*
aspirin	Prevents heart attacks. Prevents blood clots from forming by keeping platelets from sticking together.	aspirin (81 mg)	
beta-blocker drugs	Treat angina pectoris and hypertension. Beta-blocker drugs decrease the heart rate and dilate the arteries by blocking beta receptors.	atenolol (Tenormin), nadolol (Corgard), propranolol (Inderal), metoprolol (Lopressor)	
calcium channel blocker drugs	Treat angina pectoris and hypertension. Calcium channel blockers block the movement of calcium ions into myocardial cells and smooth muscle cells of the artery walls, causing the heart rate and blood pressure to decrease.	amlodipine (Norvasc), diltiazem (Cardizem), nifedipine (Adalat, Procardia), verapamil (Calan)	

Category	Indication	Examples	Word Building
digitalis drugs	Treat congestive heart failure. Digitalis drugs decrease the heart rate and strengthen the heart's contractions (see Figure 5-35 ■).	digoxin (Lanoxin)	**digitalis** (DIJ-ih-TAL-is)

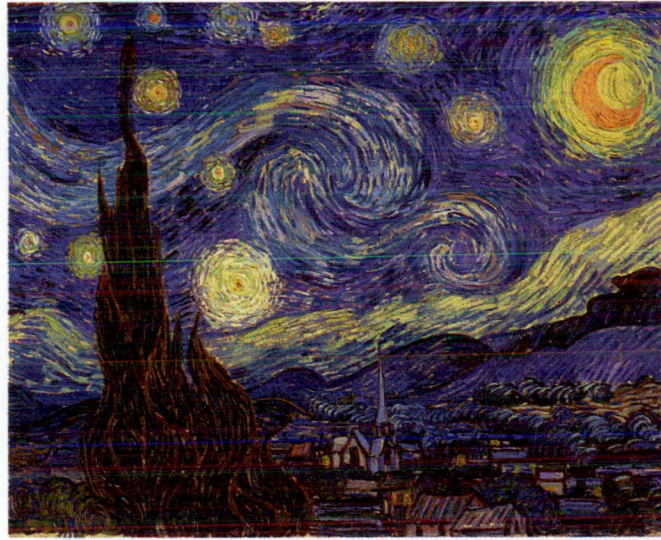

Figure 5-35 ■ The Starry Night

Vincent van Gogh's "The Starry Night" (1889) is believed by some physicians to show evidence of digitalis toxicity in the way the Dutch painter depicted yellow-green halos around the stars. Van Gogh (1853–1890) suffered from mania and epilepsy and may have been given digitalis for lack of a more specific drug therapy. Digitalis can easily reach toxic levels in the blood. Symptoms of toxicity include nausea and vomiting, decreased heart rate, and sometimes visual halos. Van Gogh may simply have painted what he actually saw because of digitalis toxicity. *Source:* Vincent van Gogh (1853-1890), "The Starry Night." 1889. Oil on canvas, 29 x 36 1/4" (73.7 x 92.1 cm). Acquired through the Lillie P. Bliss Bequest. (472.1941). The Museum of Modern Art, New York, U.S.A. Digital Image © The Museum of Modern Art/Licensed by Scala/Art Resource, NY.

Did You Know?

Digitalis drugs come from *Digitalis* (foxglove plant). Its flowers were thought to resemble fingerlike projections or digits.

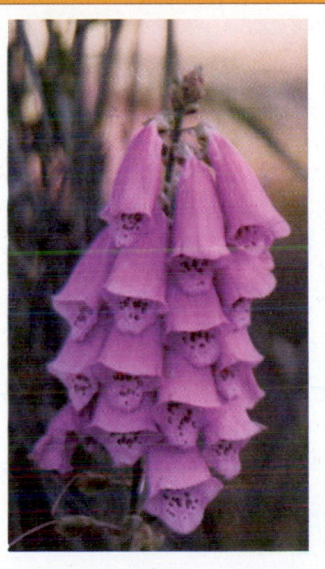

Category	Indication	Examples	Word Building
diuretic drugs	Block sodium from being absorbed from the tubule (of the nephron of the kidney) back into the blood. As the sodium is excreted in the urine, it brings water and potassium with it because of osmotic pressure. This process is known as diuresis. This decreases the volume of blood and is used to treat hypertension and congestive heart failure.	furosemide (Lasix), hydrochlorothiazide (HCTZ)	**diuretic** (DY-yoo-RET-ik) **dia-** *complete; completely through* **ur/o-** *urine; urinary system* **-etic** *pertaining to* The *a* in *dia-* is dropped when the word is formed.

Category	Indication	Examples	Word Building
drugs for cardiac arrest	Treat a nonbeating heart (asystole) by stimulating it to contract	intracardiac epinephrine (Adrenalin)	
drugs for hyperlipidemia	Treat hypercholesterolemia. They are often referred to as "statin drugs" because of the common ending of the generic drug names.	atorvastatin (Lipitor), lovastatin (Mevacor), rosuvastatin (Crestor), simvastatin (Zocor)	
nitrate drugs	Treat angina pectoris. Nitrate drugs dilate the veins (to decrease the amount of work that the heart must do) and dilate the arteries (to decrease the blood pressure)	isosorbide (Isordil), nitroglycerin (Nitro-Dur)	**nitrate** (NY-trayt)

Did You Know?

In the mid-1890s, physicians observed that the pain of angina pectoris seemed to be relieved in patients who worked in dynamite factories where nitroglycerin was an ingredient. This led to the practice of prescribing nitroglycerin for angina pectoris.

Category	Indication	Examples	Word Building
thrombolytic drugs	Treat a blood clot that is blocking blood flow through an artery. Thrombolytic drugs lyse (break apart) a clot.	alteplase (Activase), streptokinase (Streptase)	**thrombolytic** (THRAWM-boh-LIT-ik) **thromb/o-** *thrombus (blood clot)* **ly/o-** *break down; destroy* **-tic** *pertaining to*

Abbreviations

AAA	abdominal aortic aneurysm		**LVH**	left ventricular hypertrophy
ACE	angiotensin-converting enzyme		**MI**	myocardial infarction
ACS	acute coronary syndrome		**mm Hg**	millimeters of mercury
AED	automatic external defibrillator		**MR**	mitral regurgitation
AI	aortic insufficiency		**MUGA**	multiple-gated acquisition (scan)
AICD	automatic implantable cardioverter-defibrillator		**MVP**	mitral valve prolapse
AMI	acute myocardial infarction		**NSR**	normal sinus rhythm
AS	aortic stenosis		**P**	pulse (rate)
ASCVD	arteriosclerotic cardiovascular disease		**PAC**	premature atrial contraction
ASD	atrial septal defect		**PAD**	peripheral artery disease
ASHD	arteriosclerotic heart disease		**PDA**	patent ductus arteriosus
AV	atrioventricular		**PMI**	point of maximum impulse
BP	blood pressure		**PTCA**	percutaneous transluminal coronary angioplasty
BPM, bpm	beats per minute		**PVC**	premature ventricular contraction
CABG	coronary artery bypass graft		**PVD**	peripheral vascular disease
CAD	coronary artery disease		**RA**	right atrium
CCU	coronary care unit		**RBBB**	right bundle branch block
CHF	congestive heart failure		**RFA**	radiofrequency catheter ablation
CK-MB	creatine kinase–M band		**RNV**	radionuclide ventriculography
CPK-MB	creatine phosphokinase–M band		**RV**	right ventricle
CPR	cardiopulmonary resuscitation		**S$_1$**	first heart sound
CRP	C-reactive protein		**S$_2$**	second heart sound
CV	cardiovascular		**S$_3$**	third heart sound
DSA	digital subtraction angiography		**S$_4$**	fourth heart sound
ECG	electrocardiography		**SA**	sinoatrial
EKG	electrocardiography		**SBE**	subacute bacterial endocarditis
HDL	high-density lipoprotein		**SPECT**	single-photon emission computerized tomography
HTN	hypertension		**SVT**	supraventricular tachycardia
JVD	jugular venous distention		**TEE**	transesophageal echocardiography
LA	left atrium		**TPR**	temperature, pulse, and respiration
LBBB	left bundle branch block		**V fib**	ventricular fibrillation (slang)
LDH	lactic dehydrogenase		**VLDL**	very low-density lipoprotein
LDL	low-density lipoprotein		**VSD**	ventricular septal defect
LV	left ventricle		**V tach**	ventricular tachycardia (slang)
LVAD	left ventricular assist device			

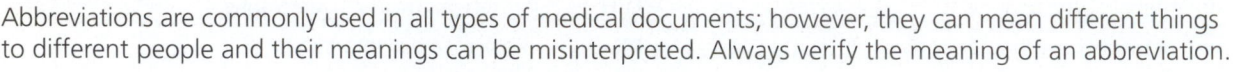

Word Alert

ABBREVIATIONS

Abbreviations are commonly used in all types of medical documents; however, they can mean different things to different people and their meanings can be misinterpreted. Always verify the meaning of an abbreviation.

RA means *right atrium,* but it also means *rheumatoid arthritis* or *room air.*

S1 means *first heart sound,* but it also means *first sacral vertebra.*

Do not confuse the abbreviation *CPR* (cardiopulmonary resuscitation) with *CRP* (C-reactive protein).

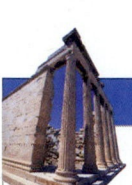

It's Greek to Me!

Did you notice that some words have two different combining forms? Combining forms from both Greek and Latin languages remain a part of medical language today.

Word	Greek	Latin	Medical Word Examples
blood vessel	angi/o-	vas/o- vascul/o-	angiography, angiogram, vasoconstriction, vasodilator vascular, vasculature
heart	card/i- cardi/o-	cor	bradycardia, endocarditis, pericarditis, cardiac, cardiology, cardiopulmonary, cardiothoracic, cor pulmonale
vein	phleb/o-	ven/o-	phlebitis, thrombophlebitis, venous, venography, venogram

CAREER FOCUS

Meet Laurie, a cardiac stress test technologist in a hospital

"Cardiology is a very important department. I use medical terminology during all aspects of my job. My daughter was born with a heart defect. Wanting to know more information about what was happening to her, I started to take a class here and a class there, and then I just wound up in a certificate program. The most rewarding part of my job is if I can get a patient through the test and at the end of the test they say, 'You made that so much easier for me.'"

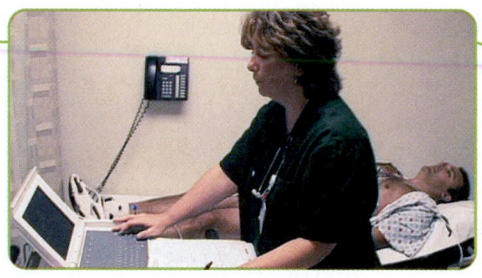

Cardiac stress test technologists are allied health professionals who perform ECGs, Holter monitor tests, and cardiac stress tests in a hospital setting or a cardiologist's office.

  Cardiologists are physicians who practice in the medical specialty of cardiology. They diagnose and treat patients with diseases of the heart and circulatory system. When cardiologists perform surgery, they are known as heart surgeons, cardiothoracic surgeons, or cardiovascular surgeons. Physicians can take additional training and become board certified in the subspecialty of pediatric cardiology. Cancerous tumors of the heart or blood vessels are treated medically by an oncologist or surgically by a cardiothoracic or cardiovascular surgeon.

technologist (tek-NAWL-oh-jist)
  techn/o- *technical skill*
  log/o- *word; the study of*
  -ist *one who specializes in*

cardiologist (KAR-dee-AWL-oh-jist)
  cardi/o- *heart*
  log/o- *word; the study of*
  -ist *one who specializes in*

myhealthprofessionskit To see Laurie's complete video profile, visit Medical Terminology Interactive at www.myhealthprofessionskit.com. Select this book, log in, and go to the 5th floor of Pearson General Hospital. Enter the Laboratory, and click on the computer screen.

CHAPTER REVIEW EXERCISES

Test your knowledge of the chapter by completing these review exercises. Use the Answer Key at the end of the book to check your answers.

Anatomy and Physiology

Matching Exercise

Match each word or phrase to its description.

1. mediastinum
2. pericardium
3. myocardium
4. ventricle
5. tricuspid valve
6. septum
7. aortic valve
8. vasculature
9. bicuspid valve
10. chordae tendineae

_____ Another name for the mitral valve

_____ Network of blood vessels related to a particular organ

_____ Dividing wall between the atria and ventricles

_____ Double-layered membrane around the heart

_____ Bottom chamber of the heart

_____ Area between the lungs that contains the heart

_____ Valve between the right atrium and right ventricle

_____ Heart muscle

_____ Valve that blood flows through as it leaves the left ventricle

_____ Ropelike strands that strengthen the tricuspid and mitral valves

True or False Exercise

Indicate whether each statement is true or false by writing T or F on the line.

1. _____ The aorta is the largest vein in the body.
2. _____ The adrenal glands secrete epinephrine, which increases the heart rate and blood pressure.
3. _____ The blood flows from the inferior vena cava to the right atrium to the right ventricle and to the pulmonary veins to the lungs.
4. _____ The refractory period is the time during which the ventricles contract.
5. _____ Little veins are known as capillaries.
6. _____ The interventricular septum is within a ventricle.
7. _____ The epicardium is the part of the pericardium that lies on the surface of the heart.
8. _____ All arteries carry blood away from the heart.
9. _____ The subclavian artery carries blood to the leg.
10. _____ The peroneal artery carries blood to the lateral aspect of the lower leg in the area of the fibula bone.
11. _____ The blood in most veins is a dark red–purple color because it has a low level of oxygen.
12. _____ The systemic circulation carries blood to the whole body with the exception of the lungs.
13. _____ Vasodilation is the opposite of vasoconstriction.

Sequencing Exercise

Beginning with blood entering the right atrium, write each structure of the circulatory system in the order in which blood moves through it.

Structure	Correct Order
aortic valve and aorta	1. <u>right atrium</u>
arteries and arterioles	2. _____
capillaries	3. _____
left atrium	4. _____
left ventricle	5. _____
lungs	6. _____
mitral valve	7. _____
pulmonary valve, pulmonary trunk, and pulmonary arteries	8. _____
pulmonary veins	9. _____
right atrium	10. _____
right ventricle	11. _____
superior and inferior venae cavae	12. _____
tricuspid valve	13. _____
venules and veins	14. _____

Circle Exercise

Circle the correct word from the choices given.

1. The great vessels include the superior and inferior venae cavae and the (**aorta, artery, mediastinum**).

2. The vascular structures of the body include all of the following *except* (**arteries, capillaries, heart valves, veins**).

3. Listening to a patient's heart sounds with a stethoscope is known as (**auscultation, diastole, repolarization**).

4. What unique structure is found only in the fetal heart? (**apex, foramen ovale, vasculature**).

5. This vein brings blood from the head to the superior vena cava: (**jugular, portal, saphenous**).

6. The (**AV node, Purkinje fiber, SA node**) is the pacemaker of the heart.

Diseases and Conditions

Matching Exercise

Match each word or phrase to its description.

1. arrhythmia
2. cardiac arrest
3. palpitation
4. cardiomegaly
5. thrombus
6. claudication
7. coarctation
8. necrosis
9. atheroma
10. tetralogy of Fallot

_____ Calf pain with peripheral artery disease
_____ Fatty deposit
_____ A dysrhythmia is categorized as this
_____ Chest sensation during premature contraction
_____ Cell death
_____ Asystole
_____ Blood clot
_____ Enlarged heart
_____ Abnormal narrowing
_____ Congenital heart defect

Circle Exercise

Circle the correct word from the choices given.

1. (**Asystole, Bradycardia, Fibrillation**) is an abnormally slow heart rate.
2. Narrowing of an artery is known as (**arteriosclerosis, endocarditis, stenosis**).
3. A weakness in the wall of an artery is known as a/an (**aneurysm, couplet, varicose vein**).
4. (**Patent foramen ovale, Heart block, Aneurysm**) is a congenital heart defect.

True or False Exercise

Indicate whether each statement is true or false by writing T or F on the line.

1. _____ Angina pectoris is chest pain that means that myocardial cells have died.
2. _____ Prolapse of a valve is when the cusps hang down and do not close completely.
3. _____ Raynaud's disease is severe vasoconstriction of the extremities triggered by cold or emotional stress.
4. _____ Hyperlipidemia includes both hypercholesterolemia and hypertriglyceridemia.
5. _____ Regurgitation is an infection of the heart caused by bacteria.
6. _____ To check for atherosclerosis in the arteries of the legs, you would feel the pulse in the radial artery.
7. _____ Auscultation is using a stethoscope to listen to the heart sounds.
8. _____ S_1 and S_2 are abnormal heart sounds.
9. _____ In a patient with right-sided congestive heart failure, the neck may show signs of jugular venous distention.
10. _____ A sphygmomanometer measures the blood pressure in millimeters of mercury (mm Hg).

Laboratory, Radiology, Surgery, and Drugs

Laboratory Test Exercise

You need to order the following laboratory tests to be done for a patient. Find each of these tests on the laboratory form and put a checkmark in the box next to it.

cardio CRP	cholesterol	HDL cholesterol	triglycerides
cardio CRP w/ lipid profile	digoxin	lipid panel	

PANELS AND PROFILES			TESTS		
968T		Lipid Panel	19687W		Bilirubin (Direct)
315F		Electrolyte Panel	265F		HBsAg
10256F		Hepatic Function Panel	51870R		HB Core Antibody
10165F		Basic Metabolic Panel	1012F		Cardio CRP
10231A		Comprehensive Metabolic Panel	23242E		GGT
10306F		Hepatitis Panel, Acute	28852E		Protein, Total
182Aaa		Obstetric Panel	141A		CBC Hemogram
18T		Chem-Screen Panel (Basic)	21105R		hCG, Qualitative, Serum
554T		Chem-Screen Panel (Basic with HDL)	10321A		ANA
7971A		Chem-Screen Panel (Basic with HDL, TIBC)	80185		Cardio CRP with Lipid Profile
TESTS			26F		PT with INR
56713E		Lead, Blood	232Aaa		UA, Dipstick
2782A		Antibody Screen	42A		CBC with Diff
3556F		Iron, TIBC	20867W		HDL Cholesterol
20933E		Cholesterol	31732E		PTT
3084111E		Uric Acid	34F		UA, Dipstick and Microscopic
53348W		Rubella Antibody	20396R		CEA
27771E		Phosphate	45443E		Hematocrit
2111600E		Creatinine	28571E		PSA, Total
29868W		Testosterone, Total	66902E		WBC count
9704F		Creatinine Clearance	20750E		Chloride
19752E		Bilirubin (Total)	7187W		Hemoglobin
30536Rrr		T3, Total	4259T		HIV-1 Antibody
687T		Protein Electrophoresis	45484R		Hemoglobin A1c
3563444R		Digoxin	67868R		Alk Phosphatase
15214R		Glucose, 2-Hour Postprandial	24984R		Iron
30502E		T3, Uptake	28512E		Sodium
7773E		Platelet Count	17426R		ALT
39685R		Dilantin (phenytoin)	**MICROBIOLOGY**		
30494R		Triglycerides	112680E		Group A Beta Strep Culture, Throat
26013E		Magnesium	5827W		Group B Beta Strep Culture, Genitals
15586R		Glucose, Fasting	49932E		Chlamydia, Endocervix/Urethra
30237W		T4, Free	6007W		Culture, Blood
28233E		Potassium	2692E		Culture, Genitals
19208W		AST	2649T		Culture, HSV
30163E		TSH	612A		Culture, Sputum
22764R		Ferritin	6262E		Culture, Throat
20008W		Calcium	6304R		Culture, Urine
54726F		Occult Blood, Stool	50286R		Gonococcus, Endocervix/Urethra
51839W		HAV Antibody, Total	6643E		Gram Stain
430A		Blood Group and Rh Type	**STOOL PATHOGENS**		
28399W		Progesterone	10045F		Culture, Stool
30262E		T4, Total	4475F		Culture, Campylobacter
20289W		Carbon Dioxide	10018T		Culture, Salmonella
1156F		RPR	86140A		E. coli Toxins
30940E		Urea Nitrogen	1099T		Ova and Parasites
17417W		Albumin	**VENIPUNCTURE**		
28423E		Prolactin	63180		Venipuncture

True or False Exercise

Indicate whether each statement is true or false by writing T or F on the line.

1. _____ Antiarrhythmic drugs are used to treat hypertension.

2. _____ Thrombolytic drugs break apart blood clots.

3. _____ An artificial valve is also known as a prosthesis.

4. _____ A stent is inserted during a MUGA scan.

5. _____ Sclerotherapy is used to treat arteriosclerosis (hardening of the arteries).

Building Medical Words

Review the Combining Forms Exercise, Combining Form and Suffix Exercise, and Multiple Combining Forms and Suffix Exercise that you already completed in the anatomy section on pages 222–224.

Combining Forms Exercise

Before you build cardiovascular words, review these additional combining forms. Next to each combining form, write its medical meaning. The first one has been done for you.

Combining Form	Medical Meaning	Combining Form	Medical Meaning
1. angin/o-	angina	16. ly/o-	
2. aneurysm/o-		17. man/o-	
3. ather/o-		18. necr/o-	
4. auscult/o-		19. palpit/o-	
5. cholesterol/o-		20. path/o-	
6. claudicat/o-		21. pat/o-	
7. ech/o-		22. rrhythm/o-	
8. electr/o-		23. scler/o-	
9. fibrill/o-		24. sphygm/o-	
10. gemin/o-		25. sten/o-	
11. idi/o-		26. tele/o-	
12. infarct/o-		27. tens/o-	
13. isch/o-		28. thromb/o-	
14. lipid/o-		29. varic/o-	
15. lumin/o-		30. vers/o-	

Related Combining Forms Exercise

Write the combining forms on the line provided. (Hint: See the It's Greek to Me feature box.)

1. Three combining forms that mean *blood vessel*. _____

2. Two combining forms that mean *heart*. _____

3. Two combining forms that mean *vein*. _____

Dividing Medical Words

Separate these words into their component parts (prefix, combining form, suffix). Note: Some words do not contain all three word parts. The first one has been done for you.

Medical Word	Prefix	Combining Form	Suffix	Medical Word	Prefix	Combining Form	Suffix
1. circulation		circulat/o-	-ion	6. bradycardia			
2. depolarization				7. aneurysmal			
3. ischemia				8. hyperlipidemia			
4. endocarditis				9. angioplasty			
5. arrhythmia				10. transluminal			

Combining Form and Suffix Exercise

Read the definition of the medical word. Select the correct suffix from the Suffix List. Select the correct combining form from the Combining Form List. Build the medical word and write it on the line. Be sure to check your spelling. The first one has been done for you.

SUFFIX LIST	COMBINING FORM LIST
-ation (a process; being or having)	aneurysm/o- (aneurysm; dilation)
-ectomy (surgical excision)	angi/o- (blood vessel; lymphatic vessel)
-ent (pertaining to)	arteri/o- (artery)
-gram (a record or picture)	ather/o- (soft, fatty substance)
-graphy (process of recording)	auscult/o- (listening)
-ion (action; condition)	cardi/o- (heart)
-itis (inflammation of; infection of)	claudicat/o- (limping pain)
-megaly (enlargement)	fibrill/o- (muscle fiber; nerve fiber)
-metry (process of measuring)	infarct/o- (area of dead tissue)
-oma (tumor; mass)	necr/o- (dead cells, tissue, or body)
-osis (condition; abnormal condition; process)	palpit/o- (to throb)
-plasty (process of reshaping by surgery)	pat/o- (to be open)
-scope (instrument used to examine)	phleb/o- (vein)
-therapy (treatment)	scler/o- (hard)
-tic (pertaining to)	sten/o- (narrowness; constriction)
-tome (instrument used to cut; area with distinct edges)	steth/o- (chest)
	tele/o- (distance)
	valvul/o- (valve)

Definition of the Medical Word

Build the Medical Word

1. Pertaining to dead cells or tissue — *necrotic*

2. Enlargement of the heart

3. Mass (composed of a) soft, fatty substance

4. Condition (of having) limping pain (in the calf of the leg)

5. Surgical excision of an aneurysm

6. Abnormal condition of narrowness or constriction (of a blood vessel)

7. Condition (of having) an area of dead tissue (in the heart)

8. Process of reshaping by surgery (of a) blood vessel

9. A process of listening (to the heart)

10. Treatment (that makes a varicose vein) hard

11. Process of measuring (the heart rate and rhythm from a) distance

12. Inflammation of or infection of a vein

13. Pertaining to (a blood vessel) to be open

14. Being or having (a very fast, uncoordinated twitching of the) muscle fibers (of the heart)

15. Process of recording (the image of a) blood vessel

16. Instrument used to cut a (heart) valve

17. Being or having (the heart) to throb (or "thump")

18. A record or picture of an artery

19. Process of reshaping by surgery (of a) valve

20. Instrument used to examine (and listen to) the chest (and heart)

Prefix Exercise

Read the definition of the medical word. Look at the medical word or partial word that is given (it already contains a combining form and a suffix). Select the correct prefix from the Prefix List and write it on the blank line. Then build the medical word and write it on the line. Be sure to check your spelling. The first one has been done for you.

PREFIX LIST

a- (away from; without)	hyper- (above; more than normal)	tachy- (fast)
bi- (two)	hypo- (below; deficient)	trans- (across; through)
brady- (slow)	peri- (around)	tri- (three)
endo- (innermost; within)	supra- (above)	

Definition of the Medical Word	Prefix	Word or Partial Word	Build the Medical Word
1. Substance in the blood of a more than normal (level) of cholesterol	hyper-	cholesterolemia	hypercholesterolemia
2. Pertaining to a fast heart (rate)	_____	cardic	_____
3. Condition of above or more than normal pressure (of the blood)	_____	tension	_____
4. Pertaining to one (normal heart contraction followed by) one (premature contraction)	_____	geminal	_____
5. Procedure to puncture (the membrane that is) around the heart	_____	cardiocentesis	_____
6. Pertaining to through the lumen or opening (in a blood vessel)	_____	luminal	_____
7. Condition of a slow heart (rate)	_____	cardia	_____
8. Substance in the blood (of a) more than normal (level of) fats	_____	lipidemia	_____
9. Pertaining to (a position) above the ventricle	_____	ventricular	_____
10. Condition (of the heart being) without a rhythm	_____	rrhythmia	_____
11. Inflammation (of the membrane that is) around the heart	_____	carditis	_____
12. Surgical excision (of plaque in the) innermost area within an artery	_____	arterectomy	_____
13. Pertaining to below (normal blood) pressure	_____	tensive	_____
14. Inflammation or infection of the innermost (lining of) the heart	_____	carditis	_____
15. Pertaining to one (normal heart contraction followed by) two (premature contractions)	_____	geminal	_____

Multiple Combining Forms and Suffix Exercise

Read the definition of the medical word. Select the correct suffix and combining forms. Then build the medical word and write it on the line. Be sure to check your spelling. The first one has been done for you.

SUFFIX LIST	COMBINING FORM LIST	
-al (pertaining to)	arteri/o- (artery)	my/o- (muscle)
-graphy (process of recording)	ather/o- (soft, fatty substance)	path/o- (disease; suffering)
-ic (pertaining to)	cardi/o- (heart)	phleb/o- (vein)
-ion (action; condition)	ech/o- (echo; sound wave)	scler/o- (hard)
-itis (inflammation of; infection of)	electr/o- (electricity)	sphygm/o- (pulse)
-meter (instrument used to measure)	idi/o- (unknown; individual)	thromb/o- (thrombus; blood clot)
-osis (condition; abnormal condition; process)	ly/o- (break down; destroy)	vers/o- (to travel; to turn)
-pathy (disease; suffering)	man/o- (thin; frenzy)	
-tic (pertaining to)		

Definition of the Medical Word

1. Abnormal condition of the artery (with) hardness

2. Pertaining to the muscle of the heart

3. Process of recording the echo of a sound wave (from the) heart

4. Pertaining to (a drug that takes) a thrombus (blood clot) and breaks it down and destroys it

5. Abnormal condition of a soft, fatty substance (as well as) hardness (in an artery)

6. Process of recording the electrical (impulses) of the heart

7. Inflammation or infection of a blood clot (in) a vein

8. Disease of the heart muscle

9. Instrument used to measure the pulse (of the blood pressure using a) thin (cuff)

10. Pertaining to an unknown (cause of a) disease

11. Action (done to the) heart to turn (it away from an arrhythmia)

Build the Medical Word

1. *arteriosclerosis* _____

2. _____

3. _____

4. _____

5. _____

6. _____

7. _____

8. _____

9. _____

10. _____

11. _____

Abbreviations

Matching Exercise

Match each abbreviation to its description.

1. LVAD   _____ "Good cholesterol," a high-density lipoprotein

2. AAA   _____ High blood pressure

3. SBE   _____ Bacterial infection inside the heart

4. CRP   _____ A type of aneurysm

5. mm Hg   _____ Test to detect inflammation in the heart

6. HTN   _____ A hole in the septum between the ventricles

7. TPR   _____ Vital signs

8. TEE   _____ Measurement of blood pressure

9. VSD   _____ Heart test that goes into the esophagus

10. HDL   _____ May be used instead of heart transplantation

Applied Skills

Plural Noun and Adjective Spelling Exercise

Read the noun and write its plural form and/or adjective form. Be sure to check your spelling. The first one has been done for you.

Singular Noun	Plural Noun	Adjective Form	Singular Noun	Plural Noun	Adjective Form
1. pericardium		pericardial	7. valve		
2. artery	_____	_____	8. aorta		_____
3. atrium	_____	_____	9. vein	_____	_____
4. ventricle	_____	_____	10. heart	_____	_____
5. septum		_____	11. artery	_____	_____
6. myocardium		_____			

Proofreading and Spelling Exercise

Read the following paragraph. Identify each misspelled medical word and write the correct spelling of it on the line provided.

The nurse used a sphigmomanometer to take the patient's blood pressure. He had hypertension in the past. He had a caroted endarterectomy because of an atherometous plaque in his artery. He has also had an arhythmia in the past with ventricular takycardia. He just developed congestive heart failure and takes a dijitalis drug for that. We are considering this patient for an angoplasty in the future to keep him from having a myocardal infarcktion. His cardiomegalee is becoming more severe.

1. _____   6. _____
2. _____   7. _____
3. _____   8. _____
4. _____   9. _____
5. _____   10. _____

You Write the Medical Report

You are a healthcare professional interviewing a patient. Listen to the patient's statements and then enter them in the patient's medical record using medical words and phrases. Be sure to check your spelling. The first one has been done for you.

1. The patient says, "Last night, I had severe pain in my chest that was like a crushing sensation and bad sweating and I felt like something really bad was happening."

   You write: Last night, the patient experienced severe ___angina pectoris___ with the pain feeling like a crushing sensation. He also had ___diaphoresis___ and a sense of doom.

2. The patient says, "Last year, I went to the emergency room and my heart rate was about 200. They brought this machine in and it had two paddles and they gave me a shock and then my heart rhythm was normal. Today, I could feel my heart do some "thumps" and then be okay. But the last time this happened, they did hook me up to those electrodes and took a tracing of my heart."

   You write: The patient states that last year she went to the emergency room with ventricular _____ with a rate of about 200. They did a _____, and her heart rhythm returned to normal. The patient says she felt some _____ today, and so we will have an _____ done in the office today.

3. The patient says, "I know I have a history of my arteries being hard and clogged with fatty stuff, but now I have this new problem and I get on-and-off pain in the calf of my leg when I try to walk very far. My podiatrist said my one toe does not get enough blood to it and the tissue might die."

   You write: The patient has a history of _____, but now she has a new problem of experiencing _____ when she tries to walk very far. Her podiatrist noted a lack of perfusion to one toe and feels it might become _____.

4. The nurse's note in the patient's medical record shows that the patient's blood pressure today is 130/88. Previous office visits have shown similar BP results. The patient says, "I am trying to stay on my low-salt diet."

You write: Based on serial blood pressure measurements today and over the past 3 months, the patient's blood pressure remains in the range of 130/88, and she now has a diagnosis of _____. She has been on a low-salt diet, and we will now add the _____ drug furosemide for treatment to lower her blood pressure.

Medical Report Exercise

This exercise contains a hospital Admission History and Physical Examination report. Read the report and answer the questions.

ADMISSION HISTORY AND PHYSICAL EXAMINATION

PATIENT NAME: COVINGTON, Victoria

HOSPITAL NUMBER: 62-700245

DATE OF ADMISSION: January 21, 20xx

HISTORY OF PRESENT ILLNESS
The patient is a 76-year-old white female who was transferred from home via ambulance to this emergency department. Apparently, the patient had just finished eating breakfast when her family noticed that she was standing in the middle of the hallway with her walker and seemed dazed. She was assisted to her bed, but rest did not improve her mental status. The family stated that she continued to be confused, incoherent, and unable to answer simple questions. At that point, the family called 911.

PAST MEDICAL HISTORY
The past medical history was obtained from the patient's daughter-in-law. The patient has a history of CHF, which has been slowly worsening over about the past 8 years. She also has a history of hypertension. The patient has been diagnosed with type 2 diabetes mellitus. The daughter-in-law remembers that the patient's last fasting blood sugar in the doctor's office last month was over 250. She is usually noncompliant with her diet, eating foods that are high in fat and calories. The patient does not take a pill or insulin for her diabetes. In the past week, the patient has had no appetite, has eaten little, but reportedly gained 2 pounds anyway. The daughter-in-law does not know the names of all of the patient's medications, except for Lasix. The patient smokes 1 pack of cigarettes per day and has done so for the past 40+ years. The patient has no known allergies.

PHYSICAL EXAMINATION
The patient is an obese female, lying in bed. She is stuporous, opening her eyes to commands but she is unable to answer questions. Heart: Regular rate and rhythm. The neck veins are slightly distended. The breath sounds reveal congestion in both lungs bilaterally. The abdomen is soft with hypoactive bowel sounds. Physical examination of the lower extremities shows severe edema in both feet and legs.

COURSE IN THE EMERGENCY DEPARTMENT
The patient was placed on a cardiac monitor and given a stat dose of intravenous Lasix. Labs were sent for CBC with WBC differential, electrolytes, CK-MB, troponin, and glucose. An arterial blood gas was drawn. Portable chest x-ray in the emergency department showed cardiomegaly with LVH. There was significant pulmonary congestion. While awaiting the results of the blood chemistries, the patient suddenly went into cardiac arrest. CPR was initiated. She responded to aggressive drug intervention, and we were able to establish a normal sinus rhythm. The patient was then transferred to the intensive care unit in critical condition, intubated, and on the ventilator.

Alfred P. Molina, M.D.

Alfred P. Molina, M.D.

APM:mtt
D: 01/21/xx
T: 01/21/xx

Word Analysis Questions

1. What is the medical abbreviation for hypertension? _____

2. The patient has hypertension. If you wanted to use the adjective form of *hypertension*, you would say, "The patient is
_____."

3. What do these abbreviations stand for?

   a. CHF _____

   b. CK-MB _____

   c. CPR _____

   d. LVH _____

4. Divide *vascular* into its two word parts and define each word part.

   Word Part   **Definition**

   _____   _____

   _____   _____

5. Divide *cardiomegaly* into its two word parts and define each word part.

   Word Part   **Definition**

   _____   _____

   _____   _____

6. Dictionary Skills

   These medical words were not covered in this chapter, but you need to know their meanings in order to understand this medical report. Look up these words in a medical or English dictionary and write their definitions.

   Word   **Definition**

   bilaterally   _____

   incoherent   _____

   stuporous   _____

Fact Finding Questions

1. What is the normal range of the heart rate in beats per minute for an adult?

   _____

2. Besides hypertension, what other two diagnoses did the patient have before this hospitalization?

   a. _____

   b. _____

3. Resuscitation was used to treat what condition? (Circle one)

   cardiomegaly   **hypertension**   **cardiac arrest**   **diabetes mellitus**

4. Circle the two tests that were done to check to see if the patient had had a myocardial infarction.

   troponin   **portable chest x-ray**   **blood glucose**   **CK-MB**   **intubation**

5. The patient had a cardiac arrest. What is the medical word for having no heart beat?

   _____

Critical Thinking Questions

1. The severe edema in the patient's lower extremities reflected backup of blood due to failure of which side of the heart?

   _____

2. The pulmonary congestion seen on the chest x-ray reflected failure of which side of the heart?

   _____

3. Lasix is a diuretic drug that removes fluid from the body by excreting it in the urine. For which of the patient's medical conditions was this drug prescribed? (Circle one)

   congestive heart failure   **lack of appetite**   **obesity**   **confusion**

4. If the patient ate little food in the past week, why did she gain 2 pounds?

   _____

Hearing Medical Words Exercise

You hear someone speaking the medical words given below. Read each pronunciation and then write the medical word it represents. Be sure to check your spelling. The first one has been done for you.

1. KAR-dee-ac   *cardiac*_____
2. AN-yoo-rizm   _____
3. KAR-dee-oh-thoh-RAS-ik _____
4. MY-oh-KAR-dee-um   _____
5. KOR-oh-nair-ee AR-ter-ee _____
6. VAY-soh-con-STRIK-shun _____

7. KAR-dee-oh-MEG-ah-lee   _____
8. aa-RITH-mee-ah   _____
9. ATH-eh-roh-skleh-ROH-sis _____
10. EK-oh-KAR-dee-oh-gram   _____
11. AN-jee-oh-PLAS-tee   _____
12. SFIG-moh-mah-NAWM-eh-ter _____

Pronunciation Exercise

Read the medical word that is given. Then review the syllables in the pronunciation. Circle the primary (main) accented syllable. The first one has been done for you.

1. cardiac (kar-dee-ac)
2. coronary (kor-oh-nair-ee)
3. vasodilation (vay-soh-dy-lay-shun)
4. cardiopulmonary (kar-dee-oh-pul-moh-nair-ee)
5. pericarditis (pair-ee-kar-dy-tis)
6. myocardial infarction (my-oh-kar-dee-al in-fark-shun)
7. fibrillation (fib-rih-lay-shun)
8. atherosclerosis (ath-eh-roh-skleh-roh-sis)
9. auscultation (aws-kul-tay-shun)
10. angioplasty (an-jee-oh-plas-tee)

Multimedia Preview

Immerse yourself in a variety of activities inside Medical Terminology Interactive. Getting there is simple:

1. Click on www.myhealthprofessionskit.com.
2. Select "Medical Terminology" from the choice of disciplines.
3. First-time users must create an account using the scratch-off code on the inside front cover of this book.
4. Find this book and log in using your username and password.
5. Click on Medical Terminology Interactive.
6. Take the elevator to the 5th Floor to begin your virtual exploration of this chapter!

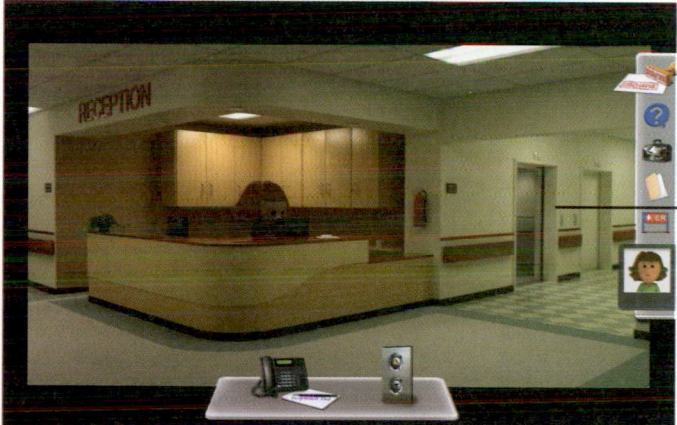 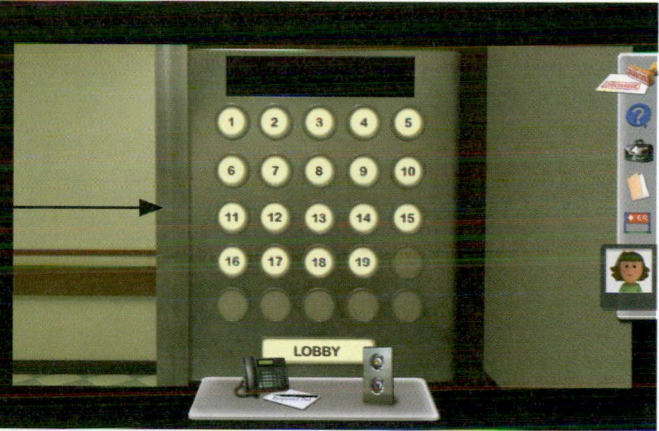

■ **Word Surgery** Are you ready for the operating room? Use your scalpel to slice each word into its component parts. Then define those parts once they're on your tray. Can you make the cut?

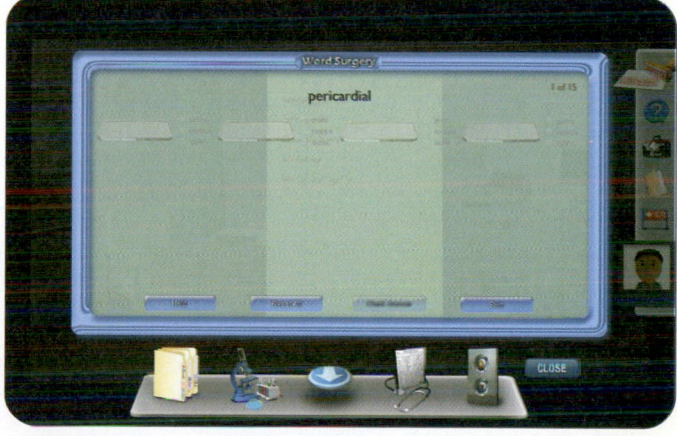

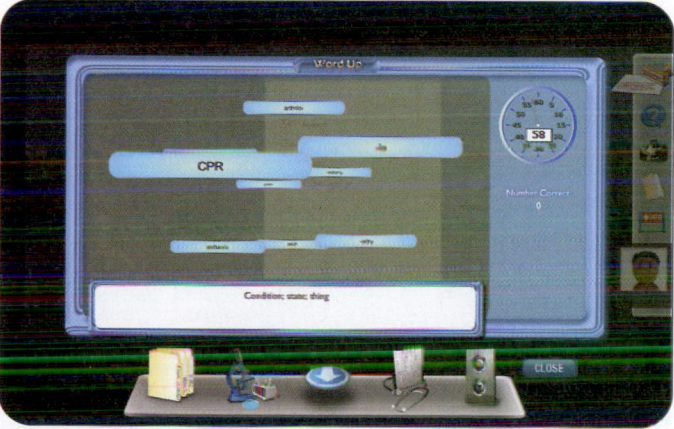

■ **Word Up!** Catch it while you can! Challenge yourself to match the definition to the corresponding word part as your choices swirl around the screen. See how many you can match up correctly before your time is up!

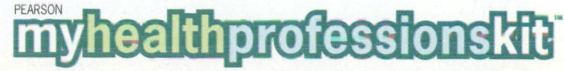

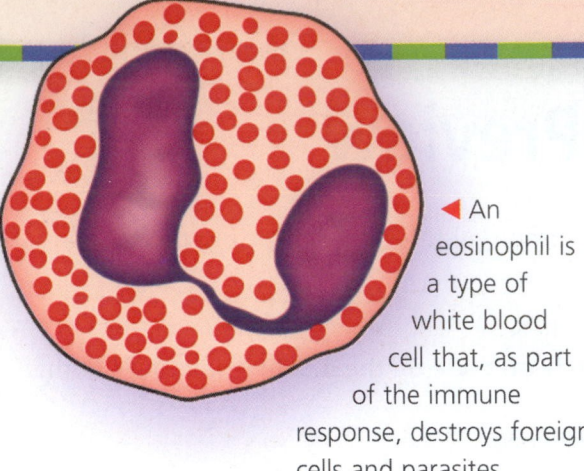

◄ An eosinophil is a type of white blood cell that, as part of the immune response, destroys foreign cells and parasites.

Dive In!

- Human blood circles the human body in about 20 seconds, traveling thousands of miles per day.

- 15 million blood cells are produced and destroyed in the body every second.

- To score an A or B (or AB or O) keep reading. In this chapter we'll explore the language that describes blood and lymphatic system structures, functions, diseases, and conditions.

- Your knowledge will be flowing once you master the language of hematology and immunology!

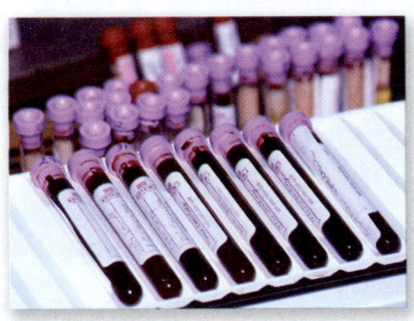

▶ Blood contains proteins that female mosquitoes need to lay their eggs. That's why only the females bite.

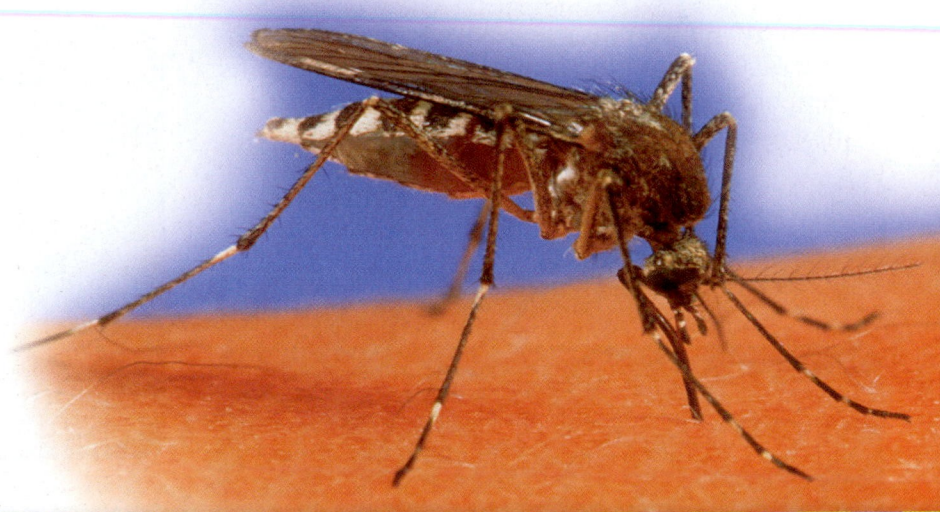

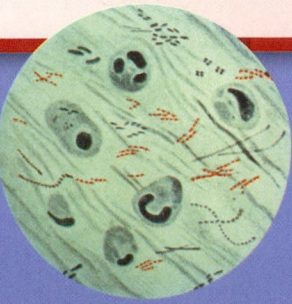

1859

Louis Pasteur suggests that microscopic organisms cause disease

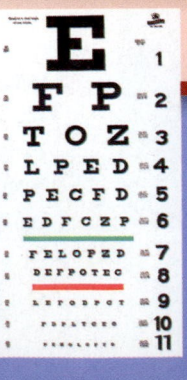

1862

Dutch physician Hermann Snellen invents the Snellen chart for testing distance vision

1864

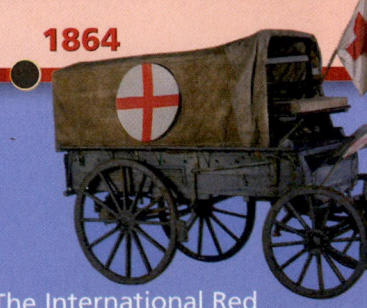

The International Red Cross is founded

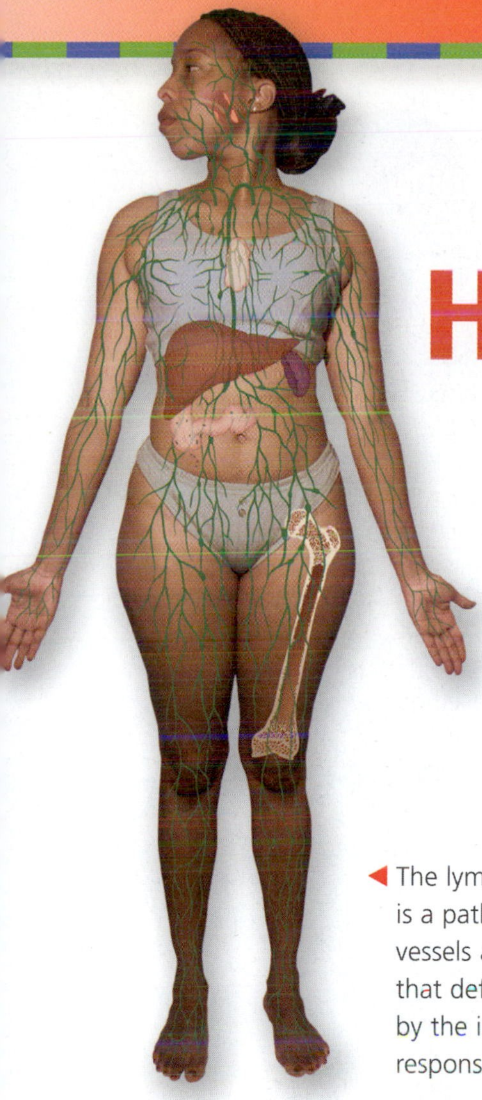

6

Hematology and Immunology

Blood and Lymphatic System

Hematology (HEE-mah-TAWL-oh-jee) is the medical specialty that studies the anatomy and physiology of the blood and uses diagnostic tests, medical and surgical procedures, and drugs to treat blood diseases.

◀ The lymphatic system is a pathway of vessels and nodes that defend the body by the immune response.

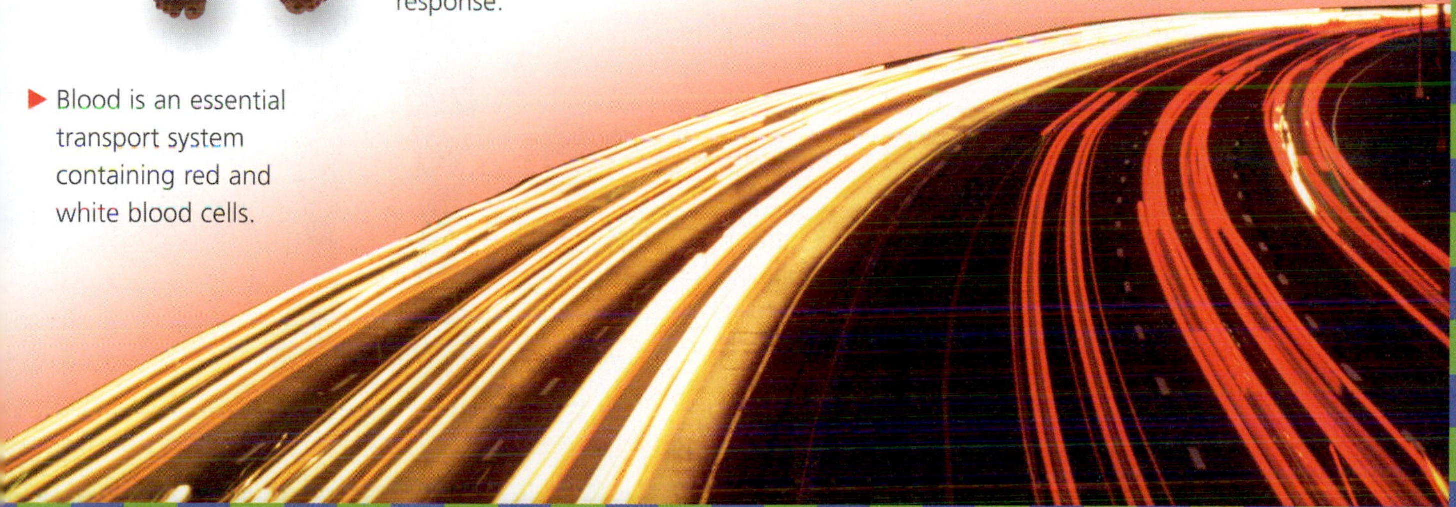

▶ Blood is an essential transport system containing red and white blood cells.

1865

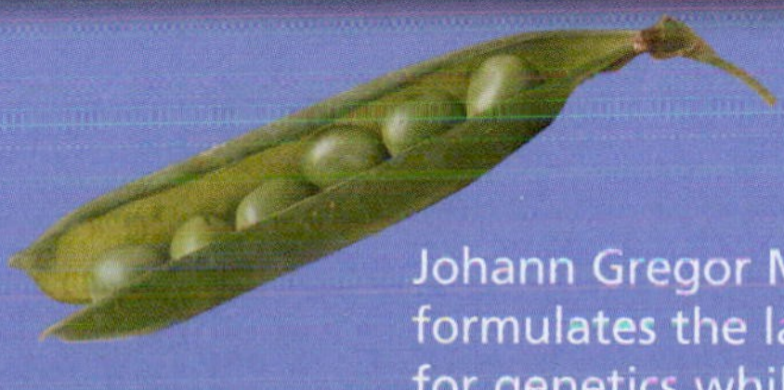

Johann Gregor Mendel formulates the laws for genetics while crossbreeding pea plants

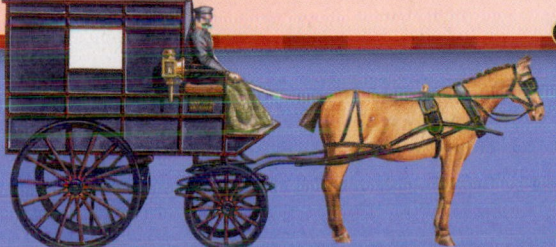

1869

The first ambulance service is established at Bellevue Hospital in New York by Dr. Edward Dalton

Measure Your Progress: Learning Objectives

After you study this chapter, you should be able to

1. Identify the structures of the blood and the lymphatic system.

2. Describe the processes of blood clotting and the immune response.

3. Describe common blood, lymphatic, and immune diseases and conditions, laboratory and diagnostic procedures, medical and surgical procedures, and drug categories.

4. Give the medical meaning of word parts related to the blood and immune system.

5. Build blood, lymph system, and immune response words from word parts and divide and define those words.

6. Spell and pronounce blood, lymph system, and immune response words.

7. Analyze the medical content and meaning of an immunology report.

8. Dive deeper into hematology and immunology by reviewing the activities at the end of this chapter and online at Medical Terminology Interactive.

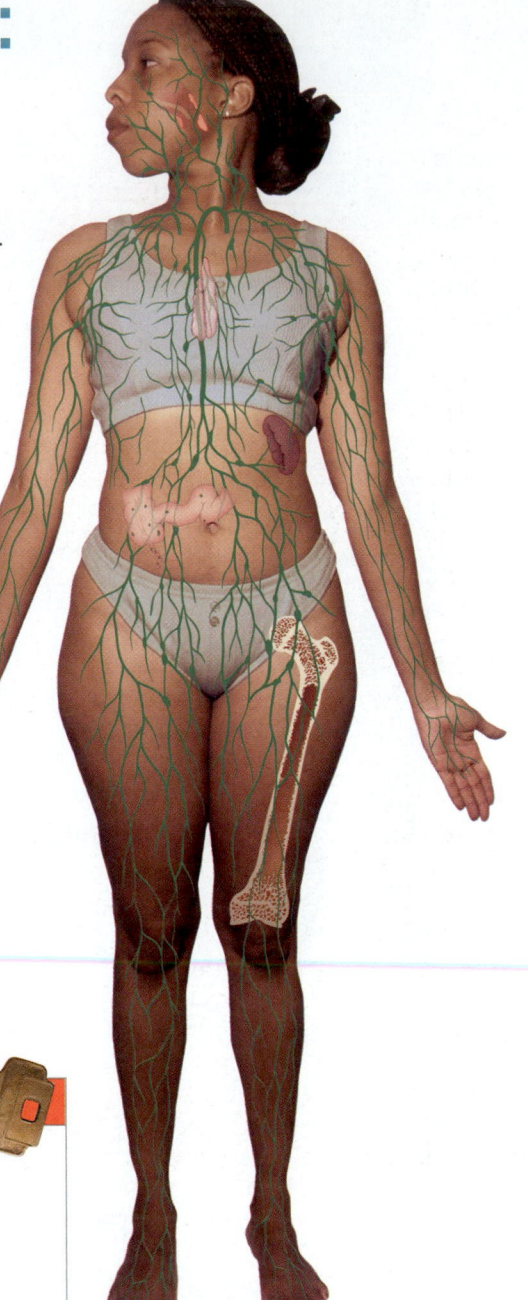

Figure 6-1 ■ **Lymphatic system.**
The lymphatic system consists of lymphatic vessels, lymph nodes, lymph fluid, lymphoid tissues, and lymphoid organs. The lymphatic system, with assistance from the blood cells, coordinates the body's immune response.

Medical Language Key

To unlock the definition of a medical word, break it into word parts. Define each word part. Put the word part meanings in order, beginning with the suffix, then the prefix (if present), then the combining form(s).

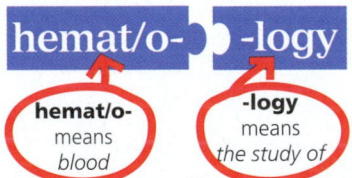

hemat/o-
means
blood

-logy
means
the study of

	Word Part	Word Part Meaning
Suffix	-logy	*the study of*
Combining Form	hemat/o-	*blood*

Hematology: *The study of the blood.*

	Word Part	Word Part Meaning
Suffix	-logy	*the study of*
Combining Form	immun/o-	*immune response*

Immunology: *The study of the immune response.*

Anatomy and Physiology

Blood is categorized as a type of connective tissue because its formed elements (blood cells and blood cell fragments) are a product of the bone marrow of the skeletal system. Blood contains blood cells and blood cell fragments, water, and other substances (proteins, clotting factors, etc.). Blood travels in the blood vessels of the cardiovascular system (discussed in "Cardiology," Chapter 5). The purpose of the blood is to transport oxygen, carbon dioxide, nutrients, and the waste products of metabolism. The blood can stop its own flow at the site of an injury. The blood also contains blood cells that function as part of the immune response of the lymphatic system.

The lymphatic system (see Figure 6-1 ■) consists of the lymphatic vessels, lymph nodes, lymph fluid, lymphoid tissues, and lymphoid organs. The lymphatic system forms a pathway throughout the body that is separate from that of the cardiovascular system; however, some cells in the blood function as part of the immune response of the lymphatic system. The purpose of the lymphatic system is to defend the body against microorganisms, foreign particles, and cancerous cells by means of the immune response.

Anatomy of the Blood

Plasma

The **plasma** is a clear, straw-colored liquid that makes up 55% of the blood (see Figure 6-2 ■). The formed elements of the blood (erythrocytes, leukocytes, thrombocytes) are suspended in the plasma. The plasma contains many different substances: amino acids, cholesterol, triglycerides, electrolytes, glucose, minerals, and vitamins; these are nutrients from digested foods. Also in the plasma are substances the body produces itself: albumin, conjugated bilirubin, unconjugated bilirubin, hormones, complement proteins, and clotting factors. Finally, the plasma contains creatinine and urea, the waste products of cellular metabolism. Plasma is about 90% water, but this percentage can change if there is a decreased intake of water or an increased loss of water (from diarrhea, increased urination, excessive sweating, etc.).

plasma (PLAZ-mah)
The combining form *plasm/o-* means *plasma*.

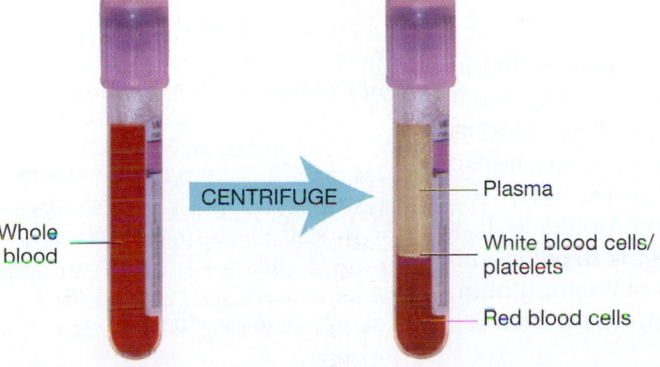

Whole blood — CENTRIFUGE →

Plasma

White blood cells/platelets

Red blood cells

Figure 6-2 ■ Plasma.

Blood is composed of plasma and formed elements (red blood cells, white blood cells, platelets). When a specimen of whole blood is placed in a centrifuge and spun quickly, the heavier parts (the formed elements) settle to the bottom, and the clear, straw-colored plasma remains on the top.

A Closer Look

Plasma proteins, primarily **albumin,** are molecules that are too large to pass through the wall of a blood vessel. They stay in the plasma and exert an osmotic pressure that keeps water in the blood from moving out into the surrounding tissues.

albumin (al-BYOO-min)

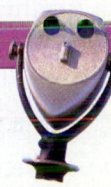

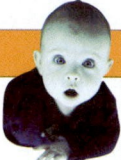

Word Alert

SOUND-ALIKE WORDS

albumen (noun) the white of an egg
Example: Albumen in egg whites is a good source of dietary protein.

albumin (noun) protein molecule in the blood
Example: Albumin is an important protein in the plasma.

Electrolytes are chemical structures that carry a positive or negative electrical charge. Electrolytes in the plasma include sodium (Na^+), potassium (K^+), chloride (Cl^-), calcium (Ca^{++}), and bicarbonate (HCO_3^-). Sodium plays an important role in maintaining the volume and pressure of the blood. Sodium, potassium, and calcium are important in the contraction of the heart and skeletal muscles. Calcium is also important during blood clotting and in the formation of bone. Bicarbonate acts as a buffer to maintain the normal pH (acidity versus alkalinity) of the blood.

Did You Know?

Blood tastes salty because the electrolytes sodium and chloride in the plasma are the same ingredients that make up table salt.

Hematopoiesis

Hematopoiesis is the process by which all of the formed elements in the plasma are produced. Hematopoiesis occurs in the red marrow of long bones or flat bones (such as the sternum, ribs, hip bones, bones of the spinal column, and bones of the legs). Every type of blood cell (erythrocyte, leukocyte) and blood cell fragment (thrombocyte) begins in the bone marrow as a very immature cell known as a **stem cell** (see Figure 6-3 ■).

Erythrocytes

Erythrocytes are the most numerous of the formed elements suspended in the plasma. An **erythrocyte** or **red blood cell (RBC)** is a round, somewhat flattened, red disk. Its depressed center (where the cell is not as thick) is paler in color (see Figure 6-4 ■). Erythrocytes are unique because, unlike other body cells, they have no cell nucleus when they are mature.

Erythrocytes contain **hemoglobin,** a red, iron-containing molecule. It is this molecule that binds to and carries oxygen from the lungs to every cell in the body. Hemoglobin bound to oxygen is known as **oxyhemoglobin.** Hemoglobin also binds to and carries carbon dioxide from the cells back to the lungs.

Erythrocytes develop in the red marrow from stem cells that become **erythroblasts** and then **normoblasts.** They are released into the blood in a slightly immature form known as **reticulocytes.** Within a day, the reticulocyte becomes a mature erythrocyte, which has no nucleus. The body produces several million erythrocytes every second. Any time the body experiences a significant blood loss, the kidneys secrete **erythropoietin,** a hormone that dramatically increases the speed at which erythrocytes are produced and become mature.

WORD BUILDING

electrolyte (ee-LEK-troh-lite)
electr/o- *electricity*
-lyte *dissolved substance*

hematopoiesis
(HEE-mah-toh-poy-EE-sis)
hemat/o- *blood*
-poiesis *condition of formation*

erythrocyte (eh-RITH-roh-site)
erythr/o- *red*
-cyte *cell*

hemoglobin (HEE-moh-GLOH-bin)
(HEE-moh-GLOH-bin)
hem/o- *blood*
glob/o- *shaped like a globe; comprehensive*
-in *a substance*

oxyhemoglobin
(AWK-see-HEE-moh-GLOH-bin)
ox/y- *oxygen; quick*
hem/o- *blood*
glob/o- *shaped like a globe; comprehensive*
-in *a substance*

erythroblast (eh-RITH-roh-blast)
erythr/o- *red*
-blast *immature cell*

normoblast (NOR-moh-blast)
norm/o- *normal; usual*
-blast *immature cell*

reticulocyte (reh-TIK-yoo-LOH-site)
reticul/o- *small network*
-cyte *cell*
A reticulocyte has a network of ribosomes in its cytoplasm.

erythropoietin
(eh-RITH-roh-POY-eh-tin)
erythr/o- *red*
-poietin *a substance that forms*
Add words to make a correct definition of *erythropoietin: a substance that forms red (blood cells).*

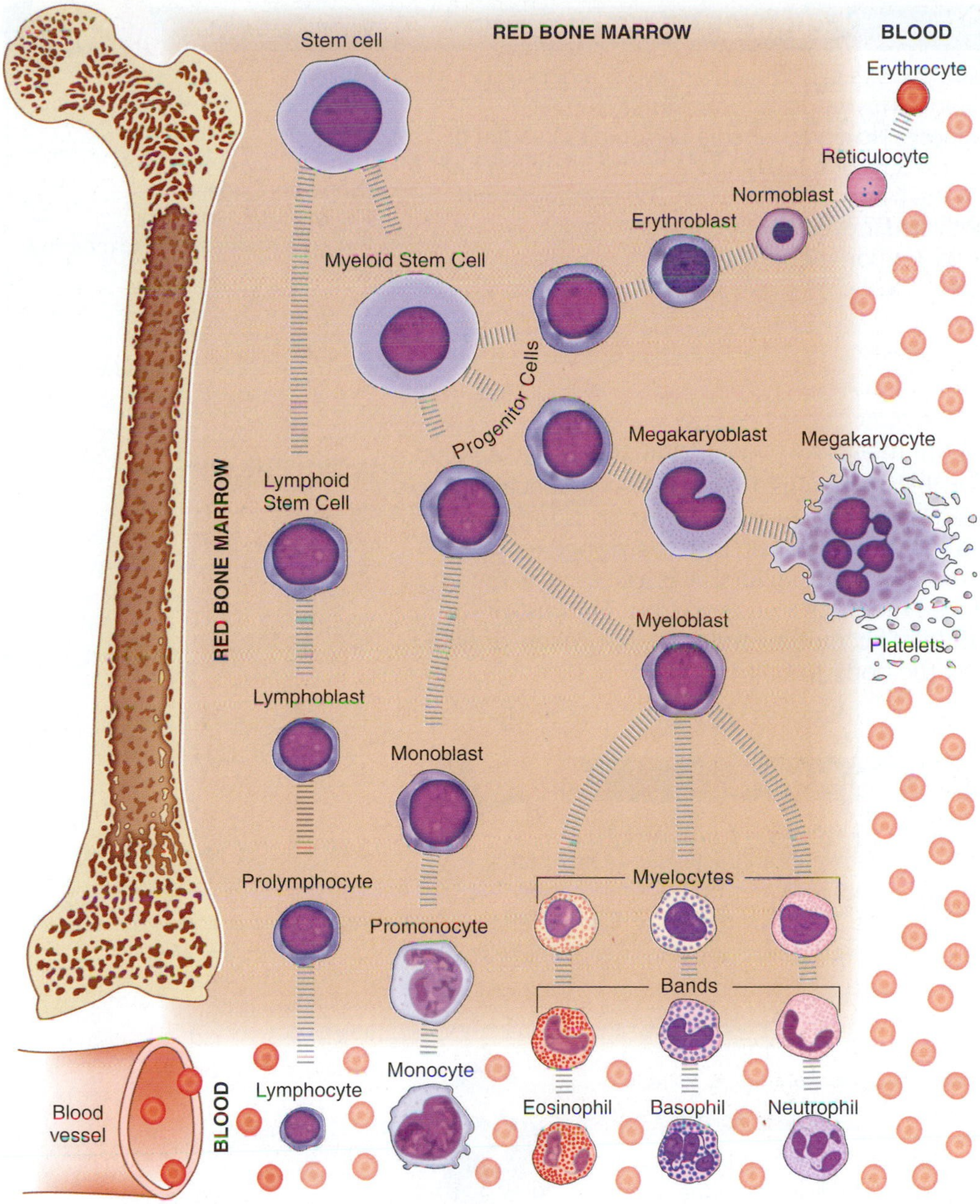

RED BONE MARROW

BLOOD

Stem cell

Erythrocyte

Reticulocyte

Normoblast

Erythroblast

Myeloid Stem Cell

Progenitor Cells

Megakaryoblast

Megakaryocyte

RED BONE MARROW

Lymphoid Stem Cell

Platelets

Myeloblast

Lymphoblast

Monoblast

Myelocytes

Prolymphocyte

Promonocyte

Bands

BLOOD

Lymphocyte

Monocyte

Eosinophil

Basophil

Neutrophil

Blood vessel

Figure 6-3 ■ **Hematopoiesis.**
All of the formed elements of the blood begin in the red bone marrow.

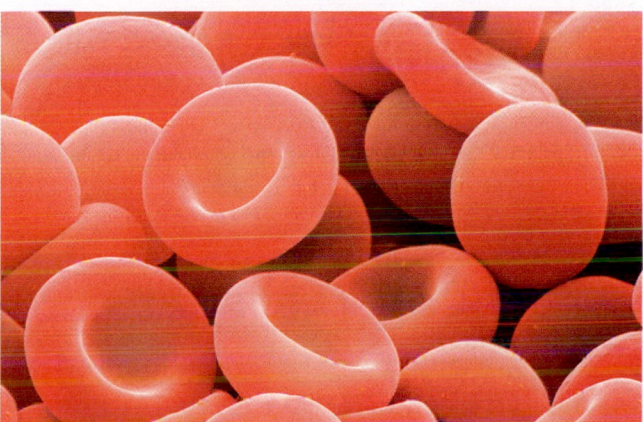

Figure 6-4 ■ **Erythrocytes.**
Notice the characteristic red color of erythrocytes (red blood cells) and their unique "donut" shape. Each erythrocyte has a depressed center and no cell nucleus.

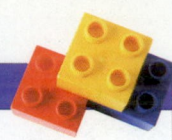

Clinical Connections

Forensic Science. When a person drowns or suffocates, there is a high level of carbon dioxide (CO_2) in the blood. This causes the skin to have a deep bluish-purple color known as cyanosis. However, when a person dies in a fire or from inhaling the fumes from car exhaust or a faulty space heater, there is a high level of carbon monoxide (CO) in the blood. Unlike oxygen and carbon dioxide, **carbon monoxide** binds so tightly and irreversibly that the hemoglobin is unable to carry any other molecule. Carbon monoxide poisoning causes a characteristic cherry red skin color.

carbon monoxide
(KAR-bon mawn-AWK-side)
Mon/o- is a combining form meaning *one; single.*

Because an erythrocyte does not have a nucleus, it is unable to divide or repair itself. It lasts 120 days and then begins to deteriorate. Specialized cells (macrophages) in the spleen engulf old erythrocytes, breaking down their hemoglobin into heme and globin molecules. Iron is stripped from the heme molecule and stored in the liver and spleen; it is released to build more erythrocytes if the diet does not contain enough iron. The rest of the heme molecule becomes bilirubin. The globin molecule is broken down into amino acids that are used by the body to build cells.

WORD BUILDING

Clinical Connections

Gastroenterology (Chapter 3). Bilirubin is used by the liver to make bile. Bilirubin is a yellow pigment that gives bile its characteristic yellow-green appearance. The combining form *rub/o-* (red) indicates that bilirubin comes from the breakdown of red blood cells, not that it is red in color. Bilirubin also plays an important role as an antioxidant, protecting body cells from damage by free radicals.

Did You Know?

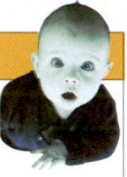

Erythrocytes and leukocytes are also known as red corpuscles and white corpuscles. *Corpuscle* is a Latin word meaning *a little body.*

Leukocytes

Leukocytes or **white blood cells (WBCs)** include five types of cells, each of which plays a unique role in the body's immune response. Leukocytes include neutrophils, eosinophils, basophils, lymphocytes, and monocytes (see Table 6-1).

You can identify each type of leukocyte by the presence or absence of granules in its cytoplasm and by the shape of its nucleus. These differences can be seen when leukocytes are stained and examined under a microscope.

Any leukocyte with large granules in its cytoplasm is categorized as a granulocyte. **Granulocytes** include neutrophils, eosinophils, and basophils. Any leukocyte with few or no granules in its cytoplasm is categorized as an agranulocyte. **Agranulocytes** include lymphocytes and monocytes.

leukocyte (LOO-koh-site)
  leuk/o- *white*
  -cyte *cell*

granulocyte (GRAN-yoo-loh-SITE)
  granul/o- *granule*
  -cyte *cell*

agranulocyte (aa-GRAN-yoo-loh-SITE)
  a- *away from; without*
  granul/o- *granule*
  -cyte *cell*

Table 6-1   Leukocyte Types and Characteristics

Leukocyte	Category	Cytoplasm	Nucleus	Function
neutrophil segmented neutrophil, segmenter, seg, polymorphonuclear leukocyte (PMN), poly	granulocyte	large, pale granules that do not stain either red or blue	three or more lobes	engulf and destroy bacteria
eosinophil eo	granulocyte	large granules that stain bright pink to red	two lobes	engulf and destroy foreign cells (pollen, animal dander, etc.) and release chemicals that kill parasites
basophil baso	granulocyte	large granules that stain dark blue to purple	more than one lobe	release histamine at the site of tissue injury, release heparin to limit the size of a forming blood clot
lymphocyte lymph	agranulocyte	few or no granules	round	engulf and destroy viruses and produce antibodies (immunoglobulins)
monocyte mono	agranulocyte	few or no granules	kidney bean–shaped	engulf and destroy micro-organisms, cancerous cells, dead leukocytes, and cellular debris

Granulocytes

1. Neutrophils are the most common leukocyte. They make up 40–60% of the leukocytes in the blood. A neutrophil has large, pale-colored granules in its cytoplasm, and its nucleus has many segments or lobes (see Figure 6-5 ■ and Table 6-1). A neutrophil is also known as a segmented neutrophil, segmenter, seg, **polymorphonuclear leukocyte (PMN),** or poly.

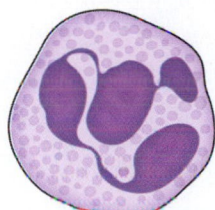

Figure 6-5 ■ Neutrophil.

A neutrophil has large granules in its cytoplasm. These granules are "neutral" in that they do not stain well with either a red, acidic dye (eosin) or with a blue, alkaline dye (hematoxylin). Neutrophils get their name from their neutral reaction to these dyes.

Neutrophils develop in the red marrow from **stem cells** that become **myeloblasts,** then **myelocytes,** and then **bands** (see Figure 6-3). A band is an immature neutrophil that has a nucleus shaped like a curved band. Bands are also known as **stabs** (the German word for *band*). There are always a few bands present in the blood, but, during severe bacterial infections, the number of bands rises as the need for more neutrophils increases.

WORD BUILDING

neutrophil (NOO-troh-fil)
  neutr/o- *not taking part*
  -phil *attraction to; fondness for*

polymorphonuclear
(PAWL-ee-MOR-foh-NOO-klee-ar)
  poly- *many; much*
  morph/o- *shape*
  nucle/o- *nucleus (of a cell)*
  -ar *pertaining to*

myeloblast (MY-eh-loh-BLAST)
  myel/o- *bone marrow; spinal cord; myelin*
  -blast *immature cell*

myelocyte (MY-eh-loh-SITE)
  myel/o- *bone marrow; spinal cord; myelin*
  -cyte *cell*

Neutrophils are blood cells, but they are also part of the immune response of the lymphatic system because they are **phagocytes** that specifically engulf and destroy bacteria. This process is known as **phagocytosis.** Neutrophils only live a few days or even just a few hours if they are actively destroying bacteria. One neutrophil can destroy about 10 bacteria before it dies.

2. Eosinophils make up just 1–4% of the leukocytes in the blood. An eosinophil has large, red-pink granules in its cytoplasm, and its nucleus has two lobes (see Figure 6-6 ■ and Table 6-1). Eosinophils are also known as eos.

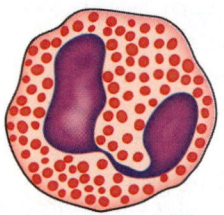

Figure 6-6 ■ Eosinophil.
An eosinophil has large granules in its cytoplasm. These granules stain bright pink to red with a red, acidic dye (eosin). Eosinophils get their name from their reaction to this dye.

Eosinophils develop in the red marrow from stem cells (see Figure 6-3). Eosinophils are blood cells, but they are also part of the immune response of the lymphatic system because they are phagocytes that specifically engulf and destroy foreign cells (pollen, animal dander, etc.) and release chemicals that kill parasites.

3. Basophils are the least common leukocyte. They make up just 0.5–1% of the leukocytes in the blood. A basophil has large, purple granules in its cytoplasm, and its nucleus has more than one lobe (see Figure 6-7 ■ and Table 6-1). Basophils are also known as basos.

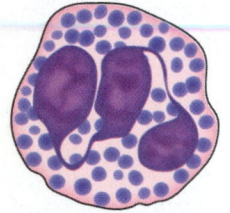

Figure 6-7 ■ Basophil.
A basophil has large granules in its cytoplasm. These granules stain dark blue to purple with a blue, alkaline dye (hematoxylin). (Something that is alkaline or is a base is the opposite of an acid.) Basophils get their name from their reaction to this dye, which is a base.

Basophils develop in the red marrow from stem cells (see Figure 6-3). Basophils are blood cells, but they are also part of the immune response of the lymphatic system because they go to the site of tissue injury and release histamine. Histamine dilates blood vessels and increases inflammation. Basophils are also part of the blood clotting process; they release heparin, an anticoagulant that limits the size of a blood clot that forms at the site of tissue injury.

Agranulocytes

1. Lymphocytes make up 20–40% of the leukocytes in the blood. Lymphocytes are the smallest leukocytes. A lymphocyte has just a thin ring of cytoplasm that contains few or no granules, and its nucleus is round and nearly fills the cell (see Figure 6-8 ■ and Table 6-1). Some lymphocytes live for just a few days, while others live for many years. Lymphocytes are also known as lymphs.

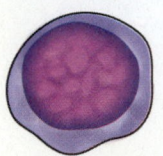

Figure 6-8 ■ Lymphocyte.
A lymphocyte has few or no granules, little cytoplasm, and a round nucleus.

WORD BUILDING

phagocyte (FAG-oh-site)
phag/o- *eating; swallowing*
-cyte *cell*

phagocytosis (FAG-oh-sy-TOH-sis)
phag/o- *eating; swallowing*
cyt/o- *cell*
-osis *condition; abnormal condition; process*

eosinophil (EE-oh-SIN-oh-fil)
eosin/o- *eosin (red acidic dye)*
-phil *attraction to; fondness for*

basophil (BAY-soh-fil)
bas/o- *base of a structure; basic (alkaline)*
-phil *attraction to; fondness for*

lymphocyte (LIM-foh-site)
lymph/o- *lymph; lymphatic system*
-cyte *cell*

Lymphocytes develop in the red marrow from stem cells that become **lymphoblasts** (see Figure 6-3). Lymphoblasts that remain in the red marrow become B lymphocytes (B cells) or NK (natural killer) cells. Other lymphoblasts migrate to the thymus (within the mediastinum), where the presence of thymosins (hormones) causes them to become T lymphocytes (T cells). Lymphocytes are blood cells, but they are also part of the immune response of the lymphatic system. They are in the lymph nodes, they produce antibodies (immunoglobulins), and they are phagocytes that specifically engulf and destroy viruses. The different types of lymphocytes and their specific functions are discussed in the section on the immune response.

2. Monocytes make up 2–4% of the leukocytes in the blood. They are the largest leukocytes. A monocyte has a large amount of cytoplasm that contains few or no granules, and its nucleus is large and kidney bean-shaped (see Figure 6-9 ■ and Table 6-1). Monocytes are also known as monos.

Monocytes develop in the red marrow from stem cells that become **monoblasts** and then mature monocytes (see Figure 6-3). Monocytes are blood cells, but they are also part of the immune response of the lymphatic system because they are phagocytes that engulf and destroy microorganisms, cancerous cells, dead leukocytes, and cellular debris. Monocytes in the lymph nodes, intestine, liver, pancreas, thymus, spleen, bone, and skin are known as **macrophages.**

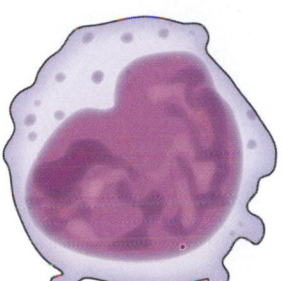

Figure 6-9 ■ Monocyte.
A monocyte has few or no granules, a large amount of cytoplasm, and a large, kidney bean–shaped nucleus.

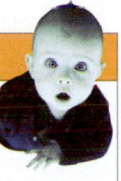

Did You Know?

Of the 5–6 quarts of blood in the body, leukocytes make up 1½ fluid ounce and thrombocytes make up only 1 teaspoonful.

Thrombocytes

A **thrombocyte** or **platelet** is different from other blood cells because it is only a cell fragment. Thrombocytes are active in the blood clotting process. Within seconds of an injury, they form clumps to decrease the loss of blood. Thrombocytes also contain some clotting factors that they release to begin the formation of a blood clot.

An individual thrombocyte begins in the red marrow as a stem cell that then becomes a **megakaryoblast** (see Figure 6-3). Then it matures into a **megakaryocyte,** a very large cell with a great deal of cytoplasm. The cytoplasm of the megakaryocyte breaks away at the edges to form cell fragments (thrombocytes) that are released into the blood. When all of the cytoplasm has broken off, the nucleus of the megakaryocyte is recycled to build other cells.

WORD BUILDING

lymphoblast (LIM-foh-blast)
  lymph/o- *lymph; lymphatic system*
  -blast *immature cell*

monocyte (MAWN-oh-site)
  mon/o- *one; single*
  -cyte *cell*
Add words to make a complete definition of *monocyte: cell (that has a) single (lobe in its nucleus).*

monoblast (MAWN-oh-blast)
  mon/o- *one; single*
  -blast *immature cell*

macrophage (MAK-roh-fayj)
  macr/o- *large*
  -phage *thing that eats*

thrombocyte (THRAWM-boh-site)
  thromb/o- *thrombus (blood clot)*
  -cyte *cell*

platelet (PLAYT-let)

megakaryoblast
(MEG-ah-KAIR-ee-oh-BLAST)
  meg/a- *large*
  kary/o- *nucleus*
  -blast *immature cell*

megakaryocyte
(MEG-ah-KAIR-ee-oh-SITE)
  meg/a- *large*
  kary/o- *nucleus*
  -cyte *cell*

Blood Type

Each person's erythrocytes have inherited genetic material that determines the blood type. The most important blood types are the ABO and Rh blood groups, although there are 22 other minor blood groups. Each blood group is named for its **antigen** (protein molecule on the cell membrane of the erythrocyte).

The **ABO blood group** contains A, B, AB, and O antigens (see Table 6-2). A person with type A blood has A antigens on their erythrocytes and so forth. A person with type O blood has neither A nor B antigens on their erythrocytes. In addition, each person's plasma contains antibodies against blood types other than its own.

The **Rh blood group** has 47 different antigens. As a group, they are known as the **Rh factor.** When these antigens are present on a person's erythrocytes, the blood type is Rh positive. When these antigens are not present, the blood type is Rh negative.

The ABO and the Rh blood groups are always considered together. For example, type A blood is either A positive (Rh positive) or A negative (Rh negative).

WORD BUILDING

antigen (AN-tih-jen)
anti- *against*
-gen *that which produces*

Table 6-2   ABO Blood Group

Blood Type	Antigen on the Erythrocyte	Antibodies in Plasma
A	A antigen	anti-B antibodies
B	B antigen	anti-A antibodies
AB	A and B antigens	none
O	none	anti-A and anti-B antibodies

Type O negative blood is known as the universal donor because it can be given to patients with any other blood type without causing a transfusion reaction (see Figure 6-10 ■).

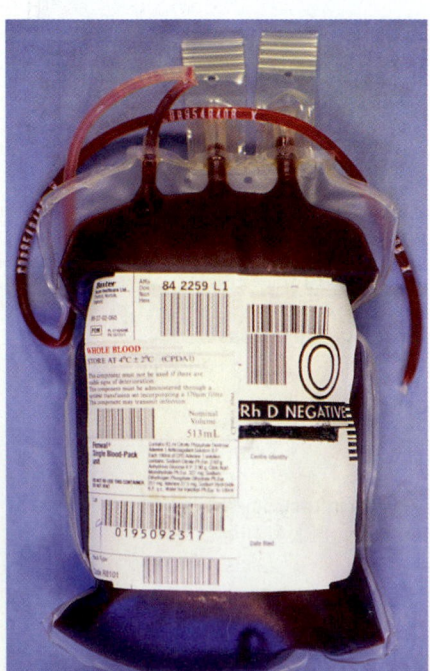

Figure 6-10 ■ Unit of blood.
This donated unit of blood is blood type O negative, the universal donor. A donated unit of blood contains 500 cc. This is nearly the same as 1 pint. That is why people talk of donating "a pint" of blood. There are approximately 10–12 pints of blood in the body.

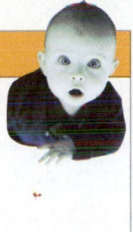

Physiology of Blood Clotting

When the body is injured, the injured blood vessel constricts to decrease the loss of blood. Thrombocytes stick to the damaged blood vessel wall and form clumps that also decrease the loss of blood. This process is known as platelet **aggregation.** The platelets also release several clotting factors. Damage to the blood vessel also activates **clotting factors** in the plasma. The clotting factors make strands of **fibrin** that trap erythrocytes and form a **thrombus** or blood clot (see Figure 6-11 ■). This process is known as **coagulation,** and the cessation of bleeding is known as **hemostasis.** The final size of a blood clot is limited by the action of heparin, a natural anticoagulant released from basophils.

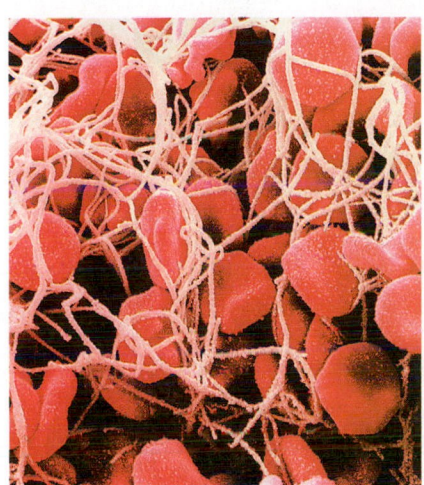

Figure 6-11 ■ **Blood clot.**
These strands of fibrin trap many erythrocytes to form a blood clot or thrombus.

All of the clotting factors must be present and be at normal levels for the blood to clot. There are 12 clotting factors (see Table 6-3), numbered as Roman numerals I through XIII (there is no factor VI). Although the clotting factors are listed in numeral order, they are not activated in this order.

Clinical Connections

Gastroenterology (Chapter 3) and Dietetics. The liver needs vitamin K in order to produce clotting factors. Vitamin K is manufactured by bacteria in the small intestine. Vitamin K is also present in leafy green vegetables, grains, and liver,

When clotting factors in the plasma are activated to form a blood clot, the fluid portion of plasma that remains is known as **serum.**

Table 6-3 Blood Clotting Factors

Factor Number and Name	Source	Word Building

I **fibrinogen**	liver	**fibrinogen** (fy-BRIN-oh-jen)
		  fibrin/o- *fibrin*
		  -gen *that which produces*

II **prothrombin**	liver	**prothrombin** (proh-THRAWM-bin)
		  pro- *before*
		  thromb/o- *thrombus (blood clot)*
		  -in *a substance*
		Prothrombin is the clotting factor that is activated just before the thrombus is formed.

III tissue factor (**thromboplastin**)	injured tissue	**thromboplastin** (THRAWM-boh-PLAS-tin)
		  thromb/o- *thrombus (blood clot)*
		  plast/o- *growth; formation*
		  -in *a substance*

IV calcium	platelets	
V prothrombin accelerator	liver	
VII prothrombin conversion accelerator	liver	
VIII antihemophilic factor	platelets	
IX plasma thromboplastin factor	liver	
X Stuart-Prower factor	liver	
XI plasma thromboplastin antecedent	liver	
XII Hageman factor	liver	
XIII fibrin-stabilizing factor	liver and platelets	

Anatomy of the Lymphatic System

Lymphatic Vessels, Lymph, and Lymph Nodes

Lymphatic vessels are similar in structure to blood vessels, but with several important differences. Lymphatic vessels have a beginning point (as tiny lymphatic capillaries in the tissues) and an end point (ducts that empty into large veins in the neck). Tissue fluid enters a lymphatic capillary and becomes **lymph** (lymphatic fluid) that then flows through the lymphatic system. Lymphatic capillaries have large openings in their walls that allow microorganisms and cancerous cells to enter. Lymphatic capillaries become larger lymphatic vessels that bring lymph to the lymph nodes. Like large veins in the cardiovascular system, large lymphatic vessels have valves that keep the lymph flowing in one direction.

WORD BUILDING

lymphatic (lim-FAT-ik)
  lymph/o- *lymph; lymphatic system*
  -atic *pertaining to*

lymph (LIMF)

Lymph nodes are encapsulated structures that are round, oval, or bean shaped. They range in size from the head of a pin to 1 inch. The lymph node filters the lymph, and then macrophages in the lymph node destroy any microorganisms or cancerous cells that are present.

Lymph nodes are grouped together in chains in areas where there is a high risk of invasion by microorganisms or cancerous cells (see Figure 6-12 ■). Lymphatic vessels end at ducts in the thoracic cavity. The right lymphatic duct receives lymph from the right side of the head, right arm, right chest, and back. The thoracic duct receives lymph from the rest of the body. Both lymphatic ducts then empty into large veins in the neck.

WORD BUILDING

node (NOHD)
Lymph gland is an alternate phrase for *lymph node,* although lymph nodes are not really glands.

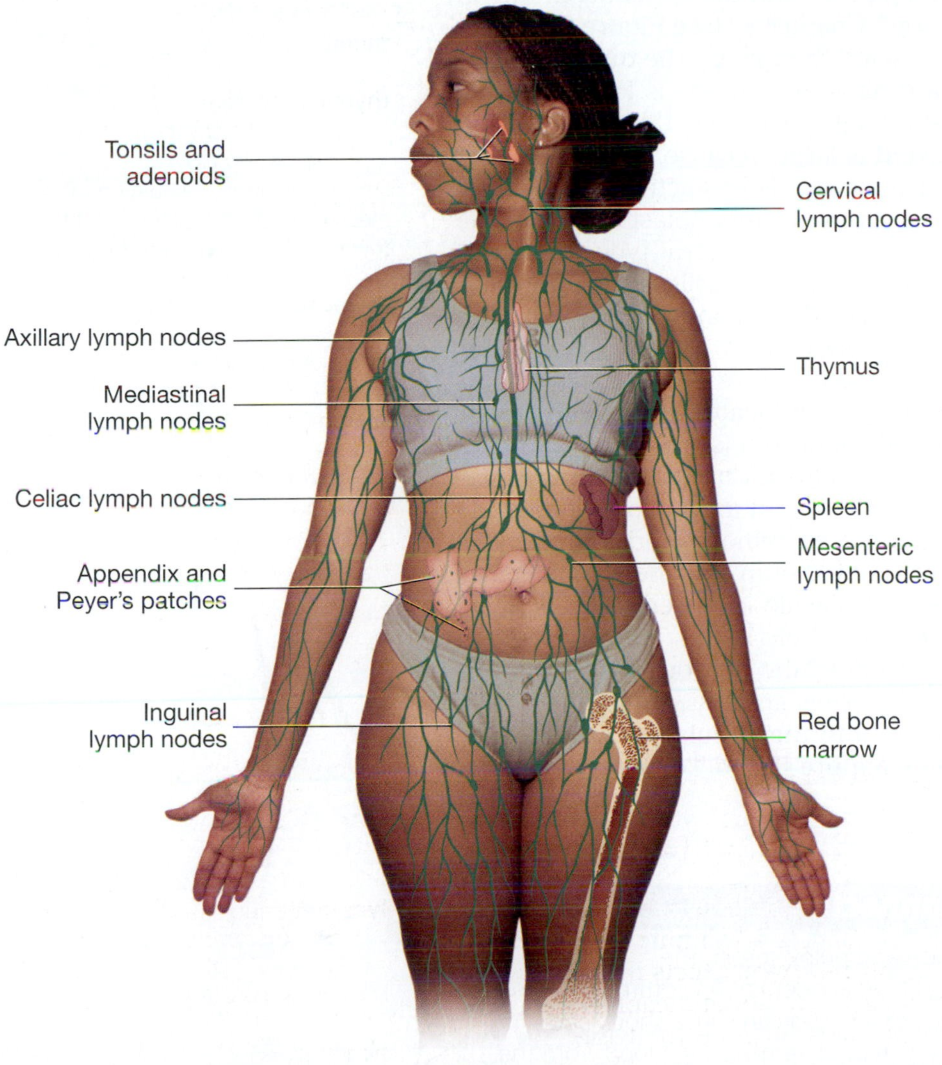

Tonsils and adenoids

Cervical lymph nodes

Axillary lymph nodes

Thymus

Mediastinal lymph nodes

Celiac lymph nodes

Spleen

Mesenteric lymph nodes

Appendix and Peyer's patches

Inguinal lymph nodes

Red bone marrow

Figure 6-12 ■ Lymphatic system.
Lymphatic capillaries in all parts of the body carry lymph to the lymph nodes where it is filtered. The lymphatic system also consists of the tonsils and adenoids in the posterior oral cavity, the thymus, the spleen, and Peyer's patches and the appendix in the intestines.

Lymphoid Tissues and Lymphoid Organs

Lymphoid tissues and lymphoid organs contain lymphocytes and macrophages that are active in the immune response. Lymphoid tissues include the tonsils and adenoids in the posterior oral cavity (discussed in "Otolaryngology," Chapter 16) and Peyer's patches and the appendix in the intestines (discussed in "Gastroenterology," Chapter 3) (see Figure 6-12).

Lymphoid organs include the thymus and the spleen. The **thymus,** a lymphoid organ with a pink color and a grainy consistency, is located within the mediastinum, posterior to the sternum (see Figure 6-12). During childhood and adolescence, the thymus gland is large because it is very active, but, during adulthood, it becomes much smaller, is less active, and most of its tissue is replaced by fat. The thymus receives lymphoblasts that migrate from the red marrow and helps them mature into several types of T lymphocytes (helper T cells, memory T cells, cytotoxic T cells, and suppressor T cells) that are part of the immune response (the *T* stands for *thymus*). The thymus is also part of the endocrine system; it secretes hormones (**thymosins**) that cause lymphoblasts to become mature T lymphocytes.

The **spleen,** a rounded lymphoid organ, is located in the left upper quadrant of the abdomen, posterior to the stomach (see Figure 6-12). The spleen is surrounded by a firm splenic capsule, but has a soft, pulpy interior. The spleen functions as part of the blood and as part of the immune response of the lymphatic system. The spleen removes old erythrocytes from the blood. It breaks down their hemoglobin into heme molecules and globin chains. Iron from the heme molecule is stored in the spleen. The spleen also acts as a storage area for whole blood. During times of danger or injury, the sympathetic division of the nervous system stimulates the adrenal glands to secrete epinephrine, and this causes the spleen to contract and release its stored blood into the circulatory system. The lymphoid tissue in the spleen contains mature B and T lymphocytes that are part of the immune response.

Clinical Connections

Sports Medicine. Because of its location and pulpy center, the spleen can rupture from sports trauma (or car accidents). A ruptured spleen spills its stored blood into the abdominal cavity. This can cause shock and death unless surgery is done to stop the bleeding, remove the blood from the abdominal cavity, and remove the damaged spleen (splenectomy).

Dermatology (Chapter 7). The skin is the body's first line of defense. Intact skin acts as a protective barrier that repels microorganisms. Openings in the skin (the nose, ears, mouth, urethra, rectum, vagina) are high-risk areas where microorganisms can enter the body, and so lymph nodes are concentrated in these areas.

Physiology of the Immune Response

The **immune response** involves a coordinated effort between the blood and the lymphatic system to destroy microorganisms that invade the body and cancerous cells that arise within the body.

The immune response begins with the detection of an invading microorganism. Microorganisms (bacteria, viruses, protozoa, fungi, yeasts, etc.) that cause disease are known as **pathogens.** Once a pathogen is detected in the blood or lymphatic system, the body attacks it in several different ways.

1. **Cytokines** are chemicals released by injured body tissues. They summon all types of leukocytes to the area.

2. **Neutrophils.** Neutrophils engulf and destroy bacteria that have been coated with antibodies.

3. **Eosinophils.** Eosinophils engulf and destroy foreign cells (pollen, animal dander, etc.) and release chemicals that destroy parasitic worms and their eggs.

4. **Basophils.** Basophils release histamine in response to microorganisms. **Histamine** dilates blood vessels and increases blood flow, which causes redness and also brings more leukocytes to the area. Histamine also changes the permeability of the blood vessel walls, allowing large protein molecules and water to leak out into the tissues; this causes edema (swelling). Redness and edema are both signs of inflammation or infection associated with the presence of microorganisms.

5. **Monocytes.** Monocytes engulf and destroy pathogens that have been coated with antibodies. They also eat dead leukocytes and cellular debris. In body tissues, a monocyte is known as a **macrophage.** It takes fragments of the pathogen it has eaten and presents them to a B cell (lymphocyte). This stimulates the B cell to become a plasma cell and make antibodies against that specific pathogen. Macrophages also produce special immune response chemicals: interferon, interleukin, and tumor necrosis factor.

   a. **Interferon** is produced by macrophages that have engulfed a virus. Interferon stimulates cells to produce an antiviral substance that prevents a virus from entering a cell and reproducing. This keeps viral infections from spreading through the body. Interferon also stimulates NK (natural killer) cells to attack viruses.

   b. **Interleukin** stimulates B and T cell lymphocytes and activates NK cells. It also produces the fever associated with inflammation and infection. An increased body temperature stimulates leukocyte activity. Interleukin is also produced by the lymphocytes themselves.

   c. **Tumor necrosis factor (TNF)** destroys **endotoxins** produced by certain bacteria. It also destroys cancer cells.

6. **Lymphocytes**

   a. **NK (natural killer) cells** are special lymphocytes that recognize a pathogen by the **antigens** on its cell wall and release chemicals to destroy it. NK cells can recognize a pathogen even before it is coated with antibodies.

   b. **B cells** (lymphocytes that matured in the red marrow) are inactive until a macrophage presents them with fragments from a pathogen.

immune (im-MYOON)

pathogen (PATH-oh-jen)
   path/o- *disease; suffering*
   -gen *that which produces*

cytokine (SY-toh-kyne)
   cyt/o- *cell*
   -kine *movement*

histamine (HIS-tah-meen)

interferon (IN-ter-FEER-on)

interleukin (IN-ter-LOO-kin)
   inter- *between*
   leuk/o- *white*
   -in *a substance*

endotoxin (EN-doh-TAWK-sin)
   endo- *innermost; within*
   tox/o- *poison*
   -in *a substance*

antigen (AN-tih-jen)
Antigen is a combination of part of the word *antibody* and the suffix *-gen* (that which produces).

Then the B cell changes into a plasma cell and produces antibodies against that pathogen. B cells also activate helper T cells.

c. **T cells** (lymphocytes that matured in the thymus) have four different subsets.

- **Helper T cells** stimulate the production of cytotoxic T cells. Helper T cells (also known as **CD4 cells** because of a protein marker on their cell membranes) also produce memory T cells.

- **Memory T cells** are created when a helper T cell is exposed to a pathogen. Memory T cells are inactive until the next time that pathogen enters the body. Then they remember the pathogen and become cytotoxic T cells.

- **Cytotoxic T cells** engulf and destroy all types of pathogens as well as body cells that have been invaded by a virus.

- **Suppressor T cells** limit the extent and duration of the immune response by inhibiting B cells and cytotoxic T cells. Suppressor T cells are also known as CD8 cells because of a special protein marker on their cell membranes.

WORD BUILDING

cytotoxic (SY-toh-TAWK-sik)
cyt/o- *cell*
tox/o- *poison*
-ic *pertaining to*

suppressor (soo-PRES-or)
suppress/o- *press down*
-or *person or thing that produces or does*

A Closer Look

There are five classes of **antibodies** or **immunonoglobulins:** immunoglobulin A (IgA), immunoglobulin D (IgD), immunoglobulin E (IgE), immunoglobulin G (IgG), and immunoglobulin M (IgM).

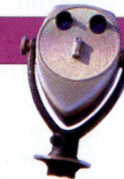

Class	Description
IgA	IgA is in body secretions (tears; saliva; mucus in the nose, lungs, and intestines) and on the surface of the skin. IgA is in colostrum, the first milk produced by a breastfeeding mother; this maternal IgA provides **passive immunity** until 18 months of age when the infant begins to make its own antibodies.
IgD	IgD is on the surface of a B cell lymphocyte and activates it to become a plasma cell.
IgE	IgE is on the surface of a basophil and causes it to release heparin and histamine during inflammatory and allergic reactions.
IgG	IgG is the most abundant of all the immunoglobulins. It provides **active immunity,** the body's response and defense against pathogens it has seen before. IgG is also the smallest immunoglobulin. It can pass from the mother's blood through the placenta, where it provides passive immunity to the fetus.
IgM	IgM is the largest immunoglobulin. It is produced the first time the body encounters a pathogen. IgM also is the immunoglobulin that reacts to incompatible blood types during a blood transfusion reaction.

immunity (im-MYOO-nih-tee)
immun/o- *immune response*
-ity *state; condition*

7. **Antibodies.** If NK cells do not immediately destroy a pathogen, then antibodies coat the pathogen (or virus-infected cell) and mark it to be destroyed. The antibody coating attracts phagocytes (neutrophils, eosinophils, lymphocytes, monocytes) to come and engulf the pathogen and destroy it. Antibodies are also known as **immunoglobulins.**

8. **Complement proteins.** Complement is a group of nine proteins (C1–C9) that activate each other. When antibodies coat a pathogen (or virus-infected cell), complement proteins attach to the antibodies and drill holes in the pathogen's cell wall.

WORD BUILDING

antibody (AN-tih-BAWD-ee)
  anti- *against*
  -body *a structure or thing*

immunoglobulin
(IM-myoo-noh-GLAWB-yoo-lin)
  immun/o- *immune response*
  globul/o- *shaped like a globe*
  -in *a substance*

complement (KAWM-pleh-ment)

Across the Life Span

Pediatrics. Childhood immunizations against measles, mumps, rubella, polio, diphtheria, pertussis, and tetanus use a vaccine made of dead or weakened pathogens or inactivated endotoxins. The vaccination causes the body to produce antibodies, and this gives active immunity without exposure to the actual disease. The meningococcal meningitis vaccine is recommended for college students living in dormitories.

Adult immunizations include annual vaccinations for influenza (the flu) and periodic boosters for tetanus.

Geriatrics. The influenza (the flu) and pneumococcal pneumonia vaccinations are recommended for older adults.

Word Alert

SOUND-ALIKE WORDS

globin   (noun)   Breakdown product of hemoglobin
            Example: The spleen breaks down old erythrocytes to form
            heme and globin molecules.

globulin   (noun)   Protein molecule in an immunoglobulin
            Example: Globulin is used by a plasma cell to build antibodies.

Vocabulary Review

Blood		
Word or Phrase	**Description**	**Combining Forms**
ABO blood group	Category that includes blood types A, B, AB, and O. Blood types are hereditary. Each blood type has **antigens** on its erythrocytes and antibodies in its plasma against other blood types.	
agranulocyte	Category of leukocytes with few or no granules in the cytoplasm. It includes lymphocytes and monocytes.	**granul/o-** *granule*
albumin	Most abundant plasma protein. Plasma proteins contribute to the osmotic pressure of the blood.	
band	Immature neutrophil in the blood. It has a nucleus shaped like a curved band. It is also known as a **stab.**	
basophil	Type of leukocyte. It is categorized as a granulocyte because granules in its cytoplasm stain dark blue to purple with basic dye. Basophils release histamine and heparin at the site of tissue injury. Basophils are also known as basos.	**bas/o-** *base of a thing; basic (alkaline)*
blood	Type of connective tissue that contains formed elements (blood cells and blood cell fragments), water, proteins, and clotting factors. The blood transports oxygen, carbon dioxide, nutrients, and waste products of metabolism.	**hem/o-** *blood* **hemat/o-** *blood*
electrolytes	Chemical structures that carry a positive or negative electrical charge: sodium (Na^+), potassium (K^+), chloride (Cl^-), calcium (Ca^{++}), and bicarbonate (HCO_3^-). They are in the plasma.	**electr/o-** *electricity*
eosinophil	Type of leukocyte. It is categorized as a granulocyte because granules in its cytoplasm stain bright pink to red with eosin dye. The nucleus has two lobes. Eosinophils are phagocytes that engulf and destroy foreign cells (pollen, animal dander, etc.). They also release chemicals to kill parasites. Eosinophils are also known as eos.	**eosin/o-** *eosin (red acidic dye)*
erythrocyte	A mature red blood cell. An **erythroblast** is a very immature form that comes from a stem cell in the red marrow. It matures into a **normoblast,** which becomes a **reticulocyte,** a nearly mature erythrocyte that is released into the blood. An erythrocyte has no nucleus. Erythrocytes contain hemoglobin.	**erythr/o-** *red* **norm/o-** *normal; usual* **reticul/o-** *small network*
erythropoietin	Hormone produced by the kidneys that increases the rate at which erythrocytes are produced and mature	**erythr/o-** *red*
granulocyte	Category of leukocytes with large granules in the cytoplasm. It includes neutrophils, eosinophils, and basophils.	**granul/o-** *granule*
hematopoiesis	Process by which blood cells are formed in the red marrow	**hemat/o-** *blood*
hemoglobin	Substance in an erythrocyte that contains a heme molecule and globin chains. The heme molecule contains iron that gives erythrocytes their red color. The compound **oxyhemoglobin** carries oxygen from the lungs to the cells and carries carbon dioxide from the cells to the lungs.	**hem/o-** *blood* **glob/o-** *shaped like a globe; comprehensive* **ox/y-** *oxygen; quick*

Word or Phrase	Description	Combining Forms
leukocyte	A white blood cell. There are five different types of mature leukocytes: neutrophils, eosinophils, basophils, lymphocytes, and monocytes.	**leuk/o-** *white*
lymphocyte	Second most abundant leukocyte, but the smallest in size. It is categorized as an agranulocyte as there are few or no granules in its cytoplasm. The cytoplasm is only a thin ring next to the round nucleus. A **lymphoblast** is an immature form that develops from a stem cell in the red marrow. Lymphocytes in the red marrow become NK cells or B lymphocytes that produce antibodies. Lymphocytes in the thymus become T lymphocytes. Lymphocytes are phagocytes that engulf and destroy viruses and produce antibodies. Lymphocytes are also known as lymphs.	**lymph/o-** *lymph; lymphatic system*
monocyte	The largest leukocyte. It is categorized as an agranulocyte as there are few or no granules in its cytoplasm. The nucleus is shaped like a kidney bean. A **monoblast** is an immature form that comes from a stem cell in the red marrow. Monocytes are phagocytes that engulf and destroy microorganisms, cancerous cells, dead leukocytes, and cellular debris. Monocytes are also known as monos. In the tissues, monocytes are known as **macrophages.**	**mon/o-** *one; single* **macr/o-** *large*
myeloblast	A very immature cell that comes from a stem cell in the red marrow. It develops into a myelocyte.	**myel/o-** *bone marrow; spinal cord; myelin*
myelocyte	Immature cell that comes from a myeloblast in the red marrow and develops into either a neutrophil, eosinophil, or basophil	**myel/o-** *bone marrow; spinal cord; myelin*
neutrophil	Most numerous type of leukocyte. It is categorized as a granulocyte because the granules in its cytoplasm do not easily stain red or blue, but remain neutral in color. The nucleus has several segmented lobes. Neutrophils are phagocytes that engulf and destroy bacteria. Neutrophils are also known as segmented neutrophils, segmenters, segs, **polymorphonuclear** leukocytes, polys, or PMNs.	**neutr/o-** *not taking part* **morph/o-** *shape* **nucle/o-** *nucleus (of a cell)*
plasma	Clear, straw-colored fluid portion of the blood that carries formed elements (blood cells and blood cell fragments) and contains dissolved substances (amino acids, cholesterol, triglycerides, electrolytes, glucose, minerals, and vitamins—nutrients from digested foods—as well as albumin, bilirubin, hormones, complement proteins, clotting factors, and the waste products of creatinine and urea—substances produced by the body).	**plasm/o-** *plasma*
Rh blood group	Category of blood type. When the Rh factor is present, the blood is Rh positive. Without the Rh factor, the blood is Rh negative.	
stem cell	Extremely immature cell in the red marrow that is the precursor to all types of blood cells	
thrombocyte	A **platelet**. A **megakaryoblast** is a very immature form that develops from a stem cell in the red marrow. A **megakaryocyte** is a very large, mature cell with an abundance of cytoplasm that breaks away in individual pieces as thrombocytes. A thrombocyte is a cell fragment that does not have a nucleus. Thrombocytes are active in the blood clotting process.	**thromb/o-** *thrombus (blood clot)* **meg/a-** *large* **kary/o-** *nucleus*

Blood Clotting

Word or Phrase	Description	Combining Forms
aggregation	Process of platelets sticking to a damaged blood vessel wall and forming clumps	**aggreg/o-** *crowding together*
clotting factors	A series of 12 substances that are released either from platelets or injured tissue or are produced by the liver. They activate each other in a series of steps that form fibrin strands that trap erythrocytes and form a blood clot.	
coagulation	Formation of a blood clot by platelets, erythrocytes, and clotting factors	**coagul/o-** *clotting*
fibrin	Strands formed by the activation of clotting factors. Fibrin traps erythrocytes to form a blood clot.	**fibr/o-** *fiber*
fibrinogen	Blood clotting factor I	**fibrin/o-** *fibrin*
hemostasis	The cessation of bleeding	**hem/o-** *blood*
prothrombin	Blood clotting factor II. It is activated just before the thrombus (blood clot) is formed.	**thromb/o-** *thrombus (blood clot)*
serum	Fluid portion of the plasma that remains after the clotting factors are activated to form a blood clot	
thromboplastin	Blood clotting factor III. It is also known as tissue factor because it is released when tissue is injured.	**thromb/o-** *thrombus (blood clot)* **plast/o-** *growth; formation*
thrombus	A blood clot	**thromb/o-** *thrombus (blood clot)*

Lymphatic System

active immunity	The body's continuing immune response and defense against pathogens it has seen before	**immun/o-** *immune response*
antibody	Produced by a B cell when it becomes a plasma cell. It is also known as an immunoglobulin.	
antigen	Protein marker on the cell membrane of an erythrocyte that indicates the blood type. Also, a protein marker on the cell wall of a pathogen or on a cancerous cell that allows the immune system to recognize it as foreign.	
B cell	Type of lymphocyte that matures in the red marrow of the bone. B cells are activated by macrophages and become plasma cells that make antibodies. B cells also activate helper T cells.	
complement proteins	Group of nine proteins in the plasma that are activated by the presence of a bacterium, virus, or parasite. They kill it by drilling holes in it. Complement proteins also cause basophils to release histamine where the tissue has been damaged.	
cytokines	Chemicals released by damaged tissues. Cytokines call leukocytes to that area.	**cyt/o-** *cell*
endotoxin	Toxic substance produced by some bacteria. It acts as a poison in the body, causing chills, fever, and shock.	**tox/o-** *poison*

Word or Phrase	Description	Combining Forms
histamine	Released by basophils. It dilates blood vessels and increases blood flow to damaged tissue, which produces redness. It also allows protein molecules to leak out of blood vessels into the tissue, which produces edema (swelling).	
IgA	Immunglobulin A. Antibody present in body secretions (tears, saliva, mucus, and breast milk) and on the surface of the skin. It gives passive immunity to a breastfeeding infant.	
IgD	Immunoglobulin D. Antibody present on the surface of B cells. It stimulates the B cell to become a plasma cell.	
IgE	Immunoglobulin E. Antibody present on the surface of basophils. It causes them to release histamine and heparin during inflammatory and allergic reactions.	
IgG	Immunoglobulin G. Antibody that is produced by plasma cells the second time a specific pathogen enters the body. IgG forms the basis for active immunity. It is the smallest of all the immunoglobulins, but also the most abundant. During pregnancy, it crosses the placenta and provides passive immunity to the fetus.	
IgM	Immunoglobulin M. Antibody that is produced by plasma cells during the initial exposure to a pathogen. IgM also reacts to incompatible blood types during a blood transfusion. It is the largest of the immunoglobulins.	
immune response	Coordinated effort between the blood and lymphatic system to identify and destroy invading microorganisms and foreign particles, or cancerous cells produced within the body	**immun/o-** *immune response*
immunoglobulins	**Antibodies.** There are five classes of immunoglobulins: IgA, IgD, IgE, IgG, and IgM.	**immun/o-** *immune response* **globul/o-** *shaped like a globe*
interferon	Substance released by macrophages that have engulfed a virus. It stimulates other cells to produce an antiviral substance that prevents the virus from entering them to reproduce itself.	
interleukin	Substance released by macrophages that stimulates B cell and T cell lymphocytes and activates NK cells. It also produces fever.	**leuk/o-** *white*
lymph	Fluid that flows through the lymphatic system	
lymph nodes	Small, encapsulated pieces of lymphoid tissue located along lymphatic vessels. Macrophages in the lymph nodes destroy microorganisms and cancerous cells in the lymph fluid. They are also known as lymph glands.	
lymphatic system	Body system that includes a network of lymphatic vessels, lymph fluid, lymph nodes, the **lymphoid organs** (thymus, spleen), and **lymphoid tissues** (tonsils and adenoids, appendix, and Peyer's patches).	**lymph/o-** *lymph; lymphatic system*
lymphatic vessels	Vessels that begin as capillaries, carry lymph, continue through lymph nodes, and empty into the right lymphatic duct or the thoracic duct	**lymph/o-** *lymph; lymphatic system*
macrophage	A large monocyte in the lymph nodes, intestine, liver, pancreas, thymus, spleen, bone, or skin	**macr/o-** *large* **phag/o-** *eating; swallowing*
natural killer (NK) cell	Type of lymphocyte that matures in the red marrow and, without the help of antibodies or complement proteins, recognizes and destroys pathogens	

Word or Phrase	Description	Combining Forms
passive immunity	Immune response and defense against pathogens that is conveyed by the mother's antibodies to the fetus via the placenta and via colostrum to the breastfeeding baby. These maternal antibodies provide protection from all the diseases the mother has had.	**immun/o-** *immune response*
pathogen	Microorganism that causes a disease. Pathogens include bacteria, viruses, and protozoa, as well as plant cells such as fungi or yeast.	**path/o-** *disease; suffering*
phagocyte	Type of leukocyte that engulfs foreign cells and cellular debris and destroys them with digestive enzymes. Phagocytes include neutrophils, eosinophils, lymphocytes, and monocytes. **Phagocytosis** is the process by which a phagocyte engulfs and destroys a pathogen.	**phag/o-** *eating; swallowing* **cyt/o-** *cell*
spleen	Lymphoid organ located in the abdominal cavity posterior to the stomach. The spleen destroys old erythrocytes, breaking their hemoglobin into heme and globin chains. It also acts as a storage area for whole blood. Its lymphoid tissue contains B cell and T cell lymphocytes.	**splen/o-** *spleen*
T cell	Type of lymphocyte that matures in the thymus. There are four subsets of T cells: helper T cells (**CD4 cells**), memory T cells, **cytotoxic** T cells, and **suppressor** T cells (CD8 cells).	**cyt/o-** *cell* **tox/o-** *poison* **suppress/o-** *press down*
thymus	Lymphoid organ in the mediastinum. As an endocrine gland, it secretes thymosins, which are hormones that cause lymphoblasts in the thymus to mature into T cell lymphocytes.	**thym/o-** *thymus; rage*
tumor necrosis factor (TNF)	Substance that destroys endotoxins produced by certain bacteria. It also destroys cancerous cells.	

Labeling Exercise

Match each anatomy word or phrase to its structure and write it in the numbered box for each figure. Be sure to check your spelling. Use the Answer Key at the end of the book to check your answers.

basophil	eosinophil	lymphocyte	monocyte	neutrophil

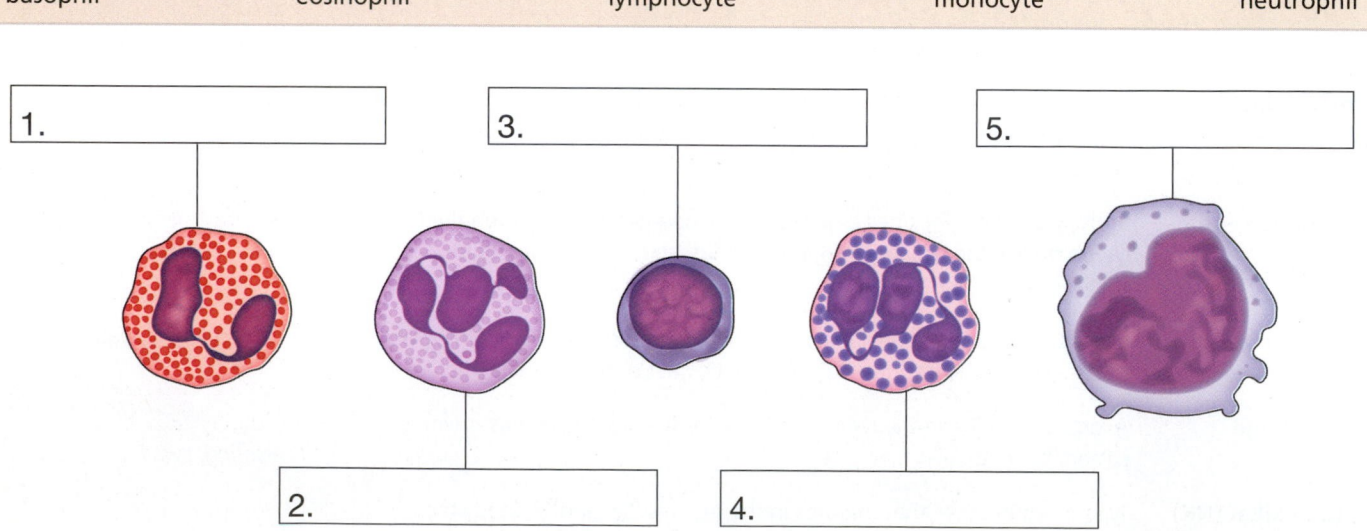

1.

2.

3.

4.

5.

appendix and Peyer's patches   cervical lymph nodes   mesenteric lymph nodes   thymus
axillary lymph nodes   inguinal lymph nodes   red bone marrow   tonsils and adenoids
celiac lymph nodes   mediastinal lymph nodes   spleen

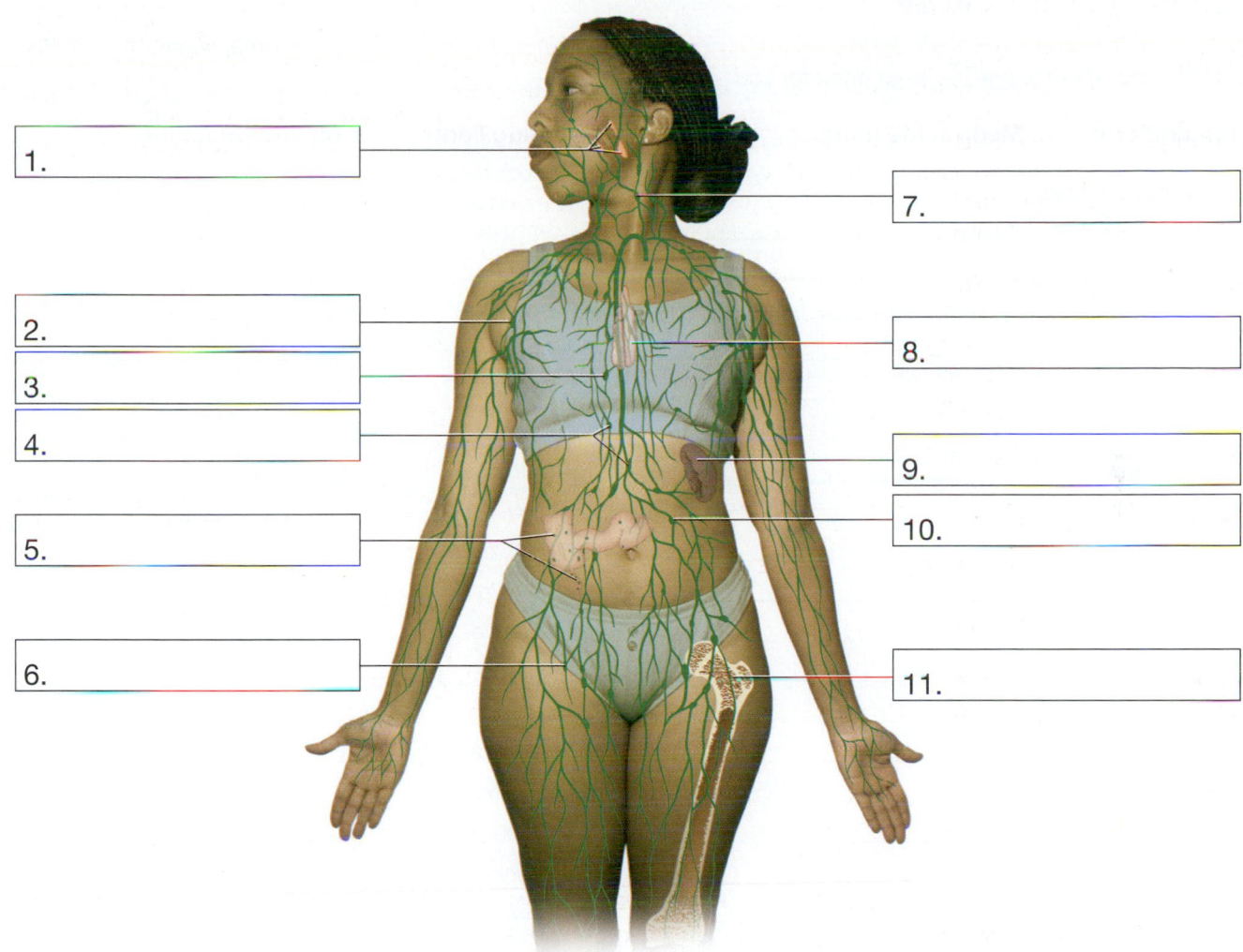

1. _____

2. _____

3. _____

4. _____

5. _____

6. _____

7. _____

8. _____

9. _____

10. _____

11. _____

Building Medical Words

Use the Answer Key at the end of the book to check your answers.

Combining Forms Exercise

Before you build blood and lymphatic system words, review these combining forms. Next to each combining form, write its medical meaning. The first one has been done for you.

Combining Form	Medical Meaning	Combining Form	Medical Meaning
1. **aggreg/o-**	crowding together	20. meg/a-	
2. bas/o-		21. mon/o-	
3. coagul/o-		22. morph/o-	
4. cyt/o-		23. myel/o-	
5. electr/o-		24. neutr/o-	
6. eosin/o-		25. norm/o-	
7. erythr/o-		26. nucle/o-	
8. fibrin/o-		27. ox/y-	
9. fibr/o-		28. path/o-	
10. glob/o-		29. phag/o-	
11. globul/o-		30. plasm/o-	
12. granul/o-		31. plast/o-	
13. hemat/o-		32. reticul/o-	
14. hem/o-		33. splen/o-	
15. immun/o-		34. suppress/o-	
16. kary/o-		35. thromb/o-	
17. leuk/o-		36. thym/o-	
18. lymph/o-		37. tox/o-	
19. macr/o-			

Combining Form and Suffix Exercise

Read the definition of the medical word. Look at the combining form that is given. Select the correct suffix from the Suffix List and write it on the blank line. Then build the medical word and write it on the line. (Remember: You may need to remove the combining vowel. Always remove the hyphens and slash.) Be sure to check your spelling. The first one has been done for you.

SUFFIX LIST

-atic (pertaining to) -ic (pertaining to) -phage (thing that eats)
-ation (a process; being or having) -ity (state; condition) -phil (attraction to; fondness for)
-blast (immature cell) -logy (the study of) -poiesis (condition of formation)
-cyte (cell) -lyte (dissolved substance) -poietin (a substance that forms)
-gen (that which produces) -oid (resembling)

Definition of the Medical Word	Combining Form	Suffix	Build the Medical Word
1. Condition of formation of blood	hemat/o-	-poiesis	hematopoiesis

(You think *condition of formation* (-poiesis) + *the blood* (hemat/o-). You change the order of the word parts to put the suffix last. You write *hematopoiesis*.)

2. White blood cell	leuk/o-		
3. Process of clotting	coagul/o		
4. Pertaining to the spleen	splen/o-		
5. Cell that eats	phag/o-		
6. Resembling the lymph or lymphatic system	lymph/o-		
7. The study of the blood	hemat/o-		
8. Substance that forms red blood cells	erythr/o-		
9. (Cell that has an) attraction to eosin (a red acidic dye)	eosin/o-		
10. That which produces disease and suffering	path/o-		
11. Cell (that helps to form) a blood clot	thromb/o-		
12. (Very) immature cell in the bone marrow	myel/o-		
13. Dissolved substance (that conducts) electricity	electr/o-		
14. State (of readiness of) the immune system	immun/o-		
15. A process of (red blood-cells) crowding together (and forming a blood clot)	aggreg/o-		
16. Pertaining to the lymph (system)	lymph/o-		
17. Cell (that has) granules (in its cytoplasm)	granul/o-		
18. Cell (that is) red	erythr/o-		
19. (Cell with) an attraction to a basic (alkaline dye)	bas/o-		
20. Thing that eats (other cells and is) large	macr/o-		

Prefix Exercise

Read the definition of the medical word. Look at the medical word or partial word that is given (it already contains a combining form and a suffix). Select the correct prefix from the Prefix List and write it on the blank line. Then build the medical word and write it on the line. Be sure to check your spelling. The first one has been done for you.

PREFIX LIST			
a- (away from; without)	endo- (innermost; within)	poly- (many; much)	pro- (before)

Definition of the Medical Word	Prefix	Word or Partial Word	Build the Medical Word
1. A substance within (some bacteria that is) poisonous (to body cells)	**endo-**)	(**toxin**	*endotoxin*
2. Cell without granules (in its cytoplasm)	_____	granulocyte	_____
3. Pertaining to a many-shaped nucleus	_____	morphonuclear	_____
4. A substance (that comes) before thrombin	_____	thrombin	_____

Multiple Combining Forms and Suffix Exercise

Read the definition of the medical word. Select the correct suffix and combining forms. Then build the medical word and write it on the line. Be sure to check your spelling. The first one has been done for you.

SUFFIX LIST	COMBINING FORM LIST	
-cyte (cell)	cyt/o- (cell)	phag/o- (eating; swallowing)
-ic (pertaining to)	globul/o- (shaped like a globe)	plast/o- (growth; formation)
-in (a substance)	immun/o- (immune response)	thromb/o- (thrombus; blood clot)
-osis (condition; abnormal condition; process)	kary/o- (nucleus)	tox/o- (poison)
	meg/a- (large)	

Definition of the Medical Word	Combining Form	Combining Form	Suffix	Build the Medical Word
1. Pertaining to a cell (that is) poison (to all pathogens)	**cyt/o-**)	(**tox/o-**)	(**-ic**	*cytotoxic*
(You think *pertaining to* (-ic) + *a cell* (cyt/o-) + *poison* (tox/o-). You change the order of the word parts to put the suffix last. You write *cytotoxic*.)				
2. A substance (needed for) thrombus (blood clot) growth and formation	_____	_____	_____	_____
3. Cell (that has a) large (amount of cytoplasm around its) nucleus	_____	_____	_____	_____
4. A substance (that is part of the) immune response (and is) shaped like a globe	_____	_____	_____	_____
5. Process of eating (done by a certain type of) cell	_____	_____	_____	_____

Diseases and Conditions

Blood

Word or Phrase	Description	Word Building
blood dyscrasia	Any disease condition involving blood cells. Treatment: Correct the underlying cause.	**dyscrasia** (dis-KRAY-zee-ah) **dys-** *painful; difficult; abnormal* **-crasia** *a mixing*
hemorrhage	Loss of a large amount of blood, externally or internally. Injury to an artery causes a forceful spurting of a large amount of bright red blood. Treatment: Tourniquet, pressure, or suturing to stop the bleeding.	**hemorrhage** (HEM-oh-rij) **hem/o-** *blood* **-rrhage** *excessive flow or discharge*
pancytopenia	Decreased numbers of all types of blood cells due to failure of the bone marrow to produce stem cells. Treatment: Correct the underlying cause.	**pancytopenia** (PAN-sy-toh-PEE-nee-ah) **pan-** *all* **cyt/o-** *cell* **-penia** *condition of deficiency*
septicemia	Severe bacterial infection of the tissues that spreads to the blood. Both the bacteria and their endotoxins cause severe systemic symptoms. It is also known as **sepsis** or **blood poisoning.** Treatment: Antibiotic drugs.	**septicemia** (SEP-tih-SEE-mee-ah) **septic/o-** *infection* **-emia** *condition of the blood; substance in the blood*

Erythrocytes

Word or Phrase	Description	Word Building
abnormal red blood cell morphology	Category that includes any type of abnormality in the size or shape of erythrocytes, such as anisocytosis, poikilocytosis, microcytic cells, or hypochromic cells. Treatment: Correct underlying cause.	**morphology** (mor-FAWL-oh-jee) **morph/o-** *shape* **-logy** *the study of*
anemia	Decrease in the number of erythrocytes or the amount of hemoglobin in each erythrocyte due to any of the following reasons. 1. Too few erythrocytes are produced because of insufficient amounts of amino acids, folic acid, iron, vitamin B_6, or vitamin B_{12}. 2. Too few erythrocytes are produced because disease, cancer, radiation therapy, or chemotherapy drugs have damaged or destroyed the red marrow. 3. There are too few erythrocytes because they have been destroyed by hemolysis or increased cell fragility. 4. There are too few erythocytes because they have been lost from the body due to hemorrhage, excessive menstruation, or chronic blood loss. Anemias can be categorized by the cause or by the size, shape, and appearance of their erythrocytes. A patient with anemia is said to be **anemic.** Treatment: Correct the underlying cause.	**anemia** (ah-NEE-mee-ah) **an-** *without; not* **-emia** *condition of the blood; substance in the blood* Add words to make a complete definition of *anemia: condition of the blood (of) not (enough red blood cells).* **anemic** (ah-NEE-mik) **an-** *without; not* **-emic** *pertaining to a condition of the blood or a substance in the blood*
aplastic anemia	Anemia caused by failure of the bone marrow to produce erythrocytes because it has been damaged by disease, cancer, radiation therapy, or chemotherapy drugs. The number of erythrocytes is decreased, but each erythrocyte is normocytic (normal in size) and normochromic (normal in color). Treatment: Blood transfusion, erythropoietin drug to stimulate erythrocyte production, or bone marrow transplantation.	**aplastic** (aa-PLAS-tik) **a-** *away from; without* **plast/o-** *growth; formation* **-ic** *pertaining to*

Word or Phrase	Description	Word Building
folic acid deficiency anemia	Anemia caused by a deficiency of folic acid in the diet. This anemia is seen in malnourished patients (older adults, those who are poor, people with alcoholism), those who have malabsorption diseases, and pregnant women. Each erythrocyte is abnormally large (**macrocytic**). Treatment: Balanced diet, folic acid supplements.	**macrocytic** (MAK-roh-SIT-ik) **macr/o-** *large* **cyt/o-** *cell* **-ic** *pertaining to*
iron deficiency anemia	Anemia caused by a deficiency of iron in the diet or by increased loss of iron due to menstruation, hemorrhage, or chronic blood loss. Each erythrocyte is **microcytic** (small in size) and **hypochromic** (pale in color) (see Figure 6-13 ■). Compare these cells to normal red blood cells (see Figure 6-4). Infant formulas include supplemental iron to prevent iron deficiency anemia. Treatment: Dietary iron supplements, correction of the cause of blood loss.	**microcytic** (MY-kroh-SIT-ik) **micr/o-** *one millionth; small* **cyt/o-** *cell* **-ic** *pertaining to* **hypochromic** (HY-poh-KROH-mik) **hypo-** *below; deficient* **chrom/o-** *color* **-ic** *pertaining to*

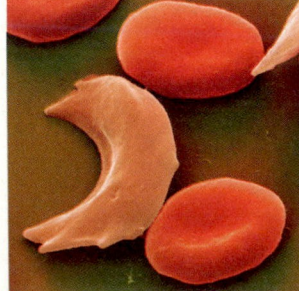

Figure 6-13 ■ Microcytic, hypochromic erythrocytes.
This blood smear shows small, pale erythrocytes that are characteristic of iron deficiency anemia.

Word or Phrase	Description	Word Building
pernicious anemia	Anemia caused by a lack of vitamin B$_{12}$ in the diet or a lack of intrinsic factor in the stomach. As a person ages, the stomach produces less hydrochloric acid and intrinsic factor; both of these must be present in order to absorb vitamin B$_{12}$. Untreated, this anemia can cause permanent damage to the nerves. Each erythrocyte is abnormally large and very immature (megaloblast). Treatment: Intramuscular injection or nasal spray of vitamin B$_{12}$ drug.	**pernicious** (per-NISH-us)
sickle cell anemia	Anemia caused by an inherited genetic abnormality of an amino acid in hemoglobin. If one amino acid is abnormal, the patient has sickle cell trait and is a carrier for sickle cell disease, but does not have the disease. If two amino acids are abnormal, the patient has sickle cell disease. In patients with sickle cell disease, when there is a low level of oxygen in the blood, an erythrocyte distorts to become a crescent or sickle shape (see Figures 6-14 ■ and 6-15 ■). Treatment: Pain medication, avoidance of situations that lower the blood oxygen level. Hydroxyurea (a drug that stimulates the production of fetal hemoglobin and erythrocytes that do not sickle).	

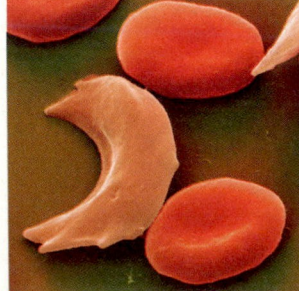

Figure 6-14 ■ Sickle cell.
The abnormal crescent shape and sharp edges of this sickled erythrocyte are very different from the smooth, rounded contour of a normal erythrocyte. Repeated sickling causes these fragile erythrocytes to have a shortened life span, resulting in anemia.

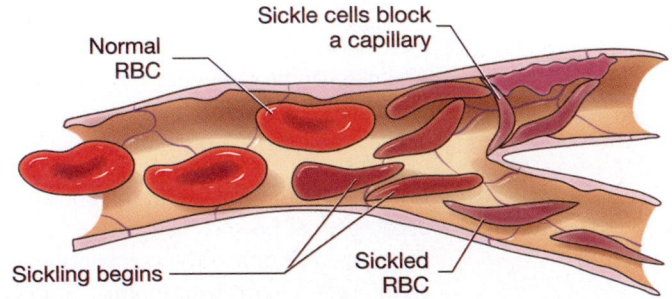

Figure 6-15 ■ Sickle cells in a capillary.
Sickle cells do not move easily through the capillaries. They become tangled and block the flow of blood, and this causes pain and blood clots, particularly in the joints and abdomen.

Word or Phrase	Description	Word Building
anisocytosis	Erythrocytes that are too large or too small. A **macrocyte** is an abnormally large erythrocyte (seen in folic acid anemia and pernicious anemia). A **microcyte** is an abnormally small erythrocyte (seen in iron deficiency anemia).	**anisocytosis** (an-EYE-soh-sy-TOH-sis) **anis/o-** unequal **cyt/o-** cell **-osis** condition; abnormal condition; process **macrocyte** (MAK-roh-site) **macr/o-** large **-cyte** cell **microcyte** (MY-kroh-site) **micr/o-** one millionth; small **-cyte** cell
poikilocytosis	Erythrocytes that vary in shape. A sickle cell is a crescent-shaped erythrocyte (seen in sickle cell anemia). Erythrocytes can also be in the shape of spheres (spherocytes), ovals, teardrops, or have spike-like projections on their surface. Treatment: None, as these are genetic defects.	**poikilocytosis** (POY-kih-loh-sy-TOH-sis) **poikil/o-** irregular **cyt/o-** cell **-osis** condition; abnormal condition; process
polycythemia vera	Increased number of erythrocytes due to uncontrolled production by the red marrow. The cause is unknown. The viscosity (thickness) of the blood increases and the blood volume is increased. There is dizziness, headache, fatigue, and splenomegaly. Patients are prone to develop blood clots and high blood pressure. Treatment: Periodic phlebotomy to remove blood to keep the blood volume and number of erythrocytes at a normal level.	**polycythemia vera** (PAWL-ee-sy-THEE-mee-ah VAIR-ah) **poly-** many; much **cyt/o-** cell **hem/o-** blood **-ia** condition; state; thing
thalassemia	Inherited genetic abnormality that affects the synthesis of the globin chains in hemoglobin. The erythrocytes are small (microcytic), pale (hypochromic), and of variable size (anisocytosis). Target cells (erythrocytes with a central dark spot) are seen. There is anemia, weakness, and splenomegaly. Thalassemia major is the severe form of the disease; thalassemia minor produces fewer symptoms and signs. Treatment: Blood transfusions.	**thalassemia** (THAL-ah-SEE-mee-ah)
transfusion reaction	Reaction that occurs when a patient receives a transfusion with an incompatible blood type. Antibodies in the patient's serum attack antigens on the erythrocytes of the donor blood, causing **hemolysis** of the donor erythrocytes—a **hemolytic reaction.** Fever, chills, and hypotension occur almost immediately. The patient has flank pain because hemolyzed erythrocytes clog the filtering membrane of the kidneys and cause kidney failure. Transfusion reactions can be fatal. Treatment: Stop the transfusion immediately and treat the patient's symptoms and signs.	**transfusion** (trans-FYOO-shun) **trans-** across; through **fus/o-** pouring **-ion** action; condition **hemolysis** (hee-MAWL-ih-sis) **hem/o-** blood **-lysis** process of breaking down or destroying **hemolytic** (HEE-moh-LIT-ik) **hem/o-** blood **ly/o-** break down; destroy **-tic** pertaining to

Leukocytes

Word or Phrase	Description	Word Building
acquired immunodeficiency syndrome (AIDS)	Severe infection caused by the human immunodeficiency virus (HIV), a retrovirus. AIDS is a sexually transmitted disease (from sexual intercourse with an infected partner), but is also transmitted by shared needles (in drug abusers), accidental needle sticks or exposure to infected blood (in healthcare workers), blood transfusions, and via the placenta to a fetus or via breast milk from an infected mother to a nursing baby. Initially, there is fever, night sweats, weight loss, enlarged lymph nodes, and diarrhea. A patient with antibodies against HIV is said to be HIV positive. HIV uses helper T cells (CD4 lymphocytes) to reproduce itself (see Figure 6-16 ■). As large numbers of helper T cells are destroyed, the action of suppressor T cells (CD8 lymphocytes) is unopposed. This suppresses the normal immune response and leaves the patient **immunocompromised** and defenseless against infection and cancer.	**immunodeficiency** (IM-myoo-noh-deh-FISH-en-see) **immun/o-** *immune response* **defici/o-** *lacking; inadequate* **-ency** *condition of being* **immunocompromised** (IM-myoo-noh-COM-proh-myzd) **immun/o-** *immune response* **compromis/o-** *exposed to danger* **-ed** *pertaining to*

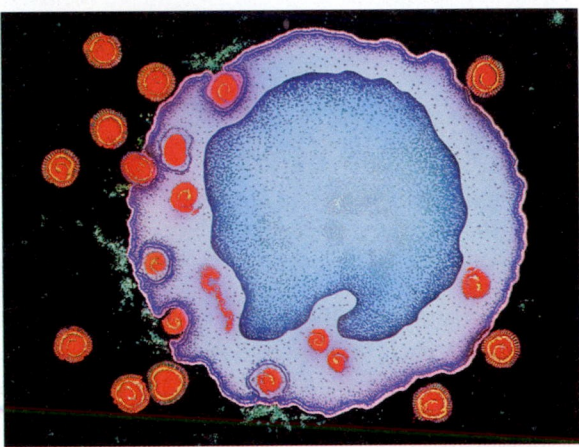

Figure 6-16 ■ Human immunodeficiency virus.

This color-enhanced photograph taken with an electron microscope shows a helper T cell (CD4 lymphocyte) being invaded by many small human immunodeficiency viruses. Like all viruses, HIV cannot reproduce itself. It must enter a lymphocyte and use that cell's DNA to replicate itself. The lymphocyte is destroyed as the new viruses are released.

A Closer Look

A diagnosis of AIDS is made when the CD4 cell count is below 200 (normal is 500–1,500 cells/mm^3) and there is an **opportunistic infection** such as *Pneumocystis jiroveci* pneumonia, oral or esophageal candidiasis (see Figure 16-16), cytomegalovirus retinitis, or unusual cancers such as Kaposi's sarcoma (see Figure 7-21). AIDS wasting syndrome is characterized by weight loss and loss of muscle mass and strength. Treatment: Antiretroviral drugs. There is no cure for AIDS. The universal symbol for AIDS is a red ribbon.

opportunistic (AWP-or-too-NIS-tik)
  opportun/o- *well timed; taking advantage of an opportunity*
  -ist *one who specializes in*
  -ic *pertaining to*

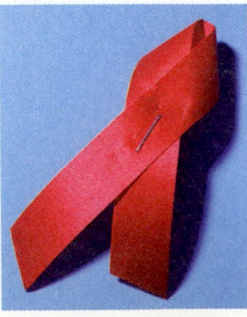

Word or Phrase	Description	Word Building

leukemia	**Cancer** of the leukocytes. Excessive numbers of leukocytes crowd out other cells in the bone marrow. There is anemia (from too few erythrocytes), easy bruising and hemorrhages (from too few thrombocytes), fever, and susceptibility to infection (from too many immature leukocytes). Leukemia is named according to the type of leukocyte that is most prevalent and whether the onset of symptoms is acute or chronic. Leukemia can be caused by exposure to radiation or toxic chemicals and drugs. Patients with chronic myelogenous leukemia have an abnormal chromosome known as the Philadelphia chromosome. Most cases of leukemia occur in persons over age 60. The most common leukemia in children is acute lymphocytic leukemia.	**leukemia** (loo-KEE-mee-ah)
		  leuk/o- *white*
		  -emia *condition of the blood; substance in the blood*
		
		cancer (KAN-ser)

	acute myelogenous leukemia (AML) has too many immature myeloblasts and myelocytes
	chronic myelogenous leukemia (CML) has too many immature myeloblasts, myelocytes, and mature neutrophils, eosinophils, and basophils
	acute lymphocytic leukemia (ALL) has too many immature lymphoblasts
	chronic lymphocytic leukemia (CLL) has too many mature lymphocytes
		myelogenous (MY-eh-LAWJ-eh-nus)
		  myel/o- *bone marrow; spinal cord; myelin*
		  gen/o- *arising from; produced by*
		  -ous *pertaining to*
		
		lymphocytic (LIM-foh-SIT-ik)
		  lymph/o- *lymph; lymphatic system*
		  cyt/o- *cell*
		  -ic *pertaining to*

	The diagnosis is made by examination of the blood (see Figure 6-17 ■) and bone marrow aspiration. Treatment: Chemotherapy drugs, radiation therapy, bone marrow or stem cell transplantation.	

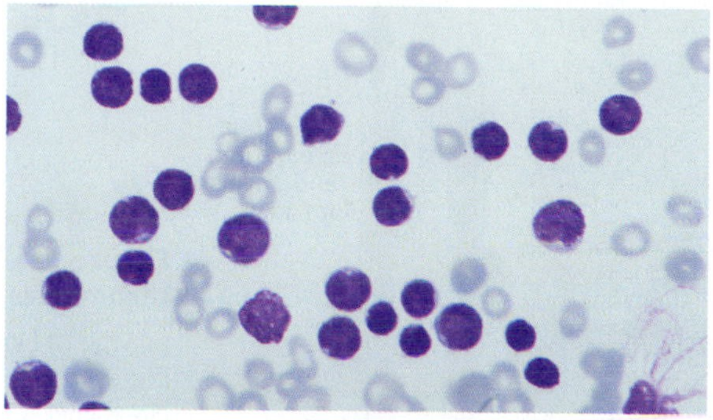

Figure 6-17 ■ **Acute lymphocytic leukemia.** This blood smear was taken from a patient with acute lymphocytic leukemia. There is a tremendous increase in the number of immature lymphoblasts with some mature lymphocytes present in the blood. The pale cells in the background are erythrocytes.

Word or Phrase	Description	Word Building

mononucleosis	Infectious disease caused by the Epstein-Barr virus (EBV). There is lymphadenopathy, fever, and fatigue. It is often called "the kissing disease" because it commonly affects young adults and is transmitted through contact with saliva that contains the virus. It is also known as "mono." Treatment: Rest. (There is no antiviral drug that is effective against mononucleosis. Antibiotic drugs are not effective against viral illnesses.)	**mononucleosis**
		(MAWN-oh-NOO-klee-OH-sis)
		  mon/o- *one; single*
		  nucle/o- *nucleus (of a cell)*
		  -osis *condition; abnormal condition; process*
		Add words to make a complete definition of *mononucleosis*: *abnormal condition of (monocytes that have) one (unlobed) nucleus.*

multiple myeloma	Cancer of the plasma cells that produce antibodies. There is weakness, anemia, and increased susceptibility to infections. Multiple tumors in the bone destroy the red marrow and cause pain, fractures, and **hypercalcemia** (as calcium is released from destroyed bone). The abnormal plasma cells produce Bence Jones protein, an abnormal immunoglobulin that can be detected in the urine. Treatment: Radiation therapy and chemotherapy drugs.	**myeloma** (MY-eh-LOH-mah)
		  myel/o- *bone marrow; spinal cord; myelin*
		  -oma *tumor; mass*
		
		hypercalcemia
		(HY-per-kal-SEE-mee-ah)
		  hyper- *above; more than normal*
		  calc/o- *calcium*
		  -emia *condition of the blood; substance in the blood*

Thrombocytes

Word or Phrase	Description	Word Building
coagulopathy	Any disease that affects the ability of the blood to clot normally. Treatment: Correct the underlying cause.	**coagulopathy** (koh-AG-yoo-LAWP-ah-thee) **coagul/o-** *clotting* **-pathy** *disease; suffering*
deep venous thrombosis (DVT)	A **thrombus** (blood clot) in one of the deep veins of the lower leg, often after surgery or in patients on bedrest. Lack of exercise causes the blood to pool in the veins (**venous stasis**) and form a blood clot (see Figure 6-18 ■). Sometimes a thrombus from a deep vein breaks free and becomes an **embolus** that travels through the circulatory system until it becomes trapped in a branch of the pulmonary artery to the lung. It blocks the blood flow, and the blood never reaches the lung to pick up oxygen. This obstruction is known as a pulmonary **embolism.** Treatment: Anticoagulant drugs to prevent another thrombus from forming; thrombolytic drugs to dissolve the embolus.	**thrombosis** (thrawm-BOH-sis) **thromb/o-** *thrombus (blood clot)* **-osis** *condition; abnormal condition; process* **thrombus** (THRAWM-bus) **thrombi** (THRAWM-by) **stasis** (STAY-sis) **embolus** (EM-boh-lus) **embolism** (EM-boh-LIZ-em) **embol/o-** *embolus (occluding plug)* **-ism** *process; disease from a specific cause*

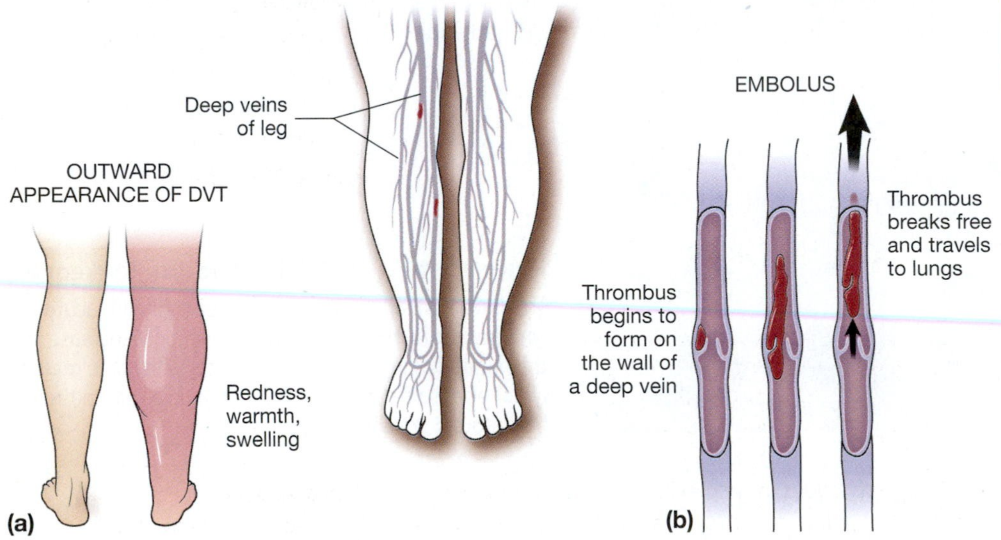

Deep veins of leg

OUTWARD APPEARANCE OF DVT

Redness, warmth, swelling

(a)

EMBOLUS

Thrombus breaks free and travels to lungs

Thrombus begins to form on the wall of a deep vein

(b)

Figure 6-18 ■ Deep venous thrombosis.
(a) When a blood clot (thrombus) forms in a deep vein, there is swelling as the blood flow is impaired, and redness and warmth as the tissues become inflamed. (b) A thrombus can become an embolus that travels to other parts of the body.

Word or Phrase	Description	Word Building
disseminated intravascular coagulation (DIC)	Severe disorder of clotting in which multiple small thrombi are formed throughout the body. These thrombi use up platelets and fibrinogen from the plasma to such an extent that there is spontaneous bleeding from the nose, mouth, IV sites, and incisions. DIC can be triggered by severe injuries, burns, cancer, or systemic infections. Treatment: Intravenous fibrinogen and platelets.	**disseminated** (dih-SEM-ih-NAYT-ed) **dissemin/o-** *widely scattered throughout the body* **-ated** *pertaining to a condition; composed of* **intravascular** (IN-trah-VAS-kyoo-lar) **intra-** *within* **vascul/o-** *blood vessel* **-ar** *pertaining to* **coagulation** (koh-AG-yoo-LAY-shun) **coagul/o-** *clotting* **-ation** *a process; being or having*

Word or Phrase	Description	Word Building
hemophilia	Inherited genetic abnormality that causes a lack or a deficiency of a specific clotting factor. The abnormal gene is carried by a female on the X chromosome, but she does not have the disease. If a male inherits the abnormal gene, it causes hemophilia. A patient who has hemophilia is a **hemophiliac**. Hemophilia A, the most common type, is due to a lack of clotting factor VIII. Hemophilia B is due to a lack of factor IX. Hemophilia C is due to a lack of factor XI. When injured, hemophiliac patients continue to bleed for long periods of time. Minor injuries produce large hematomas under the skin and bleeding inside body cavities, joints, and organs. Treatment: Intravenous administration of the specific clotting factor that is lacking.	**hemophilia** (HEE-moh-FIL-ee-ah) **hem/o-** *blood* **phil/o-** *attraction to; fondness for* **-ia** *condition; state; thing* **hemophiliac** (HEE-moh-FIL-ee-ak) **hem/o-** *blood* **phil/o-** *attraction to; fondness for* **-iac** *pertaining to*
thrombocytopenia	Deficiency in the number of thrombocytes due to exposure to radiation, chemicals, or drugs that damage stem cells in the bone marrow. It also occurs when leukemia cells crowd out the stem cells in the red marrow that produce thrombocytes. Also, some patients have antibodies that destroy their own thrombocytes. Thrombocytopenia results in small, pinpoint hemorrhages or **petechiae** and larger hemorrhages or **ecchymoses** and bruises on the skin. **Idiopathic thrombocytopenia purpura** has no identifiable cause. Treatment: Correct the underlying cause.	**thrombocytopenia** (THRAWM-boh-sy-toh-PEE-nee-ah) **thromb/o-** *thrombus (blood clot)* **cyt/o-** *cell* **-penia** *condition of deficiency* **petechiae** (peh-TEE-kee-ee) **ecchymoses** (EK-ih-MOH-seez) **idiopathic** (ID-ee-oh-PATH-ik) **idi/o-** *unknown; individual* **path/o-** *disease; suffering* **-ic** *pertaining to* **purpura** (PER-peh-rah)

Lymphatic System

Word or Phrase	Description	Word Building
graft-versus-host disease (GVHD)	Immune reaction of donor tissue or a donor organ (graft) against the patient (host). This can occur after bone marrow transplantation or any type of organ transplantation. There is a rash and fever, or it can be severe enough to cause death. Treatment: Corticosteroid drugs.	
lymphadenopathy	Enlarged lymph nodes. Lymph nodes in the neck, axillae, and groin can be felt easily if they are enlarged. A sore throat causes lymph nodes in the neck to enlarge (see Figure 6-19 ■). A severe infection or cancer will cause the lymph nodes in that area to become enlarged. Treatment: Correct the underlying cause.	**lymphadenopathy** (lim-FAD-eh-NAWP-ah-thee) **lymph/o-** *lymph; lymphatic system* **aden/o-** *gland* **-pathy** *disease; suffering*

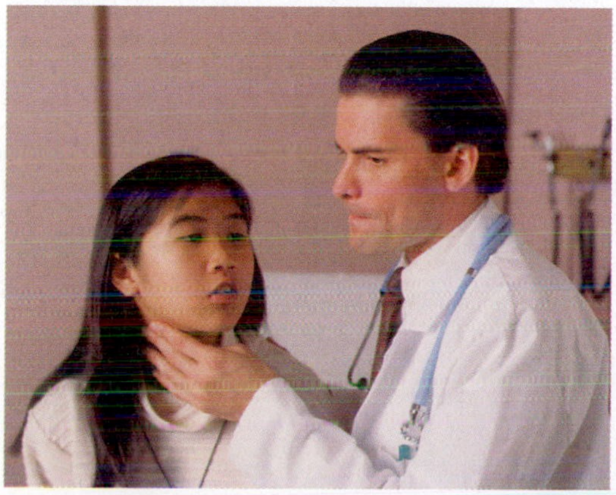

Figure 6-19 ■ Lymphadenopathy.
The physician is palpating the cervical lymph nodes of this patient. These lymph nodes trap and destroy pathogens or cancerous cells from the nose, mouth, or throat, but large numbers can overwhelm the lymph nodes and cause them to become enlarged.

Word or Phrase	Description	Word Building
lymphedema	Generalized swelling of an arm or leg that occurs after surgery when a chain of lymph nodes has been removed. Tissue fluid in that area cannot drain into the lymphatic vessels at the normal rate, and this causes edema. Treatment: Elevation of the body part to promote drainage.	**lymphedema** (LIM-fah-DEE-mah) **lymph/o-** *lymph; lymphatic system* **-edema** *swelling*
lymphoma	Cancerous tumor of lymphocytes in the lymph nodes or lymphoid tissue. A lymphoma that originates in a lymph node should not be confused with a metastasis to a lymph node from a primary site of cancer located elsewhere. Treatment: Radiation therapy, chemotherapy.	**lymphoma** (lim-FOH-mah) **lymph/o-** *lymph; lymphatic system* **-oma** *tumor; mass*
Hodgkin's lymphoma	Most common type of lymphoma. It occurs most often in young adults and is discovered on physical examination as a painless, enlarged cervical lymph node in the neck. There is fever, weakness, weight loss, and splenomegaly. A biopsy of the lymph node shows abnormal lymphocytes known as Reed-Sternberg cells. It is also known as **Hodgkin's disease.**	**Hodgkin** (HAWJ-kin)
non-Hodgkin's lymphoma	A group of more than 20 different types of lymphomas that occur in older adults and do not show Reed-Sternberg cells.	
splenomegaly	Enlargement of the spleen, as felt on palpation of the abdomen. It can be caused by mononucleosis, Hodgkin's disease, hemolytic anemia, polycythemia vera, or leukemia. Treatment: Correct the underlying cause.	**splenomegaly** (SPLEH-noh-MEG-ah-lee) **splen/o-** *spleen* **-megaly** *enlargement*
thymoma	Tumor of the thymus that is usually benign. It may cause a cough and chest pain. It is often seen in patients who already have an autoimmune disorder such as myasthenia gravis. Treatment: Thymectomy.	**thymoma** (thy-MOH-mah) **thym/o-** *thymus; rage* **-oma** *tumor; mass*

Autoimmune Disorders

autoimmune diseases	Diseases in which the body makes antibodies against its own tissues, causing pain and loss of function. The following autoimmune diseases are described in other chapters:	**autoimmune** (AW-toh-im-MYOON) **aut/o-** *self* **-immune** *immune response*

Autoimmune Disease	Area Affected
diabetes mellitus, type 1	pancreas
Graves' disease	thyroid gland
Hashimoto's thyroiditis	thyroid gland
inflammatory bowel disease	intestines
multiple sclerosis	nerves
myasthenia gravis	muscles
psoriasis	skin
rheumatoid arthritis	joints
scleroderma	skin and blood vessels
systemic lupus erythematosus	connective tissue, skin, kidneys, lungs

Laboratory and Diagnostic Procedures

Blood Cell Tests

Word or Phrase	Description	Word Building
blood type	Blood test to determine the blood type (A, B, AB, or O) and Rh factor (positive or negative) of the patient's blood. **Type and crossmatch** is done when a patient needs to receive a blood transfusion. The donor's blood was typed when it was stored in the blood bank. The patient's (recipient's) blood is then typed. The patient's plasma is mixed with the donor's red blood cells (crossmatching). If the donor's red blood cells clump together (**agglutination**), the blood types are not compatible.	**agglutination** (ah-GLOO-tih-NAY-shun) **agglutin/o-** *clumping; sticking* **-ation** *a process; being or having*
complete blood count (CBC) with differential	Group of blood tests that are performed automatically by machine to determine the number, type, and characteristics of various cells in the blood (see Table 6-4). This is also known as a "CBC with diff."	**differential** (DIF-er-EN-shal) **different/o-** *being distinct; different* **-ial** *pertaining to*

A Closer Look

A severe bacterial infection will increase the number of bands in the differential count. This is known as a **shift to the left.** It refers to a time when the differential count was done by hand with a column on the tally sheet for each type of leukocyte. While counting the leukocytes under the microscope, the laboratory technician put tally marks in the appropriate columns. The column to the far left was for bands. When there were more tally marks in that column than usual, the differential count was said to show a shift to the left.

Word or Phrase	Description	Word Building
peripheral blood smear	Blood test done manually to examine the characteristics of erythrocytes and leukocytes under the microscope. A drop of blood is spread as a thin smear on a glass slide. Then hematoxylin and eosin dyes are used to stain the blood cells. A blood smear is used to investigate abnormal blood cells discovered on the automated CBC, or a blood smear can be ordered by the physician when there is reason to suspect blood cell abnormalities.	**peripheral** (peh-RIF-eh-ral) **peripher/o-** *outer aspects* **-al** *pertaining to* *Peripheral* refers to blood that is taken from an extremity (usually by venipuncture from a vein in the arm).

Table 6-4   Complete Blood Count (CBC) with Differential

Test Name	Description	Word Building
erythrocytes (red blood cells, RBCs)	Number in millions per milliliter (mL) of blood	
hematocrit (HCT)	Percentage of RBCs in a blood sample	**hematocrit** (hee-MAT-oh-krit) **hemat/o-** *blood* **-crit** *separation of*
hemoglobin (Hgb)	Amount in grams per deciliter (g/dL) of blood	
red blood cell **indices** **mean** cell volume (MCV) mean cell hemoglobin (MCH) mean cell hemoglobin concentration (MCHC)	Average volume of one RBC Average weight of hemoglobin in one RBC Average concentration of hemoglobin in one RBC	**index** (IN-deks) **indices** (IN-dih-seez) *Index* is a Latin singular noun. Form the plural by changing *–ex* to *–ices*. **mean** (MEEN)

(continued)

Table 6-4 Complete Blood Count (CBC) with Differential (*continued*)

Test Name	Description	Word Building
leukocytes (white blood cells, WBCs)	Number in thousands per milliliter (**k**/mL) of blood	The *k* in **k**/mL stands for *kilo-*, a prefix meaning *one thousand*.

WBC differential
  neutrophils
  eosinophils
  basophils
  lymphocytes
  monocytes
	Percentage of each type of WBC per 100 WBCs	

thrombocytes (platelets)	Number in thousands per milliliter (k/mL) of blood	

Coagulation Tests

Word or Phrase	Description	Word Building
activated clotting time (ACT)	Blood test to monitor the effectiveness of the anticoagulant drug heparin when it is given in high doses. A prolonged (rather than normal) activated clotting time would be expected.	
partial thromboplastin time (PTT)	Blood test to monitor the effectiveness of the anticoagulant drug heparin when it is given in regular doses. A prolonged (rather than normal) PTT would be expected. An activated partial thromboplastin time (aPTT) test uses a chemical activator to get faster test results.	
prothrombin time (PT)	Blood test to evaluate the effectiveness of the anticoagulant drug Coumadin. A prolonged (rather than normal) PT would be expected. The **international normalized ratio (INR)** reports the PT value in a standardized way, regardless of which laboratory performed the test.	

Other Blood Tests

blood chemistries	Blood test used to determine the levels of various chemicals in the blood (see Figure 6-20 ■). These include electrolytes, albumin, total protein, ALT, AST, BUN, creatinine, bilirubin, glucose, LDH, total cholesterol, uric acid, and alkaline phosphatase. A Chem-20 includes 20 individual chemistry tests performed at the same time. This is also called a **metabolic panel.**	

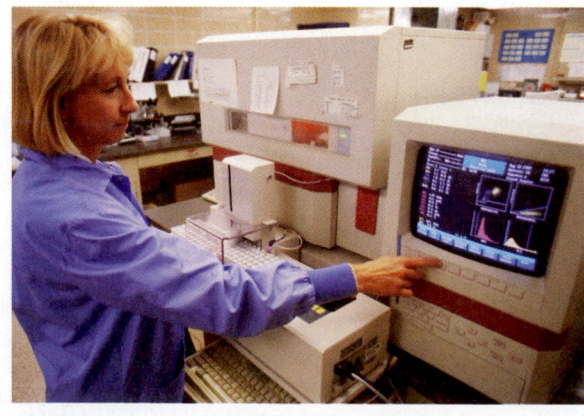

Figure 6-20 ■ Blood chemistry analyzer.
This clinical laboratory scientist is reviewing the results of a blood chemistry analysis. Multiple tests can be performed together automatically on this computerized equipment.

Word or Phrase	Description	Word Building
ferritin	Blood chemistry test that indirectly measures the amount of iron (ferritin) stored in the body by measuring the small amount that is always present in the blood. It is used to diagnose iron deficiency anemia.	**ferritin** (FAIR-ih-tin) **ferrit/o-** *iron* **-in** *a substance*
human immuno-deficiency virus (HIV) tests	Blood tests that detect infection with HIV. HIV tests are reported as either HIV negative or HIV positive.	
ELISA	First screening test done for HIV. It can be done on blood, urine, or saliva samples. The test uses two antibodies. The first binds to HIV, forming a complex; the second reacts to an enzyme in that complex. However, this test can also be positive if the patient has antibodies against lupus erythematosus, Lyme disease, or syphilis. ELISA stands for enzyme-linked immunosorbent assay. The test results are available in 1–2 weeks; however, the SUDS (Single Use Diagnostic System) test, which uses ELISA methods, is a rapid HIV test that gives results in 10 minutes. OraSure is a quick screening test done in a doctor's office or clinic to detect antibodies to HIV in the saliva.	
Western blot	Used to confirm a positive ELISA and make a diagnosis of HIV infection. A positive ELISA and a positive Western blot together are 99.9% accurate in diagnosing HIV infection.	
viral RNA load test	Measures tiny amounts of RNA (from HIV) that are in the blood during the 6 weeks before antibodies against HIV can be detected. This test is also used to monitor the progression of the disease and the patient's response to antiretroviral drugs.	
p24 antigen test	Detects p24, a protein in HIV. The results are reported as a titer. This test is also used to screen donated units of blood for HIV.	
CD4 count	Measures the number of CD4 lymphocytes (helper T cells). It is used to monitor the progression of the disease and the patient's response to antiretroviral drugs. The CD4:CD8 ratio is also monitored.	
total iron binding capacity (TIBC)	Blood chemistry test that measures the level of **transferrin,** a protein that carries iron in the blood. Used to diagnose iron deficiency anemia.	**transferrin** (trans-FAIR-in) **trans-** *across; through* **ferr/o-** *iron* **-in** *a substance*

Serum Tests

electrophoresis	Immunoglobulin electrophoresis determines the amount of each immunoglobulin (IgA, IgD, IgE, IgG, and IgM) in the blood. A sample of serum is placed in a gel with an electrical current. The immunoglobulins become charged and move toward the positive or negative electrode. Each immunoglobulin travels a different distance and direction through the gel, depending on its size and charge, and it appears as a spike in a different area on the graph paper. The size of the spike corresponds to how much immunoglobulin is present.	**electrophoresis** (ee-LEK-troh-foh-REE-sis) **electr/o-** *electricity* **phor/o-** *to bear; to carry; range* **-esis** *a process* Add words to make a complete definition of *electrophoresis: a process (of a test that uses) electricity to carry (immunoglobulins in a gel).*
MonoSpot test	Rapid test that uses the patient's serum mixed with horse erythrocytes. If the patient has infectious mononucleosis, **heterophil antibodies** in the patient's serum cause the horse's erythrocytes to clump. It is also called the **heterophil antibody test.**	**heterophil** (HET-er-oh-fil) **heter/o-** *other* **-phil** *attraction to; fondness for*

Urine Tests

Word or Phrase	Description	Word Building
Bence Jones protein	Urine test used to monitor the course of multiple myeloma. The cancerous plasma cells produce this abnormal immunoglobulin that can be detected in the urine.	
Schilling test	Urine test used to diagnose pernicious anemia. It measures the amount of radioactive vitamin B_{12} excreted in the urine. The patient swallows a capsule that contains intrinsic factor and vitamin B_{12} labeled with a radioactive tracer. The patient swallows a second capsule that contains vitamin B_{12} labeled with a different radioactive tracer but no intrinsic factor. If the patient has pernicious anemia, only the capsule that contained vitamin B_{12} and intrinsic factor will be absorbed into the blood and then excreted in the urine.	

Radiologic Procedures

color flow duplex ultrasonography	Procedure that combines a two-dimensional ultrasound image with Doppler **ultrasonography** that color-codes the images of the blood according to their velocity and direction. It shows turbulence and variation in velocity by degrees of brightness. This test is the "gold standard" for evaluating tortuous varicose veins and diagnosing deep venous thrombosis.	**ultrasonography** (UL-trah-soh-NAWG-rah-fee) **ultra-** *beyond; higher* **son/o-** *sound* **-graphy** *process of recording*
lymphangiography	Radiologic procedure in which a radiopaque contrast dye is injected into a lymphatic vessel. X-rays are taken as the dye travels through the lymphatic vessels and lymph nodes. It shows enlarged lymph nodes, lymphomas, and areas of blocked lymphatic drainage. The x-ray image is a **lymphangiogram.**	**lymphangiography** (lim-FAN-jee-AWG-rah-fee) **lymph/o-** *lymph; lymphatic system* **angi/o-** *blood vessel; lymphatic vessel* **-graphy** *process of recording*
		lymphangiogram (lim-FAN-jee-oh-gram) **lymph/o-** *lymph; lymphatic system* **angi/o-** *blood vessel; lymphatic vessel* **-gram** *a record or picture*

Medical and Surgical Procedures

Medical Procedures

Word or Phrase	Description	Word Building

bone marrow aspiration	Procedure to remove red bone marrow from the posterior iliac crest of the hip bone. This is done in patients with leukemia, lymphoma, and anemia to examine the different stages of blood cell development (stem cell to mature cell). It is also done to harvest bone marrow from a healthy donor to give to a patient who needs a bone marrow transplantation.	**aspiration** (AS-pih-RAY-shun)
		  aspir/o- *to breathe in; to suck in*
		  -ation *a process; being or having*

phlebotomy	Procedure for drawing a sample of venous blood into a vacuum tube. This is also known as **venipuncture.** The vacuum tubes have different-colored rubber stoppers that indicate which additive or anticoagulant is in the tube; this determines what blood test can be performed on the blood in that tube (see Figure 6-21 ■).	**phlebotomy** (fleh-BAW-toh-mee)
		  phleb/o- *vein*
		  -tomy *process of cutting or making an incision*
		venipuncture (VEE-nih-PUNK-chur)
		  ven/i- *vein*
		  punct/o- *hole; perforation*
		  -ure *system; result of*

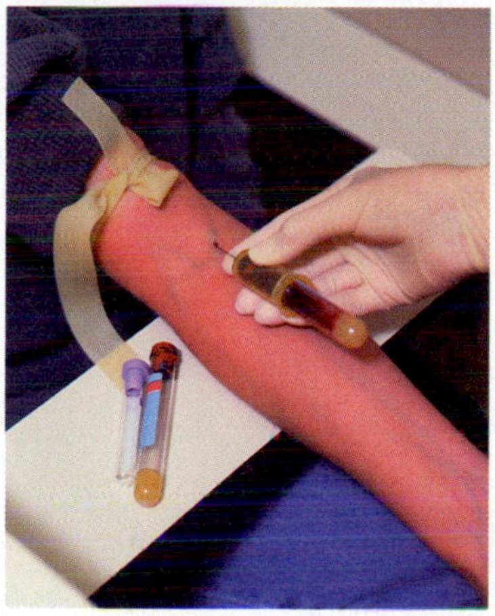

Figure 6-21 ■ Phlebotomy.
This patient is having blood drawn. The lavender-top tube is used for a complete blood count. The red-top tube is used for blood chemistry tests. The technician placed a tourniquet around the patient's upper arm to distend the veins in the lower arm. The patient's arm is supported to keep the elbow straight so that the needle goes into the lumen of the vein, not through it. A tube is placed into the plastic holder and the vacuum draws blood into the tube. The tubes of blood are sent to the laboratory for testing.

vaccination	Procedure that injects a vaccine into the body. The **vaccine** consists of killed or **attenuated** bacterial or viral cells or cell fragments. The body produces antibodies and memory B lymphocytes specific to that pathogen. If the vaccinated patient encounters that pathogen again, the patient will have mild or no symptoms of the disease. Vaccinations are routinely used to prevent diseases that could be fatal or cause serious disability (polio, diphtheria, tetanus, etc.). Immunoglobulins (antibodies) against some diseases (rabies or tetanus) can be given to provide passive immunity if the person has just been exposed. Vaccination is also known as **immunization.**	**vaccination** (VAK-sih-NAY-shun)
		  vaccin/o- *giving a vaccine*
		  -ation *a process; being or having*
		vaccine (vak-SEEN)
		attenuated (ah-TEN-yoo-AA-ted)
		  attenu/o- *weakened*
		  -ated *pertaining to a condition; composed of*
		immunization (IM-myoo-nih-ZAY-shun)
		  immun/o- *immune response*
		  -ization *process of making, creating, or inserting*

A Closer Look

The principles of vaccination were established in 1796 by Edward Jenner, an English physician. He noticed that milkmaids did not get the serious disease smallpox because they first contracted cowpox, a viral disease of cows. Jenner took fluid from the skin sores of a milkmaid with cowpox. He made cuts in the skin of a young boy and introduced the fluid, and the boy later developed cowpox. Later, Jenner gave the boy the smallpox virus, and the boy did not develop smallpox. This medical practice was successful, but it horrified people. Cartoonists drew pictures of patients with cow parts coming out of their bodies. However, several years later, most doctors were using Jenner's technique to protect their patients from smallpox.

Blood Donation and Tranfusion Procedures

Word or Phrase	Description	Word Building
blood donation	Procedure in which a unit of whole blood is collected from a donor. The unit is tested and labeled as to blood type and stored in a refrigerated blood bank. A unit of whole blood can be given as a transfusion, or the unit can be divided into its component parts (erythrocytes, platelets, plasma), and just that part can be given as a transfusion to meet the needs of a specific patient.	**donation** (doh-NAY-shun) **donat/o-** *give as a gift* **-ion** *action; condition*

Clinical Connections

Public Health. All donated blood must be tested for syphilis, hepatitis, and HIV. The Food and Drug Administration (FDA) is responsible for the safety of blood and blood products used in the United States. The FDA has banned people from donating blood if they lived in or visited Europe for a certain length of time because of the possibility of contamination with the microorganism that causes mad cow disease in cows and new variant Creutzfeldt-Jakob disease in humans, a fatal neurologic disease.

Word or Phrase	Description	Word Building
blood transfusion	Procedure in which whole blood, blood cells, or plasma is given by intravenous transfusion. Transfusions of whole blood provide a complete correction of blood loss. Packed red blood cells (PRBCs) are a concentrated preparation of RBCs in a small amount of plasma. Transfusion with PRBCs avoids fluid overload in patients with congestive heart failure or in premature infants. Platelets are given to patients with thrombocytopenia or leukemia and to cancer patients whose bone marrow is depressed after radiation therapy or chemotherapy drugs. Plasma is given to hemophiliac patients who need clotting factors.	**transfusion** (trans-FYOO-shun) **trans-** *across; through* **fus/o-** *pouring* **-ion** *action; condition*

A Closer Look

Patients scheduled to have certain types of surgery may be asked to donate a unit of their own blood in advance so they can receive it during surgery. This is known as an **autologous blood transfusion.** Also, blood in the operative field can be suctioned, collected, filtered, and returned to the patient during the surgery. At the conclusion of every surgery, the surgeon estimates the amount of blood loss and records this in the patient's operative report.

autologous (aw-TAWL-oh-gus)
aut/o- *self*
log/o- *word; the study of*
-ous *pertaining to*

Word or Phrase	Description	Word Building
bone marrow transplantation (BMT)	Procedure used to treat patients with leukemia and lymphoma. Red marrow is harvested by aspirating it from the hip bone of a matched donor. The patient is treated with chemotherapy drugs or radiation to destroy all cancerous cells (this also destroys all the cells in the red marrow). The donor marrow is then filtered and given to the patient intravenously. The donated bone marrow cells travel through the blood to the bones where they implant. After 2–4 weeks, the patient's red marrow begins to produce normal blood cells.	**transplantation** (TRANS-plan-TAY-shun) **transplant/o-** *move something to another place* **-ation** *a process; being or having*

A Closer Look

Unlike blood transfusions where donor blood and patient blood are crossmatched for compatibility of the ABO and Rh blood groups, bone marrow donors and recipient patients are matched for a different set of proteins called human leukocyte-associated (HLA) antigens. In **autologous transplants,** patients provide their own bone marrow or stem cells (which are treated to destroy any cancerous cells). In **allogeneic transplants,** patients receive bone marrow or stem cells donated by another person.	**allogeneic** (AL-oh-jeh-NEE-ik) **all/o-** *other; strange* **gene/o-** *gene* **-ic** *pertaining to* Add words to make a complete definition of *allogeneic: pertaining to (someone) other (than the patient and his or her) genes.*

Word or Phrase	Description	Word Building
plasmapheresis	Procedure in which plasma is separated from the blood cells. A donor gives a unit of blood, which is rapidly spun in a centrifuge. Centrifugal force pulls the blood cells to the bottom of the unit of blood. The plasma portion at the top is siphoned off. The blood cells are given back to the donor. Then the plasma is processed and pooled with plasma from other donors to make fresh frozen plasma, albumin, or clotting factors.	**plasmapheresis** (PLAZ-mah-feh-REE-sis) **plasm/o-** *plasma* **apher/o-** *withdrawal* **-esis** *a process*
stem cell transplantation	Medical treatment for leukemia and lymphoma. Stem cells from the patient or from a matched donor are collected. Matched stem cells from umbilical cord blood can also be used. The stem cells are given intravenously. They migrate to the red marrow and begin producing normal blood cells.	

Clinical Connections

Medical Research. In 2001, the first embryonic stem cell (see Figure 6-22 ■) was made into a mature blood cell. This ignited a controversy over the use of human embryos in stem cell research. In 2009, the first human clinical trial of embryonic stem cell therapy was done on patients with recent spinal cord injuries. Prior animal tests had shown that stem cells restored movement to rats with partially severed spinal cords.

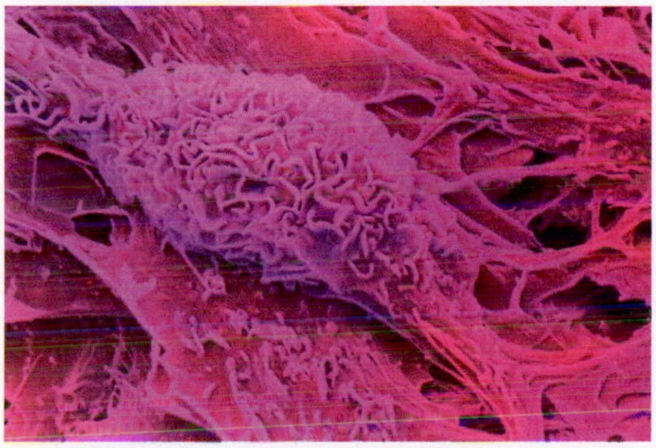

Figure 6-22 ■ Stem cell.

Surgical Procedures

Word or Phrase	Description	Word Building
lymph node biopsy	Process that uses a fine needle to aspirate material from a lymph node. The lymph node may also be completely removed by doing an **excisional biopsy.**	**biopsy** (BY-awp-see) **bi/o-** *life; living organisms; living tissue* **-opsy** *process of viewing* **excisional** (ek-SIH-shun-al) **excis/o-** *to cut out* **-ion** *action; condition* **-al** *pertaining to*
lymph node dissection	Removal of several or all of the lymph nodes in a lymph node chain during extensive surgery for cancer.	**dissection** (dy-SEK-shun) **dissect/o-** *to cut apart* **-ion** *action; condition*
splenectomy	Removal of the spleen when it has ruptured due to trauma.	**splenectomy** (spleh-NEK-toh-mee) **splen/o-** *spleen* **-ectomy** *surgical excision*

Word Alert

SOUND-ALIKE WORDS

spleen	*(noun)*	organ of the lymphatic system
splenectomy	*(noun)*	surgical removal of the spleen
splenic	*(adjective)*	pertaining to the spleen
splenomegaly	*(noun)*	enlargement of the spleen

Word or Phrase	Description	Word Building
thymectomy	Removal of the thymus because of a benign or cancerous tumor or to treat myasthenia gravis.	**thymectomy** (thy-MEK-toh-mee) **thym/o-** *thymus; rage* **-ectomy** *surgical excision*

Clinical Connections

Orthopedics (Muscular) (Chapter 9). A thymectomy is also performed in patients with the muscular disease of myasthenia gravis. This disease causes severe muscle weakness as the body's antibodies destroy acetylcholine receptors on the muscles. In these patients, the thymus contains abnormal cells that may cause this autoimmune reaction.

After a thymectomy, the level of antibodies against acetylcholine receptors falls.

Drug Categories

These categories of drugs are used to treat blood and lymphatic diseases and conditions. The most common generic and trade name drugs in each category are listed.

Category	Indication	Examples	Word Building
anticoagulant drugs	Prevent blood clots from forming by inhibiting the clotting factors (heparin drug) or by inhibiting vitamin K that is needed to make the clotting factors (warfarin drug)	heparin (subcutaneous or intravenous), warfarin (Coumadin) (oral)	**anticoagulant** (AN-tee-koh-AG-yoo-lant) (AN-tih-koh-AG-yoo-lant) **anti-** *against* **coagul/o-** *clotting* **-ant** *pertaining to*
corticosteroid drugs	Anti-inflammatory drugs that suppress the immune response and decrease inflammation. Also given to organ transplant patients to prevent rejection of the donor organ.	dexamethasone (Decadron), prednisone (Deltasone)	**corticosteroid** (KOR-tih-koh-STAIR-oyd) **cortic/o-** *cortex (outer region)* **-steroid** *steroid*
erythropoietin	Stimulates the red marrow to make erythrocytes	epoetin alfa (Epogen, Procrit)	**erythropoietin** (eh-RITH-roh-POY-eh-tin) **erythr/o-** *red* **-poietin** *a substance that forms*
immuno-suppressant drugs	Suppress the immune response. Prevent rejection of a transplanted organ.	cyclosporine (Sandimmune)	**immunosuppressant** (IM-myoo-noh-soo-PRES-ant) **immun/o-** *immune response* **suppress/o-** *press down* **-ant** *pertaining to*
nucleoside reverse transcriptase inhibitor drugs	Inhibit reverse transcriptase, an enzyme that HIV needs to reproduce itself	lamivudine (Epivir), zalcitabine (Hivid), zidovudine (Retrovir)	**nucleoside** (NOO-klee-oh-side) **transcriptase** (trans-KRIP-tays)
platelet aggregation inhibitor drugs	Prevent platelets from aggregating (clumping together), the first step in forming a blood clot	aspirin, clopidogrel (Plavix), abciximab (ReoPro)	**inhibitor** (in-HIB-ih-tor) **inhibit/o-** *block; hold back* **-or** *person or thing that produces or does*
protease inhibitor drugs	Inhibit protease, an enzyme that HIV needs to reproduce itself	indinavir (Crixivan), nelfinavir (Viracept), ritonavir (Norvir)	**protease** (PROH-tee-ace) **prote/o-** *protein* **-ase** *enzyme*
thrombolytic enzyme drugs	Break fibrin strands to dissolve blood clots that have already formed	streptokinase (Streptase). The suffix *-ase* indicates that the drug is an enzyme.	**thrombolytic** (THRAWM-boh-LIT-ik) **thromb/o-** *thrombus (blood clot)* **ly/o-** *break down; destroy* **-tic** *pertaining to*
tissue plasminogen activator (TPA) drugs	Convert plasminogen to an enzyme that breaks fibrin strands in order to dissolve a blood clot that has already formed	alteplase (Activase), reteplase (Retavase)	**plasminogen** (plaz-MIN-oh-jen)
vitamin B₁₂ drugs	Used to treat pernicious anemia. They are given by intramuscular injection or by nasal spray.	cyanocobalamin (Nascobal)	

A Closer Look

Some **antiretroviral** drugs used to treat HIV exert their action on reverse transcriptase. Reverse transcriptase in the virus tells the DNA in a human cell to make more viral RNA and more viruses. This is backward (retro-) from the normal process in which human DNA tells its own RNA what to produce.

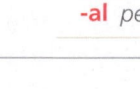

antiretroviral
(AN-tee-REH-troh-VY-ral)
(AN-tih-REH-troh-VY-ral)
anti- *against*
retro- *behind; backward*
vir/o- *virus*
-al *pertaining to*

Abbreviations

A	blood type in the ABO blood group		**IgD**	immunoglobulin D
AB	blood type in the ABO blood group		**IgE**	immunoglobulin E
AIDS	acquired immunodeficiency syndrome		**IgG**	immunoglobulin G
ALL	acute lymphocytic leukemia		**IgM**	immunoglobulin M
AML	acute myelogenous leukemia		**lymphs**	lymphocytes
B	blood type in the ABO blood group		**MCH**	mean cell hemoglobin
basos	basophils		**MCHC**	mean cell hemoglobin concentration
BMT	bone marrow transplantation		**MCV**	mean cell volume
CBC	complete blood count		**mm³**	cubic millimeter
CLL	chronic lymphocytic leukemia		**mono**	mononucleosis (slang)
CML	chronic myelogenous leukemia		**monos**	monocytes
cmm	cubic millimeter		**O**	blood type in the ABO blood group
DIC	disseminated intravascular coagulation		**PMN**	polymorphonuclear leukocyte
EBV	Epstein-Barr virus		**polys**	polymorphonuclear leukocytes
ELISA	enzyme-linked immunosorbent assay		**PRBCs**	packed red blood cells
eos	eosinophils		**pro time**	prothrombin time (slang)
GVHD	graft-versus-host disease		**PT**	prothrombin time
HCT	hematocrit		**PTT**	partial thromboplastin time
Hgb	hemoglobin		**RBC**	red blood cell
H&H	hemoglobin and hematocrit		**segs**	segmented neutrophils
HIV	human immunodeficiency virus		**TNF**	tumor necrosis factor
HLA	human leukocyte antigen		**TPA**	tissue plasminogen activator (drug)
IgA	immunoglobulin A		**WBC**	white blood cell

Word Alert

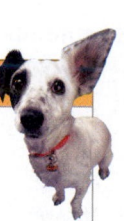

ABBREVIATIONS

Abbreviations are commonly used in all types of medical documents; however, they can mean different things to different people and their meanings can be misinterpreted. Always verify the meaning of an abbreviation.

Monos is a brief form that means *monocytes,* but the slang *mono* means *mononucleosis.*

PT means *prothrombin time,* but it also means *physical therapy* or *physical therapist.*

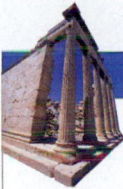

It's Greek to Me!

Did you notice that some words have two different combining forms? Combining forms from both Greek and Latin languages remain a part of medical language today.

Word	Greek	Latin	Medical Word Examples
cell	cyt/o-	cellul/o-	pancytopenia, cellular
nucleus	kary/o-	nucle/o-	megakaryocyte, polymorphonuclear
red	eosin/o-	rub/o-	eosinophil, bilirubin
	erythr/o-		erythrocyte
vein	phleb/o-	ven/o-	phlebotomy, venous

CAREER FOCUS

Meet Adriana, a phlebotomist in a hospital

"A phlebotomist's job description is to draw blood, the collection of blood. On a daily basis, I draw blood from about 30 to 50 patients. Every time it's someone different, so every time it's a different challenge. That's why I love it."

Phlebotomists are allied health professionals who use venipuncture techniques to draw blood. They follow procedures for storing and transporting blood specimens for diagnostic testing in the laboratory.

    Hematologists are physicians who practice in the medical specialty of hematology. They diagnose and treat patients with diseases of the blood. Malignancies of the blood and lymphatic system are treated medically by an oncologist or surgically by a general surgeon.

    Immunologists are physicians or they are scientists who have a Ph.D. in cellular biology or pharmacology. They practice in the medical specialty of immunology. Clinical immunologists diagnose and treat patients who have autoimmune diseases, immunodeficiency diseases, cancer, or who are undergoing transplantation (organ, bone marrow, or stem cell).

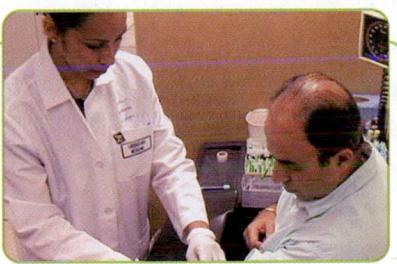

phlebotomist (fleh-BAWT-oh-mist)
  phleb/o- *vein*
  tom/o- *cut; slice; layer*
  -ist *one who specializes in*

hematologist (HEE-mah-TAWL-oh-jist)
  hemat/o- *blood*
  log/o- *word; the study of*
  -ist *one who specializes in*

immunologist
(IM-myoo-NAWL-oh-jist)
  immun/o- *immune response*
  log/o- *word; the study of*
  -ist *one who specializes in*

PEARSON myhealthprofessionskit™ To see Adriana's complete video profile, visit Medical Terminology Interactive at www.myhealthprofessionskit.com. Select this book, log in, and go to the 6th floor of Pearson General Hospital. Enter the Laboratory, and click on the computer screen.

CHAPTER REVIEW EXERCISES

Test your knowledge of the chapter by completing these review exercises. Use the Answer Key at the end of the book to check your answers.

Anatomy and Physiology

Matching Exercise

Match each word or phrase to its description.

1. albumin
2. B cell
3. bilirubin
4. eosinophil
5. erythrocyte
6. erythropoietin
7. hematopoiesis
8. hemoglobin
9. hemostasis
10. macrophage
11. lymphocyte
12. passive immunity
13. phagocytosis
14. plasma
15. stem cell
16. thrombocyte

_____ Secreted by the kidneys to increase RBCs

_____ The most immature cell in the red marrow

_____ Cell fragment

_____ Maternal antibodies cross placenta to fetus

_____ Cessation of bleeding

_____ Has granules that stain red with eosin dye

_____ Process of engulfing foreign cells

_____ Carries oxygen and carbon dioxide

_____ Red blood cell

_____ Clear yellow liquid part of the blood

_____ One of the types of agranulocytes

_____ Process by which blood cells are formed

_____ Antioxidant that protects from damage by free radicals

_____ Most abundant plasma protein

_____ Monocyte in lymph nodes that eats pathogens

_____ Lymphocyte that develops in the red marrow

True or False Exercise

Indicate whether each statement is true or false by writing T or F on the line.

1. _____ The fluid portion of the blood without the clotting factors is known as serum.

2. _____ The tonsils, adenoids, and appendix are examples of lymphoid tissues.

3. _____ IgG is the smallest immunoglobulin.

4. _____ Blood type AB negative is known as the universal donor.

5. _____ The three different categories of blood cells are erythrocytes, lymphocytes, and platelets.

6. _____ Bands are also known as segs.

7. _____ The formation of a blood clot is known as coagulation.

8. _____ Macrophages are large cells whose cytoplasm breaks off to form platelets.

9. _____ Endotoxins are poisons produced by some bacteria.

10. _____ Plasma cells produce the plasma portion of blood.

Circle Exercise

Circle the correct word from the choices given.

1. (**Blood, Serum, Thymus**) is a connective tissue that travels to every part of the body.
2. (**Hemoglobin, Platelets, Red blood cells**) are cells that have no nucleus.
3. The strong bands that trap erythrocytes to form a blood clot are known as (**antigens, fibrin, lymph nodes**).
4. Microorganisms that cause disease are known as (**antibodies, antigens, pathogens**).
5. Chemicals with a positive or negative charge are known as (**clotting factors, electrolytes, plasma proteins**).
6. (**IgA, IgD, IgM**) is the immunoglobulin present in tears, saliva, and breast milk.
7. Iron is carried in the (**globin, globulin, heme**) part of an erythrocyte.
8. The process of platelets clumping together at the site of an injury is known as (**aggregation, coagulation, hemostasis**).

Multiple Choice Exercise

Select the choice that best completes the statement.

1. Red blood cells are known by the name _____.
   - a. monocytes
   - b. lymphocytes
   - c. basophils
   - d. erythrocytes
   - e. none of the above

2. Immature forms of erythrocytes include all of the following *except* _____.
   - a. reticulocytes
   - b. myelocytes
   - c. erythroblasts
   - d. normoblasts
   - e. stem cells

3. All of the following are breakdown products of hemoglobin *except* _____.
   - a. globin chains
   - b. iron
   - c. heme
   - d. monocytes
   - e. bilirubin

4. _____ is produced by macrophages; it produces fever and stimulates the production of helper T cells.
   - a. Thymosin
   - b. Endotoxin
   - c. Interleukin
   - d. Infection
   - e. Antigen

Fill in the Blank Exercise

Answer each of these questions by filling in the correct answers in the blanks provided.

1. Name the four blood types in the ABO blood group system.

   _____   _____   _____   _____

2. Granulocytes is a category that includes which three types of white blood cells?

   _____   _____   _____

3. Give three names for a neutrophil.

   _____   _____   _____

4. Name the two lymphoid organs in the chest and abdomen.

   _____   _____

Matching Exercise

Match each word or phrase to its description.

1. lymph   _____ Limit the extent and duration of the immune response

2. CD4 cell   _____ Released from basophils

3. tumor necrosis factor   _____ Destroys cancerous cells and endotoxins produced by bacteria

4. histamine   _____ Cells that make antibodies

5. plasma cells   _____ Destroys pathogens not coated by antibodies or complement proteins

6. spleen   _____ Hormones produced by the thymus

7. suppressor T cells _____ Filters blood and removes old erythrocytes

8. NK cell   _____ Another name for lymph nodes

9. thymosins   _____ Helper T cell

10. lymph glands   _____ Fluid that flows through the lymphatic system

Diseases and Conditions

Matching Exercise

Match each word or phrase to its definition.

1. acute lymphocytic   _____ Abnormal protein in the urine seen in multiple myeloma

2. AIDS 4   _____ Caused by exposure to chemicals or radiation

3. anisocytosis   _____ Cancerous tumor in a lymph node

4. aplastic anemia   _____ Cells seen in Hodgkin's lymphoma

5. Bence Jones protein   _____ Enlargement of the spleen

6. dyscrasia 14   _____ Causes hemolysis of erythrocytes

7. hemophilia 7   _____ Genetic disease transmitted on the X chromosome of females

8. lymphoma 6   _____ Any disease condition of the blood

9. polycythemia vera 12   _____ Crescent-shaped red blood cells

10. Reed-Sternberg cells   _____ Severe bacterial infection in the blood

11. septicemia 2   _____ Sexually transmitted viral disease

12. sickle cell anemia 1   _____ Most common leukemia in childhood

13. splenomegaly 3   _____ Erythrocytes vary in size from very small to very large

14. transfusion reaction   _____ A blood clot

15. thrombus 9   _____ Blood becomes thick with erythrocytes

True or False Exercise

Indicate whether each statement is true or false by writing T or F on the line.

1. _____ Pancytopenia is a condition of decreased numbers of just platelets in the blood.

2. _____ In iron deficiency anemia, the erythrocytes are microcytic and hypochromic.

3. _____ Opportunistic infections cause diseases in people who already have hemophilia.

4. _____ Lymphadenopathy is enlarged lymph nodes.

5. _____ A low oxygen level in a person with sickle cell disease causes the red blood cells to become sickled.

6. _____ All patients with HIV also have AIDS.

7. _____ AIDS is a sexually transmitted disease that is also known as the kissing disease.

8. _____ The most common type of hemophilia is lacking blood clotting factor I.

9. _____ Petechiae are pinpoint hemorrhages in the skin.

10. _____ A thymoma is a usually benign tumor of the thymus.

Multiple Choice Exercise

Circle the choice that best answers the question or completes the statement.

1. Which of the following is an inherited genetic disease?
   - a. hemophilia
   - b. thymoma
   - c. HIV
   - d. iron deficiency anemia

2. Poikilocytosis includes all of these abnormally shaped cells *except* _____.
   - a. spherocyte
   - b. blast
   - c. target cell
   - d. sickle cell

3. Pernicious anemia is most commonly seen in _____.
   - a. children
   - b. patients with cancer
   - c. women
   - d. older adults

4. Which of the following diseases is caused by the Epstein-Barr virus (EBV)?
   - a. leukemia
   - b. anemia
   - c. mononucleosis
   - d. thalassemia

Laboratory, Radiology, Surgery, and Drugs

Circle Exercise

Circle the correct word from the choices given.

1. The physician would order a (**ferritin level, lymphangiography, type and crossmatch**) to see if a patient had iron deficiency anemia.

2. A bone marrow aspiration is done by taking red marrow from the (**blood, iliac crest, spleen**).

3. The red blood cell indices include (**HCT, MCV, WBC**).

4. The (**DNA, HCT, INR**) is given in a standardized international measurement along with the PT.

5. What test uses gel and an electric current to separate proteins? (**electrophoresis, prothrombin time, Schilling test**)

6. The (**CBC, CD4 count, heterophil antibodies test**) measures the number of helper T lymphocytes.

7. (**Anticoagulant, Antiretroviral, Thrombolytic**) drugs are used to break apart an already formed blood clot.

Matching Exercise

Match each word or phrase to its description.

1. blood smear   _____ It counts the number of different types of leukocytes

2. blood type   _____ Manual test under the microscope to look for abnormal blood cells

3. bone marrow aspiration _____ Used to diagnose mononucleosis

4. differential   _____ Done to harvest bone marrow

5. hematocrit   _____ Uses attenuated or killed bacteria

6. lymphangiography   _____ Uses dye to outline the lymphatic system

7. MonoSpot test   _____ Used to diagnose pernicious anemia

8. Schilling test   _____ Percentage of erythrocytes in a sample of blood

9. shift to the left   _____ ABO and Rh systems

10. vaccine   _____ Presence of many bands on a blood smear that indicates a severe bacterial infection

Building Medical Words

Review the Combining Forms Exercise, Combining Form and Suffix Exercise, Prefix Exercise, and Multiple Combining Forms and Suffix Exercise that you already completed in the anatomy section on pages 290–292.

Combining Forms Exercise

Before you build blood and lymphatic words, review these additional combining forms, Next to each combining form, write its medical meaning. The first one has been done for you.

Combining Form	Medical Meaning	Combining Form	Medical Meaning
1. angi/o-	blood vessel; lymphatic vessel	16. fus/o-	
2. aden/o-		17. heter/o-	
3. agglutin/o-		18. idi/o-	
4. all/o-		19. log/o-	
5. anis/o-		20. ly/o-	
6. attenu/o-		21. megal/o-	
7. aut/o-		22. micr/o-	
8. bi/o-		23. morph/o-	
9. calc/o-		24. phil/o-	
10. chrom/o-		25. phleb/o-	
11. defici/o-		26. poikil/o-	
12. dissect/o-		27. punct/o-	
13. embol/o-		28. septic/o-	
14. excis/o-		29. vaccin/o-	
15. ferrit/o-		30. ven/i-	

Prefix Exercise

Read the definition of the medical word. Look at the medical word or partial word that is given (it already contains a combining form and a suffix). Select the correct prefix from the Prefix List and write it on the blank line. Then build the medical word and write it on the line. Be sure to check you spelling. The first one has been done for you.

PREFIX LIST

a- (away from; without)	hyper- (above; more than normal)	intra- (within)	trans- (across; through)
anti- (against)	hypo- (below; deficient)	pan- (all)	

Definition of the Medical Word	Prefix	Word or Partial Word	Build the Medical Word
1. Pertaining to without growth or formation (of blood cells)	a-	plastic	aplastic
2. Pertaining to (red blood cells with) deficient (color)		chromic	
3. Condition of deficiency (of) all (blood) cells		cytopenia	
4. Action of through (a vein) pouring (in a unit of blood)		fusion	
5. Pertaining to (a drug that acts) against (blood) clotting		coagulant	
6. Condition in the blood of more than normal calcium		calcemia	
7. Pertaining to within the blood vessel		vascular	

Related Combining Forms Exercise

Write the combining forms on the line provided. (Hint: See the It's Greek to Me feature box)

1. Two combining forms that mean *cell*. _____

2. Two combining forms that mean *nucleus*. _____

3. Two combining forms that mean *vein*. _____

Combining Form and Suffix Exercise

Read the definition of the medical word. Select the correct suffix from the Suffix List. Select the correct combining form from the Combining Form List. Build the medical word and write it on the line. Be sure to check your spelling. The first one has been done for you.

SUFFIX LIST	COMBINING FORM LIST	
-ated (pertaining to a condition; composed of)	agglutin/o- (clumping; sticking)	morph/o- (shape)
-ation (a process; being or having)	attenu/o- (weakened)	myel/o- (bone marrow; spinal cord; myelin)
-cyte (cell)	aut/o- (self)	
-ectomy (surgical excision)	coagul/o- (clotting)	phleb/o- (vein)
-edema (swelling)	embol/o- (embolus; occluding plug)	septic/o- (infection)
-emia (condition of the blood)	hem/o- (blood)	splen/o- (spleen)
-immune (immune response)	leuk/o- (white)	thromb/o- (thrombus; blood clot)
-ism (process; disease from a specific cause)	lymph/o- (lymph; lymphatic system)	thym/o- (thymus)
-ization (process of making, creating, or inserting)	micr/o- (one millionth; small)	vaccin/o- (giving a vaccine)
-logy (the study of)		
-lysis (process of breaking down)		
-megaly (enlargement)		
-oma (tumor; mass)		
-osis (condition; abnormal condition)		
-pathy (disease; suffering)		
-rrhage (excessive flow or discharge)		
-tomy (process of cutting or making an incision)		

Definition of the Medical Word

1. Cell (that is an abnormally) small (red blood cell)
2. Excessive flow or discharge of blood
3. Condition of the blood (of too many) white (blood cells)
4. Process of breaking down (red) blood (cells during a transfusion reaction)
5. Disease of (blood) clotting
6. Disease from a specific cause (of an) embolus (occluding plug)
7. Tumor of a lymph node
8. Condition of the blood (having) infection
9. The study of the shape (of red blood cells)
10. Abnormal condition of (having a) thrombus (blood clot)
11. Tumor of the bone marrow
12. Process of cutting into a vein (to draw blood)
13. Process of inserting (and) giving a vaccine
14. Surgical excision of the spleen

Build the Medical Word

1. microcyte _____
2. _____
3. _____
4. _____
5. _____
6. _____
7. _____
8. _____
9. _____
10. _____
11. _____
12. _____
13. _____
14. _____

Definition of the Medical Word

Build the Medical Word

15. Swelling (because the) lymph (is not draining well)

_____

16. Immune response (directed at one's own) self (and body)

_____

17. Process of (platelets) clumping or sticking (together)

_____

18. Enlargement of the spleen

_____

19. Tumor of the thymus

_____

20. Composed of weakened (bacteria in a vaccine)

_____

Multiple Combining Forms and Suffix Exercise

Read the definition of the medical word. Select the correct suffix and combining forms. Then build the medical word and write it on the line. Be sure to check your spelling. The first one has been done for you.

SUFFIX LIST	COMBINING FORM LIST	
-ency (condition of being)	aden/o- (gland)	lymph/o- (lymph; lymphatic system)
-esis (a process)	angi/o- (blood vessel; lymphatic vessel)	ly/o- (break down; destroy)
-graphy (process of recording)	anis/o- (unequal)	mon/o- (one; single)
-ia (condition; state; thing)	cyt/o- (cell)	norm/o- (normal; usual)
-ic (pertaining to)	defici/o- (lacking; inadequate)	nucle/o- (nucleus of a cell)
-ist (one who specializes in)	electr/o- (electricity)	phil/o- (attraction to; fondness for)
-osis (condition; abnormal condition; process)	hemat/o- (blood)	phor/o- (to bear; to carry; range)
-pathy (disease; suffering)	hem/o- (blood)	poikil/o- (irregular)
-penia (condition of deficiency)	immun/o- (immune response)	punct/o- (hole; perforation)
-tic (pertaining to)	log/o- (word; the study of)	thromb/o- (thrombus; blood clot)
-ure (system; result of)		ven/i- (vein)

Definition of the Medical Word

Build the Medical Word

1. Abnormal condition of irregular (shapes of red blood) cells

_poikilocytosis_____

2. Condition (in which the) blood has a fondness (for bleeding)

_____

3. Disease of the lymph gland

_____

4. Abnormal condition (that affects monocytes that have) one (unlobed) nucleus

_____

5. Pertaining to a normal (size of red blood) cell

_____

6. Condition of deficiency (in the number of) blood clot-making cells

_____

7. Condition of being (in which the) immune response is lacking or inadequate

_____

8. A process (that uses) electricity to carry (immunoglobulins in a gel)

_____

9. Pertaining to (a drug that acts on a) thrombus to break down and destroy (it)

_____

10. Process of recording lymph and a lymphatic vessel (by using contrast dye)

_____

11. Abnormal condition of unequal (sizes of red blood) cells

_____

12. System (for creating in a) vein a hole (to withdraw blood)

_____

13. One who specializes in blood and the study of (it)

_____

Abbreviations

Matching Exercise

Match each abbreviation to its description.

1. ABO
2. CBC
3. DIC
4. EBV
5. H&H
6. HIV
7. HLA
8. PMN
9. PRBCs
10. PT
11. CML

_____ Hemoglobin and hematocrit tests

_____ Another name for a neutrophil

_____ A type of leukemia

_____ Causes AIDS

_____ Blood types that must be matched for blood transfusions

_____ Concentrated erythrocytes for transfusion

_____ Disease with both clotting and hemorrhage at the same time

_____ Common test on all blood cells

_____ Must be matched for bone marrow and organ transplantation

_____ Causes mononucleosis

_____ Test that measures coagulation time of blood

Applied Skills

Laboratory Report Exercise

Read the laboratory report and answer the questions.

ACCESSION NUMBER: 309-019   PATIENT NAME: THOMAS, Irene

LOCATION: Central Lab   PATIENT ID NUMBER: 365-14-3972

DATE DRAWN: 11/19/xx   DATE OF BIRTH: 07/29/xx

DATE RECEIVED: 11/19/xx   SEX: Female

TIME RECEIVED: 0900

TEST	Result	Normal Range	Technician
COMPLETE BLOOD COUNT (CBC)			
RBC	4.7 m/mL	4.2–5.7 m/cmm	JRT
Hemoglobin	14.7 g/dL	12.6–16.6 g/dL	JRT
Hematocrit	42.9%	38.0–50.0%	JRT
MCV	91.2 fL	80–100 fL	JRT
MCH	31.3 pg	28.0–33.0 pg	JRT
MCHC	34.3 g/dL	32–36 g/dL	JRT
WBC	7.7 k/mL	4.3–10.5 k/mL	JRT
Platelets	130 k/mL	150–450 k/mL	JRT

Fact Finding Questions

1. What is the name of the group of tests done on this patient? _____

2. What unit of measurement is used to report RBCs? _____

3. Write out this unit of measurement in words. _____

4. What individual test result was not within the normal range of values? _____

5. What does the *k* stand for in the unit of measurement k/mL? _____

Medical Report Exercise

Read this Emergency Department Report and answer the questions.

EMERGENCY DEPARTMENT REPORT

PATIENT NAME: JONES, Jerome

HOSPITAL NUMBER: 635-64-46223

DATE: November 19, 20xx

HISTORY OF PRESENT ILLNESS
This 42-year-old black male presented to the emergency room today with complaints of dysphagia, extreme weakness, fevers, diarrhea, and weight loss.

PAST MEDICAL HISTORY
He has a prior history of intravenous heroin use for many years and was diagnosed with HIV about 6 years ago. At that time, he tested HIV positive, but was asymptomatic. His CD4 count then was 500. He was subsequently lost to follow-up until recently. In the last few months, his health has deteriorated rapidly, but he refused to seek medical attention. Last month, however, he was admitted to this hospital through the emergency department in respiratory distress with a CD4 count of 100 and was diagnosed with *Pneumocystis jiroveci* pneumonia and AIDS. He was given a 14-day course of intravenous pentamidine. He was discharged on a triple-drug regimen of Retrovir, Epivir, and Sustiva. He was also given a prescription for aerosolized pentamidine to prevent future episodes of this pneumonia. Today he states that he has been noncompliant with his drug therapy, stating that he does not take his AIDS drugs on a regular basis.

PHYSICAL EXAMINATION
GENERAL: Physical examination today showed a black male appearing much older than his stated age. Temperature 101.2, pulse 100, respirations 26, blood pressure 110/76. Height: 5 feet 11 inches. Weight 128 pounds.
HEENT exam: Normocephalic, atraumatic. Eyes: Sclerae and conjunctivae pale and nonicteric. Mouth: White plaque coating on the tongue and underneath is beefy red and bleeds slightly. Neck: The neck is supple. There is cervical lymphadenopathy.
HEART: Regular rate and rhythm.
CHEST: Clear.
ABDOMEN: Soft, nontender, with normal bowel sounds.
EXTREMITIES: Wasting of the extremities. Extreme weakness with muscle strength decreased on both sides. Deep tendon reflexes intact bilaterally. The skin shows no evidence of Kaposi's sarcoma.

DIAGNOSES
1. Oral candidiasis.
2. Wasting syndrome, secondary to acquired immunodeficiency syndrome (AIDS).
3. Acquired immunodeficiency syndrome (AIDS).
4. Past history of *Pneumocystis jiroveci* pneumonia.

PLAN
Blood work was sent for CBC and differential and CD4 total count. The patient was restarted on his antiretroviral 3-drug regimen of Retrovir 300 mg b.i.d., Epivir 150 mg b.i.d., and Sustiva 600 mg q.d. h.s. He was given nystatin oral suspension 5 cc q.i.d., swish and swallow, to treat his oral infection with *Candida albicans*. He will be started on Megace oral suspension, 20 mg/0.5 cc, to stimulate his appetite and help him gain weight.

Joseph K. McAdams, M.D.

Joseph K. McAdams, M.D.

JKM:ltt
D: 11/19/xx
T: 11/19/xx

Fact Finding Questions

1. Six years ago, the patient was "asymptomatic," which means that _____.
   a. he did not have an HIV infection
   b. he did not have any symptoms of an HIV infection
   c. he was healthy

2. The patient has developed what two opportunistic infections?

   _____

   _____

3. What was the patient's CD4 count 6 years ago? _____

   What was the patient's CD4 count when he was diagnosed with AIDS? _____

   Which CD4 count is more desirable to have? _____

4. What three drugs (triple-drug regimen) were prescribed for the patient's AIDS?

   _____

   _____

   _____

5. What laboratory test was ordered to show the current number of helper T lymphocytes? _____

6. What does the physical examination show about the patient's lymph nodes in his neck? _____

Critical Thinking Questions

1. What is the probable source of the patient's HIV infection? _____

2. Which of these symptoms would be related to the patient's oral candidiasis?
   a. extreme weakness   c. dysphagia
   b. fevers   d. diarrhea

3. When the patient was admitted to the hospital last month with *Pneumocystis jiroveci* pneumonia, why was his diagnosis changed from HIV positive to AIDS? _____

4. The patient is diagnosed with wasting syndrome due to AIDS. What three pieces of information support this diagnosis?
   a. Hint: Look for a phrase at the beginning of the History of Present Illness.

   _____

   b. Hint: Look for a measurement in the "General" section of the Physical Examination.

   _____

   c. Hint: Look for a phrase in the "Extremities" section of the Physical Examination.

   _____

Hearing Medical Words Exercise

You hear someone speaking the medical words given below. Read each pronunciation and then write the medical word it represents. Be sure to check your spelling. The first one has been done for you.

1. ah-NEE-mee-ah   *anemia*
2. AW-toh-im-MYOON   _____
3. EM-boh-LIZ-em   _____
4. HEE-mah-TAWL-oh-jist   _____
5. HEM-oh-rij   _____

6. IM-myoo-noh-GLAWB-yoo-lin   _____
7. loo-KEE-mee-ah   _____
8. lim-FAN-jee-oh-gram   _____
9. MAWN-oh-noo-klee-OH-sis   _____
10. fleh-BAW-toh-mee   _____

Pronunciation Exercise

Read the medical word that is given. Then review the syllables in the pronunciation. Circle the primary (main) accented syllable. The first one has been done for you.

1. leukocyte (**loo**-koh-site)
2. erythrocyte (eh-rith-roh-site)
3. eosinophil (ee-oh-sin-oh-fil)
4. lymphatic (lim-fat-ik)
5. coagulation (koh-ag-yoo-lay-shun)

6. pathogen (path-oh-jen)
7. septicemia (sep-tih-see-mee-ah)
8. hemophilia (hee-moh-fil-ee-ah)
9. phlebotomy (fleh-baw-toh-mee)
10. splenectomy (spleh-nek-toh-mee)

Multimedia Preview

Immerse yourself in a variety of activities inside Medical Terminology Interactive. Getting there is simple:

1. Click on www.myhealthprofessionskit.com.
2. Select "Medical Terminology" from the choice of disciplines.
3. First-time users must create an account using the scratch-off code on the inside front cover of this book.
4. Find this book and log in using your username and password.
5. Click on Medical Terminology Interactive.
6. Take the elevator to the 6th Floor to begin your virtual exploration of this chapter!

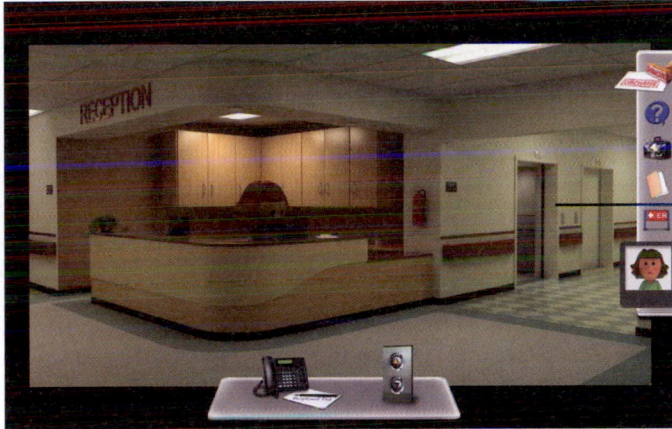 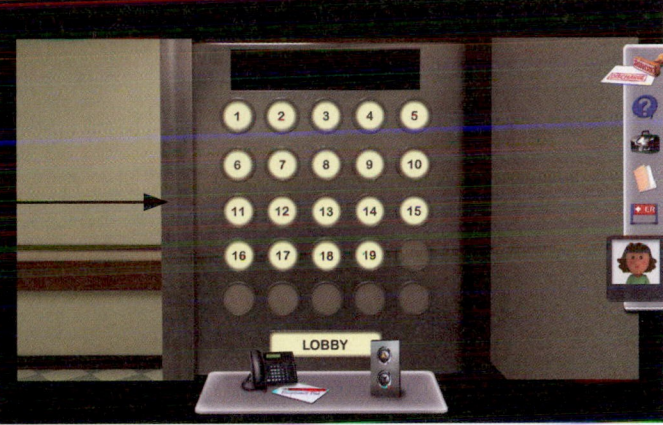

■ **Word Search**   Secret terms are hidden throughout the grid and we simply provide you with clues. Your task is to figure out what terms to find and then to seek them out. Grab a magnifying glass and your thinking cap. You'll need both!

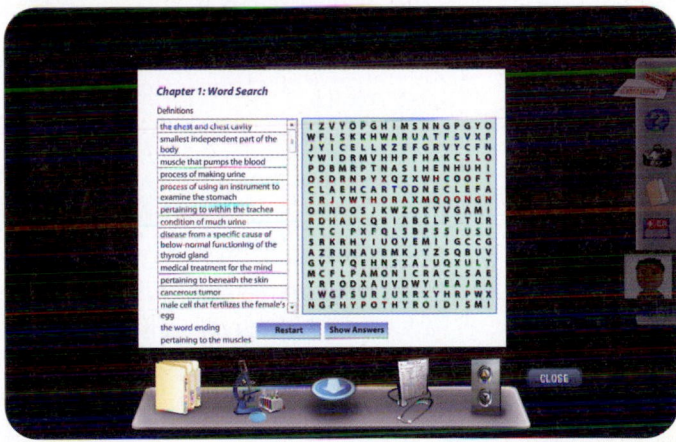

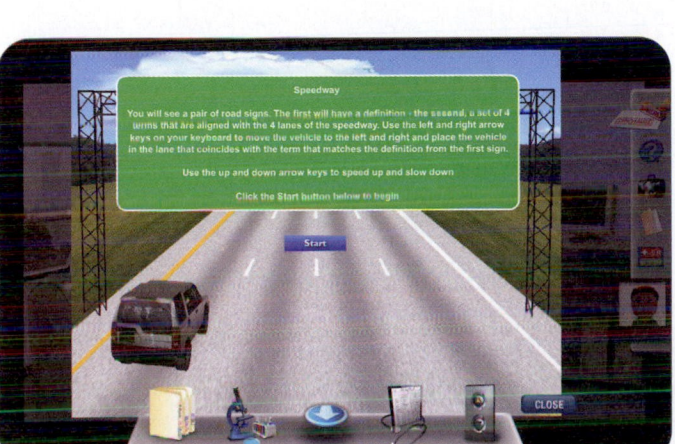

■ **Speedway**   Take a ride on the Medical Terminology superhighway. Choose a set of wheels and steer your way toward mastery by choosing the correct lanes. How fast can you accumulate 15 correct answers? Start your answers!

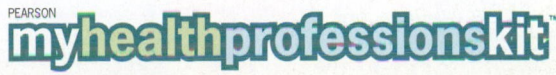

PEARSON
myhealthprofessionskit™

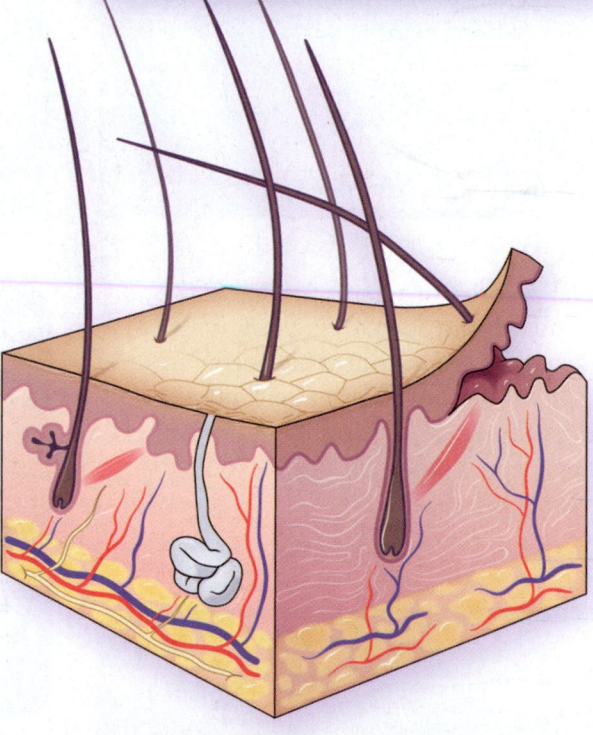

Dive In!

- There are more living organisms on the skin of a single human being than there are human beings on the surface of the earth.

- The thumbnail grows the slowest; the middle nail grows the fastest

- Ready to explore deeper layers of knowledge? In this chapter we'll explore the language that describes integumentary system structures, functions, diseases, and conditions.

- You'll move beyond scratching the surface once you master the language of dermatology!

▶ The integumentary system covers the entire surface of the body, consisting of the skin, hair, and nails in all their many variations of colors and shapes.

▶ There are many components within the epidermis and the dermis, which collectively comprise the skin.

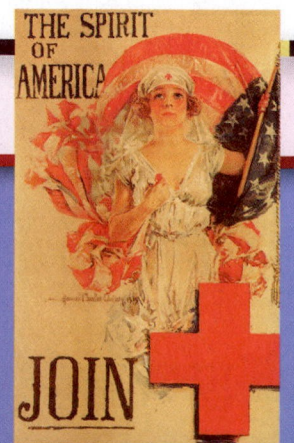

THE SPIRIT OF AMERICA

JOIN

1881

The American Red Cross is founded

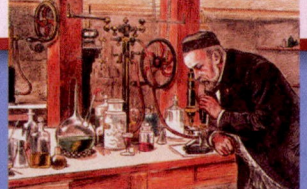

1885

Louis Pasteur develops a vaccine for rabies

1887

British physiologist Augustus Waller performs the first electrocardiography (ECG)

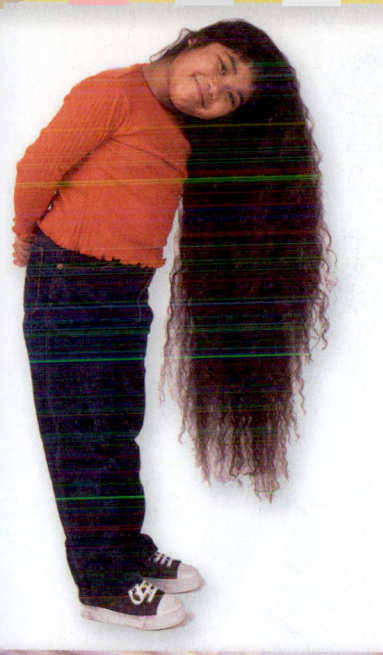

7

Dermatology

Integumentary System

Dermatology (DER-mah-TAWL-oh-jee) is the medical specialty that studies the anatomy and physiology of the integumentary system and uses diagnostic tests, medical and surgical procedures, and drugs to treat integumentary diseases.

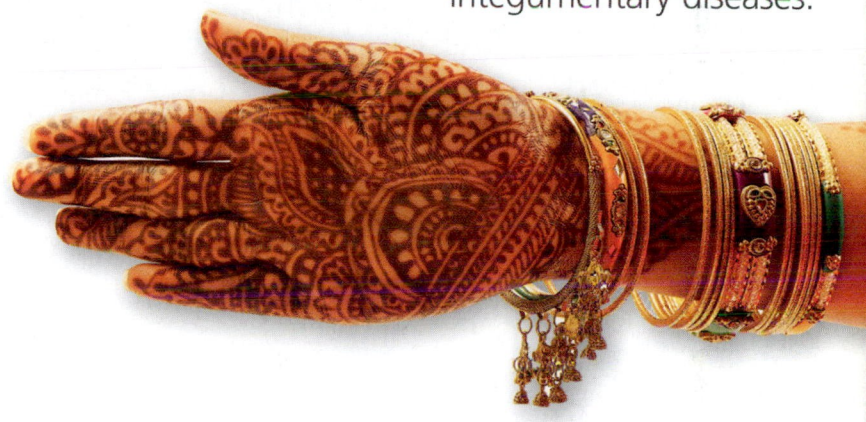

◀ ▲ Hair and skin often hold cultural meaning, and this results in many different styles around the world.

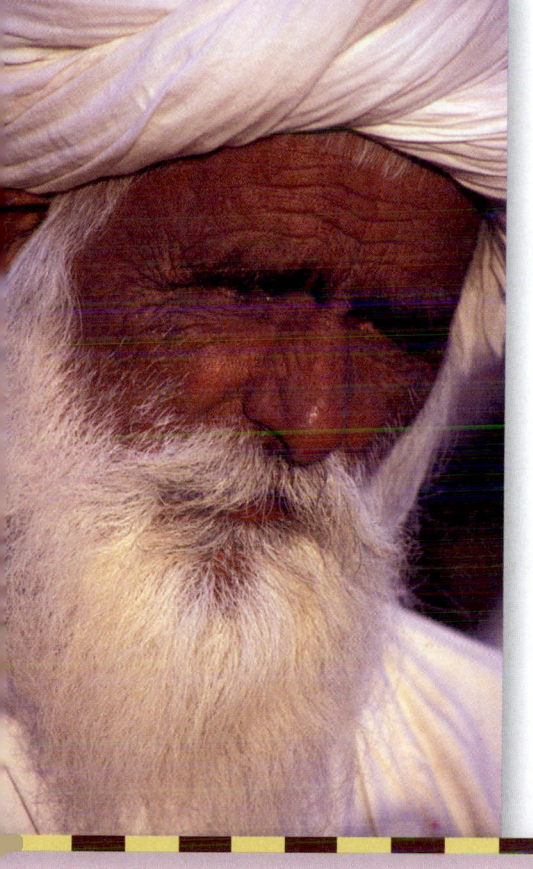

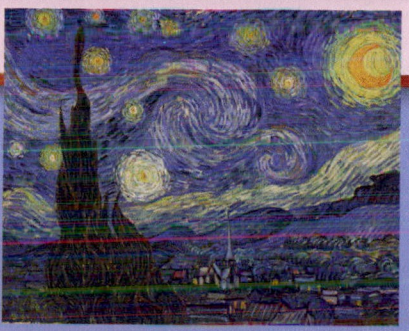

1889

"The Starry Night" is painted by Vincent van Gogh. The artist may have been suffering from digitalis overdose, the toxic effects of which are known to include visual halos around lights

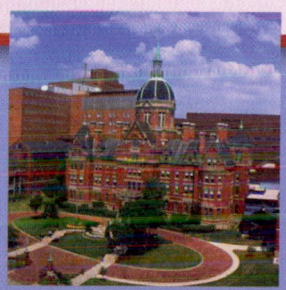

1889

The Johns Hopkins Medical School is founded in Baltimore, Maryland

Measure Your Progress: Learning Objectives

After you study this chapter, you should be able to

1. Identify the structures of the integumentary system.

2. Describe the process of an allergic reaction.

3. Describe common integumentary diseases and conditions, laboratory and diagnostic procedures, medical and surgical procedures, and drug categories.

4. Give the medical meaning of word parts related to the integumentary system.

5. Build integumentary words from word parts and divide and define integumentary words.

6. Spell and pronounce integumentary words.

7. Analyze the medical content and meaning of a dermatology report.

8. Dive deeper into dermatology by reviewing the activities at the end of this chapter and online at Medical Terminology Interactive.

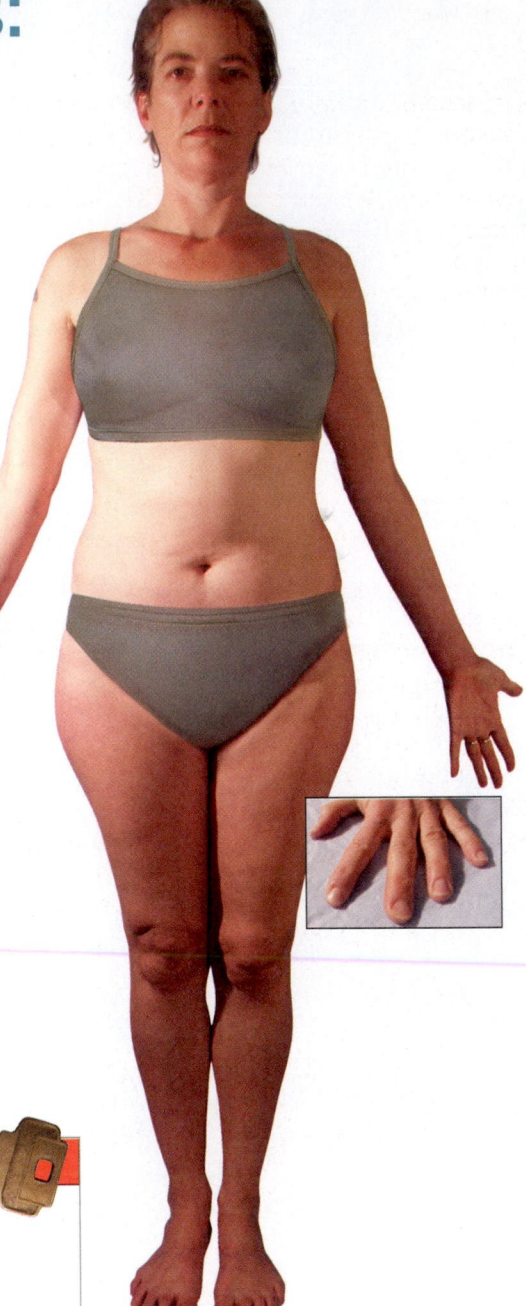

Figure 7-1 ■ **Integumentary system.**

The integumentary system covers the entire surface of the body and consists of the skin, hair, and nails.

Medical Language Key

To unlock the definition of a medical word, break it into word parts. Define each word part. Put the word part meanings in order, beginning with the suffix, then the prefix (if present), then the combining form(s).

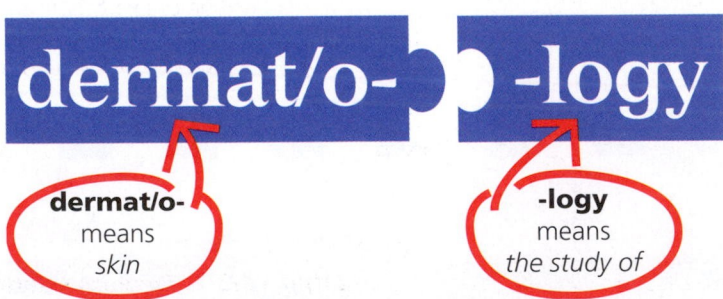

dermat/o-
means
skin

-logy
means
the study of

	Word Part	Word Part Meaning
Suffix	-logy	*the study of*
Combining Form	dermat/o-	*skin*

Dermatology: *The study of the skin (and related structures).*

Anatomy and Physiology

The **integumentary system** (see Figure 7-1 ■) is an extremely large, flat, flexible body system that covers the entire surface of the body. The integumentary system includes the skin (epidermis and dermis), sebaceous glands, sweat glands, hair, and nails. In addition, this chapter will discuss the subcutaneous tissue, a layer of connective tissue that is beneath the skin. The purpose of the integumentary system is to protect the body; it is the body's first line of defense against invading microorganisms. The sense of touch is also part of the integumentary system.

Anatomy of the Integumentary System

Skin

The skin or **integument** consists of two different layers: the epidermis and the dermis. The epidermis is categorized as **epithelium** or **epithelial tissue.** The epithelium covers the external surface of the body, but also includes the mucous membranes that line the walls of internal cavities that connect to the outside of the body. The dermis is categorized as connective tissue.

Epidermis The **epidermis** is the thin, outermost layer of the skin (see Figure 7-2 ■). The most superficial part of the epidermis contains cells that have no nuclei and are filled with **keratin,** a hard, fibrous protein. These cells form a protective layer, but they are dead cells, and so they are constantly being shed or sloughed off. This process is known as **exfoliation.** In

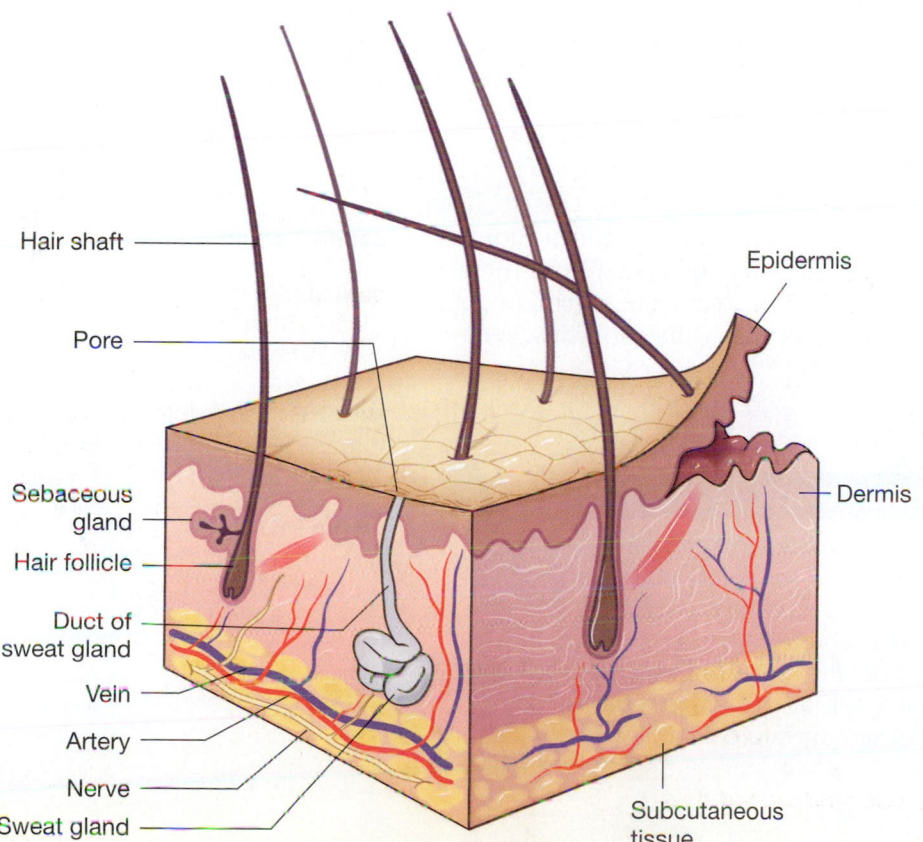

Hair shaft
Pore
Sebaceous gland
Hair follicle
Duct of sweat gland
Vein
Artery
Nerve
Sweat gland
Epidermis
Dermis
Subcutaneous tissue

WORD BUILDING

integumentary
(in-TEG-yoo-MEN-tair-ee)
   integument/o- *skin*
   -ary *pertaining to*

cutaneous (kyoo-TAY-nee-us)
   cutane/o- *skin*
   -ous *pertaining to*
Cutaneous is also the adjective form for *skin*. The combining forms *cut/i-, derm/a, dermat/o-,* and *derm/o-* also mean *skin*.

integument (in-TEG-yoo-ment)
   integu/o- *to cover*
   -ment *action; state*

epithelium (EP-ih-THEE-lee-um)
   epi- *upon; above*
   theli/o- *cellular layer*
   -um *a structure; period of time*

epithelial (EP-ih-THEE-lee-al)
   epi- *upon; above*
   theli/o- *cellular layer*
   -al *pertaining to*

epidermis (EP-ih-DER-mis)

epidermal (EP-ih-DER-mal)
   epi- *upon; above*
   derm/o- *skin*
   -al *pertaining to*

keratin (KAIR-ah-tin)
   kerat/o- *cornea (of the eye); hard, fibrous protein*
   -in *a substance*

exfoliation (eks-FOH-lee-AA-shun)
   ex- *out; away from*
   foli/o- *leaf*
   -ation *a process; being or having*
Add words to make a complete definition of *exfoliation: a process (of skin cells moving) away from (the body like a) leaf (falling off a tree).*

Figure 7-2 ■ Epidermis and dermis.
The skin is composed of the epidermis and the dermis. The epidermis contains dead protective cells on its surface and living, actively dividing cells at its base. The dermis contains hair follicles, sebaceous glands, and sweat glands. The subcutaneous tissue, a type of connective tissue, lies beneath the dermis.

contrast, the deepest part or **basal layer** of the epidermis is composed of living cells that are constantly dividing and being forced to the surface. The epidermis does not contain any blood vessels. It receives nutrients and oxygen from the blood vessels in the dermis.

The epidermis also contains **melanocytes,** pigment cells that produce **melanin,** a dark brown or black pigment. Melanin in the epidermis absorbs ultraviolet light from the sun to protect the DNA in skin cells from undergoing genetic mutations.

Did You Know?

All races have the same number of melanocytes in the skin. The differences in skin color occur because of differing levels of melanin production. Dark-skinned people produce more melanin than fair-skinned people. Albinos have a normal number of melanocytes in their skin, but the cells do not produce any melanin. Exposure to the sun's ultraviolet rays increases the rate of melanin production in all people and causes a suntan. During prolonged sun exposure, the melanin is unable to absorb all of the ultraviolet light, and the result is a sunburn.

Clinical Connections

Dietetics. The sun's ultraviolet rays convert cholesterol in the epidermis to a compound that is then made into vitamin D. The amount of vitamin D produced depends on the time of day and the season of the year. About 20–45 minutes of sunlight per week produces sufficient amounts of vitamin D. Vitamin D is stored in fat cells in the subcutaneous tissue. It helps the body absorb and use the calcium and phosphorus from foods. Vitamin D also protects the entire body against many types of cancer.

Dermis The **dermis** is a thicker layer beneath the epidermis (see Figure 7-2). It is both firm and elastic because it contains **collagen** fibers (firm, white protein) and **elastin** fibers (elastic, yellow protein). The dermis contains arteries, veins, and neurons (nerve cells), as well as hair follicles, sebaceous glands, and sweat glands.

Clinical Connections

Neurology. The neurons in the dermis are stimulated by light touch, pressure, vibration, pain, and temperature. When you touch something hot, the sensation is carried as sensory information by the neuron from the skin to the spinal cord. The spinal cord immediately sends a motor command to a muscle for you to move your hand away from the heat. This takes place without any conscious input from the brain. It is only after your hand has already moved that your brain finally receives that sensory information and thinks "That was hot!"

WORD BUILDING

basal (BAY-sal)
  bas/o- *base of a structure; basic (alkaline)*
  -al *pertaining to*

melanocyte (meh-LAN-oh-site) (MEL-ah-noh-site)
  melan/o- *black*
  -cyte *cell*
Add words to make a complete definition of *melanocyte: cell (in the skin that produces a dark brown or) black (pigment).*

melanin (MEL-ah-nin)
  melan/o- *black*
  -in *a substance*

dermis (DER-mis)

dermal (DER-mal)
  derm/o- *skin*
  -al *pertaining to*

collagen (KAWL-ah-jen)
  coll/a- *fibers that hold together*
  -gen *that which produces*

elastin (ee-LAS-tin)
  elast/o- *flexing; stretching*
  -in *a substance*

A **dermatome** is a specific area on the skin that sends sensory information to the spinal cord (see Figure 7-3 ■).

WORD BUILDING

dermatome (DER-mah-tohm)
  derm/a- *skin*
  -tome *instrument used to cut; area with distinct edges*

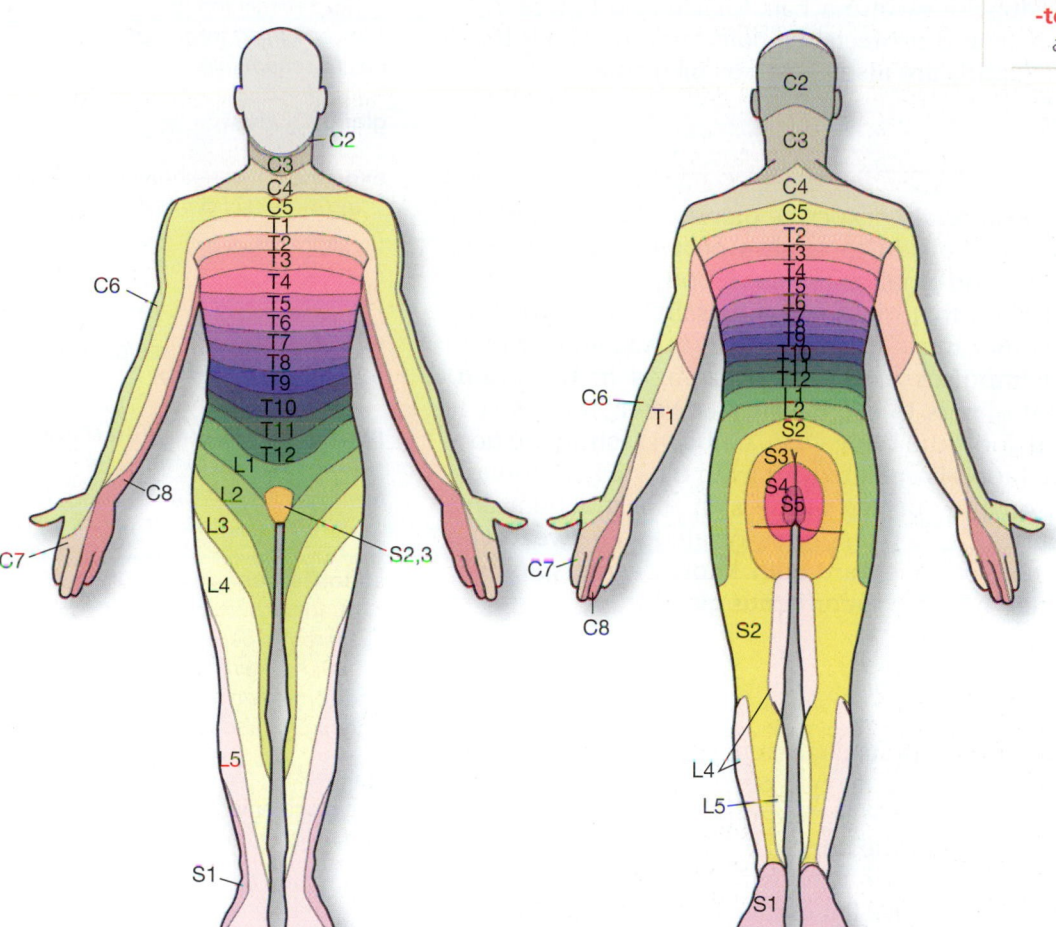

Figure 7-3 ■ Dermatomes of the body.

A dermatome is a specific area of the skin that sends sensory information through a spinal nerve to the spinal cord. Each dermatome is named according to the level at which the spinal nerve enters the spinal cord. *C* stands for the spinal cord at the level of the neck (the combining form *cervic/o-* means *neck*). *T* stands for the spinal cord at the level of the thorax. *L* stands for the spinal cord at the level of the lower back. *S* stands for the spinal cord at the level of the sacrum (last bone in the spinal column). The skin of the face sends sensory information through the cranial nerves to the brain.

A Closer Look

The skin is the body's first line of defense against disease and injury. The dead cells of the outer epidermis present a dry and slightly acidic environment that discourages the growth of microorganisms. The constant shedding of epidermal cells prevents microorganisms from multiplying and invading the dermis. Sweat and sebum (oil) contain antibodies and enzymes that kill bacteria. Normal skin flora (bacteria that are able to thrive under these conditions) do not cause disease, and they inhibit the growth of disease-causing microorganisms by competing with them for space and nutrients.

Sebaceous Glands

The **sebaceous glands** in the dermis are a type of **exocrine gland.** They secrete **sebum** through a duct that goes into a hair follicle (see Figure 7-2). Sebum consists of oil that coats and protects the hair shaft to keep it from becoming brittle. Sebaceous glands are also known as **oil glands.**

Sweat Glands

The **sweat glands** in the dermis are also exocrine glands. The sweat gland duct opens onto the surface of the skin through a pore (see Figure 7-2). Sweat contains water, sodium, and small amounts of body wastes (ammonia, creatinine, urea). It is sodium that gives sweat its salty taste. Sweating helps to regulate the body temperature. When the body is hot, temperature receptors in the skin send impulses to the hypothalamus in the brain, which then signals the sweat glands to secrete sweat. Water in the sweat evaporates from the skin and cools the body. Also, blood vessels in the dermis dilate, and heat from the blood is radiated out from the body. Although sweat is odorless, bacteria on the surface of the skin digest sebum and sweat, and their waste products cause the odor associated with sweat. The process of sweating and the sweat itself are both known as **perspiration.** The sweat glands are also known as the **sudoriferous glands.**

Hair

Hair covers most of the body, although its consistency and color vary from one part of the body to another and from one person to the next. Additional facial, axillary, and pubic hairs appear during puberty.

Each hair forms in a hair **follicle** in the dermis (see Figure 7-2). Melanocytes give color to the hair. Hair cells are filled with keratin, which makes the hair shaft strong. Usually, the hair lies flat on the surface of the skin, but when the skin is cold, a tiny erector muscle at the base of the hair follicle contracts and causes the hair to stand up (**piloerection**). The contracted muscle forms a goosebump. In furry animals, the erect hairs create an insulating layer and trap heat near the skin; but this effect is insignificant in humans.

Did You Know?

The scalp contains about 100,000 hairs. Dark hair contains melanin, but blond hair and red hair contain a variant of melanin that contains more sulfur, so the hair is more yellow or orange. As a person ages, the melanocytes stop producing melanin, and the hair appears gray or white. The hair grows fastest during the daytime and during the summer.

Nails

The nails cover and protect the distal ends of the fingers and toes because these areas are easily traumatized. Each nail consists of several parts (see Figure 7-4 ■). The outer layer—the tough, opaque **nail plate**—is composed of dead cells that contain hard keratin. The nail plate rests on the **nail bed,** a layer of living tissue that contains nerve cells and blood vessels. The blood vessels in the nail bed give the nail plate its color, normally pink (but bluish-purple if the oxygen level in the blood is low). The nail bed is also known as the quick. The **cuticle** is an edge of dead cells, arising from the skin along

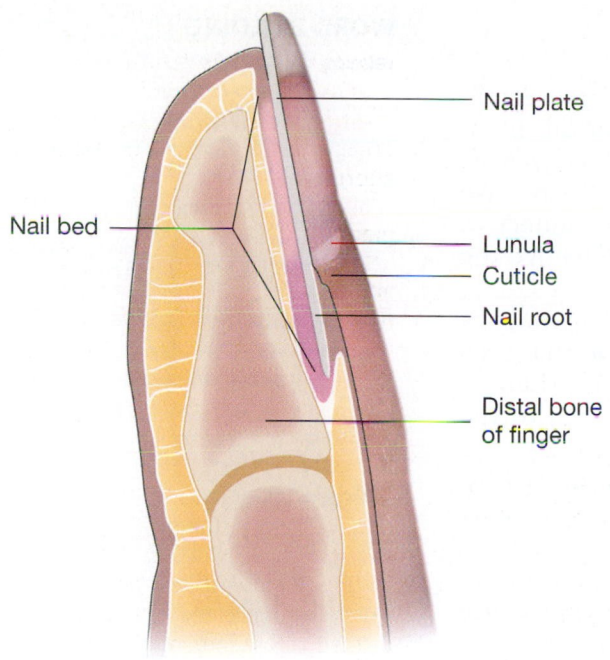

Nail plate

Nail bed

Lunula
Cuticle
Nail root

Distal bone
of finger

Figure 7-4 ■ Nail.
The nail is composed of both living and dead cells. The nail root produces keratin-containing cells that form the lunula. As the nail plate grows, these cells die and harden to form a protective covering for the distal end of the finger.

the proximal end of the nail. The cuticle is adherent to the nail plate to prevent microorganisms from gaining access to the nail root. The **lunula,** the whitish half-moon, is the visible, white part of the nail root. The **nail root,** which is located beneath the skin of the finger, produces keratin-containing cells that form the nail plate. These cells are white at first (in the lunula), but gradually become opaque as the nail plate grows. Trauma or infection of the nail root causes a misshapen nail plate.

lunula (LOO-nyoo-lah)
  lun/o- *moon*
  -ula *small thing*

Subcutaneous Tissue

The **subcutaneous tissue** is a loose, connective tissue. It is not considered to be part of the integumentary system, but because it is directly beneath the dermis of the skin, it is discussed here (see Figure 7-2). It is composed of **adipose tissue** or fat that contains **lipocytes.** These cells store fat as an energy reserve. The amount of fat in adipose tissue usually far exceeds any energy needs the body might have! The subcutaneous tissue also provides a layer of insulation to conserve internal body heat. Depending on a person's metabolism, dietary intake of sugars and fats, and the amount of fat stored in the lipocytes, the subcutaneous tissue can be thin or as thick as several inches. The subcutaneous layer also acts as a cushion to protect the bones and internal organs.

subcutaneous (SUB-kyoo-TAY-nee-us)
  sub- *below; underneath; less than*
  cutane/o- *skin*
  -ous *pertaining to*

adipose (AD-ih-pohs)
  adip/o- *fat*
  -ose *full of*

lipocyte (LIP-oh-site)
  lip/o- *lipid (fat)*
  -cyte *cell*

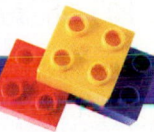

Clinical Connections

Forensic Science. Oil from the sebaceous glands leaves a fingerprint when a person touches something. Each person's fingerprints are a unique combination of whorls, loops, or arches that can be matched to fingerprints on file in a database. Cells from a hair follicle can be analyzed for DNA. Hair can be tested for evidence of toxins or poisons. White horizontal bands on the fingernails indicate arsenic poisoning. Investigators know that if a body was buried in moist dirt, the adipose tissue decomposes and forms a characteristic waxy substance known as **adipocere** (grave wax).

adipocere (AD-ih-poh-SEER)
  adip/o- *fat*
  -cere *waxy substance*

Physiology of an Allergic Reaction

An **allergy** or **allergic reaction** is a **hypersensitivity** response to certain types of antigens known as allergens. **Allergens** include cells from plant and animal sources (foods, pollens, molds, animal dander), as well as dust, chemicals, and drugs. The basis of all allergic reactions is the release of **histamine** from basophils in the blood and **mast cells** in the connective tissue. Allergic reactions anywhere in the body almost always involve the skin or mucous membranes.

A **local reaction** occurs when an allergen touches the skin or mucous membranes of a hypersensitive individual. Histamine released in that area causes inflammation and redness (erythema), swelling (edema), irritation, and itching (pruritus). Examples: Chemicals in deodorant applied to the skin or pollen in the air that enters the nose.

A **systemic reaction** occurs when allergens are inhaled by, ingested by, or injected into a hypersensitive person, causing symptoms in several body systems. Histamine constricts the bronchioles, dilates the blood vessels throughout the body, and causes hives on the skin. Examples: Inhaled pollens, molds, or dust trigger asthma attacks; ingested foods or drugs cause hives on the skin. **Anaphylaxis** is a severe systemic allergic reaction that can be life threatening. Symptoms include respiratory distress, hypotension, and shock. Examples: Eating peanuts, being stung by a bee, taking a drug that has caused a past allergic reaction, or being exposed to latex gloves are all common causes of anaphylaxis in hypersensitive individuals. This is also known as **anaphylactic shock.**

Across the Life Span

Pediatrics. The skin of an infant is smooth and very flexible. It has no wrinkles because of the large amount of elastin in the dermis and the thick layer of fat in the subcutaneous tissue. This fat layer conserves body heat and protects the internal organs as the infant learns to walk.

In persons who smoke, the nicotine in cigarettes decreases oxygen levels in the skin and destroys the collagen fibers. This causes deep wrinkles and gives a leathery quality to the skin, even in middle age.

Geriatrics. In older adults, the amount of elastin decreases, and the skin develops sags and wrinkles. The fat in the subcutaneous layer thins, the skin appears translucent, and arteries and veins—especially in the hands—become obvious. There is a simultaneous underproduction and overproduction of melanin that gives the skin a mottled, irregular appearance.

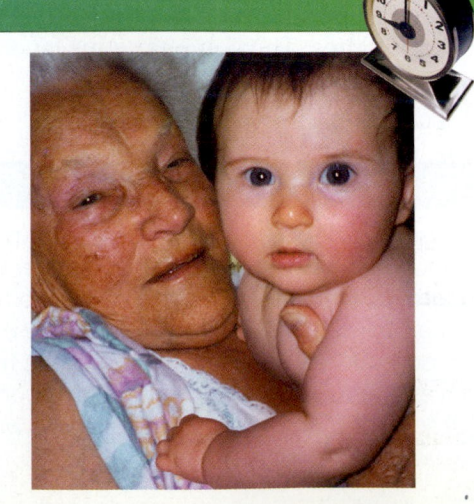

Vocabulary Review

Anatomy and Physiology

Word or Phrase	Description	Combining Forms
integumentary system	Body system that covers the entire surface of the body and consists of the skin, hair, and nails	**integument/o-** *skin*
subcutaneous tissue	Loose, connective tissue directly beneath the dermis. It is composed of **adipose tissue** that contains **lipocytes** that store fat. When a dead body is buried in moist dirt, adipose tissue becomes **adipocere.** The subcutaneous tissue is near, but not part of, the integumentary system.	**cutane/o-** *skin* **adip/o-** *fat* **lip/o-** *lipid (fat)*

Skin, Hair, and Nails

Word or Phrase	Description	Combining Forms
collagen	Firm, white protein connective tissue fibers throughout the dermis	**coll/a-** *fibers that hold together*
cutaneous	Pertaining to the skin	**cutane/o-** *skin*
cuticle	Layer of dead skin that arises from the epidermis around the proximal end of the nail. It keeps microorganisms from entering the nail root.	**cut/i-** *skin*
dermatome	Area of the skin that sends sensory information through one neuron to the spinal cord	**derm/a-** *skin*
dermis	Layer of skin under the epidermis. It contains collagen and elastin fibers. It contains arteries, veins, neurons, sebaceous glands, sweat glands, and hair follicles.	**derm/o-** *skin*
elastin	Elastic, yellow protein fibers in the dermis	**elast/o-** *flexing; stretching*
epidermis	Thin, outermost layer of skin. The most superficial part of the epidermis consists of dead cells filled with keratin. The deepest part or **basal layer** contains constantly dividing cells and melanocytes.	**derm/o-** *skin* **bas/o-** *base of a structure; basic (alkaline)*
epithelium	Tissue category that includes the epidermis and all of its structures. It also includes the mucous membranes that line the walls of internal cavities that connect to the outside of the body. It is also known as **epithelial tissue.**	**theli/o-** *cellular layer*
exfoliation	Normal process of the constant shedding of dead skin cells from the most superficial part of the epidermis	**foli/o-** *leaf*
exocrine gland	Type of gland that secretes substances through a duct. Examples: Sebaceous (oil) glands and sudoriferous (sweat) glands in the dermis.	**ex/o-** *away from; external; outward*
follicle	Site where a hair is formed. Hair follicles are located in the dermis.	**follicul/o-** *follicle (small sac)*
hair	Structure that grows as a shaft from a follicle in the dermis	**pil/o-** *hair* **trich/o-** *hair*
integument	The skin, hair, and nails	**integu/o-** *to cover*
keratin	Hard protein found in the cells of the outermost part of the epidermis and in the nails	**kerat/o-** *cornea (of the eye); hard, fibrous protein*
lipocyte	Cell in the subcutaneous tissue that stores fat	**lip/o-** *lipid (fat)*
lunula	Whitish half-moon that is under the proximal portion of the nail plate. It is the visible white part of the nail root.	**lun/o-** *moon*

Word or Phrase	Description	Combining Forms
melanocyte	Pigment-containing cell in the epidermis that produces **melanin,** a dark brown or black pigment that gives color to the skin and hair	**melan/o-** *black*
nail bed	Layer of living tissue beneath the nail plate. It is also known as the quick.	
nail plate	Hard, flat protective covering over the distal end of each finger and toe. It is composed of dead cells that contain keratin. It is also known as the nail.	**ungu/o-** *nail (fingernail or toenail)* **onych/o-** *nail (fingernail or toenail)*
nail root	Produces cells that form the lunula and nail plate	
perspiration	Process of sweating and the sweat itself. Sweat is secreted by sudoriferous glands. It contains sodium and waste products. As its water content evaporates from the skin, it cools the body.	**spir/o-** *breathe; a coil*
piloerection	Process in which an erector muscle contracts (to form a goosebump) and the body hair becomes erect when the skin is cold.	**pil/o-** *hair* **erect/o-** *to stand up*
sebaceous gland	Exocrine gland of the skin that secretes **sebum** through a duct. Sebaceous glands are in the dermis. The duct joins with a hair follicle, and sebum coats the hair shaft. It is also known as an **oil gland.**	**sebace/o-** *sebum (oil)* **seb/o-** *sebum (oil)*
skin	Tissue covering of the body that consists of two layers (epidermis and dermis). The skin is one part of the integumentary system.	**cutane/o-** *skin* **integument/o-** *skin* **derm/a-** *skin* **dermat/o-** *skin* **derm/o-** *skin*
sudoriferous gland	Exocrine gland of the skin that secretes sweat through a duct. These glands are in the dermis. The duct opens at a pore on the surface of the skin. It is also known as a **sweat gland.**	**sudor/i-** *sweat* **fer/o-** *to bear* **hidr/o-** *sweat* **diaphore/o-** *sweat*

Allergic Reaction

Word or Phrase	Description	Combining Forms
allergen	Cells from plants or animals (foods, pollens, molds, animal dander), as well as dust, chemicals, and drugs that cause an allergic reaction in a hypersensitive person	**all/o-** *other; strange*
allergic reaction	Response to an allergen in a hypersensitive person. An allergic reaction is based on the release of **histamine.** It is also known as an **allergy.**	**all/o-** *other; strange* **erg/o-** *activity; work*
anaphylaxis	Severe systemic allergic reaction characterized by respiratory distress, hypotension, and shock. It is also known as **anaphylactic shock.**	**phylact/o-** *guarding; protecting*
hypersensitivity	Individually unique response to an allergen that provokes an allergic response in some people	**sensitiv/o-** *affected by; sensitive to*
local reaction	Allergic reaction that takes place on an area of the skin that was exposed to an allergen	**loc/o-** *in one place*
mast cells	Cells in the connective tissue that release histamine during an allergic reaction	
systemic reaction	Allergic reaction that takes place throughout the body in a hypersensitive person after contact with an allergen that was ingested, inhaled, or injected	**system/o-** *the body as a whole*

Labeling Exercise

Match each anatomy word or phrase to its structure and write it in the numbered box for each figure. Be sure to check your spelling. Use the Answer Key at the end of the book to check your answers.

artery	duct of sweat gland	hair follicle	nerve	sebaceous gland	sweat gland
dermis	epidermis	hair shaft	pore	subcutaneous tissue	vein

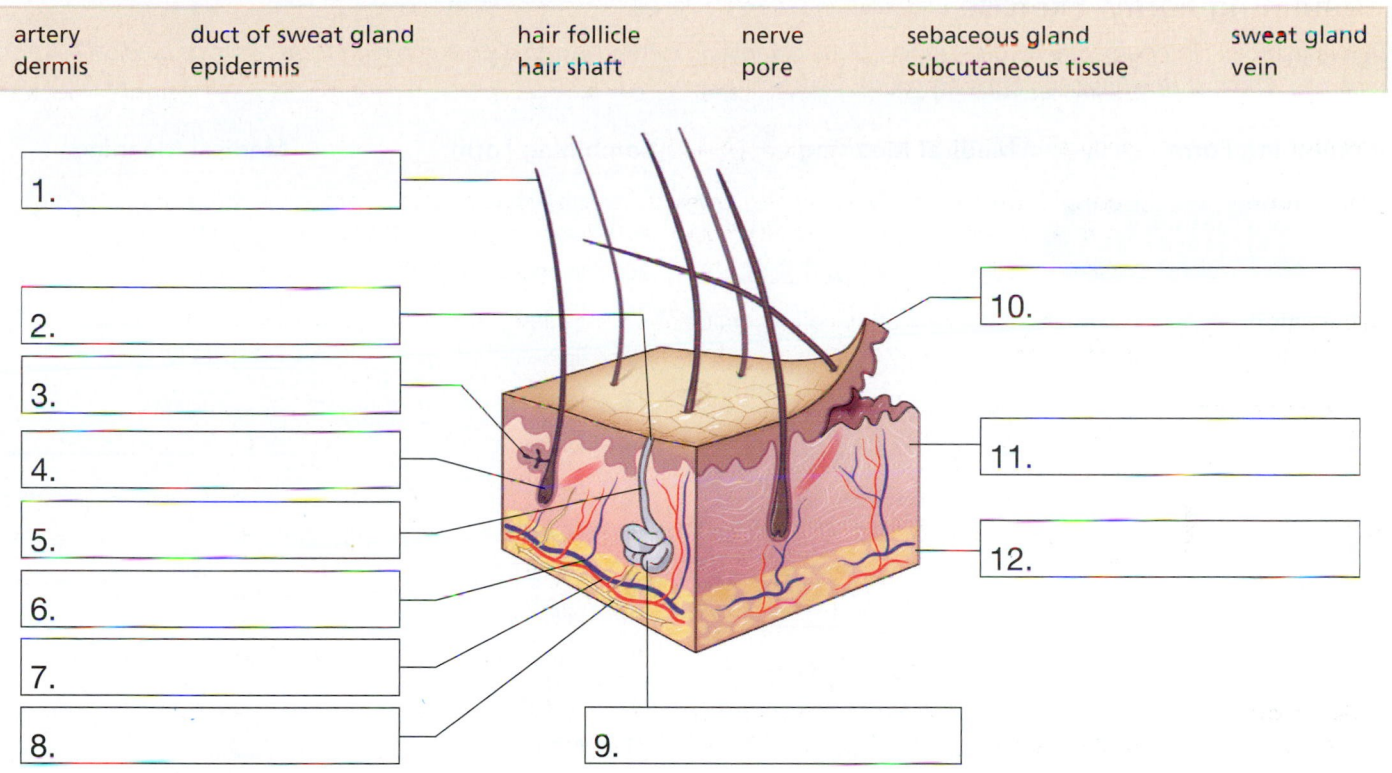

1.

2.

3.

4.

5.

6.

7.

8.

9.

10.

11.

12.

cuticle	lunula	nail bed	nail plate	nail root

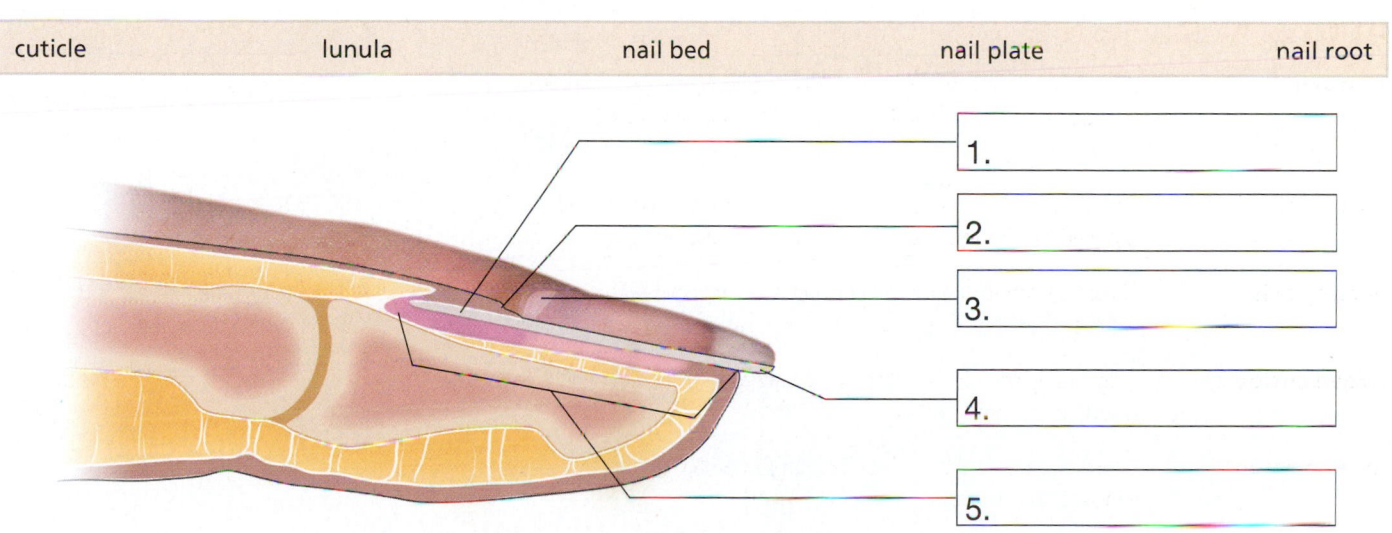

1.

2.

3.

4.

5.

Building Medical Words

Use the Answer Key at the end of the book to check your answers.

Combining Forms Exercise

Before you build integumentary words, review these combining forms. Next to each combining form, write its medical meaning. The first one has been done for you.

Combining Form	Medical Meaning	Combining Form	Medical Meaning
1. **follicul/o-**	follicle (small sac)	20. integu/o-	
2. adip/o-		21. kerat/o-	
3. all/o-		22. lip/o-	
4. bas/o-		23. loc/o-	
5. coll/a-		24. lun/o-	
6. cutane/o-		25. melan/o-	
7. cut/i-		26. onych/o-	
8. derm/a-		27. phylact/o-	
9. dermat/o-		28. pil/o-	
10. derm/o-		29. sebace/o-	
11. diaphore/o-		30. seb/o-	
12. elast/o-		31. sensitiv/o-	
13. erect/o-		32. spir/o-	
14. erg/o-		33. sudor/i-	
15. ex/o-		34. system/o-	
16. fer/o-		35. theli/o-	
17. foli/o-		36. trich/o-	
18. hidr/o-		37. ungu/o-	
19. integument/o-			

Combining Form and Suffix Exercise

Read the definition of the medical word. Look at the combining form that is given. Select the correct suffix from the Suffix List and write it on the blank line. Then build the medical word and write it on the line. (Remember: You may need to remove the combining vowel. Always remove the hyphens and slash.) Be sure to check your spelling. The first one has been done for you.

SUFFIX LIST		
-al (pertaining to)	-in (a substance)	-tome (instrument used to cut; area with distinct edges)
-ary (pertaining to)	-ment (action; state)	-ula (small thing)
-cyte (cell)	-ose (full of)	
-gen (that which produces)	-ous (pertaining to)	

Definition of the Medical Word	Combining Form	Suffix	Build the Medical Word
1. A substance that flexes and stretches	elast/o-	-in	*elastin*

(You think *a substance* (-in) + *flex and stretch* (elast/o-). You change the order of the word parts to put the suffix last. You write *elastin*.)

2. Pertaining to the nail	ungu/o-	_____	_____
3. An area with distinct edges (on the) skin	derm/a-	_____	_____
4. A substance of hard, fibrous protein	kerat/o-	_____	_____
5. That which produces fibers that hold together	coll/a-	_____	_____
6. Full of fat (tissue)	adip/o-	_____	_____
7. Cell (that makes dark brown and) black (pigment)	melan/o-	_____	_____
8. Pertaining to the skin	cutane/o-	_____	_____
9. Pertaining to sebum (oil)	sebace/o-	_____	_____
10. Cell (that stores) fat	lip/o-	_____	_____
11. Pertaining to the skin	integument/o-	_____	_____
12. Small thing (shaped like a) moon	lun/o-	_____	_____
13. State (of something that acts) to cover	integu/o-	_____	_____

Prefix Exercise

Read the definition of the medical word. Look at the medical word or partial word that is given (it already contains a combining form and a suffix). Select the correct prefix from the Prefix List and write it on the blank line. Then build the medical word and write it on the line. Be sure to check your spelling. The first one has been done for you.

PREFIX LIST			
epi- (upon; above)	ex- (out; away from)	per- (through; throughout)	sub- (below; underneath; less than)

Definition of the Medical Word	Prefix	Word or Partial Word	Build the Medical Word
1. Process (of skin cells moving) away from (the body like a) leaf	ex-	foliation	*exfoliation*
2. Pertaining to above the dermis	_____	dermal	_____
3. Pertaining to underneath the skin	_____	cutaneous	_____
4. Process of through (the skin) breathing	_____	spiration	_____

Diseases and Conditions

General

Word or Phrase	Description	Word Building
dermatitis	Any disease condition that includes inflammation or infection of the skin. Treatment: Correct the underlying cause.	**dermatitis** (DER-mah-TY-tis) **dermat/o-** *skin* **-itis** *inflammation of; infection of*
edema	Excessive amounts of fluid move from the blood into the dermis or subcutaneous tissue and cause swelling (see Figure 7-5 ■). Localized areas of edema occur with inflammation, allergic reactions, and infections. Large areas of edema occur with cardiovascular or urinary system diseases. Treatment: Correct the underlying cause.	**edema** (eh-DEE-mah)

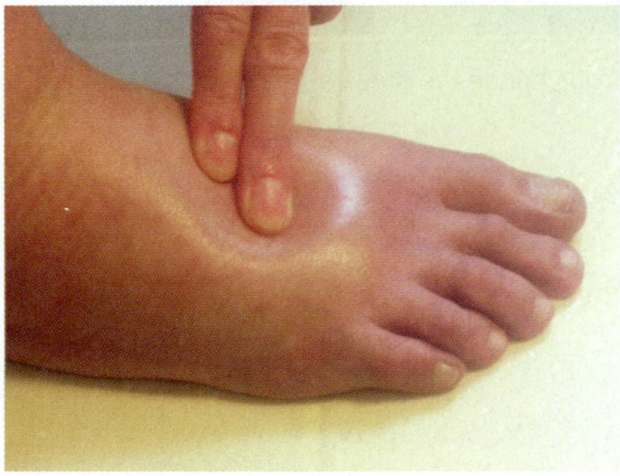

Figure 7-5 ■ Edema.

Fingertip pressure on an area of severe edema displaces the fluid and produces a deep indentation in the tissues. This is known as pitting edema.

Word or Phrase	Description	Word Building
hemorrhage	Trauma to the skin releases a small or large amount of blood. **Extravasation** is when the blood flows into the surrounding tissues. **Petechiae** are pinpoint hemorrhages in the skin from ruptured capillaries. A **contusion** is any size of hemorrhage under the skin. An **ecchymosis** is a hemorrhage under the skin that is 3 cm in diameter or larger. A contusion and an ecchymosis are both commonly known as a **bruise**. A **hematoma** is an elevated, localized collection of blood under the skin. Treatment: None.	**hemorrhage** (HEM-oh-rij) **hem/o-** *blood* **-rrhage** *excessive flow or discharge* **extravasation** (eks-TRAV-ah-SAY-shun) **extra-** *outside of* **vas/o-** *blood vessel; vas deferens* **-ation** *a process; being or having* **petechia** (peh-TEE-kee-ah) **petechiae** (peh-TEE-kee-ee) *Petechia* is a Latin singular noun. Form the plural by changing *-a* to *-ae.* **contusion** (con-TOO-zhun) **contus/o-** *bruising* **-ion** *action; condition* **ecchymosis** (EK-ih-MOH-sis) **ecchym/o-** *blood in the tissues* **-osis** *condition; abnormal condition; process* **ecchymoses** (EK-ih-MOH-seez) *Ecchymosis* is a Greek singular noun. Form the plural by changing *-is* to *-es.* **ecchymotic** (EK-ih-MAWT-ic) **hematoma** (HEE-mah-TOH-ma) **hemat/o-** *blood* **-oma** *tumor; mass*

Word or Phrase	Description	Word Building
lesion	Any area of visible damage on the skin, whether it is from disease or injury (see Figure 7-6 ■). Treatment: Correct the underlying cause.	lesion (LEE-shun)

LESION	DESCRIPTION	COLOR	CONTENTS	EXAMPLE		Word Building
Cyst	Elevated circular mound	Skin color or erythema	Semisolid or partly fluid filled	Acne sebaceous cyst		cyst (SIST)
Fissure	Small, cracklike crevice	Erythema	None; some fluid exudate	Dry, chapped skin		fissure (FISH-ur) **fiss/o-** *splitting* **-ure** *system; result of*
Macule	Flat circle	Pigmented; brown or black	None	Freckle, age spot		macule (MAK-yool)
Papule	Elevated	Skin color or erythema	Solid	Acne pimple		papule (PAP-yool)
Pustule	Elevated	White top	Pus	Acne whitehead		pustule (PUS-chool)
Scale	Flat to slightly elevated, thin flake	White	None	Dandruff, psoriasis		
Vesicle	Elevated with pointed top	Erythema; transparent top	Clear fluid	Herpes, chickenpox, shingles		vesicle (VES-ih-kl) **vesic/o-** *bladder; fluid-filled sac* **-cle** *small thing*
Wheal	Elevated with broad, flat top	Erythema; pale top	Clear fluid	Insect bites, urticaria		vesicular (veh-SIK-yoo-lar) **vesicul/o-** *bladder; fluid-filled sac* **-ar** *pertaining to* wheal (HWEEL)

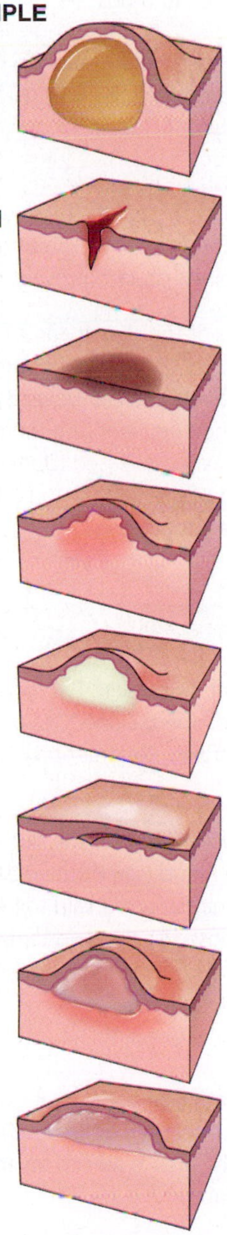

Figure 7-6 ■ Types of skin lesions.

Word or Phrase	Description	Word Building
neoplasm	Any **benign** or **malignant** new growth that occurs on or in the skin. Treatment: Excision of a benign neoplasm; excision and chemotherapy or radiation therapy for a malignant neoplasm.	neoplasm (NEE-oh-plazm) **ne/o-** *new* **-plasm** *growth; formed substance* benign (bee-NINE) malignant (mah-LIG-nant) **malign/o-** *intentionally causing harm; cancer* **-ant** *pertaining to*

Word or Phrase	Description	Word Building
pruritus	Itching. Pruritus is associated with many skin diseases. It is also part of an allergic reaction because of the release of histamine. A patient with pruritus is said to be **pruritic.** Treatment: Topical or oral antihistamine drugs or corticosteroid drugs.	**pruritus** (proo-RY-tus) **pruritic** (proo-RIT-ik) **prurit/o-** *itching* **-ic** *pertaining to*
rash	Any type of skin lesion that is pink to red, flat or raised, pruritic or non-pruritic. Certain systemic diseases (chickenpox, measles) have characteristic rashes. Treatment: Topical or oral antihistamine drugs or corticosteroid drugs.	
wound	Any area of visible damage to the skin that is caused by physical means (such as rubbing, trauma, etc.). Treatment: Apply a protective covering and topical antibiotic drug to prevent infection.	
xeroderma	Excessive dryness of the skin. It can be caused by aging, cold weather with low humidity, vitamin A deficiency, or dehydration. The level of hydration can be assessed by testing the **skin turgor.** A fold of skin pinched between the thumb and fingertips should flatten out immediately when released. Dehydration causes the skin to remain elevated (tenting of the skin) or to flatten out very slowly. Treatment: Correct the underlying cause.	**xeroderma** (ZEER-oh-DER-mah) **xer/o-** *dry* **-derma** *skin* **turgor** (TER-gor)

Changes in Skin Color

Word or Phrase	Description	Word Building
albinism	A lack of pigment in the skin, hair, and iris of the eye. This is a genetic mutation in which the melanocytes do not produce melanin. The patient is said to be an **albino.** Treatment: None.	**albinism** (AL-by-NIZ-em) **albin/o-** *white* **-ism** *process; disease from a specific cause*
cyanosis	Bluish-purple discoloration of the skin and nails due to a decreased level of oxygen in the blood (see Figure 4-10). It is caused by cardiac or respiratory disease. The patient is said to be **cyanotic.** In healthy persons, areas of skin exposed to the cold temporarily exhibit cyanosis. Treatment: Correct the underlying cause.	**cyanosis** (SY-ah-NOH-sis) **cyan/o-** *blue* **-osis** *condition; abnormal condition; process* **cyanotic** (SY-ah-NAWT-ik) **cyan/o-** *blue* **-tic** *pertaining to*
erythema	Reddish discoloration of the skin. It can be confined to one area of local inflammation or infection, or it can affect large areas of the skin surface as in sunburn. The area is said to be **erythematous.** Treatment: Correct the underlying cause.	**erythema** (AIR-eh-THEE-mah) **erythematous** (AIR-eh-THEM-eh-tus) **erythemat/o-** *redness* **-ous** *pertaining to*
jaundice	Yellowish discoloration of the skin, mucous membranes, and whites of the eyes (see Figure 3-20). It is associated with liver disease. The liver cannot process bilirubin, and high levels of unconjugated bilirubin in the blood move into the tissues and color the skin yellow. It is also known as **icterus.** The patient is said to be jaundiced or **icteric.** A patient without jaundice is said to be anicteric.	**jaundice** (JAWN-dis) **icterus** (IK-ter-us) **icteric** (ik-TAIR-ik) **icter/o-** *jaundice* **-ic** *pertaining to*

Word or Phrase	Description	Word Building
necrosis	Gray-to-black discoloration of the skin in areas where the tissue has died (see Figure 7-7 ■). **Necrotic** tissue can occur in a burn, decubitus ulcer, wound, or any tissue with a poor blood supply. Necrosis with subsequent bacterial invasion and decay is **gangrene,** and the area is said to be **gangrenous.** Treatment: Correct the underlying cause.	**necrosis** (neh-KROH-sis) **necr/o-** *dead cells, tissue, or body* **-osis** *condition; abnormal condition; process* **necrotic** (neh-KRAWT-ik) **necr/o-** *dead cells, tissue, or body* **-tic** *pertaining to* **gangrene** (GANG-green) **gangrenous** (GANG-greh-nus) **gangren/o-** *gangrene* **-ous** *pertaining to*

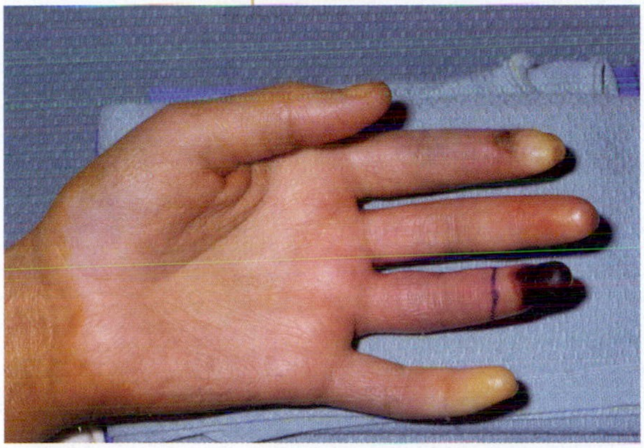

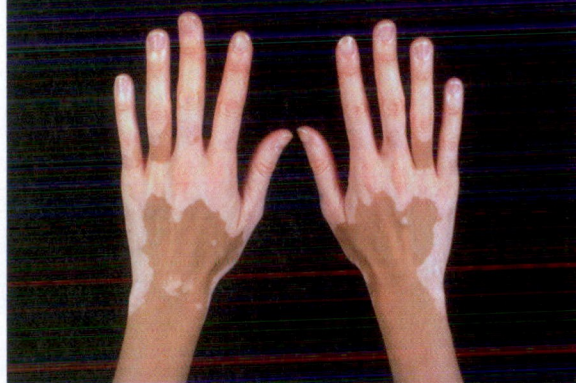

Figure 7-7 ■ Necrosis and pallor.

This patient's ring finger has necrosis and gangrene due to severe frostbite. The ring finger has been marked to show the location where an amputation will be performed. The tips of the index and little fingers show pallor, indicating poor blood flow.

Word or Phrase	Description	Word Building
pallor	Unnatural paleness due to a lack of blood supply to the tissue (see Figure 7-7). This is caused by blockage of an artery, hypotension, or severe exposure to the cold. Treatment: Correct the underlying cause.	**pallor** (PAL-or)
vitiligo	An autoimmune disease in which the melanocytes are slowly destroyed in irregular and ever-enlarging areas. There are white patches of **depigmentation** interspersed with normal skin (see Figure 7-8 ■). Treatment: None.	**vitiligo** (VIT-ih-LY-goh) **depigmentation** (dee-PIG-men-TAY-shun) **de-** *reversal of; without* **pigment/o-** *pigment* **-ation** *a process; being or having*

Figure 7-8 ■ Vitiligo.

This patient has areas of depigmentation on each hand due to vitiligo, a progressive autoimmune disease.

Clinical Connections

Obstetrics (Chapter 13). Melanocyte-stimulating hormone (from the anterior pituitary gland in the brain) can become active during pregnancy, causing dark, hyperpigmented areas on the face (**chloasma** or the mask of pregnancy) and/or a vertical dark line on the skin of the abdomen from the umbilicus downward (**linea nigra**).

Stretch marks (**striae**) in the skin of the abdomen and buttocks are the result of small tears in the dermis as the skin stretches to accommodate the pregnant uterus. These are irregular, reddened lines that later become lighter and shiny as they heal as scar tissue.

chloasma (kloh-AZ-mah)

linea nigra (LIN-ee-ah NY-grah)

striae (STRY-ee)

Skin Injuries

Word or Phrase	Description	Word Building
abrasion	Sliding injury that mechanically removes the epidermis. It is also known as a **brush burn.** Treatment: Apply a protective covering.	**abrasion** (ah-BRAY-zhun) **abras/o-** *scrape off* **-ion** *action; condition*
blister	Repetitive rubbing injury that mechanically separates the epidermis from the dermis and releases tissue fluid. A blister is a fluid-filled sac with a thin, transparent covering of epidermis. Blisters often form on the heel from walking in poorly fitting shoes or on the hand from rubbing with constant use of a tool. Treatment: Apply a protective covering before the activity.	**blister** (BLIS-ter)
burns	Heat (fire, hot objects, steam, boiling water), electrical current (lightning, electrical outlets or cords), chemicals, and radiation or x-rays (sunshine or prescribed radiation therapy) can cause a burn to the epidermis or dermis. Treatment: Topical anti-infective drugs to prevent infection. Second-degree burns over a large area and all third-degree burns require debridement and skin grafting.	
first-degree burn	This burn involves only the epidermis and causes erythema, pain, and swelling, but not blisters.	
second-degree burn	This burn involves the epidermis and the upper part of the dermis. It causes erythema, pain, and swelling. There are small blisters or larger **bullae** that form as the epidermis detaches from the dermis and the space between fills with tissue fluid (see Figure 7-9 ■). This is also known as a **partial-thickness burn.**	**bulla** (BUL-ah) **bullae** (BUL-ee) *Bulla* is a Latin singular noun. Form the plural by changing *-a* to *-ae.*

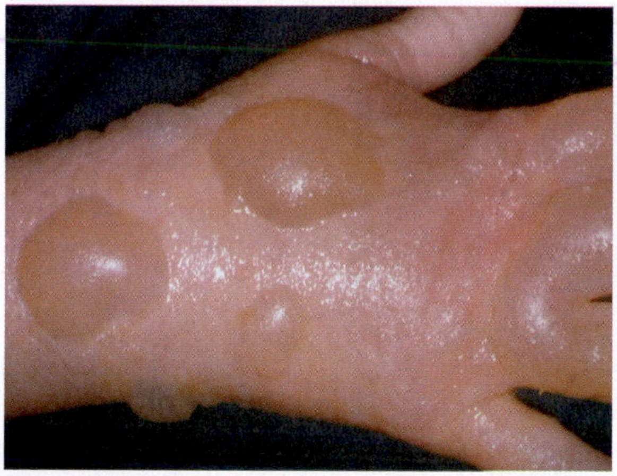

Figure 7-9 ■ Second-degree burn of the hand.
The burn caused the epidermis to separate from the dermis. Tissue fluid caused the epidermis to swell into large, fluid-filled bullae.

Word or Phrase	Description	Word Building
third-degree burn	This burn involves the epidermis and entire dermis, and sometimes the subcutaneous tissue and muscle layer beneath that may be involved. The area is black where the skin is charred. If the neurons in the dermis were destroyed, there is local **anesthesia** (no sensation of pain). This is also known as a **full-thickness burn.** An **eschar** is a thick, crusty scar of necrotic tissue that forms on a third-degree burn. Eschar is removed because it traps fluid from the burn, delays healing, and can become a source of infection.	**anesthesia** (AN-es-THEE-zee-ah) **an-** *without; not* **esthes/o-** *sensation; feeling* **-ia** *condition; state; thing* **eschar** (ES-kar)
callus	Repetitive rubbing injury that causes the epidermis to gradually thicken into a wide, elevated pad. A **corn** is a callus with a hard central area with a pointed tip that causes pain and inflammation. Treatment: Removal.	**callus** (KAL-uhs)

Word or Phrase	Description	Word Building
cicatrix	Fibrous tissue composed of collagen that forms as an injury heals. It is also known as a **scar.** A **keloid** is a very firm, abnormally large scar that is bigger than the original injury. It is caused by an overproduction of collagen (see Figure 7-10 ■). Unlike a scar, a keloid does not fade or decrease in size over time. Treatment: Surgical removal of a keloid, although they often grow back.	**cicatrix** (SIK-ah-triks) **keloid** (KEE-loyd) 　**kel/o-** *tumor* 　**-oid** *resembling*

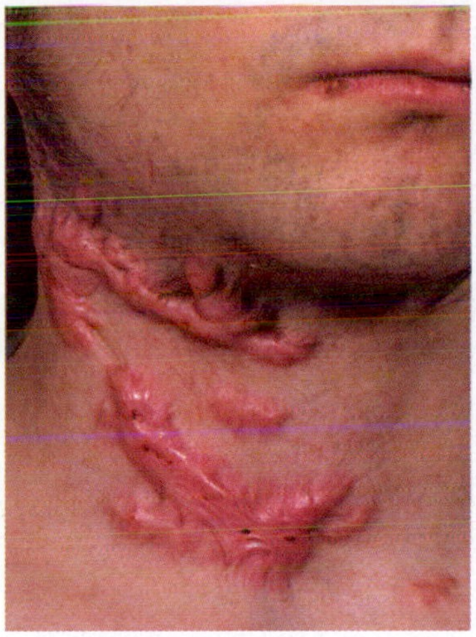

Figure 7-10 ■ Keloid.
A keloid is a scar that continues to grow until it is larger than the original injury. Depending on its location and size, a keloid can be cosmetically unacceptable.

| decubitus ulcer | Constant pressure to a particular area of the skin restricts the blood flow to those tissues. The epidermis and then dermis break down and slough off, resulting in a shallow or deep wound (see Figure 7-11 ■). Decubitus ulcers most often occur at pressure points overlying bony prominences such as the hip or sacrum. They are also known as **pressure sores** or **bed sores.** Treatment: Frequent repositioning, increased protein intake to rebuild tissue, and debridement of any necrotic tissue to promote healing. | **decubitus** (dee-KYOO-bih-tus)

decubiti (dee-KYOO-bih-tie)
Decubitus is a Latin singular noun. Form the plural by changing *–us* to *–i.*

ulcer (UL-ser) |

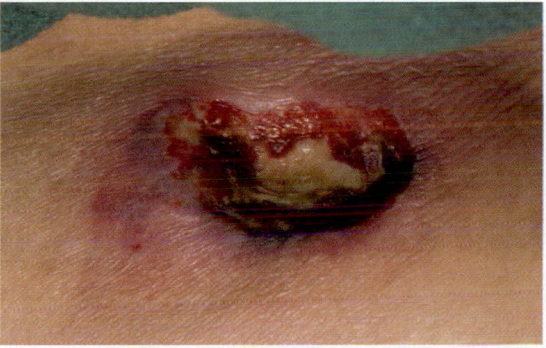

Figure 7-11 ■ Decubitus ulcer.
This stage III decubitus ulcer involves the loss of the epidermis, dermis, and subcutaneous tissue, exposing the muscle layer.

A Closer Look

Decreased fat in the subcutaneous tissue, poor nutrition, long-standing circulatory problems, and confinement to a bed or wheelchair predispose older patients to developing decubitus ulcers. Frequent repositioning of the patient and keeping the skin free of urine help prevent decubitus ulcers. The level of protein (albumin) in the blood indicates whether the patient is able to build healthy tissue and heal an existing decubitus ulcer. A low level of albumin is treated nutritionally by offering the patient high-protein snacks.

| excoriation | Superficial injury with a sharp object such as a fingernail or thorn that creates a linear scratch in the skin. Treatment: Topical antibiotic drug to prevent infection. | **excoriation** (eks-кон-ree-AA-shun)
　excori/o- *to take out skin*
　-ation *a process; being or having* |

Word or Phrase	Description	Word Building
laceration	Deep, penetrating wound. It can have clean cut or torn, ragged skin edges (see Figure 7-12 ■). Treatment: Layered closure with sutures. **Figure 7-12 ■ Laceration.** This deep laceration of the forearm was caused by a piece of glass that penetrated through the epidermis and dermis to the adipose tissue in the subcutaneous layer.	**laceration** (LAS-er-AA-shun) **lacer/o-** *a tearing* **-ation** *a process; being or having*

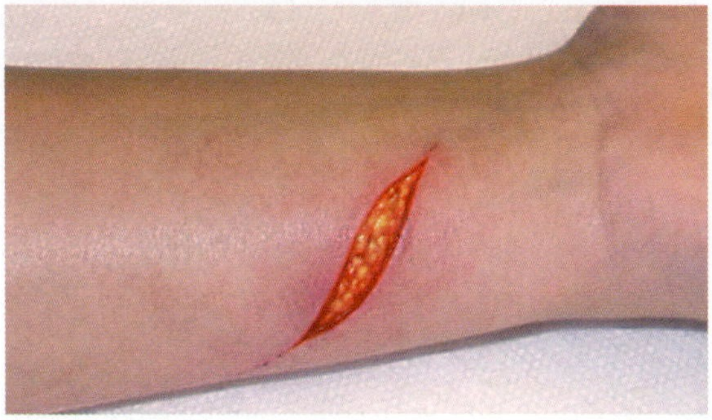

Skin Infections

Word or Phrase	Description	Word Building
abscess	Localized, pus-containing pocket caused by a bacterial infection. The infection is usually caused by *Staphylococcus aureus,* a common bacterium on the skin. A **furuncle** is a localized, elevated abscess around a hair follicle and the skin is inflamed and painful. It is also known as a **boil.** A **carbuncle** is composed of large furuncles with connecting channels through the subcutaneous tissue or to the skin surface. Treatment: Incision and drainage, oral antibiotic drugs.	**abscess** (AB-ses) **furuncle** (FYOO-rung-kl) **carbuncle** (KAR-bung-kl)
cellulitis	Spreading inflammation and infection of the connective tissues of the skin and muscle. It develops from a superficial cut, scratch, insect bite, blister, or splinter that becomes infected. The infecting bacteria produce enzymes that allow the infection to spread between the tissue layers. There is erythema (often as a red streak), warmth, and pain. Treatment: Oral antibiotic drugs.	**cellulitis** (SEL-yoo-LY-tis) **cellul/o-** *cell* **-itis** *inflammation of; infection of*
herpes	Skin infection caused by the herpes virus. There are clustered vesicles, erythema, edema, and pain. The vesicles rupture, releasing clear fluid that forms crusts. Treatment: Topical or oral antiviral drugs. **Herpes simplex virus (HSV) type 1** occurs on the lips. These lesions tend to recur during illness and stress. They are also known as **cold sores** or **fever blisters. Herpes simplex virus (HSV) type 2** is a sexually transmitted disease that causes vesicles in the genital area. These lesions tend to recur during illness and stress. This is also known as **genital herpes. Herpes whitlow** is a herpes simplex infection at the base of the fingernail from contact with herpes simplex type 1 of the mouth or type 2 of the genitals. The virus enters through a small tear in the cuticle. **Herpes varicella-zoster** causes the skin rash of chickenpox during childhood. The virus then remains dormant in the body until it is activated in later life by illness or emotional stress. Then it forms painful vesicles and crusts along a dermatome. This is also known as **shingles** (see Figure 7-13 ■).	**herpes** (HER-peez) **herpes simplex** (HER-peez SIM-pleks) **herpes whitlow** (HER-peez WHIT-loh) **herpes varicella-zoster** (HER-peez VAIR-ih-SEL-lah ZAWS-ter) **shingles** (SHING-glz)

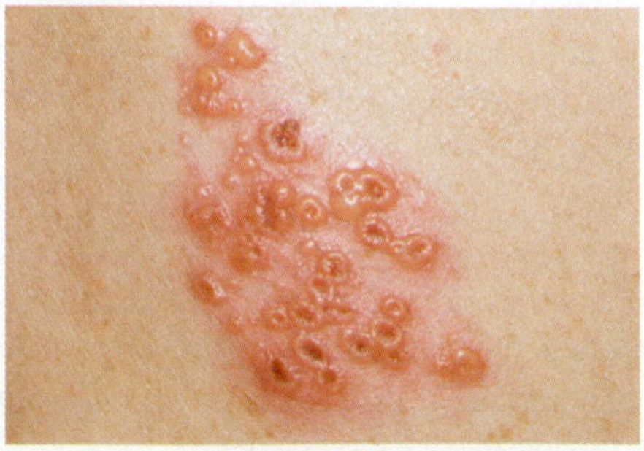

Figure 7-13 ■ Shingles.
The vesicles and crusts of shingles. The lesions occur along a dermatome.

Word or Phrase	Description	Word Building
tinea	Skin infection caused by a fungus that feeds on epidermal cells. It multiplies quickly in the warm, moist environment of body creases and areas enclosed by clothing or shoes. There is severe itching and burning with round, red, scaly lesions. Because of its round lesions, it was originally thought to be caused by a worm, and was (and still is) called **ringworm**. Tinea is named according to where it occurs on the body. **Tinea capitis** occurs on the scalp and causes hair loss. **Tinea corporis** occurs on the trunk of the body. **Tinea cruris** occurs in the groin and genital areas and is known as **jock itch. Tinea pedis** occurs on the feet and is known as **athlete's foot** (see Figure 7-14 ■). Treatment: Topical antifungal drugs.	**tinea** (TIN-ee-ah) **capitis** (KAP-ih-tis) **corporis** (KOR-por-is) **cruris** (KROOR-is) **pedis** (PEE-dis)

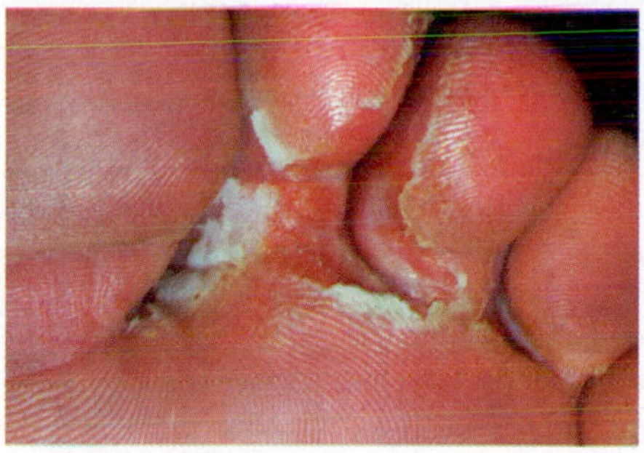

Figure 7-14 ■ Tinea pedis.
This fungal infection, also known as athlete's foot, causes severe itching and burning. The erythematous, scaly lesions become soft and white and begin to peel due to moisture between the toes.

Word or Phrase	Description	Word Building
verruca	Irregular, rough skin lesion caused by the human papillomavirus. It is usually on the hand, fingers, or the sole of the foot (plantar wart). It is also known as a **wart.** Treatment: Topical keratolytic drug to break down the keratin in the wart. Cryosurgery or electrosurgery, if needed.	**verruca** (veh-ROO-kah) **verrucae** (veh-ROO-kee) *Verruca* is a Latin singular noun. Form the plural by changing -*a* to -*ae*.

Skin Infestations

Word or Phrase	Description	Word Building
pediculosis	Infestation of lice and their eggs (nits) in the scalp, hair, eyelashes, or pubic hair. Lice are easily transmitted from one person to another by combs or hats. Treatment: Shampoo and skin lotion to kill lice.	**pediculosis** (peh-DIK-yoo-LOH-sis) **pedicul/o-** *lice* **-osis** *condition; abnormal condition; process*
scabies	Infestation of parasitic mites that tunnel under the skin and produce vesicles that are itchy. Treatment: Shampoo and skin lotion to kill mites.	**scabies** (SKAY-beez)

Allergic Skin Conditions

Word or Phrase	Description	Word Building
contact dermatitis	Local reaction to physical contact with a substance that is an allergen or an irritant. Examples: Chemicals (deodorant, soaps, detergents, makeup, urine), metals, synthetic products (latex gloves, Spandex bathing suit or girdle), plants (poison ivy), or animals (see Figure 7-15 ■). The skin becomes inflamed and irritated. Small vesicles may also appear. Treatment: Topical or oral antihistamine drug or corticosteroid drugs.	**dermatitis** (DER-mah-TY-tis) **dermat/o-** *skin* **-itis** *inflammation of; infection of*

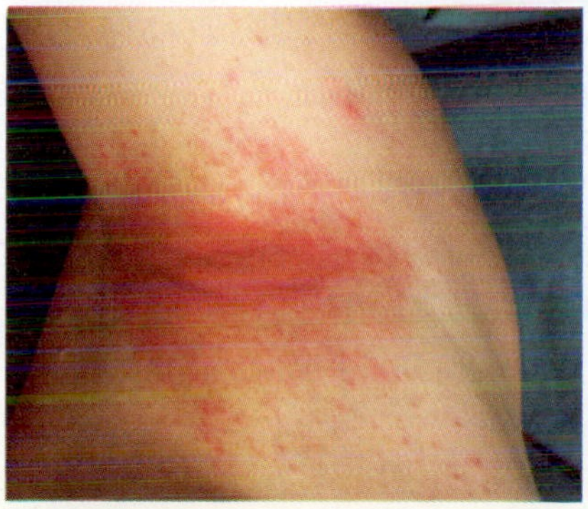

Figure 7-15 ■ Severe contact dermatitis.
This skin reaction was caused by the application of a new deodorant whose chemical ingredients caused irritation.

Word or Phrase	Description	Word Building

Clinical Connections

Infection Control. According to the National Institute for Occupational Safety and Health, there has been an increase in the number of healthcare professionals who have allergic reactions to latex rubber gloves. This causes skin rashes, hives, itching, and asthma. Nonlatex gloves should be used instead to protect and to prevent the spread of infection.

Word or Phrase	Description	Word Building
urticaria	Condition of raised areas of redness and edema that appear suddenly and may also disappear rapidly. There is itching (pruritus), and scratching tends to cause the areas to enlarge. Urticaria is caused by an allergic reaction to food, plants, animals, insect bites, or drugs. It is also known as **hives.** Each individual area is known as a **wheal.** A large wheal is a **welt.** Treatment: Topical or oral antihistamine drugs or corticosteroid drugs.	**urticaria** (ER-tih-KAIR-ee-ah) **wheal** (HWEEL)

Benign Skin Markings and Neoplasms

Word or Phrase	Description	Word Building

actinic keratoses	Raised, irregular, rough areas of skin that are dry and feel like sandpaper. These develop in middle-aged persons in areas chronically exposed to the sun. They can become squamous cell carcinoma. They are also known as **solar keratoses.** Treatment: Avoid more sun exposure.	**actinic** (ak-TIN-ik)
		  actin/o- *rays of the sun*
		  -ic *pertaining to*
		keratosis (KAIR-ah-TOH-sis)
		keratoses (KAIR-ah-TOH-seez)
		  kerat/o- *cornea (of the eye); hard, fibrous protein*
		  -osis *condition; abnormal condition; process*
		solar (SOH-lar)

freckle	**Benign,** pigmented, flat macule that develops after sun exposure. Freckles contain groups of melanocytes. Freckles fade over time without continued sun exposure.	**freckle** (FREH-kl) **benign** (bee-NINE)

hemangioma	Congenital growth composed of a mass of superficial and dilated blood vessels (see Figure 7-16 ■). Treatment: Most hemangiomas disappear without treatment by age 3.	**hemangioma** (hee-MAN-jee-OH-mah)
		  hem/o- *blood*
		  angi/o- *blood vessel; lymphatic vessel*
		  -oma *tumor; mass*

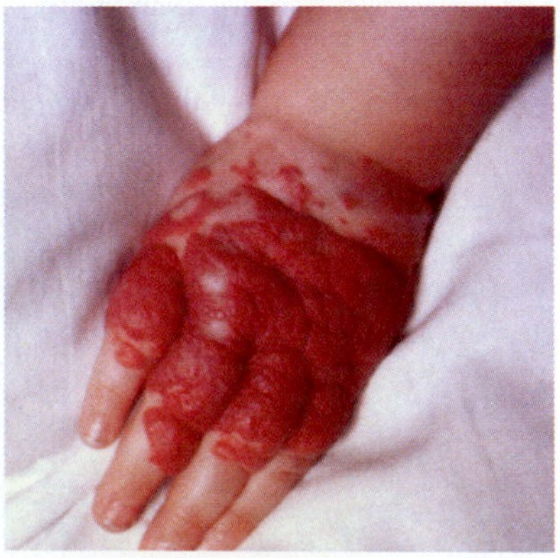

Figure 7-16 ■
Hemangioma.
The bright red color of this skin lesion comes from the large number of dilated blood vessels.

Word or Phrase	Description	Word Building

lipoma	Benign growth of adipose tissue from the subcutaneous layer. It is a soft, rounded, nontender fatty elevation in the skin. Treatment: Excision, if desired.	**lipoma** (ly-POH-mah)
		  lip/o- *lipid (fat)*
		  -oma *tumor; mass*

Word or Phrase	Description	Word Building
nevus	Benign skin lesion that is present at birth and comes in a variety of colors and shapes (see Figure 7-17 ■). **Port-wine stains** are slightly elevated, red-to-purple vascular nevi that are irregularly shaped. They can cover large areas of skin on the face and neck. Their shape and color resemble a puddle of spilled wine. They are also known as **birthmarks.** A **dysplastic nevus** has irregular edges and variations in color. It can develop into a malignant melanoma. Treatment: Excision of a mole if clothing irritates it; laser treatment to remove port-wine stains; observe a dysplastic nevus for change.	**nevus** (NEE-vus) **nevi** (NEE-vie) *Nevus* is a Latin singular noun. Form the plural by changing *–us* to *i.* **dysplastic** (dis-PLAS-tik) **dys-** *painful; difficult; abnormal* **plast/o-** *growth; formation* **-ic** *pertaining to*

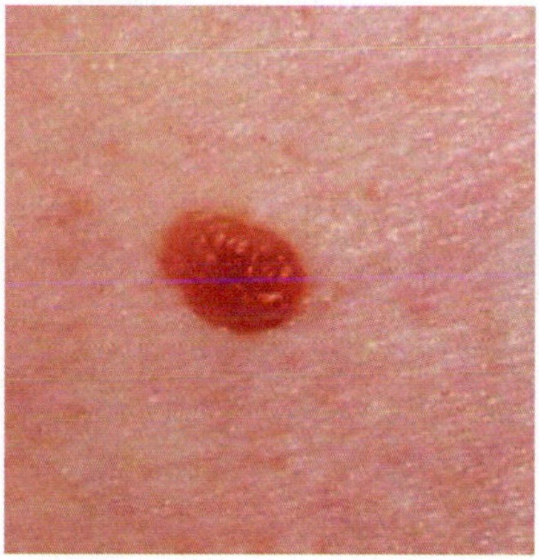

Figure 7-17 ■ Nevus.
A mole is a pigmented nevus that can be flat or round and elevated and often contains a hair.

Word or Phrase	Description	Word Building
papilloma	Small, soft, flesh-colored growth of epidermis and dermis that protrudes outwardly. It comes in a variety of shapes: irregular mounds, globes, flaps, or polyps with rounded tops on slender stalks. It occurs on the eyelid, neck, or trunk of the body. It is also known as a **skin tag.** Treatment: Removal by cryotherapy, electrocautery, or surgical excision, if desired.	**papilloma** (PAP-ih-LOH-mah) **papill/o-** *elevated structure* **-oma** *tumor; mass*
premalignant skin lesions	Abnormal skin lesions that are not yet cancerous. Over time and with continued exposure to sunlight or irritation, these lesions can become cancerous. Treatment: None; observe for changes.	**premalignant** (PREE-mah-LIG-nant) **pre-** *before; in front of* **malign/o-** *intentionally causing harm; cancer* **-ant** *pertaining to*
senile lentigo	Light-to-dark brown macules with irregular edges. They occur most often on the hands and face, areas that are chronically exposed to the sun (see Figure 7-18 ■).	**senile** (SEE-nile) **sen/o-** *old age* **-ile** *pertaining to* **lentigo** (len-TY-goh)

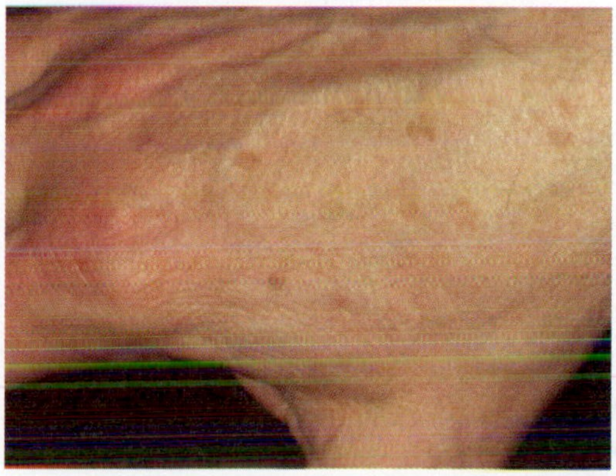

Figure 7-18 ■ Senile lentigo.
These light brown macules occur with age and are called age spots or liver spots.

Word or Phrase	Description	Word Building
syndactyly	Congenital abnormality in which the skin and soft tissues are joined between the fingers or toes (see Figure 7-19 ■). In some cases the fingernails or toenails are also joined. **Polydactyly** is a congenital abnormality in which there are extra fingers or toes. Treatment: Surgical correction, if desired. 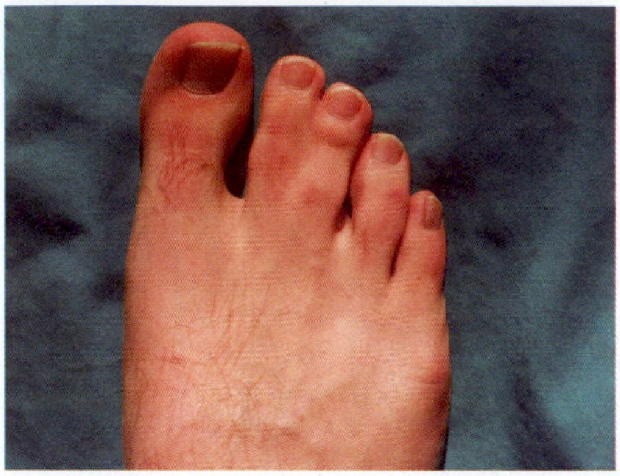 **Figure 7-19** ■ **Syndactyly.** The skin and soft tissues of the second and third toes are fused together in this patient with syndactyly.	**syndactyly** (sin-DAK-tih-lee) **syn-** *together* **-dactyly** *condition of fingers or toes* The ending *-dactyly* contains the combining form *dactyl/o-* and the one-letter suffix *–y.* **polydactyly** (PAWL-ee-DAK-tih-lee) **poly-** *many; much* **-dactyly** *condition of fingers or toes*
xanthoma	Benign growth that is a yellow nodule or plaque on the hands, elbows, knees, or feet. It is seen in patients who have a high level of lipids in the blood or have diabetes mellitus. A xanthoma that occurs on the eyelid is known as a **xanthelasma.** Treatment: Excision, if desired.	**xanthoma** (zan-THOH-mah) **xanth/o-** *yellow* **-oma** *tumor; mass* **xanthelasma** (ZAN-theh-LAZ-mah) **xanth/o-** *yellow* **-elasma** *platelike structure*

Malignant Neoplasms of the Skin

Word or Phrase	Description	Word Building
cancer of the skin	A **malignancy** in areas of the skin that are chronically exposed to ultraviolet light radiation from the sun. Skin cancer is more common in older adults (because of a lifetime of sun exposure) and in fair-skinned persons (because there is less melanin to absorb radiation). Treatment: Excision, chemotherapy drugs, photodynamic therapy.	**cancer** (KAN-ser) **malignancy** (mah-LIG-nan-see) **malign/o-** *intentionally causing harm; cancer* **-ancy** *state of*
basal cell carcinoma	Skin cancer that begins in the basal layer of the epidermis. It is the most common type of skin cancer. It often appears as a raised, pearly bump. It is a slow-growing cancer that does not metastasize to other parts of the body.	**carcinoma** (KAR-sih-NOH-mah) **carcin/o-** *cancer* **-oma** *tumor; mass*

Word or Phrase	Description	Word Building

malignant melanoma	Skin cancer that begins in melanocytes in the epidermis (see Figure 7-20 ■). It grows quickly and metastasizes to other parts of the body. Malignant melanomas have these four characteristics.
	
	A **A**symmetry. One side of the lesion has a different shape than the other side.
	B **B**order or edge is irregular or ragged.
	C **C**olor varies from black to brown (or to red) within the same lesion.
	D **D**iameter is greater than 6 mm.
		malignant (mah-LIG-nant)
		  malign/o- *intentionally causing harm; cancer*
		  -ant *pertaining to*
		
		melanoma (MEL-ah-NOH-mah)
		  melan/o- *black*
		  -oma *tumor; mass*
		Add words to make a complete definition of *melanoma: tumor (whose color is brown or) black.*

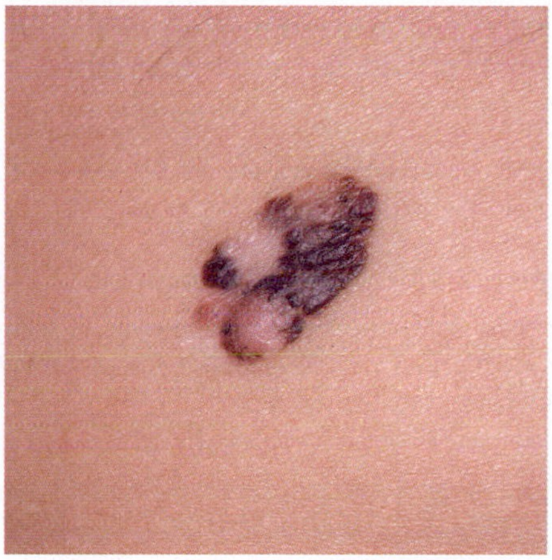

Figure 7-20 ■ Malignant melanoma.
This lesion reveals three of the four typical characteristics of a malignant melanoma: asymmetry; irregular edges; and varying shades of color. The fourth characteristic—an increase in size—would be noted over time.

Clinical Connections

Public Health. Depletion of the earth's ozone layer has led to many cases of malignant melanoma. The use of sunscreen and avoiding prolonged sun exposure, particularly during midday, helps to decrease this risk. Self-examination of the skin should be done regularly. Irregular or changing skin lesions should be examined by a dermatologist.

Word or Phrase	Description	Word Building

squamous cell carcinoma	Skin cancer that begins in the flat squamous cells of the superficial layer of the epidermis. It often begins as an actinic keratosis. It most often appears as a red bump or ulcer. It is the second most common type of skin cancer, but it grows slowly.	**squamous** (SKWAY-mus)
		  squam/o- *scalelike cell*
		  -ous *pertaining to*

Word or Phrase	Description	Word Building
Kaposi's sarcoma	Skin cancer that begins in connective tissue or lymph nodes. Tumors on the skin are elevated, irregular, and dark reddish-blue (see Figure 7-21 ■). This was once a relatively rare malignancy, but is now commonly seen in AIDS patients. Treatment: Excision of single lesions, radiation therapy for multiple lesions.	**Kaposi** (kah-POH-see) **sarcoma** (sar-KOH-mah) **sarc/o-** *connective tissue* **-oma** *tumor; mass*

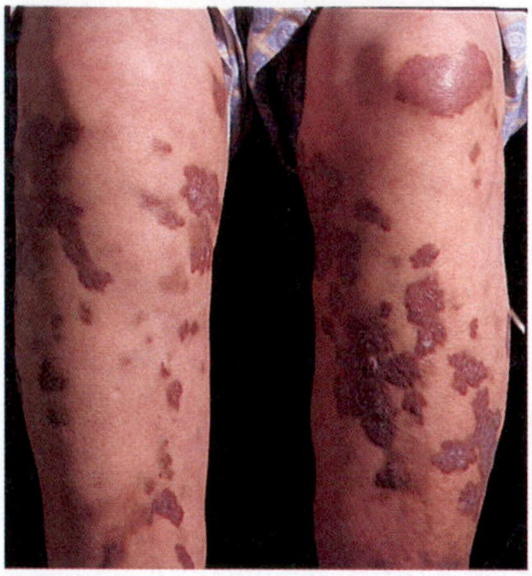

Figure 7-21 ■ Kaposi's sarcoma.
This previously rare cancer is now commonly seen in AIDS patients because of their impaired immune response. The cancer involves the skin, mucous membranes, and internal organs.

Autoimmune Diseases with Skin Symptoms

Word or Phrase	Description	Word Building
psoriasis	Autoimmune disorder that produces an excessive number of epidermal cells. The skin lesions are itchy, red, and covered with silvery scales and plaques. They usually occur on the scalp, elbows, hands, and knees (see Figure 7-22 ■). Illness and stress cause flare-ups, and psoriasis has a hereditary component. Treatment: Topical coal tar drugs, vitamin A drugs, vitamin D drugs, and corticosteroid drugs; light therapy with a psoralen drug and ultraviolet light A (PUVA).	**psoriasis** (soh-RY-ah-sis) **psor/o-** *itching* **-iasis** *state of; process of* **psoriatic** (SOH-ree-AT-ik) **psor/o-** *itching* **-iatic** *pertaining to a state or process*

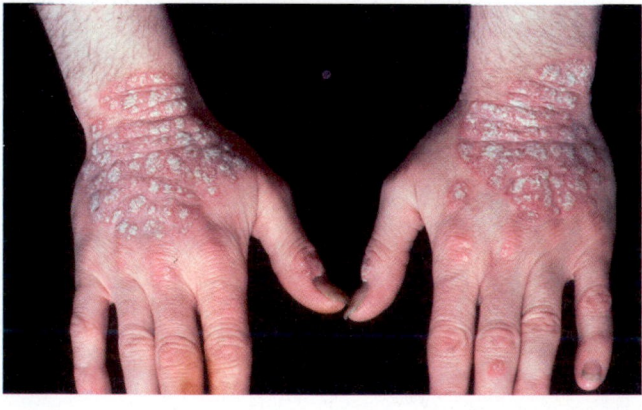

Figure 7-22 ■ Psoriasis.
Psoriasis produces characteristic elevated, erythematous lesions that are topped by silvery scales and plaques.

Word or Phrase	Description	Word Building
scleroderma	Autoimmune disorder that causes the skin and internal organs to progressively harden due to deposits of collagen. Treatment: Oral corticosteroid drugs.	**scleroderma** (SKLAIR-oh-DER-mah) **scler/o-** *hard; sclera (white of the eye)* **-derma** *skin*
systemic lupus erythematosus (SLE)	Autoimmune disorder with deterioration of collagen in the skin and connective tissues. There is joint pain, sensitivity to sunlight, and fatigue. Often there is a characteristic butterfly-shaped, erythematous rash over the bridge of the nose that spreads out over the cheeks. Treatment: Oral corticosteroid drugs.	**systemic** (sis-TEM-ik) **system/o-** *the body as a whole* **-ic** *pertaining to* **lupus erythematosus** (LOO-pus AIR-ih-THEM-ah-TOH-sus)

Diseases of the Sebaceous Glands

Word or Phrase	Description	Word Building
acne vulgaris	During puberty, the sebaceous glands produce large amounts of sebum, particularly on the forehead, nose, chin, shoulders, and back. Excess sebum builds up around the hair shaft, hardens, and blocks the follicle. The blocked secretions elevate the skin and form a reddish papule. In other hair follicles, the oily sebum traps dirt and enlarges the pore. The sebum turns black as its oil is oxidized from exposure to the air. This forms a **comedo** or **blackhead.** As bacteria feed on the sebum, they release irritating substances that produce inflammation. The bacteria also produce infection, drawing white blood cells to the area and forming pustules or **whiteheads** (see Figure 7-23 ■ and Table 7-1). In severe cystic acne, the papules enlarge to form deep, pus-filled cysts. Treatment: Topical cleansing drugs, topical or oral antibiotic drugs to kill skin bacteria; oral vitamin A–type drugs for severe cystic acne.	**acne vulgaris** (AK-nee vul-GAIR-is) **comedo** (KOH-meh-doh) (koh-MEE-doh) **comedones** (KOH-meh-dohns)

Clinical Connections

Pharmacology. Severe cystic acne is frequently treated with the vitamin A-type drug isotretinoin (Accutane). This drug has been linked to the unusual and severe side effect of suicide, and this warning must be included on the drug's package and informational insert.

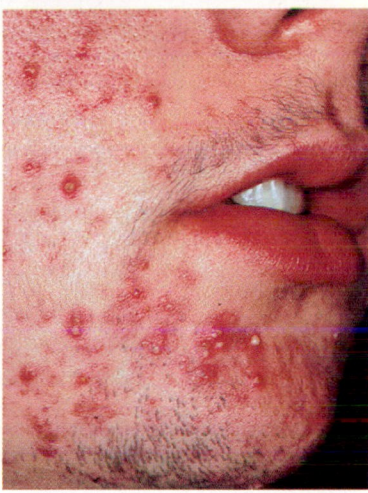

Figure 7-23 ■ Acne vulgaris.

This adolescent boy has severe acne vulgaris with papules, comedos, and pustules. Increased secretion of the sebaceous glands during puberty triggers the onset of acne vulgaris.

Word or Phrase	Description	Word Building
acne rosacea	Chronic skin condition of the face in middle-aged patients. The sebaceous glands secrete excessive amounts of sebum. There is blotchy erythema, dilated superficial blood vessels, papules, and edema that is made worse by heat, cold, stress, emotions, certain foods, alcoholic beverages, and sunlight (see Figure 7-24 ■ and Table 7-1). Men can develop **rhinophyma,** an erythematous, irregular enlargement of the nose. Treatment: Topical antibacterial and antiprotozoal drugs; laser surgery to destroy small, superficial blood vessels.	**acne rosacea** (AK-nee roh-ZAY-shee-ah) **rhinophyma** (RY-noh-FY-mah) **rhin/o-** *nose* **-phyma** *tumor; growth*

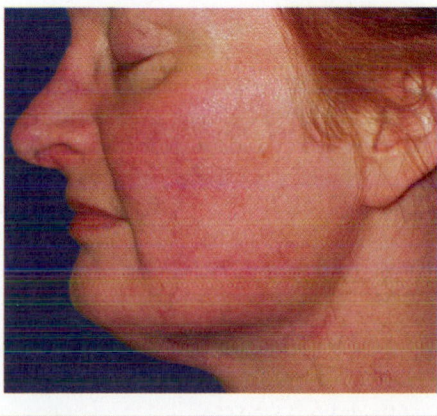

Figure 7-24 ■ Acne rosacea.

This patient's face shows the blotchy, rose-colored erythema and dilated superficial blood vessels of acne rosacea. Even the eyelids and neck are affected.

Table 7-1   Comparison of Acne Vulgaris and Acne Rosacea

	Site	Comedos	Pustules and Papules	Dilated Blood Vessels	Age
Acne vulgaris	face, shoulders, back	yes	yes	no	adolescence
Acne rosacea	face only	no	yes	yes	middle age

Word or Phrase	Description	Word Building
seborrhea	Overproduction of sebum, particularly on the face and scalp, that occurs at a time other than puberty. In seborrheic dermatitis, oily areas are interspersed with patches of dry, scaly skin and dandruff. There can also be erythema and crusty, yellow exudates. In adults, seborrheic dermatitis often appears after illness or stress. It can be caused by environmental or food allergies. It is called **cradle cap** in infants and **eczema** in children and adults. Treatment: Topical corticosteroid drugs, medicated shampoos.	**seborrhea** (SEB-oh-REE-ah) **seb/o-** *sebum (oil)* **-rrhea** *flow; discharge* **eczema** (EK-zeh-mah)

Diseases of the Sweat Glands

Word or Phrase	Description	Word Building
anhidrosis	Congenital absence of the sweat glands and inability to tolerate heat. Treatment: Avoid overheating.	**anhidrosis** (AN-hy-DROH-sis) **an-** *without; not* **hidr/o-** *sweat* **-osis** *condition; abnormal condition; process*
diaphoresis	Profuse sweating. Although a high fever, emotional stress, strenuous exercise, or the hot flashes of menopause can cause profuse sweating, these are *not* referred to as diaphoresis. Diaphoresis is caused by an underlying condition such as myocardial infarction, hyperthyroidism, hypoglycemia, or withdrawal from narcotic drugs. The patient is said to be **diaphoretic.** Treatment: Correct the underlying cause.	**diaphoresis** (DY-ah-foh-REE-sis) **diaphore/o-** *sweating* **-sis** *process; condition; abnormal condition* **diaphoretic** (DY-ah-foh-RET-ik) **diaphore/o-** *sweating* **-tic** *pertaining to*

Diseases of the Hair

Word or Phrase	Description	Word Building
alopecia	Acute or chronic loss of scalp hair. Acute alopecia can be caused by chemotherapy drugs that attack rapidly dividing cancer cells, but also affect rapidly dividing hair cells. Skin diseases of the scalp can also cause acute hair loss. Chronic hair loss usually begins in early middle age, although inherited tendencies can make it occur sooner. In men, lower testosterone levels and decreased blood flow to the scalp cause the hair follicles to shrink. The hair on the top of the scalp thins and disappears, leaving a fringe of hair at the back of the head. This is known as **male pattern baldness.** In women, menopause causes the level of estradiol from the ovaries to be lower than the male hormone androgen (produced by the adrenal cortex) and this hormonal change causes the hair to thin. Treatment: Topical drugs that dilate the arteries in the scalp or oral drugs that block the effect of DHT (substance that is increased in the balding scalp).	**alopecia** (AL-oh-PEE-shee-ah) **alopec/o-** *bald* **-ia** *condition; state; thing*

Word or Phrase	Description	Word Building
folliculitis	Inflammation or infection of the hair follicle. It occurs after shaving, plucking, or removing hair with hot wax. Treatment: Topical cortico-steroid or antibiotic drugs.	**folliculitis** (foh-LIK-yoo-LY-tis) **follicul/o-** *follicle (small sac)* **-itis** *inflammation of; infection of*
hirsutism	The presence of excessive, dark hair on the forearms and over the upper lip of a woman. It is due to too much of the male hormone androgen caused by a tumor in the adrenal cortex. Treatment: Correct the underlying cause.	**hirsutism** (HER-soo-tizm) **hirsut/o-** *hairy* **-ism** *process; disease from a specific cause*
pilonidal sinus	An abnormal passageway (**fistula**) that begins as a large, abnormal hair follicle that contains a hair that is never shed. The follicle is visible as a pit or dimple on the skin in the sacral area of the back. Irritation causes the hair follicle to become infected, eventually creating a sinus into the subcutaneous tissue, with erythema, tenderness, and purulent discharge. Treatment: Incision and drainage of the sinus.	**pilonidal** (PY-loh-NY-dal) **pil/o-** *hair* **nid/o-** *nest; focus* **-al** *pertaining to* **sinus** (SY-nus) **fistula** (FIS-tyoo-lah)

Did You Know?

Even the condition of split ends on hairs has a medical name: **schizotrichia**.	**schizotrichia** (SKIZ-oh-TRIK-ee-ah) **schiz/o-** *split* **trich/o-** *hair* **-ia** *condition; state; thing*

Diseases of the Nails

Word or Phrase	Description	Word Building
clubbing	Abnormally curved fingernails and stunted growth of the finger associated with a chronic lack of oxygen in patients with cystic fibrosis (see Figure 4-10).	
onychomycosis	Fungal infection of the fingernails or toenails. It infects the nail root and deforms the nail as it grows (see Figure 7-25 ■). Treatment: Topical or oral antifungal drugs.	**onychomycosis** (ON-ih-KOH-my-KOH-sis) **onych/o-** *nail (fingernail or toenail)* **myc/o-** *fungus* **-osis** *condition; abnormal condition; process*

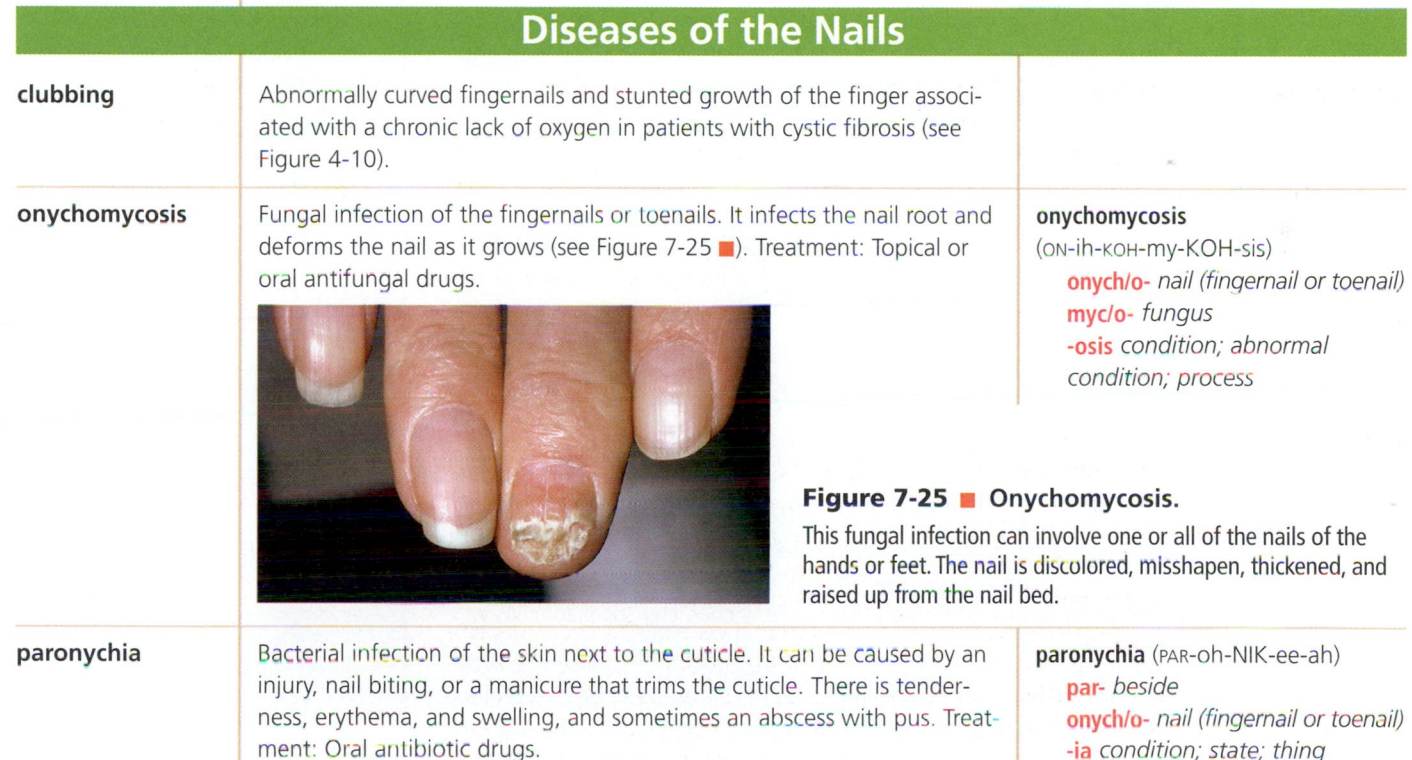

Figure 7-25 ■ Onychomycosis.
This fungal infection can involve one or all of the nails of the hands or feet. The nail is discolored, misshapen, thickened, and raised up from the nail bed.

Word or Phrase	Description	Word Building
paronychia	Bacterial infection of the skin next to the cuticle. It can be caused by an injury, nail biting, or a manicure that trims the cuticle. There is tenderness, erythema, and swelling, and sometimes an abscess with pus. Treatment: Oral antibiotic drugs.	**paronychia** (PAR-oh-NIK-ee-ah) **par-** *beside* **onych/o-** *nail (fingernail or toenail)* **-ia** *condition; state; thing*

Laboratory and Diagnostic Procedures

Word or Phrase	Description	Word Building
allergy skin testing	Antigens (animal dander, foods, plants, pollen, and so forth) in a liquid form are given by **intradermal** injections into the forearm. If the patient is allergic to a particular antigen, a wheal will form at the site of that injection (see Figure 7-26 ■). Alternatively, the antigen is scratched into the skin, and the procedure is known as a **scratch test**.	**intradermal** (IN-trah-DER-mal) **intra-** *within* **derm/o-** *skin* **-al** *pertaining to*

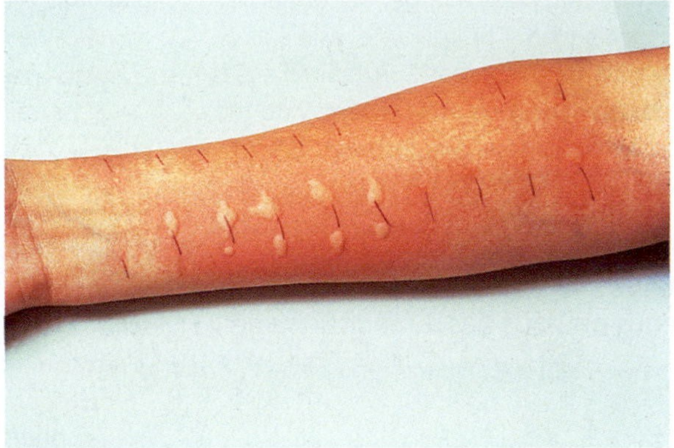

Figure 7-26 ■ **Allergy skin testing.**
This patient's forearm shows a number of wheals where the body's immune response was triggered by the injected antigen. The size of the wheal corresponds to the degree of allergy to that antigen. No wheal formation means that the patient is not allergic to that antigen.

Word or Phrase	Description	Word Building
culture and sensitivity (C&S)	A specimen of the **exudates** from an ulcer, wound, burn, or laceration or the pus from an infection is cultured in a Petri dish. The bacterium in it grows into colonies, is identified to make a diagnosis, and is tested to determine its sensitivity to specific antibiotic drugs.	**sensitivity** (SEN-sih-TIV-ih-tee) **sensitiv/o-** *affected by; sensitive to* **-ity** *state; condition* **exudate** (EKS-yoo-dayt) **exud/o-** *oozing fluid* **-ate** *composed of; pertaining to*
RAST	Blood test that measures the amount of IgE produced each time the blood is mixed with a specific allergen. It shows which of many allergens the patient is allergic to and how severe the allergy is. RAST stands for radioallergosorbent test. A newer, more sensitive test is the ImmunoCAP Specific IgE test.	
skin scraping	A skin scraping is done with the edge of a scalpel to obtain cellular material from a skin lesion. It is examined under the microscope to make a diagnosis of ringworm.	
Tzanck test	A skin scraping is done to obtain fluid from a vesicle. A smear of the fluid is placed on a slide, stained, and examined under a microscope. Herpes virus infections and shingles show characteristic giant cells with viruses in them.	**Tzanck** (TSANGK)
Wood's lamp or light	Ultraviolet light used to highlight areas of skin abnormality. In a darkened room, ultraviolet light makes vitiligo appear bright white and tinea capitus (ringworm) appear blue-green because the fungus fluoresces (glows).	

Medical and Surgical Procedures

Medical Procedures

Word or Phrase	Description	Word Building
Botox injections	Procedure in which the drug Botox is injected into the muscle to release deep wrinkle lines on the face (see Figure 7-27 ■). The drug keeps the muscle from contracting and wrinkling the skin. This treatment is only effective for several months.	**Botox** (BOH-tawks)

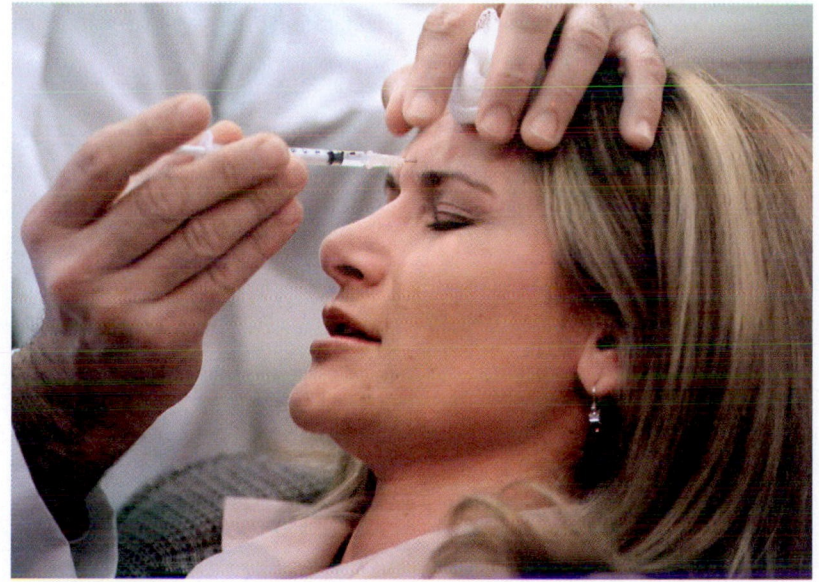

Figure 7-27 ■ Botox injection.
The drug Botox is actually a diluted neurotoxin from the bacterium *Clostridium botulinum* type A that causes food poisoning (botulism) and is present in canned goods with bulging ends.

collagen injections	Procedure in which a liquid containing collagen is injected into wrinkles or acne scars. This plumps the skin and decreases the depth of the wrinkle or scar. The collagen is from cow or human sources.	
cryosurgery	Procedure in which liquid nitrogen is sprayed or painted onto a wart, mole, or other benign lesion, or onto a small malignant lesion. The liquid nitrogen freezes and destroys the lesion.	**cryosurgery** (KRY-oh-SER-jer-ee) **cry/o-** *cold* **surg/o-** *operative procedure* **-ery** *process of*
curettage	Procedure that uses a **curet** to scrape off a superficial skin lesion. A curet is a metal instrument that ends in a small, circular or oval ring with a sharp edge. Curettage is often combined with electrodesiccation for complete removal of a lesion.	**curettage** (kyoo-reh-TAWZH) **curet** (kyoo-RET)
debridement	Procedure in which necrotic tissue is debrided (removed) from a burn, wound, or ulcer. This is done to prevent infection from developing, to assess the extent or depth of a wound, or to create a clean, raw surface that is ready to heal or receive a skin graft. Mechanical debridement consists of putting on a wet dressing, letting it dry, removing the dressing, and pulling off necrotic tissue with it. Topical enzyme drugs debride by chemically dissolving necrotic tissue. Surgical debridement is done under anesthesia using a scalpel, scissors, or curet.	**debridement** (deh-BREED-maw) *Note:* This pronunciation reflects the French origin of this word.

Word or Phrase	Description	Word Building

electrosurgery	Procedure that involves the use of electrical current to remove a nevus, wart, skin tag, or small malignant lesion. The electrical current passes through an electrode and evaporates the intracellular contents of the lesion.
	
	In **electrodesiccation,** the electrode is touched to or inserted into the skin or lesion. In **fulguration,** the electrode is held away from the skin and transmits a spark to the skin surface. **Electrosection** uses a wire loop electrode to cut out the lesion.
		electrosurgery (ee-LEK-troh-SER-jer-ee)
		   electr/o- *electricity*
		   surg/o- *operative procedure*
		   -ery *process of*
		
		electrodesiccation
		(ee-LEK-troh-DES-ih-KAY-shun)
		   electr/o- *electricity*
		   desicc/o- *to dry up*
		   -ation *a process; being or having*
		
		fulguration (FUL-gyoo-RAY-shun)
		   fulgur/o- *spark of electricity*
		   -ation *a process; being or having*
		
		electrosection (ee-LEK-troh-SEK-shun)
		   electr/o- *electricity*
		   sect/o- *to cut*
		   -ion *action; condition*

incision and drainage (I&D)	Procedure to treat a cyst or abscess. A scalpel is used to make an incision, and the fluid or pus inside is expressed manually or allowed to drain out.	**incision** (in-SIH-shun)
		   incis/o- *to cut into*
		   -ion *action; condition*

laser surgery	Procedure that uses pulses of laser light to remove birthmarks, tattoos, enlarged superficial blood vessels (of acne rosacea), or unwanted hair. A tunable laser has a specific wavelength of light that only reacts with certain colors (the dark red of a birthmark, the black pigment of a tattoo, etc.) to break up that color and the structure that contains it. Surrounding tissue of a different color is unharmed.	**laser** (LAY-zer) *Laser* is an acronym, a word made from the first letters of the phrase *light amplification by stimulated emission of radiation.*
skin examination	Procedure to examine all of the patient's skin or just one skin lesion, rash, or tumor. The dermatologist uses a lens to magnify the area (see Figure 7-28 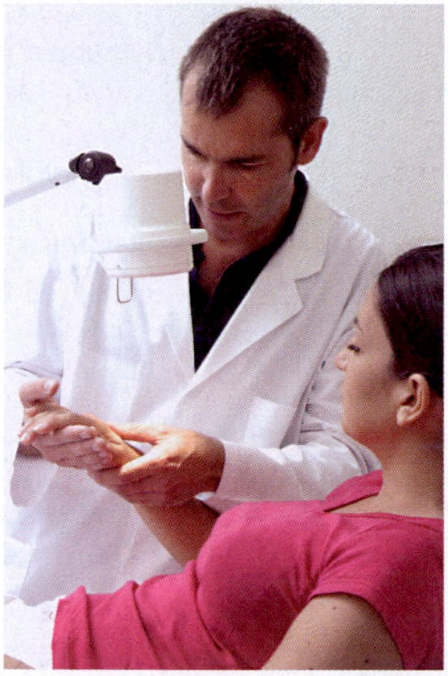 ■). **Figure 7-28** ■ **Skin examination.** This dermatologist is using a magnifying lens and strong light to examine a lesion on this patient's skin. The area may need to be biopsied to obtain a diagnosis.	

Word or Phrase	Description	Word Building
skin resurfacing	Removal of superficial and deep acne scars, fine or deep wrinkles, or tattoos, or the correction of large pores and skin tone irregularities by means of topical chemicals, abrasion, or laser treatments.	
chemical peel	Skin resurfacing that uses a chemical to remove the epidermis. The strongest chemical peels are done in surgery.	
dermabrasion	Skin resurfacing that uses a rapidly spinning wire brush or diamond surface to mechanically abrade (scrape away) the epidermis.	**dermabrasion** (DER-mah-BRAY-zhun) **derm/o-** *skin* **abras/o-** *scrape off* **-ion** *action; condition*
laser skin resurfacing	Skin resurfacing that uses a computer-controlled laser to vaporize the epidermis and some of the dermis. This promotes the regrowth of smooth skin. It is also known as a **laser peel**.	
microderm-abrasion	Skin resurfacing that uses aluminum oxide crystals to abrade and remove the epidermis to produce smoother skin	**microdermabrasion** (MY-kroh-DER-mah-BRAY-shun) **micr/o-** *one millionth; small* **derm/o-** *skin* **abras/o-** *scrape off* **-ion** *action; condition*
suturing	Procedure that uses sutures to bring the edges of the skin together after a laceration or other injury or at the end of a surgical procedure (see Figure 7-29 ■).	**suture** (SOO-chur)

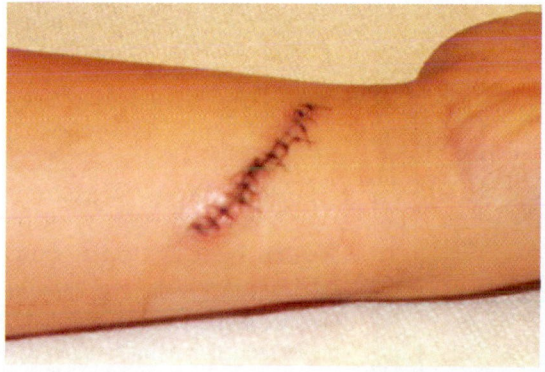

Figure 7-29 ■ Layered closure with sutures.
After an anesthetic drug was given to numb the area, this laceration in the forearm was sewn closed with two layers of sutures, the first in the deeper tissues and the second to close the skin edges. After a week, the skin sutures were removed. The deeper sutures, which were made of a material that was absorbed by the body, did not need to be removed.

Surgical Procedures

Word or Phrase	Description	Word Building
biopsy (Bx)	Procedure done in a dermatologist's office or the hospital to remove all or part of a skin lesion. The biopsy specimen is sent to the pathology department for examination and diagnosis.	**biopsy** (BY-awp-see) **bi/o-** *life; living organisms; living tissue* **-opsy** *process of viewing*
excisional biopsy	Procedure that uses a scalpel to remove an entire large lesion	**excisional** (ek-SIH-shun-al) **excis/o-** *to cut out* **-ion** *action; condition* **-al** *pertaining to*
incisional biopsy	Procedure that uses a scalpel to make an incision to remove part of a large lesion	**incisional** (in-SIH-shun-al) **incis/o-** *to cut into* **-ion** *action; condition* **-al** *pertaining to*

Word or Phrase	Description	Word Building
needle aspiration	Procedure that uses a needle to aspirate the fluid contents in a cyst	**aspiration** (AS-pih-RAY-shun) **aspir/o-** *to breathe in; to suck in* **-ation** *a process; being or having*
punch biopsy	Procedure that uses a circular metal cutter to remove a plug-shaped core that includes the epidermis, dermis, and subcutaneous tissue	
shave biopsy	Procedure that uses a scalpel or razor blade to shave off a superficial lesion in the epidermis or dermis	
dermatoplasty	Any type of plastic surgery of the skin, such as skin grafting, removal of a keloid, etc.	**dermatoplasty** (DER-mah-toh-PLAS-tee) **dermat/o-** *skin* **-plasty** *process of reshaping by surgery*
liposuction	Procedure to remove excessive adipose tissue deposits from the breasts, abdomen, hips, legs, or buttocks. A cannula inserted through a small incision is used to suction out the subcutaneous tissue (see Figure 7-30 ■). Ultrasonic-assisted liposuction uses ultrasonic waves to break up the fatty tissue before it is removed. This is also known as **suction-assisted lipectomy.**	**liposuction** (LIP-oh-SUK-shun) **lip/o-** *lipid (fat)* **suct/o-** *to suck* **-ion** *action; condition* **lipectomy** (ly-PEK-toh-mee) **lip/o-** *lipid (fat)* **-ectomy** *surgical excision*

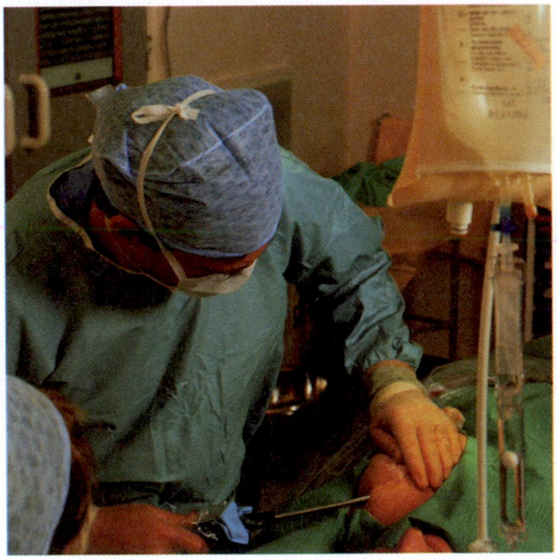

Figure 7-30 ■ Liposuction.
This surgeon is performing liposuction to reduce the size of a breast. This is a plastic surgery procedure that is known as a breast reduction or mammoplasty. Both breasts will be done to achieve a symmetrical result.

Word or Phrase	Description	Word Building
Mohs' surgery	Procedure to remove skin cancer, particularly tumors with irregular shapes and depths. An operating microscope is used during the surgery to examine each layer of excised tissue. If the tissue shows cancerous cells, more tissue is removed until no trace of cancer remains.	**Mohs'** (MOHZ)
rhytidectomy	Surgical procedure to remove wrinkles and tighten loose, aging skin on the face and neck. It is also known as a **facelift.** A **blepharoplasty,** the removal of fat and drooping skin from around the eyelids, is often done at the same time.	**rhytidectomy** (RIT-ih-DEK-toh-mee) **rhytid/o-** *wrinkle* **-ectomy** *surgical excision* **blepharoplasty** (BLEF-ah-roh-PLAS-tee) **blephar/o-** *eyelid* **-plasty** *process of reshaping by surgery*

Word or Phrase	Description	Word Building
skin grafting	Procedure that uses human, animal, or artificial skin to provide a temporary covering or a permanent layer of skin over a burn or wound (see Figure 7-31 ■). A **dermatome** is used to remove (harvest) a thin layer of skin to be used as a graft. A split-thickness skin graft contains the epidermis and part of the dermis. A full-thickness skin graft contains the epidermis and all of the dermis. Tiny holes can be cut in the skin graft to make a mesh that can stretch and cover a larger area. These holes allow tissue fluid to flow out and provide spaces into which the new skin can grow.	**dermatome** (DER-mah-tohm) **derm/a-** *skin* **-tome** *instrument used to cut; area with distinct edges*

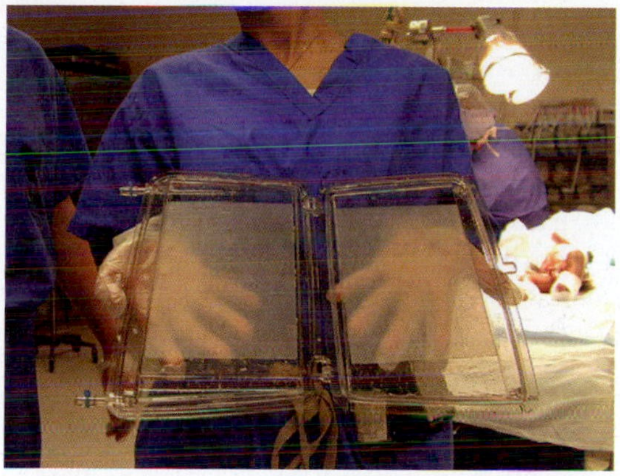

Figure 7-31 ■ Skin graft.
A skin graft is so thin that the physician's gloved hands can be seen through it. The graft is kept in a sterile container until it is applied to the patient's skin.

autograft	Skin graft that is taken from another part of the patient's own body	**autograft** (AW-toh-graft) **aut/o-** *self* **-graft** *tissue for implant or transplant*
allograft	Skin graft that is taken from a cadaver. It is frozen and stored in a skin bank until needed. This is a temporary skin graft to protect the burn and prevent infection and fluid loss.	**allograft** (AL-oh-graft) **all/o-** *other; strange* **-graft** *tissue for implant or transplant*
xenograft	Skin graft of just the dermis that is taken from an animal (pig). This is a temporary skin graft to protect the burn and prevent infection and fluid loss.	**xenograft** (ZEN-oh-graft) **xen/o-** *foreign* **-graft** *tissue for implant or transplant*
synthetic skin graft	Skin graft that is made from collagen fibers arranged in a lattice pattern. The patient's body does not reject synthetic skin, and healing skin grows into it as the graft gradually disintegrates.	

Word Alert

HOMONYMS

dermatome (noun) a specific area of the skin that sends sensory information to the spinal cord
Example: The patient had shingles on the chest and back along the T6 dermatome.

dermatome (noun) a surgical instrument used to make a shallow, continuous cut to form a skin graft
Example: After the donor site was prepped and draped, a dermatome was used to obtain a split-thickness skin graft.

Did You Know?

The skin of frogs and lizards were used as skin grafts in the 1600s.

Drug Categories

These categories of drugs are used to treat integumentary diseases and conditions. The most common generic and trade name drugs in each category are listed.

Category	Indication	Examples	Word Building
anesthetic drugs	Provide temporary numbness of the skin to treat injuries and skin diseases or to remove skin lesions. They are applied topically or injected.	lidocaine (Lidoderm, Xylocaine, Zingo)	**anesthetic** (AN-es-THET-ik) **an-** *without; not* **esthet/o-** *sensation; feeling* **-ic** *pertaining to*
antibiotic drugs	Treat bacterial infections of the skin or acne vulgaris. They are applied topically or given orally.	bacitracin, neomycin, erythromycin (Emgel, Eryderm); oral tetracycline (Sumycin)	**antibiotic** (AN-tee-by-AWT-ik) (AN-tih-by-AWT-ik) **anti-** *against* **bi/o-** *life; living organisms; living tissue* **-tic** *pertaining to*
antifungal drugs	Treat ringworm (tinea) when applied topically. Treat fungal infection of the nails when applied topically or given orally.	clotrimazole (Cruex, Desenex, Lotrimin AF), tolnaftate (Aftate, Tinactin); oral ketoconazole (Nizoral)	**antifungal** (AN-tee-FUN-gal) (AN-tih-FUN-gal) **anti-** *against* **fung/o-** *fungus* **-al** *pertaining to*
antipruritic drugs	Decrease itching. They are applied topically or given orally.	diphenhydramine (Benadryl); topical colloidal oatmeal (Aveeno)	**antipruritic** (AN-tee-proo-RIT-ik) (AN-tih-proo-RIT-ik) **anti-** *against* **prurit/o-** *itching* **-ic** *pertaining to*
antiviral drugs	Treat herpes simplex virus infections. They are applied topically or given orally.	docosanol (Abreva), acyclovir (Zovirax); oral famciclovir (Famvir)	**antiviral** (AN-tee-VY-ral) (AN-tih-VY-ral) **anti-** *against* **vir/o-** *virus* **-al** *pertaining to*
coal tar drugs	Treat psoriasis. They cause the epidermal cells to multiply more slowly and decrease itching. Coal tar is a by-product of the processing of bituminous coal. It contains more than 10,000 different chemicals. It is applied topically.	coal tar (Balnetar, Neutrogena T/Gel, Zetar)	
corticosteroid drugs	Treat skin inflammation from contact dermatitis, psoriasis, and eczema. They are applied topically or given orally.	fluocinonide (Lidex), hydrocortisone (Dermolate); oral prednisone (Deltasone)	**corticosteroid** (KOR-tih-koh-STAIR-oyd) **cortic/o-** *cortex (outer region)* **-steroid** *steroid*
drugs for alopecia	Applied topically to dilate the arteries in the scalp to increase blood flow and hair growth. Given orally to block the production of DHT.	topical minoxidil (Rogaine); oral finasteride (Propecia)	
drugs for infestations	Treat scabies (mites) and pediculosis (lice). Lotion and shampoo.	lindane, malathion (Ovide)	

Category	Indication	Examples	Word Building
photodynamic therapy (PDT)	Treats cancer of the skin with laser light and a photosensitizing drug.	porfimer (Photofrin)	**photodynamic** (FOH-toh-dy-NAM-ik) **phot/o-** *light* **dynam/o-** *power; movement* **-ic** *pertaining to*
psoralen drugs	Treat psoriasis. Psoralen sensitizes the skin to ultraviolet light therapy and it damages cellular DNA and decreases the rate of cell division. This combination is known as PUVA (psoralen drug and ultraviolet A light)	methoxsalen (Oxsoralen)	**psoralen** (SOR-ah-len)
vitamin A–type drugs	Treat acne vulgaris or severe cystic acne. They cause the epidermal cells to multiply rapidly to keep the pores from becoming clogged. Applied topically or given orally.	topical tretinoin (Retin-A); oral isotretinoin (Accutane)	

Clinical Connections

Pharmacology. Topical drugs such as creams, lotions, and ointments are absorbed into the skin for a local drug effect. Topical drug patches release small amounts of a drug over time that are absorbed through the skin and exert a systemic effect. This is the **transdermal** route. The **intradermal** route uses a needle inserted just beneath the epidermis. This is used for the Mantoux tuberculosis test and allergy testing. Other types are **hypodermic** injections because the needle goes beneath the dermis and into the subcutaneous tissue or the muscle (see Figure 7-32 ■).

topical (TOP-ih-kal)
  topic/o- *a specific area*
  -al *pertaining to*

transdermal (trans-DER-mal)
  trans- *across; through*
  derm/o- *skin*
  -al *pertaining to*

intradermal (IN-trah-DER-mal)
  intra- *within*
  derm/o- *skin*
  -al *pertaining to*

hypodermic (HY-poh-DER-mik)
  hypo- *below; deficient*
  derm/o- *skin*
  -ic *pertaining to*

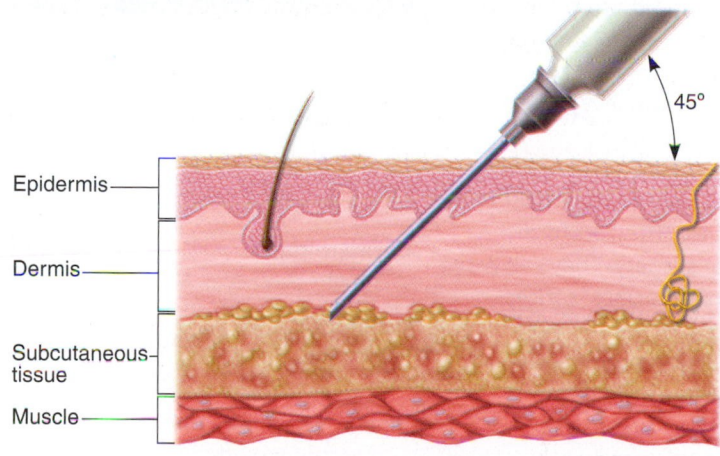

Epidermis
Dermis
Subcutaneous tissue
Muscle
45°

Figure 7-32 ■ **Subcutaneous injection.**

Abbreviations

Bx	biopsy	**PDT**	photodynamic therapy
Ca	cancer (slang)	**PUVA**	psoralen (drug and) ultraviolet A (light therapy)
C&S	culture and sensitivity	**SLE**	systemic lupus erythematosus
Derm	dermatology (slang)	**SQ***	subcutaneous
HSV	herpes simplex virus	**subcu**	subcutaneous
I&D	incision and drainage	**subQ**	subcutaneous

*According to the Joint Commission on Accreditation of Healthcare Organizations (JCAHO), this abbreviation should not be used. Because it is still used by some healthcare workers, it is included here.

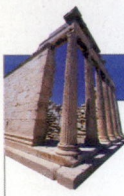

It's Greek to Me!

Did you notice that some words have two different combining forms? Combining forms from both Greek and Latin languages remain a part of medical language today.

Word	Greek	Latin	Medical Word Examples
fat	lip/o-	adip/o-	lipocyte, adipose tissue, adipocere
hair	trich/o-	hirsut/o-, pil/o-	schizotrichia, hirsutism, pilonidal cyst, piloerection
nail	onych/o-	ungu/o-	onychomycosis, ungual
skin	derm/a-, derm/o-	cutane/o-, cut/i-	dermatome, dermal, subcutaneous, cuticle
	dermat/o-	integument/o-	dermatologist, integumentary
sweat	diaphor/o-	hidr/o-, sudor/i-	diaphoresis, anhidrosis, sudoriferous gland

CAREER FOCUS

Meet Toral, a physician's assistant in a cosmetic surgeon's office

"Growing up, I always knew I would be in medicine. At first, I entertained the idea of becoming a nurse. Then I entertained the idea of becoming a physician. Being a physician's assistant allows me to see my own patients, treat and diagnose, write my own prescriptions, care for patients, and advise them. I also assist in laser procedures and all surgical procedures. Our everyday language is medical terminology—from talking to the physician, talking to your coworkers, to charting in the charts. With so many patients being Internet-savvy, they come in talking in medical terminology!"

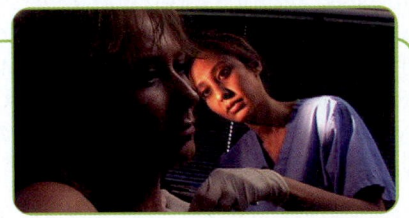

Physician's assistants are healthcare professionals who are licensed to perform basic medical care while under the supervision of a physician. They perform physical examinations, prescribe drugs, and perform minor surgery. They can assist the physician during more extensive surgery. They work in physicians' offices, clinics, and in hospitals.

Dermatologists are physicians who practice in the medical specialty of dermatology. They diagnose and treat patients with diseases of the skin. Physicians can take additional training and become board certified in the subspecialty of pediatric dermatology. Malignancies of the skin are treated medically by an oncologist or surgically by a dermatologist, a general surgeon, or plastic surgeon.

Plastic surgeons are physicians who perform plastic and reconstructive surgery to reshape the body. They remove lesions and scars and perform liposuction and other procedures that reshape the skin and subcutaneous tissue.

dermatologist
(DER-mah-TAWL-oh-jist)
 dermat/o- skin
 log/o- word; the study of
 -ist one who specializes in

plastic (PLAS-tik)
 plast/o- growth; formation
 -ic pertaining to

surgeon (SER-jun)
 surg/o- operative procedure
 -eon one who performs

PEARSON **myhealthprofessionskit**™ To see Toral's complete video profile, visit Medical Terminology Interactive at www.myhealthprofessionskit.com. Select this book, log in, and go to the 7th floor of Pearson General Hospital. Enter the Laboratory, and click on the computer screen.

CHAPTER REVIEW EXERCISES

Test your knowledge of the chapter by completing these review exercises. Use the Answer Key at the end of the book to check your answers.

Anatomy and Physiology

Matching Exercise

Match each word or phrase to its description.

1. basal layer
2. dermis
3. epidermis
4. lipocytes
5. lunula
6. integument
7. melanocytes
8. sudoriferous glands
9. allergen

_____ Consists of the epidermis, dermis, nails, and hair

_____ Outermost layer of skin

_____ Another name for sweat glands

_____ Half moon that contains keratin cells

_____ Cells that make up adipose tissue

_____ Produce brown or black pigment

_____ Deepest part of the epidermis

_____ Contains sebaceous glands and sweat glands

_____ Substance that causes an allergic reaction

Circle Exercise

Circle the correct word from the choices given.

1. The (**nail bed, nail plate, nail root**) is also known as the quick.
2. (**Collagen, Keratin, Melanin**) is a hard, fibrous protein found in the most superficial cells of the epidermis.
3. Piloerection involves contraction of the muscle around a (**dermatome, hair, lipocyte**).
4. (**Anaphylaxis, Exfoliation, Perspiration**) is the normal shedding of skin cells.
5. All of the following are changes that occur in the skin during pregnancy *except* (**dermatome, linea nigra, striae**).
6. *Ungual* is the adjective form for (**hair, nail, skin**).

True or False Exercise

Indicate whether each statement is true or false by writing T or F on the line.

1. _____ The integumentary system consists of the skin, hair, and nails.
2. _____ The epithelium is the outermost layer of the skin.
3. _____ Sebaceous glands are exocrine glands.
4. _____ Melanin is produced by melanocytes in the subcutaneous tissue.
5. _____ Sunlight on the skin helps produce vitamin D.
6. _____ Anaphylaxis is a severe, systemic allergic reaction.

Diseases and Conditions

Circle Exercise

Circle the name of the skin lesion shown in each of these illustrations.

1. This skin lesion is a (**cyst, fissure, papule, wheal**).

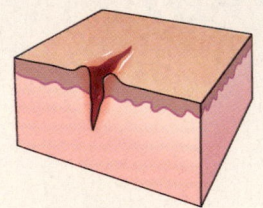

3. This skin lesion is a (**cyst, macule, scale, wheal**).

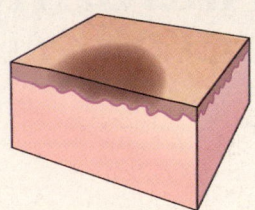

2. This skin lesion is a (**cyst, laceration, macule, vesicle**).

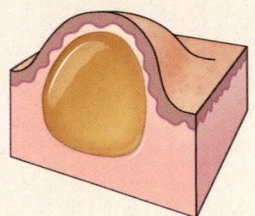

Matching Exercise

Match each word or phrase to its description.

1. abscess
2. bullae
3. callus
4. decubitus ulcers
5. dermatitis
6. diaphoresis
7. dysplastic nevus
8. hematoma
9. jaundice
10. Kaposi's sarcoma
11. onychomycosis
12. vitiligo

_____ Inflammation or infection of the skin

_____ Yellowish coloration of the skin (icterus)

_____ Localized collection of pus

_____ Often seen in AIDS patients

_____ Autoimmune disease with depigmentation patches

_____ Thickened, firm pad on the epidermis

_____ Fungal infection of the nails

_____ Present in second-degree burns

_____ Frequent repositioning avoids these

_____ Excessive sweating

_____ Collection of blood under the skin

_____ Can develop into malignant melanoma

True or False Exercise

Indicate whether each statement is true or false by writing T or F on the line.

1. _____ A neoplasm is always a malignant growth of the skin.

2. _____ Bluish discoloration of the skin from a lack of oxygen is known as a bruise.

3. _____ An abnormally enlarged scar is known as a keloid.

4. _____ Actinic keratoses are rough, raised areas due to chronic sun exposure.

5. _____ Rhinophyma is a complication of severe acne vulgaris of the nose.

6. _____ Hirsutism is a lack of hair due to aging.

7. _____ Psoriasis is treated with coal tar drugs and PUVA.

Circle Exercise

Circle the correct word from the choices given.

1. A macule is a/an (**crevice, elevated, flat**) lesion.
2. An acne whitehead is also called a (**cyst, pustule, wheal**).
3. (**Excoriation, Exfoliation, Laceration**) is a superficial linear scratch on the skin.
4. The thick, black crust over a third-degree burn is known as a/an (**cicatrix, eschar, keloid**).
5. Tinea pedis occurs on the skin of the (**feet, groin, trunk of the body**).
6. A nevus includes all of the following *except* (**birthmark, cellulitis, mole**).
7. A yellow plaque on the skin is known as a/an (**jaundice, xanthoma, scleroderma**).
8. Tinea capitis is a fungal infection of the skin that is also known as (**onychomycosis, ringworm, verruca**).

Matching Exercise

Match each word or phrase to its description.

1. chickenpox   _____ Occurs at the base of the fingernail
2. cold sores   _____ Herpes simplex type 2
3. pediculosis   _____ Infestation of parasitic mites
4. furuncle   _____ First occurrence of herpes varicella-zoster
5. herpes whitlow   _____ Second occurrence of herpes varicella-zoster
6. genital herpes   _____ Herpes simplex type 1
7. shingles   _____ Caused by the human papillomavirus
8. scabies   _____ Infestation of lice
9. verruca   _____ Caused by *Staphylococcus aureus*

Laboratory, Radiology, Surgery, and Drugs

Matching Exercise

Match each word or phrase to its description.

1. allergy skin testing   _____ Instrument used to make a skin graft
2. culture and sensitivity   _____ Uses ultrasonic waves to break up and suction fat
3. debridement   _____ Done to determine what bacterium is causing an infection
4. dermatome   _____ Procedure to remove necrotic tissue
5. liposuction   _____ Uses allergens for testing
6. Tzanck test   _____ Temporary skin graft taken from an animal
7. xenograft   _____ Examines scrapings of fluid from a vesicle

Circle Exercise

Circle the correct word from the choices given.

1. Electrosurgery includes all of the following *except* (**debridement, fulguration, electrodesiccation**).

2. (**Cryosurgery, Curettage, Incision**) uses a curet to scrape off a skin lesion.

3. Allergy skin testing uses (**hypodermic, intradermal, transdermal**) injections of allergens.

4. A surgical procedure to remove wrinkles from the face is a (**blepharoplasty, Botox injection, rhytidectomy**).

5. A/an (**dermatoplasty, excisional biopsy, incisional biopsy**) removes just a piece of a large skin lesion.

6. All of the following are skin resurfacing techniques *except* (**chemical peel, dermabrasion, incision and drainage**).

7. All of the following drugs are used to treat psoriasis *except* (**antifungal drugs, coal tar drugs, psoralen**).

Building Medical Words

Review the Combining Forms Exercise, Combining Form and Suffix Exercise, and Prefix Exercise that you already completed in the anatomy section on pages 336–337

Combining Forms Exercise

Before you build integumentary words, review these additional combining forms. Next to each combining form, write its medical meaning. The first one has been done for you.

Combining Form	Medical Meaning	Combining Form	Medical Meaning
1. abras/o-	scrape off	16. hidr/o-	
2. alopec/o-		17. kel/o-	
3. aut/o-		18. lacer/o-	
4. bi/o-		19. malign/o-	
5. blephar/o-		20. myc/o-	
6. contus/o-		21. necr/o-	
7. cry/o-		22. ne/o-	
8. cyan/o-		23. pedicul/o-	
9. erythemat/o-		24. pigment/o-	
10. esthes/o-		25. plast/o-	
11. excis/o-		26. prurit/o-	
12. exud/o-		27. psor/o-	
13. fulgur/o-		28. rhytid/o-	
14. fung/o-		29. sarc/o-	
15. hemat/o-		30. xer/o-	

Related Combining Forms Exercise

Write the combining forms on the line provided. (Hint: See the It's Greek to Me feature box.)

1. Two combining forms that mean *fat*. _____

2. Two combining forms that mean *nail*. _____

3. Three combining forms that mean *hair*. _____

4. Three combining forms that mean *sweat*. _____

5. Six combining forms that mean *skin*. _____

Combining Form and Suffix Exercise

Read the definition of the medical word. Select the correct suffix from the Suffix List. Select the correct combining form from the Combining Form List. Build the medical word and write it on the line. Be sure to check your spelling. The first one has been done for you.

SUFFIX LIST	COMBINING FORM LIST	
-ate (composed of; pertaining to)	abras/o- (scrape off)	kel/o- (tumor)
-ation (a process; being or having)	aut/o- (self)	lip/o- (lipid; fat)
-derma (skin)	bi/o- (life; living tissue)	melan/o- (black)
-ectomy (surgical excision)	blephar/o- (eyelid)	myc/o- (fungus)
-graft (tissue for implant or transplant)	contus/o- (bruising)	necr/o- (dead cells or tissue)
-ic (pertaining to)	cyan/o- (blue)	ne/o- (new)
-ion (action; condition)	derm/a- (skin)	onych/o- (nail; fingernail or toenail)
-itis (inflammation of; infection of)	dermat/o- (skin)	pedicul/o- (lice)
-oid (resembling)	erythemat/o- (redness)	prurit/o- (itching)
-oma (tumor; mass)	exud/o- (oozing fluid)	rhytid/o- (wrinkle)
-opsy (process of viewing)	fulgur/o- (spark of electricity)	xer/o- (dry)
-osis (condition; abnormal condition; process)	hemat/o- (blood)	
-ous (pertaining to)		
-plasm (growth; formed substance)		
-plasty (process of reshaping by surgery)		
-tic (pertaining to)		
-tome (instrument used to cut; area with distinct edges)		

Definition of the Medical Word

1. Process of reshaping by surgery on the skin

2. Mass of blood (under the skin)

3. Skin (that is very) dry

4. Abnormal condition of the nail having a fungus (*Hint: Use two combining forms*)

5. Condition of (the skin being) scraped off

6. Tumor (of the cell that produces the) black (pigment melanin)

7. Abnormal condition (of the skin being) blue

8. Inflammation or infection of the skin

9. Pertaining to itching

10. Tumor of fat

11. A growth (that is) new

12. Pertaining to redness (of the skin)

13. Pertaining to dead cells or tissue

14. Condition of (having) lice

15. (Scar that becomes larger until it is) resembling a tumor

16. Condition of bruising

17. Composed of oozing fluid

18. A process (on the skin that uses) a spark of electricity

19. Process of viewing (under the microscope) living tissue

20. Surgical excision of fat

21. Instrument used to cut the skin

Build the Medical Word

1. *dermatoplasty*

Definition of the Medical Word   **Build the Medical Word**

22. Process of reshaping by surgery (on the) eyelids   _____

23. Surgical excision of wrinkles   _____

24. Tissue for implant or transplant (that is taken from one's own) self   _____

Prefix Exercise

Read the definition of the medical word. Look at the medical word or partial word that is given (it already contains a combining form and a suffix). Select the correct prefix from the Prefix List and write it on the blank line. Then build the medical word and write it on the line. Be sure to check your spelling. The first one has been done for you.

PREFIX LIST		
an- (without; not)	de- (reversal of; without)	intra- (within)
anti- (against)	dys- (painful; difficult; abnormal)	pre- (before; in front of)

Definition of the Medical Word	Prefix	Word or Partial Word	Build the Medical Word
1. Pertaining to (a drug that is) against fungus	anti-	fungal	antifungal
2. Pertaining to an abnormal growth or formation	_____	plastic	_____
3. Condition (of being) without sensation or feeling	_____	esthesia	_____
4. A process (of being) without pigment (in the skin)	_____	pigmentation	_____
5. Abnormal condition (of being) without fluid (from the sweat glands)	_____	hidrosis	_____
6. Pertaining to within the skin	_____	dermal	_____
7. Pertaining to (being) before cancer	_____	malignant	_____
8. Pertaining to (a drug that is) against itching	_____	pruritic	_____

Abbreviations

Matching Exercise

Match each abbreviation to its description.

1. Bx   _____ Used to treat an abscess

2. C&S   _____ Autoimmune disease

3. HSV   _____ Can be excisional or incisional

4. I&D   _____ Causes genital herpes, cold sores, and shingles

5. PUVA   _____ Used to treat psoriasis

6. SLE   _____ Tissue beneath the dermis

7. SubQ   _____ Test to identify bacterium causing an infection and identify a drug to treat it

Applied Skills

Plural Noun and Adjective Spelling

Fill in the blanks with the correct word form. Be sure to check your spelling. The first one has been done for you.

Singular Noun	Plural Noun	Adjective
1. follicle	follicles	follicular
2. skin		
3. epidermis		
4. dermis		
5. nail		
6. epithelium		
7. vesicle		
8. pruritus		
9. cyanosis		
10. erythema		
11. icterus		
12. necrosis		
13. gangrene		
14. verruca		
15. malignancy		
16. keratosis		
17. psoriasis		
18. diaphoresis		
19. comedo		

English and Medical Word Equivalents Exercise

For each English word or phrase, write its equivalent medical word. Be sure to check your spelling. The first one has been done for you.

English Word	Medical Word
1. cradle cap	eczema
2. age spots or liver spots	
3. baldness	
4. bed sore	
5. boil	
6. brush burn	
7. hives	
8. infestation with lice	
9. infestation with mites	
10. port-wine stain	
11. ringworm	
12. skin tag	
13. wart	

Medical Report Exercise

This exercise contains an office chart note. Read the report and answer the questions.

CHART NOTE

PATIENT NAME: GUNDERSON, Denise

PATIENT NUMBER: 191-46-3985

DATE: November 19, 20xx

HISTORY

The patient has been on the antibiotic drug Zithromax for a severe skin flare-up of erythema nodosum following an untreated strep throat. This caused swelling and edema in her right foot, but it then spread to her right leg, areas on her chest, left knee, and her left foot. These areas were extremely painful, erythematous, and her right knee developed a large, painful nodule under the skin. Her right foot was so painful and edematous that it was nearly impossible for her to walk. Then the dorsum of her right foot developed cellulitis, and she was placed on the antibiotic drug Zithromax. Today, she had just taken her last scheduled dose of Zithromax when she describes that she suddenly had a very itchy scalp. When she scratched her scalp, she could feel multiple raised areas. About 20 minutes later, there were about twice as many raised areas on her scalp, and now she could see wheals on her cheeks and on her chest. When the wheals on her face became large welts, she became concerned about not being able to breathe and took two antihistamine tablets (Benadryl). One hour later, she had to take two more Benadryl. After that, the welts and itching began to subside. Although she was feeling better, she decided to come to the office today to be examined.

PHYSICAL EXAMINATION

Integumentary system: There are a few, small, scattered hives still visible on her trunk and arms. The welts on her scalp and face have completely disappeared. The cellulitis of her right foot has cleared up and the smaller nodules from the erythema nodosum have disappeared. The largest nodule over her right knee is slowly resolving.

ASSESSMENT

1. Severe urticaria, secondary to an allergic drug reaction to azithromycin (Zithromax).
2. Right foot cellulitis, resolved.
3. Resolving erythema nodosum following an untreated strep throat.

PLAN

A note has been made in the patient's medical record that she is allergic to Zithromax. The acute phase of this allergic reaction is past. The patient has been instructed to never take that antibiotic drug again. Follow-up as needed for her resolving erythema nodosum.

Bonnie R. Grant, M.D.

Bonnie R. Grant, M.D.

BRG: smt
D: 11/19/xx
T: 11/19/xx

Word Analysis Questions

1. Divide *cellulitis* into word parts and define each word part.

   Word Part   **Definition**

   _____   _____

   _____   _____

2. The patient has erythema on her legs. If you wanted to use the adjective form of *erythema*, you would say, "She has _____ areas on her legs."

Fact Finding Questions

1. What is the medical word for *itching*? _____

2. Circle the word that means reddened: (**edematous, erythematous, flare-up**)

3. Which are larger—welts or wheals? _____

4. In the Physical Examination section of this chart note, which body system is examined? _____

5. The patient's urticaria was due to a (**cellulitis, drug reaction, strep throat**).

Critical Thinking Skills

1. What four symptoms of urticaria did this patient have?

   _____

   _____

   _____

   _____

2. What skin condition did the patient develop after having an untreated strep throat? _____

On the Job Challenge Exercise

On the job, you will encounter new medical words. Practice your medical dictionary skills by looking up the medical words in bold and writing their definitions on the lines provided.

OFFICE CHART NOTE

This 11-year-old young lady was brought in by her mother. The mother states that the patient continually bites her fingernails despite all attempts to discourage her. Her fingernails are always bitten to the quick, and the skin around them is frequently bloody. The patient states she is unable to stop. When the mother stepped out of the examining room, the patient became tearful as she related pressure at school and an impending divorce between her parents.

On examination, the fingernails show evidence of chronic biting, right hand greater than left. The patient is right handed. Examination of the feet also shows evidence of nail biting. There is erythema and swelling of the tissue along the medial nail groove of her right great toe where the nail was bitten away and is growing back but is ingrown. The skin on the lower arms bilaterally shows aggressive scratching of small, isolated insect bites. The scalp shows some small, patchy areas where there is an absence of hair. The patient admits to some hair-pulling.

DIAGNOSES

1. **Onychophagia.**

2. **Onychocryptosis.**

3. **Trichotillomania.**

Plan: The medial side of the nail on the right great toe was trimmed with clippers. The patient's mother was given a prescription for a 7-day course of an antibiotic drug. The patient's mother was also given a referral for the patient to see a child psychologist for counseling.

---

1. onychophagia _____

2. onychocryptosis _____

3. trichotillomania _____

Hearing Medical Words Exercise

You hear someone speaking the medical words given below. Read each pronunciation and then write the medical word it represents. Be sure to check your spelling. The first one has been done for you.

1. AK-nee vul-GAIR-is   *acne vulgaris*
2. AN-ah-fih-LAK-sis   _____
3. BLEF-ah-roh-PLAS-tee   _____
4. KRY-oh-SER-jer-ee   _____
5. SY-ah-NOH-sis   _____

6. deh-BREED-maw   _____
7. DER-mah-TAWL-oh-jist   _____
8. AIR-eh-THEM-ah-tus   _____
9. proo-RY-tus   _____
10. soh-RY-ah-sis   _____

Pronunciation Exercise

Read the medical word that is given. Then review the syllables in the pronunciation. Circle the primary (main) accented syllable. The first one has been done for you.

1. abrasion (ah-(bray)-zhun)
2. adipose (ad-ih-pohs)
3. alopecia (al-oh-pee-shee-ah)
4. biopsy (by-awp-see)
5. cellulitis (sel-yoo-ly-tis)

6. hematoma (hee-mah-toh-mah)
7. liposuction (lip-oh-suk-shun)
8. neoplasm (nee-oh-plazm)
9. psoriasis (soh-ry-ah-sis)
10. subcutaneous (sub-kyoo-tay-nee-us)

Multimedia Preview

Immerse yourself in a variety of activities inside Medical Terminology Interactive. Getting there is simple:

1. Click on www.myhealthprofessionskit.com.
2. Select "Medical Terminology" from the choice of disciplines.
3. First-time users must create an account using the scratch-off code on the inside front cover of this book.
4. Find this book and log in using your username and password.
5. Click on Medical Terminology Interactive.
6. Take the elevator to the 7th Floor to begin your virtual exploration of this chapter!

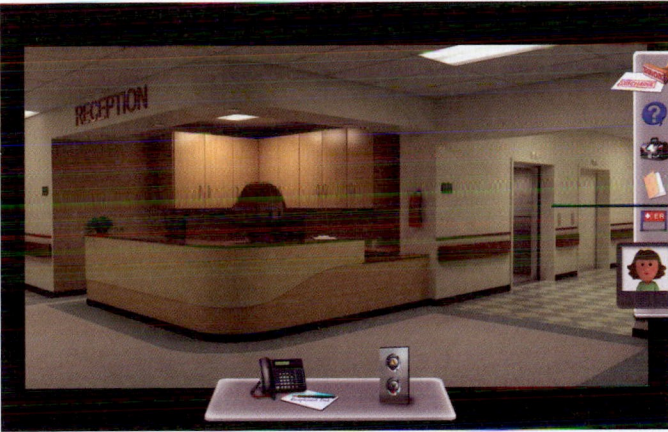
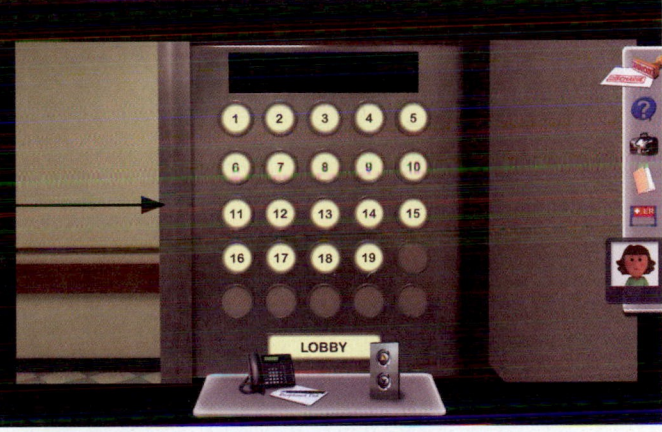

■ **Strikeout**   Click on the alphabet tiles to fill in the empty squares in the word or phrase to complete the sentence. This game quizzes your vocabulary and spelling. But choose your letters carefully because three strikes and you're out!

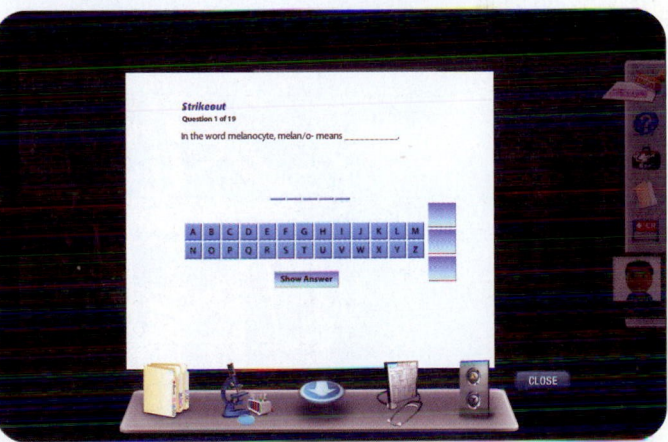

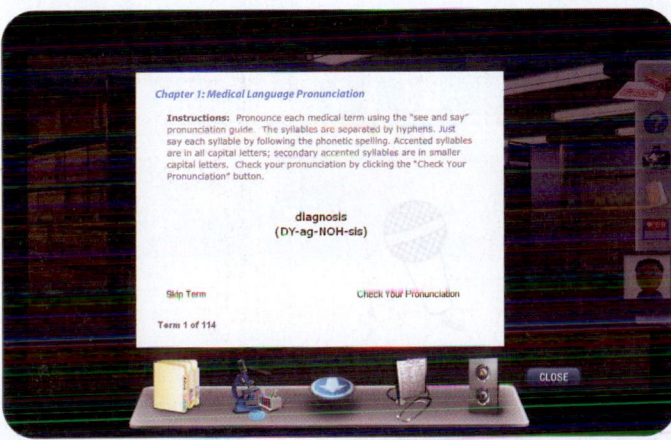

■ **Medical Language Pronunciation**   When using medical language, correct pronunciation is key! Carefully listen to a pronounced medical word and then practice pronouncing it yourself.

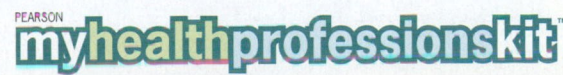

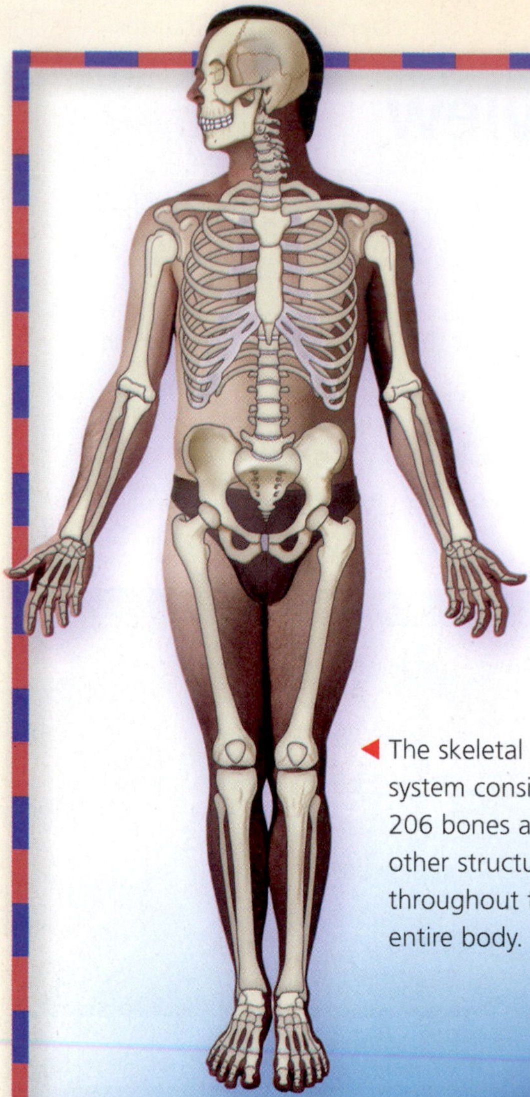

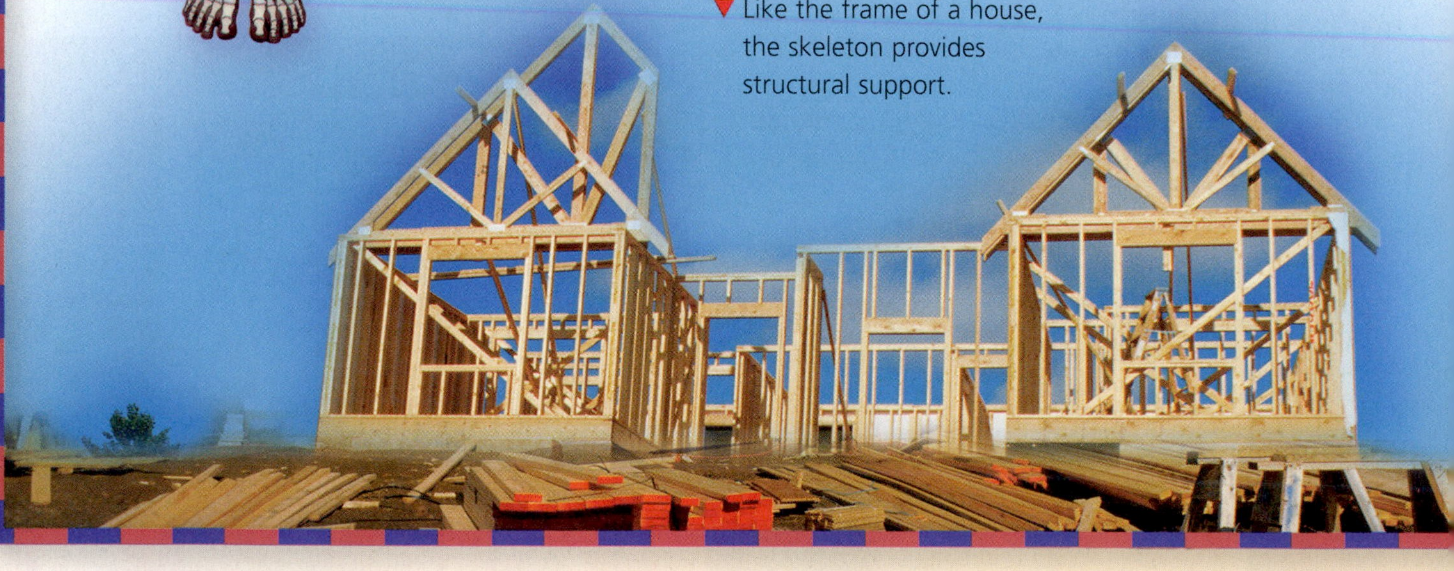

Dive In!

- Babies are born with about 100 more bones than adults.
- Humans and giraffes have the same number of bones in their necks.
- Do you want to discover some more hard facts? In this chapter, we'll explore the language that describes skeletal system structures, functions, diseases, and conditions.
- You'll have structure and support once you master the language of the skeletal system!

◀ The skeletal system consists of 206 bones and other structures throughout the entire body.

▼ Like the frame of a house, the skeleton provides structural support.

Medicine Through HISTORY

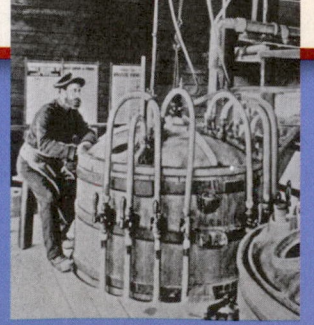

1895

Nitroglycerin is first prescribed to treat angina when workers in a dynamite factory experience relief of their chest pain. Nitroglycerin is an ingredient in dynamite

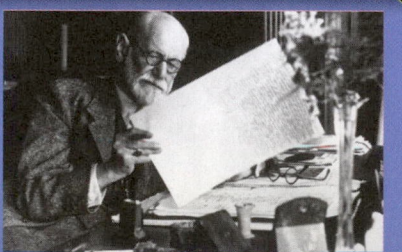

1896

Freud first uses the term psychoanalysis

8

Orthopedics

Skeletal System

Orthopedics (OR-thoh-PEE-diks) is the medical specialty that studies the anatomy and physiology of the skeletal and muscular systems and uses diagnostic tests, medical and surgical procedures, and drugs to treat skeletal and muscular diseases. In this chapter, you will study orthopedics from the perspective of the skeletal system. In Chapter 9, you will study the muscular system.

▶ Bones come in a variety of shapes and sizes, and are composed of exterior and interior structures.

▶ Breaking news…injuries do occur, but so does the healing process.

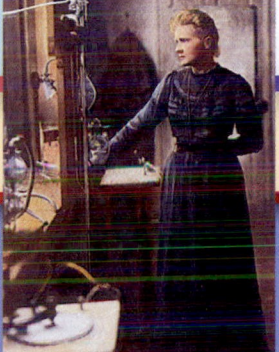

Marie Curie discovers radioactivity as she works with radium

1898

1899

Aspirin is introduced by Bayer, a German company

1899

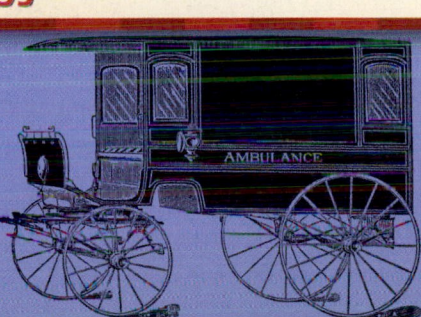

First motorized ambulance company begins in Ohio

Measure Your Progress: Learning Objectives

After you study this chapter, you should be able to

1. Identify the structures of the skeletal system.

2. Describe the process of growth.

3. Describe common skeletal diseases and conditions, laboratory and diagnostic procedures, medical and surgical procedures, and drug categories.

4. Give the medical meaning of word parts related to the skeletal system.

5. Build skeletal words from word parts and divide and define skeletal words.

6. Spell and pronounce skeletal words.

7. Analyze the medical content and meaning of an orthopedic report.

8. Dive deeper into orthopedics (skeletal) by reviewing the activities at the end of this chapter and online at Medical Terminology Interactive.

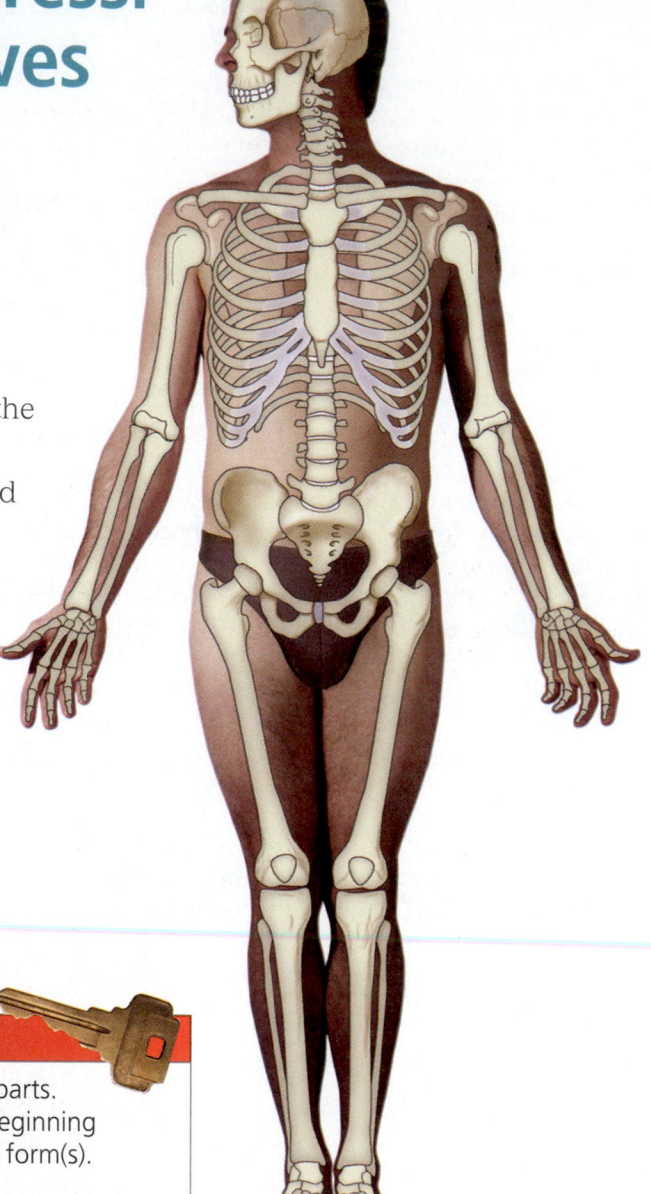

Figure 8-1 ■ **The skeletal system.**
The skeletal system is a widespread, connected system that consists of 206 bones and other structures. It stretches throughout the body from the top of the head to the tips of the fingers and toes.

Medical Language Key

To unlock the definition of a medical word, break it into word parts. Define each word part. Put the word part meanings in order, beginning with the suffix, then the prefix (if present), then the combining form(s).

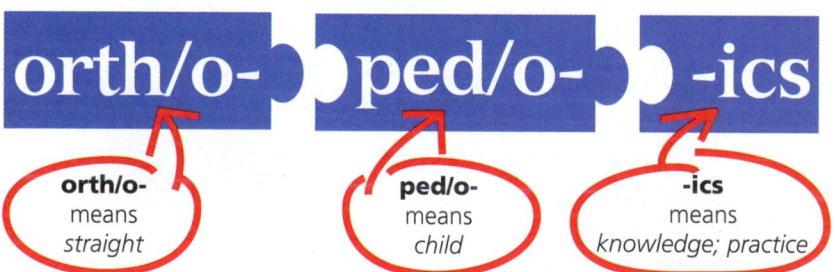

orth/o-
means
straight

ped/o-
means
child

-ics
means
knowledge; practice

	Word Part	Word Part Meaning
Suffix	-ics	*knowledge; practice*
Combining Form	orth/o-	*straight*
Combining Form	ped/o-	*child*

Orthopedics: *The knowledge and practice (of producing) straight(ness of the bones and muscles in a) child (or other person).*
Orthopedics can also be spelled *orthopaedics*. Many hospitals retain this spelling in the title *Department of Orthopaedics*, although others do not.

Anatomy and Physiology

The **skeletal system** is the **bony** framework on which the body is built. The **skeleton** is composed of 206 bones as well as cartilage and ligaments (see Figure 8-1 ■). The purpose of the skeletal system is to provide structural support for the body, work with the muscles to maintain body posture and produce movement, and protect the body's internal organs. The skeletal system is also known as the **skeletomuscular system** or **musculoskeletal system** because of the close working relationship between the bones and muscles.

Anatomy of the Skeletal System

Axial and Appendicular Skeleton

The skeleton can be divided into two areas: the axial skeleton and the appendicular skeleton. The **axial skeleton** forms the central bony structure of the body around which other parts move. It consists of the bones of the head, chest, and back. The **appendicular skeleton** consists of the bones of the shoulders, upper extremities, hips, and lower extremities.

Bones of the Head

The **skull** is the bony structure of the head. It includes both the cranium and facial bones.

Cranium   The **cranium** is the domelike bone at the top of the head. Within the cranium is the **cranial cavity,** which contains the brain and other structures. There are 8 bones in the cranium (see Figure 8-2 ■ and

WORD BUILDING

skeletal (SKEL-eh-tal)
  skelet/o- *skeleton*
  -al *pertaining to*

bony (BOH-nee)
Osseous and *osteal* are also adjectives for *bone*. The combining forms *osse/o-* and *oste/o-* mean *bone.*

skeleton (SKEL-eh-ton)

skeletomuscular
(SKEL-eh-toh-MUS-kyoo-lar)
  skelet/o- *skeleton*
  muscul/o- *muscle*
  -ar *pertaining to*

musculoskeletal
(MUS-kyoo-loh-SKEL-eh-tal)
  muscul/o- *muscle*
  skelet/o- *skeleton*
  -al *pertaining to*

axial (AK-see-al)
  axi/o- *axis*
  -al *pertaining to*

appendicular (AP-en-DIK-yoo-lar)
  appendicul/o- *limb; small attached part*
  -ar *pertaining to*

skull (SKUHL)

cranium (KRAY-nee-um)

cranial (KRAY-nee-al)
  crani/o- *cranium (skull)*
  -al *pertaining to*

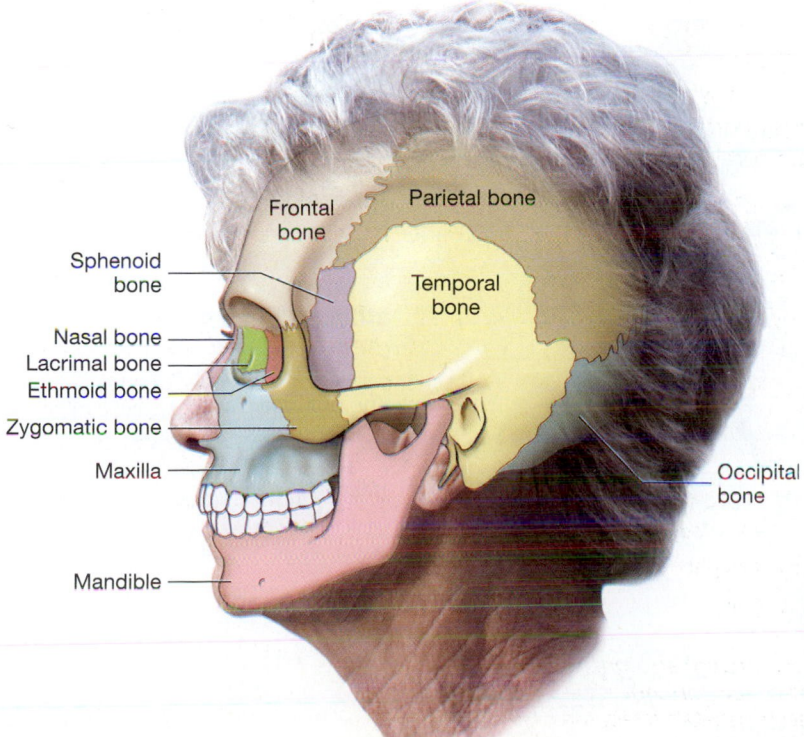

Frontal bone
Parietal bone
Sphenoid bone
Temporal bone
Nasal bone
Lacrimal bone
Ethmoid bone
Zygomatic bone
Maxilla
Mandible
Occipital bone

Figure 8-2 ■ Side view of the cranium and facial bones.

The frontal bone, parietal bone, occipital bone, temporal bone, sphenoid bone, and ethmoid bone form the side of the cranium. From the side, these facial bones are visible: nasal bone, lacrimal bone, zygomatic bone, maxilla, and mandible.

see Figure 8-3 ■). A **suture** is the line where one cranial bone meets another. The **frontal bone** forms the forehead and top of the cranium and ends at the coronal suture (see Figure 8-14). The **parietal bones** form the upper sides and upper posterior part of the cranium. Between these bones is the **sagittal suture,** which runs from front to back. The **occipital bone** forms the posterior base of the cranium. It contains the **foramen magnum,** a large, round opening through which the spinal cord passes to join the brain. The **temporal bones** form the lower sides of the cranium. Each temporal bone contains an opening for the external ear canal. The **mastoid process** is a projection from the temporal bone just behind the ear. The inferior temporal bone ends in the sharp **styloid process,** a point of attachment for tendons to the muscles of the tongue and pharynx and for ligaments to the hyoid bone in the throat. The **sphenoid bone,** a large, irregularly shaped bone, forms part of the central base and sides of the cranium and the posterior walls of the eye sockets. The sphenoid bone has bony projections where the tendons of muscles attach that move the soft palate and lower jaw. A bony cup in the sphenoid bone holds the pituitary gland (discussed in "Endocrinology," Chapter 14). The **ethmoid bone** forms the posterior nasal septum that divides the nasal cavity into right and left sides and forms the medial walls of the eye sockets. The frontal bone, sphenoid bones, and ethmoid bones all contain hollow sinuses (discussed in "Otolaryngology," Chapter 16).

Facial Bones   The facial bones support the tissues of the face (the nose, cheeks, and lips) and protect the eyes and internal structures of the nose, mouth, and upper throat. There are 12 bones in the face (see Figures 8-2 and 8-3). The **nasal bones** form the bridge of the nose and the roof of the

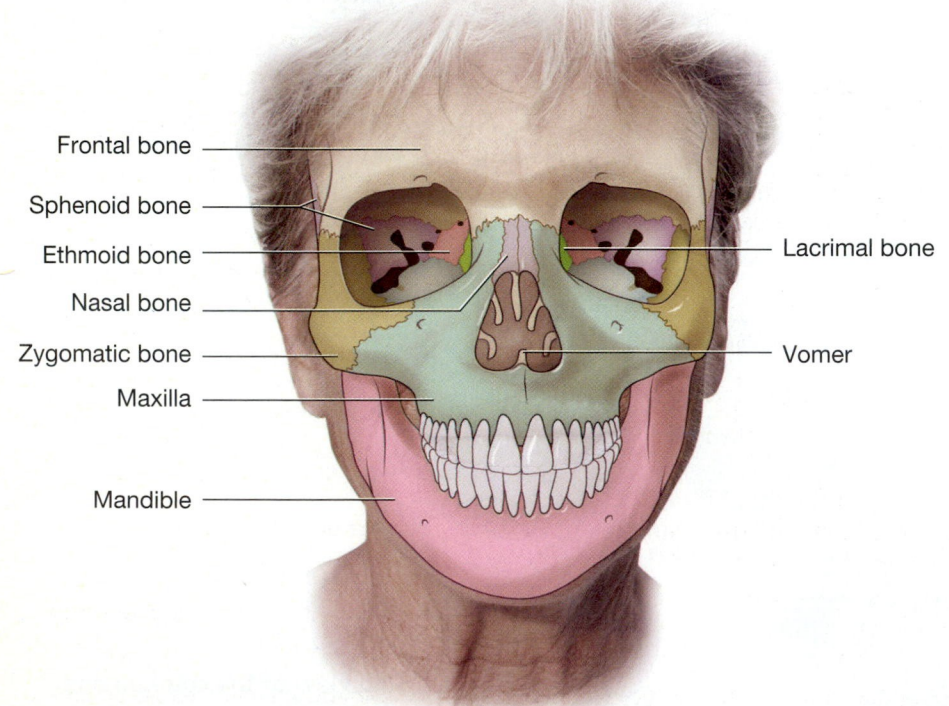

Frontal bone
Sphenoid bone
Ethmoid bone
Nasal bone
Zygomatic bone
Maxilla
Mandible
Lacrimal bone
Vomer

Figure 8-3 ■ Front view of the cranium and facial bones.
The facial bones connect to each other and to the bones of the cranium.

WORD BUILDING

suture (SOO-chur)

frontal (FRUN-tal)
  front/o- *front*
  -al *pertaining to*

parietal (pah-RY-eh-tal)
  pariet/o- *wall of a cavity*
  -al *pertaining to*

sagittal (SAJ-ih-tal)
  sagitt/o- *going from front to back*
  -al *pertaining to*

occiptal (awk-SIP-ih-tal)
  occipit/o- *occiput (back of the head)*
  -al *pertaining to*

foramen magnum
(foh-RAY-min MAG-num)

temporal (TEM-poh-ral)
  tempor/o- *temple (side of the head)*
  -al *pertaining to*

mastoid (MAS-toyd)
  mast/o- *breast; mastoid process*
  -oid *resembling*
This rounded, downward-pointing bone was thought to resemble a breast.

process (PRAW-ses)

styloid (STY-loyd)
  styl/o- *stake*
  -oid *resembling*

sphenoid (SFEE-noyd)
  sphen/o- *wedge shape*
  -oid *resembling*

ethmoid (ETH-moyd)
  ethm/o- *sieve*
  -oid *resembling*
The ethmoid bone has many small, hollow spaces like a sieve.

nasal (NAY-zal)
  nas/o- *nose*
  -al *pertaining to*

nasal cavity. The **vomer** is a narrow wall of bone that forms the inferior part of the nasal septum and continues posteriorly to join the sphenoid bone. The **lacrimal bones** are small, flat bones within the eye sockets, near the lacrimal (tear) glands. Each **zygoma** or **zygomatic bone** forms each cheek bone and the edge of the eye socket. The **maxilla** is the upper jaw bone. It contains the roots of the upper teeth. The maxilla contains two **maxillary bones** that are fused at the midline. The **palatine bones** are small, flat bones that form the posterior hard palate. The **mandible** is the lower jaw bone. It is the only moveable bone in the skull. The roots of the lower teeth are in the mandible. Each side of the mandible ends in two bony tips; one tip is under the zygoma, while the other tip forms a moveable joint (the temporomandibular joint) with the temporal bone just in front of the ear.

Clinical Connections

Neonatology. When a fetus is in the uterus, the bones of the cranium have large areas of fibrous connective tissue between them. These are **fontanels** (laypersons call these "soft spots") (see Figure 8-4 ■). Fontanels allow the cranial bones to move toward each other as the head is compressed and the fetus passes through the birth canal and to move away from each other as the brain grows during childhood. The bony edges finally fuse together at a suture line, and the cranial bones become immobile in early adulthood.

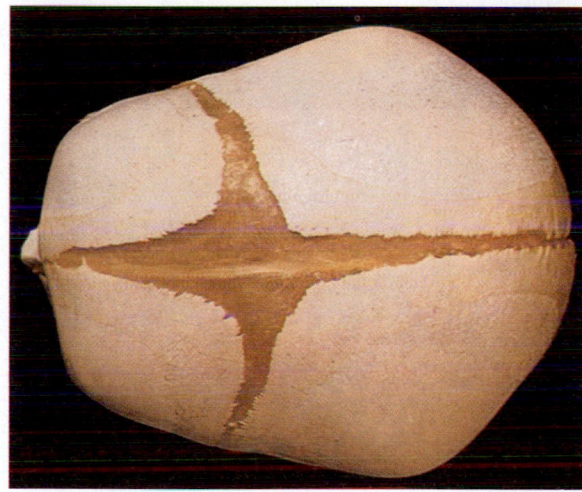

Figure 8-4 ■ Fontanel.
This fetal cranium shows a large open space (the anterior fontanel) between the two frontal bones (that have not yet fused into one bone) and the parietal bones. The translucent yellow membrane in the fontanel is fibrous connective tissue.

Other Bones of the Head   There are also three tiny bones in each middle ear: the malleus, incus, and stapes. Collectively, these are known as the **ossicles** or the ossicular chain because they are arranged in a row. They are active in the process of hearing (discussed in "Otolaryngology," Chapter 16).

The **hyoid bone** is a flat, U-shaped bone in the anterior neck. It does not touch any other bones. It is attached to tendons of muscles that go to the tongue and larynx.

Bones of the Chest

The chest contains the **thorax** or **rib cage** (see Figure 8-5 ■). Within the thorax is the **thoracic cavity**, which contains the heart, lungs, and other structures. The **sternum** or **breast bone** is in the center of the anterior thorax. It consists of the triangular-shaped **manubrium**, the body of the sternum, and the posterior tip or **xiphoid process.**

There are 12 pairs of **ribs**. Rib pairs 1–7 (true ribs) are attached to the spinal column posteriorly and to the sternum anteriorly by **costal cartilage**. Cartilage is a smooth, firm, but flexible connective tissue. The **costochondral joint** is where the cartilage meets the rib. Rib pairs 8–10 (false ribs) are attached to the spinal column posteriorly, but are only indirectly attached to the sternum by long lengths of costal cartilage. Rib pairs 11 and 12 (floating ribs) are attached to the spinal column posteriorly but are not attached to the sternum.

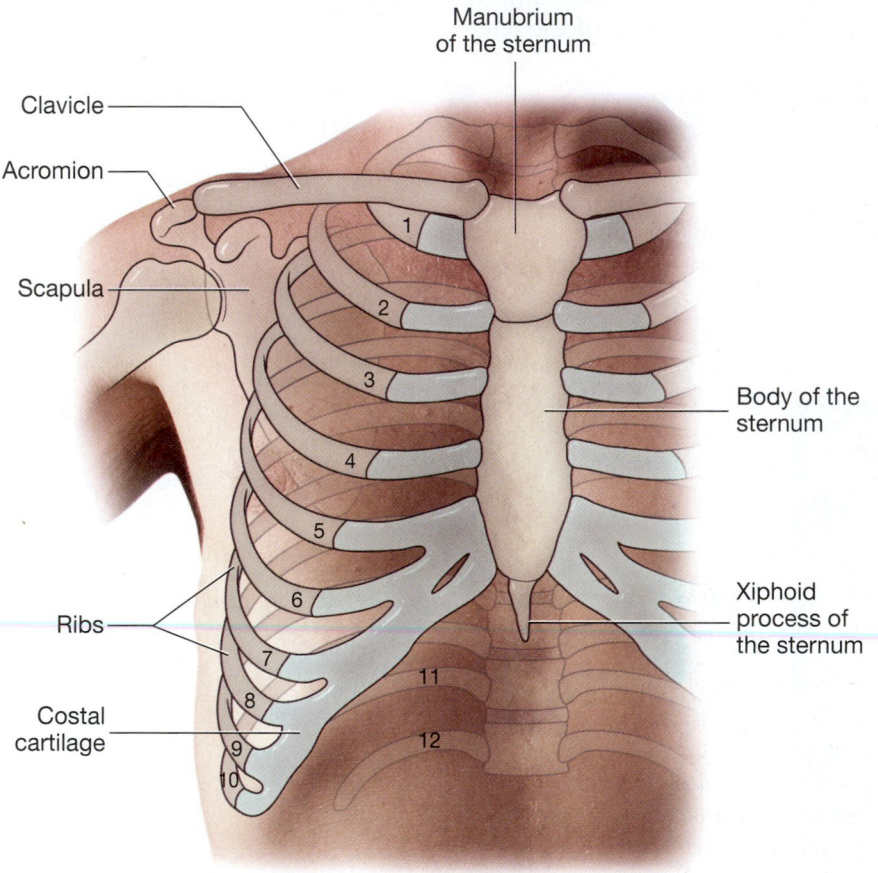

Figure 8-5 ■ Bones of the chest and shoulder.

The sternum and ribs form the thorax, a bony cage that protects the heart and lungs. The clavicle and scapula are part of the bones of each shoulder.

Bones of the Back

The **spine** or **backbone** is a vertical column of bones. It is also known as the **spinal column** or **vertebral column** (see Figure 8-6 ■). The spinal column supports the weight of the head, neck, and trunk of the body and protects the spinal cord.

The spinal column is composed of 24 individual vertebrae, plus the sacrum and coccyx. It is divided into five regions: the cervical vertebrae, the thoracic vertebrae, the lumbar vertebrae, the sacrum, and the coccyx. The **cervical vertebrae** (C1–C7) are in the neck. The first cervical vertebra (C1, the **atlas**) is directly below the occipital bone of the cranium. Its

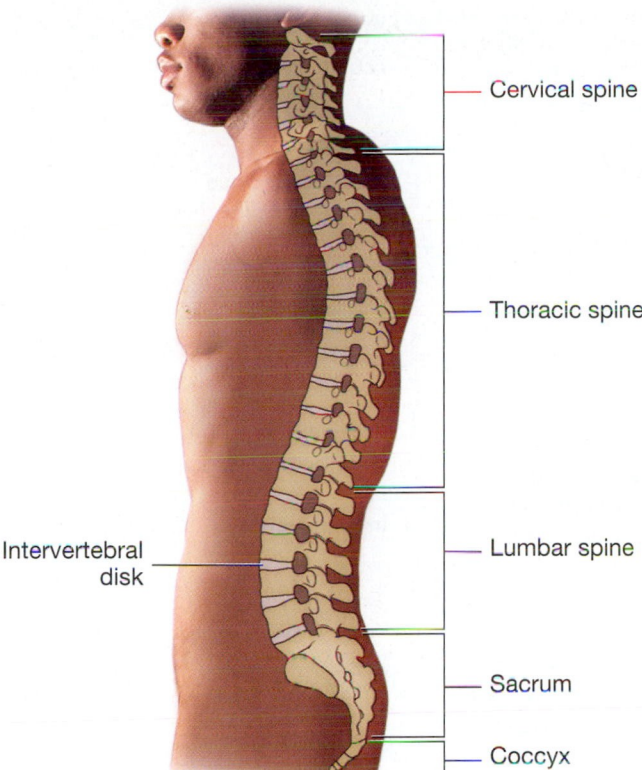

Cervical spine

Thoracic spine

Intervertebral disk

Lumbar spine

Sacrum

Coccyx

Figure 8-6 ■ **Bones of the spinal column.**

The spinal column consists of five regions: cervical vertebrae, thoracic vertebrae, lumbar vertebrae, and the sacrum and coccyx. Notice how the vertebrae become progressively larger from top to bottom as they bear more and more of the weight of the body.

appearance is different from the other cervical vertebrae because it must form a joint that allows the head to move up and down. The second cervical vertebra (C2, the **axis**) fits into the atlas to form a joint that allows the head to move from side to side. The **thoracic vertebrae** (T1–T12) are in the chest. Each thoracic vertebra joins with one of the 12 pairs of ribs. The **lumbar vertebrae** (L1–L5) are in the lower back. The lumbar vertebrae are larger than the cervical or thoracic vertebrae because they bear the weight of the head, neck, and trunk of the body. The **sacrum** is a group of five fused vertebrae that are not individually numbered, except for the first sacral vertebra (S1). The sacrum joins with the hip bones in the posterior pelvis. The **coccyx** or **tail bone** is a group of several small, fused vertebrae that also are not individually numbered.

WORD BUILDING

axis (AK-sis)

thoracic (thoh-RAS-ik)
 thorac/o- *thorax (chest)*
 -ic *pertaining to*

lumbar (LUM-bar)
 lumb/o- *lower back; area between the ribs and pelvis*
 -ar *pertaining to*

sacrum (SAY-krum)

sacral (SAY-kral)
 sacr/o- *sacrum*
 -al *pertaining to*

coccyx (KAWK-siks)

coccygeal (kawk-SIJ-ee-al)
 coccyg/o- *coccyx (tail bone)*
 -eal *pertaining to*

Did You Know?

Atlas was the name given to the mythological Greek god who was forced to hold the world on his shoulders. A person's head was imagined as a round globe and therefore the first vertebra was named the *atlas*.

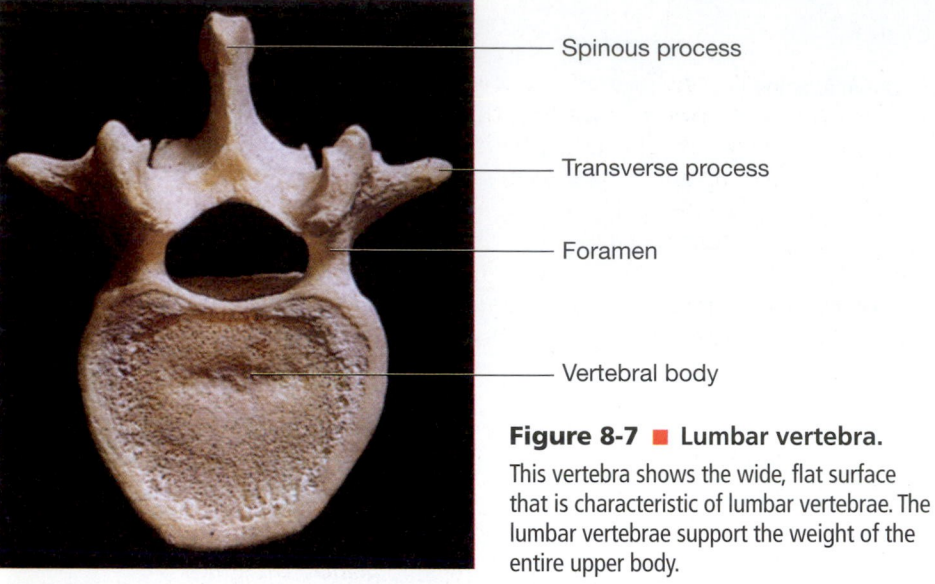

Spinous process

Transverse process

Foramen

Vertebral body

Figure 8-7 ■ Lumbar vertebra.
This vertebra shows the wide, flat surface that is characteristic of lumbar vertebrae. The lumbar vertebrae support the weight of the entire upper body.

Many of the vertebrae share common features (see Figure 8-7 ■): a vertebral body (circular, flat area), a **spinous process** (a long, bony projection that juts out in the midline along a person's back), two **transverse processes** (bony projections to each side), and a vertebral **foramen** (the hole through which the spinal cord passes). The spinous and transverse processes are points of attachment for tendons for the spinal muscles. Between most vertebrae are **intervertebral disks.** The outer wall of each disk is fibrocartilage, and the inside is filled with **nucleus pulposus,** a gelatinous substance. The disks act as cushions to absorb the impact during body movements.

WORD BUILDING

spinous (SPY-nus)
  spin/o- *spine; backbone*
  -ous *pertaining to*

process (PRAW-ses)

transverse (trans-VERS)
  trans- *across; through*
  -verse *to travel; to turn*

foramen (foh-RAY-min)

intervertebral (IN-ter-VER-teh-bral)
  inter- *between*
  vertebr/o- *vertebra*
  -al *pertaining to*

disk (DISK)
Some medical dictionaries prefer the spelling *disc.*

nucleus pulposus
(NOO-klee-us pul-POH-sis)
The nucleus is the central part of a structure. *Pulposis* refers to the pulpy consistency of the contents within the intervertebral disk.

Did You Know?

Andreas Vesalius (1514–1564) was born in Belgium and was educated in medical universities in France and Italy. At that time, medical textbooks contained almost no illustrations. He studied and illustrated a human skeleton by taking down a dead body after a public hanging and dissecting it. His masterpiece, *De Humani Corporis Fabrica* (*The Structure of the Human Body*), was published in 1543. Its illustrations showed dissected bodies in natural poses with scenery in the background. These beautiful, highly detailed, anatomically correct, and occasionally whimsical illustrations educated a new generation of physicians (see Figure 8-8 ■).

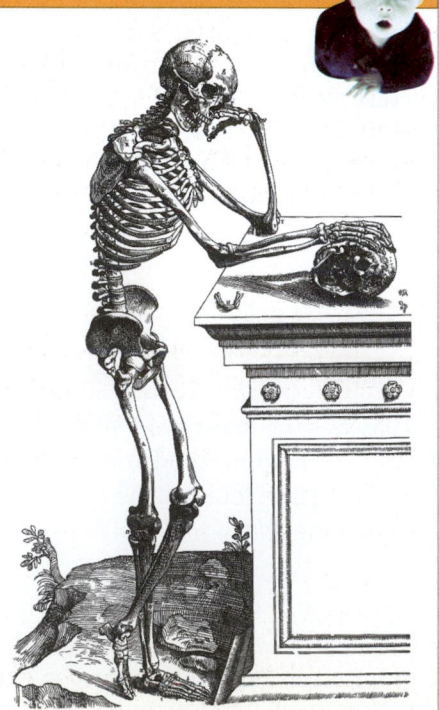

Figure 8-8 ■ The skeleton.
An anatomical illustration of the skeleton by Andreas Vesalius.

Bones of the Shoulders

The shoulder bones include a clavicle and a scapula on the right and the left sides (see Figures 8-5 and 8-9 ■). The **clavicle** or **collar bone** is a thin, rodlike bone on each side of the anterior neck. It connects to the manubrium of the sternum and laterally to the scapula. The **scapula** or shoulder blade is a triangular-shaped bone on either side of the spinal column in the upper back. It has a long, bony blade across its upper half that ends in a flat projection (the **acromion**) that connects to the clavicle. The **glenoid fossa,** a shallow depression, is where the head of the humerus (upper arm bone) joins the scapula to make the shoulder joint.

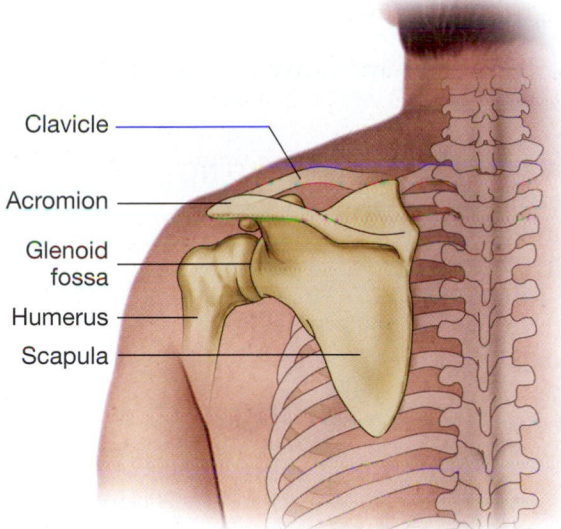

Clavicle
Acromion
Glenoid fossa
Humerus
Scapula

Figure 8-9 ■ Bones of the shoulder.

This posterior view shows the scapula joining the humerous (upper arm bone) at the glenoid fossa. The acromion of the scapula is connected to the clavicle. The scapula itself is not connected to the ribs or vertebral column. This allows it to move freely in several directions as the shoulder moves.

Bones of the Upper Extremities

Upper and Lower Arm   The upper extremity consists of the upper arm and lower arm (forearm) (see Figure 8-10 ■). The **humerus** is the long bone in the upper arm. The head of the humerus fits into the glenoid fossa of the scapula to form the shoulder joint. At its distal end, the humerus joins with both the radius and the ulna to form the elbow joint.

Did You Know?

The "funny bone" is not a bone at all. The ulnar nerve travels across a rounded, bony projection (medial epicondyle) on the distal humerus. When you accidentally bump this area, you hit the ulnar nerve and send a shock wave (that is in no way "funny") through your entire upper extremity.

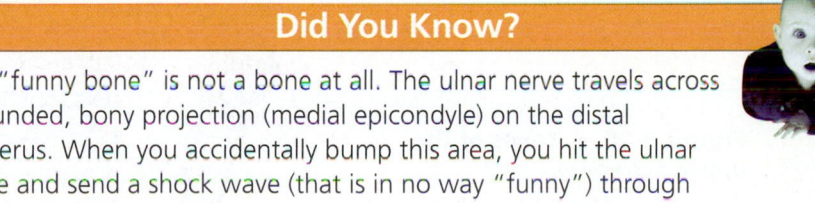

The **radius** is one of the two bones in the forearm. It lies on the thumb side of the forearm. At its distal end, it connects to the bones of the wrist. The **ulna** lies on the little finger side of the forearm. At its proximal end is the **olecranon,** a large, square projection that forms the point of the elbow. At its distal end, the ulna connects to the bones of the wrist.

WORD BUILDING

clavicle (KLAV-ih-kl)

clavicular (klah-VIK-yoo-lar)
  clavicul/o- *clavicle (collar bone)*
  -ar *pertaining to*

scapula (SKAP-yoo-lah)

scapulae (SKAP-yoo-lee)
Scapula is a Latin singular noun. Form the plural by changing *-a* to *-ae.*

scapular (SKAP-yoo-lar)
  scapul/o- *scapula (shoulder blade)*
  -ar *pertaining to*

acromion (ah-KROH-mee-on)

glenoid (GLEH-noyd)
  glen/o- *socket of a joint*
  -oid *resembling*

fossa (FAW-sah)

humerus (HYOO-mer-us)

humeri (HYOO-mer-eye)
Humerus is a Latin singular noun. Form the plural by changing *-us* to *-i.*

humeral (HYOO-mer-al)
  humer/o- *humerus (upper arm bone)*
  -al *pertaining to*

radius (RAY-dee-us)

radii (RAY-dee-eye)
Radius is a Latin singular noun. Form the plural by changing *-us* to *-i.*

radial (RAY-dee-al)
  radi/o- *radius (forearm bone); x-rays; radiation*
  -al *pertaining to*
Select the correct combining form meaning to get the definition of *radial: pertaining to the radius (forearm bone).*

ulna (UL-nah)

ulnae (UL-nee)
Ulna is a Latin singular noun. Form the plural by changing *-a* to *-ae.*

ulnar (UL-nar)
  uln/o- *ulna (forearm bone)*
  -ar *pertaining to*

olecranon (oh-LEK-rah-non)

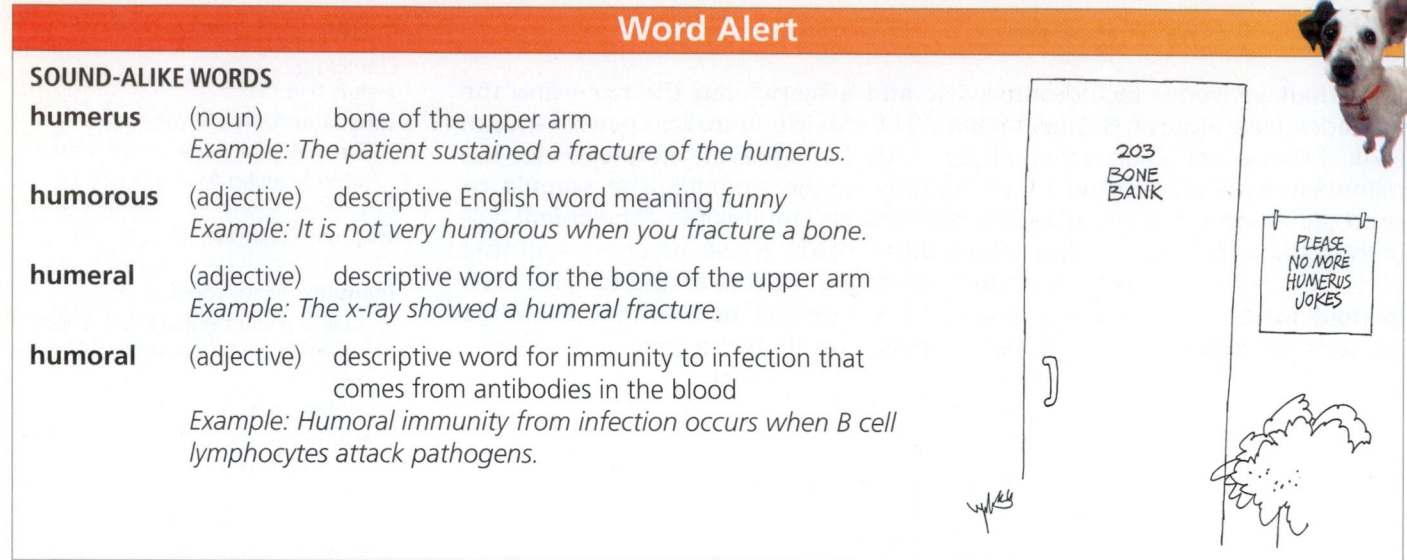

Word Alert

SOUND-ALIKE WORDS

humerus   (noun)   bone of the upper arm
Example: The patient sustained a fracture of the humerus.

humorous   (adjective)   descriptive English word meaning *funny*
Example: It is not very humorous when you fracture a bone.

humeral   (adjective)   descriptive word for the bone of the upper arm
Example: The x-ray showed a humeral fracture.

humoral   (adjective)   descriptive word for immunity to infection that comes from antibodies in the blood
Example: Humoral immunity from infection occurs when B cell lymphocytes attack pathogens.

Wrist, Hand, and Fingers   The wrist contains eight small **carpal bones** arranged in two rows (see Figure 8-10). One row connects to the radius and ulna. The other row connects to the bones of the hand. Each hand contains five individual **metacarpal bones,** one for each finger. Each finger contains three individual **phalangeal bones** or **phalanges** (except the thumb, which contains two), arranged end to end. The distal **phalanx** is the final bone at the very tip of each finger. The fingers are also known as **digits** or **rays.** The metacarpophalangeal (MCP) joint is between a metacarpal bone of the hand and a phalanx. The distal interphalangeal (DIP) joint is between the last two phalanges.

WORD BUILDING

carpal (KAR-pal)
carp/o- wrist
-al pertaining to

metacarpal (MET-ah-KAR-pal)
meta- after; subsequent to; transition; change
carp/o- wrist
-al pertaining to
Select the correct combining form meaning to get the definition of *metacarpal: pertaining to (bones that are) after or subsequent to the wrist.*

phalangeal (fah-LAN-jee-al)
phalang/o- phalanx (finger or toe)
-eal pertaining to

phalanges (fah-LAN-jeez)
Phalanx is a Greek singular noun. Form the plural by changing *-x* to *-ges.*

phalanx (FAY-langks)
The combining form *dactyl/o-* also means *finger or toe.*

digit (DIJ-it)

ray (RAY)
The rays or digits extend outward from the hand like the rays of the sun.

Glenoid fossa
Humerus
Medial epicondyle
Radius
Ulna
Carpal bones
Metacarpal bones
Phalanges

Figure 8-10 ■ Bones of the upper extremity.
The humerus of the upper arm joins with both the radius and the ulna, the bones of the forearm. The radius and ulna rotate around each other to allow the hand to turn palm up or palm down. The carpal bones in the wrist are connected to the metacarpal bones in the hand. Each finger contains three phalangeal bones; the thumb contains only two.

Bones of the Hips

The **pelvis** includes the hip bones as well as the sacrum and coccyx of the spinal column. The hip bones include an ilium, ischium, and pubis on each side of the spinal column (see Figure 8-11 ■). The **ilium,** the most superior of the hip bones, has a broad, flaring rim known as the **iliac crest.** Posteriorly, each ilium joins to the sacrum. The ilium contains the **acetabulum** (the deep socket of the hip joint). The **ischium** is the most inferior of the hip bones. Each ischium is one of the "seat bones" that you sit on, and it contains a large opening that is covered by a fibrous membrane and is the point of attachment for tendons of some muscles of the hip. The **pubis** or **pubic bone,** a small bridgelike bone, is the most anterior of the hip bones. Its two halves meet in the midline, where they form the **pubic symphysis,** a nearly immobile joint that has a cartilage pad between the bone ends. The pubis also forms the inferior part of the acetabulum.

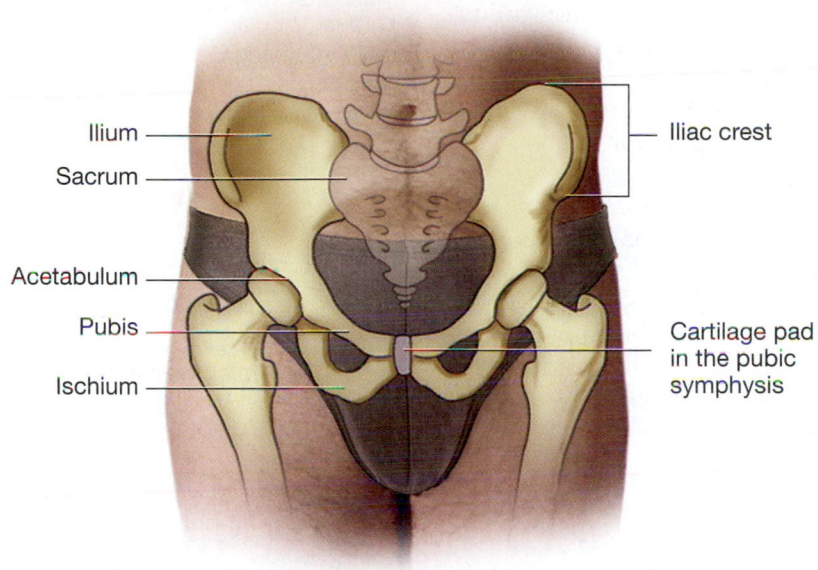

Ilium

Sacrum

Acetabulum

Pubis

Ischium

Iliac crest

Cartilage pad
in the pubic
symphysis

Figure 8-11 ■ Bones of the hip.
The ilium, ischium, and pubis on each side of the hip flow into each other without visible sutures or joints. However, the main part of each bone can be identified according to bony landmarks.

WORD BUILDING

pelvis (PEL-vis)

pelvic (PEL-vik)
  pelv/o- *pelvis (hip bone; renal pelvis)*
  -ic *pertaining to*

ilium (IL-ee-um)
Ilium is a Latin singular noun. There are two ilia, but the plural form is seldom used.

iliac (IL-ee-ak)
  ili/o- *ilium (hip bone)*
  -ac *pertaining to*

acetabulum (AS-eh-TAB-yoo-lum)

acetabular (AS-eh-TAB-yoo-lar)
  acetabul/o- *acetabulum (hip socket)*
  -ar *pertaining to*

ischium (IS-kee-um)
Ischium is a Latin singular noun. There are two ischia, but the plural form is seldom used.

ischial (IS-kee-al)
  ischi/o- *ischium (hip bone)*
  -al *pertaining to*

pubis (PYOO-bis)

pubic (PYOO-bik)
  pub/o- *pubis (hip bone)*
  -ic *pertaining to*

symphysis (SIM-fih-sis)
  sym- *together; with*
  -physis *state of growing*

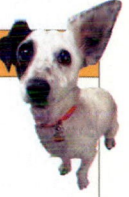

Word Alert

SOUND-ALIKE WORDS

ilium (noun) the superior flaring part of the hip bone
          Example: During the car accident, she sustained a hip fracture that involved the ilium.

ileum (noun) the third part of the small intestine
          Example: Inflammation in the ileum can also extend to other parts of the small bowel.

ileus (noun) abnormal absence of contractions in the small intestine
          Example: A postoperative ileus can occur after extensive abdominal surgery.

Bones of the Lower Extremities

Upper and Lower Leg   The lower extremity consists of the upper leg (thigh) and the lower leg (see Figure 8-12 ■). The **femur** or **thigh bone** is the long bone in the upper leg. The head of the femur fits into the acetabulum to form the hip joint.

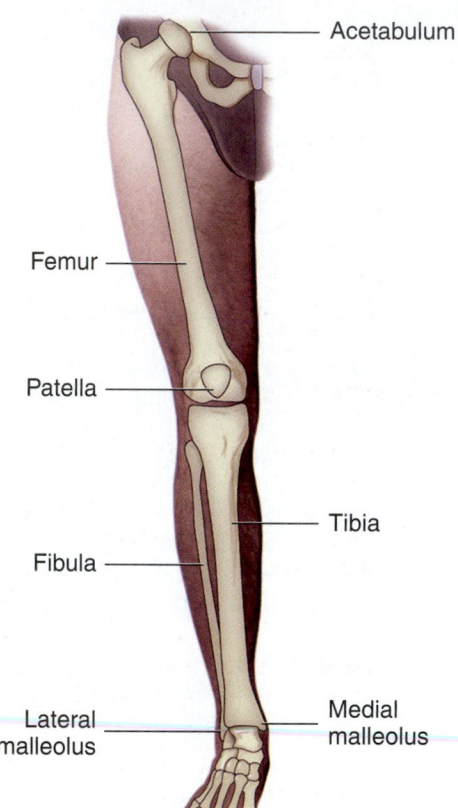

Acetabulum

Femur

Patella

Tibia

Fibula

Lateral malleolus

Medial malleolus

Figure 8-12 ■ Bones of the lower extremity.

The femur of the upper leg joins the tibia of the lower leg to support the weight of the body. The fibula, the smaller of the two bones in the lower leg, is on the little toe side. The patella is a small, round bone that protects the anterior knee joint.

The **tibia** or **shin bone** is the large bone on the medial side of the lower leg. At its distal end, it has a bony prominence known as the **medial malleolus.** The **fibula** is the very thin bone on the lateral side of the lower leg. Its proximal end connects to the tibia, not to the femur, and it is not a weight-bearing bone in the leg. Its distal end has a bony prominence known as the **lateral malleolus.** The malleoli are often mistakenly called the ankle bones. The **patella** or **kneecap** is a small, round bone anterior to the knee joint. It is most prominent in thin people and when the knee is partially bent.

Ankle, Foot, and Toes   Each ankle contains seven **tarsal bones** (see Figure 8-13 ■). The talus is the first tarsal bone, and the **calcaneus** or **heel bone** is the largest tarsal bone. The midfoot contains five **metatarsal bones,** one for each toe. The instep or arch of the foot contains both tarsal bones and metatarsal bones. Each toe or digit contains three phalangeal bones or phalanges (except the great toe, which contains two). The distal phalanx is at the very tip of the toe. The toes are also known as rays. The great toe is known as the **hallux.**

WORD BUILDING

femur (FEE-mur)

femora (FEM-oh-rah)
Femur is a Latin singular noun. The plural form is *femora*.

femoral (FEM-oh-ral)
  femor/o- *femur (thigh bone)*
  -al *pertaining to*

tibia (TIB-ee-ah)

tibiae (TIB-ee-ee)
Tibia is a Latin singular noun. Form the plural by changing *-a* to *-ae*.

tibial (TIB-ee-al)
  tibi/o- *tibia (shin bone)*
  -al *pertaining to*

malleolus (mah-LEE-oh-lus)

malleoli (mah-LEE-oh-lie)
Malleolus is a Latin singular noun. Form the plural by changing *-us* to *-i*.

fibula (FIB-yoo-lah)

fibulae (FIB-yoo-lee)
Fibula is a Latin singular noun. Form the plural by changing *-a* to *-ae*.

fibular (FIB-yoo-lar)
  fibul/o- *fibula (lower leg bone)*
  -ar *pertaining to*
The combining form *perone/o-* also means *fibula*.

patella (pah-TEL-ah)

patellae (pah-TEL-ee)
Patella is a Latin singular noun. Form the plural by changing *-a* to *-ae*.

patellar (pah-TEL-ar)
  patell/o- *patella (kneecap)*
  -ar *pertaining to*

tarsal (TAR-sal)
  tars/o- *ankle*
  -al *pertaining to*

calcaneus (kal-KAY-nee-us)

calcaneal (kal-KAY-nee-al)
  calcane/o- *calcaneus (heel bone)*
  -al *pertaining to*

metatarsal (MET-ah-TAR-sal)

hallux (HAL-uks)

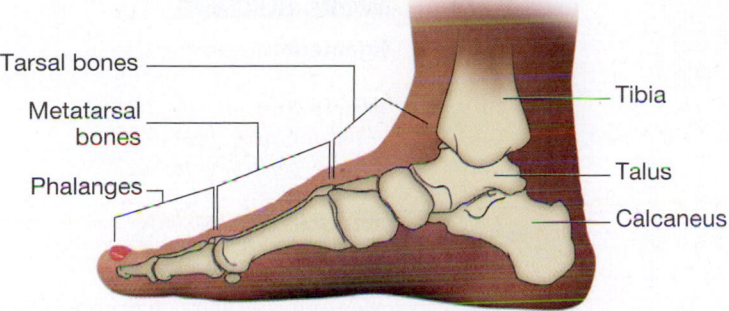

Figure 8-13 ■ Bones of the ankle and foot.
The tarsal bones in the ankle are connected to the metatarsal bones in the midfoot. Each toe contains three phalangeal bones; the great toe or hallux contains only two. In all, each foot contains 26 bones and 150 ligaments.

Joints, Cartilage, and Ligaments

A **joint** or **articulation** is where two bones come together. There are three types of joints: suture, symphysis, and synovial.

1. A **suture joint** between two cranial bones is immovable and contains no cartilage (see Figure 8-14 ■).
2. A **symphysis joint**, such as the pubic symphysis or the joints between the vertebrae, is a slightly moveable joint with a fibrocartilage pad or disk between the bones (see Figures 8-6 and 8-11).
3. A **synovial joint** is a fully moveable joint (see Figure 8-15 ■). There are two kinds of synovial joints: hinge joints (the elbow and the knee) that allow motion in two directions and ball-and-socket joints (the shoulder and the hip) that allow motion in many directions. A synovial joint joins two bones whose ends are covered with **articular cartilage.**

WORD BUILDING

joint (JOYNT)

articulation (ar-TIK-yoo-LAY-shun)
 articul/o- *joint*
 -ation *a process; being or having*
The combining form *arthr/o-* also means *joint.*

synovial (sih-NOH-vee-al)
 synovi/o- *synovium (membrane)*
 -al *pertaining to*

articular (ar-TIK-yoo-lar)
 articul/o- *joint*
 -ar *pertaining to*

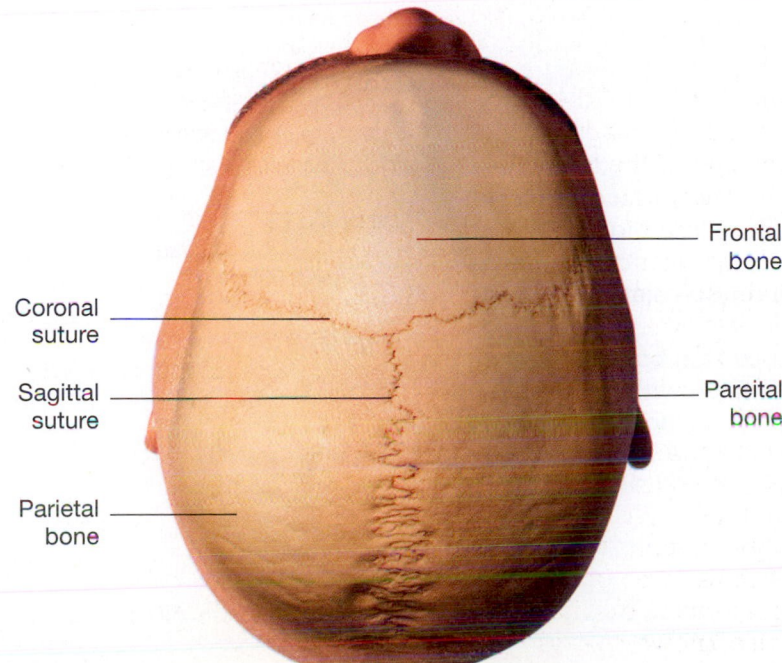

Figure 8-14 ■ Suture joint.
In an adult, the coronal suture is an immoveable joint that joins the frontal and parietal bones. The parietal suture joins the two parietal bones on either side of the cranium. A suture is not a straight line as the two bones grow together faster in some areas than in others.

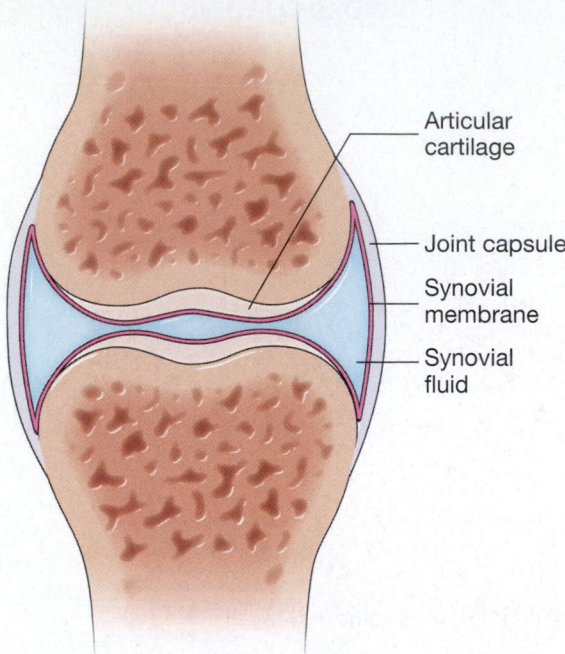

Articular cartilage

Joint capsule

Synovial membrane

Synovial fluid

Figure 8-15 ■ Synovial joint.
Synovial joints are fully moveable joints that have a joint capsule and a synovial membrane that makes synovial fluid. Hinge joints (the elbows and the knees) allow motion in two directions. Ball-and-socket joints (the shoulders and the hips) allow motion in many directions.

Ligaments are strong fibrous bands of connective tissue that hold the two bones together in a synovial joint. The entire joint is encased in a **joint capsule** that has a fibrous outer layer and an inner membrane. This inner **synovial membrane** produces **synovial fluid,** a clear, thick fluid that lubricates the joint. A **meniscus** is a special crescent-shaped cartilage pad found in some synovial joints, such as the knee.

The Structure of Bone

Bone or **osseous tissue** is a type of connective tissue. The surface of a bone is covered with **periosteum,** a thick, fibrous membrane (see Figure 8-16 ■). A long bone such as the humerus or femur has a straight shaft or **diaphysis** and two widened ends or **epiphyses.** It is at the **epiphysial plates** that bone growth takes place.

Along the diaphysis is a layer of dense compact **cortical bone** for weight bearing. Inside this is the **medullary cavity,** which is filled with yellow bone marrow that contains fatty tissue. In each epiphysis is **cancellous bone** or spongy bone. It is less dense than compact bone, and the spaces in it are filled with red bone marrow.

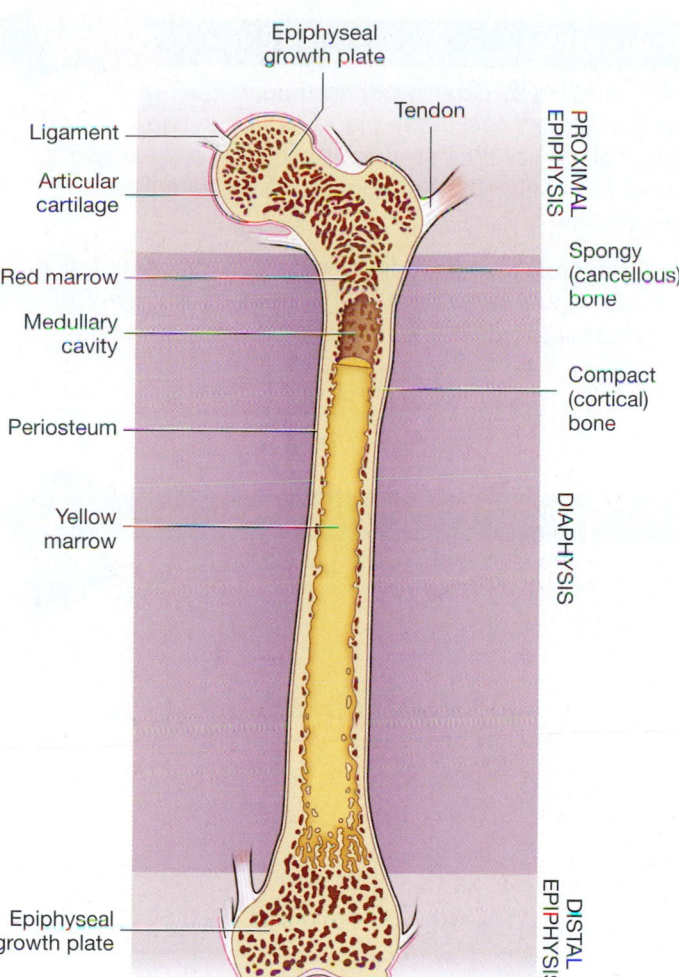

Epiphyseal growth plate

Tendon

PROXIMAL EPIPHYSIS

Ligament

Articular cartilage

Red marrow

Spongy (cancellous) bone

Medullary cavity

Compact (cortical) bone

Periosteum

DIAPHYSIS

Yellow marrow

Epiphyseal growth plate

DISTAL EPIPHYSIS

WORD BUILDING

Figure 8-16 ■ Structure of a bone.
A long bone has a diaphysis (shaft) and epiphyses (ends). The internal structure has areas of dense cortical bone for weight bearing, a medullary cavity that contains yellow marrow, and bone ends of cancellous bone filled with red marrow that produces blood cells.

Clinical Connections

Hematology and Immunology (Chapter 6). Red bone marrow produces stem cells that eventually mature, become erythrocytes, leukocytes, etc., and enter the blood. Red bone marrow is found in the ends of the long bones and in the skull, clavicles, sternum, ribs, vertebrae, and hip bones.

Physiology of Bone Growth

Ossification is the gradual replacing of cartilage with bone that takes place during childhood and adolescence. In addition, new bone is formed along the epiphysial growth plates at the ends of long bones as the body grows taller. Although mature bone is a hard substance, it is also a living tissue that undergoes change. About 10% of the entire skeleton is broken down and rebuilt each year. This process occurs in areas that are damaged or subjected to mechanical stress. **Osteoclasts** break down areas of old or damaged bone. **Osteoblasts** deposit new bone tissue in those areas. **Osteocytes** maintain and monitor the mineral content (calcium, phosphorus) of the bone. Almost all of the body's calcium is stored in the bones, but calcium is also needed to help the heart and skeletal muscles contract. Calcium comes from the diet but also as osteoclasts break down old or damaged bone the calcium in that bone is released into the blood.

ossification (AWS-ih-fih-KAY-shun)
ossificat/o- *changing into bone*
-ion *action; condition*

osteoclast (AWS-tee-oh-klast)
oste/o- *bone*
-clast *cell that breaks down substances*

osteoblast (AWS-tee-oh-blast)
oste/o- *bone*
-blast *immature cell*

osteocyte (AWS-tee-oh-site)
oste/o- *bone*
-cyte *cell*

Clinical Connections

Endocrinology (Chapter 14). The calcium level in the blood is controlled by parathyroid hormone secreted by the parathyroid glands. Parathyroid hormone raises the calcium level in the blood by stimulating osteoclasts to break down more bone. Calcitonin from the thyroid gland has the opposite effect, and so these two hormones constantly balance the amount of calcium in the blood. Estradiol and other hormones stimulate bone formation. Growth hormone from the pituitary gland influences the rate of bone growth.

Space Medicine. Astronauts who live in a weightless environment for prolonged periods of time are in danger of losing bone mass. The lack of weight-bearing stress on the bones decreases new bone formation while bone breakdown continues at its normal rate. The astronauts have regular exercise programs that include resistance exercises that exert force on the bones.

Across the Life Span

Pediatrics. During birth, it is not unusual for the clavicle to break as the baby goes through the birth canal. This fracture does not need to be treated, as it heals by itself within a matter of days because of the high rate of bone growth in babies. Babies are born without kneecaps! These bones develop between 2 and 6 years of age. From infancy through puberty, new bone formation exceeds bone breakdown, as cartilage is continuously replaced by mature bone. The height and weight of a child is an important indicator of health. These measurements are taken at regular intervals by the pediatrician and recorded on a standardized pediatric growth chart in the child's medical record (see Figure 8-17 ■).

During adulthood, the rate of new bone formation equals the rate of bone breakdown. In all stages of life, formation of new bone is dependent on having enough calcium and phosphorus in the diet.

Geriatrics. In older adults, the rate of bone breakdown exceeds that of new bone formation, and the bones become fragile and prone to fracture. Patients confined to bed who are unable to do any weight-bearing exercise to stimulate new bone formation have an increased rate of bone loss.

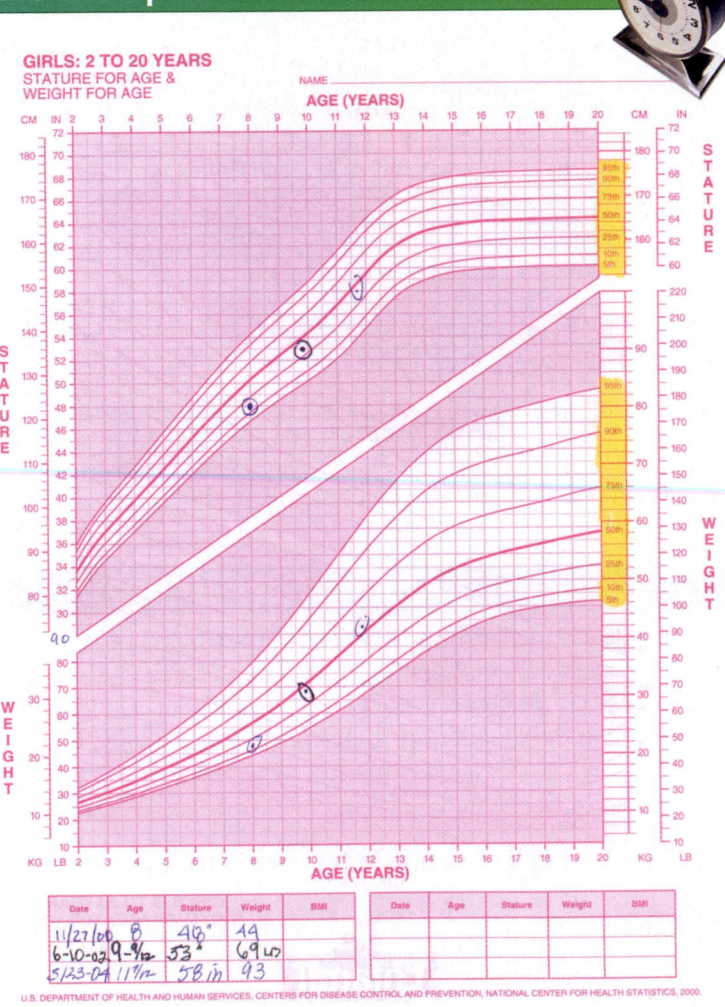

Figure 8-17 ■ Pediatric growth chart.
This chart tracks height and weight for girls ages 2–20 years and assigns percentiles. On the initial visit to her pediatrician, this 8-year-old child had a diagnosis of malnutrition and was in about the 15th percentile for both height (stature) and weight. After 3 years of good nutrition, her most recent visit at age 11 years, 7 months, shows that she is now in about the 40th percentile for height and about the 55th percentile for weight.

Vocabulary Review

Anatomy and Physiology

Word or Phrase	Description	Combining Forms
appendicular skeleton	The bones of the shoulders, upper extremities, hips, and lower extremities	**appendicul/o-** limb; small attached part
axial skeleton	The bones of the head, chest, and back	**axi/o-** axis
bones	The 206 individual pieces of the skeleton. Bone is also known as **osseous tissue.** Bony and osteal are also adjectives.	**osse/u-** bone **oste/o-** bone
skeletal system	Body system that consists of all of the bones, ligaments, and joints in the body	**skelet/o-** skeleton
skeletomuscular system	The combined systems of the bones and muscles. The bones provide support for the muscles, and the muscles enable the bones to move. It is also known as the **musculoskeletal system.**	**skelet/o-** skeleton **muscul/o-** muscle
skeleton	Bony framework of the body that consists of all the bones	**skelet/o-** skeleton

Bones of the Head

coronal suture	Immoveable suture between the frontal bone and the parietal bones of the cranium	**coron/o-** structure that encircles like a crown
cranium	Domelike bone at the top of the head that contains the **cranial cavity** and the brain and other structures	**crani/o-** cranium (skull)
ethmoid bone	Bone that forms the posterior nasal septum and the medial walls of the eye sockets. It contains many tiny hollow areas that are the ethmoid sinus.	**ethm/o-** sieve
fontanel	Soft spot on a baby's head where the cranial sutures are still open and there is only fibrous connective tissue	
foramen	A hole in a bone. The **foramen magnum** is the largest. The spinal cord passes through it to join with the brain. There is a foramen in each vertebra where the spinal cord passes through. There are small foramina in the bones where blood vessels go through to the bone marrow.	
frontal bone	Bone that forms the forehead and front of the cranium and ends at the coronal suture. It contains the frontal sinuses.	**front/o-** front
hyoid bone	A U-shaped bone in the anterior neck that anchors the muscles of the tongue and larynx	**hy/o-** U-shaped structure
lacrimal bones	Facial bones within the eye socket. They are small, flat bones near the lacrimal glands, which produce tears.	**lacrim/o-** tears
mandible	Facial bone that forms the lower jaw and contains the roots of the lower teeth. It is the only moveable bone in the skull and forms a joint just in front of the ear with the temporal bone (the temporomandibular joint).	**mandibul/o-** mandible (lower jaw)
maxillary bones	Facial bones that form the immoveable upper jaw, the inferior edges of the eye sockets, and the anterior part of the hard palate. They support the nose and lips and contain the roots of the upper teeth and the maxillary sinuses. The two fused maxillary bones are the **maxilla.**	**maxill/o-** maxilla (upper jaw)

Word or Phrase	Description	Combining Forms
nasal bones	Facial bones that form the bridge of the nose and the roof of the nasal cavity	**nas/o-** *nose*
occipital bone	Bone that forms the posterior base of the cranium. It contains the large opening, the foramen magnum.	**occipit/o-** *occiput (back of the head)*
ossicles	Three tiny bones in the middle ear that function in the process of hearing. They are also known as the ossicular chain.	
palatine bones	Facial bones that are small and flat and form the posterior hard palate	**palat/o-** *palate*
parietal bones	Bones that form the upper sides and upper back of the cranium. They join at the sagittal suture.	**pariet/o-** *wall of a cavity*
sagittal suture	Immoveable suture between the two parietal bones on the right and left sides of the cranium	**sagitt/o-** *going from front to back*
skull	Bony structure of the head that consists of the cranium and facial bones	
sphenoid bone	Large, irregular bone that forms the central base of the cranium and the posterior walls of the eye sockets. It contains the sphenoid sinuses. A bony cup in the sphenoid bone holds the pituitary gland.	**sphen/o-** *wedge shape*
temporal bones	Bones that form the lower sides of the cranium. They contain the openings for the external ear canals. Bony landmarks include the **mastoid process** behind the ear and the pointed **styloid process,** a site of attachment for tendons to the muscles of the tongue and pharynx and for ligaments to the hyoid bone.	**tempor/o-** *temple (side of the head)* **mast/o-** *breast; mastoid process* **styl/o-** *stake*
vomer	Facial bone that forms the inferior part of the nasal septum and continues posteriorly to join the sphenoid bone	
zygoma	Facial bone that forms the lateral edge of the eye socket and the cheek bone	

Bones of the Chest

costal cartilage	Firm, but flexible segments of connective tissue that join the ribs to the sternum. The area where the costal cartilage meets the rib is the **costochondral joint.**	**cost/o-** *rib* **chondr/o-** *cartilage* **cartilagin/o-** *cartilage*
ribs	Twelve pairs of bones that form the sides of the thorax. There are true ribs, false ribs, and floating ribs.	**cost/o-** *rib*
sternum	Vertical bone of the anterior thorax to which the clavicle and ribs are attached. It is also known as the **breast bone.** The **manubrium** is the triangular-shaped superior part of the sternum, while the **xiphoid process** is the inferior pointed tip.	**stern/o-** *sternum (breast bone)* **xiph/o-** *sword*
thorax	Bony cage of the chest that contains the **thoracic cavity** with the heart, lungs, and other structures. It is also known as the **rib cage.**	**thorac/o-** *thorax (chest)*

Bones of the Back

Word or Phrase	Description	Combining Forms
cervical vertebrae	Vertebrae C1–C7 of the spinal column in the neck. C1 is the **atlas**; C2 is the **axis.**	**cervic/o-** *neck; cervix*
coccyx	Group of several small, fused vertebrae inferior to the sacrum. It is also known as the **tail bone.**	**coccyg/o-** *coccyx (tail bone)*
intervertebral disk	Circular disk between two vertebrae. It consists of an outer wall of fibrocartilage and an inner gelatinous substance, the **nucleus pulposus** that acts as a cushion.	**vertebr/o-** *vertebra*
lumbar vertebrae	Vertebrae L1–L5 of the spinal column in the lower back	**lumb/o-** *lower back; area between the ribs and pelvis*
sacrum	Group of five fused vertebrae inferior to the lumbar vertebrae	**sacr/o-** *sacrum*
spine	Bony vertical column of vertebrae. It is also known as the **spinal column**, **vertebral column,** or **backbone**. It is divided into five regions: cervical vertebrae, thoracic vertebrae, lumbar vertebrae, sacrum, and coccyx. *Spine* also refers to a bony projection, such as the spinous process on a vertebra.	**spin/o-** *spine; backbone* **vertebr/o-** *vertebra*
thoracic vertebrae	Vertebrae T1–T12 of the spinal column in the area of the chest	**thorac/o-** *thorax (chest)*
vertebrae	Bony structure in the spine. Most vertebrae have a vertebral body (flat, circular area), **spinous process** (bony projection along the midback), two **transverse processes** (bony projections to the side), and a **foramen** (hole where the spinal cord passes through).	**vertebr/o-** *vertebra* **spondyl/o-** *vertebra* **spin/o-** *spine; backbone*

Bones of the Shoulders

acromion	Flat, bony projection of the scapula where it connects to the clavicle	
clavicle	Horizontal rodlike bone along each shoulder. It joins with the manubrium of the sternum and the acromion of the scapula. It is also known as the **collar bone.**	**clavicul/o-** *clavicle (collar bone)*
glenoid fossa	Shallow depression in the scapula where the head of the humerus joins the scapula to make the shoulder joint	**glen/o-** *socket of a joint*
scapula	Triangular-shaped bone on each side of the upper back. It is also known as the **shoulder blade.** It contains the **acromion.**	**scapul/o-** *scapula (shoulder blade)*

Bones of the Upper Extremities

carpal bones	The eight small bones of the wrist joint	**carp/o-** *wrist*
humerus	Long bone of the upper arm. The head of the humerus fits into the glenoid fossa of the scapula to make the shoulder joint.	**humer/o-** *humerus (upper arm bone)*
metacarpal bones	The five long bones of the hand, one corresponding to each finger. They are distal to the wrist bones.	**carp/o-** *wrist*
olecranon	Large, square, bony projection on the proximal ulna that forms the point of the elbow	

Word or Phrase	Description	Combining Forms
phalanx	One of the individual bones of a finger or toe. A finger or toe is a **digit** or a **ray.**	**phalang/o-** *phalanx (finger or toe)* **dactyl/o-** *finger or toe*
radius	Forearm bone located along the thumb side of the lower arm	**radi/o-** *radius (forearm bone); x-rays; radiation*
ulna	Forearm bone located along the little finger side of the lower arm	**uln/o-** *ulna (forearm bone)*

Bones of the Hips

Word or Phrase	Description	Combining Forms
acetabulum	Cup-shaped deep socket in the hip bone that is formed by the ilium and the pubic bone. It is where the head of the femur fits to make the hip joint.	**acetabul/o-** *acetabulum (hip socket)*
ilium	Most superior hip bone. It has a broad, flaring **iliac crest.** Posteriorly, each ilium joins the sacrum. The ilium contains the acetabulum, the deep socket of the hip joint.	**ili/o-** *ilium (hip bone)*
ischium	Most inferior hip bone. Each ischium is one of the "seat bones."	**ischi/o-** *ischium (hip bone)*
pelvis	The hip bones as well as the sacrum and coccyx of the spinal column	**pelv/o-** *pelvis (hip bone; renal pelvis)*
pubis	Small bridgelike bone that is the most anterior hip bone. The **pubic symphysis** is a nearly immobile joint between the two **pubic bones.**	**pub/o-** *pubis (hip bone)*

Bones of the Lower Extremities

Word or Phrase	Description	Combining Forms
calcaneus	Largest of the ankle bones. It is also known as the **heel bone.**	**calcane/o-** *calcaneus (heel bone)*
femur	Long bone of the upper leg. It is also known as the **thigh bone.** The head of the femur fits into the acetabulum to make the hip joint.	**femor/o-** *femur (thigh bone)*
fibula	Smaller of the two bones in the lower leg, located on the little toe side. The adjectives *fibular* and *peroneal* mean *fibula.*	**fibul/o-** *fibula (lower leg bone)* **perone/o-** *fibula (lower leg bone)*
hallux	The great toe	
malleolus	Bony projection of the distal tibia (**medial malleolus**) or the fibula (**lateral malleolus**). Often mistakenly called the ankle bones.	
metatarsal bones	The five long bones of the midfoot, one corresponding to each toe. They are distal to the ankle bones.	**tars/o-** *ankle*
patella	Thick, round bone anterior to the knee joint. It is also known as the **kneecap.**	**patell/o-** *patella (kneecap)*
phalanx	(See previous section)	
tarsal bones	The seven bones in the ankle joint. The first is the tarsus; the largest is the calcaneus.	**tars/o-** *ankle*
tibia	Larger of the two bones of the lower leg and located on the great toe side of the lower leg. It is also known as the **shin bone.**	**tibi/o-** *tibia (shin bone)*

Joints, Cartilage, and Ligaments

Word or Phrase	Description	Combining Forms
articular cartilage	Cartilage that covers the bone ends in a synovial joint	**articul/o-** *joint* **cartilagin/o-** *cartilage*
joint	Area where two bones come together. It is also known as an **articulation.** There are three types of joints: suture, symphysis, and synovial.	**articul/o-** *joint* **arthr/o-** *joint*
ligament	Fibrous bands that hold two bone ends together in a synovial joint	**ligament/o-** *ligament*
meniscus	Crescent-shaped cartilage pad found in some synovial joints such as the knee	
suture joint	Immovable joint between two cranial bones. This joint contains no cartilage.	
symphysis joint	Slightly movable joint between the two pubic bones (the pubic symphysis) or between the vertebrae. This joint contains a fibrocartilage pad or a disk.	
synovial joint	A fully moveable joint. There are two types: hinge joint (the elbow and the knee) and ball-and-socket joint (the shoulder and the hip). Ligaments hold the bone ends together. The entire joint is enclosed in a joint capsule. The inner surface of the joint capsule is lined by a **synovial membrane** that produces **synovial fluid** to lubricate the joint.	**synovi/o-** *synovium (membrane)*

Bone Structure and Bone Growth

Word or Phrase	Description	Combining Forms
cancellous bone	Spongy bone in the epiphyses of long bones. Its spaces are filled with red bone marrow that makes blood cells. It is also found in the skull, clavicles, sternum, ribs, vertebrae, and hip bones.	**cancell/o-** *lattice structure*
cortical bone	Dense, compact, weightbearing bone along the diaphysis or shaft of a long bone	**cortic/o-** *cortex (outer region)*
diaphysis	The straight shaft of a long bone	**diaphys/o-** *shaft of a bone*
epiphysis	One of the two widened ends of a long bone. It contains the **epiphysial plate** where bone growth takes place.	**epiphys/o-** *growth area at the end of a long bone*
medullary cavity	Cavity within the shaft (diaphysis) of a long bone. It contains yellow bone marrow (fatty tissue).	**medull/o-** *medulla (inner region)*
ossification	Process by which cartilage is changed into bone from infancy through adolescence	**ossificat/o-** *changing into bone*
osteoblast	Bone cell that forms new bone or rebuilds bone	**oste/o-** *bone*
osteoclast	Bone cell that breaks down old or damaged areas of bone	**oste/o-** *bone*
osteocyte	Bone cell that maintains and monitors the mineral content (calcium, phosphorus) of bone	**oste/o-** *bone*
periosteum	Thick, fibrous membrane that covers the outer surface of a bone	**oste/o-** *bone*

Labeling Exercise

Match each anatomy word or phrase to its structure and write it in the numbered box for each figure. Be sure to check your spelling. Use the Answer Key at the end of the book to check your answers.

coronal suture	frontal bone	mandible	nasal bone	parietal bone	temporal bone
ethmoid bone	lacrimal bone	maxilla	occipital bone	sphenoid bone	zygomatic bone

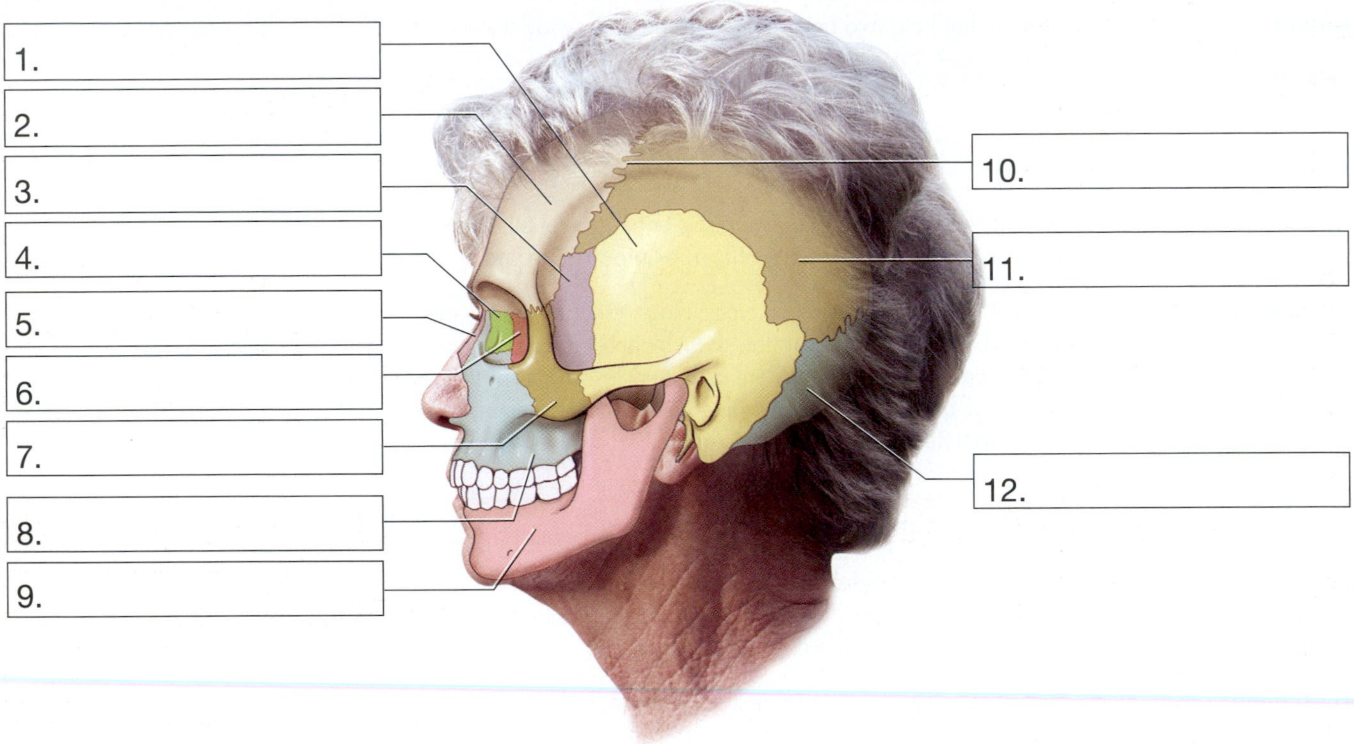

1.

2.

3.

4.

5.

6.

7.

8.

9.

10.

11.

12.

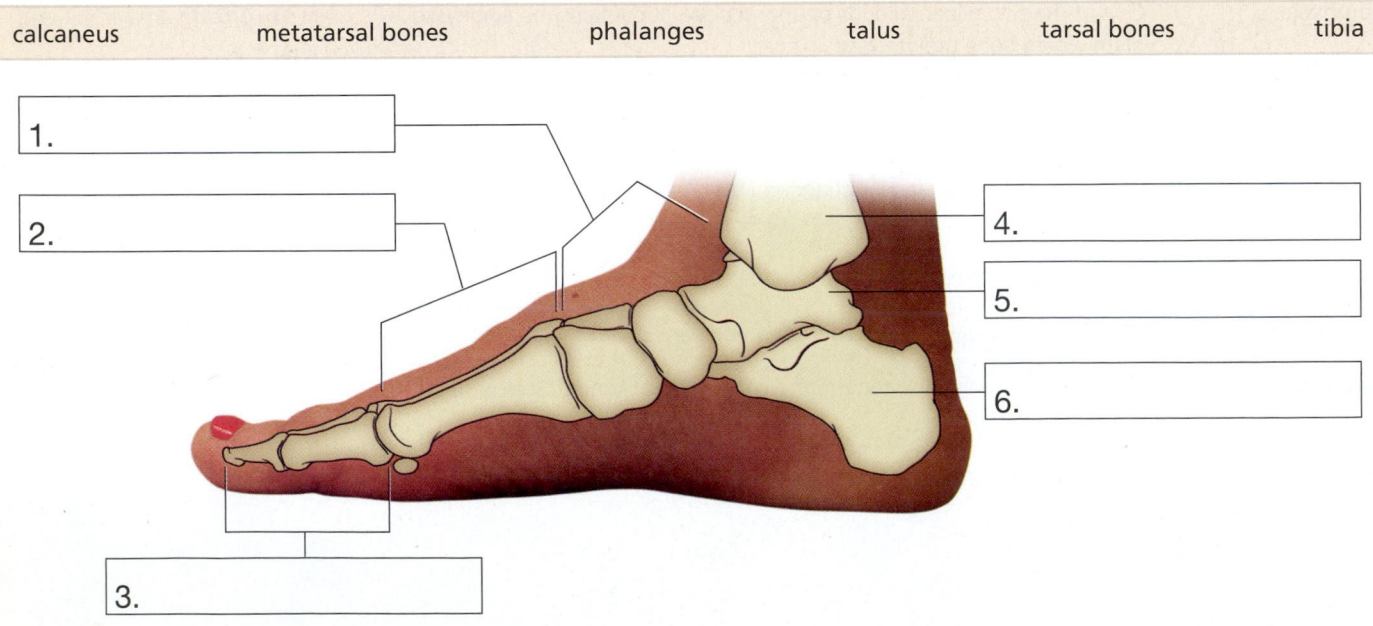

calcaneus	metatarsal bones	phalanges	talus	tarsal bones	tibia

1.

2.

3.

4.

5.

6.

carpal bones	glenoid fossa	patella	scapula
clavicle	humerus	phalanges	sternum
coccyx	ilium	pubis or pubic bone	tibia
costal cartilage	ischium	radius	ulna
femur	manubrium	rib	vertebra
fibula	metacarpal bones	sacrum	xiphoid process

1.

2.

3.

4.

5.

6.

7.

8.

9.

10.

11.

12.

13.

14.

15.

16.

17.

18.

19.

20.

21.

22.

23.

24.

Building Medical Words

Use the Answer Key at the end of the book to check your answers.

Combining Forms Exercise

Before you build skeletal words, review these combining forms. Next to each combining form, write its medical meaning. The first one has been done for you.

Combining Form	Medical Meaning	Combining Form	Medical Meaning
1. **acetabul/o-**	acetabulum (hip socket)	30. maxill/o-	
2. appendicul/o-		31. nas/o-	
3. arthr/o-		32. occipit/o-	
4. articul/o-		33. osse/o-	
5. calcane/o-		34. ossificat/o-	
6. carp/o-		35. oste/o-	
7. cartilagin/o-		36. palat/o-	
8. cervic/o-		37. pariet/o-	
9. chondr/o-		38. patell/o-	
10. clavicul/o-		39. pelv/o-	
11. cost/o-		40. perone/o-	
12. crani/o-		41. phalang/o-	
13. dactyl/o-		42. pub/o-	
14. diaphys/o-		43. radi/o-	
15. epiphys/o-		44. sacr/o-	
16. ethm/o-		45. scapul/o-	
17. femor/o-		46. skelet/o-	
18. fibul/o-		47. sphen/o-	
19. front/o-		48. spin/o-	
20. glen/o-		49. spondyl/o-	
21. humer/o-		50. stern/o-	
22. hy/o-		51. synovi/o-	
23. ili/o-		52. tars/o-	
24. ischi/o-		53. tempor/o-	
25. lacrim/o-		54. thorac/o-	
26. ligament/o-		55. tibi/o-	
27. lumb/o-		56. uln/o-	
28. mandibul/o-		57. vertebr/o-	
29. mast/o-		58. xiph/o-	

Combining Form and Suffix Exercise

Read the definition of the medical word. Look at the combining form that is given. Select the correct suffix from the Suffix List and write it on the blank line. Then build the medical word and write it on the line. (Remember: You may need to remove the combining vowel. Always remove the hyphens and slash.) Be sure to check your spelling. The first one has been done for you.

SUFFIX LIST

-al (pertaining to)	-cyte (cell)	-ion (action; condition)
-ar (pertaining to)	-eal (pertaining to)	-oid (resembling)
-ation (a process; being or having)	-ic (pertaining to)	-ous (pertaining to)
-clast (cell that breaks down substances)		

Definition of the Medical Word	Combining Form	Suffix	Build the Medical Word
1. Pertaining to the cranium	crani/o-	-al	cranial

(You think *pertaining to* (-al) + *the cranium* (crani/o-). You change the order of the word parts to put the suffix last. You write *cranial*.)

Definition of the Medical Word	Combining Form	Suffix	Build the Medical Word
2. Pertaining to the thorax	thorac/o-		
3. Pertaining to the ribs	cost/o-		
4. Pertaining to the mandible	mandibul/o-		
5. Pertaining to a ligament	ligament/o-		
6. Pertaining to the pelvis	pelv/o-		
7. Pertaining to a finger or toe	phalang/o-		
8. Pertaining to bone	osse/o-		
9. Being or having a joint	articul/o-		
10. Cell that breaks down bone	oste/o-		
11. Pertaining to the vertebra	vertebr/o-		
12. Pertaining to the lower back	lumb/o-		
13. Pertaining to the ulna	uln/o-		
14. Pertaining to the fibula	fibul/o-		
15. Action of changing into bone	ossificat/o-		
16. (A bone) resembling a sieve	ethm/o-		
17. Pertaining to the sternum	sterno-		
18. Pertaining to the neck	cervic/o-		
19. Pertaining to the clavicle	clavicul/o-		
20. Pertaining to the humerus	humer/o-		
21. Pertaining to the pubis	pub/o-		
22. Pertaining to the wrist	carp/o-		
23. Pertaining to the kneecap	patell/o-		
24. Cell (that maintains the mineral content of) bone	oste/o-		

Diseases and Conditions

Diseases of the Bones and Cartilage

Word or Phrase	Description	Word Building

avascular necrosis	Death of cells in the epiphysis of a long bone, often the femur. This is caused by an injury, fracture, or dislocation that damages nearby blood vessels or by a blood clot that interrupts the blood supply to the bone. Treatment: Surgery to remove the dead bone, then a bone graft. For large areas of avascular necrosis, joint replacement surgery is done.	**avascular** (aa-VAS-kyoo-lar)
		   a- *away from; without*
		   vascul/o- *blood vessel*
		   -ar *pertaining to*
		
		necrosis (neh-KROH-sis)
		   necr/o- *dead cells, tissue, or body*
		   -osis *condition; abnormal condition; process*

bone tumor	**Osteoma** is a benign tumor of the bone. **Osteosarcoma** is a malignant bone tumor in which osteoblasts, the cells that form new bone, multiply uncontrollably. It is also known as **osteogenic sarcoma.** **Ewing's sarcoma** is a malignant bone tumor that occurs mainly in young men. Treatment: Surgical excision of the tumor or amputation of the limb followed by radiation therapy or chemotherapy.	**osteoma** (AWS-tee-OH-mah)
		   oste/o- *bone*
		   -oma *tumor; mass*
		
		osteosarcoma (AWS-tee-oh-sar-KOH-mah)
		   oste/o- *bone*
		   sarc/o- *connective tissue*
		   -oma *tumor; mass*
		
		osteogenic (AWS-tee-oh-JEN-ik)
		   oste/o- *bone*
		   gen/o- *arising from; produced by*
		   -ic *pertaining to*
		
		Ewing (YOO-ing)

chondroma	Benign tumor of the cartilage. Treatment: Excision, if large.	**chondroma** (con-DROH-mah)
		   chondr/o- *cartilage*
		   -oma *tumor; mass*

chondromalacia patellae	Abnormal softening of the patella because of thinning and uneven wear. The thigh muscle pulls the patella in a crooked path that wears away the underside of the bone. Treatment: Strengthening of the thigh muscle to correct the direction of its contraction.	**chondromalacia** (CON-droh-mah-LAY-shee-ah)
		   chondr/o- *cartilage*
		   malac/o- *softening*
		   -ia *condition; state; thing*
		
		patellae (pah-TEL-ee)

Word or Phrase	Description	Word Building

fracture	Broken bone due to an accident, injury, or disease process. Fractures are categorized according to how the bone breaks (see Figure 8-18 ■ and Table 8-1). A fracture caused by force or torsion during an accident or sports activity is a **stress fracture.** A fracture caused by a disease process such as osteoporosis, bone cancer, or metastases to the bone is a **pathologic fracture.** Fractures that are allowed to heal without treatment often show malunion or **malalignment** of the fracture fragments. Treatment: Closed reduction and manipulation to align the fracture pieces, application of a cast. Surgery: Open reduction and internal fixation using wires, pins, screws, or plates.
	
	Figure 8-18 ■ **Bone fracture.**
	This x-ray shows an oblique fracture of the fibula of the lower leg.
		fracture (FRAK-chur)
		  fract/o- *break up*
		  -ure *system; result of*
		
		pathologic (PATH-oh-LAWJ-ik)
		  path/o- *disease; suffering*
		  log/o- *word; the study of*
		  -ic *pertaining to*
		
		malalignment (MAL-ah-LINE-ment)
		  mal- *bad; inadequate*
		  align/o- *arranged in a straight line*
		  -ment *action; state*

Table 8-1   Fracture Names and Descriptions

Fracture Name	Description	Illustration	Word Building
closed fracture	Any fracture in which the bone does not break through the overlying skin		
open fracture	Any fracture in which the bone breaks through the overlying skin. It is also known as a **compound fracture.**		
nondisplaced fracture	Broken bone ends remain in their normal anatomical alignment		**nondisplaced** (non-dis-PLAYSD) The prefix *non-* means *not.* The prefix *dis-* means *away from.*
displaced fracture	Broken bone ends are pulled out of their normal anatomical alignment		**displaced** (dis-PLAYSD)

(continued)

Table 8-1 Fracture Names and Descriptions (*continued*)

Fracture name	Description	Illustration	Word Building
Colles' fracture	Distal radius is broken by falling onto an outstretched hand	Colles' fracture	**Colles' fracture** (KOH-leez)
comminuted fracture	Bone is crushed into several pieces	Comminuted fracture	**comminuted** (COM-ih-NYOO-ted) **comminut/o-** *break into small pieces* **-ed** *pertaining to*
compression fracture	Vertebrae are compressed together when a person falls onto the buttocks or when a vertebra collapses in on itself because of disease	[[Insert UNF 8-1 Compression fracture	**compression** (com-PRESH-un) **compress/o-** *press together* **-ion** *action; condition*
depressed fracture	Cranium is fractured inward toward the brain	Depressed fracture	**depressed** (dee-PRESD) **depress/o-** *press down* **-ed** *pertaining to*
greenstick fracture	Bone is broken on only one side. This occurs in children because part of the bone is still flexible cartilage.	Greenstick fracture	
hairline fracture	Very thin fracture line with the bone pieces still together. It is difficult to detect except on an x-ray.	Hairline fracture	

Table 8-1   Fracture Names and Descriptions   (*continued*)

Fracture name	Description	Illustration	Word Building
oblique fracture	Bone is broken on an oblique angle	Oblique fracture	**oblique** (awb-LEEK)
spiral fracture	Bone is broken in a spiral because of a twisting force	Spiral fracture	**spiral** (SPY-ral) **spir/o-** *breathe; a coil* **-al** *pertaining to*
transverse fracture	Bone is broken in a transverse plane perpendicular to its long axis	Transverse fracture	**transverse** (trans-VERS) **trans-** *across; through* **-verse** *to travel; to turn* The ending -*verse* contains the combining form *vers/o-* (to travel; to turn) and the one-letter suffix –*e*.

Word or Phrase	Description	Word Building
osteomalacia	Abnormal softening of the bones due to a deficiency of vitamin D or inadequate exposure to the sun. In children, this causes rickets with bone pain and fractures. Treatment: Vitamin D supplements, sun exposure.	**osteomalacia** (AWS-tee-oh-mah-LAY-shee-ah) **oste/o-** *bone* **malac/o-** *softening* **-ia** *condition; state; thing*
osteomyelitis	Infection in the bone and the bone marrow. Bacteria enter the bone following an open fracture, crush injury, or surgical procedure. Treatment: Antibiotic drugs.	**osteomyelitis** (AWS-tee-oh-my-LIE-tis) **oste/o-** *bone* **myel/o-** *bone marrow; spinal cord; myelin* **-itis** *inflammation of; infection of* Select the correct combining form meaning to get the definition of *osteomyelitis*: *inflammation or infection of the bone and bone marrow.*

Word or Phrase	Description	Word Building
osteoporosis	Abnormal thinning of the bone structure. When bone breakdown exceeds new bone formation, calcium and phosphorus are lost, and the bone becomes osteoporotic (porous) with many small areas of **demineralization** (see Figure 8-19 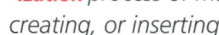). This can cause a compression fracture as a vertebra collapses in on itself. The vertebral column decreases in height, the patient becomes shorter, and there is an abnormal curvature of the upper back and shoulders (dowager's hump). Osteoporosis can also cause a spontaneous fracture (pathologic fracture) of the hip or femur. Sometimes it is unclear whether an older patient fell and fractured the bone or whether the osteoporotic bone itself spontaneously fractured and caused the patient to fall. Osteoporosis occurs in postmenopausal women and older men. Estradiol in women stimulates bone formation, and loss of estradiol at menopause leads to osteoporosis. A lack of dietary calcium and a lack of exercise contribute to the process. Treatment: Bone density test for diagnosis; drugs that decrease the rate of bone resorption or drugs that activate estradiol receptors, and calcium supplements.	**osteoporosis** (AWS-tee-oh-poh-ROH-sis) **oste/o-** *bone* **por/o-** *small openings; pores* **-osis** *condition; abnormal condition; process* **demineralization** (dee-MIN-er-al-ih-ZAY-shun) **de-** *reversal of; without* **mineral/o-** *mineral; electrolyte* **-ization** *process of making, creating, or inserting*

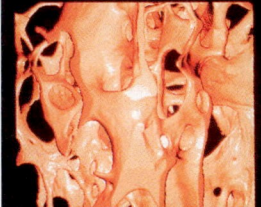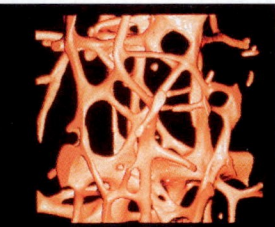

Figure 8-19 ■ **Normal bone versus bone with osteoporosis.**

The bone on the left shows normal mineralization and density. The bone on the right shows demineralization, large holes, and loss of density. This bone would be extremely prone to fracture.

Diseases of the Vertebrae

ankylosing spondylitis	Chronic inflammation of the vertebrae that leads to fibrosis, restriction of movement, and stiffening of the spine. Treatment: Nonsteroidal anti-inflammatory drugs.	**ankylosing** (ANG-kih-LOH-sing) **ankyl/o-** *fused together; stiff* **-osing** *a condition of doing* **spondylitis** (SPAWN-dih-LY-tis) **spondyl/o-** *vertebra* **-itis** *inflammation of; infection of*
kyphosis	Abnormal, excessive, posterior curvature of the thoracic spine (see Figure 8-20 ■). It is also known as **humpback** or **hunchback.** The back is said to have a **kyphotic** curvature. **Kyphoscoliosis** is a complex curvature with components of both kyphosis and scoliosis. Treatment: Back brace or surgery to fuse and straighten the spine.	**kyphosis** (ky-FOH-sis) **kyph/o-** *bent; humpbacked* **-osis** *condition; abnormal condition; process* **kyphotic** (ky-FAWT-ik) **kyph/o-** *bent; humpbacked* **-tic** *pertaining to* **kyphoscoliosis** (KY-foh-SKOH-lee-OH-sis) **kyph/o-** *bent; humpbacked* **scoli/o-** *curved; crooked* **-osis** *condition; abnormal condition; process*

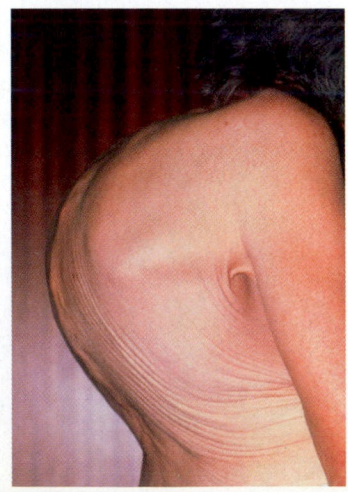

Figure 8-20 ■ **Kyphosis.**

This patient has extreme kyphosis of the upper back.

Word or Phrase	Description	Word Building
lordosis	Abnormal, excessive, anterior curvature of the lumbar spine. It is also known as **swayback.** The back is said to have a **lordotic** curvature. Treatment: Back brace or surgery to fuse and straighten the spine.	**lordosis** (lor-DOH-sis) **lord/o-** *swayback* **-osis** *condition; abnormal condition; process* **lordotic** (lor-DAWT-ik) **lord/o-** *swayback* **-tic** *pertaining to*
scoliosis	Abnormal, excessive, C-shaped or S-shaped lateral curvature of the spine (see Figure 8-21 ■). The back is said to have a **scoliotic** curvature. A **dextroscoliosis** curves to the patient's right, while a **levoscoliosis** curves to the patient's left. Scoliosis can be congenital but most often the cause is unknown. It develops during childhood and may continue to progress during adolescence. It impairs movement, posture, and breathing. An x-ray is used to determine the number of degrees in the curvature. Treatment: Back brace or surgery to fuse and straighten the spine. **Clinical Connections** **Public Health.** Scoliosis screening is routinely done by a school nurse for all elementary school children. The child's back is observed while standing and then while bending over. Some cases of scoliosis become more apparent with bending over as one side of the back becomes noticeably higher and one scapula sticks out. **Figure 8-21 ■ Scoliosis.** This patient with moderate scoliosis of the spine to the left shows the characteristic tilt to the shoulders and hips and a difference in arm lengths.	**scoliosis** (SKOH-lee-OH-sis) **scoli/o-** *curved; crooked* **-osis** *condition; abnormal condition; process* **scoliotic** (SKOH-lee-AWT-ik) **scoli/o-** *curved; crooked* **-tic** *pertaining to* **dextroscoliosis** (DEKS-troh-SKOH-lee-OH-sis) **dextr/o-** *right* **scoli/o-** *curved; crooked* **-osis** *condition; abnormal condition; process* **levoscoliosis** (LEE-voh-SKOH-lee-OH-sis) **lev/o-** *left* **scoli/o-** *curved; crooked* **-osis** *condition; abnormal condition; process*
spondylolisthesis	Degenerative condition of the spine in which one vertebra moves anteriorly over another vertebra and slips out of proper alignment due to degeneration of the intervertebral disk. It can occur because of a sports injury or a compression fracture of the vertebra from osteoporosis. Treatment: Back brace or surgery to relieve a pinched spinal nerve. Analgesic drugs, nonsteroidal anti-inflammatory drugs. Intra-articular injection of a corticosteroid drug.	**spondylolisthesis** (SPAWN-dih-LOH-lis-THEE-sis) **spondyl/o-** *vertebra* **-olisthesis** *abnormal condition with slipping*

Diseases of the Joints and Ligaments

Word or Phrase	Description	Word Building
arthralgia	Pain in the joint from injury, inflammation, or infection from various causes. Treatment: Correct the underlying cause.	**arthralgia** (ar-THRAL-jee-ah) **arthr/o-** *joint* **alg/o-** *pain* **-ia** *condition; state; thing*
arthropathy	Disease of a joint from any cause. Treatment: Correct the underlying cause.	**arthropathy** (ar-THRAWP-ah-thee) **arthr/o-** *joint* **-pathy** *disease; suffering*
dislocation	Displacement of the end of a bone from its normal position within a joint. This is usually caused by injury or trauma. **Congenital dislocation of the hip (CDH)** is present at birth because the acetabulum is poorly formed or the ligaments are loose. Treatment: Manipulate and return the bone to its normal position. Congenital dislocation of the hip is treated with a splint or with surgery to correct the shape of the acetabulum or looseness of the ligaments.	**dislocation** (DIS-loh-KAY-shun) **dis-** *away from* **locat/o-** *a place* **-ion** *action; condition* **congenital** (con-JEN-ih-tal) **congenit/o-** *present at birth* **-al** *pertaining to*

Word or Phrase	Description	Word Building

gout	Metabolic disorder that occurs most often in men. There is a high level of uric acid in the blood. An acute attack causes sudden, severe pain as uric acid moves from the blood into the soft tissues and forms masses of crystals known as **tophi**. Historically, patients with gout have been pictured with throbbing big toes, although tophi can also form in the hands. Tophi in the joints causes **gouty arthritis.** Treatment: Avoid foods that increase the uric acid level. Drugs to decrease the uric acid level.	**gout** (GOWT)
		tophus (TOH-fus)
		tophi (TOH-fie)
		Tophus is a Latin singular noun. Form the plural by changing *-us* to *-i*.
		gouty (GOW-tee)
		arthritis (ar-THRY-tis)
		  arthr/o- *joint*
		  -itis *inflammation of; infection of*

hemarthrosis	Blood in the joint cavity from blunt trauma or a penetrating wound. It also occurs spontaneously in hemophiliac patients. Treatment: Temporary immobilization of the joint, aspiration of blood from the joint cavity, corticosteroid drugs. Surgery: Arthroscopy.	**hemarthrosis** (HEE-mar-THROH-sis)
		  hem/o- *blood*
		  arthr/o- *joint*
		  -osis *condition; abnormal condition; process*

Lyme disease	Arthritis caused by a bacterium in the bite of an infected deer tick. There is an erythematous rash that expands outward for several weeks (bull's-eye rash) but is not itchy; there is joint pain, fever, chills, and fatigue. If untreated, Lyme disease can cause severe fatigue and affect the nervous system (numbness, severe headache) and the heart. Treatment: Antibiotic drugs.	**Lyme** (LIME)

osteoarthritis	Chronic inflammatory disease of the joints, particularly the large weight-bearing joints (knees, hips) and joints that move repeatedly (shoulders, neck, hands). Osteoarthritis usually begins in middle age, but can develop sooner in a joint that has been overused or subjected to trauma. There is joint pain and stiffness. There is inflammation from constant wear and tear, and this is worsened if the patient is overweight. The normally smooth cartilage becomes roughened and then wears away in spots (see Figure 8-22 ■). The bone ends rub against each other, causing additional inflammation and **crepitus,** a grinding sound. New bone sometimes forms abnormally as an **osteophyte,** a sharp bone spur that causes pain. This condition is also known as **degenerative joint disease (DJD).** Treatment: Analgesic drugs, nonsteroidal anti-inflammatory drugs. Intra-articular injection of a corticosteroid drug.	**osteoarthritis** (AWS-tee-oh-ar-THRY-tis)
		  oste/o- *bone*
		  arthr/o- *joint*
		  -itis *inflammation of; infection of*
		crepitus (KREP-ih-tus)
		osteophyte (AWS-tee-oh-fite)
		  oste/o- *bone*
		  -phyte *growth*
		degenerative (dee-JEN-er-ah-tiv)
		  de- *reversal of; without*
		  gener/o- *production; creation*
		  -ative *pertaining to*

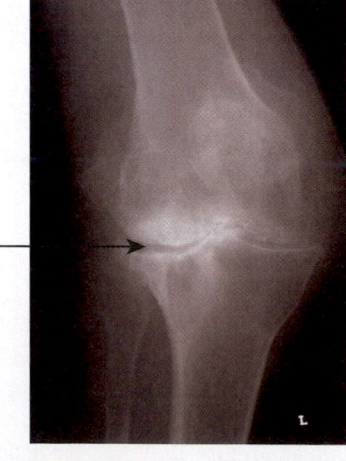

Figure 8-22 ■ Osteoarthritis.
This patient's knee shows loss of the articular cartilage and narrowing of the joint space between the bone ends. This finding is characteristic of degenerative joint disease.

Word or Phrase	Description	Word Building
rheumatoid arthritis	Acute and chronic inflammatory disease of connective tissues, particularly of the joints. It is an autoimmune disease in which the patient's own antibodies attack cartilage and connective tissues. Patients are usually young to middle-aged females. There is redness and swelling of the joints, most often of the hands and feet. The joint cartilage is slowly destroyed by inflammation. The symptoms flare and subside over time, and there is progressive deformity of the joints (see Figure 8-23 ■). Treatment: Corticosteroid drugs. Surgery: Joint replacement surgery.	**rheumatoid** (ROO-mah-toyd) **rheumat/o-** *watery discharge* **-oid** *resembling* **arthritis** (ar-THRY-tis) **arthr/o-** *joint* **-itis** *inflammation of; infection of*

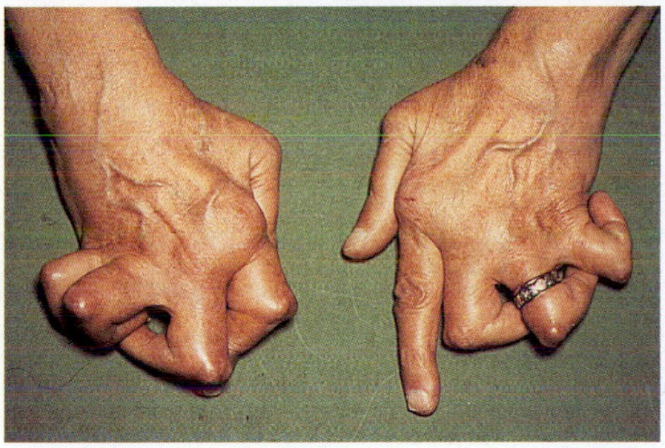

Figure 8-23 ■ Rheumatoid arthritis.
This patient has severe joint deformities of the hands that are characteristic of rheumatoid arthritis.

Word or Phrase	Description	Word Building
sprain	Overstretching or tearing of a ligament. Treatment: Rest or surgery to repair the ligament.	**sprain** (SPRAYN)
torn meniscus	Tear of the cartilage pad of the knee because of an injury. Treatment: Arthroscopy and repair.	**meniscus** (meh-NIS-kus)

Diseases of the Bony Thorax

Word or Phrase	Description	Word Building
pectus excavatum	Congenital deformity of the bony thorax in which the sternum, particularly the xiphoid process, is bent inward, creating a hollow depression in the anterior chest. Treatment: Surgery, if severe.	**pectus excavatum** (PEK-tus EKS-kah-VAH-tum)

Diseases of the Bones of the Legs and Feet

Word or Phrase	Description	Word Building
genu valgum	Congenital deformity in which the knees are rotated toward the midline and are abnormally close together and the lower legs are bent laterally. This is also known as **knock-knee.** Treatment: Surgical correction, if severe.	**genu valgum** (JEE-noo VAL-gum)
genu varum	Congenital deformity in which the knees are rotated laterally away from each other and the lower legs are bent toward the midline. This is also known as **bowleg.** Treatment: Surgical correction, if severe.	**genu varum** (JEE-noo VAR-um)

Word or Phrase	Description	Word Building
hallux valgus	Deformity in which the great toe is angled laterally toward the other toes (see Figure 8-24 ■). Often a **bunion** develops at the base of the great toe with swelling and inflammation. This is a common deformity seen in women who wear pointy-toed shoes. Treatment: Wear wide-toed shoes; bunionectomy.	**hallux valgus** (HAL-uks VAL-gus) **bunion** (BUN-yun)

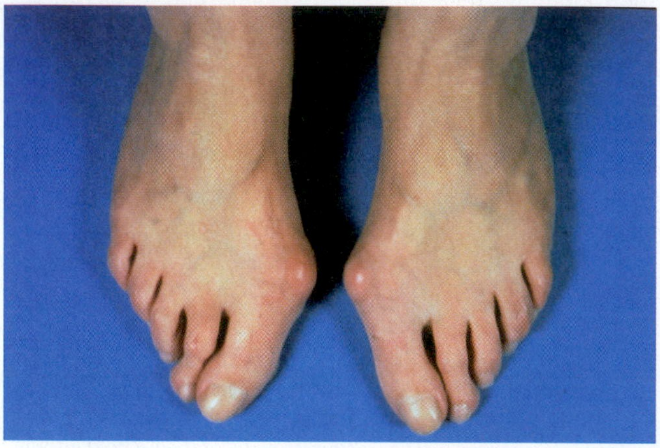

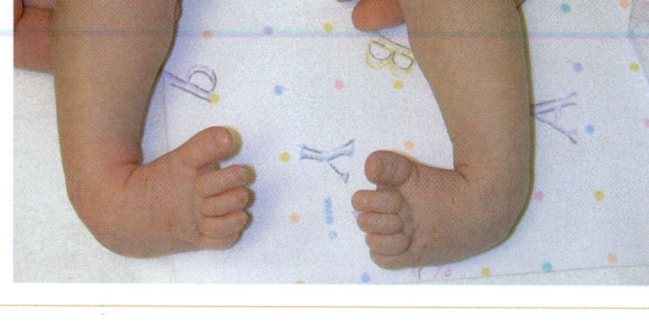

Figure 8-24 ■ Bilateral hallux valgus.
The great toes are angled away from the midline, and there are reddened, enlarged bunions on the medial side of each foot.

Word or Phrase	Description	Word Building
talipes equinovarus	Congenital deformity in which the foot is pulled downward and toward the midline. This is also known as **clubfoot.** One or both feet can be affected (see Figure 8-25 ■). Treatment: Casts applied to progressively straighten the foot. Surgical correction for severe cases.	**talipes equinovarus** (TAY-lih-peez ee-ĸwy-noh-VAIR-us)

Figure 8-25 ■ Bilateral clubfeet.
This infant was born with bilateral clubfeet. Although all newborns' feet are rotated medially due to the confining environment of the uterus, the feet can easily be moved into an anatomically correct position. In talipes equinovarus, the position of the feet cannot be corrected and does not correct itself over time.

Laboratory and Diagnostic Procedures

Laboratory Tests

Word or Phrase	Description	Word Building
rheumatoid factor (RF)	Blood test that is positive in patients with rheumatoid arthritis	
uric acid	Blood test that has an elevated level in patients with gout and gouty arthritis	**uric acid** (YOO-rik AS-id)

Radiology and Nuclear Medicine Procedures

Word or Phrase	Description	Word Building
arthrography	Procedure that uses a radiopaque contrast dye that is injected into a joint. It coats and outlines the bone ends and joint capsule. An x-ray or CT scan is then taken. MRI arthrography uses a strong magnetic field to align protons in the atoms of the patient's body. The protons emit signals to form a series of thin, successive images or "slices" of the joint. An MRI can be done with or without contrast dye. The x-ray, CT, or MRI image is an **arthrogram.**	**arthrography** (ar-THRAWG-rah-fee) **arthr/o-** *joint* **-graphy** *process of recording* **arthrogram** (AR-throh-gram) **arthr/o-** *joint* **-gram** *a record or picture*
bone density tests	Procedure that measures the bone mineral density (BMD) to determine if demineralization from osteoporosis has occurred (see Figure 8-26 ■). The heel or wrist bone can be tested, but the hip and spine bones give a more accurate result. There are two types of bone density tests: **DEXA (or DXA) scan** and **quantitative computerized tomography (QCT)**. This is also known as **bone densitometry.** A DEXA scan uses two x-ray beams with different energy levels to create a two-dimensional image. This scan can detect as little as a 1% loss of bone. Quantitative computerized tomography uses an x-ray beam and a CT scan to create a three-dimensional image. QCT is able to measure the density of both cancellous and cortical bone. Cancellous bone is the first to be affected by osteoporosis and the first to respond to therapy.	**DEXA scan** (DEK-sah) *DEXA stands for dual-energy x-ray absorptiometry.* **tomography** (toh-MAWG-rah-fee) **tom/o-** *cut; slice; layer* **-graphy** *process of recording* **densitometry** (DEN-sih-TAWM-eh-tree) **densit/o-** *density* **-metry** *process of measuring*

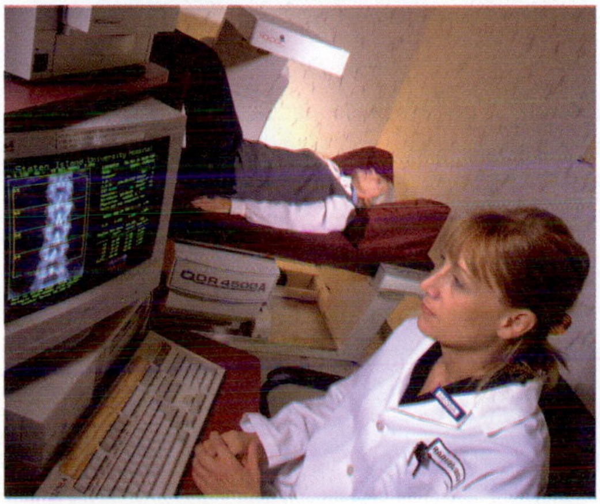

Figure 8-26 ■ **Bone density test.**
This patient is having a bone mineral density test performed, and the technician is viewing the results on the computer screen.

Did You Know?

A standard x-ray is not used to measure bone density, because you must lose at least 30% of your bone mass before the loss can be detected on an x-ray image. Both older men and postmenopausal women lose bone mass. After menopause, a woman can lose 1–2 percent of her bone mass each year.

Word or Phrase	Description	Word Building
bone scintigraphy	Nuclear medicine procedure in which a phosphate compound (DPD or MDP) is tagged with the radioactive tracer technetium-99m. This is injected intravenously and is taken up into the bone. A gamma scintillation camera detects gamma rays from the radioactive tracer. Areas of increased uptake ("hot spots") indicate arthritis, fracture, osteomyelitis, cancerous tumors of the bone, or areas of bony metastasis. The nuclear medicine image is a **scintigram.**	**scintigraphy** (sin-TIG-rah-fee) **scint/i-** *point of light* **-graphy** *process of recording* **scintigram** (SIN-tih-gram) **scint/i-** *point of light* **-gram** *a record or picture*
x-ray	Procedure that uses x-rays to diagnose bony abnormalities in any part of the body. X-rays are the primary means for diagnosing fractures, dislocations, and bone tumors.	**x-ray** (EKS-ray)

Medical and Surgical Procedures

Medical Procedures

Word or Phrase	Description	Word Building
cast	Procedure in which a cast of plaster or fiberglass is applied around a fractured bone and adjacent areas to immobilize the fracture in a fixed position to facilitate healing (see Figures 8-27 ■ and 8-28 ■). For fractures of the leg, the physician may order the patient to be nonweight bearing (putting no weight on the affected leg), toe touch (partial weight bearing), or full weight bearing (with a walking cast). Patients with leg casts are instructed in the use of crutches.	**cast** (KAST)

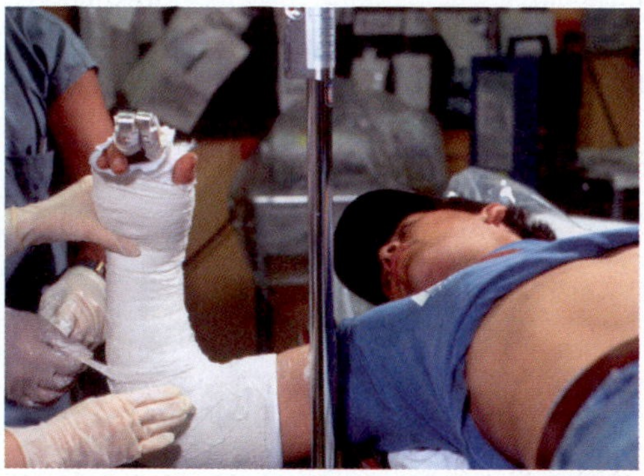

Figure 8-27 ■ Application of a cast.
This patient sustained several fractures during a dirt-bike accident. His two fractured fingers were placed in an aluminum buddy splint to immobilize them, while his fractured wrist (Colles' fracture) was placed in a long-arm cast.

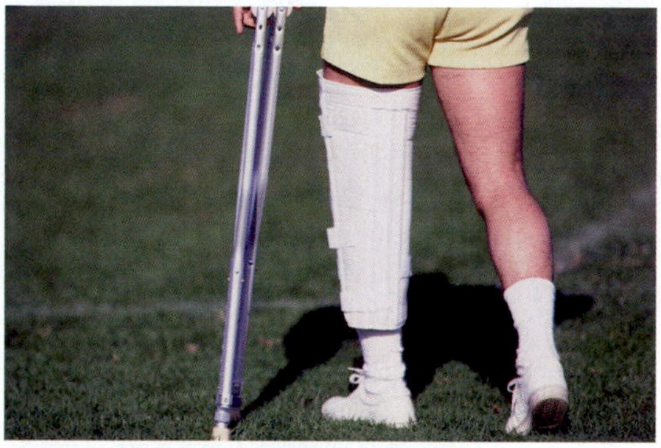

Figure 8-28 ■ Cast and crutches.
A leg cylinder cast is used to treat fractures of the knee or immobilize the knee after extensive surgery.

Word or Phrase	Description	Word Building
closed reduction	Procedure in which manual manipulation of a displaced fracture is performed so that the bone ends go back into normal alignment without the need for surgery	**reduction** (ree-DUK-shun) **reduct/o-** *to bring back; decrease* **-ion** *action; condition*
extracorporeal shock wave therapy (ESWT)	Procedure in which sound waves originating outside the body (extracorporeal) are used to break up bony spurs and treat other minor but painful problems of the foot	**extracorporeal** (EKS-trah-kor-POH-ree-al) **extra-** *outside of* **corpor/o-** *body* **-eal** *pertaining to*
goniometry	Procedure in which a **goniometer** is used to measure the range of movement (ROM) of a joint (see Figure 8-29 ■)	**goniometry** (GOH-nee-AWM-eh-tree) **goni/o-** *angle* **-metry** *process of measuring* **goniometer** (GOH-nee-AWM-eh-ter) **goni/o-** *angle* **-meter** *instrument used to measure*

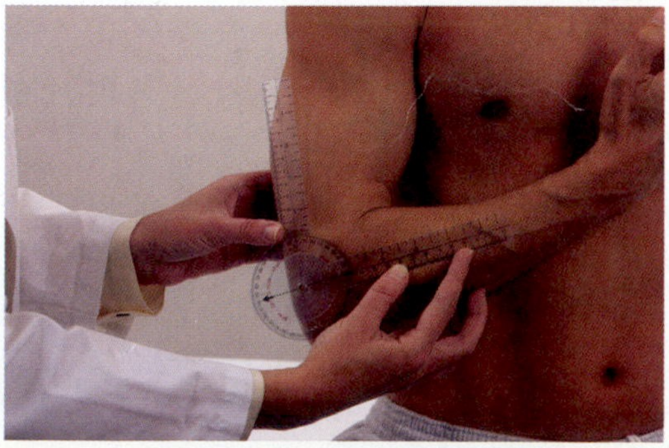

Figure 8-29 ■ Goniometer.
The two arms of the goniometer are positioned to correspond to body parts on either side of the joint. A scale on the goniometer measures (in degrees) how much motion of the joint is possible.

Word or Phrase	Description	Word Building
orthosis	Orthopedic device such as a brace, splint, or collar that is used to immobilize or correct an orthopedic problem. It is often custom made to fit the patient.	**orthosis** (or-THOH-sis) **orth/o-** *straight* **-osis** *condition; abnormal condition; process*
physical therapy	Procedure that uses active or passive exercises to improve a patient's range of motion, joint mobility, strength, and balance while walking	**physical** (FIZ-ih-kal) **physic/o-** *body* **-al** *pertaining to* **therapy** (THAIR-ah-pee) The combining form *therap/o-* means *treatment.*
prosthesis	Orthopedic device such as an artificial leg that is used by a patient who has had an amputation of a limb (see Figure 8-30 ■). It is known as a **prosthetic device.** An artificial joint is also considered to be a prosthetic device.	**prosthesis** (praws-THEE-sis) **prosthetic** (praws-THET-ik) **prosthet/o-** *artificial part* **-ic** *pertaining to*

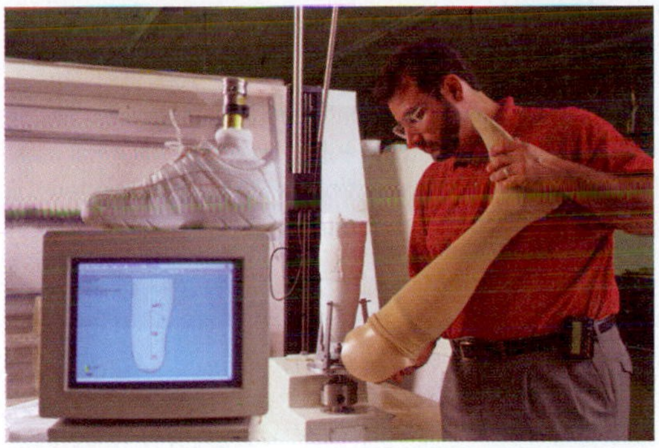

Figure 8-30 ■ Leg prosthesis.
This person is a prosthetist. He uses computer-aided design to create an artificial leg. It is built according to the patient's height and weight (to match the unamputated leg) and according to where the leg was amputated.

Word or Phrase	Description	Word Building
traction	Procedure that uses a weight to pull the bone ends of a fracture into correct alignment. Skin traction uses elastic wraps, straps, halters, or skin adhesives connected to a pulley and a weight. Skeletal traction uses pins, wires, or tongs inserted into the bone during surgery. Halo traction uses pins inserted into the cranium and attached to a circular metal frame that forms a halo around the patient's head. Bars connect the halo to a rigid vest that immobilizes the chest and back while exerting upward traction on the head to straighten a fracture of the spine.	**traction** (TRAK-shun) **tract/o-** *pulling* **-ion** *action; condition*

Surgical Procedures

Word or Phrase	Description	Word Building
amputation	Procedure to remove all or part of an extremity because of trauma or circulatory disease. A below-the-knee amputation (BKA) is performed at the level of the tibia and fibula. An above-the-knee amputation (AKA) is performed at the level of the femur. A muscle flap is wrapped over the end of the amputated limb to provide a cushion and some bulk so that the patient can be fitted with an artificial limb (prosthesis). A patient who has had an amputation is an **amputee.**	**amputation** (AM-pyoo-TAY-shun) **amputat/o-** *to cut off* **-ion** *action; condition* **amputee** (AM-pyoo-tee) **amput/o-** *to cut off* **-ee** *person who is the object of an action*
arthrocentesis	Procedure to remove an accumulation of fluid in a joint by using a needle inserted into the joint space	**arthrocentesis** (AR-throh-sen-TEE-sis) **arthr/o-** *joint* **-centesis** *procedure to puncture*
arthrodesis	Procedure to fuse the bones in a degenerated, unstable joint	**arthrodesis** (AR-throh-DEE-sis) **arthr/o-** *joint* **-desis** *procedure to fuse together*

Word or Phrase	Description	Word Building
arthroscopy	Procedure that uses an **arthroscope** inserted into the joint to visualize the inside of the joint and its structures (see Figure 8-31 ■). Other instruments can be inserted through the arthroscope to scrape or cut damaged cartilage or smooth sharp bone edges. **Figure 8-31** ■ **Arthroscopic surgery.** The skin around the patient's elbow was scrubbed with an orange antiseptic solution prior to surgery. The arthroscope was inserted into the elbow joint through a surgically created portal (opening in the skin). Other portals were used to insert instruments or remove fluid. A fiberoptic light and a magnifying lens on the arthroscope allow the surgeon to see inside of the joint, and the image is also displayed on a monitor in the operating room.	**arthroscopy** (ar-THRAWS-koh-pee) **arthr/o-** *joint* **-scopy** *process of using an instrument to examine* **arthroscope** (AR-throh-skohp) **arthr/o-** *joint* **-scope** *instrument used to examine* **arthroscopic** (ar-throh-SKAW-pik) **arthr/o-** *joint* **scop/o-** *examine with an instrument* **-ic** *pertaining to*
bone graft	Procedure that uses whole bone or bone chips to repair fractures with extensive bone loss or defects due to bone cancer. Bone taken from the patient's own body is an **autograft.** Frozen or freeze-dried bone taken from a cadaver is an **allograft.**	**graft** (GRAFT) **autograft** (AW-toh-graft) **aut/o-** *self* **-graft** *tissue for implant or transplant* **allograft** (AL-oh-graft) **all/o-** *other; strange* **-graft** *tissue for implant or transplant*
bunionectomy	Procedure to remove the prominent part of the metatarsal bone that is causing a bunion	**bunionectomy** (BUN-yun-EK-toh-mee) **bunion/o-** *bunion* **-ectomy** *surgical excision*
cartilage transplantation	Procedure that is an alternative to a total knee replacement. It is used to treat middle-aged adults (as opposed to older adults) with degenerative joint disease of the knee who have an active lifestyle.	**transplantation** (TRANS-plan-TAY-shun) **transplant/o-** *move something to another place* **-ation** *a process; being or having*

Did You Know?

Active people walk 1–3 million steps each year! The average person walks 4 miles each day. Wear and tear on the knee joints can result in the need for a cartilage transplant or a total knee replacement.

external fixation	Procedure used to treat a complicated fracture. An external fixator orthopedic device has metal pins that are inserted into the bone on either side of the fracture and connected to a metal frame. This immobilizes the fracture. A similar device is used to perform a **leg lengthening** to treat a congenitally short leg, but that device has screws that are turned each day to pull the bone and lengthen it.	**external** (eks-TER-nal) **extern/o-** *outside* **-al** *pertaining to* **fixation** (fik-SAY-shun) **fixat/o-** *to make stable or still* **-ion** *action; condition*

Word or Phrase	Description	Word Building
joint replacement surgery	Procedure to replace a joint that has been destroyed by disease or osteoarthritis. A metal or plastic joint prosthesis is inserted (see Figure 8-32 ■). This surgery is done on the hips as a **total hip replacement (THR),** or on the knees, shoulders, or even on the small joints of the fingers. For a total hip replacement, the head of the femur is sawn off. The stem (long metal projection) of the prosthesis is hammered into the cut end of the femur. The head (ball) of the prosthesis is matched to the size of the patient's acetabulum. The cup of the prosthesis is used to replace the acetabulum, and the ball is inserted into the cup. This is also known as an **arthroplasty.**	**arthroplasty** (AR-throh-PLAS-tee) **arthr/o-** *joint* **-plasty** *process of reshaping by surgery*

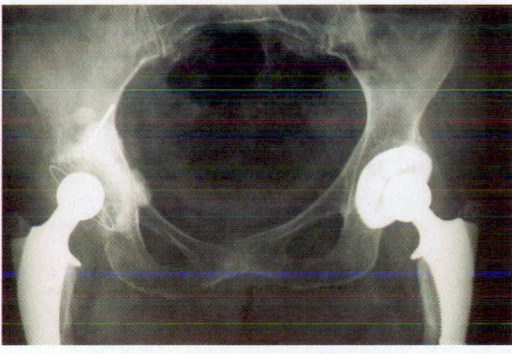

Figure 8-32 ■ Hip prostheses.

This patient has had two total hip replacement surgeries and received a different style of hip prosthesis each time. The metal components of a prosthesis stand out clearly on an x-ray.

Word or Phrase	Description	Word Building
open reduction and internal fixation (ORIF)	Procedure to treat a complicated fracture. An incision is made at the fracture site, the fracture is reduced (realigned), and an internal fixation procedure is done using screws, nails, or plates to hold the fracture fragments in correct anatomical alignment (see Figure 8-33 ■).	**reduction** (ree-DUK-shun) **reduct/o-** *to bring back; decrease* **-ion** *action; condition*

Did You Know?

Orthopedic surgery is not unlike carpentry. Surgical orthopedic instruments include hammers, nails, screws, metal plates, chisels, mallets, gouges, and saws. An **osteotome** is used to cut bone. A **rongeur** is a forceps that is used to remove small bone fragments.

osteotome (AWS-tee-oh-tohm)
oste/o- *bone*
-tome *instrument used to cut; area with distinct edges*

rongeur (rawn-ZHER)

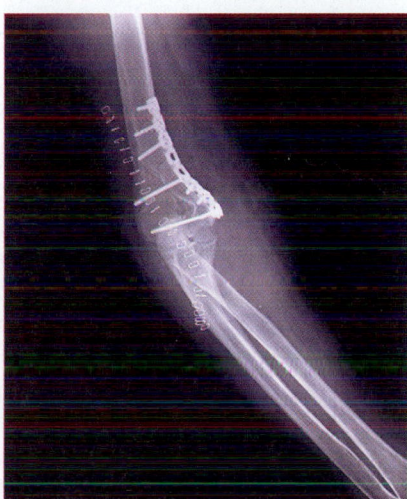

Figure 8-33 ■ Orthopedic plate and screws.

This fracture of the humerus was surgically repaired with an open reduction and internal fixation using a metal plate, three short nails, and two long nails to stabilize the bone fragments.

Drug Categories

These categories of drugs are used to treat skeletal diseases and conditions. The most common generic and trade name drugs in each category are listed.

Category	Indication	Examples	Word Building

analgesic drugs	Over-the-counter drugs aspirin and acetaminophen decrease inflammation and pain. They are used to treat minor injuries and osteoarthritis. Prescription narcotic drugs are used to treat severe pain.	aspirin (Bayer, Ecotrin), acetaminophen (Tylenol); prescription narcotic drugs: meperidine (Demerol), oxycodone (OxyContin), morphine sulfate (MS Contin)	**analgesic** (AN-al-JEE-zik)
			   an- *without; not*
			   alges/o- *sensation of pain*
			   -ic *pertaining to*

bone resorption inhibitor drugs	Inhibit osteoclasts from breaking down bone. They are used to prevent and treat osteoporosis.	alendronate (Fosamax), ibandronate (Boniva), zoledronic acid (Reclast, Zometa)	**resorption** (ree-SORP-shun)
			   re- *again and again; backward; unable to*
			   sorb/o- *to suck up*
			   -tion *a process; being or having*
			The *b* in *sorb/o-* (absorb) is changed to a *p*.

corticosteroid drugs	Decrease severe inflammation. They are given orally to treat osteoarthritis and rheumatoid arthritis. Some are given by **intra-articular** injection into the joint.	dexamethasone (Decadron), hydrocortisone (Cortef, Solu-Cortef), prednisone (Deltasone, Meticorten); intra-articular injection: betamethasone (Celestone), methylprednisolone (Depo-Medrol), triamcinolone (Aristospan, Kenalog)
		Note: This is often referred to as a "cortisone shot," even though it is actually one or several corticosteroid drugs.
			corticosteroid (KOR-tih-koh-STAIR-oyd)
			   cortic/o- *cortex (outer region)*
			   -steroid *steroid*
			
			intra-articular (IN-trah-ar-TIK-yoo-lar)
			   intra- *within*
			   articul/o- *joint*
			   -ar *pertaining to*

gold compound drugs	Inhibit the immune response that attacks the joints and connective tissue in patients with rheumatoid arthritis. These drugs actually contain gold.	auranofin (Ridaura), aurothioglucose (Solganal)	

nonsteroidal anti-inflammatory drugs (NSAIDs)	Decrease inflammation and pain. They are used to treat osteoarthritis and orthopedic injuries. Celebrex is a COX-2 inhibitor drug, a type of NSAID that blocks the COX-2 enzyme that produces prostaglandins that cause pain.	celecoxib (Celebrex), diclofenac (Cataflam, Voltaren), ibuprofen (Advil, Motrin), naproxen (Aleve, Naprosyn)	**nonsteroidal** (NON-stair-OY-dal)
			   non- *not*
			   steroid/o- *steroid*
			   -al *pertaining to*
			
			anti-inflammatory (AN-tee-in-FLAM-ah-TOR-ee)
			   anti- *against*
			   inflammat/o- *redness and warmth*
			   -ory *having the function of*

Abbreviations

AKA	above-the-knee amputation
AP	anteroposterior
BKA	below-the-knee amputation
BMD	bone mineral density
C1–C7	cervical vertebrae
Ca	calcium
CDH	congenital dislocation of the hip
DEXA, DXA	dual-energy x-ray absorptiometry
DIP	distal interphalangeal (joint)
DJD	degenerative joint disease
ESWT	extracorporeal shock wave therapy
Fx	fracture
L1–L5	lumbar vertebrae
LLE	left lower extremity
LUE	left upper extremity
MCP	metacarpophalangeal (joint)

NSAID	nonsteroidal anti-inflammatory drug
OA	osteoarthritis
ORIF	open reduction and internal fixation
ortho	orthopedics (slang)
P	phosphorus
PIP	proximal interphalangeal (joint)
PT	physical therapy or physical therapist
QCT	quantitative computerized tomography
RA	rheumatoid arthritis
RF	rheumatoid factor
RLE	right lower extremity
ROM	range of motion
RUE	right upper extremity
S1	first sacral vertebra
T1–T12	thoracic vertebrae
THR	total hip replacement
tib-fib	tibia-fibula (slang)

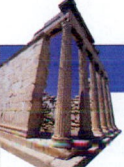

Word Alert

ABBREVIATIONS

Abbreviations are commonly used in all types of medical documents; however, they can mean different things to different people and their meanings can be misinterpreted. Always verify the meaning of an abbreviation.

AKA means *above-the-knee amputation*, but it also means the English phrase *also known as*.

Ca means *calcium*, but it also means *cancer*.

OA means *osteoarthritis*, but it also means *Overeaters Anonymous*.

P means *phosphorus*, but it also means *para* (the number of births a woman has had).

RA means *rheumatoid arthritis*, but it also means *right atrium* (of the heart) or *room air*.

It's Greek To Me!

Did you notice that some words have two different combining forms? Combining forms from both Greek and Latin languages remain a part of medical language today.

Word	Greek	Latin	Medical Word Examples
bone	oste/o-	osse/o-	osteoarthritis, osseous
bent, crooked, stiff	ankyl/o-	scoli/o-	ankylosing, scoliosis
cartilage	chondr/o-	cartilagin/o-	costochondral, cartilaginous
fibula	perone/o-	fibul/o-	peroneal, fibular
joint	arthr/o-	articul/o-	arthroscopy, articulation
vertebra	spondyl/o-	vertebr/o-	spondylolisthesis, vertebral

CAREER FOCUS

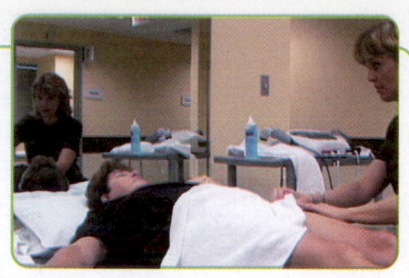

Meet Sara, a physical therapist in an outpatient physical therapy department

"I always knew I wanted to work in health care. My mom was a nurse. I became aware of other careers in health care, and physical therapy was one of them. It sounded interesting to me, and I enjoyed anatomy. We use a lot of medical terminology on the job, in our daily practice, and particularly in our documentation. That's the way we communicate with physicians, other healthcare providers, and our patients or clients."

Physical therapists are allied health professionals who develop treatment and rehabilitation plans based on a physician's order. However, in most states, physical therapists have the option to practice with or without a physician referral. Physical therapists use strengthening exercises and assistive devices (crutches, canes, wheelchairs, and so forth) to help patients improve and maintain maximum balance and mobility without surgery. They work in hospitals, outpatient clinics, rehabilitation centers, nursing homes, home health agencies, and sports and fitness facilities; many physical therapists have their own private practice. Most physical therapy programs award a doctoral degree.

   Orthopedists (or orthopaedists) are physicians who practice in the medical specialty of orthopedics. They diagnose and treat patients with skeletal and muscular problems. Orthopedists are physicians who have an M.D. (doctor of medicine) degree and have graduated from a school of medicine. When orthopedists perform surgery, they are known as orthopedic surgeons. **Rheumatologists** are physicians who specialize in treating inflammatory and degenerative diseases of the joints. Physicians can take additional training and become board certified in the subspecialty of pediatric orthopedics. Malignancies of the skeletomuscular system are treated medically by an oncologist or surgically by an orthopedic surgeon.

physical (FIZ-ih-kal)
   physic/o- *body*
   -al *pertaining to*

therapist (THAIR-ah-pist)
   therap/o- *treatment*
   -ist *one who specializes in*

orthopedist (OR-thoh-PEE-dist)
   orth/o- *straight*
   ped/o- *child*
   -ist *one who specializes in*

rheumatologist
(ROO-mah-TAWL-oh-jist)
   rheumat/o- *watery discharge*
   log/o- *word; the study of*
   -ist *one who specializes in*

CHAPTER REVIEW EXERCISES

Test your knowledge of the chapter by completing these review exercises. Use the Answer Key at the end of the book to check your answers.

Anatomy and Physiology

Matching Exercise

Match each word or phrase to its description.

1. acetabulum	_____	Cell that breaks down bone
2. calcaneus	_____	Cranial suture that names the plane that divides the body into anterior and posterior parts
3. carpal bones	_____	Cranial bone that forms the posterior base of the head
4. coronal	_____	Facial bone that moves up and down when you chew
5. diaphysis	_____	Pointed tip at the end of the sternum
6. humerus	_____	Opening where the spinal cord goes through the spinal column bones
7. ilium	_____	Contains the glenoid fossa area of the shoulder joint
8. ligaments	_____	Fibrous bands that connect bone to bone
9. mandible	_____	Bone of the upper arm
10. medial malleolus	_____	Lower arm bone that is on the same side as the thumb
11. occipital	_____	The bones of the wrist
12. osteoclast	_____	Another name for a finger
13. radius	_____	Part of the hip bone where the head of the femur rests
14. ray	_____	Bony projection on the distal tibial bone
15. scapula	_____	The heel bone
16. symphysis	_____	Slightly moveable joint that joins the two pubic bones
17. vertebral foramen	_____	Shaft of a long bone
18. xiphoid process	_____	One of the hip bones

Circle Exercise

Circle the correct word from the choices given.

1. The bone of the upper arm is the (**acetabulum, fibula, humerus**).
2. Replacing cartilage with hard bone is the process of (**articulation, costochondral, ossification**).
3. The hip bone that has a large crest on it is the (**ilium, intervertebral disk, ischium**).
4. Cells that maintain the minerals in the bones are (**osteoblasts, osteoclasts, osteocytes**).
5. The tarsal bones are in the (**ankle, elbow, hand**).
6. If you hit your "funny bone," you would have hit the nerve that runs across the (**glenoid fossa, lateral malleolus, medial epicondyle**).
7. The olecranon is located in the (**ankle, elbow, hip**).
8. (**Parietal, Periosteum, Peroneal**) is the adjective for *fibula*.
9. The (**clavicle, coccyx, cranium**) is another name for the collar bone.

True or False Exercise

Indicate whether each statement is true or false by writing T or F on the line.

1. _____ The parietal and temporal bones are in the cranium.
2. _____ The olecranon is a large, square bony projection off the ulna.
3. _____ The humorous is the name of the upper arm bone.
4. _____ The adjective form for *rib* is *costal.*
5. _____ The fibula is in the lower leg on the side of the little toe.
6. _____ The patella is a small bone that protects the knee joint.

Diseases and Conditions

True or False Exercise

Indicate whether each statement is true or false by writing T or F on the line.

1. _____ An arthroscope and a rongeur are surgical instruments.
2. _____ A sprain is the overstretching or tearing of a ligament.
3. _____ An osteoma is a malignant tumor of the bone.
4. _____ A Colles' fracture is often caused by a car accident.
5. _____ Osteoporosis can occur in both men and women.
6. _____ Scoliosis is an abnormal posterior curvature of the thoracic spine.
7. _____ Blood in the joint is known as hemarthrosis.
8. _____ Osteoarthritis is an autoimmune disease in which the body attacks its own cartilage.
9. _____ Pectus excavatum is another name for clubfoot.

Matching Exercise

Match each word or phrase to its description.

1. comminuted	_____ Wear and tear disease of the joints
2. osteomyelitis	_____ Screening is done for this deformity in schoolchildren
3. spondylolisthesis	_____ Pain in the joints
4. arthropathy	_____ Infection in the bone and bone marrow
5. compound	_____ Malignant tumor of the bone
6. osteoarthritis	_____ Fracture where the bone is crushed into several pieces
7. arthralgia	_____ Fracture where the bone breaks the overlying skin
8. scoliosis	_____ One vertebra slips anteriorly over another due to degeneration
9. osteosarcoma	_____ General word for disease of a joint

Circle Exercise

Circle the correct word from the choices given.

1. Infection in the bone and bone marrow is known as (**osteoarthritis, osteomyelitis, osteoporosis**).
2. An injury that disrupts the blood flow to a bone might cause (**ankylosing spondylitis, avascular necrosis, bone tumor**).
3. (**Demineralization, Levoscoliosis, Malalignment**) is seen in patients with osteoporosis.
4. Trauma or hemophilia can cause (**chondromalacia, hemarthrosis, scoliosis**).
5. A bony abnormality that affects the thorax is (**gout, lordosis, pectus excavatum**).

6. Spondylolisthesis involves slipping of the (**joints, sutures, vertebrae**).

7. A (**comminuted, hairline, transverse**) fracture is when the bone is crushed into several pieces.

Laboratory, Radiology, Surgery, and Drugs

Circle Exercise

Circle the correct word from the choices given.

1. The degree of joint movement is measured with a/an (**arthroscope, goniometer, osteotome**).

2. A patient with an amputated limb would be fitted with a (**brace, cast, prosthesis**).

3. A surgical procedure to fuse a degenerated, unstable joint is known as an (**allograft, arthrocentesis, arthrodesis**).

4. Gold compound drugs are used to treat (**fractures, osteoarthritis, rheumatoid arthritis**).

5. Rheumatoid factor can be identified by (**arthroscopy, a blood test, an x-ray**).

6. A DEXA scan is also known as (**bone densitometry, bone graft, uric acid**).

7. A radiologic procedure that uses contrast dye injected into a joint is (**arthrography, closed reduction, traction**).

8. An orthopedic device like a brace or splint is known as a/an (**cast, external fixation, orthosis**).

9. A transplant of bone from a cadaver is known as a/an (**allograft, arthroscopy, autograft**).

10. To diagnose rheumatoid arthritis, the physician would check the (**bone density, rheumatoid factor, uric acid**).

Building Medical Words

Review the Combining Forms Exercise and Combining Form and Suffix Exercise that you already completed in the anatomy section on pages 398–399.

Combining Forms Exercise

Before you build skeletal words, review these additional combining forms. Next to each combining form, write its medical meaning. The first one has been done for you.

Combining Form	Medical Meaning	Combining Form	Medical Meaning
1. alg/o-	pain	16. lev/o-	
2. alges/o-		17. locat/o-	
3. align/o-		18. lord/o-	
4. amputat/o-		19. malac/o-	
5. amput/o-		20. mineral/o-	
6. bunion/o-		21. myel/o-	
7. comminut/o-		22. orth/o-	
8. congenit/o-		23. path/o-	
9. dextr/o-		24. ped/o-	
10. disk/o-		25. physic/o-	
11. fract/o-		26. por/o-	
12. gener/o-		27. prosthet/o-	
13. goni/o-		28. sarc/o-	
14. hem/o-		29. scoli/o-	
15. kyph/o-		30. vascul/o-	

Related Combining Forms Exercise

Write the combining forms on the line provided. (Hint: See the It's Greek to Me feature box.)

1. Two combining forms that mean *bone*. _____

2. Two combining forms that mean *cartilage*. _____

3. Two combining forms that mean *joint*. _____

4. Two combining forms that mean *vertebra*. _____

5. Two combining forms that mean *fibula*. _____

Combining Form and Suffix Exercise

Read the definition of the medical word. Select the correct suffix from the Suffix List. Select the correct combining form from the Combining Form List. Build the medical word and write it on the line. Be sure to check your spelling. The first one has been done for you.

SUFFIX LIST	COMBINING FORM LIST	
-al (pertaining to)	amput/o- (to cut off)	goni/o- (angle)
-desis (procedure to fuse together)	arthr/o- (joint)	kyph/o- (bent; humpbacked)
-ectomy (surgical excision)	bunion/o- (bunion)	lord/o- (swayback)
-ed (pertaining to)	chondr/o- (cartilage)	oste/o- (bone)
-ee (person who is the object of an action)	comminut/o- (break into small pieces)	prosthet/o- (artificial part)
-ic (pertaining to)	congenit/o- (present at birth)	spondyl/o- (vertebra)
-itis (inflammation of; infection of)	densit/o- (density)	
-meter (instrument used to measure)		
-metry (process of measuring)		
-olisthesis (abnormal condition with slipping)		
-oma (tumor; mass)		
-osis (condition; abnormal condition; process)		
-pathy (disease; suffering)		
-scope (instrument used to examine)		

Definition of the Medical Word   **Build the Medical Word**

1. Disease of a joint   arthropathy _____

2. Tumor of the cartilage   _____

3. Abnormal condition of humpback (posterior curvature of the spine) _____

4. Inflammation of a joint   _____

5. Pertaining to (a condition that is) present at birth   _____

6. Process of measuring (the bone) density   _____

7. Tumor of the bone   _____

8. Pertaining to an artificial part (arm or leg)   _____

9. Instrument used to measure the angle (between two body parts)   _____

10. Surgical excision of a bunion   _____

11. Procedure to fuse together a joint   _____

12. Instrument used to examine a joint   _____

13. Person who is the object of an action (that is) to cut off (a body part)   _____

14. Pertaining to break into small pieces   _____

15. Abnormal condition with slipping (of one) vertebra (onto the next)   _____

16. Abnormal condition of swayback   _____

Prefix Exercise

Read the definition of the medical word. Look at the medical word or partial word that is given (it already contains a combining form and suffix.) Select the correct prefix from the Prefix List and write it on the blank line. Then build the medical word and write it on the line. Be sure to check your spelling. The first one has been done for you.

PREFIX LIST

a- (away from; without)
an- (without; not)

de- (reversal of; without)
dis- (away from)

intra- (within)
mal- (bad; inadequate)

Definition of the Medical Word	Prefix	Word or Partial Word	Build the Medical Word
1. Pertaining to without blood vessels (and blood to a bone)	a-	vascular	avascular
2. Process of making (the bone to be) without minerals	_____	mineralization	_____
3. Pertaining to within the joint	_____	articular	_____
4. Action of (moving a bone) away from (its normal) place	_____	location	_____
5. State of (a bone being in a) bad arrangement in a straight line	_____	alignment	_____
6. Pertaining to (being) without production (of bone)	_____	generative	_____
7. Pertaining to (a drug that makes you be) without pain	_____	algesic	_____

Multiple Combining Forms and Suffix Exercise

Read the definition of the medical word. Select the correct suffix and combining forms. Then build the medical word and write it on the line. Be sure to check your spelling. The first one has been done for you.

SUFFIX LIST

-ia (condition; state; thing)
-ics (knowledge; practice)
-itis (inflammation of; infection of)
-oma (tumor; mass)
-osis (condition; abnormal condition; process)

COMBINING FORM LIST

alg/o- (pain)
arthr/o- (joint)
chondr/o- (cartilage)
dextr/o- (right)
hem/o- (blood)
lev/o- (left)
malac/o- (softening)
myel/o- (bone marrow; spinal cord)

orth/o- (straight)
oste/o- (bone)
ped/o- (child)
por/o- (small openings; pores)
sarc/o- (connective tissue)
scoli/o- (curved; crooked)

Definition of the Medical Word

1. Abnormal condition of a left-(turning) curved (back).
2. Condition of cartilage softening
3. Abnormal condition of bone (having) small openings
4. The knowledge and practice (of producing) straight(ness of the bones and muscles in a) child (or other person)
5. Abnormal condition of blood in the joint
6. Abnormal condition of right-(turning) curved (back)
7. Condition of joint pain
8. Inflammation of the bone and bone marrow
9. Tumor of the bone and connective tissue

Build the Medical Word

1. levoscoliosis
2. _____
3. _____
4. _____
5. _____
6. _____
7. _____
8. _____
9. _____

Dividing Medical Words

Separate these words into their component parts (prefix, combining form, suffix). Note: Some words do not contain all three word parts. The first one has been done for you.

Medical Word	Prefix	Combining Form	Suffix	Medical Word	Prefix	Combining Form	Suffix
1. osteocyte	_____	_oste/o-_	_-cyte_	6. avascular	_____	_____	_____
2. intervertebral	_____	_____	_____	7. scoliosis	_____	_____	_____
3. metatarsal	_____	_____	_____	8. malalignment	_____	_____	_____
4. phalangeal	_____	_____	_____	9. arthrography	_____	_____	_____
5. densitometry	_____	_____	_____	10. demineralization	_____	_____	_____

Test Yourself

Three of these words are related in some way to each other. Define each word. Then circle the word that is not related.

1. osteoblast _____

2. osteoclast _____

3. osteocyte _____

4. osteophyte _____

Abbreviations

Matching Exercise

Match each abbreviation to its description.

1. NSAID   _____ Uses sound to break up bony spurs in the foot

2. RLE   _____ An autoimmune disease of the joints

3. ESWT   _____ Also known as osteoarthritis

4. ROM   _____ Right leg

5. DJD   _____ Joint between the metacarpal bone and the phalanx

6. RA   _____ Drug that treats inflammation

7. MCP   _____ Ability of a limb to move normally

Applied Skills

Plural Noun and Adjective Spelling Exercise

Read the noun and write the plural form and/or adjective form. Be sure to check your spelling. The first one has been done for you.

Singular Noun	Plural Noun	Adjective
1. cranium		cranial
2. mandible		
3. thorax		
4. rib		
5. vertebra		
6. phalanx		
7. ilium		
8. fibula		
9. patella		
10. scapula		

English and Medical Word Equivalents Exercise

For each English word, write its equivalent medical word. Be sure to check your spelling. The first one has been done for you.

English Word	Medical Word	English Word	Medical Word
1. top of the skull	cranium	12. thigh bone	
2. cheek bone		13. kneecap	
3. soft spot		14. shin bone	
4. upper jaw		15. heel bone	
5. lower jaw		16. hunchback	
6. shoulder blade		17. swayback	
7. breast bone		18. bowleg	
8. collar bone		19. knock-knee	
9. point of the elbow		20. clubfoot	
10. finger or toe		21. bone spur	
11. tail bone		22. great toe/big toe	

Medical Report Exercise

This exercise contains a physician's office chart note. Read the report and answer the questions.

CHART NOTE

PATIENT NAME: LOWE, James

RECORD NUMBER: 63-1004

DATE: November 19, 20xx

HISTORY
This is a 24-year-old male who has been having problems with intermittent low back pain for several years now. He leads an active lifestyle and his job requires him to do a lot of lifting and walking. The pain is getting worse, and he would like to get some definitive treatment at this time. He has been told in the past by a physician that his pelvis is tilted up on the left. However, he does not believe this was ever diagnosed as a leg-length discrepancy. He denies any radiation of the pain to his buttocks or legs and he says he has not noticed any tingling in his lower extremities.

PHYSICAL EXAMINATION
Left leg: The leg length from the iliac crest to the medial malleolus is 106 cm. Right leg: The leg length from the iliac crest to the medial malleolus is 103 cm. Examination of his back reveals diffuse tenderness over the spinous processes in the lumbar region. I also noticed a dextroscoliosis in the lower thoracic region, which seemed to be significant. Neurologically, the patient had normal reflexes and normal strength in the lower extremities.

ASSESSMENT
Chronic back pain due to a significant leg-length discrepancy. He also has a dextroscoliosis, although the exact number of degrees of the curvature was not measured.

PLAN
1. Refer to an orthopedist for a definitive diagnosis and measurement of the scoliosis.
2. Prescription for Motrin 600 mg tablet, 1 tablet 3 times a day.

Samantha P. Campbell, M.D.

Samantha P. Campbell, M.D.

SPC: lcc
D: 11/19/xx
T: 11/19/xx

Word Analysis Questions

1. Divide *dextroscoliosis* into its three word parts and define each word part.

   Word Part   **Definition**

   _____   _____

   _____   _____

   _____   _____

2. The adjective *spinal* refers to the spine or backbone while the adjective *spinous* refers to a bony process. **True**   **False**

3. Divide *orthopedist* into its three word parts and define each word part.

Word Part	Definition
_____	_____
_____	_____
_____	_____

Fact Finding Questions

1. The medial malleolus is located on the distal end of what bone? _____

2. Which leg was shorter, the patient's right leg or left leg? _____

3. The spinous processes are located on what bones? _____

4. What is the single-letter designation for the bones of the spine in the lumbar region? _____

Critical Thinking Questions

1. Which way did the patient's spine curve? To the right or to the left?

   _____

2. What category of drugs does Motrin belong to? What drug action does it have?

   _____

3. What will the orthopedist measure that this physician did not measure during the office visit?

   _____

On the Job Challenge Exercise

On the job, you will often have to talk with patients and explain medical words to them. Give the meanings of these sound-alike phrases.

1. closed fracture _____

2. closed reduction of a fracture _____

3. open fracture _____

4. open reduction and internal fixation of a fracture _____

Hearing Medical Words Exercise

You hear someone speaking the medical words given below. Read each pronunciation and then write the medical word it represents. Be sure to check your spelling. The first one has been done for you.

1. ar-THRY-tis   arthritis_____   6. MUS-kyoo-loh-SKEL-eh-tal   _____

2. ar-THRAWG-rah-fee   _____   7. OR-thoh-PEE-dist   _____

3. con-DROH-mah   _____   8. AWS-tee-oh-poh-ROH-sis   _____

4. COM-ih-nyoo-ted FRAK-chur _____   9. FAY-langks   _____

5. DEKS-troh-SKOH-lee-OH-sis _____   10. praws-THEE-sis   _____

Pronunciation Exercise

Read the medical word that is given. Then review the syllables in the pronunciation. Circle the primary (main) accented syllable. The first one has been done for you.

1. amputation (am-pyoo-(tay)-shun)
2. arthralgia (ar-thral-jee-ah)
3. arthroscopy (ar-thraws-koh-pee)
4. cartilaginous (kar-tih-laj-ih-nus)
5. hemarthrosis (hee-mar-throh-sis)
6. humeral (hyoo-mer-al)
7. kyphosis (ky-foh-sis)
8. mandibular (man-dib-yoo-lar)
9. metacarpal (met-ah-kar-pal)
10. osteoarthritis (aws-tee-oh-ar-thry-tis)

Multimedia Preview

Immerse yourself in a variety of activities inside Medical Terminology Interactive. Getting there is simple:

1. Click on www.myhealthprofessionskit.com.
2. Select "Medical Terminology" from the choice of disciplines.
3. First-time users must create an account using the scratch-off code on the inside front cover of this book.
4. Find this book and log in using your username and password.
5. Click on Medical Terminology Interactive.
6. Take the elevator to the 8th Floor to begin your virtual exploration of this chapter!

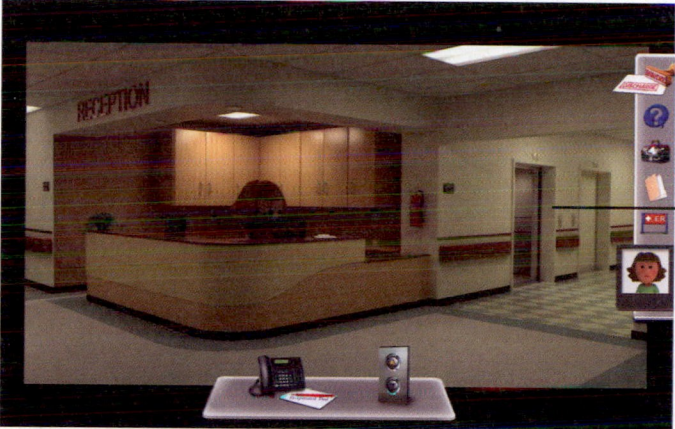 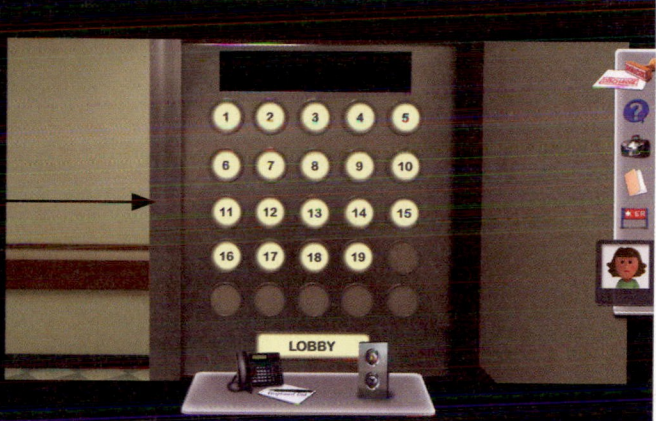

■ **Show and Spell**   We're all mixed up, but maybe you can help. Unscramble the letters to form a word that matches the definition provided. When you finish, you'll be dizzy with delight.

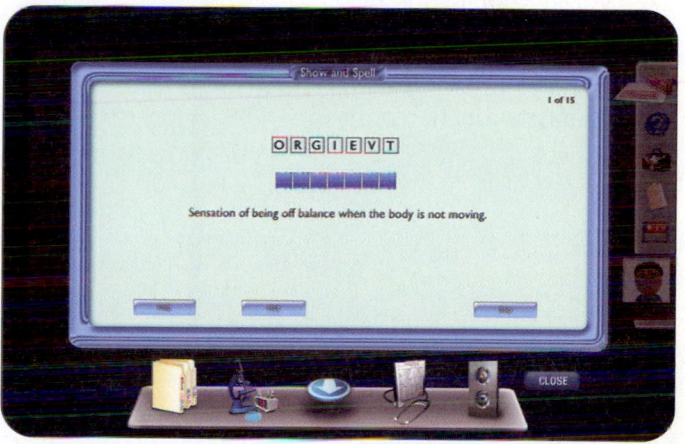

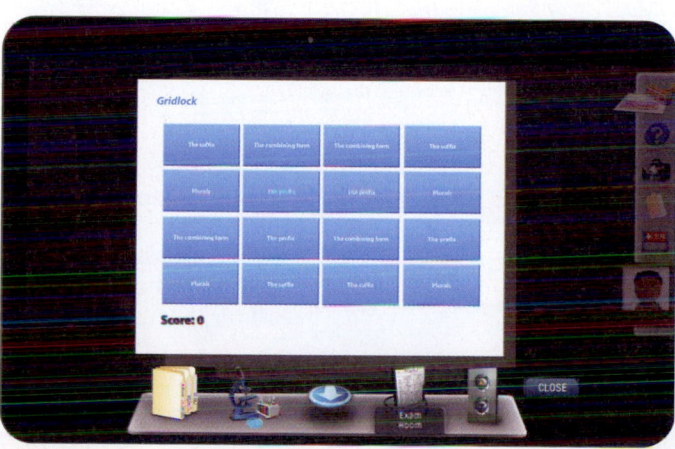

■ **Gridlock**   Are you a Jeopardy! champ? Prove your quiz show smarts by clicking here to answer the medical terminology questions hidden beneath the tiles. Get them all right to clear the grid.

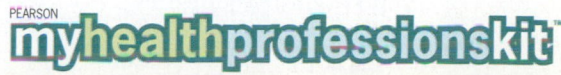

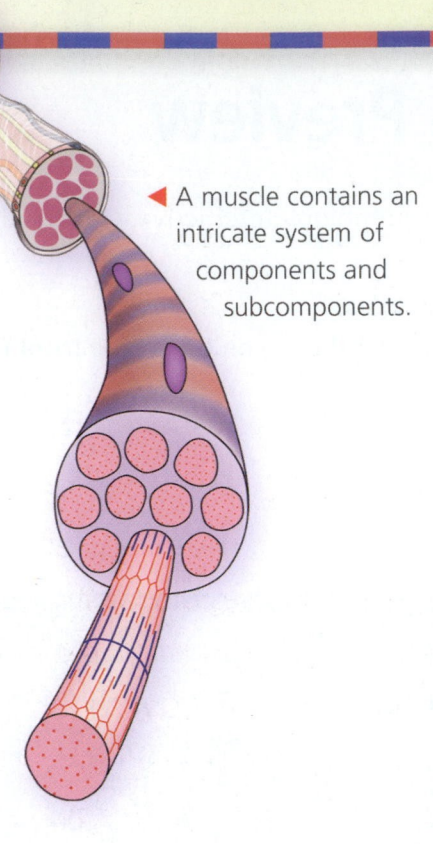

◄ A muscle contains an intricate system of components and subcomponents.

Dive In!

- Smiling uses fewer muscles than frowning.
- The human body has fewer muscles in it than a caterpillar has.
- You sit on your largest muscle, the gluteus maximus.
- Ready to stretch and exercise your mind more? In this chapter we'll explore the language that describes muscular system structures, functions, diseases, and conditions.
- You'll be ready to flex your wits once you master the language of the muscular system!

▶ The combination of movement, strength, and coordination represents muscle function at its best.

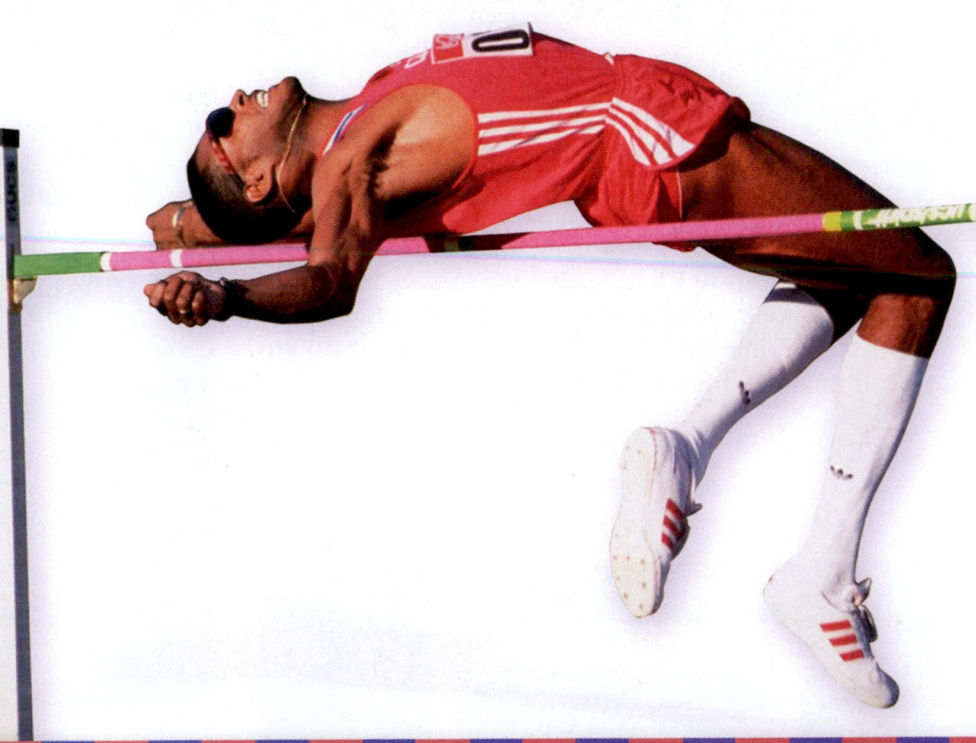

Medicine Through HISTORY

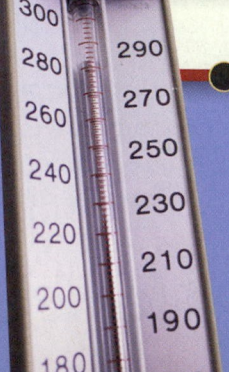

1896

The sphygmomanometer, a device for measuring the blood pressure, is invented by S. Riva-Rocci, an Italian physician

1900

Dr. Walter Reed discovers that mosquitos transmit yellow fever

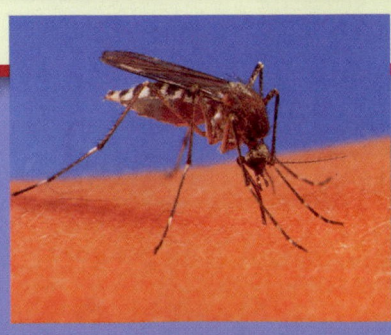

9

Orthopedics

Muscular System

Orthopedics (OR-thoh-PEE-diks) is the medical specialty that studies the anatomy and physiology of the muscular and skeletal systems and uses diagnostic tests, medical and surgical procedures, and drugs to treat muscular and skeletal diseases. In Chapter 8, you studied orthopedics from the perspective of the skeletal system. In this chapter, you will study the muscular system.

◄ The muscular system is the engine that moves the bony framework of the body.

► Like yarn, muscles are composed of fibers made up of even thinner strands wrapped around each other.

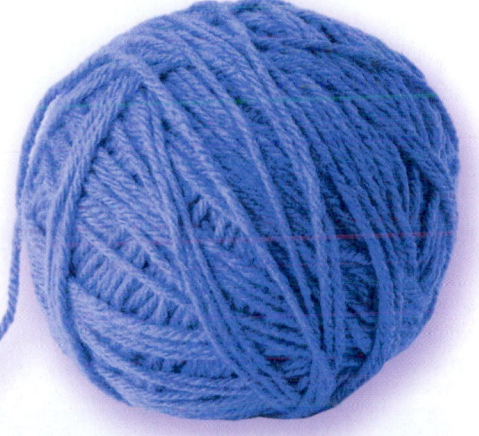

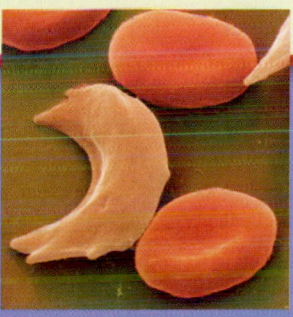

1904

"An apple a day keeps the doctor away." First uttered by J.T. Stinson while addressing the St. Louis Exposition, it becomes a well-known expression

1904

The sickle cells of sickle cell anemia are first seen under the microscope

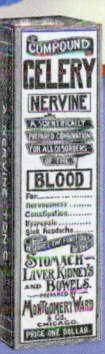

1906

The Pure Food and Drug Act is the first federal drug law. It prohibits mislabeling of the ingredients in drugs

Measure Your Progress: Learning Objectives

After you study this chapter, you should be able to

1. Identify the structures of the muscular system.

2. Describe how muscles contract and produce movement.

3. Describe common muscular diseases and conditions, laboratory and diagnostic procedures, medical and surgical procedures, and drug categories.

4. Give the medical meaning of word parts related to the muscular system.

5. Build muscular words from word parts and divide and define muscular words.

6. Spell and pronounce muscular words.

7. Analyze the medical content and meaning of an orthopedic report.

8. Dive deeper into orthopedics (muscular) by reviewing the activities at the end of this chapter and online at Medical Terminology Interactive.

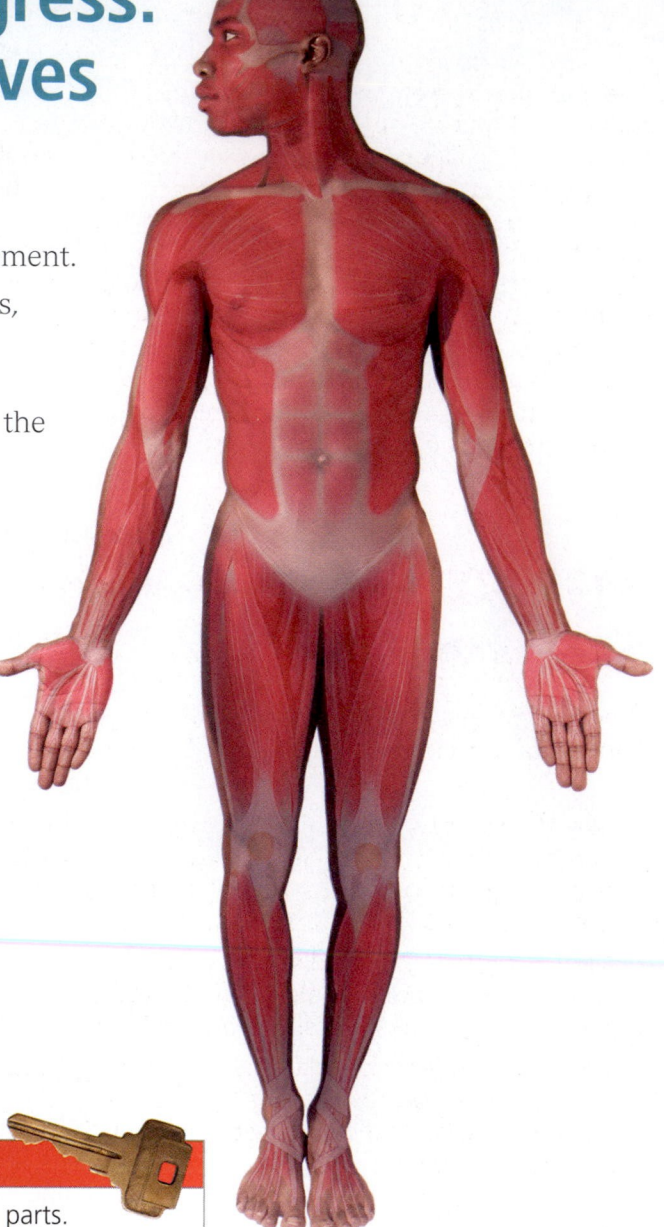

Figure 9-1 ■ **Muscular system.**
The muscular system is a widespread body system that consists of the voluntary skeletal muscles and other structures throughout the body.

Medical Language Key

To unlock the definition of a medical word, break it into word parts. Define each word part. Put the word part meanings in order, beginning with the suffix, then the prefix (if present), then the combining form(s).

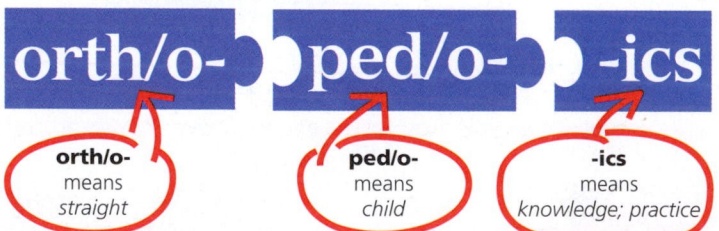

orth/o- means *straight*

ped/o- means *child*

-ics means *knowledge; practice*

	Word Part	Word Part Meaning
Suffix	-ics	*knowledge; practice*
Combining Form	orth/o-	*straight*
Combining Form	ped/o-	*child*

Orthopedics: *The knowledge and practice (of producing) straight(ness of the bones and muscles in a) child (or other person).*

Anatomy and Physiology

The **muscular system** is the engine that moves the bony framework of the body (see Figure 9-1 ■). There are approximately 700 skeletal muscles in the body, as well as tendons and other structures of the muscular system. The contours of some skeletal muscles are visible under the skin; their size and movement are particularly visible when they contract. Others are located more deeply, and their movements are not visible, although they may be felt. The purpose of the muscular system is to produce body movement. All of the muscles of the body (or the muscles in a particular part of the body) are referred to as the **musculature**. The muscular system is also known as the **musculoskeletal system** because of the close relationship between the muscles and the bones. Without the muscles, the bones would not be able to move and, without the bones, the muscles would lack support.

Anatomy of the Muscular System

Types of Muscles

There are three types of muscles: skeletal muscles, the cardiac muscle, and smooth muscles (see Figure 9-2 ■).

- **Skeletal muscles:** Skeletal muscles provide the means by which the body can move. Skeletal muscles are **voluntary muscles** that contract and relax in response to conscious thought. They are **striated** and show bands of color when seen under a microscope.
- **Cardiac muscle:** The cardiac muscle of the heart pumps blood through the circulatory system. It is an involuntary muscle that is not under conscious control. The heart was discussed in "Cardiology," Chapter 5.
- **Smooth muscles:** Smooth muscles are involuntary, nonstriated muscles. They form a continuous, thin layer around many organs and structures (blood vessels, bronchi, intestines, etc.). Smooth muscles are discussed in various chapters.

WORD BUILDING

muscle (MUS-el)

muscular (MUS-kyoo-lar)
  muscul/o- *muscle*
  -ar *pertaining to*
The combining forms *my/o-* and *myos/o-* also mean *muscle*.

musculature (MUS-kyoo-LAH-chur)
  muscul/o- *muscle*
  -ature *system composed of*

musculoskeletal
(MUS-kyoo-loh-SKEL-eh-tal)
  muscul/o- *muscle*
  skelet/o- *skeleton*
  -al *pertaining to*

voluntary (VAWL-un-TAIR-ee)
  volunt/o- *done of one's own free will*
  -ary *pertaining to*

striated (STRY-aa-ted)

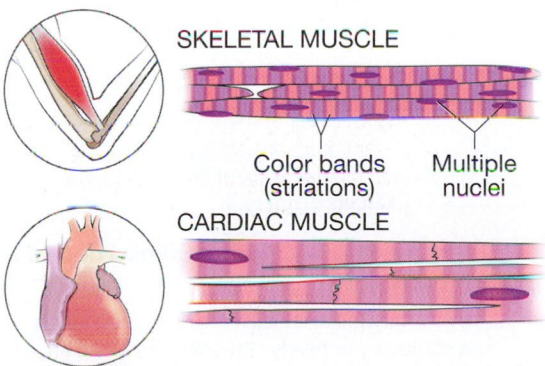

SKELETAL MUSCLE

Color bands (striations)   Multiple nuclei

CARDIAC MUSCLE

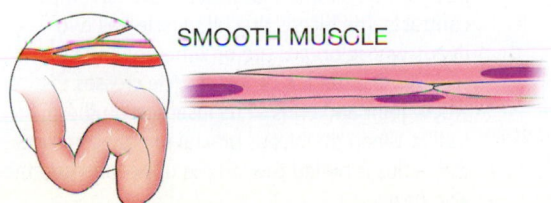

SMOOTH MUSCLE

Figure 9-2 ■ Types of muscle.
There are three types of muscles—skeletal muscles, the cardiac muscle, and smooth muscles. Each has a different appearance under a microscope. Note the very pronounced color bands (striations) and multiple nuclei in each skeletal muscle cell. Cardiac muscle cells have less pronounced bands, and nonstriated smooth muscle cells have no bands.

Of the three types of muscles, only skeletal muscle belongs to the muscular system. In the rest of this chapter, the word *muscle* should be understood to mean *skeletal muscle*.

Muscle Origins, Insertions, and Related Structures

A muscle is attached to a bone by a **tendon,** a cordlike, nonelastic, white fibrous band of connective tissue (see Figure 9-3 ■). The **origin** or beginning of a muscle is where its tendon is attached to a stationary or nearly stationary bone (see Figure 9-4 ■). The **insertion** or ending of a muscle is where its tendon is attached to the bone that moves when the muscle contracts and relaxes. The **belly** of a muscle is where its mass is the greatest, usually midway between the origin and insertion. From its attachment to a bone, the tendon and its muscle often travel across a joint; this is the joint that will move when the muscle contracts.

A **bursa,** a thin sac of synovial membrane filled with synovial fluid, acts as a cushion to reduce friction where a tendon rubs against the bone in a

WORD BUILDING

tendon (TEN-dun)
  tendin/o- *tendon*
  -ous *pertaining to*
The combining forms *tendon/o-* and *ten/o-* also mean *tendon.*

origin (OR-ih-jin)

insertion (in-SER-shun)
  insert/o- *to put in; introduce*
  -ion *action; condition*

bursa (BER-sah)

bursae (BER-see)
Bursa is a Latin singular noun. Form the plural by changing *-a* to *-ae.*

bursal (BER-sal)
  burs/o- *bursa*
  -al *pertaining to*

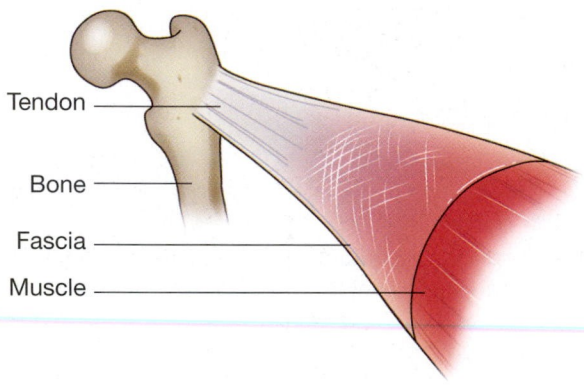

Tendon
Bone
Fascia
Muscle

Figure 9-3 ■ Tendon.
At their origins and insertions, most muscles are attached to the bone by a tendon. As the muscle transitions to the tendon, the red color of the muscle is replaced by the white color of the tendon. The fascia that envelops the muscle also merges with the tendon.

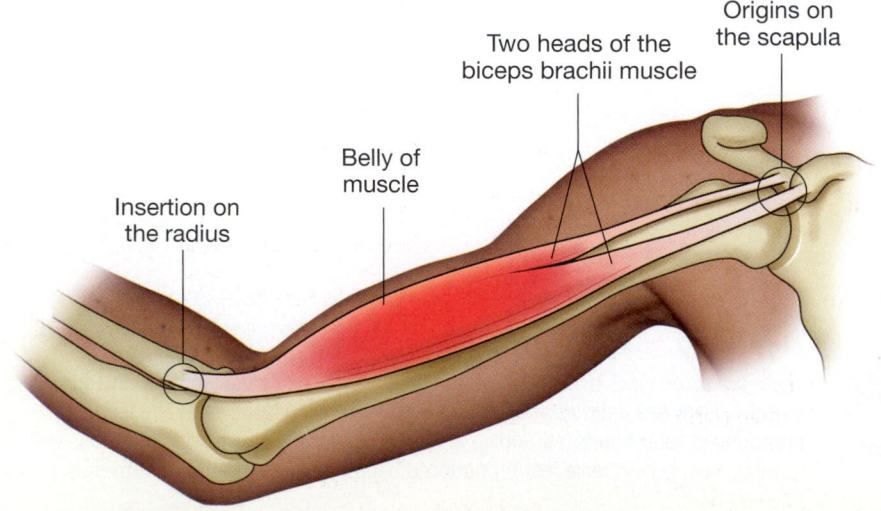

Origins on the scapula

Two heads of the biceps brachii muscle

Belly of muscle

Insertion on the radius

Figure 9-4 ■ Origin and insertion of a muscle.

Every muscle has at least one point of origin on a stationary or nearly stationary bone and an insertion on a bone that moves when the muscle contracts. The biceps brachii muscle has two heads whose origins are on different parts of the scapula. The tendon of this muscle crosses the elbow joint and ends at its insertion on the radius. When the biceps brachii muscle contracts, the radius is pulled toward the upper arm and the arm flexes.

joint. Each muscle is wrapped in **fascia,** a thin connective tissue that joins with the tendon (see Figure 9-3). An **aponeurosis** is a flat, wide, white fibrous sheet of connective tissue, sometimes composed of several tendons, that attaches a flat muscle to a bone or to other, deeper muscles (see Figures 9-9, 9-11, and 9-14). A **retinaculum** is a nearly translucent band of fibrous tissue and fascia that holds down the tendons that cross the wrist and ankle (see Figures 9-12, 9-13, and 9-15).

Muscle Names

Muscle names can seem complex because they are in Latin, but you will recognize some of the Latin words because they relate to the bones you studied in Chapter 8. Other Latin words become familiar because they consistently describe where the muscle is located, its shape, its size, or what action it performs (see Table 9-1).

WORD BUILDING

fascia (FASH-ee-ah)

fascial (FASH-ee-al)
  fasci/o- *fascia*
  -al *pertaining to*

aponeurosis (AP-oh-nyoo-ROH-sis)

retinaculum (RET-ih-NAK-yoo-lum)

Table 9-1   Muscle Names and Their Meanings

Muscle Name	What the Muscle Name Tells You	Word Building

biceps brachii	Shape: One end divides into two parts or heads (*biceps*)
	Location: Arm (*brachii*)
		biceps (BY-seps)
		  bi- *two*
		  -ceps *head*
		brachii (BRAY-kee-eye)

brachioradialis	Location: Radial bone (*radi/o-*) in the arm (*brachi/o-*)	**brachioradialis** (BRAY-kee-oh-RAY-dee-AL-is)
		  brachi/o- *arm*
		  radi/o- *radius (forearm bone); x-rays; radiation*
		  -alis *pertaining to*

extensor digitorum	Action: Extends
	Location: Digits (*digitorum*)
		extensor (eks-TEN-sor)
		  extens/o- *straightening*
		  -or *person or thing that produces or does*
		digitorum (DIJ-ih-TOR-um)

flexor hallucis brevis	Action: Flexes
	Location: Big toe (*hallux*)
	Size: Short (*brevis*)
		flexor (FLEK-sor)
		  flex/o- *bending*
		  -or *person or thing that produces or does*
		hallucis (HAL-yoo-sis)
		brevis (BREV-is)

gluteus maximus	Location: Buttocks (*gluteus*) Size: Large (*maximus*)	**gluteus** (gloo-TEE-us) **maximus** (MAK-sih-mus)
rectus abdominis	Orientation: Straight up and down (*rectus*) Location: Abdomen (*abdominis*)	**rectus** (REK-tus) **abdominis** (ab-DAWM-ih-nis)

temporalis	Location: Temporal bone (*temporalis*) of the cranium	**temporalis** (TEM-poh-RAY-lis)
		  tempor/o- *temple (side of the head)*
		  -alis *pertaining to*

triceps brachii	Shape: One end divides into three parts or heads (*triceps*)
	Location: Arm (*brachii*)
		triceps (TRY-seps)
		  tri- *three*
		  -ceps *head*

Types of Muscle Movement

Muscles function in antagonistic pairs to produce movement. When the first muscle contracts, the second muscle relaxes to allow the movement or it partially contracts to control the movement. Flexion and extension, abduction and adduction, rotation to the right and to the left, supination and pronation, and eversion and inversion are opposite movements that are controlled by muscle pairs (see Figures 9-5 ■ through 9-8 ■ and Table 9-2).

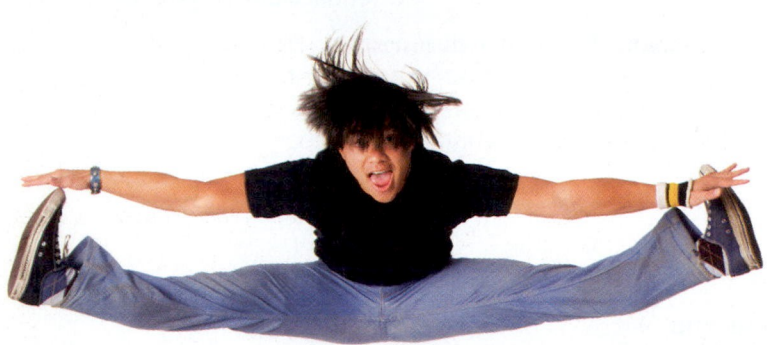

Figure 9-5 ■ Extension, abduction, and dorsiflexion.
This dancer has his arms and legs extended and abducted. His feet are in dorsiflexion.

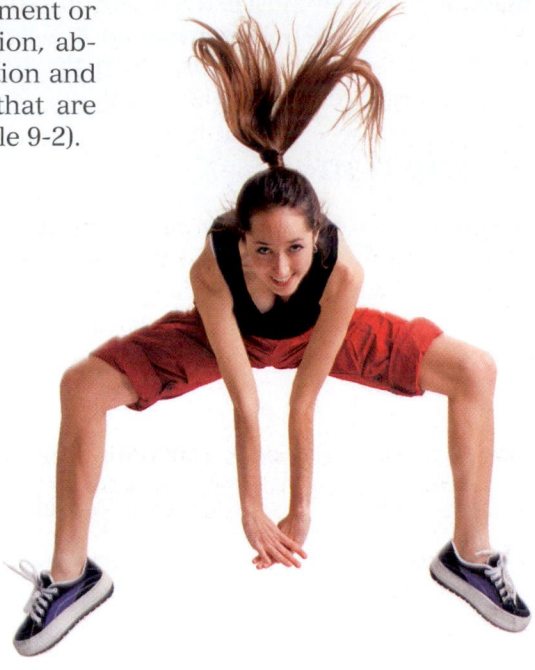

Figure 9-6 ■ Extension, adduction, pronation, abduction, flexion, and plantar flexion.
This dancer has her arms extended and adducted, with her hands in pronation. Her thighs are abducted, and her knees flexed. Her feet are in plantar flexion.

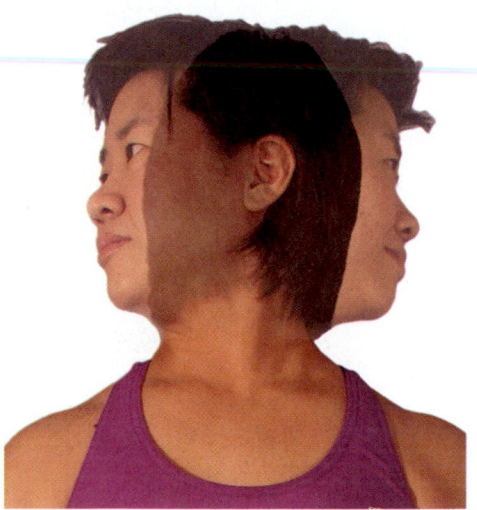

Figure 9-7 ■ Rotation.
The head rotates to the right and left around its axis, which is the vertebral column.

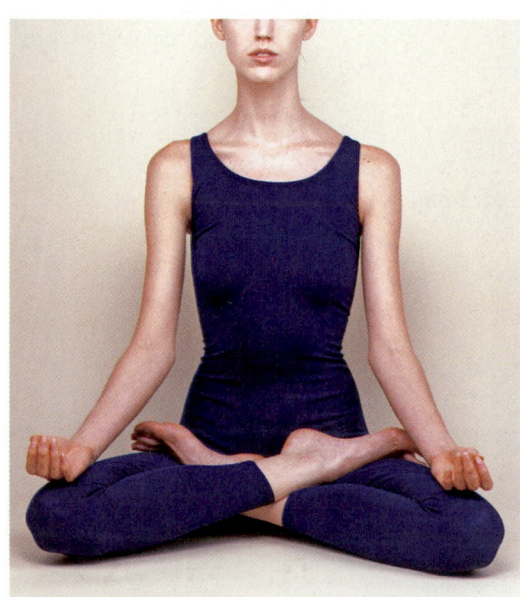

Figure 9-8 ■ Extension, supination, abduction, flexion, and inversion.
This person is in a yoga position with her arms extended, her hands in supination, her thighs abducted, and her knees flexed. Her feet are in inversion.

Table 9-2   Types of Muscle Movement

Movement	Description	Muscle Type	Word Building

flexion	Bending a joint to decrease the angle between two bones or two body parts. (*Note:* Plantar flexion of the foot causes the toes to point downward. Dorsiflexion of the foot causes the toes to point upward.)	**flexor**	**flexion** (FLEK-shun)
			  flex/o- *bending*
			  -ion *action; condition*
			flexor (FLEK-sor)
			  flex/o- *bending*
			  -or *person or thing that produces or does*

extension	Straightening and extending a joint to increase the angle between two bones or two body parts	**extensor**	**extension** (eks-TEN-shun)
			  extens/o- *straightening*
			  -ion *action; condition*
			extensor (eks-TEN-sor)
			  extens/o- *straightening*
			  -or *person or thing that produces or does*

abduction	Moving a body part away from the midline of the body	**abductor**	**abduction** (ab-DUK-shun)
			  ab- *away from*
			  duct/o- *bring; move; a duct*
			  -ion *action; condition*
			abductor (ab-DUK-tor)
			  ab- *away from*
			  duct/o- *bring; move; a duct*
			  -or *person or thing that produces or does*

adduction	Moving a body part toward the midline of the body	**adductor**	**adduction** (ad-DUK-shun)
			  ad- *toward*
			  duct/o- *bring; move; a duct*
			  -ion *action; condition*
			adductor (ad-DUK-tor)
			  ad- *toward*
			  duct/o- *bring; move; a duct*
			  -or *person or thing that produces or does*

rotation	Moving a body part around its axis	**rotator**	**rotation** (roh-TAY-shun)
			  rotat/o- *rotate*
			  -ion *action; condition*
			rotator (ROH-tay-tor)
			  rotat/o- *rotate*
			  -or *person or thing that produces or does*

supination	Turning the palm of the hand anteriorly or upward. (*Note:* Here, *lying on the back* refers to the back of the hand.)	**supinator**	**supination** (soo-pih-NAY-shun)
			  supinat/o- *lying on the back*
			  -ion *action; condition*
			supinator (SOO-pih-NAY-tor)
			  supinat/o- *lying on the back*
			  -or *person or thing that produces or does*

pronation	Turning the palm of the hand posteriorly or downward. (*Note:* Here, *face down* refers to the face of the palm.)	**pronator**	**pronation** (proh-NAY-shun)
			  pronat/o- *face down*
			  -ion *action; condition*
			pronator (proh-NAY-tor)
			  pronat/o- *face down*
			  -or *person or thing that produces or does*

(continued)

Table 9-2 Types of Muscle Movement *(continued)*

Movement	Description	Muscle Type	Word Building

eversion	Turning a body part outward and toward the side	evertor	**eversion** (ee-VER-zhun)
			  e- *without; out*
			  vers/o- *to travel; to turn*
			  -ion *action; condition*
			
			evertor (ee-VER-tor)
			  e- *without; out*
			  vert/o- *to travel; to turn*
			  -or *person or thing that produces or does*

inversion	Turning a body part inward	invertor	**inversion** (in-VER-zhun)
			  in- *in; within; not*
			  vers/o- *to travel; to turn*
			  -ion *action; condition*
			
			invertor (in-VER-tor)
			  in- *in; within; not*
			  vert/o- *to travel; to turn*
			  -or *person or thing that produces or does*

Muscles of the Head and Neck

The most important muscles of the head and neck are described in this section (see Figure 9-9 ■).

- **Frontalis:** Moves the forehead to raise the eyebrows or wrinkle the skin
- **Temporalis:** Moves the mandible (lower jaw) upward and backward
- **Orbicularis oculi:** Closes the eyelids or presses them together
- **Orbicularis oris:** Closes the lips or presses them together
- **Masseter:** Moves the mandible (lower jaw) upward
- **Buccinator:** Moves the cheeks
- **Sternocleidomastoid:** Bends the head toward the sternum (flexion) and turns the head to either side (rotation)
- **Platysma:** Moves the mandible (lower jaw bone) down

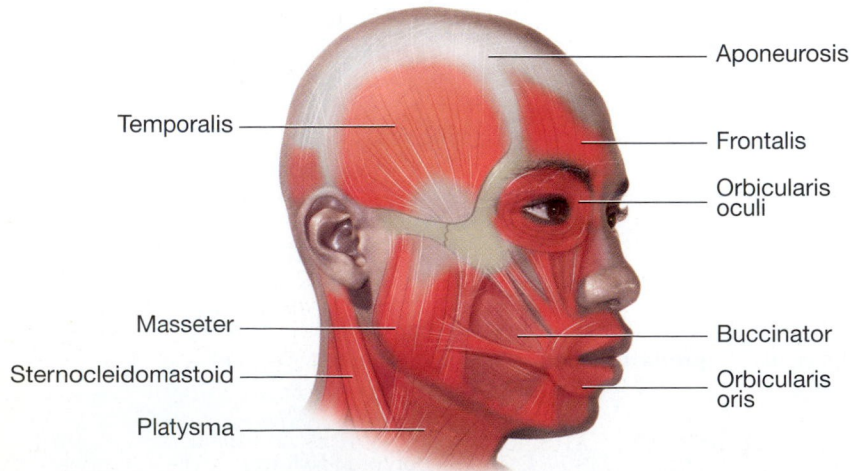

Figure 9-9 ■ Muscles of the head and neck.
These muscles contract and relax when you close your eyes, make facial expressions, chew food, etc.

WORD BUILDING

frontalis (frun-TAY-lis)
  front/o- *front*
  -alis *pertaining to*

temporalis (TEM-poh-RAY-lis)
  tempor/o- *temple (side of the head)*
  -alis *pertaining to*

orbicularis (or-BIK-yoo-LAIR-is)
  orbicul/o- *small circle*
  -aris *pertaining to*

oculi (AWK-yoo-lie)

oris (OR-is)

masseter (MAS-eh-ter)
  masset/o- *chewing*
  -er *person or thing that produces or does*

buccinator (BUK-sih-NAY-tor)
  buccinat/o- *cheek*
  -or *person or thing that produces or does*

sternocleidomastoid
(STER-noh-KLY-doh-MAS-toyd)
  stern/o- *sternum (breast bone)*
  cleid/o- *clavicle (collar bone)*
  mast/o- *breast; mastoid process*
  -oid *resembling*

platysma (plah-TIZ-mah)

Muscles of the Shoulders, Chest, and Back

The most important muscles of the shoulders, chest, and back are described in this section (see Figures 9-10 ■ and 9-11 ■).

- **Deltoid:** Raises the arm and moves the arm away from the body (abduction)
- **Pectoralis major:** Moves the arm anteriorly and medially across the chest (adduction)
- **Intercostal muscles:** Muscle pairs between the ribs; one contracts during inspiration to spread the ribs apart; the other contracts during forced expiration, coughing, or sneezing to pull the ribs together.
- **Trapezius:** Raises the shoulder, pulls the shoulder blades together, elevates the clavicle. Turns the head from side to side (rotation). Moves the head posteriorly (extension).
- **Latissimus dorsi:** Moves the arm posteriorly and medially toward the spinal column (adduction)

WORD BUILDING

deltoid (DEL-toyd)
  delt/o- *triangle*
  -oid *resembling*
In the Greek alphabet, the capital letter *delta* is in the shape of a triangle.

pectoralis (PEK-toh-RAY-lis)
  pector/o- *chest*
  -alis *pertaining to*

intercostal (IN-ter-KAWS-tal)
  inter- *between*
  cost/o- *rib*
  -al *pertaining to*

trapezius (trah-PEE-zee-us)
This muscle resembles a trapezoid, a geometric figure that has two parallel sides and two nonparallel sides.

latissimus (lah-TIS-ih-mus)

dorsi (DOR-sigh)

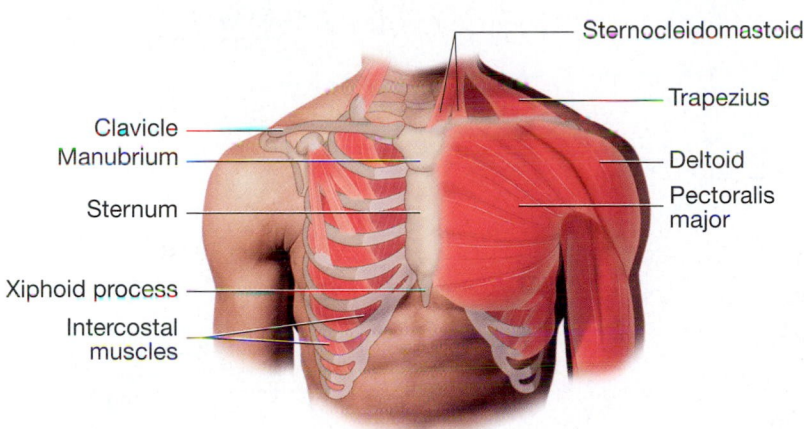

Figure 9-10 ■ **Muscles of the shoulders and chest.**
These muscles contract and relax when you raise your arms, move your arms and shoulders toward the midline to hug someone you love, or rotate your arms inwardly.

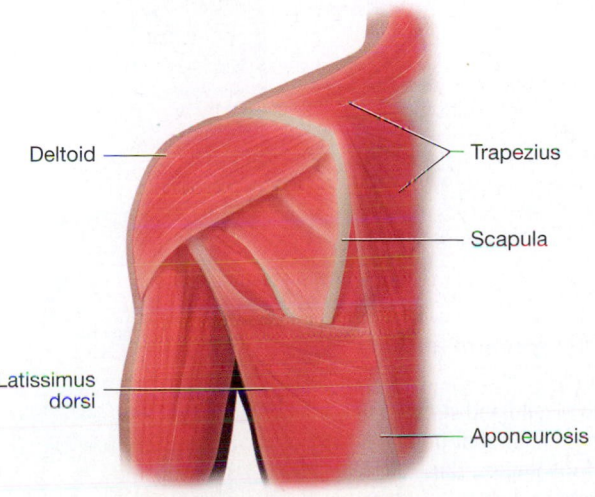

Figure 9-11 ■ **Muscles of the shoulder and back.**
These muscles contract and relax when you shrug your shoulders or pull your shoulder blades together to sit up straight. They also pull your head backward and to the side, and turn your trunk to the right or left.

Muscles of the Upper Extremity

The most important muscles of the arm and hand are described in this section (see Figures 9-12 ■ and 9-13 ■).

- **Biceps brachii:** Bends the upper arm toward the shoulder (flexion) and bends the lower arm toward the upper arm (flexion).
- **Triceps brachii:** Straightens the lower arm (extension)
- **Brachioradialis:** Bends the lower arm toward the upper arm (flexion)
- **Thenar muscles:** Bend the thumb (flexion) and move it toward the palm (adduction)

Biceps brachii

Brachioradialis

Flexor muscles of the fingers

Flexor retinaculum

Thenar muscles

Triceps brachii

Extensor muscles of the fingers

Extensor retinaculum

ANTERIOR VIEW

POSTERIOR VIEW

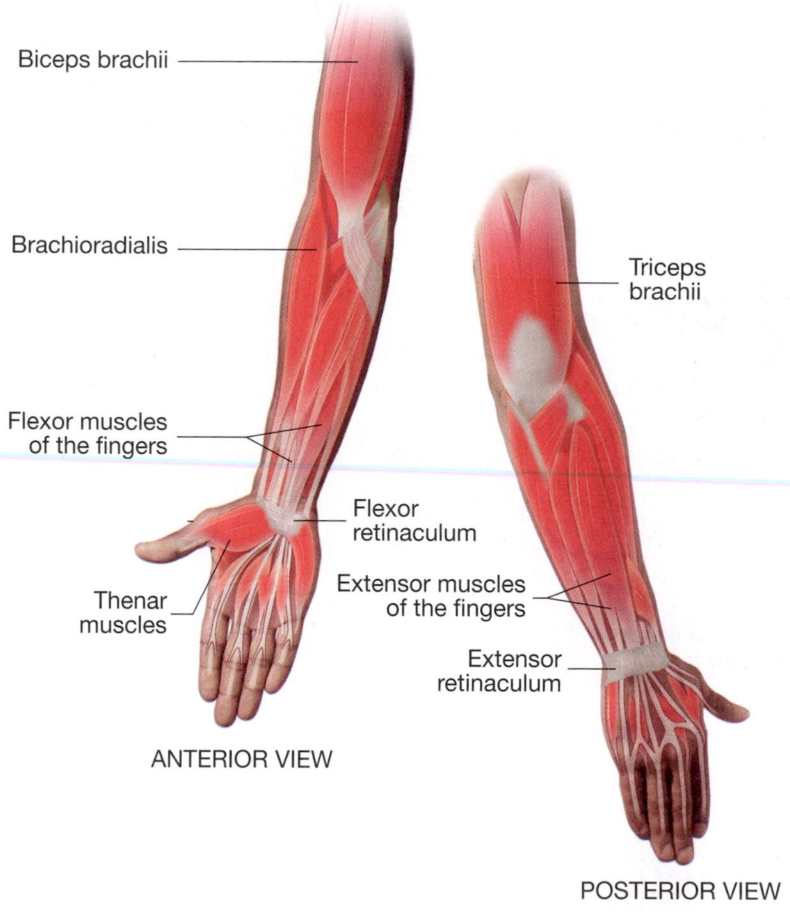

Figure 9-12 ■ Muscles of the upper extremity.
These muscles contract and relax when you lift a heavy box, straighten your arms to do a handstand, shake hands, make a fist, or play the piano.

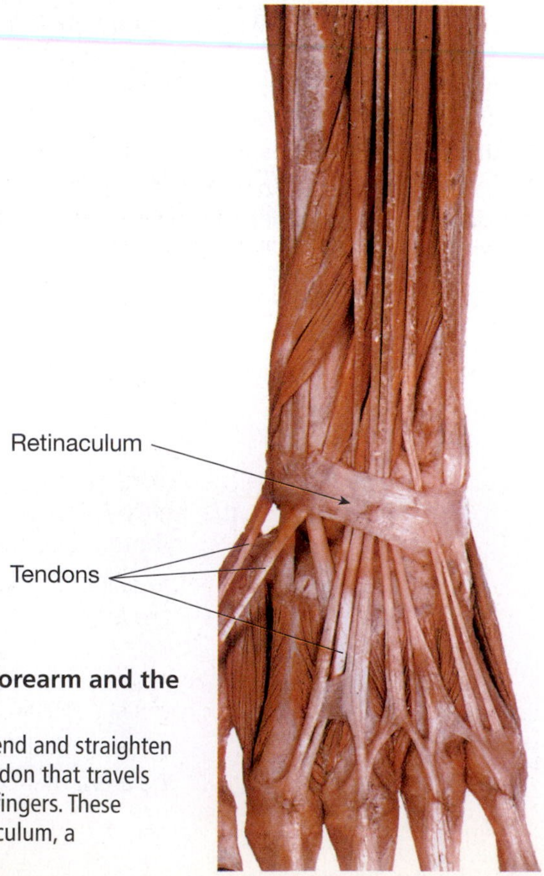

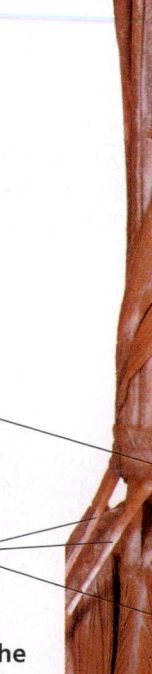

Retinaculum

Tendons

Figure 9-13 ■ Muscles of the forearm and the retinaculum.
Muscles in the forearm contract to extend and straighten the fingers. Each muscle has a long tendon that travels across the wrist to one or more of the fingers. These tendons are held in place by the retinaculum, a translucent, horizontal band of tissue.

Muscles of the Abdomen

The most important muscles of the abdomen are described in this section (see Figure 9-14 ■).

- **External abdominal oblique:** Bends the upper body forward (flexion), rotates the side of the body medially, and compresses the side of the abdominal wall
- **Internal abdominal oblique:** Bends the upper body forward (flexion), rotates the side of the body medially, and compresses the side of the abdominal wall
- **Rectus abdominis:** Bends the upper body forward (flexion) and compresses the anterior abdominal wall

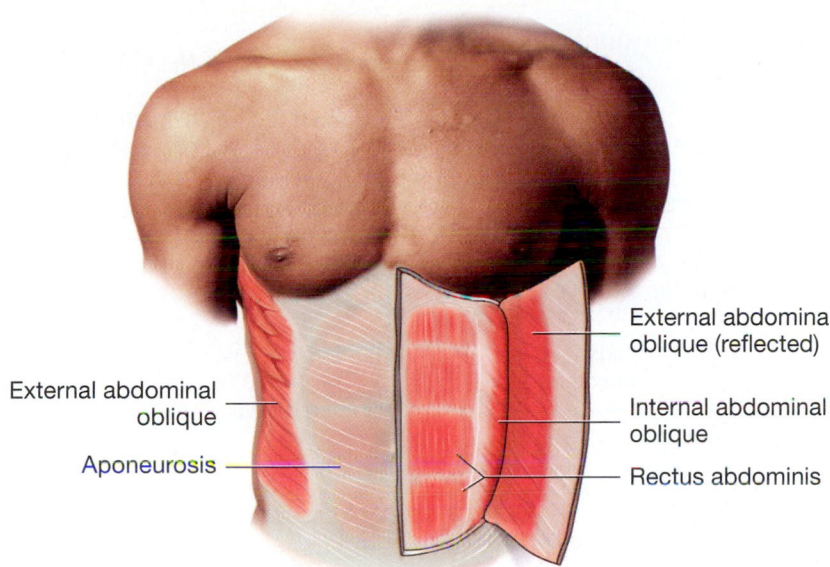

External abdominal oblique

Aponeurosis

External abdominal oblique (reflected)

Internal abdominal oblique

Rectus abdominis

Figure 9-14 ■ Muscles of the abdomen.

These muscles contract and relax when you rotate the trunk of your body from side to side, flatten your abdomen, bend forward, or do a sit-up.

WORD BUILDING

external (eks-TER-nal)
  extern/o- *outside*
  -al *pertaining to*

abdominal (ab-DAWM-ih-nal)
  abdomin/o- *abdomen*
  -al *pertaining to*

oblique (awb-LEEK)

internal (in-TER-nal)
  intern/o- *inside*
  -al *pertaining to*

rectus (REK-tus)

abdominis (ab-DAWM-ih-nis)

Word Alert

SOUND-ALIKE WORDS

rectus	(noun)	Latin word meaning *straight*. The segments of the rectus abdominis muscle are in a straight row, top to bottom, on the abdomen.
		Example: When the rectus abdominis muscle contracts, it pulls the chest toward the legs.
rectum	(noun)	Straight part of the large intestine that comes after the curving S-shaped sigmoid colon
		Example: Digested food travels through the colon, through the rectum, through the anus, and is then expelled from the body.

Muscles of the Lower Extremity

The most important muscles of the buttocks, leg, and foot are described in this section (see Figure 9-15 ■).

Anterior Leg

- **Rectus femoris:** Bends the upper leg toward the abdomen (flexion); straightens the lower leg (extension)
- **Sartorius:** Bends the upper leg toward the abdomen (flexion) and rotates it laterally
- **Vastus lateralis and vastus medialis:** Bend the upper leg toward the abdomen (flexion); straighten the lower leg (extension)
- **Peroneus longus:** Raises the lateral edge of the foot (eversion) and bends the foot downward (plantar flexion)
- **Tibialis anterior:** Bends the foot up toward the leg (dorsiflexion)

WORD BUILDING

rectus (REK-tus)

femoris (FEM-oh-ris)

sartorius (sar-TOR-ee-us)

vastus lateralis (VAS-tus LAT-er-AL-is)

vastus medialis (VAS-tus MEE-dee-AL-is)

peroneus (PAIR-oh-NEE-us)

peroneal (PAIR-oh-NEE-al)
  perone/o- *fibula (lower leg bone)*
  -al *pertaining to*
Peroneal is the adjective form for *fibula*.

longus (LONG-us)

tibialis (TIB-ee-AL-is)
  tibi/o- *tibia (shin bone)*
  -alis *pertaining to*

anterior (an-TEER-ee-or)
  anter/o- *before; front part*
  -ior *pertaining to*

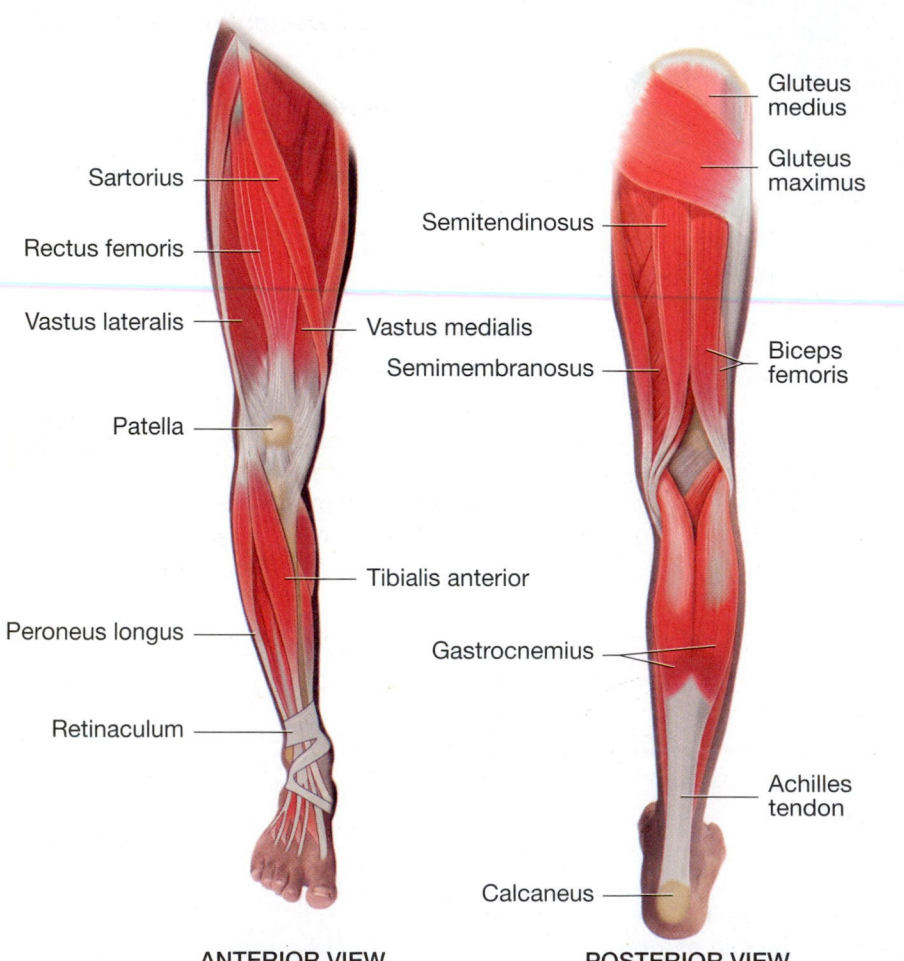

Sartorius
Rectus femoris
Vastus lateralis
Patella
Peroneus longus
Retinaculum
Vastus medialis
Semimembranosus
Tibialis anterior

ANTERIOR VIEW

Gluteus medius
Gluteus maximus
Semitendinosus
Biceps femoris
Gastrocnemius
Achilles tendon
Calcaneus

POSTERIOR VIEW

Figure 9-15 ■ Muscles of the lower extremity.
The muscles of the legs and buttocks contract and relax when you move your legs in any direction, bend your knees, walk on your toes, climb the stairs, or get up from a sitting position.

Posterior Leg

- **Gluteus maximus:** Moves the upper leg posteriorly and rotates it laterally
- **Biceps femoris:** Moves the upper leg posteriorly (extension) and bends the lower leg toward the buttocks (flexion)
- **Semitendinosus and semimembranosus:** Move the upper leg posteriorly (extension), bend the lower leg toward the buttocks (flexion), and rotate the leg medially
- **Gastrocnemius:** Bends the foot downward (plantar flexion) and lets you stand on tiptoe

Quadriceps femoris is a collective name for the group of four muscles—the rectus femoris, vastus lateralis, vastus intermedius (beneath the vastus lateralis), and vastus medialis—on the anterior upper leg. The tendons of the four heads of these muscles join together and insert on the tibia. These muscles straighten the lower leg (extension).

Hamstrings is a collective name for the group of three muscles—the biceps femoris, semitendinosus, and semimembranosus—on the posterior upper leg. These muscles move the upper leg posteriorly and bend the lower leg toward the buttocks (flexion).

WORD BUILDING

gluteus (gloo-TEE-us)

maximus (MAK-sih-mus)

biceps (BY-seps)
  bi- *two*
  -ceps *head*

femoris (FEM-oh-ris)

semitendinosus
(SEM-eye-TEN-dih-NOH-sus)

semimembranosus
(SEM-eye-MEM-brah-NOH-sus)

gastrocnemius
(GAS-trawk-NEE-mee-us)
  gastr/o- *stomach*
  -cnemius *leg*
The gastrocnemius muscle is shaped somewhat like a stomach filled with food, which may be how it got its name.

quadriceps (KWAD-rih-seps)
  quadri- *four*
  -ceps *head*

Did You Know?

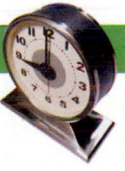

The gastrocnemius muscle has its insertion through the calcaneal tendon to the calcaneus (heel bone). This tendon is also known as the Achilles tendon in reference to Achilles, the mythical Greek hero of Homer's *Iliad* who was wounded in the heel, his only vulnerable spot.

Across the Life Span

Pediatrics. Babies are evaluated by the pediatrician on their ability to attain developmental milestones. A 1-month-old baby can lift its head only briefly. By 3 months of age, a baby has developed the muscular coordination to turn over in bed. One of the next developmental milestones is being able to lift up the head and chest (see Figure 9-16 ■).

Geriatrics. Throughout life, regular exercise is an important part of wellness and physical fitness. Aging and chronic disease can limit mobility and decrease muscle strength. The size and strength of the muscles decrease over time. There is less flexibility because elastic muscle tissue is replaced by fibrous connective tissue, but active exercise helps maintain muscle strength and flexibility.

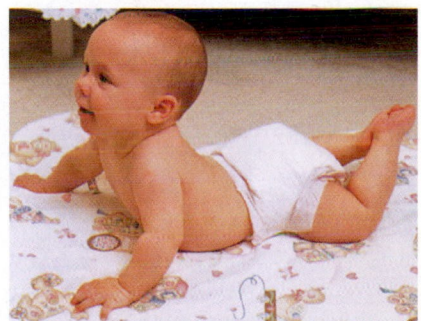

Figure 9-16 ■ Growth and development milestones.
This baby is able to lift his head and support his entire upper body with his arms, an activity that requires strength and coordination in the muscles of the neck, shoulders, and arms.

Physiology of a Muscle Contraction

A **muscle** is composed of several muscle fascicles, each of which is individually wrapped in fascia within the muscle (see Figure 9-17 ■). Each **muscle fascicle** is a bundle of individual muscle fibers. These muscle fibers run parallel to each other so that, when they contract, they all pull in the same direction. A **muscle fiber** (which is actually one long muscle cell) has hundreds of nuclei along its length to speed up the chemical processes that must occur before it can contract. Each muscle fiber is composed of **myofibrils** that contain thin strands of the protein actin and thick strands of the protein myosin that give skeletal muscle its characteristic striated (striped) appearance under the microscope (see Figure 9-2). Actin and myosin are the basis of a muscle contraction at the microscopic level.

A muscle contracts in response to an electrical impulse from a nerve. On a microscopic level, each muscle fiber is connected to a single nerve cell at a **neuromuscular junction.** The nerve cell releases the **neurotransmitter acetylcholine,** a chemical messenger that changes the permeability of the muscle fiber and allows sodium ions to flow into the muscle fiber. This releases calcium ions from their storage site within the muscle fiber. Calcium then causes the thin strands (actin) to slide between the thick strands (myosin), which shortens the muscle and produces a muscle **contraction.** The muscle eventually relaxes when acetylcholine is inactivated by an enzyme and the calcium ions are pumped back into their storage site.

Even when not actively moving, your muscles are in a state of mild, partial contraction because of nerve impulses from the brain and spinal cord. This produces muscle tone that keeps the muscles firm and ready to act. This is the only aspect of muscle activity that is not under conscious control.

WORD BUILDING

fascicle (FAS-ih-kl)
  fasci/o- *fascia*
  -cle *small thing*

myofibril (MY-oh-FY-bril)
  my/o- *muscle*
  fibr/o- *fiber*
  -il *a thing*

neuromuscular
(NYOOR-oh-MUS-kyoo-lar)
  neur/o- *nerve*
  muscul/o- *muscle*
  -ar *pertaining to*

neurotransmitter
(NYOOR-oh-TRANS-mit-er)
(NYOOR-oh-trans-MIT-er)
  neur/o- *nerve*
  transmitt/o- *to send across or through*
  -er *person or thing that produces or does*

acetylcholine (AS-eh-til-KOH-leen)

contraction (con-TRAK-shun)
  contract/o- *pull together*
  -ion *action; condition*

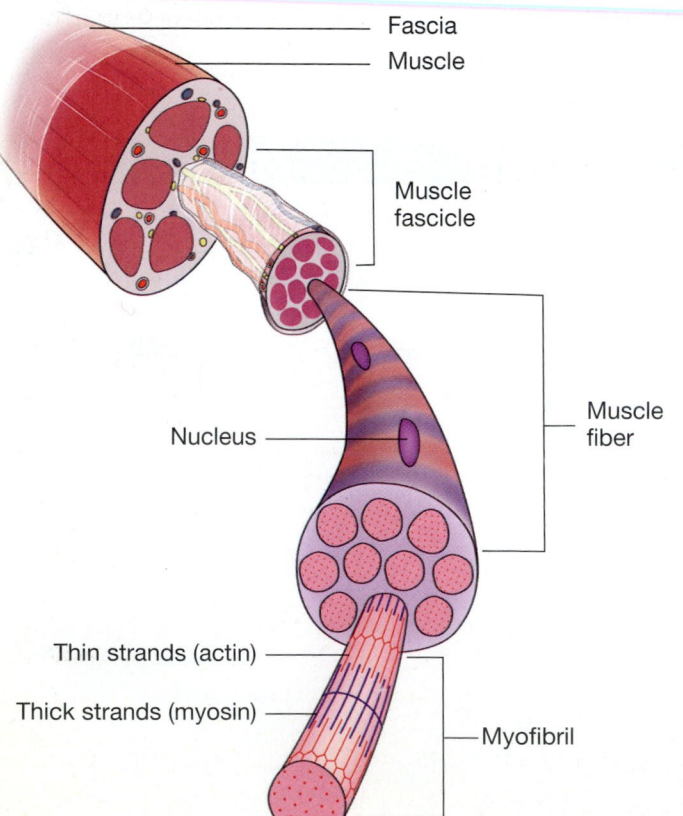

Fascia
Muscle

Muscle fascicle

Muscle fiber

Nucleus

Thin strands (actin)

Thick strands (myosin)

Myofibril

Figure 9-17 ■ Parts of a muscle.

A muscle is composed of muscle fascicles. Around each fascicle are arteries, veins, nerves, and fascia. Each fascicle contains several muscle fibers (muscle cells). Within each muscle fiber are myofibrils that contain thin strands of actin and thick strands of myosin.

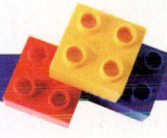

Clinical Connections

Sports Medicine. Professional athletes depend on their muscles to help them win. The muscle fibers of a marathon runner are different from those of a sprinter. Marathon runners have mostly slow-twitch muscle fibers that can contract many times without becoming fatigued. Sprinters have fast-twitch muscle fibers that can contract very quickly and repeatedly, but soon become tired. Because of the effect of the male hormone testosterone, men have larger muscles than women and a bulkier musculature, but vigorous weight training can increase the size of a muscle (**muscle hypertrophy**) in either sex. Bodybuilders work to enlarge, define, and sculpt their muscles (see Figure 9-18 ■). Some athletes try to enhance their performance with the use of illicit drugs, particularly anabolic steroid drugs that add bulk to the muscles.

hypertrophy (hy-PER-troh-fee)
hyper- *above; more than normal*
-trophy *process of development*
The ending -*trophy* contains the combining form *troph/o-* and the one-letter suffix –*y.*

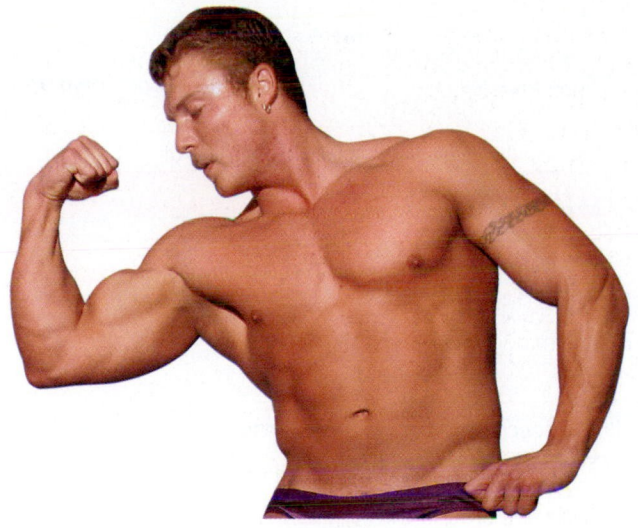

Figure 9-18 ■ Muscle strength and size.
This bodybuilder has highly developed muscles: the biceps brachii of the flexed right arm, the deltoid muscle of the shoulder, and the well-defined pectoral muscle of the chest. The individual segments of the rectus abdominis muscles can be seen on either side of the umbilicus.

Vocabulary Review

Anatomy and Physiology

Word or Phrase	Description	Combining Forms
muscle	Structure that produces movement of the body	**muscul/o-** *muscle* **my/o-** *muscle* **myos/o-** *muscle*
muscular system	Provides movement for the body in conjunction with support from the bones. It is also known as the **musculoskeletal system.**	**muscul/o-** *muscle* **skelet/o-** *skeleton*
musculature	Group of skeletal muscles in one body part or the muscles in the body as a whole	**muscul/o-** *muscle*
skeletal muscle	One of three types of muscles in the body, but the only one that is under **voluntary** control. Skeletal muscles move bones. Skeletal muscles contract and relax in response to conscious thought.	**skelet/o-** *skeleton* **volunt/o-** *done of one's own free will*

Muscle Structures

aponeurosis	Flat, wide, white sheet of fibrous connective tissue that attaches a muscle to a bone or other structure	
belly of the muscle	Area of greatest mass, usually the center of the muscle midway between the origin and insertion	
bursa	Sac of synovial membrane that contains synovial fluid. It decreases friction where a tendon rubs against a bone near a synovial joint.	**burs/o-** *bursa*
fascia	Thin connective tissue sheet around each muscle fascicle and around the muscle itself. It merges to become part of the tendon.	**fasci/o-** *fascia*
insertion	Where the tendon of a muscle ends on a bone that moves as the muscle contracts or relaxes	**insert/o-** *to put in; introduce*
origin	Where the tendon of a muscle begins and is attached to a stationary or nearly stationary bone	
retinaculum	Thin, nearly translucent band of fibrous tissue and fascia that holds down tendons that cross the wrist and ankle	
tendon	Cordlike white band of nonelastic fibrous connective tissue that attaches a muscle to a bone	**tendin/o-** *tendon* **tendon/o-** *tendon* **ten/o-** *tendon*

Muscle Movements

abduction	Moving a body part away from the midline. It is the opposite of adduction. An **abductor** is a muscle that produces abduction when it contracts.	**duct/o-** *bring; move; a duct*
adduction	Moving a body part toward the midline. It is the opposite of abduction. An **adductor** is a muscle that produces adduction when it contracts.	**duct/o-** *bring; move; a duct*
eversion	Turning a body part outward and toward the side. It is the opposite of inversion. An **evertor** is a muscle that produces eversion when it contracts.	**vers/o-** *to travel; to turn* **vert/o-** *to travel; to turn*

Word or Phrase	Description	Combining Forms
extension	Straightening and extending a joint to increase the angle between two bones or two body parts. It is the opposite of flexion. An **extensor** is a muscle that produces extension when it contracts.	**extens/o-** *straightening*
flexion	Bending of a joint to decrease the angle between two bones or two body parts. It is the opposite of extension. A **flexor** is a muscle that produces flexion when it contracts.	**flex/o-** *bending*
inversion	Turning a body part inward. It is the opposite of eversion. An **invertor** is a muscle that produces inversion when it contracts.	**vers/o-** *to travel; to turn* **vert/o-** *to travel; to turn*
pronation	Turning the palm of the hand posteriorly or downward. It is the opposite of supination. A **pronator** is a muscle that produces pronation when it contracts.	**pronat/o-** *face down*
rotation	Moving a body part around its axis. A **rotator** is a muscle that produces rotation when it contracts.	**rotat/o-** *rotate*
supination	Turning the palm of the hand anteriorly or upward. It is the opposite of pronation. A **supinator** is a muscle that produces supination when it contracts.	**supinat/o-** *lying on the back*

Muscles of the Head and Neck

Word or Phrase	Description	Combining Forms
buccinator muscle	Muscle of the side of the face that moves the cheek	**buccinat/o-** *cheek*
frontalis muscle	Muscle of the forehead that moves the forehead skin and eyebrows	**front/o-** *front*
masseter muscle	Muscle of the side of the face that moves the mandible upward	**masset/o-** *chewing*
orbicularis oculi muscle	Muscle around the eye that closes the eyelids	**orbicul/o-** *small circle*
orbicularis oris muscle	Muscle around the mouth that closes the lips	**orbicul/o-** *small circle*
platysma muscle	Muscle of the neck that moves the mandible down	
sternocleido-mastoid muscle	Muscle of the neck that bends the head toward the sternum (flexion) and turns the head to either side (rotation). Its origin is at two muscle heads on the sternum and clavicle. Its insertion is at the mastoid process of the temporal bone behind the ear.	**stern/o-** *sternum (breast bone)* **cleid/o-** *clavicle (collar bone)* **mast/o-** *breast; mastoid process*
temporalis muscle	Muscle of the side of the head that moves the mandible upward and backward	**tempor/o-** *temple (side of the head)*

Muscles of the Shoulders, Chest, and Back

Word or Phrase	Description	Combining Forms
deltoid muscle	Muscle of the shoulder that raises the arm and moves the arm away from the body (abduction)	**delt/o-** *triangle*
intercostal muscles	Muscles between the ribs that work in pairs to spread the ribs apart during inspiration and move the ribs together during forced expiration, coughing, or sneezing	**cost/o-** *rib*
latissimus dorsi muscle	Muscle of the back that moves the arm posteriorly and medially toward the spinal column (adduction)	

Word or Phrase	Description	Combining Forms
pectoralis major muscle	Muscle of the chest that moves the arm anteriorly and medially across the chest (adduction)	**pector/o-** *chest*
trapezius muscle	Muscle of the shoulder that raises the shoulder, pulls the shoulder blades together, and elevates the clavicle. It turns the head from side to side (rotation) and moves the head posteriorly (extension).	

Muscles of the Upper Extremity

Word or Phrase	Description	Combining Forms
biceps brachii muscle	Muscle of the anterior upper arm that bends the upper arm toward the shoulder (flexion) and bends the lower arm toward the upper arm (flexion). One end of the muscle is divided into two heads.	
brachioradialis muscle	Muscle of the anterior lower arm that bends the lower arm toward the upper arm (flexion)	**brachi/o-** *arm* **radi/o-** *radius (forearm bone); x-rays; radiation*
extensor digitorum muscle	Muscle that extends the fingers or toes	**extens/o-** *straightening*
thenar muscles	Group of muscles in the hand that bends the thumb (flexion) and moves it toward the palm (adduction)	**then/o-** *thumb*
triceps brachii muscle	Muscle of the posterior upper arm that straightens the lower arm (extension). One end is divided into three heads.	

Muscles of the Abdomen

Word or Phrase	Description	Combining Forms
external abdominal oblique muscle	Muscle of the abdomen that bends the upper body forward (flexion), rotates the side of the body medially, and compresses the side of the abdominal wall. The **internal abdominal oblique muscle** lies directly beneath it and performs the same movements, but its muscle fibers are oriented in the opposite direction.	**extern/o-** *outside* **abdomin/o-** *abdomen* **intern/o-** *inside*
rectus abdominis muscle	Muscle of the abdomen that bends the upper body forward (flexion) and compresses the anterior abdominal wall	

Muscles of the Lower Extremity

Word or Phrase	Description	Combining Forms
biceps femoris muscle	Muscle of the posterior upper leg that moves the upper leg posteriorly (extension) and bends the lower leg toward the buttocks (flexion). One end of the muscle is divided into two heads.	
flexor hallucis brevis muscle	Muscle that flexes the big toe (hallux)	**flex/o-** *bending*
gastrocnemius muscle	Muscle of the posterior lower leg that bends the foot downward (plantar flexion) and lets you stand on tiptoe	**gastr/o-** *stomach* *Note: The shape of this muscle is somewhat like a stomach filled with food.*
gluteus maximus muscle	Muscle of the buttocks that moves the upper leg posteriorly and rotates it laterally	

Word or Phrase	Description	Combining Forms
hamstrings	Group of muscles in the posterior aspect of the upper leg that moves the upper leg posteriorly and bends the lower leg toward the buttocks (flexion). It includes the biceps femoris, semitendinosus, and semimembranosus muscles.	
peroneus longus muscle	Muscle of the lateral lower leg that raises the lateral edge of the foot (eversion) and bends the foot downward (plantar flexion)	**perone/o-** *fibula (lower leg bone)*
quadriceps femoris	Group of muscles in the anterior and lateral upper leg that straightens the lower leg (extension). It includes the rectus femoris, vastus lateralis, vastus intermedius, and vastus medialis muscles.	
rectus femoris muscle	Muscle of the anterior upper leg that bends the upper leg toward the abdomen (flexion) and straightens the lower leg (extension)	
sartorius muscle	Muscle of the anterior upper leg that bends the upper leg toward the abdomen (flexion) and rotates it laterally	
semitendinosus muscle	Muscle of the posterior upper leg that moves the upper leg posteriorly (extension), bends the lower leg toward the buttock (flexion), and rotates the leg medially. The **semimembranosus muscle** has the same action.	
tibialis anterior muscle	Muscle of the anterior lower leg that bends the foot up toward the leg (dorsiflexion)	**tibi/o-** *tibia (shin bone)* **anter/o-** *before; front part*
vastus lateralis muscle	Muscle of the anterior upper leg that bends the upper leg toward the abdomen (flexion) and straightens the lower leg (extension). The **vastus medialis muscle** has the same action.	

Muscle Contraction

Word or Phrase	Description	Combining Forms
acetylcholine	Neurotransmitter that initiates a muscle contraction	
contraction	Shortening of the length of all the muscle fibers and of the muscle itself. It is the opposite of relaxation.	**contract/o-** *pull together*
fascicle	A bundle composed of many muscle fibers. It is surrounded by fascia. Many fascicles grouped together form a muscle.	**fasci/o-** *fascia*
hypertrophy	An increase in the size of a muscle	**troph/o-** *development*
muscle fiber	One muscle cell. So named because it stretches over a long distance.	
myofibril	Section of a muscle fiber that contains thin strands (**actin**) and thick strands (**myosin**) that give it its characteristic **striated** appearance under a microscope	**my/o-** *muscle* **fibr/o-** *fiber*
neuromuscular junction	Area on a single muscle fiber where a nerve cell connects to it	**neur/o-** *nerve* **muscul/o-** *muscle*
neurotransmitter	Chemical messenger between a nerve cell and a muscle fiber	**neur/o-** *nerve* **transmitt/o-** *to send across or through*

Labeling Exercise

Match each anatomy word or phrase to its structure and write it in the numbered box for each figure. Be sure to check your spelling. Use the Answer Key at the end of the book to check your answers.

| abduction and extension | flexion | flexion and adduction | rotation | slight flexion |

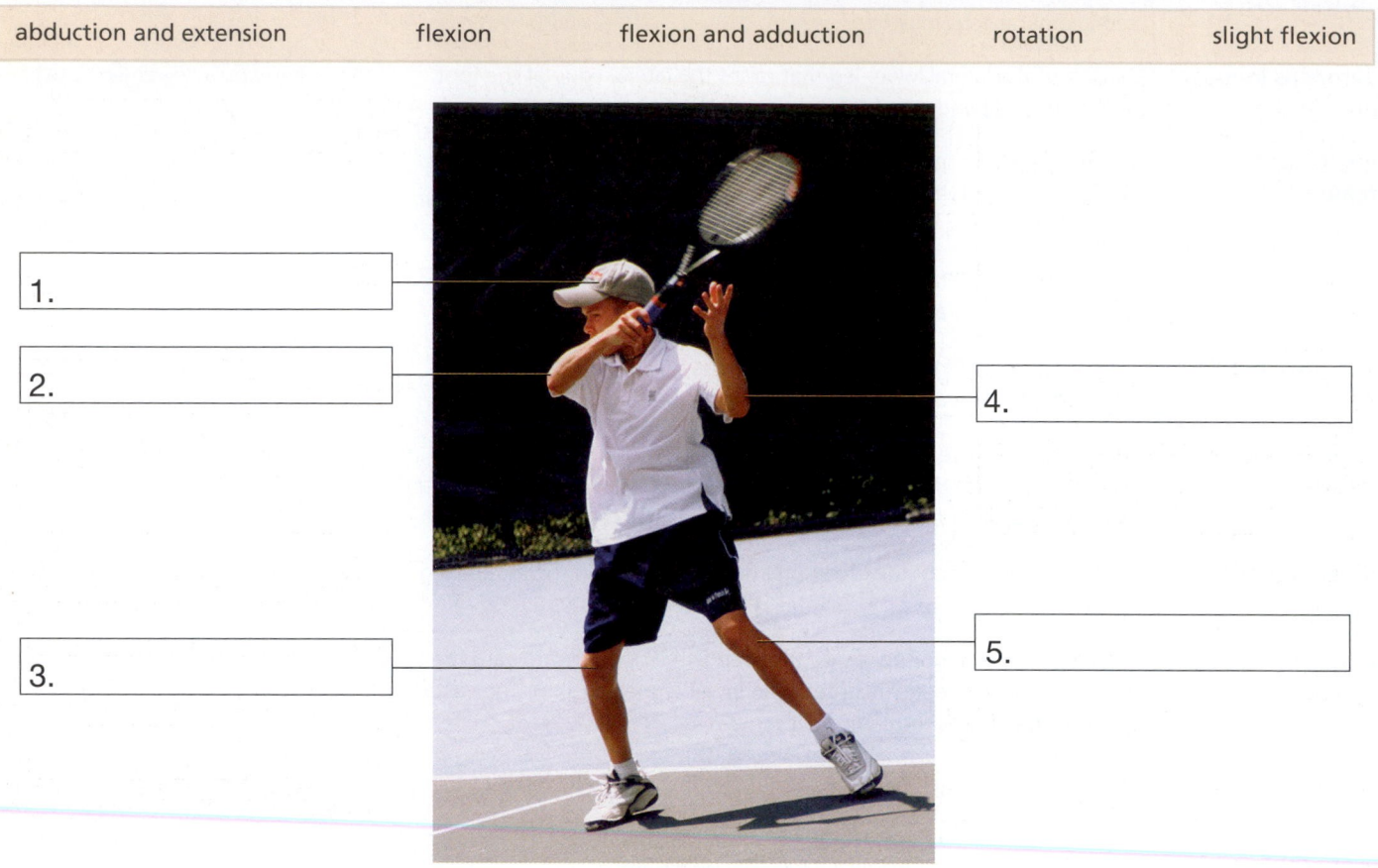

1.

2.

3.

4.

5.

biceps brachii muscle
brachioradialis muscle
deltoid muscle
frontalis muscle
gastrocnemius muscle

gluteus maximus muscle
latissimus dorsi muscle
masseter muscle
pectoralis major muscle

peroneus longus muscle
rectus abdominis muscle
rectus femoris muscle
sternocleidomastoid muscle

temporalis muscle
tibialis anterior muscle
trapezius muscle
triceps brachii muscle

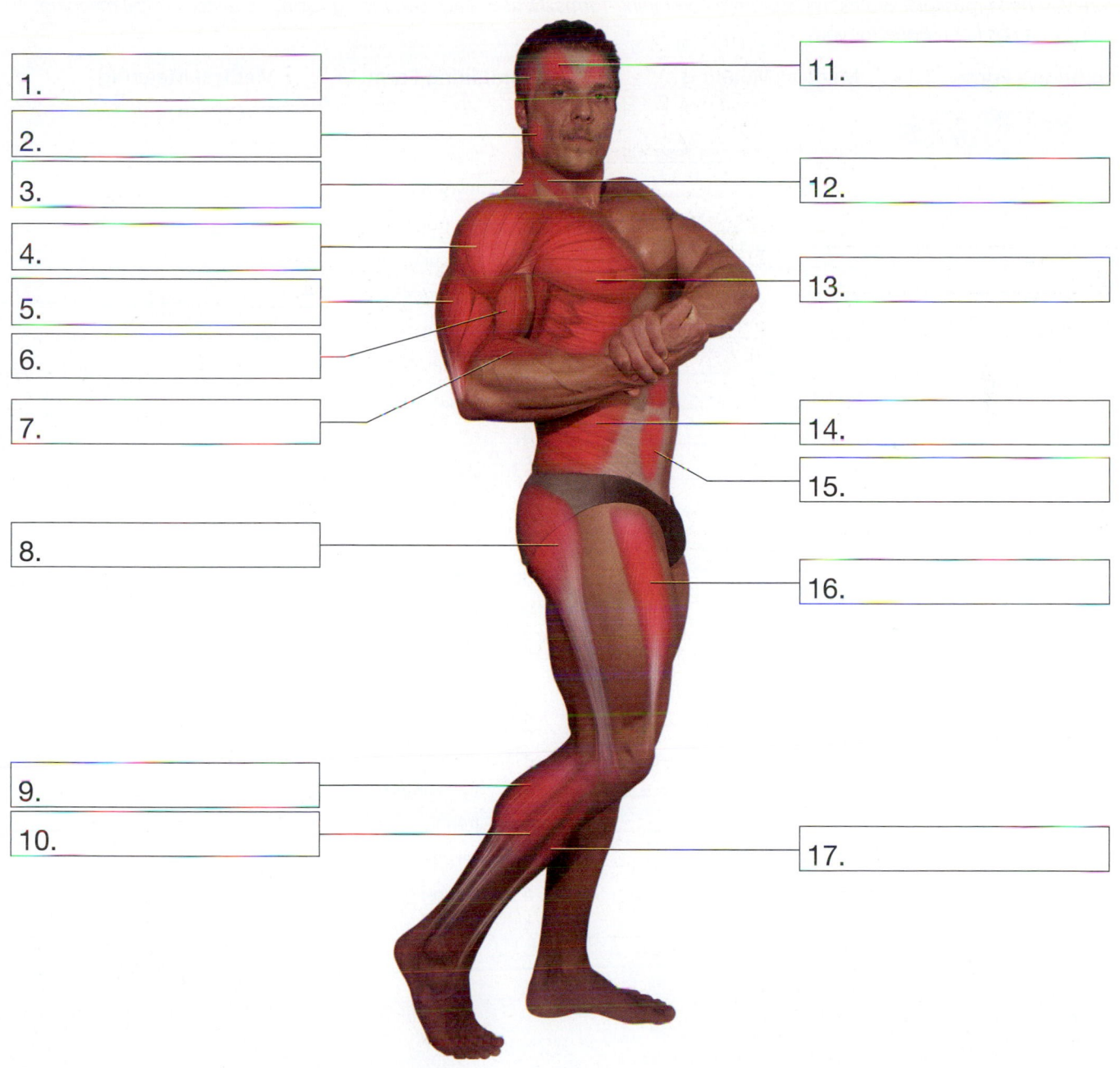

1.

2.

3.

4.

5.

6.

7.

8.

9.

10.

11.

12.

13.

14.

15.

16.

17.

Building Medical Words

Use the Answer Key at the end of the book to check your answers.

Combining Forms Exercise

Before you build muscular words, review these combining forms. Next to each combining form, write its medical meaning. The first one has been done for you.

Combining Form	Medical Meaning	Combining Form	Medical Meaning
1. **volunt/o-**	*done of one's own free will*	24. my/o-	
2. abdomin/o-		25. myos/o-	
3. anter/o-		26. neur/o-	
4. brachi/o-		27. orbicul/o-	
5. buccinat/o-		28. pector/o-	
6. burs/o-		29. perone/o-	
7. cleid/o-		30. pronat/o-	
8. contract/o-		31. radi/o-	
9. cost/o-		32. rotat/o-	
10. delt/o-		33. skelet/o-	
11. duct/o-		34. stern/o-	
12. extens/o-		35. supinat/o-	
13. extern/o-		36. tempor/o-	
14. fasci/o-		37. tendin/o-	
15. fibr/o-		38. tendon/o-	
16. flex/o-		39. ten/o-	
17. front/o-		40. then/o-	
18. gastr/o-		41. tibi/o-	
19. insert/o-		42. transmitt/o-	
20. intern/o-		43. troph/o-	
21. masset/o-		44. vers/o-	
22. mast/o-		45. vert/o-	
23. muscul/o-			

Combining Form and Suffix Exercise

Read the definition of the medical word. Look at the combining form that is given. Select the correct suffix from the Suffix List and write it on the blank line. Then build the medical word and write it on the line. (Remember: You may need to remove the combining vowel. Always remove the hyphens and slash.) Be sure to check your spelling. The first one has been done for you.

SUFFIX LIST

-al (pertaining to)	-ary (pertaining to)	-oid (resembling)
-alis (pertaining to)	-ature (system composed of)	-or (person or thing that produces or does)
-ar (pertaining to)	-er (person or thing that produces or does)	-ous (pertaining to)
-aris (pertaining to)	-ion (action; condition)	

Definition of the Medical Word	Combining Form	Suffix	Build the Medical Word
1. Thing that produces or does (make something) rotate	**rotat/o-**	**-or**	rotator

(You think *thing that produces or does* (-or) + *rotate* (rotat/o-). You change the order of the word parts to put the suffix last. You write *rotator*.)

2. Pertaining to a tendon	tendin/o-	_____	_____
3. Pertaining to a muscle	muscul/o-	_____	_____
4. Action of bending	flex/o-	_____	_____
5. Pertaining to the fascia	fasci/o-	_____	_____
6. System composed of muscles	muscul/o-	_____	_____
7. (Muscle) resembling a triangle	delt/o-	_____	_____
8. Pertaining to (being) done of one's own free will	volunt/o-	_____	_____
9. Thing that produces or does chewing	masset/o-	_____	_____
10. Pertaining to a small circle (of muscle)	orbicul/o-	_____	_____
11. (Muscle name that means) pertaining to the chest	pector/o-	_____	_____
12. Action of lying on the back (of the hand)	supinat/o-	_____	_____
13. Action (as a muscle) pulls together	contract/o-	_____	_____

Diseases and Conditions

Diseases of the Muscles

Word or Phrase	Description	Word Building
atrophy	Loss of muscle bulk in one or more muscles. It is caused by a lack of use or by malnutrition, or it can occur in any part of the body that is paralyzed because the muscles receive no electrical impulses from the nerves. The muscle is **atrophic.** It is also known as **muscle wasting.** Treatment: Correct the underlying cause.	**atrophy** (AT-roh-fee) **a-** *away from; without* **-trophy** *process of development* The ending of *–trophy* contains the combining form *troph/o-* and the one-letter suffix *–y.* **atrophic** (ah-TROF-ik) **a-** *away from; without* **troph/o-** *development* **-ic** *pertaining to*
avulsion	Condition in which the muscle tears away from the tendon or the tendon tears away from the bone. Treatment: Surgical repair (myorrhaphy or tenorrhaphy).	**avulsion** (ah-VUL-shun) **a-** *away from; without* **vuls/o-** *to tear* **-ion** *action; condition*
compartment syndrome	The result of a severe blunt or crushing injury that causes bleeding in the muscles of the leg. The fascia acts as a compartment, holding in the accumulating blood. The increased pressure causes muscle and nerve damage and tissue death. Treatment: Fasciotomy to allow the blood and fluid to drain out.	
contracture	Inactivity or paralysis coupled with continuing nerve impulses can cause an arm or leg muscle to become progressively flexed and drawn into a position where it becomes nearly immovable (see Figure 9-19 ■). Treatment: Muscle relaxant drugs, range of motion (ROM) exercises.	**contracture** (con-TRAK-chur) **contract/o-** *pull together* **-ure** *system; result of*

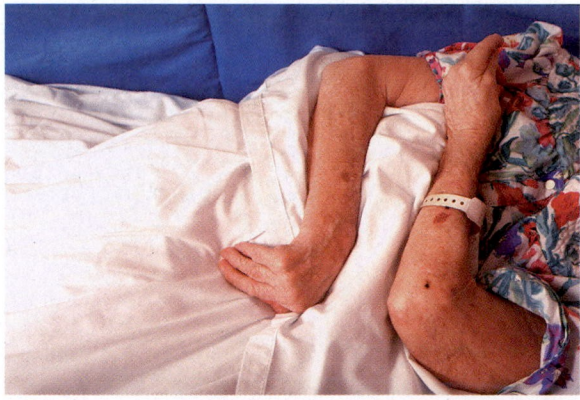

Figure 9-19 ■ **Muscle contracture.**
This elderly woman has severe arthritis and is a patient in a long-term care facility. She has developed contractures of the arms and wrists, which could have been prevented by proper body positioning and regular range of motion exercises.

Word Alert

SOUND-ALIKE WORDS

contraction   (noun)   the normal tensing and shortening of a muscle in response to a nerve impulse
Example: It requires a strong, sustained contraction of the arm muscles to lift a heavy box.

contracture   (noun)   abnormal, fixed position in which the muscle is permanently flexed
Example: Range of motion exercises help prevent a contracture from occurring.

Word or Phrase	Description	Word Building

fibromyalgia	Pain located at specific trigger points in the muscles of the neck, back, or hips. The trigger points are tender to the touch and feel firm. The cause is not known, but may be related to an overreaction to painful stimuli with a possible history of prior injury or a genetic predisposition. Fibromyalgia is associated with disturbed sleep patterns and sometimes depression. Treatment: Analgesic drugs, muscle relaxant drugs, massage, and trigger point injections with a local anesthetic drug.	**fibromyalgia** (FY-broh-my-AL-jee-ah) (FY-broh-my-AL-jah)
		  fibr/o- *fiber*
		  my/o- *muscle*
		  alg/o- *pain*
		  -ia *condition; state; thing*

hyperextension–hyperflexion injury	Injury that occurs during a car accident as a person's head snaps forward and then backward. This causes a muscle strain or muscle tear, as well as damage to the nerves. It is also known as **acceleration–deceleration injury** or **whiplash.** Treatment: Soft cervical collar to support the neck, rest, analgesic drugs, nonsteroidal anti-inflammatory drugs.	**hyperextension** (HY-per-eks-TEN-shun)
		  hyper- *above; more than normal*
		  extens/o- *straightening*
		  -ion *action; condition*
		
		hyperflexion (HY-per-FLEK-shun)
		  hyper- *above; more than normal*
		  flex/o- *bending*
		  -ion *action; condition*

muscle contusion	Condition in which blunt trauma causes some bleeding in the muscle but does not break the skin. It is also known as a **bruise.** Treatment: Analgesic drugs.	**contusion** (con-TOO-shun)
		  contus/o- *bruising*
		  -ion *action; condition*

muscle spasm	Painful but temporary condition with a sudden, severe, involuntary, and prolonged contraction of a muscle, often in the legs. It can be brought on by overexercise. It is also known as a **muscle cramp. Torticollis** is a painful spasm of the muscles on one side of the neck. It is also known as **wryneck.** Treatment: Massage, muscle relaxant drugs, analgesic drugs.	**spasm** (SPAZM)
		
		torticollis (TOR-tih-KOL-is)
		  tort/i- *twisted position*
		  -collis *condition of the neck*

muscle strain	Overstretching of a muscle, often due to physical overexertion. This causes **inflammation,** pain, swelling, and bruising as capillaries in the muscle tear. It is also known as a **pulled muscle.** Treatment: Rest, analgesic drugs, nonsteroidal anti-inflammatory drugs.	**strain** (STRAYN)
		
		inflammation (IN-flah-MAY-shun)
		  inflammat/o- *redness and warmth*
		  -ion *action; condition*

muscular dystrophy	Genetic inherited disease due to a mutation of the gene that makes the muscle protein dystrophin. Without dystrophin, the muscles weaken and then atrophy. It begins in early childhood with weakness in the lower extremities and then the upper extremities (see Figure 9-20 ■). The most common and most severe form is **Duchenne's muscular dystrophy;** Becker's muscular dystrophy is a milder form. Weakness of the diaphragm with an inability to breathe is the most frequent cause of death. Treatment: Supportive care.	**dystrophy** (DIS-troh-fee)
		  dys- *painful; difficult; abnormal*
		  -trophy *process of development*
		
		Duchenne (doo-SHAYN)

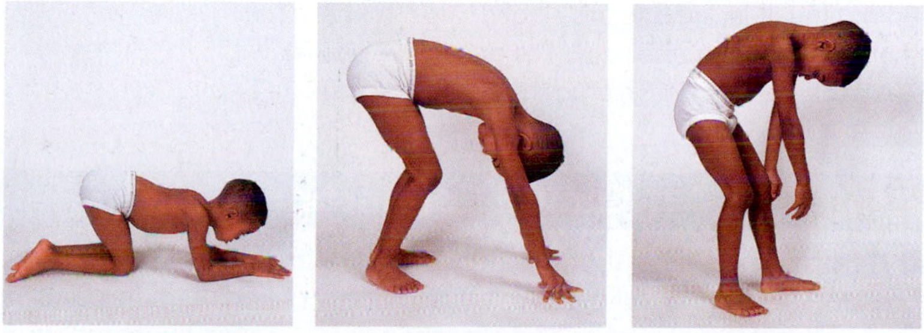

Figure 9-20 ■ Muscular dystrophy.
Weakness of the muscles in the legs causes this patient with muscular dystrophy to stand up in a way that is characteristic of this disease. The legs and arms must work together to raise the body. Because muscular dystrophy is a progressive disease, this patient soon may not be able to walk at all.

Word or Phrase	Description	Word Building
myalgia	Pain in one or more muscles due to injury or muscle disease. **Polymyalgia** is pain in several muscle groups. Treatment: Analgesic drugs, massage.	**myalgia** (my-AL-jee-ah) (my-AL-jah) **my/o-** *muscle* **alg/o-** *pain* **-ia** *condition; state; thing* **polymyalgia** (PAWL-ee-my-AL-jee-ah) (PAWL-ee-my-AL-jah) **poly-** *many; much* **my/o-** *muscle* **alg/o-** *pain* **-ia** *condition; state; thing*
myasthenia gravis	Abnormal and rapid fatigue of the muscles, particularly in the muscles of the face, where there is **ptosis** (drooping) of the eyelids. The weakness worsens during the day, but is relieved by rest. The body produces antibodies against its own acetylcholine receptors on the muscle fibers. The antibodies destroy many of the receptors. There are normal levels of acetylcholine, but too few receptors remain to produce a sustained muscle contraction. Treatment: Thymectomy to remove the thymus; drugs that prolong the action of acetylcholine. Plasmapheresis to remove antibodies from the blood.	**myasthenia gravis** (MY-as-THEE-nee-ah GRAV-is) **my/o-** *muscle* **asthen/o-** *lack of strength* **-ia** *condition; state; thing* **ptosis** (TOH-sis)
myopathy	Category that includes many different diseases of the muscles. Treatment: Correct the underlying cause.	**myopathy** (my-AWP-ah-thee) **my/o-** *muscle* **-pathy** *disease; suffering*
myositis	Inflammation of a muscle with localized swelling and tenderness. It can be caused by injury or strain. **Polymyositis** is a chronic, progressive disease that causes widespread inflammation of muscles with weakness and fatigue. The cause is unknown, although it may be an autoimmune disease. **Dermatomyositis** causes a skin rash as well as muscle weakness and inflammation. Treatment: Analgesic drugs, nonsteroidal anti-inflammatory drugs, corticosteroid drugs.	**myositis** (MY-oh-SY-tis) **myos/o-** *muscle* **-itis** *inflammation of; infection of* **polymyositis** (PAWL-ee-MY-oh-SY-tis) **poly-** *many; much* **myos/o-** *muscle* **-itis** *inflammation of; infection of* **dermatomyositis** (DER-mah-toh-MY-oh-SY-tis) **dermat/o-** *skin* **myos/o-** *muscle* **-itis** *inflammation of; infection of*
repetitive strain injury (RSI)	Condition affecting the muscles, tendons, and sometimes the nerves. It occurs as a result of trauma caused by repetitious movements over an extended period of time. It includes tennis elbow, carpal tunnel syndrome, and other disorders. It is also known as **cumulative trauma disorder (CTD).** Treatment: Rest, analgesic drugs, nonsteroidal anti-inflammatory drugs.	

Clinical Connections

Occupational Health. The Occupational Safety and Health Administration (OSHA) educates healthcare professionals about workplace-related injuries. Lifting, carrying, pulling, or pushing something heavy and not using proper body mechanics can cause injury as can repetitive motions done constantly, such as typing on a computer.

Word or Phrase	Description	Word Building

rhabdomyoma	**Benign** tumor that arises from muscle. Treatment: Surgical excision.	**rhabdomyoma** (RAB-doh-my-OH-mah)
		   rhabd/o- *rod shaped*
		   my/o- *muscle*
		   -oma *tumor; mass*
		Note: The immature muscle cells in this tumor are shaped like a rod.
		benign (bee-NINE)

rhabdomyo-sarcoma	Cancerous tumor that arises from muscle. This **malignancy** usually occurs in children and young adults. Treatment: Surgical excision, chemotherapy, and radiation therapy.	**rhabdomyosarcoma**
		(RAB-doh-MY-oh-sar-KOH-mah)
		   rhabd/o- *rod shaped*
		   my/o- *muscle*
		   sarc/o- *connective tissue*
		   -oma *tumor; mass*
		malignancy (mah-LIG-nan-see)
		   malign/o- *intentionally causing harm; cancer*
		   -ancy *state of*

rotator cuff tear	Tear in the rotator muscles of the shoulder that surround the head of the humerus. These muscles help to abduct the arm. The tear can result from acute trauma or repetitive overuse, particularly involving motions in which the arm is above the head. Treatment: Surgical repair.	

Clinical Connections

Forensic Science. Rigor mortis is not a muscle disease of the living, but rather a normal condition of the muscles that occurs several hours after death. As each muscle fiber dies, its stored calcium is released and this causes the muscle fiber—and then each muscle of the body— to contract. The muscle fiber is no longer able to pump calcium ions back into the storage site, and so the muscles remain contracted for about 72 hours until the muscle fibers begin to decompose. This is also known as **postmortem rigidity.** Forensic scientists use rigor mortis to help determine the time of death.

rigor mortis (RIG-or MOR-tis)

postmortem (pohst-MOR-tem)

Movement Disorders

ataxia	Incoordination of the muscles during movement, particularly incoordination of the gait. It is caused by diseases of the brain or spinal cord, cerebral palsy, or an adverse reaction to a drug. The patient is **ataxic.** Treatment: Correct the underlying cause. Leg braces or crutches, if needed.	**ataxia** (ah-TAK-see-ah)
		   a- *away from; without*
		   tax/o- *coordination*
		   -ia *condition; state; thing*
		ataxic (ah-TAK-sik)
		   a- *away from; without*
		   tax/o- *coordination*
		   -ic *pertaining to*

bradykinesia	Abnormally slow muscle movements or a decrease in the number of spontaneous muscle movements. It is usually associated with Parkinson's disease, a neurologic disease of the brain. Treatment: Drugs for Parkinson's disease.	**bradykinesia** (BRAD-ee-kin-EE-zee-ah)
		   brady- *slow*
		   kines/o- *movement*
		   -ia *condition; state; thing*

Word or Phrase	Description	Word Building
dyskinesia	Abnormal motions that occur because of difficulty controlling the voluntary muscles. Attempts at movement become tics, muscle spasms, muscle jerking (**myoclonus**), or slow, wandering, purposeless writhing of the hand (**athetoid movements**) in which some muscles of the fingers are flexed and others are extended. It is associated with neurologic disorders (Parkinson's disease, Huntington's chorea, cerebral palsy, etc.). Treatment: Correct the underlying cause.	**dyskinesia** (DIS-kih-NEE-zee-ah) **dys-** *painful; difficult; abnormal* **kines/o-** *movement* **-ia** *condition; state; thing* Select the correct prefix meaning to get the definition of *dyskinesia*: *condition of abnormal movement.* **myoclonus** (MY-oh-KLOH-nus) **my/o-** *muscle* **-clonus** *condition of rapid contracting and relaxing* **athetoid** (ATH-eh-toyd) **athet/o-** *without position or place* **-oid** *resembling*

Clinical Connections

Neurology (Chapter 10). Cerebral palsy is caused by a lack of oxygen to parts of a fetus' brain before or during birth. The extent of the symptoms varies, but can include spastic muscles; dyskinesia; lack of coordination in walking, eating, and talking; or even muscle paralysis.

Word or Phrase	Description	Word Building
hyperkinesis	An abnormally increased amount of muscle movements. Restlessness. It can be a side effect of some drugs. Treatment: Correct the underlying cause.	**hyperkinesis** (HY-per-kih-NEE-sis) **hyper-** *above; more than normal* **-kinesis** *condition of movement*
restless legs syndrome (RLS)	An uncomfortable restlessness and twitching of the muscles of the legs, particularly the calf muscles, along with an indescribable tingling, aching, or crawling-insect sensation. This usually occurs at night and can interfere with sleep. The exact cause is unknown. Treatment: The drug Requip, which stimulates dopamine receptors in the brain. Tranquilizer drugs may be of some help.	
tremor	Small, involuntary, sometimes jerky, back-and-forth movements of the hands, neck, jaw, or extremities. These are continuous and cannot be controlled by the patient. It is usually associated with essential familial tremor, an inherited condition. Treatment: Beta-blocker drugs.	**tremor** (TREM-or)

Diseases of the Bursa, Fascia, or Tendon

Word or Phrase	Description	Word Building
bursitis	Inflammation of the bursal sac because of repetitive muscle contractions or pressure on the bone underneath the bursa. It can occur with any joint that has a bursa, but most often occurs in the shoulders and knees. Prolonged periods of kneeling cause bursitis known as **housemaid's knee.** Treatment: Rest, analgesic drugs, nonsteroidal anti-inflammatory drugs.	**bursitis** (ber-SY-tis) **burs/o-** *bursa* **-itis** *inflammation of; infection of*
Dupuytren's contracture	Progressive disease in which the fascia in the palm of the hand becomes thickened and shortened, causing a contracture and flexion deformity of the fingers. Treatment: Surgery (fasciectomy).	**Dupuytren** (DOO-pyoo-tren) **contracture** (con-TRAK-chur) **contract/o-** *pull together* **-ure** *system; result of*
fasciitis	Inflammation of the fascia around a muscle. Plantar fasciitis is inflammation of the fascia on the bottom of the foot that is caused by excessive running or exercise. There is aching or stabbing pain around the heel. It is the most common cause of heel pain. Treament: Analgesic drugs, nonsteroidal anti-inflammatory drugs. Injection into the fascia of a corticosteroid drug.	**fasciitis** (FAS-ee-EYE-tis) **fasci/o-** *fascia* **-itis** *inflammation of; infection of*

Word or Phrase	Description	Word Building
ganglion	Semisolid or fluid-containing cyst that develops on a tendon, often in the wrist, hand, or foot. A ganglion is a rounded lump under the skin and may or may not be painful (see Figure 9-21 ■). Treatment: Needle aspiration of fluid from the ganglion or surgical removal (ganglionectomy).	**ganglion** (GANG-glee-on)

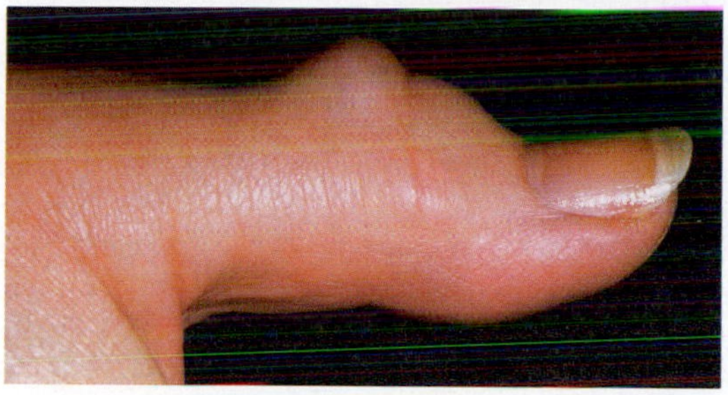

Figure 9-21 ■ **Ganglion.**
This patient has a semisolid ganglion on the extensor tendon of the digit. Even after a ganglionectomy is done to surgically remove it, it may recur.

Word or Phrase	Description	Word Building
pitcher's elbow	Inflammation and pain of the flexor and pronator muscles of the forearm where their tendons originate on the medial epicondyle of the humerus (by the elbow joint). This is an overuse injury caused by repeated flexing of the wrist while the fingers tightly grasp. It is also known as **golfer's elbow** or **medial epicondylitis.** Treatment: Rest, analgesic drugs, nonsteroidal anti-inflammatory drugs.	
shin splints	Pain and inflammation of the tendons of the flexor muscles of the lower leg over the anterior tibia (shin bone). It is an overuse injury common to athletes who run. Treatment: Rest, analgesic drugs, nonsteroidal anti-inflammatory drugs.	
tendonitis	Inflammation of any tendon from injury or overuse. Treatment: Rest, analgesic drugs, nonsteroidal anti-inflammatory drugs.	**tendonitis** (TEN-doh-NY-tis) **tendon/o-** *tendon* **-itis** *inflammation of; infection of* *Tendinitis* is also an acceptable spelling.
tennis elbow	Inflammation and pain of the extensor and supinator muscles where their tendons originate on the lateral epicondyle of the humerus (by the elbow joint). It is an overuse injury caused by repeated extension and supination of the wrist. It is also known as **lateral epicondylitis.** Treatment: Rest, analgesic drugs, nonsteroidal anti-inflammatory drugs.	
tenosynovitis	Inflammation and pain due to overuse of a tendon and inability of the synovium to produce enough lubricating fluid. Treatment: Rest, analgesic drugs, nonsteroidal anti-inflammatory drugs.	**tenosynovitis** (TEN-oh-SIN-oh-VY-tis) **ten/o-** *tendon* **synov/o-** *synovium (membrane)* **-itis** *inflammation of; infection of*

Laboratory and Diagnostic Procedures

Blood Tests

Word or Phrase	Description	Word Building

acetylcholine receptor antibody test	Detects antibodies that the body produces against its own acetylcholine receptors. It is used to diagnose myasthenia gravis.	**antibody** (AN-tee-BAWD-ee) (AN-tih-BAWD-ee)
		   anti- *against*
		   -body *a structure or thing*

creatine phosphokinase (CPK-MM)	Measures the level of serum CPK-MM, an isoenzyme found in the muscles. A high blood level of CPK-MM is present in various diseases, particularly muscular dystrophy, in which muscle tissue is being destroyed.	**creatine phosphokinase** (KREE-ah-teen FAWS-foh-KY-nays)

Muscle Tests

electromyography (EMG)	Procedure to diagnose muscle disease or nerve damage. A needle electrode inserted into a muscle records electrical activity as the muscle contracts and relaxes. The electrical activity is displayed as waveforms on a screen and recorded on paper as an **electromyogram.**	**electromyography** (ee-LEK-troh-my-AWG-rah-fee)
		   electr/o- *electricity*
		   my/o- *muscle*
		   -graphy *process of recording*
		
		electromyogram (ee-LEK-troh-MY-oh-gram)
		   electr/o- *electricity*
		   my/o- *muscle*
		   -gram *a record or picture*

Tensilon test	Diagnostic procedure in which the drug Tensilon is given to confirm a diagnosis of myasthenia gravis. The drug blocks the enzyme that breaks down acetylcholine, and patients with myasthenia gravis show temporarily increased muscle strength during the test.	**Tensilon** (TEN-sih-lawn)

Medical and Surgical Procedures

Medical Procedures

Word or Phrase	Description	Word Building
braces and adaptive devices	A brace is an orthopedic device that supports a body part that has weak muscles. It keeps the body part in anatomical alignment while still permitting movement (see Figure 9-22 ■). An adaptive or assistive device increases mobility or independence by helping a physically challenged patient to perform activities of daily living (ADLs). Examples of adaptive devices: a grasper to extend the reach, spoons that can be attached to the wrist, and extra-large pens that can be easily grasped. **Did You Know?** The Americans with Disabilities Act (ADA) of 1990 is a federal law that prohibits discrimination against disabled persons. It provides guidelines and requirements for accommodating persons with disabilities at work and in public buildings and transportation vehicles. Instead of *handicapped*, the correct phrase is *physically challenged*.	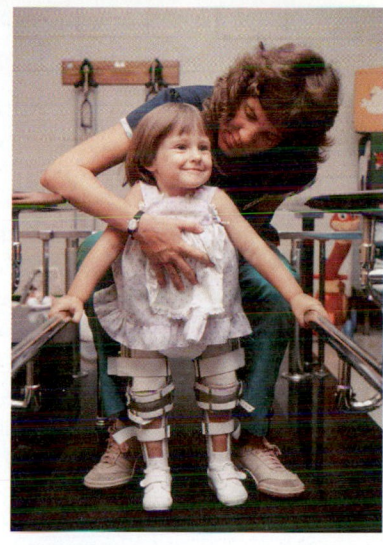 **Figure 9-22 ■ Braces.** Braces provide support and stability when the muscles are weak or uncoordinated. The physical therapist is assisting this young child to walk with leg braces that are held on by Velcro straps.
deep tendon reflexes (DTR)	Tapping briskly on a tendon causes an involuntary, automatic contraction of the muscle connected to that tendon. This tests whether the muscular-nervous pathway is functioning normally. This test can be done in several places, but the most common site is at the knee (see Figure 9-23 ■). It is also known as the **knee jerk** or **patellar reflex.**	**reflex** (REE-fleks)

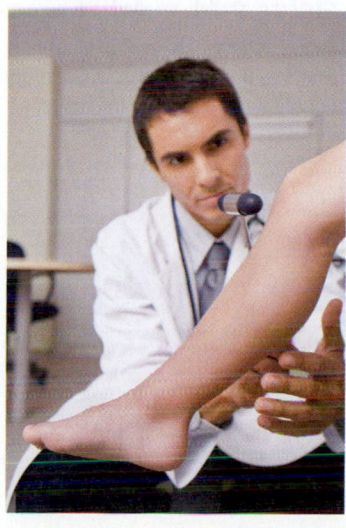

Figure 9-23 ■ Deep tendon reflex.
A percussion hammer with a rounded rubber end is used to tap just below the patella on the combined tendons of the quadriceps femoris muscle group. A normal response is a sudden involuntary contraction of the muscles that briskly extends the lower leg. The response in both legs is tested and compared.

Word or Phrase	Description	Word Building

Word Alert

SOUND-ALIKE WORDS

reflex   (noun)   involuntary, automatic response of the muscular–nervous pathway

Example: The patient's knee jerk reflex was equal and symmetrical bilaterally.

reflux   (noun)   backward flowing of fluid

Example: Acid reflux from the stomach can cause inflammation and ulcers in the esophagus.

Word or Phrase	Description	Word Building
muscle strength test	Procedure used to test the **motor strength** of certain muscle groups. For muscles in the legs and feet, the physician presses against the lower leg or foot and asks the patient to extend the leg or flex the foot upward. For shoulder muscles, the physician presses down and the patient tries to shrug the shoulders. For muscles in the hand, the patient grasps two of the physician's fingers and squeezes them as tightly as possible. Muscle strength is measured on a scale of 0 to 5, with 5 being normal strength and 0 being an inability to move the muscles being tested.	**motor** (MOH-tor) **mot/o-** *movement* **-or** *person or thing that produces or does*
rehabilitation exercises	Physical therapy that includes exercises to increase muscle strength and improve coordination and balance. It is prescribed as part of a rehabilitation plan. In active exercise, the patient exercises without assistance (see Figure 9-24 ■). In passive exercise, a physical therapist or nurse performs range of motion (ROM) exercises for a patient who is unable to move. This does not build muscle strength, but it does decrease stiffness and spasticity and prevent contractures. **Figure 9-24 ■ Active exercise.** These patients are part of a friendly and supportive physical therapy group. Even patients confined to wheelchairs benefit from regular exercise.	**rehabilitation** (REE-hah-BIL-ih-TAY-shun) **re-** *again and again; backward; unable to* **habilitat/o-** *give ability* **-ion** *action; condition* Select the correct prefix meaning to get the definition of *rehabilitation*: *action of again and again (exercises) to give ability.* During rehabilitation, exercises are repeated again and again.
trigger point injections	Procedure to treat fibromyalgia. A combination of a local anesthetic drug and a corticosteroid drug are injected into each trigger point to relieve pain and decrease inflammation.	

Surgical Procedures

Word or Phrase	Description	Word Building
fasciectomy	Procedure to partially or totally remove the fascia that is causing Dupuytren's contracture	**fasciectomy** (FASH-ee-EK-toh-mee) **fasci/o-** *fascia* **-ectomy** *surgical excision*
fasciotomy	Procedure to cut the fascia and release pressure from built-up blood and tissue fluid in a patient with compartment syndrome	**fasciotomy** (FASH-ee-AW-toh-mee) **fasci/o-** *fascia* **-tomy** *process of cutting or making an incision*
ganglionectomy	Procedure to remove a ganglion from a tendon	**ganglionectomy** (GANG-glee-oh-NEK-toh-mee) **ganglion/o-** *ganglion* **-ectomy** *surgical excision*
muscle biopsy	Procedure performed to diagnose muscle weakness that could be caused by many different muscular diseases. An incision is made in the muscle and a piece of tissue is removed; this is an **incisional biopsy** or open biopsy. Alternatively, a needle is inserted and some muscle tissue is aspirated through the needle; this is a closed biopsy.	**biopsy** (BY-awp-see) **bi/o-** *life; living organisms; living tissue* **-opsy** *process of viewing* **incisional** (in-SIH-shun-al) **incis/o-** *to cut into* **-ion** *action; condition* **-al** *pertaining to*
myorrhaphy	Procedure to suture together a torn muscle after an injury	**myorrhaphy** (my-OR-ah-fee) **my/o-** *muscle* **-rrhaphy** *procedure of suturing*
tenorrhaphy	Procedure to suture together a torn tendon after an injury	**tenorrhaphy** (teh-NOR-ah-fee) **ten/o-** *tendon* **-rrhaphy** *procedure of suturing*
thymectomy	Excision of the thymus gland. It is used to treat patients with myasthenia gravis because, after a thymectomy, the patient produces fewer antibodies against acetylcholine receptors.	**thymectomy** (thy-MEK-toh-mee) **thym/o-** *thymus; rage* **-ectomy** *surgical excision* Select the correct combining form meaning to get the definition of *thymectomy: surgical excision of the thymus.*

Drug Categories

These categories of drugs are used to treat muscular diseases and conditions. The most common generic and trade name drugs in each category are listed.

Category	Indication	Examples	Word Building
analgesic drugs	Over-the-counter drugs aspirin and acetaminophen decrease inflammation and pain. They are used to treat minor injuries, muscle strains, tendonitis, bursitis, and muscle overuse. Prescription narcotic drugs are used to treat chronic, severe pain.	aspirin (Bayer, Ecotrin), acetaminophen (Tylenol). Prescription narcotic drugs: meperidine (Demerol), oxycodone (OxyContin), morphine sulfate (MS Contin)	**analgesic** (AN-al-JEE-zik) **an-** *without; not* **alges/o-** *sensation of pain* **-ic** *pertaining to*
beta-blocker drugs	Block the action of epinephrine to suppress essential familial tremor	propranolol (Inderal)	
corticosteroid drugs	Decrease inflammation. They are given orally to treat severe inflammation. Some are injected into the fascia.	dexamethasone (Decadron), hydrocortisone (Cortef, Solu-Cortef), prednisone (Deltasone, Meticorten) Injection into the fascia: betamethasone (Celestone), methylprednisolone (Depo-Medrol), triamcinolone (Aristospan, Kenalog). *Note:* This is often referred to as a "cortisone shot," even though it is actually one or several corticosteroid drugs.	**corticosteroid** (KOR-tih-koh-STAIR-oyd) **cortic/o-** *cortex (outer region)* **-steroid** *steroid*
dopamine stimulant drugs	Stimulate dopamine receptors to treat restless legs syndrome	ropinirole (Requip)	
drugs for fibromyalgia	Include an oral muscle relaxant drug (cyclobenzaprine), injected local anesthetic drugs (lidocaine, procaine), and oral pregabalin.	cyclobenzaprine (Flexeril), lidocaine (Xylocaine), pregabalin (Lyrica), procaine (Novacaine)	
drugs for myasthenia gravis	Inhibit an enzyme that breaks down acetylcholine	neostigmine (Prostigmin), pyridostigmine (Mestinon)	
muscle relaxant drugs	Relieve muscle spasm and stiffness. They are used to treat muscle strains. They are also used to treat muscle spasms in patients with multiple sclerosis, cerebral palsy, and stroke.	carisoprodol (Soma), cyclobenzaprine (Flexeril), methocarbamol (Robaxin)	**relaxant** (ree-LAK-sant) **relax/o-** *relax* **-ant** *pertaining to*

Category	Indication	Examples	Word Building
neuromuscular blocker drugs	Block acetylcholine receptors to prevent muscle contraction. They are used during surgery to produce muscle relaxation, particularly during abdominal surgery to allow visualization of the organs in the abdominal cavity.	atracurium (Tracrium)	**neuromuscular** (NYOOR-oh-MUS-kyoo-lar) **neur/o-** *nerve* **muscul/o-** *muscle* **-ar** *pertaining to*
nonsteroidal anti-inflammatory drugs (NSAIDs)	Decrease inflammation and pain. They are used to treat minor injuries, muscle strains, tendonitis, bursitis, and muscle overuse. Celebrex is a COX-2 inhibitor drug, a type of NSAID that blocks the COX-2 enzyme that produces prostaglandins that cause pain.	celecoxib (Celebrex), diclofenac (Cataflam, Voltaren), ibuprofen (Advil, Motrin), naproxen (Aleve, Naprosyn)	**nonsteroidal** (NON-stair-OY-dal) **non-** *not* **steroid/o-** *steroid* **-al** *pertaining to* **anti-inflammatory** (AN-tee-in-FLAM-ah-TOR-ee) **anti-** *against* **inflammat/o-** *redness and warmth* **-ory** *having the function of*

Clinical Connections

Pharmacology. Some drugs are administered by **intramuscular (IM) injection.** Intramuscular injections are given in a large muscle that is not near a large artery, vein, or nerve. In adults, these sites include the deltoid muscle (lateral upper arm), the vastus lateralis (anterolateral thigh), the gluteus medius muscle (lateral hip), and the gluteus maximus (upper outer quadrant of the buttocks). In infants, the only suitable site for an intramuscular injection is in the anterolateral thigh (see Figure 9-25 ■).

intramuscular (IN-trah-MUS-kyoo-lar)
intra- *within*
muscul/o- *muscle*
-ar *pertaining to*

injection (in-JEK-shun)
inject/o- *insert; put in*
-ion *action; condition*

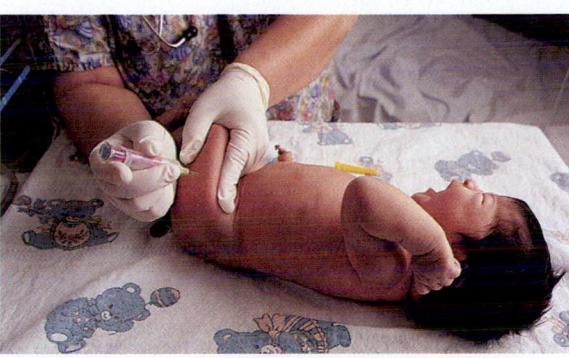

Figure 9-25 ■ Intramuscular injection.
The thigh muscles are the largest muscles in a baby's body, and infant immunizations are injected there.

Abbreviations

ADA	Americans with Disabilities Act		**OOB**	out of bed
ADLs	activities of daily living		**ortho**	orthopedics (slang)
COTA	certified occupational therapy assistant		**OSHA**	Occupational Safety and Health Administration
CPK-MM	creatine phosphokinase (MM bands)		**OT**	occupational therapy or occupational therapist
CTD	cumulative trauma disorder		**PM&R**	physical medicine and rehabilitation
D.C.	Doctor of Chiropracty or Chiropractic Medicine		**PT**	physical therapy or physical therapist
DTRs	deep tendon reflexes		**rehab**	rehabilitation (slang)
EMG	electromyography		**RICE**	rest, ice, compression, and elevation
IM	intramuscular		**RLE**	right lower extremity
LLE	left lower extremity		**ROM**	range of motion
LUE	left upper extremity		**RUE**	right upper extremity
MD	muscular dystrophy		**RSI**	repetitive strain injury
NSAID	nonsteroidal anti-inflammatory drug			

Word Alert

ABBREVIATIONS

Abbreviations are commonly used in all types of medical documents; however, they can mean different things to different people and their meanings can be misinterpreted. Always verify the meaning of an abbreviation.

ADA means *Americans with Disabilities Act*, but it also means *American Diabetes Association*, *American Dental Association*, or *American Dietetic Association*.

MD means *muscular dystrophy*, but it also means *macular degeneration* or *Doctor of Medicine (M.D.)*.

ROM means *range of motion*, but it also means *rupture of membranes* (prior to delivery of a baby).

It's Greek to Me!

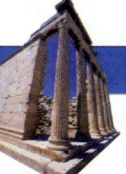

Did you notice that some words have two different combining forms? Combining forms from both Greek and Latin languages remain a part of medical language today.

Word	Greek	Latin	Medical Word Examples
muscle	my/o-	muscul/o-, myos/o-	fibromyalgia, muscular, myositis
tendon	ten/o-	tendin/o-, tendon/o-	tenorrhaphy, tendinous, tendonitis

CAREER FOCUS

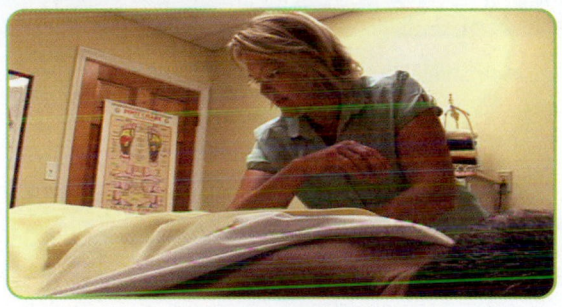

Meet Iris, a massage therapist

"I became a massage therapist because I wanted to help people. I get to see clients that I can honestly say I enjoy, and to see the progress of them, physically—and emotionally, sometimes—is very rewarding. Massage therapy is basically known for its relaxation qualities, but more and more people are understanding that it increases circulation, increases range of motion, and reduces pain. I personally use a lot of medical terminology. I use the names of muscles—origins and insertions. The education involved with massage therapy begins with intense anatomy and physiology. There's a lot of ethics training, a lot of training in dealing with people."

Massage therapists are allied health professionals who use pressure and manipulation of the muscles and soft tissues to relieve stress and prevent or treat muscular injuries. Massage therapists work in athletic clubs, resorts, chiropractic or orthopedic offices, or in their own private offices.

Osteopaths, Doctors of **Osteopathy or Osteopathic Medicine** (D.O.), can diagnose and treat any patient that an orthopedist with an M.D. can treat, but they base their treatment on osteopathy, the study of how to prevent and treat diseases by using proper nutrition and keeping the body structures in a normal anatomical relationship.

Chiropractors, Doctors of **Chiropracty** or **Chiropractic Medicine** (D.C.), diagnose and treat patients with injuries involving the bones, muscles, and nerves by manipulating the alignment of the vertebral column.

Podiatrists, Doctors of **Podiatry** or **Podiatric Medicine** (D.P.M.), diagnose and treat medical and surgical conditions of the foot. **Physiatrists** are physicians who specialize in physical medicine and rehabilitation. **Physiatry** is the medical specialty that diagnoses and treats musculoskeletal diseases and acute and chronic pain by using the physical properties of cold, heat, light, and water in conjunction with exercise and some drugs. It is also known as the field of **physical medicine and rehabilitation (PM&R). Sports medicine** encompasses the prevention, treatment, and rehabilitation of musculoskeletal injuries from sports, as well as athletic training and endurance, biomechanics, nutrition, and psychology. A physician (M.D.) or Doctor of Osteopathy can take additional training and become board certified in physical medicine and rehabilitation or in sports medicine.

---

therapist (THAIR-ah-pist)
  therap/o- treatment
  -ist one who specializes in

osteopath (AW-stee-oh-path)
  oste/o- bone
  -path disease; suffering

osteopathy (AWS-tee-AWP-ah-thee)
  oste/o- bone
  -pathy disease; suffering

chiropractor (KY-roh-PRAK-tor)
  chir/o- hand
  pract/o- medical practice
  -or person or thing that produces or does
Add words to make a complete definition of *chiropractor: person who does (manipulation and alignment of the body by using the) hands (to perform) medical practice.*

chiropractic (KY-roh-PRAK-tic)
  chir/o- hand
  pract/o- medical practice
  -ic pertaining to

podiatrist (poh-DY-ah-trist)
  pod/o- foot
  iatr/o- physician; medical treatment
  -ist one who specializes in

podiatry (poh-DY-ah-tree)
  pod/o- foot
  -iatry medical treatment

podiatric (POH-dee-AT-rik)
  pod/o- foot
  iatr/o- physician; medical treatment
  -ic pertaining to

physiatrist (fih-ZY-ah-trist)
  physi/o- physical function
  iatr/o- physician; medical treatment
  -ist one who specializes in

physiatry (fih-ZY-ah-tree)
  physi/o- physical function
  -iatry medical treatment

PEARSON myhealthprofessionskit™ To see Iris's complete video profile, visit Medical Terminology Interactive at www.myhealthprofessionskit.com. Select this book, log in, and go to the 9th floor of Pearson General Hospital. Enter the Laboratory, and click on the computer screen.

CHAPTER REVIEW EXERCISES

Test your knowledge of the chapter by completing these review exercises. Use the Answer Key at the end of the book to check your answers.

Anatomy and Physiology

Fill in the Blank Exercise

Fill in the blank with the correct word from the word list.

biceps brachii muscle	gluteus maximus muscle	pectoralis major muscle	sternocleidomastoid muscle
biceps femoris muscle	latissimus dorsi muscle	rectus abdominis muscle	tibialis anterior muscle
deltoid muscle	masseter muscle	rectus femoris muscle	trapezius muscle
gastrocnemius muscle			

1. Posterior aspect of lower leg _____

2. On the chest by the sternum _____

3. Triangular muscle on the shoulder _____

4. Side of the back _____

5. Anterior aspect of upper leg _____

6. Anterior neck to behind the ear _____

7. Anterior aspect of upper arm _____

8. Anterior aspect of the lower leg _____

9. On either side of the midline of the abdomen _____

10. Shoulder, back of neck, and down the center of the back _____

11. On the side of the face _____

12. Large muscle in the buttocks _____

13. Posterior aspect of upper leg _____

Circle Exercise

Circle the correct word from the choices given.

1. The (**belly, insertion, origin**) is where the muscle is attached to a stationary bone.

2. The (**aponeurosis, bursa, fascia**) is a flat, wide, white sheet of fibrous connective tissue that attaches a muscle to a bone.

3. The (**muscle, musculature, musculus**) is a group of muscles in one body part.

4. Skeletal muscle is (**involuntary, nonstriated, striated**).

5. Hallux means (**big toe, short in length, three**).

6. The (**deltoid, pectoralis, rectus**) muscle is shaped like a triangle.

7. The prefix (**bi-, quadri-, tri-**) means *three*.

Matching Exercise

Match each word or phrase to its description.

1. acetylcholine
2. actin and myosin
3. aponeurosis
4. calcium ion
5. contraction
6. fascia
7. fascicle
8. muscle fiber
9. neuromuscular junction
10. origin
11. striated
12. tendon

_____ Characteristic of skeletal muscle

_____ Muscle becomes shorter

_____ A neurotransmitter

_____ Area where a nerve cell ends and a muscle fiber begins

_____ Electrolyte that plays a role in muscle contraction

_____ A single cell in a muscle

_____ Thin connective tissue wrapped around a muscle

_____ Beginning of a muscle

_____ Thin and thick strands of protein that slide together as the muscle contracts

_____ Several muscle fibers

_____ Sheet of fibrous tissue that holds muscle to bone

_____ Fibrous cord that holds muscle to bone

Recall and Describe Exercise

In your own words, describe what happens when the stated action occurs to the body part given below.

1. Abduction of the arm _____

2. Extension of the knee _____

3. Pronation of the hand _____

4. Rotation of the head _____

5. Flexion of the knee _____

6. Dorsiflexion of the foot _____

Diseases and Conditions

Matching Exercise

Match each word or phrase to its description or synonym.

1. acceleration–deceleration injury
2. ataxia
3. atrophy
4. contusion
5. cumulative trauma disorder
6. muscular dystrophy
7. polymyalgia
8. torticollis
9. tremor

_____ Wryneck

_____ Incoordination of muscle movement

_____ Bruise

_____ Pain in many muscle groups

_____ Small, involuntary muscle movements

_____ Duchenne's is one type

_____ Repetitive strain injury

_____ Whiplash

_____ Muscle wasting

True or False Exercise

Indicate whether each statement is true or false by writing T or F on the line.

1. _____ Myalgia means inflammation in a muscle.
2. _____ Muscular dystrophy is a genetic disorder.
3. _____ Involuntary muscle jerking is known as bradykinesia.
4. _____ Muscle wasting is also known as muscle atrophy.
5. _____ The two types of muscular dystrophy are Duchenne's and Dupuytren's.
6. _____ Patients with fibromyalgia may also develop rigor mortis.
7. _____ Myasthenia gravis is caused by antibodies that destroy acetylcholine receptors.
8. _____ Golfer's elbow is a type of overuse injury that is similar to pitcher's elbow.
9. _____ A contracture is a fixed state of flexion of a muscle.
10. _____ Muscular dystrophy causes pain at certain trigger points.

Circle Exercise

Circle the correct word from the choices given.

1. (**Ataxia, Atrophy, Contracture**) is a type of movement disorder.
2. A ganglion develops on a (**muscle, nerve, tendon**).
3. A slow, writhing movement of the hand is described as (**athetoid, myalgia, tendonitis**).
4. An injury in which the muscle is torn away from the tendon is a/an (**avulsion, compartment syndrome, contusion**).
5. Which is not a type of muscular dystrophy? (**Becker's, Duchenne's, Dupuytren's**)
6. A (**ganglion, rhabdomyosarcoma, tenosynovitis**) is a malignant tumor of the muscle.

Laboratory, Surgery, and Drugs

Multiple Choice

Circle the best answer.

1. A ganglionectomy is a procedure to surgically remove a _____.
   a. ganglion
   b. fascia
   c. muscle
   d. tendon

2. All of the following are sports-related injuries *except* _____.
   a. shin splints
   b. golfer's elbow
   c. rigor mortis
   d. lateral epicondylitis

3. In which of the following is a piece of muscle tissue removed and examined?
   a. muscle biopsy
   b. trigger point injections
   c. electromyography
   d. CPK-MM

4. Which of the following is a procedure that may need to be performed after a laceration of the hand?
   a. Tensilon test
   b. tenorrhaphy
   c. trigger point injection
   d. muscle biopsy

5. Which of the following is a category of drugs used to relieve muscle spasm?
   a. neuromuscular blocker drugs
   b. muscle relaxant drugs
   c. analgesic drugs
   d. nonsteroidal anti-inflammatory drugs

Circle Exercise

Circle the correct word from the choices given.

1. Trigger point injections are used to treat (**bursitis, fibromyalgia, tendonitis**).

2. Exercises where the therapist moves the extremity for the patient are (**active, passive, rehabilitation**) exercises.

3. A (**muscle biopsy, tenorrhaphy, thymectomy**) is used to treat myasthenia gravis.

4. Surgical procedure to remove a piece of muscle for examination is a/an (**fasciotomy, incisional biopsy, tenorrhaphy**).

Building Medical Words

Review the Combining Forms Exercise and Combining Form and Suffix Exercise that you already completed in the anatomy section on page 450–451.

Combining Forms Exercise

Before you build muscular words, review these additional combining forms. Next to each combining form, write its medical meaning. The first one has been done for you.

Combining Form	Medical Meaning	Combining Form	Medical Meaning
1. alges/o-	sensation of pain	11. iatr/o-	
2. alg/o-		12. inflammat/o-	
3. asthen/o-		13. kines/o-	
4. athet/o-		14. pod/o-	
5. chir/o-		15. rhabd/o-	
6. contus/o-		16. synov/o-	
7. dermat/o-		17. tax/o-	
8. electr/o-		18. therap/o-	
9. ganglion/o-		19. tort/i-	
10. habilitat/o-		20. vuls/o-	

Dividing Medical Words

Separate these words into their component parts (prefix, combining form, suffix). Note: Some words do not contain all three word parts. The first one has been done for you.

Medical Word	Prefix	Combining Form	Suffix	Medical Word	Prefix	Combining Form	Suffix
1. abduction	ab-	duct/o-	-ion	6. gastrocnemius			
2. atrophic				7. myositis			
3. bradykinesia				8. ganglionectomy			
4. deltoid				9. rehabilitation			
5. fascial				10. tenorrhaphy			

Combining Form and Suffix Exercise

Read the definition of the medical word. Select the correct suffix from the Suffix List. Select the correct combining form from the Combining Form List. Build the medical word and write it on the line. Be sure to check your spelling. The first one has been done for you.

SUFFIX LIST	COMBINING FORM LIST	
-clonus (condition of rapid contracting and relaxing) -collis (condition of the neck) -ectomy (surgical excision) -ion (action; condition) -itis (inflammation of; infection of) -oid (resembling) -pathy (disease; suffering) -rrhaphy (procedure of suturing) -tomy (process of cutting or making an incision) -ure (system; result of)	athet/o- (without position or place) burs/o- (bursa) contract/o- (pull together) contus/o- (bruising) fasci/o- (fascia) ganglion/o- (ganglion)	inflammat/o- (redness and warmth) my/o- (muscle) myos/o- (muscle) tendon/o- (tendon) ten/o- (tendon) tort/i- (twisted position)

Definition of the Medical Word

Build the Medical Word

1. Surgical excision of the fascia

   <u>fasciectomy</u>

2. Disease of the muscles

3. Condition of redness and warmth (in a muscle)

4. Result of (a muscle being) pulled together (permanently)

5. Inflammation or infection of the fascia

6. Resembling (purposeless writhing of the muscles) without position or place

7. Process of cutting or making an incision in the fascia

8. Condition of bruising

9. Condition of rapid contracting and relaxing of a muscle

10. Inflammation of a muscle

11. Procedure of suturing a tendon

12. Inflammation of a tendon

13. Surgical excision of a ganglion

14. Procedure of suturing a muscle

15. Inflammation or infection of a bursa

16. Condition of the neck (being in a) twisted position

Prefix Exercise

Read the definition of the medical word. Look at the medical word or partial word that is given (it already contains a combining form and a suffix.) Select the correct prefix from the Prefix List and write it on the blank line. Then build the medical word and write it on the line. Be sure to check your spelling. The first one has been done for you.

PREFIX LIST

a- (away from; without)	dys- (painful; difficult; abnormal)	inter- (between)	re- (again and again;
an- (without; not)	hyper- (above; more than	intra- (within)	backward; unable to)
brady- (slow)	normal)	poly- (many; much)	

Definition of the Medical Word	Prefix	Word or Partial Word	Build the Medical Word
1. Action of again and again giving ability	re-	habilitation	rehabilitation
2. Pertaining to within a muscle	_____	muscular	_____
3. Condition of slow movement	_____	kinesia	_____
4. Condition of (being) without coordination	_____	taxia	_____
5. Action of more than normal straightening	_____	extension	_____
6. Pertaining to (muscles) between the ribs	_____	costal	_____
7. Pertaining to (muscles being) without development	_____	trophic	_____
8. Condition in many muscles of pain	_____	myalgia	_____
9. Condition (of the muscle or tendon) away from (the bone) to tear	_____	vulsion	_____
10. Condition of abnormal movements	_____	kinesia	_____
11. Inflammation or infection of many muscles	_____	myositis	_____
12. Pertaining to (a drug that makes you be) without pain	_____	algesic	_____

Multiple Combining Forms and Suffix Exercise

Read the definition of the medical word. Select the correct suffix and combining forms. Then build the medical word and write it on the line. Be sure to check your spelling. The first one has been done for you.

SUFFIX LIST	COMBINING FORM LIST	
-al (pertaining to)	alg/o- (pain)	myos/o- (muscle)
-alis (pertaining to)	brachi/o- (arm)	neur/o- (nerve)
-ar (pertaining to)	dermat/o- (skin)	pod/o- (foot)
-ia (condition; state; thing)	electr/o- (electricity)	radi/o- (radius; forearm bone)
-ist (one who specializes in)	fibr/o- (fiber)	rhabd/o- (rod shaped)
-itis (inflammation of; infection of)	iatr/o- (physician; medical treatment)	skelet/o- (skeleton)
-graphy (process of recording)	muscul/o- (muscle)	synov/o- (synovium membrane)
-oma (tumor; mass)	my/o- (muscle)	ten/o- (tendon)

Definition of the Medical Word

Build the Medical Word

1. Pertaining to the muscles and skeleton

   musculoskeletal _____

2. Pertaining to (a muscle of the) arm and radius (bone)

   _____

3. Pertaining to nerves and muscles

   _____

4. Inflammation or infection of the skin and muscle

   _____

5. Condition (in which) fibers in the muscles (cause) pain
   (Hint: Use three combining forms.)

   _____

Definition of the Medical Word

Build the Medical Word

6. Process of recording electricity in a muscle

_____

7. (Benign) tumor (with cells) shaped like a rod (that occurs in a) muscle

_____

8. Inflammation or infection of the tendon and synovial membrane

_____

9. One who specializes in (treating the) foot (and is a) physician

_____

Abbreviations

Define and Match Exercise

Give the definition for each abbreviation. Then match it to its correct description.

1. EMG _____   _____ Stimulates a muscle with electricity

2. ADLs _____   _____ An arm

3. NSAID _____   _____ Does strengthening exercises and uses assistive devices

4. RUE _____   _____ Progressive muscle weakness beginning in childhood

5. OT _____   _____ Tasks at home and on the job

6. MD _____   _____ A drug route

7. IM _____   _____ Drug for muscle pain and inflammation

Applied Skills

Proofreading and Spelling Exercise

Read the following paragraph. Identify each misspelled medical word and write the correct spelling of it on the line provided.

Orothopedics is the study of the bones and muscles. A tendin connects the bone to the muscle and the facsia around it. The rectis femoris is in the leg. Fibromialgia has pain at trigger points, while bersitis is inflammation of a fluid-filled sac. A ganglian forms on a tendon. A muscle biopsee is used to diagnose muscular dystrophee. A tenorhaphy sews together a tendon after an injury.

1. _____   6. _____

2. _____   7. _____

3. _____   8. _____

4. _____   9. _____

5. _____   10. _____

English and Medical Word Equivalents Exercise

For each English word, write its equivalent medical word. Be sure to check your spelling. The first one has been done for you.

English Word	Medical Word	English Word	Medical Word
1. housemaid's knee	<u>bursitis</u>	5. whiplash	_____
2. muscle wasting	_____	6. bruise	_____
3. wryneck	_____	7. pitcher's elbow	_____
4. pulled muscle	_____	8. tennis elbow	_____

Medical Report Exercise

This exercise contains two related reports: a hospital Operative Report and a Pathology Report. Read both reports and answer the questions.

OPERATIVE REPORT

PATIENT NAME: PHELPS, George R.

HOSPITAL NUMBER: 42-51-55

DATE OF OPERATION: November 19, 20xx

PREOPERATIVE DIAGNOSIS: Myopathy of undetermined etiology.

POSTOPERATIVE DIAGNOSIS: Myopathy of undetermined etiology.

PROCEDURE: Right quadriceps muscle biopsy.

ANESTHESIA: Xylocaine 1% local anesthetic with I.V. sedation.

SPECIMEN: Muscle biopsy x3.

COMPLICATIONS: None.

CLINICAL HISTORY: The patient is a 68-year-old male who has had progressive lower back and right leg weakness for approximately 6 months. He notes difficulty climbing stairs or getting up from a chair or bed. He moves slowly. There is mild eyelid ptosis noted.

OPERATIVE TECHNIQUE: After the induction of I.V. sedation, the right thigh skin was prepped with Betadine and draped in the usual fashion. After infiltration with local anesthesia, a longitudinal incision was made over the anterolateral aspect of the thigh. The incision was deepened through subcutaneous tissue to the quadriceps fascia, which was incised. Three muscle specimens were obtained for biopsy as per Armed Forces Institute of Pathology (AFIP) protocol. A core of muscle, approximately the thickness of a pencil, was submitted for the first biopsy. Then 2 muscle segments were grasped with biopsy clamps and excised. Pressure was held over the muscle for hemostasis. The wound was irrigated with warm saline solution, and the fascia was reapproximated with 2 interrupted sutures of #2-0 Vicryl. The subcutaneous and subcuticular tissues were approximated with interrupted sutures of #3-0 Vicryl. The skin was approximated with skin staples. A sterile dressing was applied. The patient was transferred to the recovery room in stable condition. Blood loss during the procedure was minimal.

Jamison R. Smith, M.D.

Jamison R. Smith, M.D.

JRS:srd
D: 11/19/xx
T: 11/19/xx

PATHOLOGY REPORT

PATIENT NAME: PHELPS, George R.

HOSPITAL NUMBER: 42-51-55

DATE: November 19, 20xx

OPERATION PERFORMED: Right quadriceps muscle biopsy.

CLINICAL HISTORY: Myopathy.

GROSS SPECIMEN: Received on ice are 3 specimen jars. One is a porcelain jar labeled "without a clamp, for freezing" and it contains a fragment of red-tan muscle wrapped in gauze, 1.2 × 1.0 × 0.7 cm. There are also 2 glass jars. One is labeled "formalin" and within the jar is a large clamp with a fragment of red-tan muscle, 2.2 × 1.3 × 1.3 cm. The other jar is labeled "glutaraldehyde" and contains a small clamp to which is attached a fragment of red-tan muscle measuring about 1.8 × 2.0 × 1.3 cm. All 3 containers are sent on ice to the Armed Forces Institute of Pathology for processing and diagnosis.

MICROSCOPIC SPECIMEN: Biopsy of right quadriceps muscle. Await forthcoming report from the Armed Forces Institute of Pathology.

Ralph A. Stanley, M.D.
_____
Ralph A. Stanley, M.D.

RAS:drc
D: 11/19/xx
T: 11/19/xx

Word Analysis Questions

1. Divide *myopathy* into its two word parts and define each word part.

   Word Part   **Definition**

   _____   _____

   _____   _____

2. Divide *etiology* into its two word parts and define each word part.

   Word Part   **Definition**

   _____   _____

   _____   _____

3. Divide *biopsy* into its two word parts and define each word part.

   Word Part   **Definition**

   _____   _____

   _____   _____

4. Use your medical dictionary to look up the definition of these words.

   glutaraldehyde _____

   protocol _____

Fact Finding Questions

1. What operative procedure was performed?

   _____

2. In what muscle group was this procedure done?

   _____

3. Where is that muscle group located?

   _____

4. How many specimens were taken?

   _____

5. What two ADLs does the report specifically mention that the patient had difficulty doing before surgery?

   _____

   _____

6. What color is the muscle biopsy specimen?

   _____

7. What was this patient's postoperative diagnosis?

   _____

Critical Thinking Skills

1. In what order were these structures encountered when the incision was performed?
   a. Quadriceps muscle, skin, fascia, subcutaneous tissue
   b. Skin, subcutaneous tissue, fascia, quadriceps muscle
   c. Fascia, skin, subcutaneous tissue, quadriceps muscle
2. Formalin and glutaraldehyde are _____.
   a. used to prep and drape the skin
   b. used as preservatives for biopsy specimens
   c. local anesthetic drugs

On the Job Challenge

1. On the job, you will often encounter new medical words. Practice your medical dictionary skills by looking up *muscle* and *musculus* (the Latin word for *muscle*). Which entry has subentries with a full description of each muscle?

   _____

2. Also look up *tendon* and *tendo* (the Latin word for *tendon*). Are these complete lists of all the tendons in the body? Circle the correct answer: **Yes   No**

3. What other anatomical structure might lend its name to a tendon?

   _____

Hearing Medical Words Exercise

You hear someone speaking the medical words given below. Read each pronunciation and then write the medical word it represents. Be sure to check your spelling. The first one has been done for you.

1. BER-sah   <u>bursa</u>
2. AT-roh-fee   _____
3. BRAD-ee-kin-EE-zee-ah   _____
4. ee-LEK-troh-my-AWG-rah-fee   _____
5. FASH-ee-ah   _____
6. GAS-trawk-NEE-mee-us MUS-el   _____
7. my-AL-jee-ah   _____
8. poh-DY-ah-trist   _____
9. REE-hah-BIL-ih-TAY-shun   _____
10. teh-NOR-ah-fee   _____

Pronunciation Exercise

Read the medical word that is given. Then review the syllables in the pronunciation. Circle the primary (main) accented syllable. The first one has been done for you.

1. abduction (ab-(duk)-shun)
2. atrophy (at-roh-fee)
3. chiropractor (ky-roh-prak-tor)
4. fibromyalgia (fy-broh-my-al-jah)
5. hypertrophy (hy-per-troh-fee)
6. intramuscular (in-trah-mus-kyoo-lar)
7. musculoskeletal (mus-kyoo-loh-skel-eh-tal)
8. sterncleidomastoid (ster-noh-kly-doh-mas-toyd)

Multimedia Preview

Immerse yourself in a variety of activities inside Medical Terminology Interactive. Getting there is simple:

1. Click on www.myhealthprofessionskit.com.
2. Select "Medical Terminology" from the choice of disciplines.
3. First-time users must create an account using the scratch-off code on the inside front cover of this book.
4. Find this book and log in using your username and password.
5. Click on Medical Terminology Interactive.
6. Take the elevator to the 9th Floor to begin your virtual exploration of this chapter!

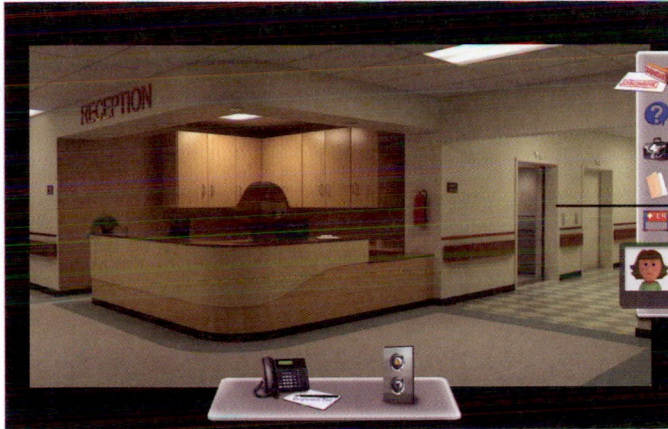
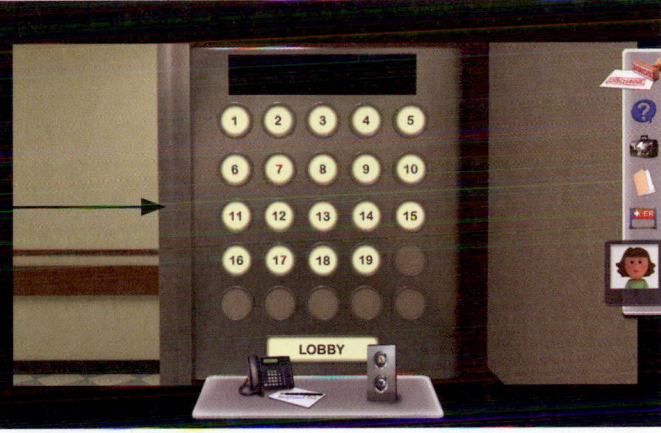

■ **Beat the Clock**   Challenge the clock by testing your medical terminology smarts against time. Click here for a game of knowledge, spelling, and speed. Can you correctly answer 20 questions before the final tick?

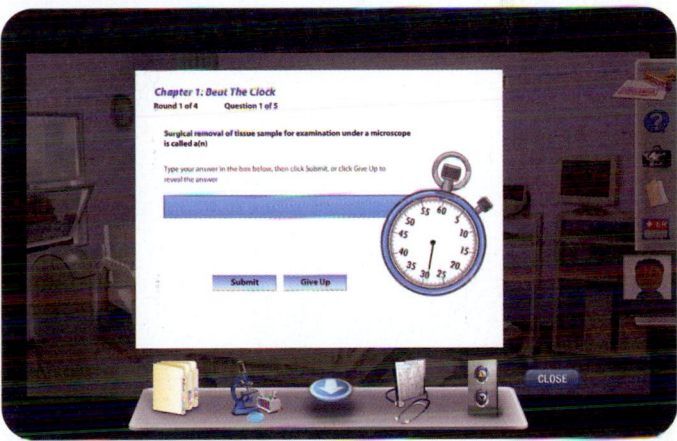

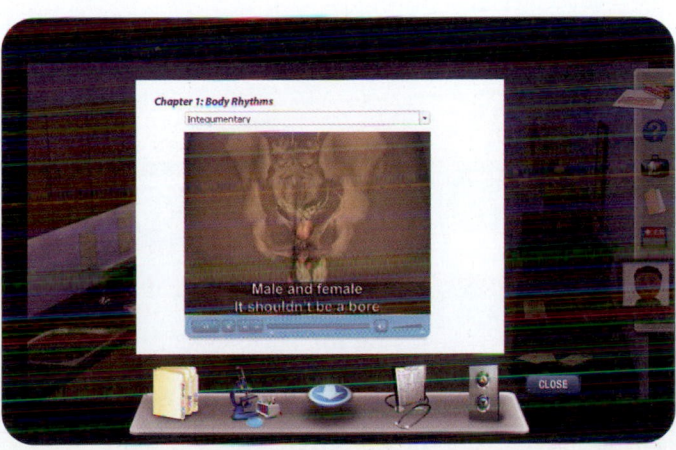

■ **Body Rhythms**   Sing along and learn! We've created a series of original music videos that correspond to each body system. They might not make it to MTV but they'll help you remember basic anatomy and give you a fun study break at the same time.

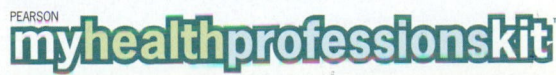

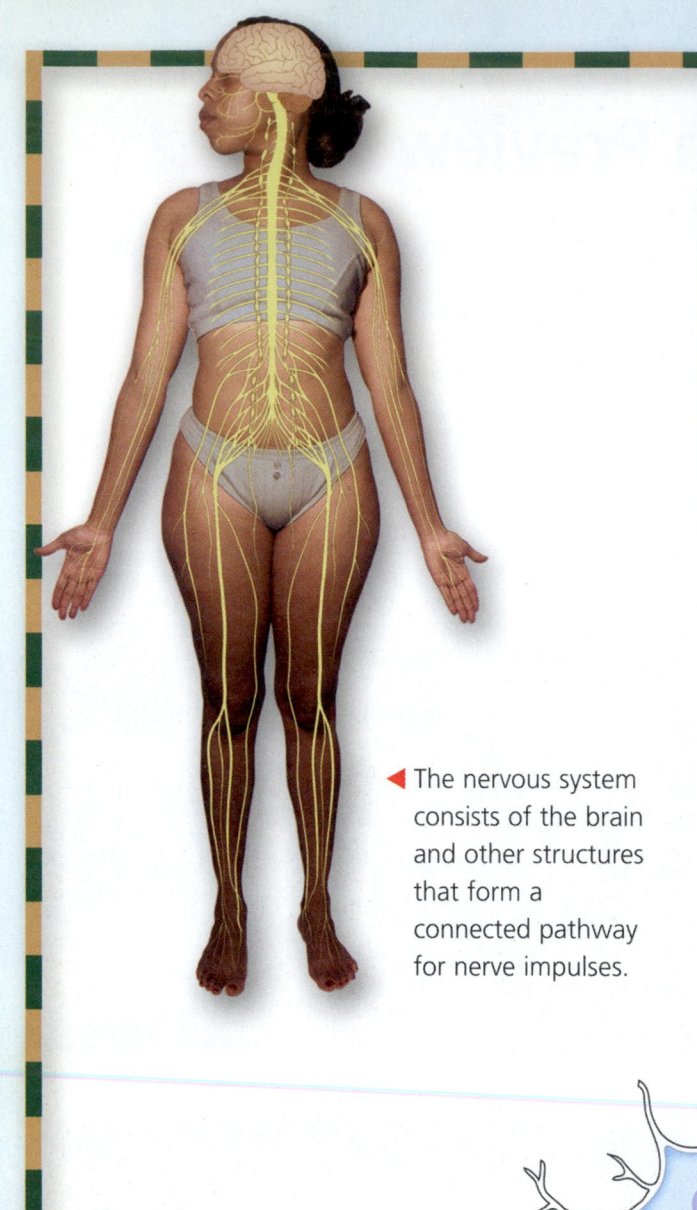

◀ The nervous system consists of the brain and other structures that form a connected pathway for nerve impulses.

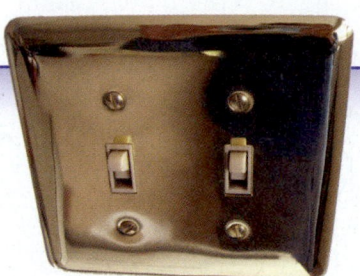

Dive In!

- There are more nerve cells in the human brain than stars in the Milky Way.
- Albert Einstein's brain was found to be no larger than average.
- Do you have the impulse to learn more? In this chapter we'll explore the language that describes nervous system structures, functions, diseases, and conditions.
- You'll get the message once you master the language of neurology!

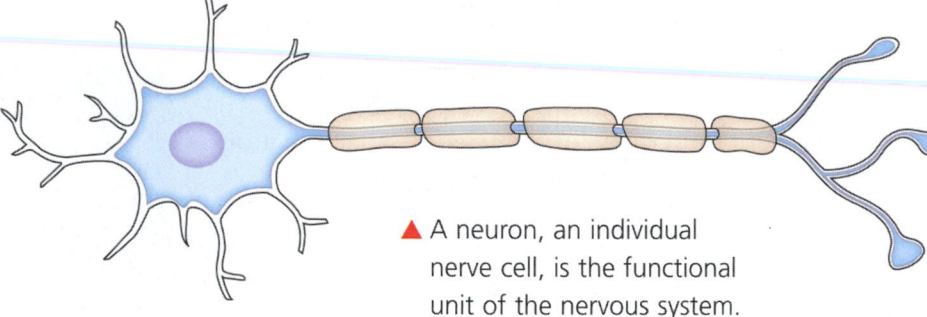

▲ A neuron, an individual nerve cell, is the functional unit of the nervous system.

1912

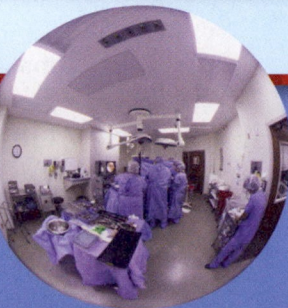

Vitamin A is identified

1913

The American College of Surgeons (ACS) is founded

1913

The x-ray tube is invented by a researcher at General Electric

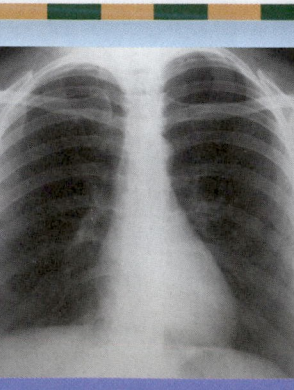

10 Neurology
Nervous System

Neurology (nyoo-RAWL-oh-jee) is the medical specialty that studies the anatomy and physiology of the nervous system and uses diagnostic tests, medical and surgical procedures, and drugs to treat nervous system diseases.

▲ Like a computer motherboard, the nervous system processes, interprets, and sends electrical impulses to control body functions.

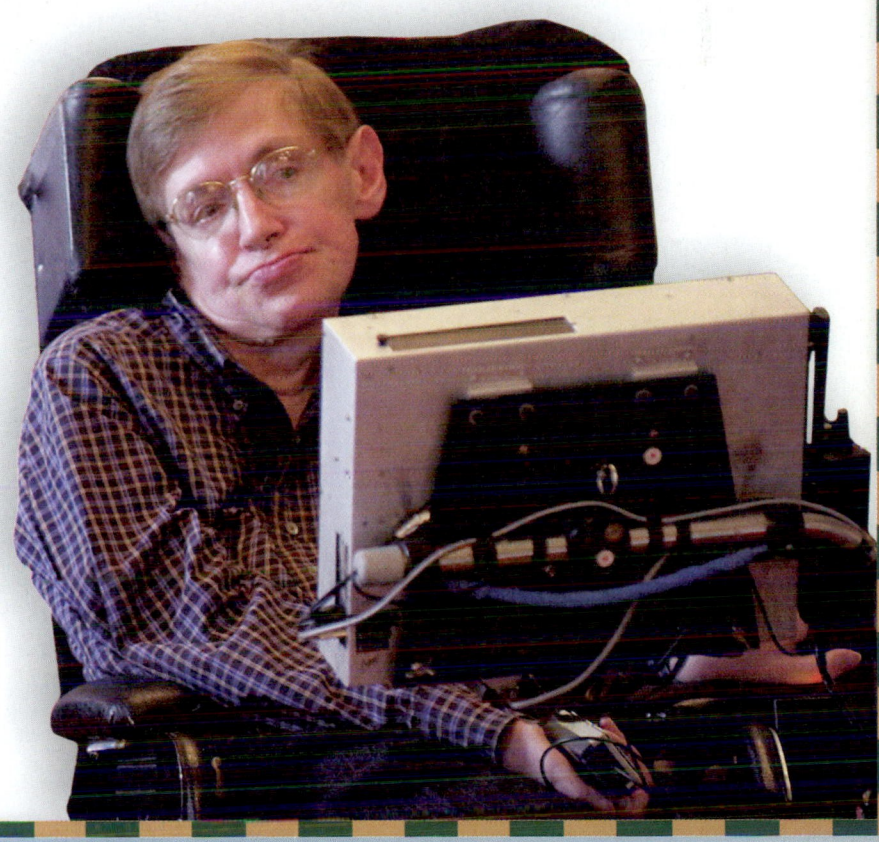

▶ Since 1963, preeminent physicist Stephen Hawking has had a neuromuscular dystrophy that is similar to ALS, a disease of the nervous system that paralyzes motor functions but does not affect mental capacity.

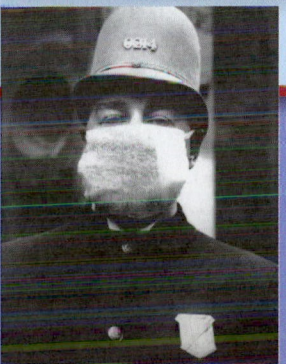

1918

Influenza kills 15 million people around the world

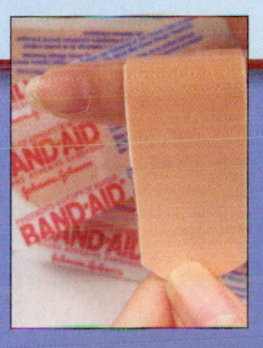

1920

The Band-Aid is invented by an employee of Johnson & Johnson Company

Measure Your Progress: Learning Objectives

After you study this chapter, you should be able to

1. Identify the structures of the nervous system.

2. Describe the process of nerve transmission.

3. Describe common nervous system diseases and conditions, laboratory and diagnostic procedures, medical and surgical procedures, and drug categories.

4. Give the medical meaning of word parts related to the nervous system.

5. Build nervous system words from word parts and divide and define words.

6. Spell and pronounce nervous system words.

7. Analyze the medical content and meaning of a neurology report.

8. Dive deeper into neurology by reviewing the activities at the end of this chapter and online at Medical Terminology Interactive.

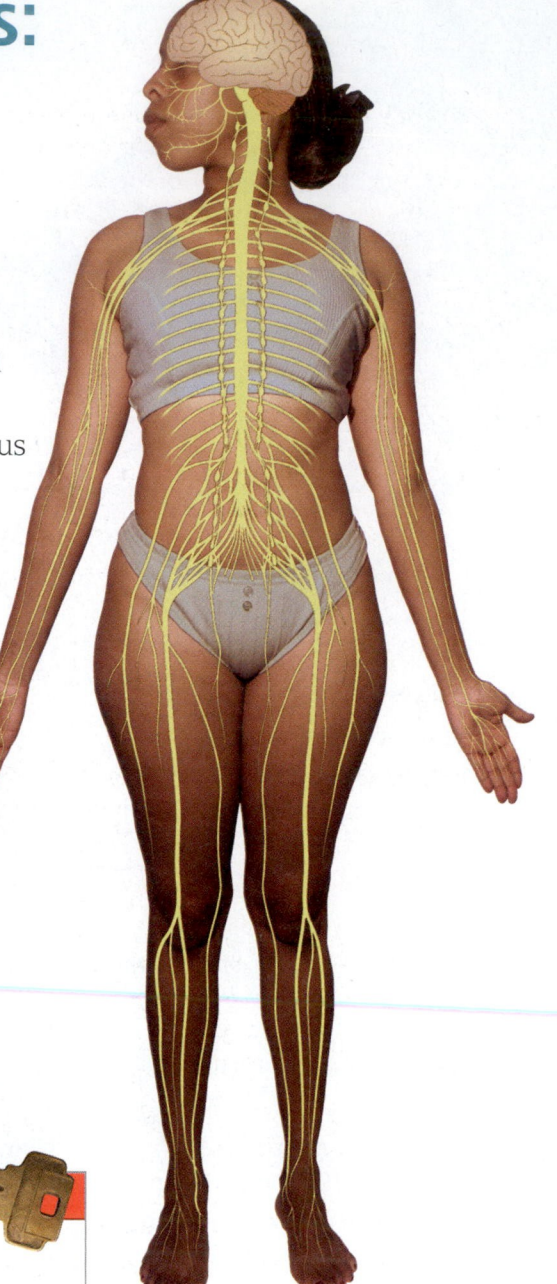

Figure 10-1 ■ **Nervous system.**

The nervous system is a widespread body system that consists of the brain, spinal cord, and nerves that form a connected pathway along which nerve impulses travel throughout the body.

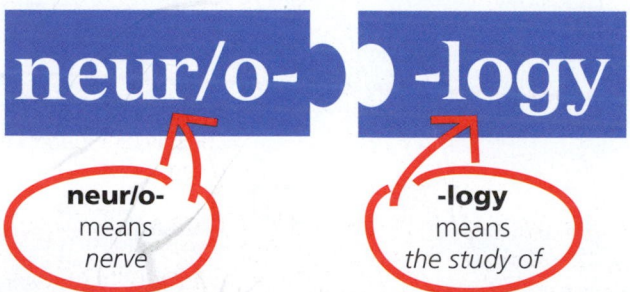

Medical Language Key

To unlock the definition of a medical word, break it into word parts. Define each word part. Put the word part meanings in order, beginning with the suffix, then the prefix (if present), then the combining form(s).

neur/o- ● -logy

neur/o- means *nerve*

-logy means *the study of*

	Word Part	Word Part Meaning
Suffix	-logy	*the study of*
Combining Form	neur/o-	*nerve*

Neurology: *The study of the nerves (and related structures).*

Anatomy and Physiology

The **nervous system** is a body system that is found in every part of the body from the head to the tips of the fingers and toes (see Figure 10-1 ■). The nervous system is divided into the central nervous system (CNS) and the peripheral nervous system (see Figure 10-2 ■). The **central nervous system** contains the brain and the spinal cord. The **peripheral nervous system** contains the cranial nerves and the spinal nerves. The peripheral nervous system can also be further divided into the autonomic nervous system (which includes the parasympathetic and sympathetic divisions) and the somatic nervous system.

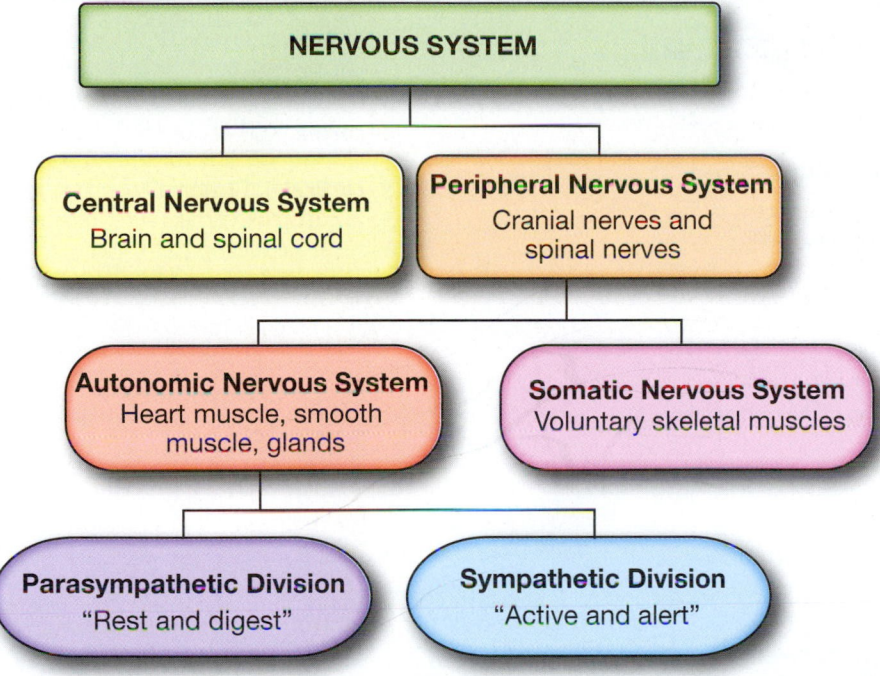

Figure 10-2 ■ **Divisions of the nervous system.**
The two main divisions of the nervous system are the central nervous system and the peripheral nervous system. The peripheral nervous system contains other subdivisions.

Anatomy of the Central Nervous System

Brain

The **brain** is the largest part of the central nervous system. It is located within the bony **cranium** and fills the **cranial cavity.** The brain consists of the cerebrum (and its lobes), the thalamus, hypothalamus, ventricles, brainstem, and cerebellum. The brain is surrounded by the meninges, three layers of membranes (see the following section on Meninges).

Cerebrum The largest and most obvious part of the brain is the **cerebrum** (see Figures 10-3 ■, 10-4 ■, and 10-5 ■). The surface of the cerebrum has elevated folds (**gyri**) and narrow grooves (**sulci**). The **cerebral cortex** or gray matter is the outermost layer of the cerebrum

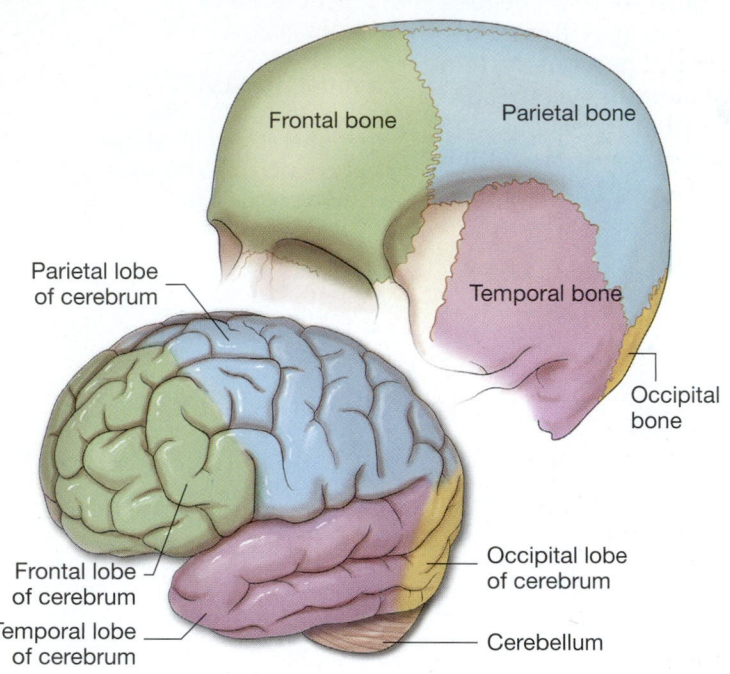

Figure 10-3 ■ **Lobes of the cerebrum.**

Each lobe of the cerebrum takes its name from the bone of the cranium that lies above it.

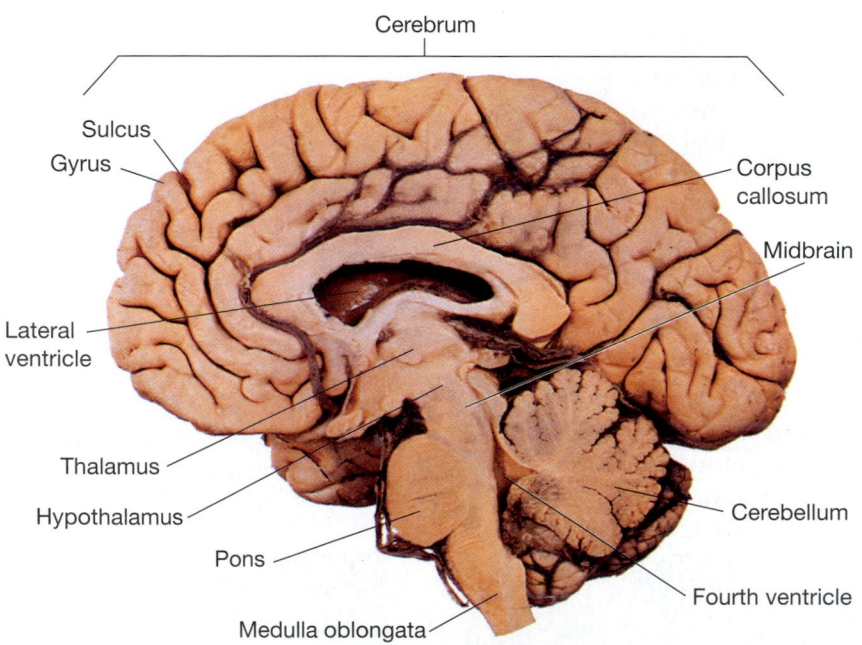

Figure 10-4 ■ **Midline cut section of the brain.**

This cut section shows the right half of the brain. The large size of the cerebrum is seen in comparison to the cerebellum and other structures. Many gyri and sulci are visible on the surface of the cerebrum. The lateral ventricle, thalamus, hypothalamus, midbrain, pons, and medulla oblongata are seen.

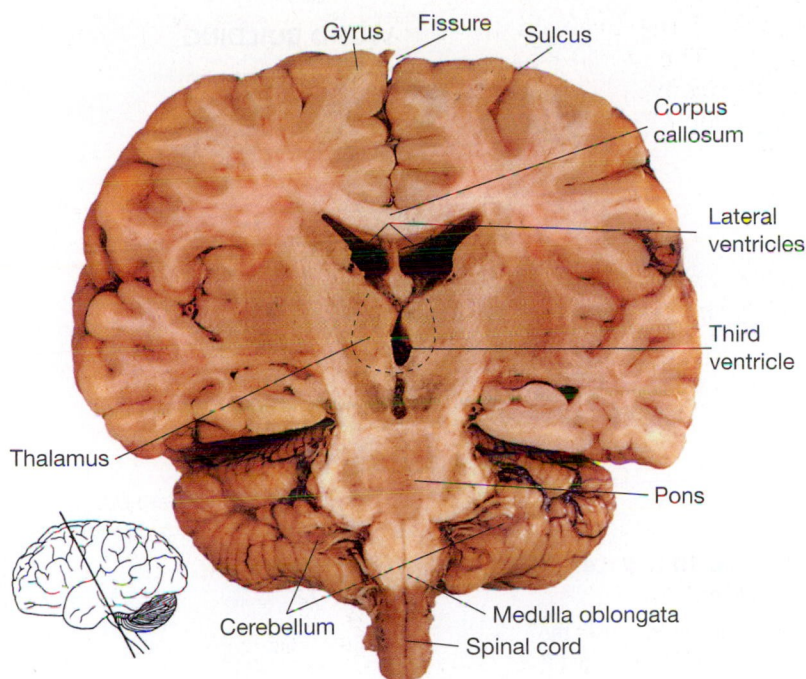

Gyrus Fissure Sulcus

Corpus callosum

Lateral ventricles

Third ventricle

Thalamus

Pons

Cerebellum

Medulla oblongata

Spinal cord

Figure 10-5 ■ Posterior half of the brain.
The anterior part of the cerebrum has been removed. The fissure that divides the right and left hemispheres of the cerebrum can be seen at the top. The corpus callosum is the white connecting bridge between the hemispheres. The right and left lateral ventricles and the small, central third ventricle can be seen. The medulla oblongata, the most posterior part of the brainstem, merges with the spinal cord.

that follows the curves of the gyri and sulci (see Figure 10-7). The gray matter is composed of the cell bodies of neurons. Beneath the gray matter, the white matter of the cerebrum is composed of the axons of neurons. Most of these axons are covered by a fatty, white insulating layer of myelin (that increases the speed at which electrical impulses travel), and it is the myelin that gives the white color to the white matter of the cerebrum.

There is a very deep, anterior-to-posterior **fissure** in the superior surface of the cerebrum. It divides the cerebrum into right and left halves. Each half of the cerebrum is a **hemisphere.** The only connection between the right and left hemispheres is the **corpus callosum.** This connecting arch of neurons deep within the brain allows the two hemispheres to communicate with each other and coordinate their activities. The hemisphere on one side of the brain receives sensory information from the other side of the body and sends motor commands to that side. In general, the right hemisphere of the brain plays an important role in recognizing faces, patterns, and three-dimensional structures. The right hemisphere also analyzes the emotional content of words but not the actual words. The left hemisphere of the brain performs mathematical and logical reasoning and problem solving (see Figure 10-6 ■) and coordinates the recall of memories. It also contains the speech center and is important in language skills.

Each hemisphere of the cerebrum is divided into sections or **lobes.** Each lobe has the same name as the cranial bone that is above it (see Figure 10-3). The lobes of the right and left hemispheres have the following functions.

WORD BUILDING

fissure (FISH-ur)
  fiss/o- splitting
  -ure system; result of

hemisphere (HEM-ih-sfeer)
  hemi- one half
  -sphere sphere; ball
The ending *-sphere* contains the combining form *spher/o-* and the one-letter suffix *-e.*

corpus callosum
(KOR-pus kah-LOH-sum)

lobe (LOHB)

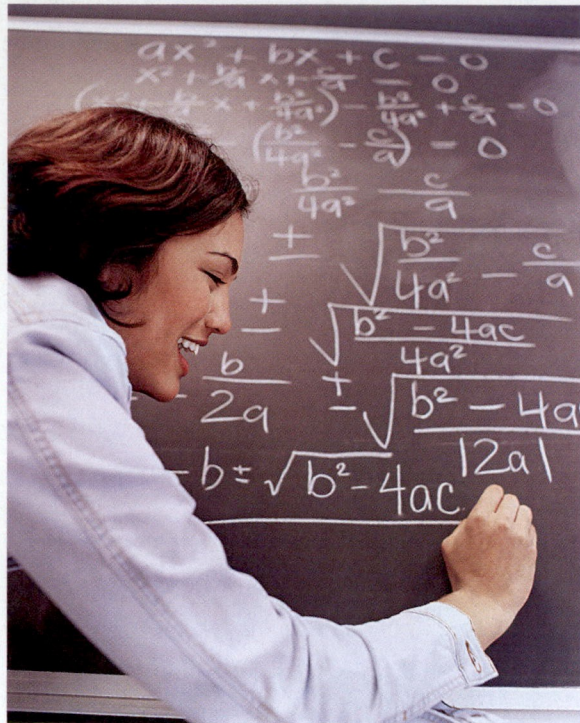

Figure 10-6 ■ Left-brain thinking.

Left-brain thinking uses the left hemisphere, the site of mathematical and logical reasoning.

Frontal Lobe

- Originates conscious thought and intelligence
- Predicts future events and the benefits or consequences of actions
- Coordinates and analyzes information coming from other lobes of the cerebrum
- Exerts conscious, voluntary control over the skeletal muscles
- Coordinates the muscles of the mouth, lips, tongue, pharynx, and larynx to produce speech. This is done in the **speech center,** which is only in the left frontal lobe.

Parietal Lobe

- Analyzes sensory information about touch, temperature, vibration, and pain. This information comes from receptors in the skin, joints, and muscles and is analyzed by the **somatosensory** area of the parietal lobe.
- Analyzes sensory information about taste. This information comes from taste receptors in the tongue and throat and is analyzed by the **gustatory cortex** of the parietal lobe.

Temporal Lobe

- Analyzes sensory information about hearing. This information comes from receptors in the cochlea of the inner ear and is analyzed by the **auditory cortex** of the temporal lobe. (The auditory cortex of the right temporal lobe analyzes sensory information from the left ear, and the auditory cortex of the left temporal lobe analyzes sensory information from the right ear.)
- Analyzes sensory information about smells. This information comes from olfactory receptors in the nose and is analyzed by the **olfactory cortex** of the temporal lobe.

WORD BUILDING

frontal (FRUN-tal)
  front/o- *front*
  -al *pertaining to*

parietal (pah-RY-eh-tal)
  pariet/o- *wall of a cavity*
  -al *pertaining to*

somatosensory
(soh-MAH-toh-SEN-soh-ree)
  somat/o- *body*
  sens/o- *sensation*
  -ory *having the function of*
The combining forms *esthes/o-* and *esthet/o-* also mean *sensation; feeling.*

gustatory (GUS-tah-TOR-ee)
  gustat/o- *the sense of taste*
  -ory *having the function of*

temporal (TEM-poh-ral)
  tempor/o- *temple (side of the head)*
  -al *pertaining to*

auditory (AW-dih-TOR-ee)
  audit/o- *the sense of hearing*
  -ory *having the function of*

olfactory (ol-FAK-toh-ree)
  olfact/o- *the sense of smell*
  -ory *having the function of*

Occipital Lobe

- Analyzes sensory information about vision. This information comes from receptors in the retina of the eye and is analyzed by the **visual cortex** of the occipital lobe. (The visual cortex of the right occipital lobe analyzes sensory information from some parts of both eyes, and the visual cortex of the left occipital lobe analyzes sensory information from the other parts of both eyes, and this gives us three-dimensional vision.)

Thalamus   The **thalamus** is located near the center of the cerebrum (see Figures 10-4 and 10-5). Its two lobes form the walls of the third ventricle. The thalamus acts as a relay station, receiving sensory information (sight, hearing, taste, smell, and touch) from the cranial nerves and the spinal nerves and sending it (1) to the midbrain (that generates motor commands if the sensory information suggests an immediate danger) and (2) to the cerebrum (that analyzes sensory information, compares it with memories, and uses it to plan future actions). The thalamus is also part of the limbic system that deals with emotions (discussed in "Psychiatry," Chapter 17).

Hypothalamus   The **hypothalamus,** as its name indicates, is located below the thalamus (see Figure 10-4). It forms the floor and part of the walls of the third ventricle, and it has a stalk of blood vessels and nerves that connects it to the pituitary gland. The hypothalamus functions as part of both the endocrine system and the nervous system. As part of the endocrine system, the hypothalamus produces hormones that control the functions of the anterior pituitary gland; it also produces other hormones that are stored in and released by the posterior pituitary gland (discussed in "Endocrinology," Chapter 14). As part of the nervous system, the hypothalamus coordinates the activities of the pons and medulla oblongata, which control the heart rate, blood pressure, and respiratory rate. The hypothalamus also regulates body temperature, sensations of hunger and thirst, and the circadian (24-hour) rhythm of the body. The hypothalamus also plays a role in emotions and the sexual drive (discussed in "Psychiatry," Chapter 17).

Ventricles   The **ventricles** are four interconnected cavities within the brain. The largest of these are the lateral ventricles, two C-shaped cavities, one in each hemisphere in the cerebrum (see Figures 10-4 and 10-5). The third ventricle, a narrow central cavity, lies between the two lobes of the thalamus. The fourth ventricle is a long, narrow cavity that connects to the spinal canal. The **ependymal cells** that line the ventricles produce **cerebrospinal fluid (CSF),** a clear, colorless fluid that cushions and protects the brain and contains glucose and other nutrients. Cerebrospinal fluid flows through the ventricles, into the spinal cavity, then back toward the brain, and through the subarachnoid space in the meninges where it is absorbed into the blood of large veins.

Brainstem   The **brainstem** (see Figures 10-4 and 10-5) is a column of tissue that begins in the center of the brain and continues inferiorly until it meets the spinal cord. It is composed of the midbrain, the pons, and the medulla oblongata.

The **midbrain** is the most superior part of the brainstem. It keeps the mind conscious. It coordinates immediate reflex responses to things you see or hear (such as a child suddenly crossing in front of your car or a very loud noise). It maintains muscle tone and the position of the extremities so that you do not have to consciously think about them. It contains the

WORD BUILDING

occipital (awk-SIP-ih-tal)
 occipit/o- *occiput (back of the head)*
 -al *pertaining to*

visual (VIH-shoo-al)
 vis/o- *sight; vision*
 -al *pertaining to*

thalamus (THAL-ah-mus)

thalamic (thah-LAM-ik)
 thalam/o- *thalamus*
 -ic *pertaining to*

hypothalamus (HY-poh-THAL-ah-mus)

hypothalamic (HY-poh-thah-LAM-ik)
 hypo- *below; deficient*
 thalam/o- *thalamus*
 -ic *pertaining to*

ventricle (VEN-trih-kl)

ventricular (ven-TRIK-yoo-lar)
 ventricul/o- *ventricle (lower heart chamber; chamber in the brain)*
 -ar *pertaining to*

ependymal (eh-PEN-dy-mal)
 ependym/o- *cellular lining*
 -al *pertaining to*

cerebrospinal (seh-REE-broh-SPY-nal)
(SAIR-eh-broh-SPY-nal)
 cerebr/o- *cerebrum (largest part of the brain)*
 spin/o- *spine; backbone*
 -al *pertaining to*

brainstem (BRAYN-stem)

substantia nigra, a gray-to-black pigmented area that produces the neuro-transmitter dopamine that regulates muscle tone.

The **pons** is a relay station that links nerve impulses from the spinal cord to the midbrain, hypothalamus, thalamus, and cerebrum.

The **medulla oblongata** is the most inferior part of the brainstem. It contains the respiratory centers that automatically set the respiratory rate, and other centers that control the heart rate. (In the medulla oblongata, nerve tracts cross, and nerve impulses from the right side of the body are relayed to the left side of the cerebrum, and vice versa.)

Cerebellum   The **cerebellum** is the separate rounded section of the brain that lies inferior and posterior to the cerebrum (see Figures 10-3, 10-4, and 10-5). The cerebellum receives sensory information about muscle tone and the position of the body and uses this to help maintain balance. It receives information from the cerebrum about motor commands sent to the body to produce movements and then makes minor adjustments to coordinate those movements.

Meninges   The brain is surrounded by the **meninges,** three separate membrane layers (see Figure 10-7 ■). The outermost membrane (beneath the bony cranium) is the **dura mater,** a tough, fibrous layer that protects the brain. The second layer is the **arachnoid.** Beneath the arachnoid is the **subarachnoid space,** which is filled with cerebrospinal fluid and contains large, branching fibers that connect the arachnoid to the pia mater beneath it. The innermost layer is the **pia mater,** a thin, delicate membrane next to the brain that contains a spider-weblike network of small blood vessels.

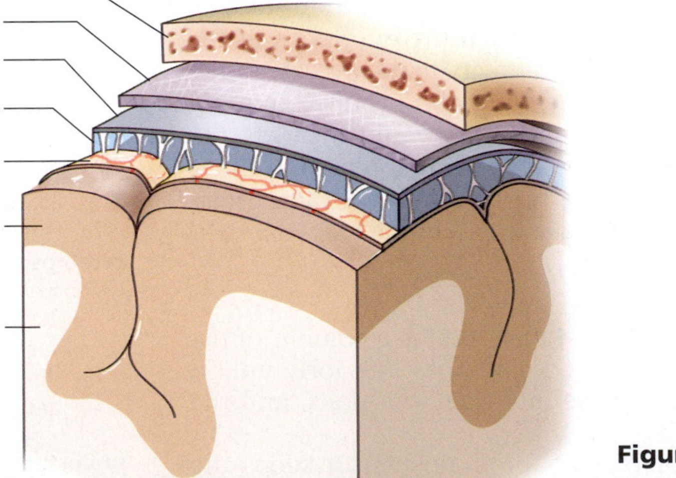

Cranium
Dura mater
Arachnoid
Cerebrospinal fluid
(in subarachnoid space)
Pia mater
Gray matter of
the cerebrum
White matter of
the cerebrum

WORD BUILDING

substantia nigra
(sub-STAN-shee-ah NY-grah)

pons (PAWNZ)

medulla (meh-DUL-ah)
(meh-DOOL-ah)

oblongata (AWB-long-GAW-tah)

cerebellum (SAIR-eh-BEL-um)

cerebellar (SAIR-eh-BEL-ar)
 cerebell/o- *cerebellum (posterior part of the brain)*
 -ar *pertaining to*

meninges (meh-NIN-jeez)
Meninx, the singular form, is seldom used.

meningeal (meh-NIN-jee-al)
(MEN-in-JEE-al)
 mening/o- *meninges*
 -eal *pertaining to*
The combining form *meningi/o-* also means *meninges.*

dura mater (DOO-rah MAY-ter)
(DOO-rah MAH-ter)

dural (DOO-ral)
 dur/o- *dura mater*
 -al *pertaining to*

arachnoid (ah-RAK-noyd)
 arachn/o- *spider; spider web*
 -oid *resembling*

subarachnoid (SUB-ah-RAK-noyd)
 sub- *below; underneath; less than*
 arachn/o- *spider; spider web*
 -oid *resembling*

pia mater (PY-ah MAY-ter)
(PEE-ah MAH-ter)

Figure 10-7 ■ Meninges.

The three membrane layers of the dura mater, arachnoid, and pia mater make up the meninges. Between the arachnoid and the pia mater is the subarachnoid space, which is filled with cerebrospinal fluid.

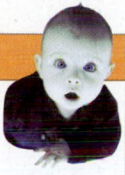

Spinal Cord

The **spinal cord** is part of the central nervous system. The spinal cord is a long, narrow column of neural tissue within the **spinal cavity** or **spinal canal.** At its superior end, the spinal cord joins the medulla oblongata of the brain. The spinal cord extends to the level of the second lumbar vertebra in the spinal column. There, at its inferior end, the spinal cord becomes a group of nerve roots known as the **cauda equina.** The spinal cord is protected because it is within the central opening (foramen) of each bony vertebra (see Figure 10-8 ■). The spinal cord is also protected and nourished by the meninges, which continue in an uninterrupted fashion from around the brain. A narrow canal at the center of the spinal cord is lined with ependymal cells that also produce cerebrospinal fluid. There is one difference between the meninges around the brain and those around the spinal cord: between the dura mater and the bony vertebrae is the **epidural space,** an area that is unique to the spinal cord. This space is filled with fatty tissue and blood vessels.

The gray matter of the spinal column is composed of the cell bodies of neurons in the spinal cord and spinal nerves. The white matter of the spinal column is composed of the axons of neurons bundled together as an ascending tract that carries sensory information from a sensory spinal nerve to the brain or as a descending tract that carries motor commands from the brain to a motor spinal nerve connected to a muscle.

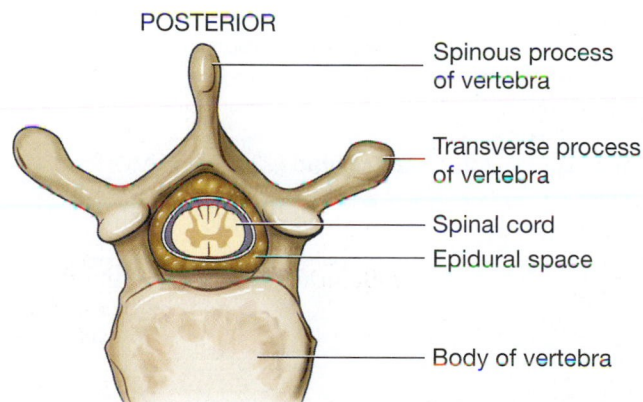

POSTERIOR

Spinous process of vertebra

Transverse process of vertebra

Spinal cord

Epidural space

Body of vertebra

Figure 10-8 ■ Spinal cord.
The spinal cord passes through the foramen of each vertebra. It is protected by the bony foramen as well as by the dura mater of the meninges.

Anatomy of the Peripheral Nervous System

Cranial Nerves

The **cranial nerves** are part of the peripheral nervous system (see Table 10-1). There are 12 pairs of cranial nerves. Each pair consists of a cranial nerve to the right side of the body and a cranial nerve to the left side of the body. Each pair of cranial nerves has a name that reflects its location or function. Some cranial nerves receive **sensory** information from the body (e.g., visual images, sounds, smells, tastes, touch, pressure, vibration, temperature, pain, or position). Other cranial nerves send **motor** commands from the brain to voluntary muscles (e.g., to move the face, head, and neck) or to involuntary muscles (e.g., to slow the heart rate, to cause peristalsis in the digestive tract, to cause the bronchioles to constrict, to cause the lacrimal or salivary glands to secrete tears or saliva). Some cranial nerves carry both sensory and motor nerve impulses.

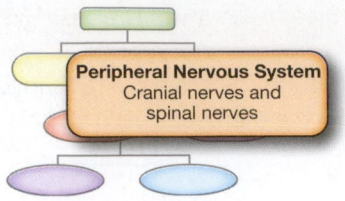

Peripheral Nervous System
Cranial nerves and spinal nerves

WORD BUILDING

cranial (KRAY-nee-al)
  crani/o- *cranium (skull)*
  -al *pertaining to*

sensory (SEN-soh-ree)
  sens/o- *sensation*
  -ory *having the function of*

motor (MOH-tor)
  mot/o- *movement*
  -or *person or thing that produces or does*

Table 10-1　Cranial Nerves

Cranial Nerve	Type of Nerve	Function	Location	Word Building

I olfactory nerve	sensory	Receives sensory information about smells from olfactory receptors in the nose	Begins at receptors in the nose
			Goes to the olfactory bulb (and on to the olfactory cortex) in the temporal lobe
				olfactory (ol-FAK-toh-ree)
				  olfact/o- *the sense of smell*
				  -ory *having the function of*

II optic nerve	sensory	Receives sensory information about light, dark, and color from rods and cones in the retina of the eye	Begins at receptors in the retina
			Goes to the optic chiasm in the brain
				optic (AWP-tik)
				  opt/o- *eye; vision*
				  -ic *pertaining to*

III oculomotor nerve	motor	Sends motor commands to four of the extraocular muscles to move the eye
		Sends motor commands to move the eyelid and to move muscles of the iris to increase or decrease the diameter of the pupil
			Begins in the midbrain (of the brainstem)
			Goes to four of the six extraocular muscles around the eye
			Goes to the eyelid
			Goes to the iris
				oculomotor (AWK-yoo-loh-MOH-tor)
				  ocul/o- *eye*
				  mot/o- *movement*
				  -or *person or thing that produces or does*

IV trochlear nerve	motor	Sends motor commands to one of the extraocular muscles to move the eye	Begins in the midbrain (of the brainstem)
			Goes to one of the extraocular muscles around the eye
				trochlear (TROH-klee-ar)
				  trochle/o- *structure shaped like a pulley*
				  -ar *pertaining to*
				At the top of the bony eye socket, there is a loop of ligament that is attached to bone at both ends. When a nerve impulse from the trochlear nerve stimulates the superior oblique muscle, it contracts, pulling its tendon through the loop like the rope of a pulley, and this moves the eye.

Table 10-1   Cranial Nerves   (continued)

Cranial Nerve	Type of Nerve	Function	Location	Word Building
V trigeminal nerve	**sensory**	Receives sensory information about touch, temperature, vibration, and pain from the skin of the forehead, eyelids, eyebrows, face, nose, and lips, and from the nasal cavity, oral cavity, gums, teeth, tongue, and palate	Begins at receptors in the skin and mucous membranes of those areas Goes to the pons (of the brainstem)	**trigeminal** (try-JEM-ih-nal) **tri-** *three* **gemin/o-** *set or group* **-al** *pertaining to* The trigeminal nerve is composed of three different branches: the ophthalmic, maxillary, and mandibular nerves.
	motor	Sends motor commands to move the muscles for chewing	Begins in the pons (of the brainstem) Goes to the lower jaw (mandibular branch of the nerve)	
VI abducens nerve	**motor**	Sends motor commands to one of the extraocular muscles to move the eye	Begins in the pons (of the brainstem) Goes to one of the extraocular muscles around the eye	**abducens** (ab-DOO-senz)
VII facial nerve	**sensory**	Receives sensory information about taste (sweet, sour, bitter, etc.) from taste receptors in the front of the tongue	Begins at receptors in the tongue Goes to the pons (of the brainstem)	**facial** (FAY-shal) **faci/o-** *face* **-al** *pertaining to*
	motor	Sends motor commands to move the facial muscles Contracts the lacrimal glands to secrete tears Contracts the submandibular and sublingual salivary glands to secrete saliva	Begins in the pons (of the brainstem) Goes to the facial muscles Goes to the muscles in the lacrimal glands Goes to the muscles in the submandibular and sublingual salivary glands	
VIII vestibulocochlear nerve	**sensory**	Receives sensory information about sounds (loudness and pitch) from the cochlea (in the inner ear) Receives sensory information from the semicircular canals about the position of the head to keep the balance of the body	Begins at receptors in the vestibule (entrance to the cochlea) and in the semicircular canals in the inner ear Goes to the pons and medulla oblongata (of the brainstem)	**vestibulocochlear** (ves-TIB-yoo-loh-KOH-klee-ar) **vestibul/o-** *vestibule (entrance)* **cochle/o-** *cochlea (of the inner ear)* It is also known as the **auditory nerve.** **auditory** (AW-dih-TOR-ee) **audit/o-** *the sense of hearing* **-ory** *having the function of*

(continued)

Table 10-1 Cranial Nerves *(continued)*

Cranial Nerve	Type of Nerve	Function	Location	Word Building
IX glossopharyn-geal nerve	sensory	Receives sensory information about taste (sweet, sour, bitter, etc.) from taste receptors at the back of the tongue, palate, and pharynx Receives sensory information about the blood pressure and the levels of oxygen and carbon dioxide in arterial blood from pressure receptors in the carotid artery	Begins at receptors in the tongue, palate, and pharynx Begins at receptors in the carotid artery Goes to the medulla oblongata (of the brainstem)	**glossopharyngeal** (GLAWS-oh-phah-RIN-jee-al) **gloss/o-** *tongue* **pharyng/o-** *pharynx (throat)* **-eal** *pertaining to*
	motor	Sends motor commands to move the muscles involved in swallowing Contracts the parotid gland to secrete saliva	Begins in the medulla oblongata (of the brainstem) Goes to muscles in the pharynx and parotid gland	
X vagus nerve	sensory	Receives sensory information about taste (sweet, sour, bitter, etc.) from taste receptors in the soft palate and pharynx Receives sensory information about touch, temperature, vibration, and pain from receptors in the ear, diaphragm, and organs in the thoracic cavity and abdominopelvic cavity	Begins at receptors in the soft palate and pharynx Begins at receptors in the skin and smooth muscles Goes to the medulla oblongata (of the brainstem)	**vagus** (VAY-gus) **vagal** (VAY-gal) **vag/o-** *wandering; vagus nerve* **-al** *pertaining to* The vagus nerve travels farther into the body than any cranial nerve.
	motor	Sends motor commands to slow the heart rate Contracts smooth muscle around the bronchi Contracts smooth muscle in the gastrointestinal tract to produce peristalsis	Begins in the medulla oblongata (of the brainstem) Goes to the heart muscle and involuntary smooth muscles around the bronchi, blood vessels, esophagus, stomach, and intestines	
XI accessory nerve	motor	Sends motor commands to move the muscles involved in swallowing Moves the vocal cords Moves the muscles of the neck and upper back	Begins in the medulla oblongata (of the brainstem) Goes to muscles in the pharynx, larynx, neck, and upper back	**accessory** (ak-SES-oh-ree) **access/o-** *supplemental or contributing part* **-ory** *having the function of* The accessory nerve has two branches that supplement the work of the vagus nerve.
XII hypoglossal nerve	motor	Sends motor commands to move the tongue	Begins in the medulla oblongata (of the brainstem) Goes to the muscles of the tongue	**hypoglossal** (HY-poh-GLAWS-al) **hypo-** *below; deficient* **gloss/o-** *tongue* **-al** *pertaining to*

Spinal Nerves

WORD BUILDING

The **spinal nerves** are part of the peripheral nervous system because they are found in the periphery of the body (those parts away from the center). There are 31 pairs of spinal nerves that originate at regular intervals along the spinal cord. Each pair consists of a spinal nerve to the right side of the body and a spinal nerve to the left side of the body. Each pair of spinal nerves is named according to the vertebra next to it.

Each spinal nerve has two different groups of nerve roots that connect it to the spinal cord: dorsal nerve roots and ventral nerve roots (see Figure 10-9 ■).

spinal (SPY-nal)
spin/o- *spine; backbone*
-al *pertaining to*

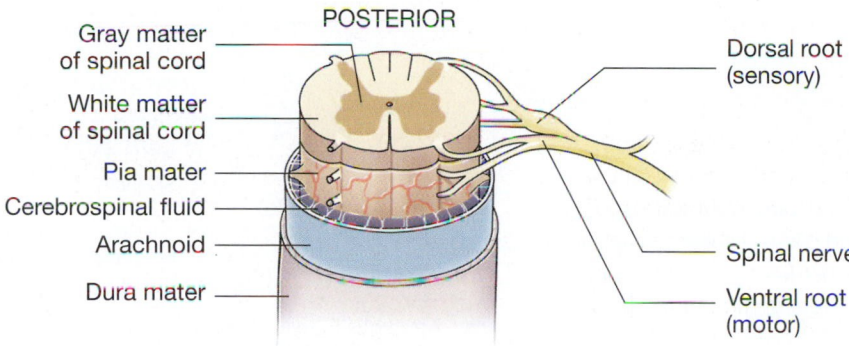

Figure 10-9 ■ Spinal nerves.
The spinal nerves originate at regular intervals along the spinal column. Each spinal nerve consists of dorsal nerve roots that receive sensory information from the body and ventral nerve roots that carry motor commands to the body.

The posterior or **dorsal nerve roots** receive sensory information (touch, pressure, vibration, temperature, pain, and body position) from the skin. Each dorsal nerve root receives sensory information from a specific area of the skin known as a dermatome (discussed in "Dermatology," Chapter 7) (see Figure 7-3). Dermatomes are important in the diagnosis of nerve injuries because they correlate a specific spinal nerve and its dermatome to an area of the skin where there is loss of sensation or movement. The dorsal nerve roots also receive sensory information from the muscles and joints.

The anterior or **ventral nerve roots** carry motor commands from the spinal cord to skeletal muscles and involuntary smooth muscles within organs, glands, and other structures.

Dorsal nerve roots and their spinal nerve are categorized as an **afferent nerve** because they carry nerve impulses to the spinal cord. Ventral nerve roots and their spinal nerve are categorized as an **efferent nerve** because they carry nerve impulses from the spinal cord to the body.

A **reflex** is a rapid, involuntary muscle reaction that is controlled by the spinal cord. The spinal cord reacts immediately to certain types of sensory information (sudden pain or when a physician uses a percussion hammer to tap on a tendon and that stretches a muscle) (see Figure 9-23). For example, accidentally placing your hand on a hot stove causes you to pull your hand away, even before your brain understands what is wrong. Sensory information from a spinal nerve in the hand reached the spinal cord, and the spinal cord immediately sent a motor command to muscles to make you move your hand. This circuit is known as a **reflex arc.** Later, the sensory information is analyzed by the brain, and you say "Ouch."

dorsal (DOR-sal)
dors/o- *back; dorsum*
-al *pertaining to*

nerve root (NERV ROOT)
The combining forms *radicul/o-* and *rhiz/o-* also mean *spinal nerve root.*

ventral (VEN-tral)
ventr/o- *front; abdomen*
-al *pertaining to*

afferent (AF-eh-rent)
affer/o- *bring toward the center*
-ent *pertaining to*

efferent (EF-eh-rent)
effer/o- *go out from the center*
-ent *pertaining to*

reflex (REE-fleks)

Neurons and Neuroglia

All of the structures of the nervous system are composed of neural tissue. **Neural tissue** is made up of two categories of cells: neurons and neuroglia.

A **neuron,** an individual nerve cell, is the functional unit of the nervous system. **Nerves** are bundles of individual nerve cells (neurons).

Neuroglia are the other category of neural tissue. Neuroglia do not generate or conduct electrical impulses like neurons do. However, their role in the function of the nervous system is very important. Neuroglia perform specialized tasks to help neurons do their work (see Table 10-2). Cancers of the nervous system arise from the neuroglia, not from the neurons.

WORD BUILDING

neural (NYOOR-al)
  neur/o- *nerve*
  -al *pertaining to*

neuron (NYOOR-on)
  neur/o- *nerve*
  -on *a substance; structure*

nerve (NERV)
The combining forms *nerv/o-* and *neur/o-* mean *nerve.*

neuroglia (nyoo-ROH-glee-ah)
  neur/o- *nerve*
  -glia *cells that provide support*

Table 10-2   Neuroglia

Cell Name	Cell Description and Function	Word Building

astrocytes	Cells with branches that radiate outward like a star. They support the dendrites of neurons and connect them to capillaries. Astrocytes form the blood–brain barrier that keeps certain harmful substances in the blood from getting to the brain.	**astrocyte** (AS-troh-site)
		  astr/o- *starlike structure*
		  -cyte *cell*

ependymal cells	Cells that line the ventricles of the brain, the spinal cavity, and the narrow, central canal within the spinal cord and produce cerebrospinal fluid	**ependymal** (ep-EN-dih-mal)
		  ependym/o- *cellular lining*
		  -al *pertaining to*

microglia	Cells that move throughout the tissues of the brain and spinal cord. They engulf and destroy dead tissue and pathogens (bacteria, viruses, etc.). Microglia are the smallest of all the neuroglia.	**microglia** (my-KROHG-lee-ah)
		  micr/o- *one millionth; small*
		  -glia *cells that provide support*

oligodendroglia	Cells that provide structural support and produce myelin that surrounds the larger axons of neurons in the brain and spinal cord	**oligodendroglia** (OL-ih-GOH-den-DROHG-lee-ah)
		  olig/o- *scanty; few*
		  dendr/o- *branching structure*
		  -glia *cells that provide support*
		Add words to make a complete definition of *oligodendroglia: cells that provide support (to a neuron but have) few branching structures.*

Schwann cells	Cells that produce myelin that surrounds the larger axons of neurons of the cranial nerves and the spinal nerves	**Schwann** (SHVAHN)

Somatic Nervous System

The **somatic nervous system** controls the voluntary movements of skeletal muscles. Cranial nerves and spinal nerves send nerve impulses as motor commands to skeletal muscles and cause them to contract. These motor commands are the result of conscious thoughts in the brain, and the movements produced are voluntary movements. For example, if you decide to open this book and begin studying, your brain sends nerve impulses as motor commands through specific spinal nerves to the skeletal muscles in your arms and hands, and you open the book and find the correct page. Then your brain sends nerve impulses as motor commands through specific cranial nerves to the extraocular muscles of the eyes, and your eyes move across the page as you read.

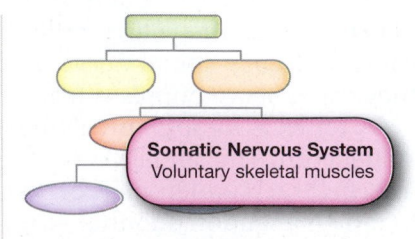

Somatic Nervous System
Voluntary skeletal muscles

somatic (soh-MAT-ik)
  somat/o- *body*
  -ic *pertaining to*

Autonomic Nervous System

The **autonomic nervous system** controls the involuntary contractions of cardiac muscle in the heart, as well as smooth muscles around organs, glands, and other structures. The autonomic nervous system can be further broken down into two divisions: the parasympathetic division and the sympathetic division.

The **parasympathetic division** is active when the body is sleeping, resting, eating, or doing light activity (so-called "rest and digest" activities). The neurotransmitter of the parasympathetic division is acetylcholine. The action of the parasympathetic division and acetylcholine is to

- Decrease the heart rate, blood pressure, and metabolic rate
- Increase or decrease the diameter of the pupils in response to changing levels of light
- Increase peristalsis in the gastrointestinal tract
- Cause the secretion of saliva, digestive enzymes, and insulin
- Prepare the body for sexual activity
- Contract the bladder for urination.

The **sympathetic division** is active when the body is active or exercising. The neurotransmitter of the sympathetic division is norepinephrine. The action of the sympathetic division and norepinephrine is to

- Increase mental alertness
- Dilate the pupils to increase the amount of light entering the eye to optimize vision
- Increase the heart rate and metabolic rate
- Cause the smooth muscles in the arteries to contract to raise the blood pressure
- Cause the smooth muscles in the bronchioles to relax to increase air flow to the lungs
- Increase the respiratory rate
- Cause the skeletal muscles and liver to release glycogen (stored glucose) to meet increased energy needs.

During stress, anxiety, fear, or anger, the hypothalamus sends nerve impulses to the sympathetic division which then stimulates the adrenal medulla to secrete the hormone epinephrine into the blood to prepare the body for more intense activity as in "fight or flight."

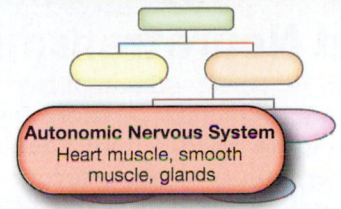

Physiology of a Neuron and Neurotransmitters

A neuron consists of three parts: dendrites, the cell body, and an axon (see Figure 10-10 ■). The **dendrites** are multiple branching structures at the beginning of the neuron. The cell body contains the **nucleus** of the neuron, which directs cellular activities. The cell body also contains **cytoplasm;** structures in the cytoplasm produce neurotransmitters as well as energy for the neuron. The **axon** is an elongated extension of cytoplasm at the end of the neuron. At the tip of the axon are vesicles that

WORD BUILDING

dendrite (DEN-dryt)
  dendr/o- *branching structure*
  -ite *thing that pertains to*

nucleus (NYOO-klee-us)

cytoplasm (SY-toh-plasm)
  cyt/o- *cell*
  -plasm *growth; formed substance*

axon (AK-sawn)

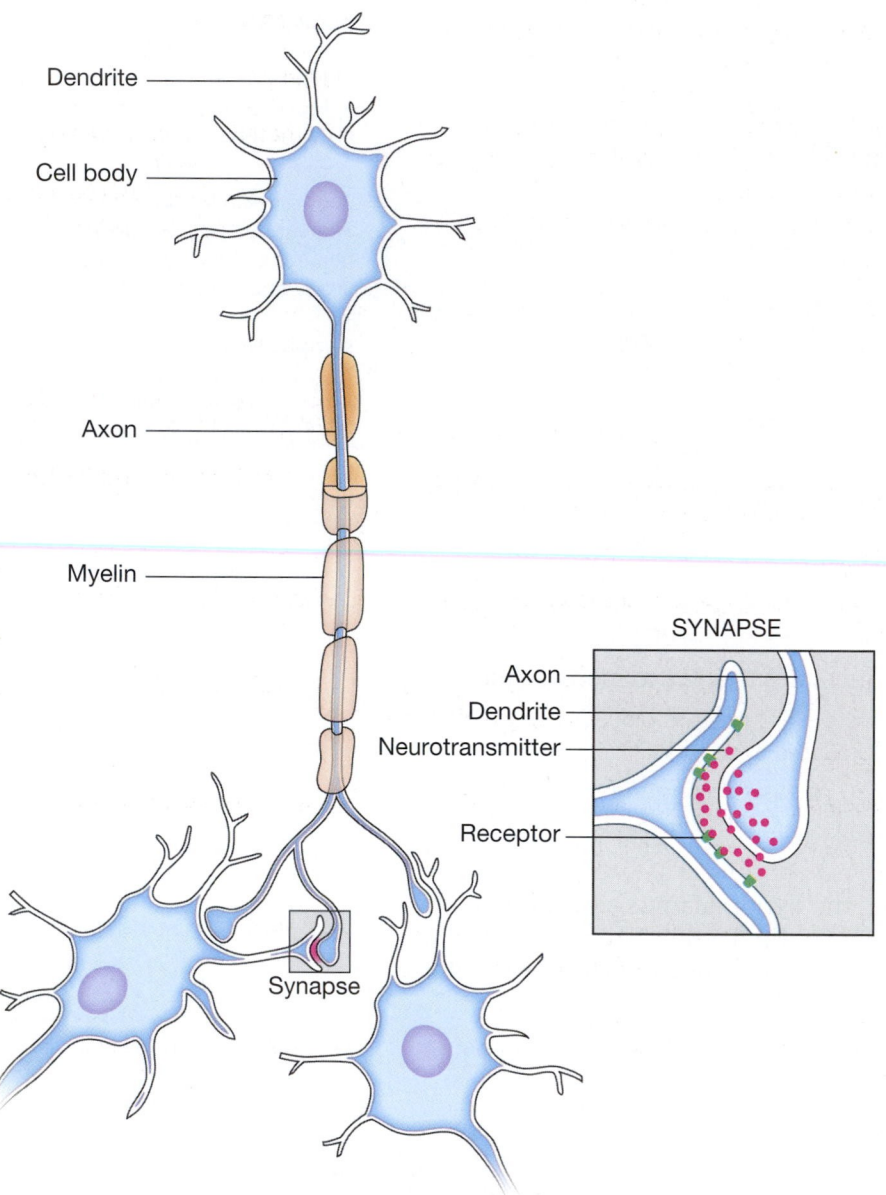

Dendrite

Cell body

Axon

Myelin

Synapse

SYNAPSE

Axon
Dendrite
Neurotransmitter
Receptor

Figure 10-10 ■ **Neuron.**
A neuron consists of several dendrites, a cell body, and an axon. The dendrites receive nerve impulses from other neurons. The cell body contains the nucleus of the neuron. The axon transmits nerve impulses to other neurons (or to a muscle fiber, to a cell in an organ, or to a cell in a gland).

store a neurotransmitter. The axon of one neuron does not connect directly to the dendrites of the next neuron. Instead, there is a space or **synapse** between the two neurons. There is also a synapse between a neuron and other structures, such as the cell of a muscle, organ, or gland.

A neuron is able to (1) generate an electrical impulse when stimulated, (2) conduct that electrical impulse throughout its length, and (3) change that electrical impulse into a chemical substance (neurotransmitter). An electrical impulse is relayed from one neuron to the next neuron in the following way. An electrical impulse travels along the dendrite, cell body, and to the end of the axon. The electrical impulse cannot travel across the synapse, and so vesicles in the axon release a **neurotransmitter** stored inside of them. The neurotransmitter is a chemical messenger that travels across the synapse and binds with a **receptor** on the cell membrane of a dendrite of the next neuron (or the cell membrane of a muscle, organ, or gland). This causes a change in the cell membrane that produces an electrical impulse that travels along that dendrite, etc. All of these events happen in a fraction of a second. The presence of myelin dramatically increases the speed at which an electrical impulse can travel along the axon. Larger axons are covered by a fatty, white insulating layer of **myelin** and are said to be myelinated. Smaller axons do not have myelin.

There are many different neurotransmitters in the nervous system. The most common ones are described in Table 10-3.

WORD BUILDING

synapse (SIN-aps)

neurotransmitter
(NYOOR-oh-TRANS-mit-er)
  neur/o- *nerve*
  transmitt/o- *to send across or through*
  -er *person or thing that produces or does*

receptor (ree-SEP-tor)
  recept/o- *receive*
  -or *person or thing that produces or does*

myelin (MY-eh-lin)

myelinated (MY-eh-lih-NAYT-ed)
  myelin/o- *myelin*
  -ated *pertaining to a condition; composed of*

Table 10-3   Neurotransmitters

Neurotransmitter	Location	Word Building
acetylcholine	Neurotransmitter in synapses between neurons of the parasympathetic division. It is also in the somatic nervous system in synapses between a motor neuron and a voluntary skeletal muscle.	**acetylcholine** (AS-ee-til-KOH-leen)
dopamine	In the brain in synapses between neurons in the cerebral cortex, hypothalamus, midbrain, and limbic system	**dopamine** (DOH-pah-meen)
endorphins	In the brain in synapses between neurons in the hypothalamus, thalamus, and brainstem. Endorphins are neuromodulators, one of several natural pain relievers produced by the brain.	**endorphins** (en-DOR-finz)
epinephrine	Secreted by the adrenal medulla and released into the blood. It stimulates neurons in the sympathetic division during times of anxiety, fear, or anger to prepare the body for "fight or flight."	**epinephrine** (EP-ih-NEF-rin)
norepinephrine	Major neurotransmitter of the sympathetic division. It is also found in synapses between neurons in the cerebral cortex, hypothalamus, cerebellum, brainstem, and spinal cord.	**norepinephrine** (NOR-ep-ih-NEF-rin)
serotonin	In synapses between neurons of the limbic system, hypothalamus, cerebellum, and spinal cord	**serotonin** (SAIR-oh-TOH-nin)

Vocabulary Review

Anatomy and Physiology

Word or Phrase	Description	Combining Forms
afferent nerves	Nerves that carry sensory nerve impulses from the body to the brain (or from the body to the spinal cord)	**affer/o-** *bring toward the center*
autonomic nervous system	Division of the peripheral nervous system that carries nerve impulses to the heart, involuntary smooth muscles, and glands. It includes the parasympathetic division and the sympathetic division.	**autonom/o-** *independent; self-governing*
central nervous system	Division of the nervous system that includes the brain and the spinal cord	**nerv/o-** *nerve*
efferent nerves	Nerves that carry motor nerve impulses from the brain to the body (or from the spinal cord to the body)	**effer/o-** *go out from the center*
nervous system	Body system that consists of the brain, spinal cord, cranial nerves, and spinal nerves. It receives nerve impulses from the body and sends nerve impulses to the body. It includes the central nervous system and the peripheral nervous system. The nervous system is made of **neural tissue**.	**nerv/o-** *nerve* **neur/o-** *nerve*
parasympathetic division	Division of the autonomic nervous system. It uses the neurotransmitter acetylcholine. It directs the activity of the heart, involuntary smooth muscles, and glands while the body is at rest.	**pathet/o-** *suffering*
peripheral nervous system	Division of the nervous system that includes the cranial nerves and the spinal nerves	**peripher/o-** *outer aspects*
receptor	Structure on the cell membrane of a dendrite (or on a muscle, organ, or gland) where a neurotransmitter binds	**recept/o-** *receive*
reflex	Involuntary muscle reaction that is controlled by the spinal cord. In response to sudden pain or muscle stretch, the spinal cord immediately sends a command to move. All of this takes place without conscious thought or processing by the brain. The entire circuit that the nerve impulse travels is also known as a **reflex arc**.	
somatic nervous system	Division of the peripheral nervous system that controls the movements of voluntary skeletal muscles	**somat/o-** *body*
sympathetic division	Division of the autonomic nervous system. It uses the neurotransmitter norepinephrine. It directs the activity of the heart, involuntary muscles, and glands during times of increased activity. During danger or stress ("fight or flight"), it stimulates the adrenal medulla to release the hormone epinephrine into the blood.	**pathet/o-** *suffering*

Brain

Word or Phrase	Description	Combining Forms
arachnoid	Thin, middle layer of the meninges that contains a spider-weblike network of fibers that go into the subarachnoid space	**arachn/o-** *spider; spiderweb*
auditory cortex	Area in the temporal lobe of the cerebrum that analyzes sensory information from receptors in the cochlea to give the sense of hearing	**audit/o-** *the sense of hearing*
brain	Largest organ of the nervous system. It is part of the central nervous system and is located in the cranial cavity.	**encephal/o-** *brain*

Word or Phrase	Description	Combining Forms
brainstem	Most inferior part of the brain that joins with the spinal cord. It is composed of the midbrain, pons, and medulla oblongata.	
cerebellum	Small, rounded structure that is the most posterior part of the brain. It monitors muscle tone and position and coordinates new muscle movements.	cerebell/o- cerebellum (posterior part of the brain)
cerebral cortex	The outermost surface of the cerebrum. It consists of gray matter that contains the cell bodies of neurons.	cortic/o- cortex (outer region)
cerebrospinal fluid	Clear, colorless fluid that circulates through the subarachnoid space, around the brain, through the ventricles, and through the spinal cavity. It cushions and protects the brain and contains glucose and other nutrients. It is produced by the ependymal cells that line the ventricles in the brain and are in the central canal in the spinal cord.	cerebr/o- cerebrum (largest part of the brain) spin/o- spine; backbone
cerebrum	The largest and most visible part of the brain. Its surface contains gyri and sulci, and it is divided into two hemispheres.	cerebr/o- cerebrum (largest part of the brain)
corpus callosum	Connecting band of neurons between the two hemispheres of the cerebrum that allows them to communicate and coordinate their activities	
cranial cavity	Hollow cavity inside the cranium that contains the brain	crani/o- cranium (skull) cav/o- hollow space
cranium	Rounded dome of bone at the top of the skull	crani/o- cranium (skull)
dura mater	Tough, outermost layer of the meninges. The dura mater lies just beneath the bones of the cranium and within the foramen of each vertebra.	dur/o- dura mater
fissure	Deep division that runs in an anterior-to-posterior direction through the cerebrum and divides it into right and left hemispheres	fiss/o- splitting
frontal lobe	Lobe of the cerebrum that predicts future events and consequences. Exerts conscious control over the skeletal muscles. Contains the gustatory cortex for the sense of taste.	front/o- front
gustatory cortex	Area in the frontal lobe of the cerebrum that analyzes sensory information from taste receptors in the tongue to give the sense of taste	gustat/o- the sense of taste
gyrus	One of many large elevated folds of brain tissue on the surface of the cerebrum with smaller folds on the cerebellum. In between each gyrus is a sulcus (groove).	
hemisphere	One half of the cerebrum. The right hemisphere recognizes patterns and three-dimensional structures (including faces) and the emotions of words. The left hemisphere deals with mathematical and logical reasoning, analysis, and interpreting sights, sounds, and sensations. The left hemisphere is active in reading, writing, and speaking.	
hypothalamus	Area in the center of the brain just below the thalamus that coordinates the activities of the pons and medulla oblongata. It also controls heart rate, blood pressure, respiratory rate, body temperature, sensations of hunger and thirst, and the circadian rhythm. It also produces hormones as part of the endocrine system; it has a stalk of tissue that connects it to the pituitary gland of the endocrine system.	thalam/o- thalamus
lobe	Large area of the cerebrum. Each lobe is named for the bone of the cranium that is above it: frontal lobe, parietal lobe, temporal lobe, and occipital lobe.	

Word or Phrase	Description	Combining Forms
medulla oblongata	Most inferior part of the brainstem that joins to the spinal cord. It relays nerve impulses from the cerebrum to the cerebellum. It contains the respiratory centers. Cranial nerves IX through XII originate here.	
meninges	Three separate membranes that envelope and protect the entire brain and spinal cord. The meninges include the dura mater, arachnoid, and pia mater.	**mening/o-** *meninges* **meningi/o-** *meninges*
midbrain	Most superior part of the brainstem. It keeps the mind conscious, coordinates immediate responses, and maintains muscle tone and body position. It contains the substantia nigra. Cranial nerves III and IV originate here.	
occipital lobe	Lobe of the cerebrum that receives and analyzes sensory information from the eyes. Contains the visual cortex for the sense of sight.	**occipit/o-** *occiput (back of the head)*
olfactory cortex	Area in the temporal lobe of the cerebrum that analyzes sensory information from receptors in the nose to give the sense of smell	**olfact/o-** *the sense of smell*
parietal lobe	Lobe of the cerebrum that receives and analyzes sensory information about temperature, touch, pressure, vibration, and pain from the skin and internal organs	**pariet/o-** *wall of a cavity*
pia mater	Thin, delicate, innermost layer of the meninges. It covers the surface of the brain and contains many small blood vessels.	
pons	Middle area of the brainstem that relays nerve impulses from the spinal cord to the midbrain, hypothalamus, thalamus, and cerebrum. Cranial nerves V through VII originate here.	
somatosensory area	Area of the parietal lobe of the cerebrum that analyzes sensory information (touch, temperature, vibration, and pain) from receptors in the skin, joints, and muscles	**somat/o-** *body* **esthes/o-** *sensation; feeling* **esthet/o-** *sensation; feeling*
subarachnoid space	Space beneath the arachnoid layer of the meninges. It is filled with cerebrospinal fluid.	**arachn/o-** *spider; spider web*
substantia nigra	A darkly pigmented area in the midbrain of the brainstem that produces the neurotransmitter dopamine	
sulcus	Groove between two gyri on the surface of the cerebrum and cerebellum	
temporal lobe	Lobe of the cerebrum that analyzes sensory information. It contains the auditory cortex for the sense of hearing and the olfactory cortex for the sense of smell.	**tempor/o-** *temple (side of the head)*
thalamus	Area in the center of the brain that acts as a relay station. It takes sensory nerve impulses from the body and sends them to areas in the cerebrum.	**thalam/o-** *thalamus*
ventricle	One of four hollow chambers in the brain that contains cerebrospinal fluid. The two lateral ventricles are in the right and left hemispheres of the cerebrum. The small third ventricle is between the two lobes of the thalamus. The long, narrow fourth ventricle connects to the spinal cavity.	**ventricul/o-** *ventricle (lower heart chamber; chamber in the brain)*
visual cortex	Area in the occipital lobe of the cerebrum that analyzes sensory information from receptors in the retina of each eye to give the sense of sight	**vis/o-** *sight; vision*

Spinal Cord

Word or Phrase	Description	Combining Forms
cauda equina	Group of nerve roots that begin where the spinal cord ends and continue inferiorly within the spinal cavity. They look like the tail (cauda) of a horse (equine).	
epidural space	Area between the dura mater and the vertebral body. It is filled with fatty tissue and blood vessels.	**dur/o-** *dura mater*
spinal cavity	Hollow cavity within each vertebra. It contains the spinal cord. It also known as the **spinal canal.**	**spin/o-** *spine; backbone* **cav/o-** *hollow space*
spinal cord	Part of the central nervous system. It begins at the medulla oblongata of the brain and extends down the back within the spinal cavity. It ends at lumbar vertebra L2 and separates into nerve roots (cauda equina).	**spin/o-** *spine; backbone* **myel/o-** *bone marrow; spinal cord; myelin*

Cranial Nerves

Word or Phrase	Description	Combining Forms
abducens nerve	Cranial nerve VI. Movement of the eye.	
accessory nerve	Cranial nerve XI. Movement of the muscles for swallowing, the vocal cords, and muscles of the neck and upper back. Two of its nerve branches also assist the vagus nerve.	**access/o-** *supplemental or contributing part*
cranial nerves (I–XII)	Twelve pairs of nerves that originate in the brain. They carry **sensory** nerve impulses to the brain or **motor** nerve impulses from the brain.	**crani/o-** *cranium (skull)* **sens/o-** *sensation* **mot/o-** *movement*
facial nerve	Cranial nerve VII. Sense of taste from the front of the tongue. Control of the salivary and lacrimal glands. Movement of the facial muscles.	**faci/o-** *face*
glossopharyngeal nerve	Cranial nerve IX. Sense of taste from the back of the tongue. Movement of the muscles for swallowing. It controls the parotid salivary glands.	**gloss/o-** *tongue* **pharyng/o-** *pharynx (throat)*
hypoglossal nerve	Cranial nerve XII. Movement of the tongue.	**gloss/o-** *tongue*
oculomotor nerve	Cranial nerve III. Movement of the eyeball, eyelids, and iris (to change the diameter of the pupil).	**ocul/o-** *eye* **mot/o-** *movement*
olfactory nerve	Cranial nerve I. Sense of smell.	**olfact/o-** *the sense of smell*
optic nerve	Cranial nerve II. Sense of vision.	**opt/o-** *eye; vision*
trigeminal nerve	Cranial nerve V. Sensation in the eyelids, scalp, face, lips, and tongue. Movement of the muscles for chewing. It consists of three branches: ophthalmic nerve, maxillary nerve, mandibular nerve.	**gemin/o-** *set or group*
trochlear nerve	Cranial nerve IV. Movement of the eyeball.	**trochle/o-** *structure shaped like a pulley*
vagus nerve	Cranial nerve X. Sensation of taste from the soft palate and throat. Sensation in the ears, diaphragm, and the internal organs of the chest and abdomen. It controls the beating of the heart and the smooth muscles in the bronchi and GI tract.	**vag/o-** *wandering; vagus nerve*
vestibulocochlear nerve	Cranial nerve VIII. Sense of hearing and balance. It is also known as the **auditory nerve.**	**vestibul/o-** *vestibule (entrance)* **cochle/o-** *cochlea (of the inner ear)* **audit/o-** *the sense of hearing*

Spinal Nerves

Word or Phrase	Description	Combining Forms
dorsal nerve roots	Group of spinal nerve roots that enter the posterior (dorsal) part of the spinal cord and carry sensory nerve impulses from the body to the spinal cord	dors/o- back; dorsum radicul/o- spinal nerve root rhiz/o- spinal nerve root
spinal nerves	Thirty-one pairs of nerves. Each pair joins the spinal cord in the area between two vertebrae. An individual spinal nerve consists of dorsal nerve roots and ventral nerve roots.	spin/o- spine; backbone
ventral nerve roots	Group of spinal nerve roots that exit from the anterior (ventral) part of the spinal cord and carry motor nerve impulses to the body	ventr/o- front; abdomen

Neurons

axon	Part of the neuron that is a single, elongated branch at the opposite end from the dendrites. It conducts the electrical impulse and releases neurotransmitters into the synapse. Larger axons are covered by an insulating layer of myelin.	
cytoplasm	Area in the cell body of a neuron that contains structures that produce neurotransmitters and energy for the neuron	cyt/o- cell
dendrite	Multiple branches at the beginning of a neuron that receive a neurotransmitter and convert it to an electrical impulse	dendr/o- branching structure
myelin	Fatty sheath around a larger axon. It is an insulating layer that is important for the conduction of electrical impulses. An axon with myelin is said to be myelinated. Myelin around larger axons in the brain and spinal cord is produced by oligodendroglia. Myelin around larger axons in the cranial and spinal nerves is produced by the Schwann cells.	myelin/o- myelin
nerve	A bundle of individual neurons	nerv/o- nerve
neuron	An individual nerve cell. The functional part of the nervous system.	neur/o- nerve
nucleus	Structure in the cell body of a neuron that directs cellular activities	
synapse	Space between the axon of one neuron and the dendrites of the next neuron. Space between the axon of a neuron and the cells of a muscle, organ, or gland.	

Neuroglia

astrocyte	Star-shaped cell that provides structural support for neurons, connects them to capillaries, and forms the blood–brain barrier	astr/o- starlike structure
ependymal cells	Specialized cells that line the walls of the ventricles, spinal cavity, and the central canal within the spinal cord and produce cerebrospinal fluid	ependym/o- cellular lining
microglia	Cells that move, engulf, and destroy pathogens anywhere in the central nervous system	micr/o- one millionth; small
neuroglia	Cells that hold neurons in place and perform specialized tasks. Neuroglia include astrocytes, ependymal cells, microglia, oligodendroglia, and Schwann cells.	neur/o- nerve

Word or Phrase	Description	Combining Forms
oligodendroglia	Cells that form the myelin sheath around larger axons in the brain and spinal cord. These cells have few branching structures.	**olig/o-** *scanty; few* **dendr/o-** *branching structure*
Schwann cells	Cells that form the myelin sheath around larger axons of the cranial and spinal nerves	

Neurotransmitters

acetylcholine	Neurotransmitter in synapses between neurons of the parasympathetic division. It is also in synapses between motor neurons and voluntary skeletal muscles in the somatic nervous system.	
dopamine	Neurotransmitter in the synapses between neurons in the cerebral cortex, hypothalamus, and limbic system in the brain	
endorphins	Neuromodulators that are one of several natural pain relievers produced by the brain	
epinephrine	Neurotransmitter secreted by the adrenal medulla and released into the blood. It stimulates the body to prepare for "fight or flight."	
neurotransmitter	Chemical messenger that travels across the synapse between neurons	**neur/o-** *nerve* **transmitt/o-** *to send across or through*
norepinephrine	Neurotransmitter of the sympathetic division	
serotonin	Neurotransmitter in synapses between neurons in the limbic system, hypothalamus, cerebellum, and spinal cord	

Labeling Exercise

Match each anatomy word or phrase to its structure and write it in the numbered box for each figure. Be sure to check your spelling. Use the Answer Key at the end of the book to check your answers.

cerebellum	frontal lobe	occipital lobe	parietal lobe	temporal lobe

1.

2.

3.

4.

5.

arachnoid
cranium
dura mater

gray matter of the cerebrum (cortex)
pia mater

subarachnoid space
white matter of the cerebrum

1.

2.

3.

4.

5.

6.

7.

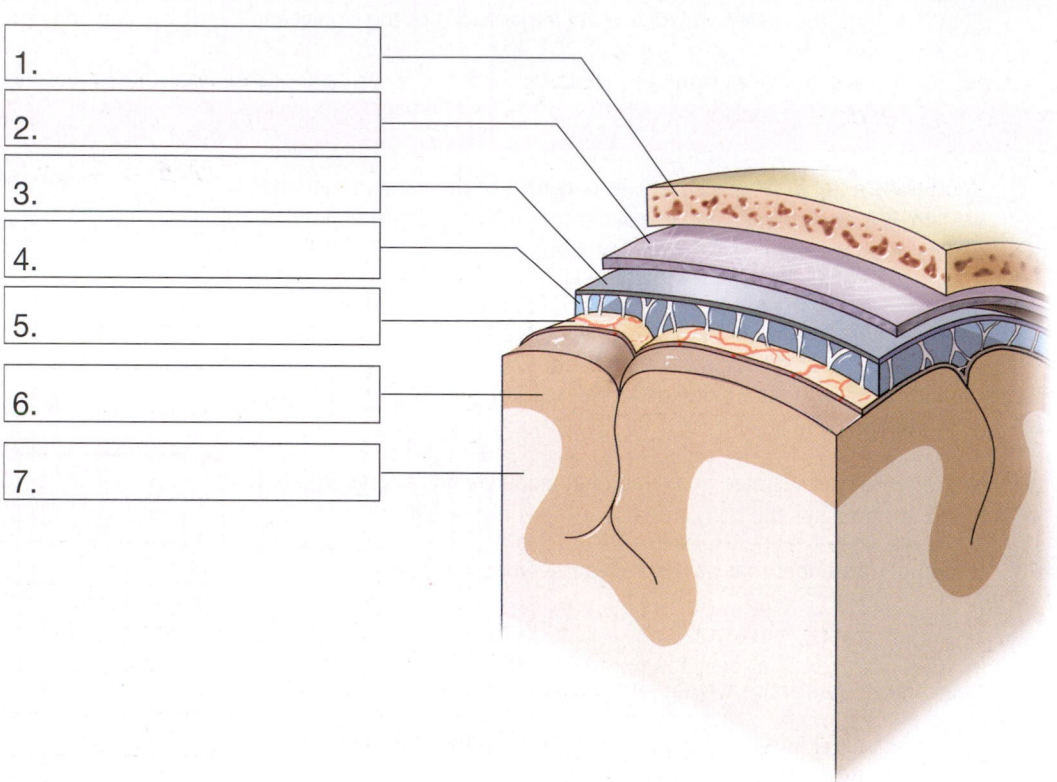

cerebellum
cerebrum

corpus callosum
fourth ventricle

gyrus
hypothalamus

lateral ventricle
medulla oblongata

midbrain
pons

sulcus
thalamus

1.

2.

3.

4.

5.

6.

7.

8.

9.

10.

11.

12.

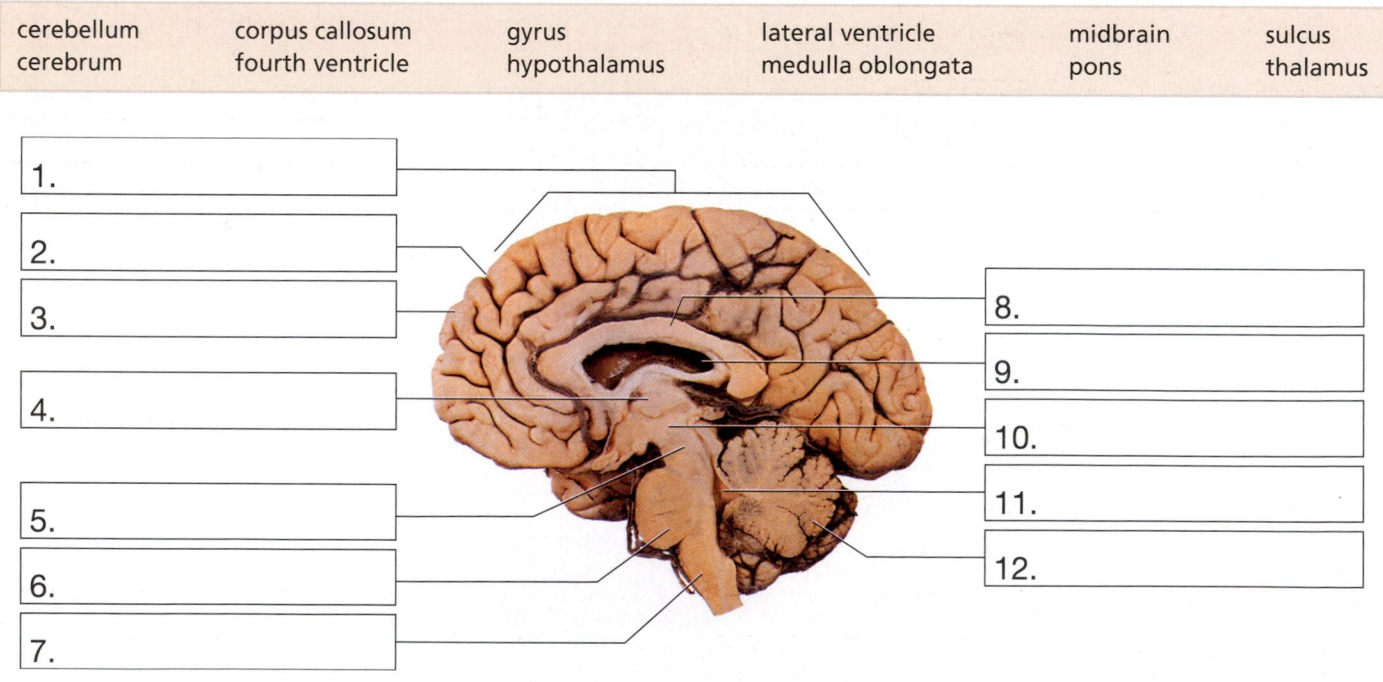

Building Medical Words

Use the Answer Key at the end of the book to check your answers.

Combining Forms Exercise

Before you build nervous system words, review these combining forms. Next to each combining form, write its medical meaning. The first one has been done for you.

Combining Form	Medical Meaning	Combining Form	Medical Meaning
1. **gemin/o-**	set or group	31. mot/o-	
2. access/o-		32. myelin/o-	
3. affer/o-		33. myel/o-	
4. arachn/o-		34. nerv/o-	
5. astr/o-		35. neur/o-	
6. audit/o-		36. occipit/o-	
7. autonom/o-		37. ocul/o-	
8. cav/o-		38. olfact/o-	
9. cerebell/o-		39. olig/o-	
10. cerebr/o-		40. opt/o-	
11. cochle/o-		41. pariet/o-	
12. cortic/o-		42. pathet/o-	
13. crani/o-		43. peripher/o-	
14. cyt/o-		44. pharyng/o-	
15. dendr/o-		45. radicul/o-	
16. dors/o-		46. recept/o-	
17. dur/o-		47. rhiz/o-	
18. effer/o-		48. sens/o-	
19. encephal/o-		49. somat/o-	
20. ependym/o-		50. spin/o-	
21. esthes/o-		51. tempor/o-	
22. esthet/o-		52. thalam/o-	
23. faci/o-		53. transmitt/o-	
24. fiss/o-		54. trochle/o-	
25. front/o-		55. vag/o-	
26. gloss/o-		56. ventricul/o-	
27. gustat/o-		57. ventr/o-	
28. meningi/o-		58. vestibul/o-	
29. mening/o-		59. vis/o-	
30. micr/o-			

Combining Form and Suffix Exercise

Read the definition of the medical word. Look at the combining form that is given. Select the correct suffix from the Suffix List and write it on the blank line. Then build the medical word and write it on the line. (Remember: You may need to remove the combining vowel. Always remove the hyphens and slash.) Be sure to check your spelling. The first one has been done for you.

SUFFIX LIST

-al (pertaining to)	-ent (pertaining to)	-or (person or thing that produces
-ar (pertaining to)	-glia (cells that provide support)	or does)
-ated (pertaining to a condition;	-ic (pertaining to)	-ory (having the function of)
composed of)	-ite (thing that pertains to)	-ous (pertaining to)
-cyte (cell)	-oid (resembling)	-ure (system; result of)
-eal (pertaining to)	-on (a substance; structure)	

Definition of the Medical Word	Combining Form	Suffix	Build the Medical Word
1. (Division of the nervous system) pertaining to the body	somat/o-	-ic	*somatic*

(You think *pertaining to* (-ic) + *the body* (somat/o-). You change the order of the word parts to put the suffix last. You write *somatic*.)

Definition of the Medical Word	Combining Form	Suffix	Build the Medical Word
2. Pertaining to the cerebrum	cerebr/o-	_____	_____
3. Pertaining to the top of the skull	crani/o-	_____	_____
4. Pertaining to the nerves	nerv/o-	_____	_____
5. Having the function of hearing	audit/o-	_____	_____
6. Pertaining to the ventricles (in the brain)	ventricul/o-	_____	_____
7. Resembling a spider web	arachn/o-	_____	_____
8. Pertaining to the meninges	mening/o-	_____	_____
9. Cell shaped like a star	astr/o-	_____	_____
10. Pertaining to the spine	spin/o-	_____	_____
11. Thing that pertains to a branching structure	dendr/o-	_____	_____
12. Pertaining to going out from the center	effer/o-	_____	_____
13. (Something that is the) result of splitting	fiss/o-	_____	_____
14. Pertaining to the outer aspects of the body	peripher/o-	_____	_____
15. Pertaining to the thalamus	thalam/o-	_____	_____
16. Having the function of sensation	sens/o-	_____	_____
17. (Person or) thing that (produces or) does receive	recept/o-	_____	_____
18. Composed of myelin	myelin/o-	_____	_____
19. Pertaining to independent or self-governing	autonom/o-	_____	_____
20. Structure of a (single) nerve (cell)	neur/o-	_____	_____
21. Pertaining to the temple	tempor/o-	_____	_____
22. Having the function of the sense of smell	olfact/o-	_____	_____
23. Pertaining to the cerebellum	cerebell/o-	_____	_____
24. Cells that support nerves	neur/o-	_____	_____
25. Pertaining to the dura mater	dur/o-	_____	_____
26. Pertaining to the back of the head	occipit/o-	_____	_____

Prefix Exercise

Read the definition of the medical word. Look at the medical word or partial word that is given (it already contains a combining form and a suffix). Select the correct prefix from the Prefix List and write it on the blank line. Then build the medical word and write it on the line. Be sure to check your spelling. The first one has been done for you.

PREFIX LIST		
epi- (upon; above)	hypo- (below; deficient)	sym- (together; with)
hemi- (one half)	sub- (below; underneath; less than)	tri- (three)

Definition of the Medical Word	Prefix	Word or Partial Word	Build the Medical Word
1. Pertaining to with suffering	**sym-**	**pathetic**	sympathetic
2. Structure below the thalamus	_____	thalamus	_____
3. Pertaining to above the dura mater	_____	dural	_____
4. Underneath the arachnoid	_____	arachnoid	_____
5. One half of a ball or sphere (like the brain)	_____	sphere	_____
6. (Cranial nerve) pertaining to three in a set or group	_____	geminal	_____
7. (Cranial nerve whose branches go) below the tongue	_____	glossal	_____

Diseases and Conditions

Brain

Word or Phrase	Description	Word Building
amnesia	Partial or total (global) loss of memory of recent or remote (past) experiences. It is often a consequence of brain injury or a stroke that damages the hippocampus where long-term memories are stored and processed. Treatment: None.	**amnesia** (am-NEE-zee-ah)

anencephaly	Rare congenital condition in which some or all of the cranium and cerebrum are missing in a newborn. The newborn breathes because the respiratory centers in the medulla oblongata are present, but only survives a few hours or days. Treatment: None.	**anencephaly** (AN-en-SEF-ah-lee)
		  an- *without; not*
		  -encephaly *condition of the brain*
		The ending *-encephaly* contains the combining form *encephal/o-* and the one-letter suffix *-y.*

aphasia	Loss of the ability to communicate verbally or in writing. Aphasia can occur with head trauma, a stroke, or Alzheimer's disease when there is injury to the areas of the brain that deal with language and the interpretation of sounds and symbols. Patients with aphasia are said to be **aphasic. Expressive aphasia** is the inability to verbally express thoughts. **Receptive aphasia** is the inability to understand the spoken or written word. Patients with both types are said to have **global aphasia.** Limited impairment that involves some difficulty speaking or understanding words is known as **dysphasia.** Treatment: Correct the underlying cause.	**aphasia** (ah-FAY-zee-ah)
		  a- *away from; without*
		  phas/o- *speech*
		  -ia *condition; state; thing*
		
		aphasic (ah-FAY-sik)
		  a- *away from; without*
		  phas/o- *speech*
		  -ic *pertaining to*
		
		expressive (eks-PREH-siv)
		  express/o- *communicate*
		  -ive *pertaining to*
		
		receptive (ree-SEP-tiv)
		  recept/o- *receive*
		  -ive *pertaining to*
		
		global (GLOH-bal)
		  glob/o- *shaped like a globe; comprehensive*
		  -al *pertaining to*
		
		dysphasia (dis-FAY-zee-ah)
		  dys- *painful; difficult; abnormal*
		  phas/o- *speech*
		  -ia *condition; state; thing*

arteriovenous malformation (AVM)	Abnormality in which arteries in the brain connect directly to veins (rather than to capillaries), forming an abnormal twisted nest of blood vessels. An AVM can rupture and cause a stroke. Treatment: Focused beam radiation to destroy the AVM or embolization to block blood flow to the AVM; surgical excision, if needed.	**arteriovenous** (ar-TEER-ee-oh-VEE-nus)
		  arteri/o- *artery*
		  ven/o- *vein*
		  -ous *pertaining to*
		
		malformation (MAL-for-MAY-shun)
		  mal- *bad; inadequate*
		  format/o- *structure; arrangement*
		  -ion *action; condition*

Word or Phrase	Description	Word Building

brain tumor	**Benign** or **malignant** tumor of any area of the brain. Brain tumors arise from the neuroglia or meninges, rather than from neurons themselves. They are named according to the type of cell from which they originated (see Table 10-4). Malignant brain tumors can also be secondary tumors that metastasized from a primary malignant tumor elsewhere in the body. Because the cranium is rigid, the enlarging bulk of a benign or malignant tumor causes increased **intracranial pressure (ICP)**, cerebral edema, and sometimes seizures (see Figure 10-11 ■). The pressure compresses and destroys brain tissue. Treatment: Surgery to remove or debulk the tumor; chemotherapy drugs or radiation therapy for malignant tumors.	**benign** (bee-NINE)
		
		malignant (mah-LIG-nant)
		   malign/o- *intentionally causing harm; cancer*
		   -ant *pertaining to*
		
		intracranial (IN-trah-KRAY-nee-al)
		   intra- *within*
		   crani/o- *cranium (skull)*
		   -al *pertaining to*

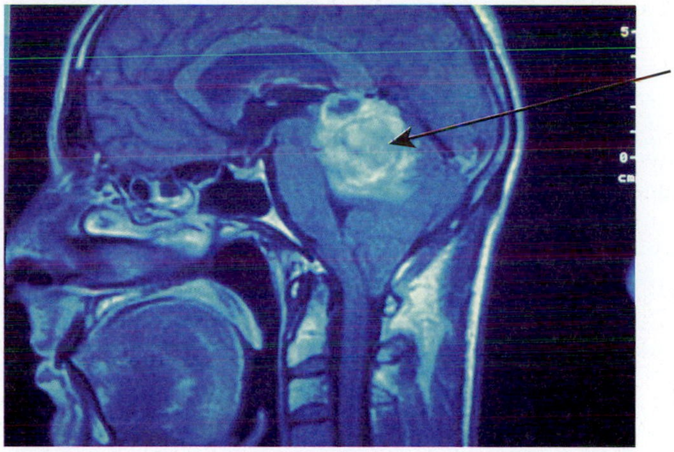

Figure 10-11 ■ Glioma.
This patient's MRI scan of the brain shows a large glioma that is pressing on the cerebellum.

Word or Phrase	Description	Word Building

cephalalgia	Pain in the head. It is commonly known as a **headache.** It can be caused by eyestrain, muscle tension in the face or neck, generalized infections such as the flu, migraine headaches, sinus infections, hypertension, or by more serious conditions such as head trauma, meningitis, or brain tumors. Treatment: Correct the underlying cause.	**cephalalgia** (SEF-al-AL-jee-ah)
		   cephal/o- *head*
		   alg/o- *pain*
		   -ia *condition; state; thing*

cerebral palsy (CP)	Cerebral palsy is caused by a lack of oxygen to parts of the fetus' brain during birth. The result can include spastic muscles; lack of coordination in walking, eating, and talking; muscle paralysis; seizures; or mental retardation. Treatment: Braces, muscle relaxant drugs.	**cerebral** (SAIR-eh-bral) (seh-REE-bral)
		   cerebr/o- *cerebrum (largest part of the brain)*
		   -al *pertaining to*
		
		palsy (PAWL-zee)

Table 10-4 Types of Brain Tumors

Brain Tumor	Characteristic	Originating Cell or Structure	Word Building
astrocytoma	malignant	astrocyte in the cerebrum	**astrocytoma** (AS-troh-sy-TOH-mah) **astr/o-** *starlike structure* **cyt/o-** *cell* **-oma** *tumor; mass*
ependymoma	benign	ependymal cells that line the ventricles	**ependymoma** (eh-PEN-dih-MOH-mah) **ependym/o-** *cellular lining* **-oma** *tumor; mass*
glioblastoma multiforme	malignant	immature astrocyte in the cerebrum	**glioblastoma multiforme** (GLY-oh-blas-TOH-mah MUL-tih-FOR-may) **gli/o-** *cells that provide support* **blast/o-** *immature; embryonic* **-oma** *tumor; mass*
glioma (see Figure 10-11)	benign or malignant	any neuroglial cell	**glioma** (gly-OH-mah) **gli/o-** *cells that provide support* **-oma** *tumor; mass*
lymphoma	malignant	microglia in the cerebrum	**lymphoma** (lim-FOH-mah) **lymph/o-** *lymph; lymphatic system* **-oma** *tumor; mass*
meningioma	benign	meninges around the brain or spinal cord	**meningioma** (meh-NIN-jee-OH-mah) **meningi/o-** *meninges* **-oma** *tumor; mass*
oligodendroglioma	malignant	oligodendroglia in the cerebrum	**oligodendroglioma** (OL-ih-goh-den-DROH-gly-OH-mah) **olig/o-** *scanty; few* **dendr/o-** *branching structure* **gli/o-** *cells that provide support* **-oma** *tumor; mass*
schwannoma	benign	Schwann cells near the cranial or spinal nerves	**schwannoma** (shwah-NOH-mah)

Word or Phrase	Description	Word Building
cerebrovascular accident (CVA)	Disruption or blockage of blood flow to the brain, which causes tissue death and an area of necrosis known as an **infarct**. This can be caused by an embolus, arteriosclerosis, or hemorrhage. An embolus is a thrombus (blood clot) that forms in the heart or aorta because of arteriosclerosis, breaks free, travels through the blood, and becomes lodged in a small artery to the brain. Hemorrhage occurs when high blood pressure causes an artery to rupture or when an aneurysm ruptures. A CVA is also known as a **stroke** or **brain attack**. A **transient ischemic attack (TIA)**, a temporary lack of oxygenated blood to an area of the brain, is like a CVA, but its effects last only 24 hours. A **reversible ischemic neurologic deficit (RIND)** is a TIA whose effects last for several days. TIAs and RINDs are precursors to an impending CVA. A cerebrovascular accident on the left side of the brain affects the right side of the body and vice versa (see Figure 10-12 ■).	**cerebrovascular** (SAIR-eh-broh-VAS-kyoo-lar) (seh-REE-broh-VAS-kyoo-lar) **cerebr/o-** *cerebrum (largest part of the brain)* **vascul/o-** *blood vessel* **-ar** *pertaining to* **infarct** (IN-farkt) **infarction** (in-FARK-shun) **infarct/o-** *area of dead tissue* **-ion** *action; condition* **ischemia** (is-KEE-mee-ah) **isch/o-** *keep back; block* **-emia** *condition of the blood; substance in the blood* **ischemic** (is-KEE-mik) **isch/o-** *keep back; block* **-emic** *pertaining to a condition of the blood or a substance in the blood* **neurologic** (NYOOR-oh-LAWJ-ik) **neur/o-** *nerve* **log/o-** *word; the study of* **-ic** *pertaining to* **deficit** (DEF-ih-sit) **hemiparesis** (HEM-ee-pah-REE-sis) (HEM-ee-PAIR-eh-sis) **hemi-** *one half* **-paresis** *condition of weakness* **hemiplegia** (HEM-ee-PLEE-jee-ah) **hemi-** *one half* **pleg/o-** *paralysis* **-ia** *condition; state; thing* **hemiplegic** (HEM-ee-PLEE-jik) **hemi-** *one half* **pleg/o-** *paralysis* **-ic** *pertaining to*

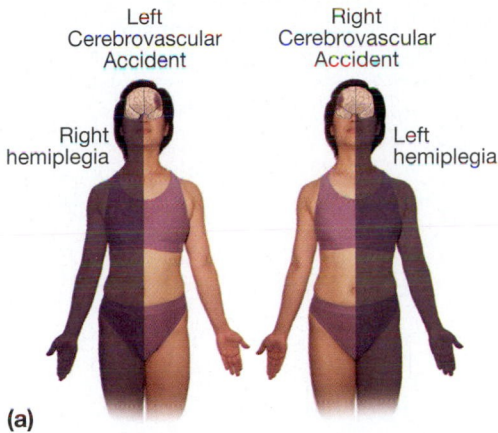

Left Cerebrovascular Accident — Right hemiplegia

Right Cerebrovascular Accident — Left hemiplegia

(a)

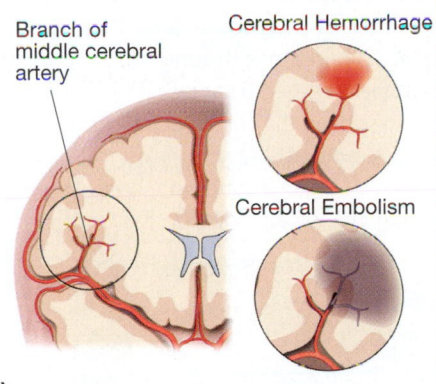

Branch of middle cerebral artery

Cerebral Hemorrhage

Cerebral Embolism

(b)

Figure 10-12 ■ Cerebrovascular accident.

(a) A cerebrovascular accident on the left side of the brain affects the right side of the body and vice versa. (b) A hemorrhage of an aneurysm disrupts blood flow to the brain and causes a cerebrovascular accident. An embolus blocks blood flow to the brain and causes a cerebrovascular accident.

The severity of the CVA depends on how much brain tissue is damaged. **Hemiparesis** is muscle weakness on one side of the body. **Hemiplegia** is paralysis on one side of the body, and the patient is said to be **hemiplegic** (see Figure 10-13 ■). A CVA can also cause amnesia, aphasia, dysphasia, or dysphagia (difficulting swallowing). Treatment: Thrombolytic drugs to break up an embolus that is occluding the artery. Surgery: Carotid endarterectomy, aneurysm clipping, or aneurysmectomy to prevent a CVA.

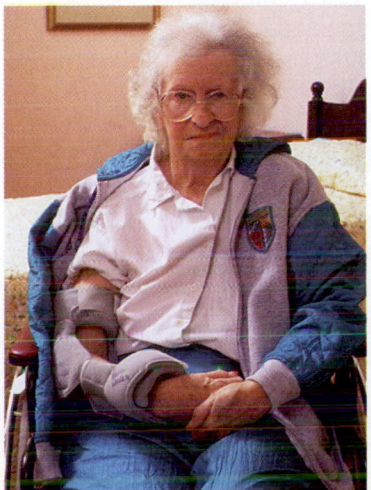

Figure 10-13 ■ Patient with a cerebrovascular accident.

This patient had a cerebrovascular accident on the left side of her brain that has paralyzed the right side of her body. Notice the drooping of the right side of her mouth and her right shoulder. The elbow and wrist of her right arm are covered with protective padding. She is using her good left hand to hold her right hand in her lap and move her right arm from time to time.

Word or Phrase	Description	Word Building

coma	Deep state of unconsciousness and unresponsiveness caused by trauma or disease in the brain, metabolic imbalance with accumulation of waste products (hepatic coma), or a deficiency of glucose in the blood (hypoglycemia). The patient is said to be **comatose.** Treatment: Correct the underlying cause.
	
	  Brain death is a condition in which there is irreversible loss of all brain function as confirmed by an electroencephalogram (EEG) that is flat, showing no brain wave activity of any kind for 30 minutes.
		coma (KOH-mah)
		comatose (KOH-mah-tohs)
		  comat/o- *unconsciousness*
		  -ose *full of*

concussion	Traumatic injury to the brain that results in an immediate loss of consciousness that continues for a brief or prolonged period of time (see Figure 10-14 ■). Even after consciousness returns, the patient must be watched closely for signs of a slowly enlarging hemorrhage in the brain. These signs include sleepiness or irritability, a vacant stare, slowness in answering questions, inability to follow commands, disorientation to time and place, slurred speech, or a lack of coordination. A **contusion** is a traumatic injury to the brain or spinal cord. There is no loss of consciousness, but there is bruising with some bleeding in the tissues. **Shaken baby syndrome** is caused by an adult vigorously shaking an infant in anger or to discipline the child. Because the infant's head is large and the neck muscles are weak, severe shaking causes the head to whip back and forth. This can cause a contusion, concussion, hemorrhaging, mental retardation, coma, or even death.	**concussion** (con-KUH-shun)
		  concuss/o- *violent shaking or jarring*
		  -ion *action; condition*
		contusion (con-TOO-shun)
		  contus/o- *bruising*
		  -ion *action; condition*

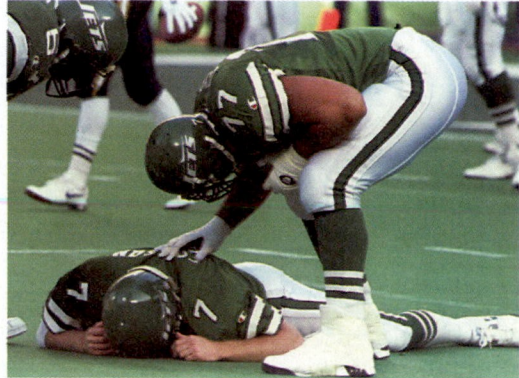

Figure 10-14 ■ Concussion.
Although football helmets are padded and constructed to protect the head, this player has sustained a concussion with loss of consciousness. Repeated concussions can result in developing Alzheimer's disease in middle age.

Clinical Connections

Public Health. New variant **Creutzfeldt-Jakob disease,** a fatal neurologic disorder, is caused by a prion (a small infectious protein particle). This disease is contracted from cows infected with mad cow disease (bovine spongiform encephalopathy). It was first discovered in British cows. It is transmitted to cows when they eat animal feed contaminated with the processed spinal cords and brains of infected cows. All such animal feed has been banned in the United States. The disease can be transmitted to humans who eat meat from the infected cows. People who have lived or traveled extensively in England are even prohibited from donating blood to prevent possible transmission of this disease.

Creutzfeldt-Jakob
(KROITS-felt YAH-kohp)

Word or Phrase	Description	Word Building
dementia	Disease of the brain in which many neurons in the cerebrum die, the cerebral cortex shrinks in size, and there is progressive deterioration in mental function (see Figures 10-15 ■ and 10-16 ■). At first, there is a gradual decline in mental abilities, with forgetfulness, inability to learn new things, inability to perform daily activities, and difficulty making decisions. The patient uses the wrong words and is unable to comprehend what others say. This becomes progressively more severe over time and includes inability to care for personal needs, inability to recognize friends and family, and complete memory loss. Psychiatric symptoms of depression, anxiety, impulsiveness, and combativeness can also occur. Dementia is most often associated with old age (**senile dementia**) and the cumulative effect of multiple small cerebrovascular accidents (**multi-infarct dementia**). Dementia can also be caused by brain trauma, chronic alcoholism or drug abuse, or chronic neurodegenerative diseases such as multiple sclerosis, Parkinson's disease, and Huntington's chorea. However, the most common cause of dementia is Alzheimer's disease. **Alzheimer's disease** is a hereditary dementia that is known to run in families with inherited mutations on chromosomes 1, 14, and 21. At autopsy, the neurons show characteristic **neurofibrillary tangles** that distort the cells. There are also microscopic **senile plaques.** The brain also has a decreased level of the neurotransmitter acetylcholine. Alzheimer's disease that occurs in late middle age or later is a form of senile dementia. Alzheimer's disease that occurs in early middle age is known as early-onset Alzheimer's disease or **presenile dementia.** Treatment: Drugs that inhibit the enzyme that breaks down acetylcholine.	**dementia** (deh-MEN-shee-ah) **de-** *reversal of; without* **ment/o-** *mind; chin* **-ia** *condition; state; thing* Select the correct combining form meaning to get the definition of *dementia: condition (of being) without the mind.* **senile** (SEE-nile) **sen/o-** *old age* **-ile** *pertaining to* **Alzheimer** (AWLZ-hy-mer) **neurofibrillary** (NYOOR-oh-FIB-rih-LAIR-ee) **neur/o-** *nerve* **fibrill/o-** *muscle fiber; nerve fiber* **-ary** *pertaining to* **plaque** (PLAK) **presenile** (pree-SEE-nile) **pre-** *before; in front of* **sen/o-** *old age* **-ile** *pertaining to*

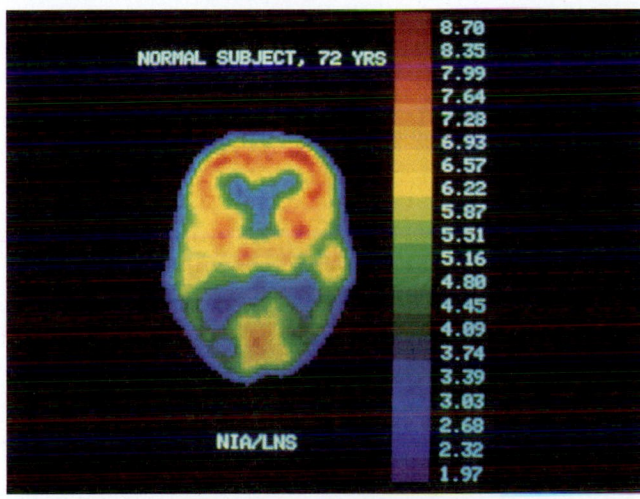
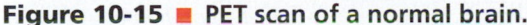

Figure 10-15 ■ PET scan of a normal brain.

A PET scan shows the metabolic activity of the brain. This patient's scan shows large, symmetrical areas of metabolism and active brain cells. The bar at the right correlates colors on the scan with numerical measurements for the amount of metabolic activity. Areas with the highest metabolic activity appear yellow to red.

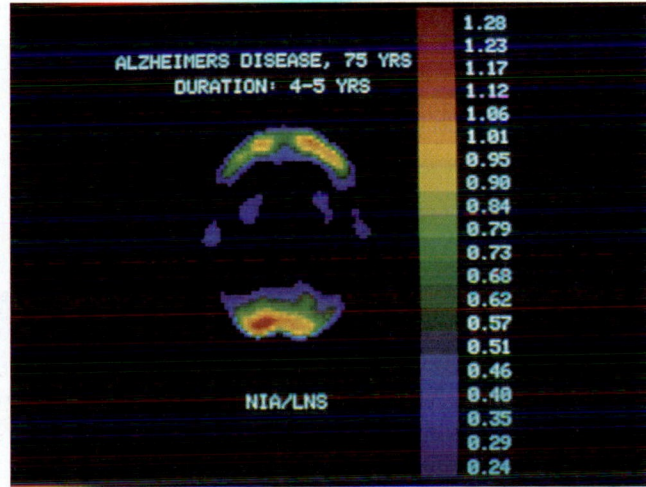

Figure 10-16 ■ PET scan of the brain in a patient with Alzheimer's disease.

Notice the large areas that are without any evidence of metabolism or brain cell activity.

Word or Phrase	Description	Word Building

Down syndrome	Congenital genetic defect in which there are three of chromosome 21, instead of the normal two. This defect affects every cell in the body, but is most obvious as mild-to-severe **mental retardation** and characteristic physical features of a thick, protruding tongue, short fingers, and a single transverse crease on the palm of the hand (see Figure 10-17 ■)	**mental** (MEN-tal)
		  ment/o- *mind; chin*
		  -al *pertaining to*
		retardation (REE-tar-DAY-shun)
		  retard/o- *slow down; delay*
		  -ation *a process; being or having*

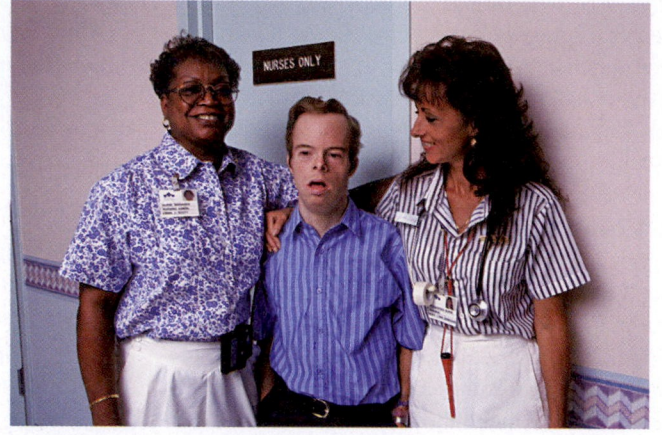

Figure 10-17 ■ Down syndrome.
This patient with Down syndrome shows the characteristic facial features (eyes and tongue) that accompany mental retardation.

dyslexia	Difficulty reading and writing words even though visual acuity and intelligence are normal (see Figure 10-18 ■). Dyslexia tends to run in families and is more prevalent in left-handed persons and in males. It is caused by an abnormality in the occipital lobe of the cerebrum that interprets moving visual images (as the eye moves quickly across the page). A person with dyslexia is said to be **dyslexic.** Treatment: Educational techniques that help a child learn to compensate or overcome this difficulty.	**dyslexia** (dis-LEK-see-ah)
		  dys- *painful; difficult; abnormal*
		  lex/o- *word*
		  -ia *condition; state; thing*
		dyslexic (dis-LEK-sik)
		  dys- *painful; difficult; abnormal*
		  lex/o- *word*
		  -ic *pertaining to*

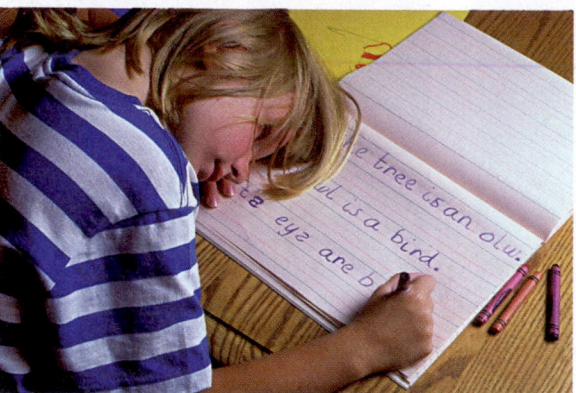

Figure 10-18 ■ Dyslexia.
A patient with dyslexia may write certain alphabet letters backwards or may change the order of the letters in a word.

encephalitis	Inflammation and infection of the brain caused by a virus. Herpes simplex virus is the most common cause of encephalitis, but others include herpes zoster virus, West Nile virus, and cytomegalovirus. There is fever, headache, stiff neck, lethargy, vomiting, irritability, and **photophobia.** Treatment: Corticosteroid drugs to decrease inflammation of the brain. Only encephalitis caused by the herpes virus responds to antiviral drugs. Antibiotic drugs are not effective against viruses.	**encephalitis** (en-SEF-ah-LY-tis)
		  encephal/o- *brain*
		  -itis *inflammation of; infection of*
		photophobia (FOH-toh-FOH-bee-ah)
		  phot/o- *light*
		  phob/o- *fear; avoidance*
		  -ia *condition; state; thing*

Word or Phrase	Description	Word Building

epilepsy	Recurring condition in which a group of neurons in the brain spontaneously sends out electrical impulses in an abnormal, uncontrolled way. These impulses spread from neuron to neuron. The type and extent of the symptoms depend on the number and location of the affected neurons. It is also known as **seizures** or **convulsions**. A patient with epilepsy is said to be **epileptic.** There are four common types of epilepsy (see Table 10-5). With each type of epilepsy, the patient displays a specific EEG pattern during a seizure (see Figure 10-19 ■). A seizure can be triggered by a flashing light, stress, lack of sleep, alcohol or drugs, or the cause can be unknown. Before the onset of a seizure, some epileptic patients experience an **aura,** a visual, olfactory, sensory, or auditory sign (flashing lights, strange odor, tingling, or buzzing sound) that warns them of an impending seizure. After a tonic-clonic seizure, the patient experiences sleepiness and confusion. This is known as the **postictal state.** Over time, seizures can cause memory loss and personality changes. **Status epilepticus** is a state of prolonged continuous seizure activity or frequently repeated individual seizures that occur without the patient regaining consciousness. Treatment: Antiepileptic drugs. Sometimes surgery, if a tumor or a specific area of the brain is causing the seizures.	**epilepsy** (EP-ih-LEP-see)
		
		 seizure (SEE-zher)
		
		 convulsion (con-VUL-shun)
		   convuls/o- *seizure*
		   -ion *action; condition*
		
		 epileptic (EP-ih-LEP-tik)
		   epilept/o- *seizure*
		   -ic *pertaining to*
		
		 aura (AW-rah)
		
		 postictal (post-IK-tal)
		   post- *after; behind*
		   ict/o- *seizure*
		   -al *pertaining to*
		
		 status epilepticus
		 (STAT-us EP-ih-LEP-tih-kus)

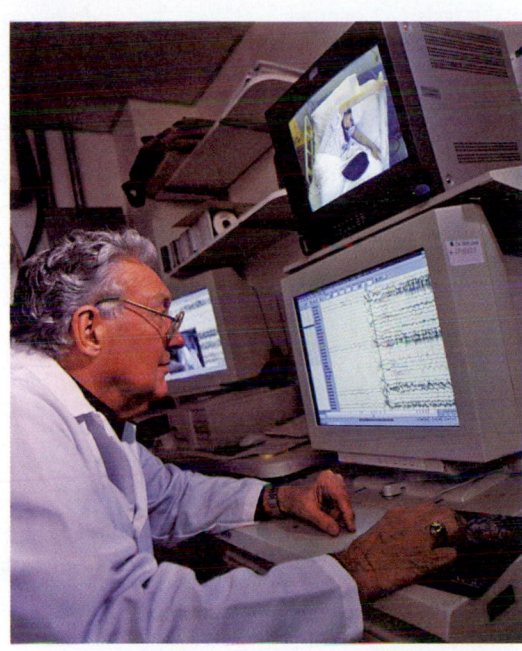

Figure 10-19 ■ Epilepsy.

This physician is monitoring a patient who is having a seizure. The computer screen at the top shows the patient, who is in a hospital bed while having a seizure. The computer screen at the bottom shows the patient's brain waves as they change from normal to abnormal with the onset of the seizure. The characteristic movements of the patient while having the seizure and the specific EEG pattern will lead to a diagnosis of the type of seizure disorder that the patient has.

Table 10-5 Seizures

Type of Seizure	Description	Word Building
tonic-clonic (grand mal)	Unconsciousness with excessive motor activity. The body alternates between excessive muscle tone with rigidity (tonic) and jerking muscle contractions (clonic) in the extremities, with tongue biting and sometimes incontinence. It lasts 1–2 minutes.	**tonic** (TAWN-ik) **ton/o-** *pressure; tone* **-ic** *pertaining to* **clonic** (CLAWN-ik) **clon/o-** *rapid contracting and relaxing* **-ic** *pertaining to* **grand mal** (GRAN MAWL)
absence (petit mal)	Impaired consciousness with slight or no muscle activity. Muscle tone is retained and the patient does not fall down, but is unable to respond to external stimuli. It can include vacant staring, repetitive blinking, or facial tics. It lasts 5–15 seconds, after which the patient resumes activities and is unaware of the seizure. A patient can have many absence seizures during the course of a day.	**absence** (AB-sens) **petit mal** (peh-TEE MAWL)
complex partial (psychomotor)	Some degree of impairment of consciousness. Involuntary contractions of one or several muscle groups. There can be **automatisms** such as lip smacking or repetitive muscle movements. It lasts 1–2 minutes.	**psychomotor** (SY-koh-MOH-tor) **psych/o-** *mind* **mot/o-** *movement* **-or** *person or thing that produces or does* **automatism** (aw-TAW-mah-tizm)
simple partial (focal motor)	No impairment of consciousness. The patient is aware of the seizure but is unable to stop the involuntary motor activity such as jerking of one hand or turning of the head. There can also be sensory hallucinations. Lasts 1–2 minutes.	**focal** (FOH-kal) **foc/o-** *point of activity* **-al** *pertaining to*

Word or Phrase	Description	Word Building
hematoma	Localized collection of blood that forms in the brain because of the rupture of an artery or vein. This can be caused by trauma to the cranium or the rupture of an intracranial aneurysm. An **intraventricular hematoma** occurs within one of the ventricles. A **subdural hematoma** forms between the dura mater and the arachnoid (see Figure 10-20 ■). Treatment: Surgery to remove the hematoma.	**hematoma** (HEE-mah-TOH-mah) **hemat/o-** *blood* **-oma** *tumor; mass* **intraventricular** (IN-trah-ven-TRIK-yoo-lar) **intra-** *within* **ventricul/o-** *ventricle (lower heart chamber; chamber in the brain)* **-ar** *pertaining to* **subdural** (sub-DOO-ral) **sub-** *below; underneath; less than* **dur/o-** *dura mater* **-al** *pertaining to*

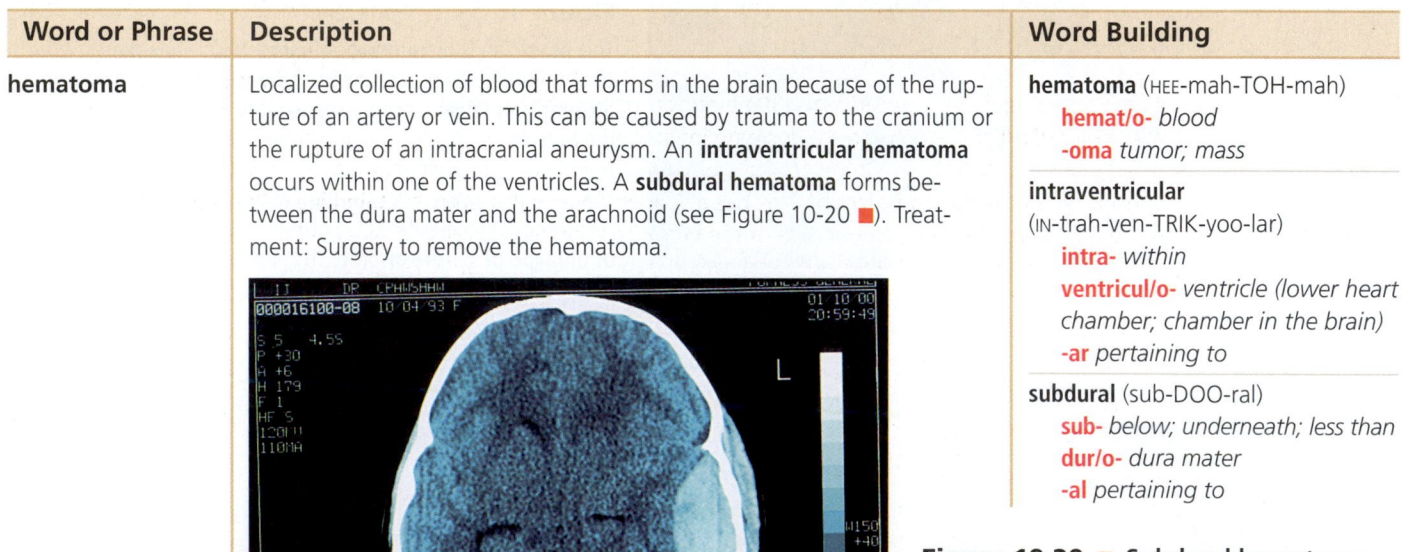

Figure 10-20 ■ Subdural hematoma.
This patient developed a subdural hematoma after trauma to the side of the head. Also notice the hematoma of the scalp where blood has collected between the cranium and the skin. An MRI scan shows both hematomas and the extent of the compression of the brain.

Word or Phrase	Description	Word Building
Huntington's chorea	Progressive inherited degenerative disease of the brain that begins in middle age. It is characterized by dementia with irregular spasms of the extremities and face (chorea), alternating with slow writhing movements of the hands and feet (athetosis). Treatment: None.	**Huntington** (HUN-ting-ton) **chorea** (kor-EE-ah)
hydrocephalus	Condition in which an excessive amount of cerebrospinal fluid is produced or the flow of cerebrospinal fluid is blocked. Intracranial pressure builds up, distends the ventricles in the brain, and compresses the brain tissue (see Figure 10-21 ■). Hydrocephalus is most often associated with the congenital conditions of meningocele or myelomeningocele (see Figure 10-23), although it can occur in adults (normal pressure hydrocephalus) when the cerebrospinal fluid is not absorbed back into the blood. Untreated hydrocephalus causes a grossly enlarged head and mental retardation. The patient is said to be **hydrocephalic.** A layman's phrase for this condition is "water on the brain." Treatment: Placement of a ventriculoperitoneal shunt to move excess cerebrospinal fluid from the cranial cavity to the peritoneal cavity.	**hydrocephalus** (HY-droh-SEF-ah-lus) **hydr/o-** *water; fluid* **-cephalus** *head* **hydrocephalic** (HY-droh-sih-FAL-ik) **hydr/o-** *water; fluid* **cephal/o-** *head* **-ic** *pertaining to*

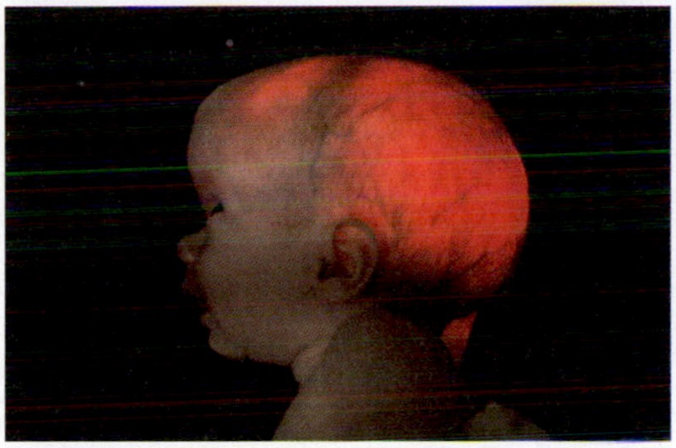

Figure 10-21 ■ Hydrocephalus.
This infant has pronounced hydrocephalus. A light shown on the cranium reveals large areas of illumination where the enlarged ventricles are filled with cerebrospinal fluid and the more dense brain tissue has been pushed aside.

Word or Phrase	Description	Word Building
meningitis	Inflammation and infection of the meninges of the brain or spinal cord caused by a bacterium or virus. There is fever, headache, **nuchal rigidity** (stiff neck with pain and inability to touch the chin to the chest), lethargy, vomiting, irritability, and sensitivity to light (photophobia). Treatment: Vaccination to prevent bacterial meningitis in susceptible groups (particularly college students); antibiotic drugs to treat bacterial meningitis. Corticosteroid drugs to decrease inflammation.	**meningitis** (MEN-in-JY-tis) **mening/o-** *meninges* **-itis** *inflammation of; infection of* **nuchal** (NOO-kal) **nuch/o-** *neck* **-al** *pertaining to*
migraine headache	Specific type of recurring headache that has a sudden onset with severe, throbbing pain, often on just one side of the head. This is often accompanied by nausea and vomiting and sensitivity to light (photophobia). Migraines are caused by a constriction of the arteries in the brain followed by a sudden dilation (which causes pain), accompanied by the release of neuropeptides by the trigeminal nerve (which causes inflammation). Treatment: Drugs that keep the blood vessels from dilating to prevent or treat a migraine.	**migraine** (MY-grayn)

Word or Phrase	Description	Word Building
narcolepsy	Brief, involuntary episodes of falling asleep during the daytime while engaged in activity. The patient is not unconscious and can be aroused, but is unable to keep from falling asleep. There is a hereditary component to narcolepsy, and it may be an autoimmune disorder. There is also an underlying abnormality of REM sleep. Treatment: Central nervous system stimulant drugs.	**narcolepsy** (NAR-koh-LEP-see) **narc/o-** *stupor; sleep* **-lepsy** *seizure*
Parkinson's disease	Chronic, degenerative disease due to an imbalance in the levels of the neurotransmitters dopamine and acetylcholine in the brain. There is muscle rigidity and tremors. In the later stages, it is difficult for the patient to initiate voluntary movements except with effort and concentration (see Figure 10-22 ■). There is also a mask-like facial expression, shuffling gait, or inability to ambulate. Treatment: Drugs that balance the level of the neurotransmitters by increasing the amount of dopamine or inhibiting the action of acetylcholine in the brain.	**Parkinson** (PAR-kin-son)

Figure 10-22 ■ Parkinson's disease.

Parkinson's patients boxing legend Mohammad Ali and actor Michael J. Fox talk with each other before testifying at a Senate hearing on Parkinson's disease research. Muhammad Ali has had Parkinson's disease for many years, as evidenced by his advanced symptoms of an expressionless face and difficulty initiating movement of his hands.

Word or Phrase	Description	Word Building
syncope	Temporary loss of consciousness. A **syncopal episode** is one in which the patient becomes lightheaded and then faints and remains unconscious briefly. It is most often caused by carotid artery stenosis and plaque that block blood flow or by cardiac arrhythmias that decrease blood flow to the brain.	**syncope** (SIN-koh-pee) **syncopal** (SIN-koh-pal) **syncop/o-** *fainting* **-al** *pertaining to*

Spinal Cord

Word or Phrase	Description	Word Building
neural tube defect	Congenital abnormality of the neural tube (embryonic structure that becomes the fetal brain and spinal cord). The vertebrae form incompletely (**spina bifida**), and there is an abnormal opening in the vertebral column through which the spinal cord and nerves may protrude to the outside of the body. This defect is covered only by the meninges (see Figure 10-23 ■).	**neural** (NYOOR-al) **neur/o-** *nerve* **-al** *pertaining to* **spina bifida** (SPY-nah BIF-ih-dah)

(continued)

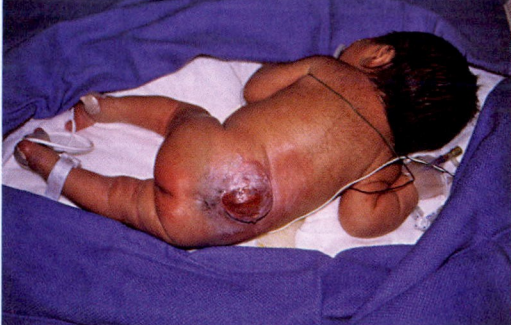

Figure 10-23 ■ Meningocele.

Meningocele with the meninges in the hernia sac. The delicate tissues of the meningocele can be traumatized easily, allowing infection to enter and travel to the brain. Therefore, the meningocele is surgically closed shortly after birth.

Word or Phrase	Description	Word Building
neural tube defect (*continued*)	A **meningocele** is the protrusion of the meninges through the defect. A **meningomyelocele** is the protrusion of the meninges and the spinal cord; it is also known as **myelomeningocele.** Children with meningocele or meningomyelocele may also have hydrocephalus. The amount of spinal cord involvement determines the degree of impairment of muscle control of the legs and bladder and bowel function. A sample of amniotic fluid taken during the pregnancy shows an elevated level of alpha fetoprotein. Treatment: Surgery to close the defect immediately after birth because of the risk of infection. The surgery is not able to restore impaired function to the muscles. The hydrocephalus is treated separately.	**meningocele** (meh-NING-goh-seel) **mening/o-** *meninges* **-cele** *hernia* **meningomyelocele** (meh-NING-goh-MY-loh-seel) **mening/o-** *meninges* **myel/o-** *bone marrow; spinal cord; myelin* **-cele** *hernia* Select the correct combining form meaning to get the definition of *meningomyelocele: hernia of the meninges and spinal cord.* **myelomeningocele** (MY-loh-meh-NING-goh-seel) **myel/o-** *bone marrow; spinal cord; myelin* **mening/o-** *meninges* **-cele** *hernia*

Clinical Connections

Dietetics. A folic acid supplement taken during pregnancy greatly reduces the risk of neural tube defects. Folic acid is present in prenatal vitamins and in enriched cereals and breads.

Word or Phrase	Description	Word Building
radiculopathy	Acute or chronic condition that occurs because of a tumor, arthritis, or a **herniated nucleus pulposus (HNP)** (when the contents of an intervertebral disk are forced out through a weak area in the disk wall). Any of these press on nearby spinal nerve roots (see Figure 10-24 ■). An HNP usually involves a lumbar disk and is often caused by heavy lifting and poor body mechanics. It is also known as a **slipped disk.** There is pain, numbness, and paresthesias along the dermatome for that spinal nerve. It is also known as **sciatica** because the pain is often from compression of several branches of the sciatic nerve whose nerve roots come from L4, L5, and the sacrum. Treatment: Anti-inflammatory drugs, bed rest, traction to the spine, physical therapy; injection into the nerve root of a corticosteroid drug to decrease inflammation. Surgery: Rhizotomy, diskectomy, or laminectomy.	**radiculopathy** (rah-DIK-yoo-LAWP-oh-thee) **radicu/lo-** *spinal nerve root* **-pathy** *disease; suffering* **herniated** (HER-nee-AA-ted) **herni/o-** *hernia* **-ated** *pertaining to a condition; composed of* **nucleus pulposus** (NOO-klee-us pul-POH-sus) **sciatica** (sy-AT-ih-kah)

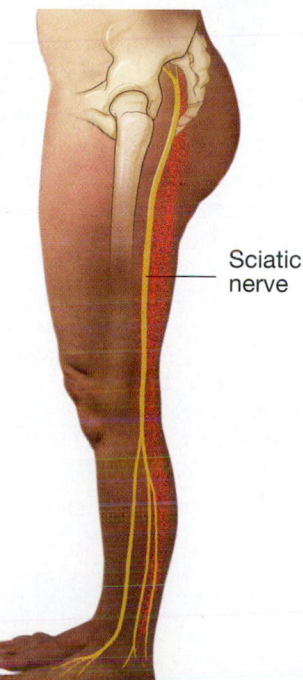

Sciatic nerve

Figure 10-24 ■ Radiculopathy.
The path of the sciatic nerve in the leg. A herniated nucleus pulposus presses on the sciatic nerve. The resulting area of pain, numbness, and tingling in the leg is shown in red.

Word or Phrase	Description	Word Building
spinal cord injury (SCI)	Trauma to the spinal cord with a partial or complete **transection** of the cord. This interrupts nerve impulses to particular dermatomes, causing partial or complete anesthesia (loss of sensation) and **paralysis** (an inability to voluntarily move the muscles). An injury to the lower spinal cord causes **paraplegia** with paralysis of the legs (see Figure 10-25 ■). A patient with paraplegia is known as a **paraplegic.** An injury to the upper spinal cord causes **quadriplegia** with paralysis of all four extremities. A patient with quadriplegia is known as a **quadriplegic.** Without nerve impulses, the muscles lose their tone and firmness and eventually atrophy. This is known as **flaccid paralysis.** However, the reflex arc of the lower spinal cord often remains intact and, in response to pain or a full bladder, the spinal cord below the injury will send nerve impulses that cause the muscles to spasm. This is known as **spastic paralysis.** The bladder may also contract spontaneously, causing incontinence. Treatment: After a suspected spinal cord injury, the patient is carefully transported to the hospital on a rigid spinal board, with a cervical collar in place, and with the head taped to the board to prevent any movement of the head, neck, or back that might further injure the spinal cord; traction to the skull to align the vertebrae; surgery may be needed to fuse damaged vertebrae; corticosteroid drugs to decrease spinal cord inflammation; passive range-of-motion exercises, splints, muscle relaxant drugs.	**transection** (tran-SEK-shun) **trans-** *across; through* **sect/o-** *to cut* **-ion** *action; condition* The duplicate *s* is omitted. **paralysis** (pah-RAL-ih-sis) **para-** *beside; apart from; two parts of a pair; abnormal* **-lysis** *process of breaking down or destroying* Select the correct combining form meaning to get the definition of *paralysis: process of breaking down (paralyzing) two parts of a pair (of arms or legs).* **paraplegia** (PAIR-ah-PLEE-jee-ah) **para-** *beside; apart from; two parts of a pair; abnormal* **pleg/o-** *paralysis* **-ia** *condition; state; thing* **paraplegic** (PAIR-ah-PLEE-jik) **para-** *beside; apart from; two parts of a pair; abnormal* **pleg/o-** *paralysis* **-ic** *pertaining to* **quadriplegia** (KWAH-drih-PLEE-jee-ah) **quadri-** *four* **pleg/o-** *paralysis* **-ia** *condition; state; thing* Add words to make a complete definition of *quadriplegia: condition (in which all) four (extremities have) paralysis.* **quadriplegic** (KWAH-drih-PLEE-jik) **quadri-** *four* **pleg/o-** *paralysis* **-ic** *pertaining to* **flaccid** (FLAS-id) (FLAK-sid) **spastic** (SPAS-tic) **spast/o-** *spasm* **-ic** *pertaining to*

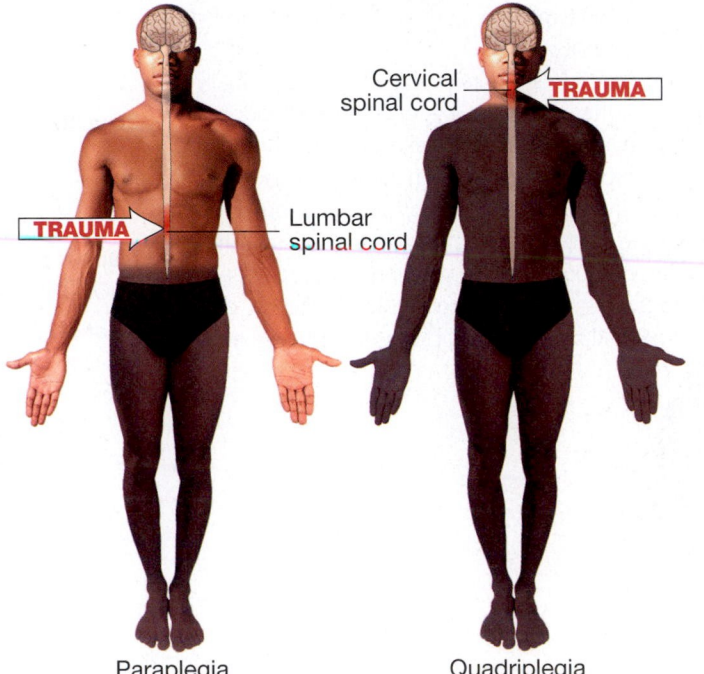

Cervical spinal cord   TRAUMA

Lumbar spinal cord   TRAUMA

Paraplegia   Quadriplegia

Figure 10-25 ■ Spinal cord injury.
The level of the spinal cord where an injury occurs and whether the spinal cord was partially or completely transected determines how much of the body is affected and to what extent. Paraplegia affects the lower body and the legs. Quadriplegia affects the body from the neck down and all four extremities.

Nerves

Word or Phrase	Description	Word Building
amyotrophic lateral sclerosis (ALS)	Chronic, progressive disease of the motor nerves coming from the spinal cord. There is muscle wasting and spasms, with eventual paralysis of all the muscles, including the swallowing and respiratory muscles. There is no damage to the sensory nerves and so sensation remains intact. Some cases of ALS are caused by the lack of an enzyme, which is an inherited defect; but in most cases the cause is not known. It is also known as Lou Gehrig's disease after the famous baseball player who developed the disease in the late 1930s. Treatment: Supportive care.	**amyotrophic** (ah-MY-oh-TROH-fik) **a-** *away from; without* **my/o-** *muscle* **troph/o-** *development* **-ic** *pertaining to* **sclerosis** (skleh-ROH-sis) **scler/o-** *hard; sclera (white of the eye)* **-osis** *condition; abnormal condition; process*
anesthesia	Condition in which sensation of any type, including touch, pressure, proprioception, or pain, has been lost. Local areas of anesthesia can occur temporarily when your hand goes numb from pressing on a nerve in your arm as you sleep. Third-degree burns cause permanent anesthesia of the damaged skin. Permanent anesthesia along a dermatome can occur after a spinal cord injury. Temporary therapeutic anesthesia to relieve pain can be produced in specific regions by injecting an **anesthetic drug** under the skin, near a nerve root, or into the epidural space in the spinal cavity. Unconsciousness is accompanied by an inability to perceive any sensation, and this is the basis for the use of drugs that induce general anesthesia prior to a surgical procedure. Treatment: Correct the underlying cause.	**anesthesia** (AN-es-THEE-zee-ah) **an-** *without; not* **esthes/o-** *sensation; feeling* **-ia** *condition; state; thing* **anesthetic** (AN-es-THET-ik) **an-** *without; not* **esthet/o-** *sensation; feeling* **-ic** *pertaining to*
Bell's palsy	Weakness, drooping, or actual paralysis of one side of the face because of inflammation of the facial nerve (cranial nerve VII) (see Figure 10-26 ■). It can be caused by a viral infection, possibly herpesvirus. The condition usually lasts a month and then disappears. Treatment: Corticosteroid drugs.	**palsy** (PAWL-zee)

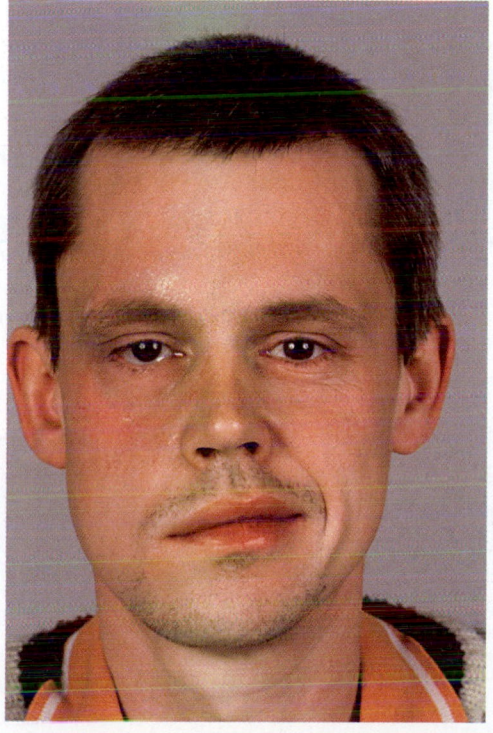

Figure 10-26 ■ **Bell's palsy.**
This patient with Bell's palsy has paralysis of the facial nerve on the right side of his face, as shown by drooping of his cheek and lips.

Word or Phrase	Description	Word Building
carpal tunnel syndrome (CTS)	Chronic condition caused by repetitive motions of the hand and wrist, often from constant typing or data entry. There is tingling in the hand because of inflammation and swelling of the tendons that go through the carpal tunnel of the wrist bones to reach the hand. This swelling compresses the median nerve. Bending or extending the wrist for 60 seconds (Phalen's maneuver) aggravates the pain and is a positive diagnostic test. Treatment: Rest, splinting the wrist, use of a special split keyboard that positions the wrists, physical therapy; surgery, if needed.	**carpal** (KAR-pal) **carp/o-** *wrist* **-al** *pertaining to*
Guillain-Barré syndrome	Autoimmune disorder in which the body makes antibodies against myelin. There is acute inflammation of the peripheral nerves, loss of myelin with interruption of nerve conduction, muscle weakness, and changes in sensation (paresthesias). This disease is caused by a triggering event such as an infection (often a viral respiratory illness), stress, or trauma. The muscle weakness begins in the legs and then rapidly involves the entire body. The patient may even temporarily require respiratory support until the inflammation subsides. Guillain-Barré does not recur, and the patient recovers some or all neurologic function over a period of days to months. Treatment: Corticosteroid drugs to treat inflammation.	**Guillain-Barré** (GEE-yah bah-RAY)
hyperesthesia	Condition in which there is an abnormally heightened awareness and sensitivity to touch and increased response to painful stimuli. Treatment: A variety of drugs (antidepressants, tranquilizers) are used and are somewhat effective.	**hyperesthesia** (HY-per-es-THEE-zee-ah) **hyper-** *above; more than normal* **esthes/o-** *sensation; feeling* **-ia** *condition; state; thing*
multiple sclerosis (MS)	Chronic, progressive, degenerative autoimmune disease in which the body makes antibodies against myelin. There is acute inflammation of the nerves and loss of myelin (**demyelination**) with interruption of nerve conduction in the brain and spinal cord. The areas of demyelination eventually become scar tissue that is hard. These areas are known as plaque and can be seen on MRI scans of the brain. This disease can be caused by a triggering event such as a viral infection. Patients are typically in their 20s to early middle age. There is double vision, nystagmus, large muscle weakness, uncoordinated gait, spasticity, early fatigue after repeated muscle contractions, tremors, paresthesias, and later, inability to walk and sometimes dementia. Heat, stress, and fatigue temporarily worsen the condition. There can be periodic remissions in which there is some improvement, followed by exacerbations or flare-ups, but always with worsening of the condition over time. Treatment: Corticosteroid drugs, muscle relaxant drugs.	**sclerosis** (skleh-ROH-sis) **scler/o-** *hard; sclera (white of the eye)* **-osis** *condition; abnormal condition; process* Select the correct combining form and suffix meanings to get the definition of *sclerosis:* an abnormal condition of hard(ness). **demyelination** (dee-MY-eh-lin-AA-shun) **de-** *reversal of; without* **myelin/o-** *myelin* **-ation** *a process; being or having*
neuralgia	Pain along the path of a nerve and its branches that is caused by an injury. Neuralgia can cause mild-to-severe pain. **Trigeminal neuralgia,** also known as **tic douloureux,** is characterized by episodes of brief but severe, stabbing pain (like an electrical shock) on one or both sides of the face or jaw along the distribution of the trigeminal nerve (cranial nerve V). **Causalgia** is severe, burning pain along a nerve and its branches. **Complex regional pain syndrome (CRPS)** consists of causalgia with hyperesthesia, changes in skin color and temperature, and swelling. Treatment: Anti-inflammatory drugs, topical anesthetic drugs, corticosteroid drugs, antidepressant drugs, anticonvulsant drugs, skeletal muscle relaxant drugs, nerve blocks, TENS unit, and physical therapy.	**neuralgia** (nyoo-RAL-jee-ah) **neur/o-** *nerve* **alg/o-** *pain* **-ia** *condition; state; thing* **trigeminal** (try-JEM-ih-nal) **tri-** *three* **gemin/o-** *set or group* **-al** *pertaining to* **tic douloureux** (TIK doo-loo-ROO) **causalgia** (kaw-ZAL-jee-ah) **caus/o-** *burning* **alg/o-** *pain* **-ia** *condition; state; thing*

(continued)

Word or Phrase	Description	Word Building
neuralgia *(continued)*	<table><tr><td>**Clinical Connections**</td></tr><tr><td>**Dermatology (Chapter 7).** Shingles is a painful skin condition caused by the herpes zoster virus, the virus that causes chickenpox in children. The virus remains dormant in the body until later in life when a stress triggers it to erupt. It affects nerves and the skin in the distribution of the dermatomes of those nerves and causes redness, pain, and vesicles. Lingering, chronic pain from shingles is known as postherpetic neuralgia. Treatment: Antiviral drugs.</td></tr></table>	
neuritis	Inflammation or infection of a nerve. **Polyneuritis** is a generalized inflammation of many nerves in one part of the body or all the nerves in the body. Treatment: Correct the underlying cause; analgesic drugs, anti-inflammatory drugs, corticosteroid drugs, or antibiotic drugs.	**neuritis** (nyoo-RY-tis) **neur/o-** *nerve* **-itis** *inflammation of; infection of* **polyneuritis** (PAWL-ee-nyoo-RY-tis) **poly-** *many; much* **neur/o-** *nerve* **-itis** *inflammation of; infection of*
neurofibromatosis	Hereditary disease with multiple benign fibrous tumors (**neurofibromata**) that arise from the peripheral nerves. These are most noticeable on the skin, but they can also be present anywhere in the body—on the internal organs and even in the eye. They range in size from small nodules to large tumors. It is also known as **von Recklinghausen's disease.**	**neurofibromatosis** (NYOOR-oh-fy-BROH-mah-TOH-sis) **neur/o-** *nerve* **fibr/o-** *fiber* **-omatosis** *abnormal condition of multiple tumors or masses* **neurofibroma** (NYOOR-oh-fy-BROH-mah) **neur/o-** *nerve* **fibr/o-** *fiber* **-oma** *tumor; mass* Neurofibroma is a Greek singular noun. Form the plural by changing *-oma* to *-omata*. **von Recklinghausen** (vawn REK-ling-HOW-sen)
neuroma	Benign tumor of a nerve or any of the specialized cells of the nervous system. A **Morton's neuroma** specifically forms from repetitive damage to the nerve that is near the metatarsophalangeal joints between the ball of the foot and the toes. Treatment: Surgical excision.	**neuroma** (nyoo-ROH-mah) **neur/o-** *nerve* **-oma** *tumor; mass*
neuropathy	General category for any type of disease or injury to a nerve. Treatment: Correct the underlying cause.	**neuropathy** (nyoo-RAWP-ah-thee) **neur/o-** *nerve* **-pathy** *disease; suffering*
	<table><tr><td>**Clinical Connections**</td></tr><tr><td>**Endocrinology (Chapter 14). Diabetic neuropathy** is a chronic, slowly progressive condition that affects the peripheral nerves in diabetic patients. It is caused by a lack of blood flow (arteriosclerosis) to the nerves. There is severe pain and a loss of sensation and sense of position. Treatment: Treat the diabetes mellitus.</td></tr></table>	**diabetic** (DY-ah-BET-ik) **diabet/o-** *diabetes* **-ic** *pertaining to* **neuropathy** (nyoo-RAWP-ah-thee) **neur/o-** *nerve* **-pathy** *disease; suffering*

Word or Phrase	Description	Word Building
paresthesia	Condition in which abnormal sensations such as tingling, burning, or pinpricks are felt on the skin (see Figure 10-27 ■). Paresthesias are often the result of chronic nerve damage from a pinched nerve or diabetic neuropathy. Treatment: Correct the underlying cause. **There's relief for pain like this. Ask your doctor about Lyrica.** LYRICA PREGABALIN C Designed for Relief	**paresthesia** (PAIR-es-THEE-zee-ah) **para-** beside; apart from; two parts of a pair; abnormal **esthes/o-** sensation; feeling **-ia** condition; state; thing The final *a* in the prefix *para-* is omitted when the word *paresthesia* is formed. Select the correct prefix meaning to get the definition of *paresthesia: condition of abnormal sensation or feeling.* **Figure 10-27** ■ **Paresthesias.** This drug advertisement graphically shows the sensation that some patients have with paresthesias: a stabbing pain or shooting sensation. Other symptoms include burning pain, tingling, or numbness. Other advertisements for this drug show ants crawling on the feet or thumbtacks pricking the feet.

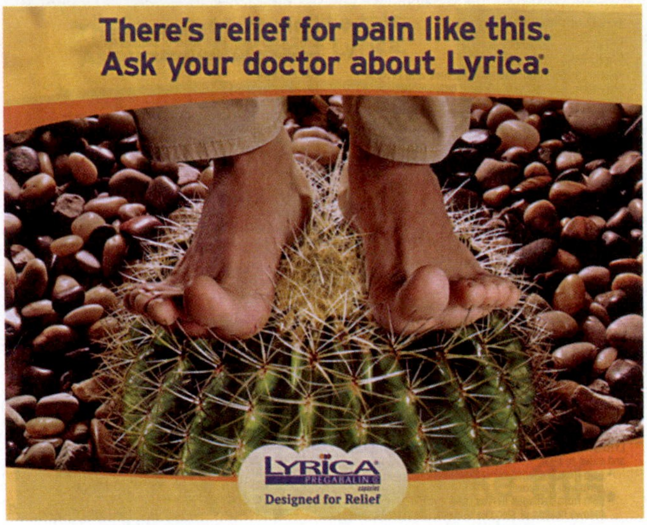

Laboratory and Diagnostic Procedures

Laboratory Tests

Word or Phrase	Description	Word Building
alpha fetoprotein (AFP)	Chemistry test performed on a sample of amniotic fluid taken from the uterus by amniocentesis (see Figure 13-27) during pregnancy. It is used to diagnose a neural tube defect in the fetus before birth. The fetal liver makes alpha fetoprotein, and small amounts are normally present in the amniotic fluid. However, an increased level indicates that alpha fetoprotein is leaking into the amniotic fluid through a myelocele or meningomyelocele.	**alpha fetoprotein** (AL-fah FEE-toh-PROH-teen)
cerebrospinal fluid (CFS) examination	Laboratory test that visually examines the CSF for clarity and color, microscopically for cells, and chemically for proteins and other substances. Normal CSF is clear and colorless. CSF with a pink or reddish tint contains a large number of red blood cells, and this indicates bleeding in the brain from a stroke or trauma. Cloudy CSF contains a large number of white blood cells, and this indicates an infection such as encephalitis or meningitis. An elevated level of protein indicates infection or the presence of a tumor. The presence of oligoclonal bands points to multiple sclerosis. Myelin-basic protein is elevated in multiple sclerosis and amyotrophic lateral sclerosis.	

Radiologic and Nuclear Medicine Procedures

Word or Phrase	Description	Word Building
cerebral angiography	Procedure in which a radiopaque contrast dye is injected into the carotid arteries, and an x-ray is taken to visualize the arterial circulation in the brain (see Figure 10-28 ■). This is done to show an aneurysm, stenosis, plaque in the arteries, or a tumor. A tumor is seen as an interwoven collection of new blood vessels, or it can be seen indirectly when it distorts normal anatomy and forces the arteries into abnormal positions. It is also known as **arteriography.** The x-ray image is an **angiogram** or an **arteriogram.** 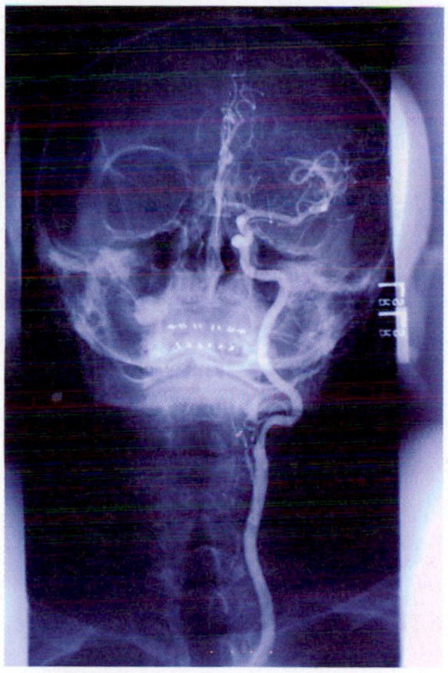 **Figure 10-28 ■ Arteriogram.** The injected dye clearly outlines the patient's left carotid artery and its many smaller branches within the cranial cavity. There is no evidence of carotid artery plaques or cerebral aneurysm.	**angiography** (AN-jee-AWG-rah-fee) 　**angi/o-** *blood vessel; lymphatic vessel* 　**-graphy** *process of recording* **angiogram** (AN-jee-oh-gram) 　**angi/o-** *blood vessel; lymphatic vessel* 　**-gram** *a record or picture* **arteriography** (ar-TEER-ee-AWG-rah-fee) 　**arteri/o-** *artery* 　**-graphy** *process of recording* **arteriogram** (ar-TEER-ee-oh-gram) 　**arteri/o-** *artery* 　**-gram** *a record or picture*
computed axial tomography (CAT, CT)	Procedure that uses x-rays to create many individual, closely spaced images ("slices"). CT scans are used to view the cranium, brain, vertebral column, and spinal cord. Radiopaque contrast dye can be injected to provide more detail.	**axial** (AK-see-al) 　**axi/o-** *axis* 　**-al** *pertaining to* **tomography** (toh-MAWG-rah-fee) 　**tom/o-** *cut; slice; layer* 　**-graphy** *process of recording*
Doppler ultrasonography	Procedure that uses ultrasound (high-frequency sound waves) to produce a two-dimensional image to visualize areas of stenosis and plaque and turbulence in the blood flow in the carotid arteries (see Figure 5-25). This is also known as a **carotid duplex scan.**	**carotid** (kah-RAWT-id) **duplex** (DOO-pleks)
magnetic resonance imaging (MRI)	Procedure that uses a magnetic field and radiowaves to align the protons in the body and cause them to emit signals that create an image. Magnetic resonance imaging is a type of tomography that creates images as many individual "slices." MRI scans are used to view the cranium, brain, vertebral column, and spinal cord (see Figure 10-11). Radiopaque contrast dye can be injected to provide more detail.	**magnetic** (mag-NET-ik) 　**magnet/o-** *magnet* 　**-ic** *pertaining to* **resonance** (REZ-oh-nans)
myelography	Procedure in which a radiopaque contrast dye is injected into the subarachnoid space at the level of the L3 and L4 vertebrae. The contrast dye outlines the spinal cavity and shows spinal nerves, nerve roots, and intervertebral disks, as well as tumors, herniated disks, or obstructions within the cavity. The x-ray image is a **myelogram.** Because a myelogram can cause the side effect of a severe headache, an MRI scan of the spine is more often done.	**myelography** (MY-eh-LAWG-rah-fee) 　**myel/o-** *bone marrow; spinal cord; myelin* 　**-graphy** *process of recording* **myelogram** (MY-eh-LOH-gram) 　**myel/o-** *bone marrow; spinal cord; myelin* 　**-gram** *a record or picture*

Word or Phrase	Description	Word Building
positron emission tomography (PET) scan	Procedure that uses a radioactive substance that emits positrons. This substance is combined with glucose molecules and injected intravenously. As the glucose is metabolized, the radioactive substance emits positrons, and these form gamma rays that are detected by a gamma camera. The camera produces an image that reflects the amount of metabolism in that area (see Figure 10-15). An area of increased metabolism can be due to a cancerous tumor. Areas of decreased metabolism can be due to Alzheimer's disease, Parkinson's disease, or epilepsy (see Figure 10-16).	**positron** (PAWZ-ih-trawn) **emission** (ee-MISH-un) **emiss/o-** *to send out* **-ion** *action; condition* **tomography** (toh-MAWG-rah-fee) **tom/o-** *cut; slice; layer* **-graphy** *process of recording*
skull x-ray	Procedure in which a plain film (without contrast dye) is taken of the skull. An x-ray can show fractures of the bones of the skull but cannot clearly show the soft tissues of the brain or the blood vessels.	

Other Diagnostic Tests

electroencepha-lography (EEG)	Diagnostic procedure to record the electrical activity of the brain (see Figure 10-29 ■). Multiple electrodes are placed on the scalp overlying specific lobes of the brain. The electrodes are attached to lead wires to an **electroencephalograph,** a machine that records brain waves. The computerized recording of the brain waves is an **electroencephalogram.** There are four types of normal brain waves (named for letters of the Greek alphabet): alpha, beta, delta, and theta. The patterns of brain waves in each of the two hemispheres of the cerebrum are compared for symmetry. A difference between the two hemispheres suggests a tumor or injury. The presence of abnormal waves suggests encephalopathy or dementia. Brain waves during an epileptic seizure show specific patterns that are used to diagnose the particular type of epilepsy. In order to induce an epileptic seizure during the EEG, the patient may look at flashing lights or have a sleep-deprived EEG recording. An EEG is also done as part of a polysomnography to diagnose sleep disorders and also as part of evoked potential testing. 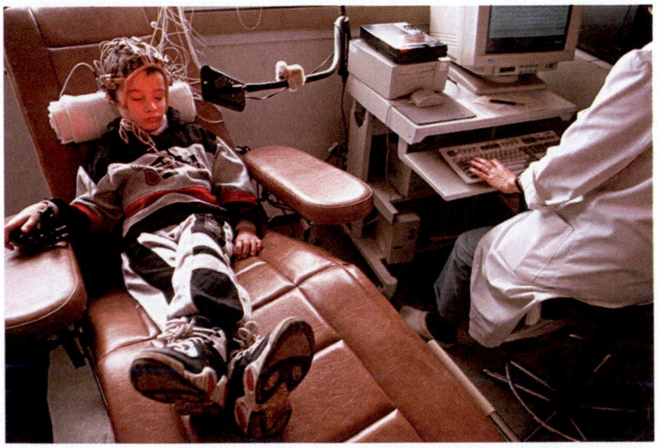	**electroencephalography** (ee-LEK-troh-en-SEF-ah-LAWG-rah-fee) **electr/o-** *electricity* **encephal/o-** *brain* **-graphy** *process of recording* **electroencephalograph** (ee-LEK-troh-en-SEF-ah-loh-graf) **electr/o-** *electricity* **encephal/o-** *brain* **-graph** *instrument used to record* **electroencephalogram** (ee-LEK-troh-en-SEF-ah-loh-gram) **electr/o-** *electricity* **encephal/o-** *brain* **-gram** *a record or picture*

Figure 10-29 ■ **Electroencephalography (EEG).**
This boy is having an EEG done to diagnose what type of epileptic seizures he is having. Electrodes on his scalp pick up the electrical impulses of brain waves and display them on the computer screen.

Word or Phrase	Description	Word Building

evoked potential testing	Procedure in which an EEG is used to record changes in brain waves that occur following various stimuli. It is used to evaluate the potential ability of a particular nervous pathway to conduct nerve impulses. A stimulus is presented to evoke (stimulate) a response, and this procedure is also called evoked response testing. For a **visual evoked potential (VEP)** or **visual evoked response (VER),** the patient watches a TV monitor that displays rapidly alternating checkerboard patterns. This evaluates nerve pathways from the eye to the cerebrum. For a **brainstem auditory evoked potential (BAEP)** or **brainstem auditory evoked response (BAER),** the patient has on headphones and listens to a series of clicks in one ear and then the other. This evaluates nerve pathways from the ears to the cerebrum. For a **somatosensory evoked potential (SSEP)** or **somatosensory evoked response (SSER),** a small electrical impulse is administered to the arm or leg. This evaluates nerve pathways from the extremities to the cerebrum. These tests are particularly helpful with patients who are too young or are unable to respond to standard vision and hearing tests. These tests are also used to detect subtle abnormalities in patients with multiple sclerosis, head trauma, or spinal cord injury. The patient cannot voluntarily alter the response to these tests.	**evoked** (ee-VOKED)
		
		potential (poh-TEN-shal)
		    potent/o- *being capable of doing*
		    -al *pertaining to*
		
		somatosensory (soh-MAH-toh-SEN-soh-ree)
		    somat/o- *body*
		    sens/o- *sensation*
		    -ory *having the function of*

nerve conduction study	Procedure to measure the speed at which an electrical impulse travels along a nerve. An electrical impulse through an electrode applied to the skin is used to stimulate a peripheral nerve. Another electrode a measured distance away records how long it takes for the electrical impulse to reach it. This test is usually performed in conjunction with electromyography to help differentiate between weakness due to nerve disorders versus weakness due to muscle disorders.	**conduction** (con-DUK-shun)
		    conduct/o- *carrying; conveying*
		    -ion *action; condition*

polysomnography	Multifaceted test to diagnose the underlying conditions that can cause insomnia, sleep disruption, sleep apnea, or narcolepsy. Electrodes on the face and head and various other monitors are used to record the patient's EEG, eye movements, muscle activity, heartbeat, and respirations during sleep. It is also known as a **sleep study.**	**polysomnography** (PAWL-ee-sawm-NAWG-rah-fee)
		    poly- *many; much*
		    somn/o- *sleep*
		    -graphy *process of recording*
		Add words to make a complete definition of *polysomnography*: *process of recording many (of the body's activities that occur during) sleep.*

Medical and Surgical Procedures

Medical Procedures

Word or Phrase	Description	Word Building
Babinski's sign	Neurologic test in which the end of the metal handle of a percussion hammer is used to firmly stroke the lateral sole of the foot from the heel to the toes. A normal test (negative Babinski) produces a downward curling of the toes. An abnormal test (positive Babinski) produces extension of the great toe and lateral fanning of the other toes (see Figure 10-30 ■). A positive Babinski indicates injury to the parietal lobe of the cerebrum or to the spinal nerves. **Figure 10-30 ■ Positive Babinski's sign.** This patient has a positive (abnormal) Babinski's sign with extension of the great toe and fanning of the other toes laterally.	**Babinski** (bah-BIN-skee)
Glasgow Coma Scale (GCS)	Numerical scale that measures the depth of a coma. The total score ranges from 1 to 15 and is the sum of individual scores for eye opening, motor response, and verbal response following a painful stimulus (such as pressure on the nailbed or on the supraorbital ridge over the eye). For example, if a patient opens his eyes to a verbal command, has confused answers, and withdraws from the painful stimulus, his GCS would be Eyes (3) + Verbal (4) + Motor (4) = 11.	**Glasgow** (GLAS-goh)

lumbar puncture (LP)	Procedure to obtain cerebrospinal fluid (CSF) for testing. It is also known as a **spinal tap.** The patient is positioned on the side with the upper legs flexed toward the chest. This curves the spine and widens the space between the spinous processes of two vertebrae, allowing accurate positioning of the spinal needle (see Figure 10-31 ■). A needle is inserted in the space between the L3–4 or L4–5 vertebrae and into the subarachnoid space. Cerebrospinal fluid flows through the needle and is collected and sent to the laboratory. Before the spinal needle is removed, a calibrated **manometer** (a thin tube) can be attached to measure the intracranial pressure as the CSF rises in the manometer.	**lumbar** (LUM-bar)
		  lumb/o- *lower back; area between the ribs and pelvis*
		  -ar *pertaining to*
		
		puncture (PUNGK-chur)
		  punct/o- *hole; perforation*
		  -ure *system; result of*
		
		manometer (mah-NAWM-eh-ter)
		  man/o- *thin; frenzy*
		  -meter *instrument used to measure*

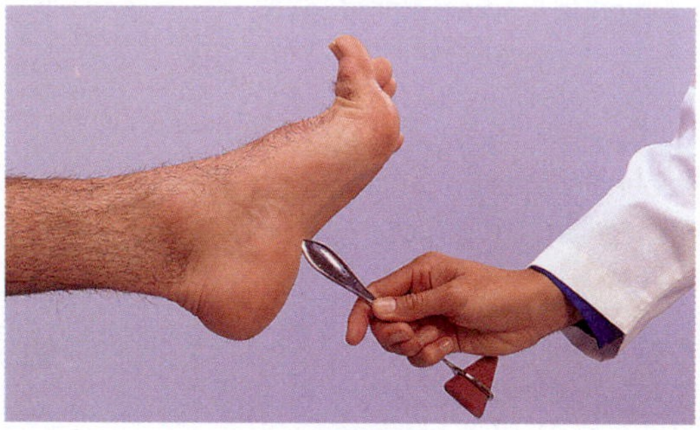

Word or Phrase	Description	Word Building

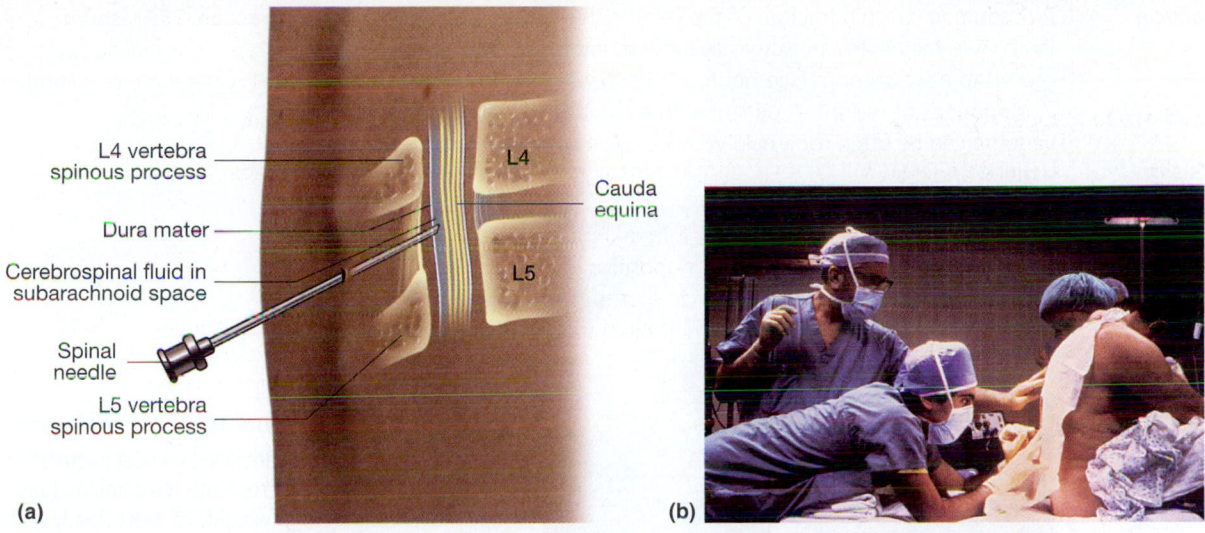

L4 vertebra
spinous process

L4

Cauda
equina

Dura mater

Cerebrospinal fluid in
subarachnoid space

L5

Spinal
needle

L5 vertebra
spinous process

(a)

(b)

Figure 10-31 ■ Lumbar puncture.

(a) For a lumbar puncture, the needle is inserted into the subarachnoid space where there is cerebrospinal fluid. (b) This patient is having a lumbar puncture. In this case, an upright position is being used, but this older patient does not have much flexibility of the spine and is only able to flex the head and shoulders forward. One physician is helping the patient to maintain this position while the other physician inserts the spinal needle. A white sterile drape covers the patient's back except for a round opening in the drape where the needle is inserted.

Word or Phrase	Description	Word Building
mini mental status examination (MMSE)	Tests the patient's concrete and abstract thought processes and long- and short-term memory. The patient is asked to state his/her name, the date, and where he/she is. If the answers are all correct, the patient is said to be oriented to person, time, and place (oriented x3). The patient is asked to perform simple mental arithmetic, recall objects or words, name the current president and recent past presidents, spell a word backwards, and give the meaning of a proverb. A full mental status examination is done during a psychiatric evaluation (discussed in "Psychiatry," Chapter 17).	**mental** (MEN-tal) **ment/o-** *mind; chin* **-al** *pertaining to*
neurologic examination	Tests coordination, sensation, balance, and gait. Coordination tests: (1) Rapid alternating movements. The patient taps the tip of the index finger against the thumb as rapidly as possible. (2) Finger-to-nose test. With eyes closed, the patient touches the tip of the index finger to the nose. (3) The patient touches the nose, then touches the physician's finger as it moves to various locations, then touches the nose again. (4) Heel-to-shin test: The patient puts the heel of one foot onto the opposite leg and then runs it from the knee down the shin to the toes. Sensation tests: (1) With the patient's eyes closed, the skin is touched in various places with a cotton swab (to test light touch), a vibrating tuning fork (to test vibration), and the point of a pin (pinprick to test pain). One or two pins are used to see if the patient can distinguish the number of things touching the skin (two-point discrimination). (2) The patient's toe or finger is moved up and down and the patient is asked to identify the direction (to test body position and **proprioception**). Balance tests: (1) **Romberg test.** The patient stands with the feet together and the eyes closed. In a normal test, the patient does not sway excessively or lose balance. The Romberg test is also known as the **station test.** Gait tests: (1) The manner of walking is assessed for a normal arm swing and stride. (2) The patient is asked to walk across the room in a heel-to-toe fashion. The patient is asked to walk on the toes, on the heels, and then hop in place on each foot.	**proprioception** (PROH-pree-oh-SEP-shun) *Proprioception* comes from the combining form *propri/o-* (*one's own self*), part of the word *receptor,* and the suffix *-tion* (*a process; being or having*). **Romberg** (RAWM-berg)

Word or Phrase	Description	Word Building
spinal traction	Procedure in which a fracture of the vertebra is immobilized while it heals. Two metal pins are surgically inserted into the cranium and attached to a set of tongs (see Figure 10-32 ■) with a rope and pulley and 7–10 pounds of weight. A patient with a partially healed fracture of the vertebra can be fitted for a halo vest with pins in the cranium attached to a metal ring (halo).	**traction** (TRAK-shun) **tract/o-** *pulling* **-ion** *action; condition*

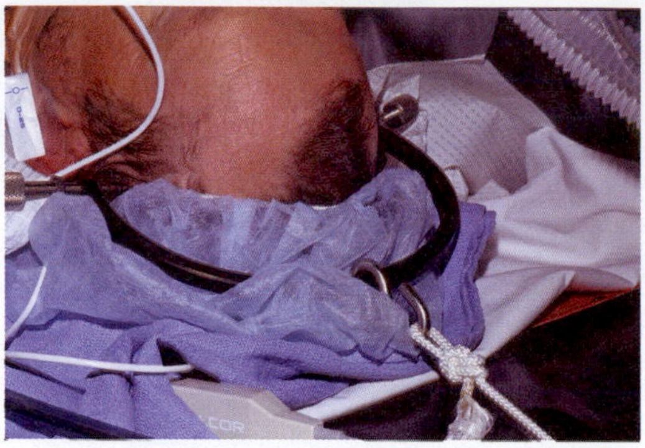

Figure 10-32 ■ Spinal traction with tongs.
This patient's spine is immobilized while a fractured vertebra heals. Notice the pins inserted into the cranium, tongs, and the rope that is connected to weights to exert steady and constant traction.

Word or Phrase	Description	Word Building
transcutaneous electrical nerve stimulation (TENS) unit	Procedure that uses an electrical device to control chronic pain. A battery produces regular, preset electrical impulses that travel through wires to electrodes on the skin. These impulses block the transmission of pain sensations to the brain. The impulses also stimulate the body to produce its own natural pain-relieving endorphins.	**transcutaneous** (TRANS-kyoo-TAY-nee-us) **trans-** *across; through* **cutane/o-** *skin* **-ous** *pertaining to*

Surgical Procedures

Word or Phrase	Description	Word Building
biopsy	Procedure to remove a tumor or mass from the brain or other part of the nervous system. In an **excisional biopsy,** the entire tumor or mass is removed and sent to the laboratory for microscopic examination to determine if it is benign or malignant. Even a benign tumor must be totally removed because it causes increasing intracranial pressure in the inflexible bony cranium.	**biopsy** (BY-awp-see) **bi/o-** *life; living organisms; living tissue* **-opsy** *process of viewing* **excisional** (ek-SIH-shun-al) **excis/o-** *to cut out* **-ion** *action; condition* **-al** *pertaining to*
carotid endarterectomy	Procedure to remove plaque from the carotid artery. This opens up the lumen of the artery, restores blood flow to the brain, and decreases the possibility of a stroke.	**endarterectomy** (END-ar-ter-EK-toh-mee) **endo-** *innermost; within* **arter/o-** *artery* **-ectomy** *surgical excision*
craniotomy	Surgical incision into the cranium to expose the brain tissue. A craniotomy is the first phase of any type of brain surgery (i.e., evacuation of a subdural hematoma or excising a brain tumor).	**craniotomy** (KRAY-nee-AW-toh-mee) **crani/o-** *cranium (skull)* **-tomy** *process of cutting or making an incision*
diskectomy	Surgical excision of part or all of the herniated nucleus pulposus from an intervertebral disk. This relieves pressure on the adjacent dorsal nerve roots and relieves the pain.	**diskectomy** (dis-KEK-toh-mee) **disk/o-** *disk* **-ectomy** *surgical excision*

Word or Phrase	Description	Word Building
laminectomy	Surgical excision of the lamina (the flat area of the arch of the vertebra). Removal of this bony segment relieves pressure on the dorsal nerve roots and relieves pain from a herniated nucleus pulposus.	**laminectomy** (LAM-ih-NEK-toh-mee) **lamin/o-** *lamina (flat area on the vertebra)* **-ectomy** *surgical excision*

Clinical Connections

Pain Management. This subspecialty for treating chronic or severe pain is shared by both neurology and anesthesiology. Pain management procedures include a dorsal nerve root injection into an area where a nerve is compressed. Surgical treatment includes a **rhizotomy,** an incision to cut spinal nerve roots. The dorsal (sensory) nerve roots can be cut to relieve severe pain. The ventral (motor) nerve roots can be cut to relieve severe muscle spasticity and spasm.	**rhizotomy** (ry-ZAW-toh-mee) **rhiz/o-** *spinal nerve root* **-tomy** *process of cutting or making an incision*

Word or Phrase	Description	Word Building
stereotactic neurosurgery	Procedure that uses three dimensions to excise a tumor deep within the cerebrum. A CT or MRI scan is used to show the tumor in three dimensions and give its precise coordinates. The patient's head is fixed in a stereotactic apparatus that guides the position of an electrode in the brain. Then heat, cold, or high-energy gamma rays are used to destroy the tumor.	**stereotactic** (STAIR-ee-oh-TAK-tik) **stere/o-** *three dimensions* **tact/o-** *touch* **-ic** *pertaining to* **neurosurgery** (NYOO-roh-SER-jer-ee) **neur/o-** *nerve* **surg/o-** *operative procedure* **-ery** *process of*
ventriculo-peritoneal shunt	Procedure to insert a plastic tube to connect the ventricles of the brain to the peritoneal cavity. The shunt continuously removes excess cerebrospinal fluid associated with hydrocephalus.	**ventriculoperitoneal** (ven-TRIK-yoo-loh-PAIR-ih-toh-NEE-al) **ventricul/o-** *ventricle (lower heart chamber; chamber in the brain)* **peritone/o-** *peritoneum* **-eal** *pertaining to* **shunt** (SHUNT)

Drug Categories

These categories of drugs are used to treat neurologic diseases and conditions. The most common generic and trade name drugs in each category are listed.

Category	Indication	Examples	Word Building
analgesic drugs	Aspirin, nonsalicylate drugs such as acetaminophen, and nonsteroidal anti-inflammatory drugs are used to treat mild-to-moderate pain. **Narcotic** drugs are used to treat severe, chronic pain.	acetaminophen (Tylenol), aspirin (Bayer, Empirin), ibuprofen (Advil, Motrin), naproxen (Aleve, Naprosyn). Narcotic drugs: fentanyl (Actiq, Duragesic), meperidine (Demerol), morphine (MS Contin), oxycodone (OxyContin), propoxyphene (Darvon)	**analgesic** (AN-al-JEE-zik) **an-** *without; not* **alges/o-** *sensation of pain* **-ic** *pertaining to* **narcotic** (nar-KAWT-ik) **narc/o-** *stupor; sleep* **-tic** *pertaining to*

Category	Indication	Examples	Word Building
antiepileptic drugs	Prevent the seizures of epilepsy. They are also known as **anticonvulsant drugs.**	ethosuximide (Zarontin), phenytoin (Dilantin), topiramate (Topamax), valproic acid (Depakene, Depakote)	**antiepileptic** (AN-tee-EP-ih-LEP-tik) (AN-tih-EP-ih-LEP-tik) **anti-** *against* **epilept/o-** *seizure* **-ic** *pertaining to* **anticonvulsant** (AN-tee-con-VUL-sant) (AN-tih-con-VUL-sant) **anti-** *against* **convuls/o-** *seizure* **-ant** *pertaining to*
corticosteroid drugs	Suppress inflammation in chronic pain conditions and multiple sclerosis. They are used to treat swelling and edema in the brain or spinal cord following traumatic injury or stroke.	dexamethasone (Decadron), prednisone (Deltasone, Meticorten)	**corticosteroid** (KOR-tih-koh-STAIR-oyd) **cortic/o-** *cortex (outer region)* **-steroid** *steroid*
drugs for Alzheimer's disease	Inhibit an enzyme that breaks down acetylcholine	donepezil (Aricept), rivastigmine (Exelon), tacrine (Cognex)	
drugs for neuralgia and neuropathy	Work in various ways to treat the many different causes of neuralgia and neuropathy. These drugs are classified as anticonvulsant drugs. Antianxiety and antidepressant drugs are also used.	gabapentin (Neurontin), pregabalin (Lyrica)	
drugs for Parkinson's disease	Stimulate dopamine receptors, inhibit the action of acetylcholine, or inhibit the enzyme that metabolizes the drug levodopa (this allows more levodopa to reach the brain)	amantadine (Symmetrel), benztropine (Cogentin), Duodopa (combination of carbidopa and levodopa), entacapone (Comtan), ropinirole (Requip)	

Clinical Connections

Pharmacology. Patients who take drugs to treat Parkinson's disease can develop a tolerance to the drug and require higher and higher doses. However, the higher doses produce more side effects. When the drug dose can no longer be increased, or the side effects of a high dose become intolerable, the physician will place the patient on a drug holiday. When the drug is restarted at a lower dose, it is effective.

Abbreviations

AFP	alpha fetoprotein	**HNP**	herniated nucleus pulposus
ALS	amyotrophic lateral sclerosis	**ICP**	intracranial pressure
AVM	arteriovenous malformation	**LP**	lumbar puncture
BAEP	brainstem auditory evoked potential	**MRI**	magnetic resonance imaging
BAER	brainstem auditory evoked response	**MS***	multiple sclerosis
CNS	central nervous system	**NICU**	neurologic intensive care unit
CP	cerebral palsy	**PET**	positron emission tomography
CRPS	chronic regional pain syndrome	**RIND**	reversible ischemic neurologic deficit
CSF	cerebrospinal fluid	**SCI**	spinal cord injury
CT	computed tomography	**SSEP**	somatosensory evoked potential
CTS	carpal tunnel syndrome	**SSER**	somatosensory evoked response
CVA	cerebrovascular accident	**TENS**	transcutaneous electrical nerve stimulation (unit)
EEG	electroencephalography	**TIA**	transient ischemic attack
END	electroneurodiagnostic (technician)	**VEP**	visual evoked potential
GCS	Glasgow Coma Scale (or Score)	**VER**	visual evoked response

*According to the Joint Commission on Accreditation of Healthcare Organizations (JCAHO) and the Institute for Safe Medication Practices (ISMP), this abbreviation should not be used. However, because it is still used by some healthcare providers, it is included here.

Word Alert

ABBREVIATIONS

Abbreviations are commonly used in all types of medical documents; however, they can mean different things to different people and their meanings can be misinterpreted. Always verify the meaning of an abbreviation.

CP means *cerebral palsy,* but it also means *cardiopulmonary.*

CNS means *central nervous system,* but it can be confused with the sound-alike abbreviation *C&S,* which means *culture and sensitivity.*

HNP means *herniated nucleus pulposus,* but it can be confused with the sound-alike abbreviation *H&P,* which means *history and physical (examination).*

MS means *multiple sclerosis,* but it also means the drugs *morphine sulfate* or *magnesium sulfate.*

NICU means *neurologic intensive care unit,* but it also means *neonatal intensive care unit.*

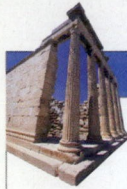

It's Greek To Me!

Did you notice that some words have two different combining forms? Combining forms from both Greek and Latin languages remain a part of medical language today.

Word	Greek	Latin	Medical Word Examples
mind	psych/o-	ment/o-	psychomotor, dementia
nerve	neur/o-	nerv/o-	neuron, nervous system
seizure	epilept/o-	convuls/o-	epileptic, convulsion
		ict/o-	postictal
sensation	esthes/o-	sens/o-	paresthesia, sensory nerve
spinal nerve root	rhiz/o-	radicul/o-	rhizotomy, radiculopathy
spine, spinal cord	myel/o-	spin/o-	myelomeningocele, spinal

CAREER FOCUS

Meet Amelia, a pharmacy technician

"Here in the hospital pharmacy, I have the responsibility of making IVs and filling orders. I deliver med carts; I deliver patient meds. I do expiration dates—pulling all expired drugs off the shelf, and I also get to work with wonderful pharmacists. Even though I initial all the drug orders that I fill, they cannot leave the pharmacy until the pharmacist has checked off on them. The best part of my job is meeting different people. I enjoy helping people and making someone's day a little better."

Pharmacy technicians are allied health professionals who assist pharmacists in their work. Pharmacy technicians provide pharmacy services to home health, long-term care, and outpatient facilities, and to hospitals. They also work in retail pharmacies (drug stores).

    Neurologists are physicians who practice in the medical specialty of neurology. They diagnose and treat patients with diseases of the nervous system.

    Neurosurgeons perform surgery on the brain, spinal cord, and nerves. Physicians can take additional training and become board certified in the subspecialty of pediatric neurology.

    Malignancies of the nervous system are treated medically by an oncologist or surgically by a neurosurgeon.

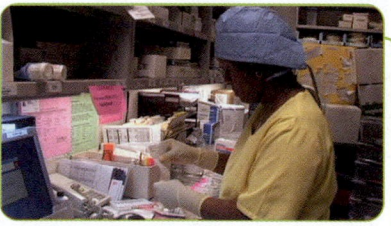

pharmacy (FAR-mah-see)

technician (tek-NISH-un)
  techn/o- *technical skill*
  -ician *skilled professional or expert*

neurologist (nyoo-RAWL-oh-jist)
  neur/o- *nerve*
  log/o- *word; the study of*
  -ist *one who specializes in*

neurosurgeon (NYOOR-oh-SER-jun)
  neur/o- *nerve*
  surg/o- *operative procedure*
  -eon *one who performs*

PEARSON myhealth**professionskit** To see Amelia's complete video profile, visit Medical Terminology Interactive at www.myhealthprofessionskit.com. Select this book, log in, and go to the 10th floor of Pearson General Hospital. Enter the Laboratory, and click on the computer screen.

CHAPTER REVIEW EXERCISES

Test your knowledge of the chapter by completing these review exercises. Use the Answer Key at the end of the book to check your answers.

Anatomy and Physiology

Matching Exercise

Match each word or phrase to its description.

1. axon
2. cauda equina
3. corpus callosum
4. cranial nerves
5. cranium
6. dermatome
7. epinephrine
8. gustatory cortex
9. medulla oblongata
10. neurotransmitter
11. reflex
12. Schwann
13. subarachnoid space
14. synapse
15. ventricles

_____ Hormone from the adrenal medulla that acts with the sympathetic division of the nervous system

_____ Four hollow chambers within the brain that contain CSF

_____ Between the pons and the spinal cord

_____ Cells that make myelin around axons of cranial nerves and spinal nerves

_____ Involuntary muscle reaction controlled by the spinal cord

_____ There are 12 pairs of them

_____ Nerve roots that come out of the inferior end of the spinal cord

_____ Part of the neuron that may be myelinated

_____ Space between the axon of one neuron and the dendrite of the next neuron

_____ Area that contains cerebrospinal fluid in the meninges

_____ Area of the cerebrum that receives sensory impulses from the taste receptors

_____ Area of the skin that supplies sensory information to a specific spinal nerve

_____ Dome-shaped bone of the skull

_____ Chemical messenger

_____ Band of neurons that connects the two hemispheres of the cerebrum

Circle Exercise

Circle the correct word from the choices given.

1. The (**axon, cerebellum, cerebrum**) is divided into two hemispheres.
2. The olfactory cortex receives sensory impulses from the (**ears, eyes, nose**).
3. The most delicate of the meninges and the one that is closest to the brain is the (**arachnoid, dura mater, pia mater**).
4. The functional unit of the nervous system is the (**nephron, nerve, neuron**).
5. In the majority of people, the (**cerebellum, gyrus, left hemisphere of the cerebrum**) performs math, analysis, and logical thinking.
6. The hypothalamus is located (**above, below, beside**) the thalamus.
7. The (**auditory, oculomotor, trigeminal**) cranial nerve controls eye movements.
8. The neurotransmitter that goes between a neuron and a voluntary skeletal muscle is (**acetylcholine, dopamine, endorphins**).

True or False Exercise

Indicate whether each statement is true or false by writing T or F on the line.

1. _____ The autonomic nervous system is composed of the central nervous system and the peripheral nervous system.
2. _____ Efferent nerves carry nerve impulses away from the brain or spinal cord.
3. _____ After a nerve impulse passes through the cell body, it then goes to the dendrites.
4. _____ The occipital lobe is a lobe of the cerebellum that is directly beneath the occipital bone of the cranium.
5. _____ The peripheral nervous system consists of the cranial nerves and spinal nerves.
6. _____ The hypothalamus functions as part of the nervous system and endocrine system.
7. _____ Cranial nerve X (vagus nerve) is the only cranial nerve that goes into the thoracic and abdominal cavities.
8. _____ Endorphins are the body's own natural pain relievers.

Fill in the Blank Exercise

Write the correct answers in the blanks provided.

1. Name the three layers that comprise the meninges.

   _____

   _____

   _____

2. Rounded tissue folds in the cerebral cortex are known as _____ and the narrow grooves between the folds are known as _____.
3. Medical name for one half of the cerebrum _____
4. The _____ cells that line the ventricles produce cerebrospinal fluid.
5. The _____ regulates sensations of hunger and thirst as well as the body's 24-hour circadian rhythm.

Multiple Choice Exercise

Circle the best answer from the choices given.

1. Sensory information consists of all of the following *except* _____.
   a. pain
   b. sounds
   c. motor commands
   d. temperature
2. _____ are cells that are small and move around the brain and spinal cord to engulf and destroy dead tissue and pathogens.
   a. Microglia
   b. Axons
   c. Cerebrospinal fluid
   d. Dorsal nerve roots
3. The division of the nervous system that is active in the "fight or flight" response is the _____.
   a. central nervous system
   b. peripheral nervous system
   c. brain
   d. sympathetic nervous system

Diseases and Conditions

True or False Exercise

Indicate whether each statement is true or false by writing T *or* F *on the line.*

1. _____ Causalgia is a severe, burning type of neuralgia.

2. _____ A neural tube defect can result in multiple sclerosis.

3. _____ A hematoma is a type of brain tumor.

4. _____ Presenile dementia is another name for early-onset Alzheimer's disease.

5. _____ Photophobia and throbbing pain are symptoms of a migraine headache.

6. _____ A TIA and a RIND are types of cerebrovascular accidents.

7. _____ Mad cow disease can be transmitted to humans as new variant Creutzfeldt-Jakob disease.

8. _____ The incidence of myelomeningocele can be greatly decreased if the mother takes a folic acid supplement while she is pregnant.

Circle Exercise

Circle the correct word from the choices given.

1. (**Amnesia, Myelomeningocele, Shingles**) is a painful skin condition caused by herpes zoster infection of a nerve.

2. Prior to the onset of a seizure, a patient may experience a/an (**aura, coma, polyneuritis**).

3. (**Dyslexia, Status epilepticus, Subdural hematoma**) is caused by trauma to the head.

4. An imbalance of dopamine and acetylcholine in the brain is associated with (**Down syndrome, multiple sclerosis, Parkinson's disease**).

5. Abnormal burning or tingling sensations on the skin are (**neuritis, paralysis, paresthesias**).

Fill in the Blank Exercise

Fill in the blank with the correct word from the word list.

amnesia	hydrocephalus	multiple sclerosis	nuchal rigidity	status epilepticus
aphasia	mental retardation	narcolepsy	sciatica	syncope
concussion				

1. Symptoms caused by progressive demyelination _____

2. Head trauma with loss of consciousness _____

3. Involuntary falling asleep during the day _____

4. Enlarged head because of excess CSF _____

5. Continuous seizure activity _____

6. Partial or total loss of memory _____

7. Radiculopathy in the lumbar area _____

8. Down syndrome _____

9. Stiff neck associated with meningitis _____

10. Inability to communicate verbally _____

11. Temporary loss of consciousness with fainting _____

Multiple Choice Exercise

Circle the correct word from the choices given.

1. All of the following are congenital disorders *except* _____.
   - a. cerebral palsy
   - b. hemiplegia
   - c. myelomeningocele
   - d. anencephaly

2. Alzheimer's disease is diagnosed at autopsy by the presence of _____.
   - a. demyelinization
   - b. coma
   - c. hydrocephalus
   - d. neurofibrillary tangles

3. All of the following are types of epilepsy *except* _____.
   - a. petit mal
   - b. complex partial
   - c. absence
   - d. aura

4. Neurofibromatosis is also known as _____.
   - a. Lou Gehrig's disease
   - b. Down syndrome
   - c. von Recklinghausen's disease
   - d. Parkinson's disease

Laboratory, Radiology, Surgery, Drugs

True or False Exercise

Indicate whether each statement is true or false by writing T or F on the line.

1. _____ Antiepileptic drugs are also known as anticonvulsant drugs.
2. _____ A patient with a partially healed vertebral fracture can be fitted for a halo vest to provide spinal traction.
3. _____ A laminectomy is a surgical procedure to remove plaque from a carotid artery.
4. _____ A TENS unit is used during a sleep study.
5. _____ An electroencephalography records brain wave patterns.
6. _____ Testing the patient's proprioception is testing an awareness of body position.
7. _____ A skull x-ray will show a fractured cranium as well as plaques in the cerebral arteries.

Matching Exercise

Match each word or phrase to its description.

1. PET scan   _____ Tests patient's balance with the eyes closed
2. vision test   _____ Passing this test shows normal function of cranial nerve II (optic nerve)
3. hearing test   _____ Patient's manner of walking
4. Babinski's sign   _____ Shows areas of decreased brain metabolism
5. oriented x3   _____ Passing this test shows normal function of the cranial nerve VIII (vestibulocochlear nerve)
6. mini mental status exam _____ Abnormal upward extension of big toe and fanning of other toes
7. gait   _____ Patient can state his name, the date, where he is
8. pinprick   _____ Test to detect numbness on the skin
9. Romberg test   _____ Proverbs, counting backwards, recall of objects, names of presidents

Fill in the Blank Exercise

Fill in the blank with the correct word from the word list.

alpha fetoprotein	EEG	PET scan	rhizotomy
corticosteroid drug	myelography	polysomnography	spinal tap

1. Used to treat edema of the brain or spinal cord after injury _____

2. Uses dye to outline the spinal cord and nerves_____

3. Indicates the presence of a neural tube defect_____

4. Surgical procedure to cut spinal nerve roots_____

5. Used to diagnose the type of epilepsy _____

6. Shows patterns of metabolism in the brain _____

7. Sleep study _____

8. Lumbar puncture _____

Building Medical Words

Review the Combining Forms Exercise, Combining Form and Suffix Exercise, and Prefix Exercise that you already completed in the anatomy section on pages 503–505.

Combining Forms Exercise

Before you build nervous system words, review these additional combining forms. Next to each combining form, write its medical meaning. The first one has been done for you.

Combining Form	Medical Meaning	Combining Form	Medical Meaning
1. alg/o-	pain	16. ict/o-	
2. bi/o-		17. infarct/o-	
3. caus/o-		18. lex/o-	
4. cephal/o-		19. log/o-	
5. clon/o-		20. ment/o-	
6. comat/o-		21. narc/o-	
7. concuss/o-		22. phas/o-	
8. convuls/o-		23. phob/o-	
9. cyt/o-		24. phot/o-	
10. disk/o-		25. pleg/o-	
11. electr/o-		26. somn/o-	
12. epilept/o-		27. surg/o-	
13. fibr/o-		28. syncop/o-	
14. hemat/o-		29. ton/o-	
15. hydr/o-		30. vascul/o-	

Related Combining Forms Exercise

Write the combining forms on the line provided. (Hint: See the It's Greek to Me feature box.)

1. Two combining forms that mean *mind*. _____

2. Two combining forms that mean *nerve*. _____

3. Two combining forms that mean *spinal nerve root*. _____

4. Two combining forms that mean *sensation*. _____

5. Two combining forms that mean *spine or spinal cord*. _____

6. Three combining forms that mean *seizure*. _____

Combining Form and Suffix Exercise

Read the definition of the medical word. Select the correct suffix from the Suffix List. Select the correct combining form from the Combining Form List. Build the medical word and write it on the line. Be sure to check your spelling. The first one has been done for you.

SUFFIX LIST	COMBINING FORM LIST	
-al (pertaining to)	bi/o- (life; living organisms; living tissue)	hemat/o- (blood)
-cele (hernia)	clon/o- (rapid contracting and relaxing)	hydr/o- (water; fluid)
-cephalus (head)	comat/o- (unconsciousness)	infarct/o- (area of dead tissue)
-ectomy (surgical excision)	concuss/o- (violent shaking or jarring)	mening/o- (meninges)
-graphy (process of recording)	convuls/o- (seizure)	myel/o- (bone marrow; spinal cord;
-ic (pertaining to)	crani/o- (cranium; skull)	myelin)
-ion (action; condition)	disk/o- (disk)	narc/o- (stupor; sleep)
-itis (inflammation of; infection of)	encephal/o- (brain)	neur/o- (nerve)
-lepsy (seizure)	ependym/o- (cellular lining)	radicul/o- (spinal nerve root)
-oma (tumor; mass)	epilept/o- (seizure)	rhiz/o- (spinal nerve root)
-opsy (process of viewing)	gli/o- (cells that provide support)	syncop/o- (fainting)
-ose (full of)		
-pathy (disease; suffering)		
-tomy (process of cutting or making an incision)		

Definition of the Medical Word

Build the Medical Word

1. Pertaining to the mind

    <u>mental</u>

2. Pertaining to (a person with a condition of) seizures

3. Mass of blood

4. Inflammation or infection of a nerve

5. Process of (removing and) viewing living tissue

6. Process of cutting and making an incision into the cranium

7. Inflammation or infection of the meninges

8. Seizure(-like state of being unable to keep from going to) sleep

9. (Condition of the) head (of having too much cerebrospinal) fluid

10. Pertaining to rapid contracting and relaxing (during a seizure)

11. Condition (caused by) violent shaking or jarring (of the head)

12. Tumor of the cellular lining (in the ventricle of the cerebrum)

13. Condition (that results in an) area of dead tissue

14. Process of recording (an image using contrast dye) of the spinal cord

Definition of the Medical Word

Build the Medical Word

15. Disease of the nerves

16. Process of cutting the spinal nerve root

17. Action or condition of (having) a seizure

18. Inflammation or infection of the brain

19. (Condition of a person being) full of unconsciousness

20. Tumor (in the brain composed of) cells that provide support

21. Pertaining to fainting

22. Hernia of the meninges (to the outside of the body)

23. Disease of the spinal nerve root

24. Tumor of a nerve

25. Surgical excision of (an intervertebral) disk

Prefix Exercise

Read the definition of the medical word. Look at the medical word or partial word that is given (it already contains a combining form and a suffix). Select the correct prefix from the Prefix List and write it on the blank line. Then build the medical word and write it on the line. Be sure to check your spelling. The first one has been done for you.

PREFIX LIST		
a- (away from; without)	dys- (painful; difficult; abnormal)	poly- (many; much)
an- (without; not)	hemi- (one half)	post- (after; behind)
anti- (against)	hyper- (above; more than normal)	quadri- (four)
de- (reversal of; without)	intra- (within)	sub- (below; underneath)

Definition of the Medical Word	Prefix	Word or Partial Word	Build the Medical Word
1. Pertaining to within the ventricle	intra-	ventricular	intraventricular
2. State (of being) without the mind	_____	mentia	_____
3. Pertaining to (the time) after a seizure	_____	ictal	_____
4. State of (being) without sensation or feeling	_____	esthesia	_____
5. Inflammation of many nerves	_____	neuritis	_____
6. Pertaining to (a drug that is) against seizures	_____	convulsant	_____
7. Pertaining to (having a) difficult (time with) words	_____	lexic	_____
8. Pertaining to within the cranium	_____	cranial	_____
9. State (of being) without speech	_____	phasia	_____
10. Pertaining to one half (of the body having) paralysis	_____	plegic	_____
11. Pertaining to underneath the dura mater	_____	dural	_____
12. Condition of four (extremities having) paralysis	_____	plegia	_____
13. Process of recording many (types of tests during) sleep	_____	somnography	_____
14. State of more than normal (response to) sensations or feelings	_____	esthesia	_____
15. Condition of difficult speech (after a stroke)	_____	phasia	_____

Multiple Combining Forms and Suffix Exercise

Read the definition of the medical word. Select the correct suffix and combining forms. Then build the medical word and write it on the line. Be sure to check your spelling. The first one has been done for you.

SUFFIX LIST	COMBINING FORM LIST	
-ar (pertaining to)	alg/o- (pain)	log/o- (word; the study of)
-cele (hernia)	astr/o- (starlike structure)	mening/o- (meninges)
-ery (process of)	caus/o- (burning)	myel/o- (bone marrow; spinal cord; myelin)
-gram (a record or picture)	cephal/o- (head)	neur/o- (nerve)
-ia (condition; state; thing)	cerebr/o- (cerebrum)	phot/o- (light)
-ic (pertaining to)	cyt/o- (cell)	phob/o- (fear; avoidance)
-oma (tumor; mass)	electr/o- (electricity)	surg/o- (operative procedure)
-omatosis (abnormal condition of multiple tumors)	encephal/o- (brain)	vascul/o- (blood vessels)
	fibr/o- (fiber)	

Definition of the Medical Word

Build the Medical Word

1. Pertaining to nerves and the study of them

    neurologic _____

2. Condition (in which) light (causes) fear or avoidance

    _____

3. Hernia of the spinal cord and the meninges (to the outside of the body)

    _____

4. Condition of burning pain

    _____

5. Abnormal condition of multiple tumors of the nerve that are fibrous

    _____

6. A record or picture of the electricity (brain waves) in the brain

    _____

7. Condition of the nerves (having) pain

    _____

8. Process of a nerve (or brain) operative procedure

    _____

9. Pertaining to the cerebrum and blood vessels

    _____

10. Tumor composed of starlike structure cells

    _____

11. Condition of the head (having) pain

    _____

Abbreviations

Matching Exercise

Match each abbreviation to its description.

1. ALS   _____ Presses on spinal nerve roots

2. CP   _____ Congenital disorder from lack of oxygen to the fetal brain

3. CSF   _____ Lou Gehrig's disease

4. CVA   _____ Can result in paraplegia or quadriplegia

5. EEG   _____ Also known as a spinal tap

6. HNP   _____ Circulates through the subarachnoid space

7. LP   _____ Test that records brain wave patterns

8. SCI   _____ A stroke

Applied Skills

Proofreading and Spelling Exercise

Read the following paragraph. Identify each misspelled medical word and write the correct spelling of it on the line.

A patient might need nurosurgery because of a subdural hematomma or a tumor such as a menengioma. A cerebrohvascular accident is a stroke or brain attack and is from an infarkt. An ordinary headache is cephalalga, while having half of the body paralysed from a stroke is called hemeplegia. A seizure or a convulsion is known as epilepsee. Inflammation of many individual nerves is polyneuritus. The study of the brain and spinal cord and nerves is neurology.

1. _____   6. _____
2. _____   7. _____
3. _____   8. _____
4. _____   9. _____
5. _____   10. _____

Medical Report Exercise

This exercise contains a neurologic office consultation. Read the report and answer the questions that follow.

Neurologic Associates
Centennial Medical Building, Suite 312
5005 Frankstown Road
Pittsburgh, PA 15237

November 19, 20xx

Marshall Gibbons, M.D.
Primary Care Associates
19 Walker Avenue
Middletown, PA 15222

Re: JENCKS, Justine

Dear Dr. Gibbons:

I saw your patient, Justine Jencks, in neurologic consultation on November 19, 20xx. She is a 38-year-old, right-handed Caucasian female who has complained of intermittent dizziness and other symptoms for the past year. She reports temporary dizziness with hyperextension of the neck when raising her hands above her head to reach a high shelf or hang drapes. Two months ago, the patient had an acute episode in which she awoke with a sense of doom, headache, profuse perspiration, nausea, paresthesias of the fingers, dizziness, tachycardia, and felt the room was spinning. On the way to the emergency room, her husband commented about their dogs, but she could only remember her older dog and had no recollection of having another dog. In the emergency room, she commented to the nurse that she felt like her "blood pressure was zero." When asked about her last menstrual period, she felt that she might be pregnant but could not explain why she felt this way. On the mini mental status exam, she could not name the current and most recent presidents but was otherwise oriented x3. She was able to count back by serial 7s. The physical examination in the emergency room was essentially negative. Her blood pressure and blood sugar results were normal.

The patient has a past history that is significant for possible MS. This was tentatively diagnosed 10 years ago. At that time, laboratory test results were inconclusive: visual evoked responses were abnormal, but the CFS showed no oligoclonal bands and an MRI scan of the brain was read as negative. At that time, her symptoms included extreme muscle weakness. She could only walk a short distance by using a wide-based gait for stability. This initial episode lasted 2 months and then the symptoms gradually resolved.

(continued)

She does not routinely have headaches. She denies ever having had seizures. She denies any smell or taste disturbances. She denies difficulty swallowing. She has no speech difficulties and is able to relate her medical history easily.

Examination of cranial nerves V through XII was normal. Examination of the motor system revealed normal muscle strength. Babinski was negative. Sensory examination to light touch, pinprick, vibration, position, and 2-point discrimination was normal. Cerebellar functions in the form of finger-to-nose and heel-to-shin tests were normal. Gait was normal. Romberg's sign was negative. There was marked muscle spasm of the trapezius muscles bilaterally and limitation of neck motion laterally to the right and rotationally to the left.

Several of the patient's complaints could be due to a vestibular migraine, but the episode with the 2-hour alteration in memory is problematic and may suggest a TIA. She has some typical migraine symptoms, but the dizziness points to a vestibular focus to the migraine. Because of the past history of possible MS, I will have her undergo an MRI scan with contrast to pinpoint any demyelinization that has occurred since her last MRI. I have also ordered a carotid arteriography to rule out blockage of the carotid arteries.

After these tests are obtained, I will follow up with her in about 3 weeks to review the test results.

Thank you for referring this interesting and delightful patient to me.

Sincerely yours,

Renworth R. Pitman, M.D.

Rentworth R. Pitman, M.D.

RRP: sct
D: 11/19/xx
T: 11/19/xx

Word Analysis Questions

1. Divide *neurologic* into its three word parts and define each word part.

Word Part	Definition
_____	_____
_____	_____
_____	_____

2. Divide *paresthesia* into its three word parts and define each word part.

Word Part	Definition
_____	_____
_____	_____
_____	_____

3. What is the abbreviation for *visual evoked response?* _____

4. Divide *arteriography* into its two word parts and define each word part.

Word Part	Definition
_____	_____
_____	_____

Fact Finding Questions

1. Two months ago, what symptom did the patient experience in her fingers? _____

2. Define these neurologic abbreviations.

   MS _____

   TIA _____

   CSF _____

3. The sensory examination consisted of five separate tests. Name them.

   a. _____

   b. _____

   c. _____

   d. _____

   e. _____

4. The mini mental status examination mentions what three mental status tests?

   a. _____

   b. _____

   c. _____

5. Which test showed that the patient's balance was intact? (**Babinski, Romberg, serial 7s**)

6. Which of the patient's symptoms is directly related to the nervous system? (**nausea, paresthesias, tachycardia**)

7. The carotid arteriography will be done to look for evidence of what disease? (**blockage of the artery, demyelination, muscle weakness**)

8. If present, oligoclonal bands are found in what body fluid? _____

Critical Thinking Questions

1. When the patient could remember the name of her older dog but not the name of her newest dog, this would be described as which of the following?

   a. Impairment of both remote and recent memory

   b. Impairment of remote memory; recent memory intact

   c. Remote memory intact; impairment of recent memory

2. A specimen of the patient's CSF was tested in the laboratory. What medical procedure was done to obtain that specimen?

   _____

3. The finger-to-nose and heel-to-shin tests are used to test what function? (**coordination, eye sight, memory**)

4. If the carotid arteriography showed a blockage of those arteries, this would relate to which of the patient's symptoms? (**alteration in memory, multiple sclerosis, wide-based gait**)

5. If the MRI with contrast does show areas of demyelination, what diagnosis would that confirm?

   _____

Dividing Medical Words

Separate these words into their component parts (prefix, combining form, suffix). Note: Some words do not contain all three word parts. The first one has been done for you.

Medical Word	Prefix	Combining Form	Suffix	Medical Word	Prefix	Combining Form	Suffix
1. aphasia	a-	phas/o-	-ia	6. meningioma	___	___	___
2. dementia	___	___	___	7. narcolepsy	___	___	___
3. epidural	___	___	___	8. neuroglia	___	___	___
4. hypothalamic	___	___	___	9. postictal	___	___	___
5. intracranial	___	___	___	10. subdural	___	___	___

Hearing Medical Words Exercise

You hear someone speaking the medical words given below. Read each pronunciation and then write the medical word it represents. Be sure to check your spelling. The first one has been done for you.

1. SEE-zher   _seizure_
2. SEF-al-AL-jee-ah   _____
3. KRAY-nee-AW-toh-mee   _____
4. HEM-ee-PLEE-jik   _____
5. MY-grayn   _____
6. IN-trah-KRAY-nee-al   _____
7. awk-SIP-ih-tal   _____
8. SIN-koh-pee   _____
9. MEN-in-JY-tis   _____
10. KOH-mah-tohs   _____

Pronunciation Exercise

Read the medical word that is given. Then review the syllables in the pronunciation. Circle the primary (main) accented syllable. The first one has been done for you.

1. nervous (⟨ner⟩-vus)
2. anesthesia (an-es-thee-zee-ah)
3. aphasic (ah-fay-sik)
4. astrocytoma (as-troh-sy-toh-mah)
5. hydrocephalus (hy-droh-sef-ah-lus)
6. infarct (in-farkt)
7. meninges (meh-nin-jeez)
8. paralysis (pah-ral-ih-sis)
9. sciatica (sy-at-ih-kah)
10. syncope (sin-koh-pee)

Multimedia Preview

Immerse yourself in a variety of activities inside Medical Terminology Interactive. Getting there is simple:

1. Click on www.myhealthprofessionskit.com.
2. Select "Medical Terminology" from the choice of disciplines.
3. First-time users must create an account using the scratch-off code on the inside front cover of this book.
4. Find this book and log in using your username and password.
5. Click on Medical Terminology Interactive.
6. Take the elevator to the 10th Floor to begin your virtual exploration of this chapter!

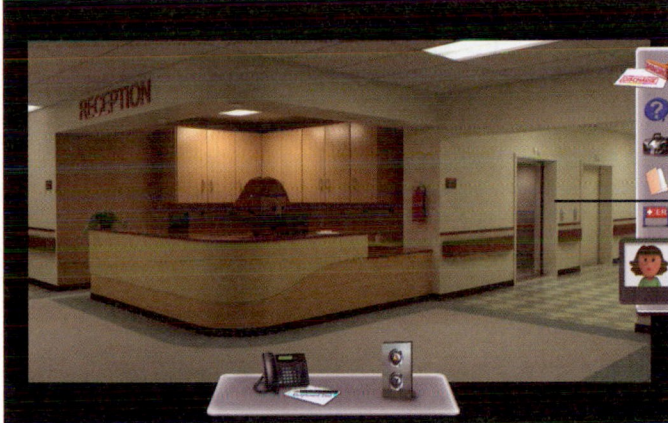 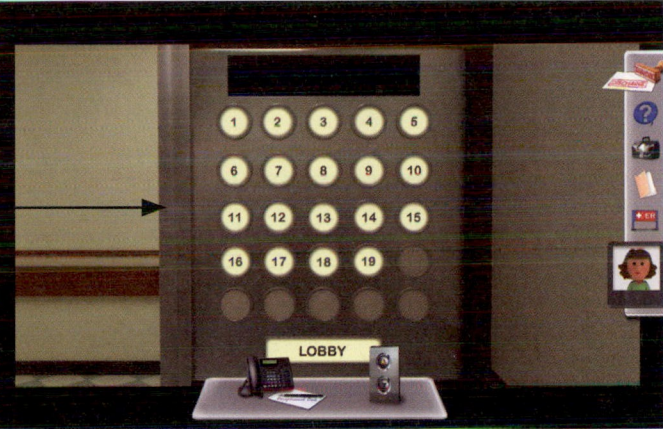

■ **Strikeout**   Click on the alphabet tiles to fill in the empty squares in the word or phrase to complete the sentence. This game quizzes your vocabulary and spelling. But choose your letters carefully because three strikes and you're out!

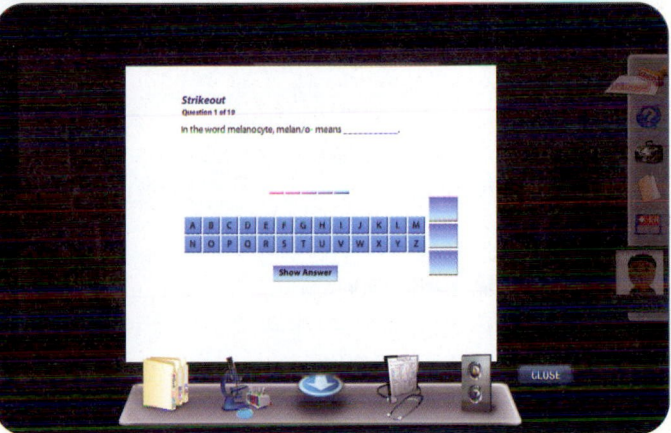

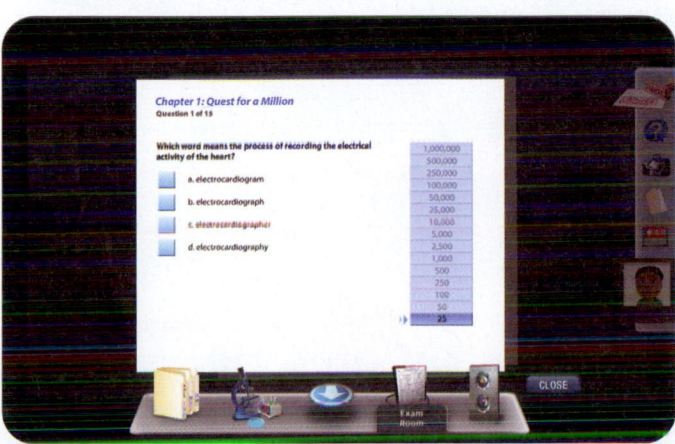

■ **Quest for a Million**   Who wants to win a million points? If it's you, then click on this game to begin your challenge. If you correctly answer 15 questions in a row, then you're a winner. But be very careful, because one wrong response will take you back down to zero.

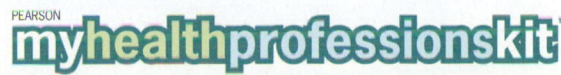

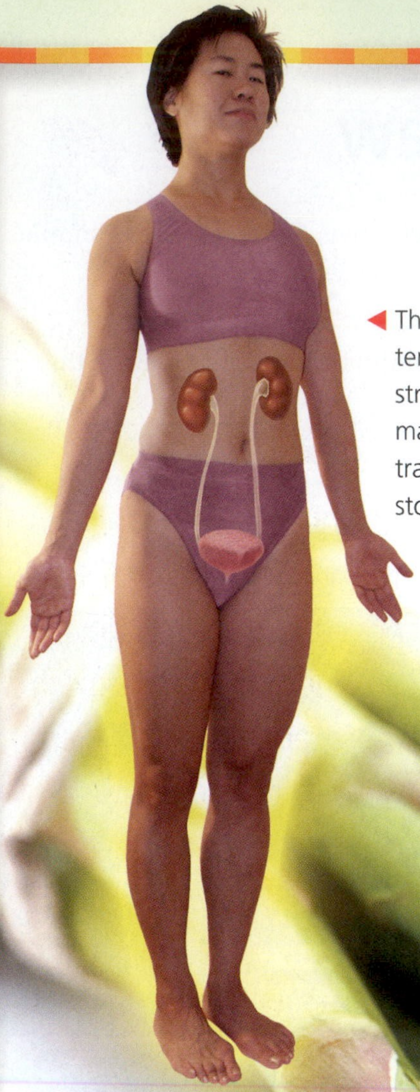

◄ The urinary system consists of structures that manufacture, transport, and store urine.

Dive In!

- Drinking urine is part of many non-traditional remedies, especially in Ayurvedic medicine.
- Don Winfield of Ontario, Canada, has produced and passed over 4,500 kidney stones since his condition began in 1986.
- Don't let these facts go to waste. In this chapter we'll explore the language that describes urinary system structures, functions, diseases, and conditions.
- You'll be relieved once you master the language of urology!

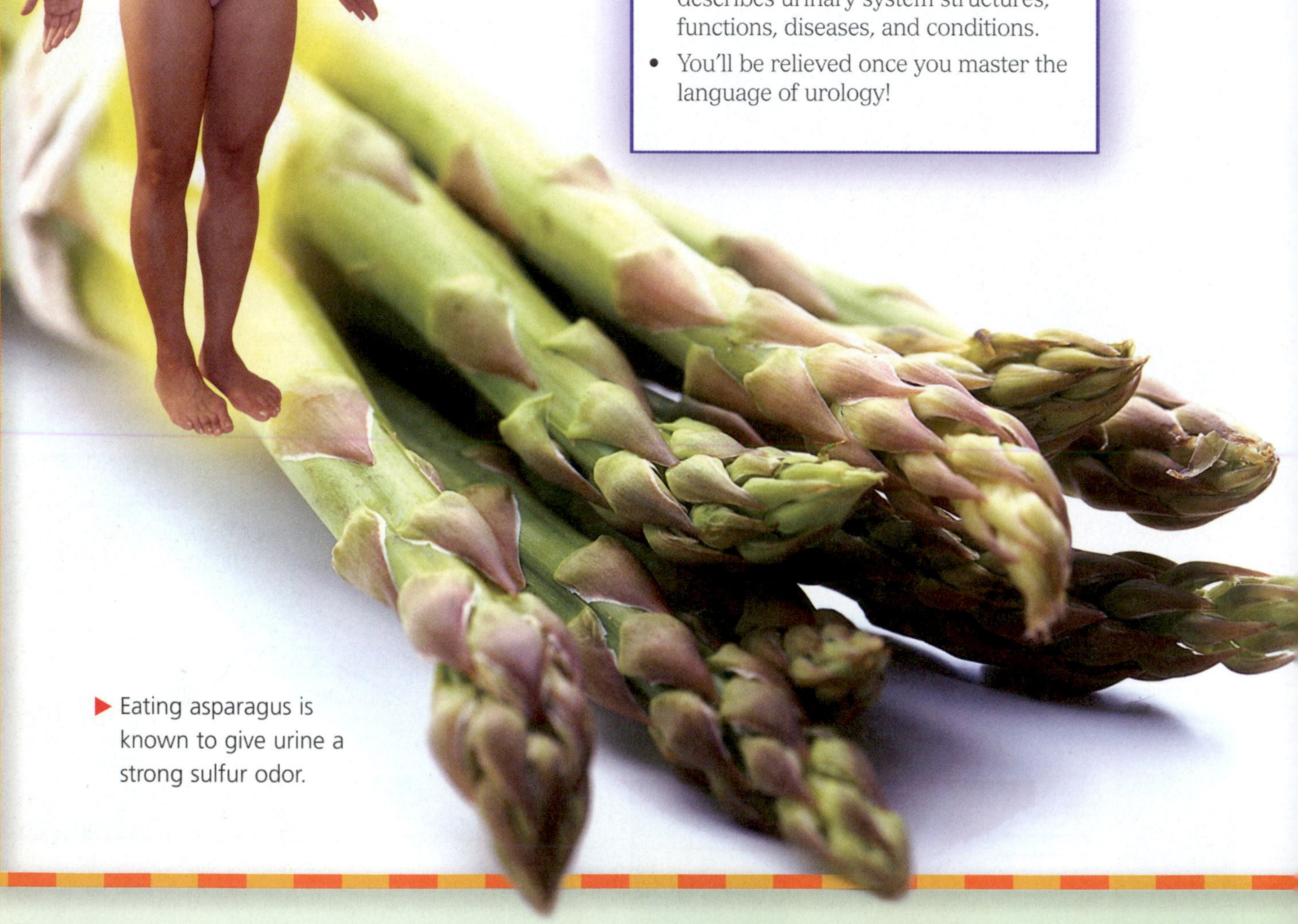

► Eating asparagus is known to give urine a strong sulfur odor.

1921

1921

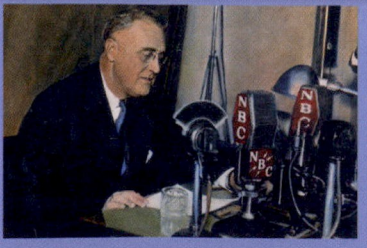

Medicine Through HISTORY

Franklin Delano Roosevelt, age 39, contracts polio and is partially paralyzed from the waist down. He goes on to become the 32nd President from 1933-1945, and is active in forming the March of Dimes foundation

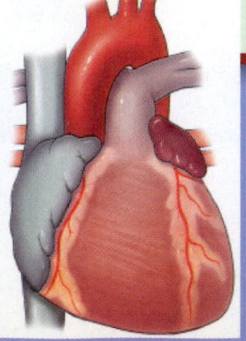

Heart disease becomes the number one cause of death

11
Urology
Urinary System

Urology (yoo-RAWL-oh-jee) is the medical specialty that studies the anatomy and physiology of the urinary system and uses diagnostic tests, medical and surgical procedures, and drugs to treat urinary diseases.

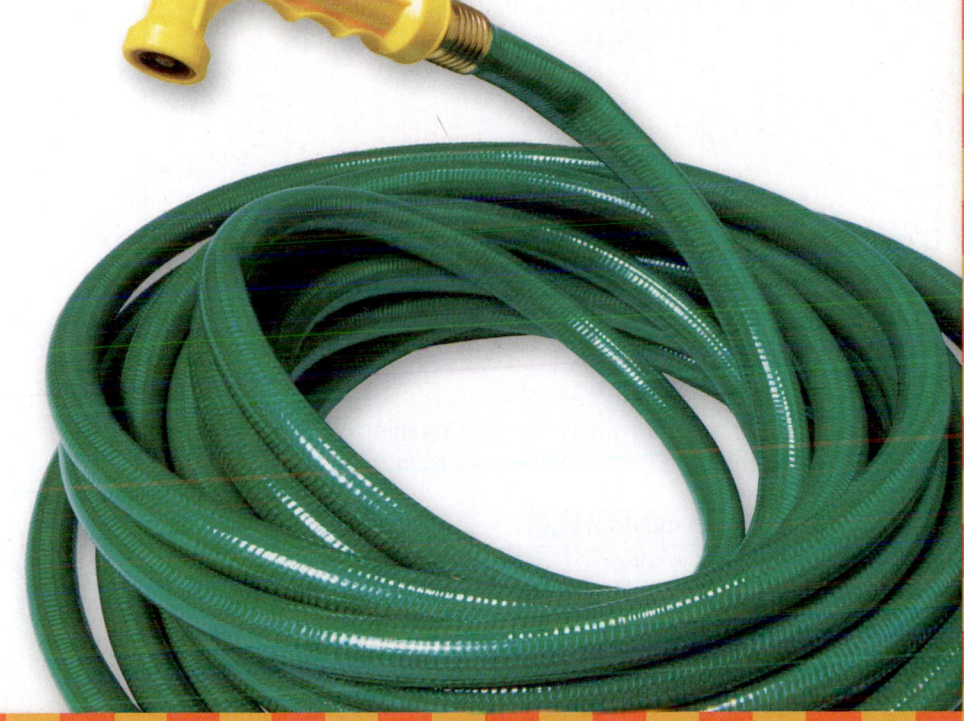

▲ The nephron is a microscopic structure that is the site of urine production in the kidney.

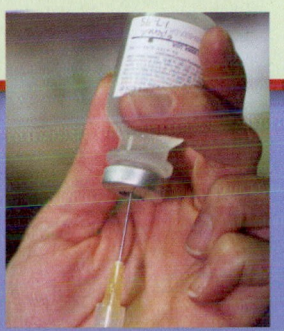

1922

Researchers Frederick Banting and Charles Best extract insulin and inject it to treat a patient with diabetes mellitus

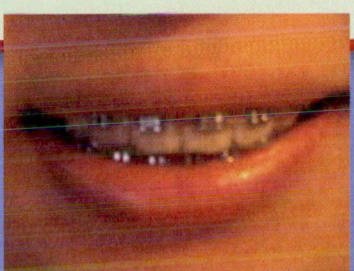

1922

Dr. Edward Angle invents the bracket system for braces to straighten teeth

Measure Your Progress: Learning Objectives

After you study this chapter, you should be able to

1. Identify the structures of the urinary system.

2. Describe the process of urine production and excretion.

3. Describe common urinary diseases and conditions, laboratory and diagnostic procedures, medical and surgical procedures, and drug categories.

4. Give the medical meaning of word parts related to the urinary system.

5. Build urinary words from word parts and divide and define urinary words.

6. Spell and pronounce urinary words.

7. Analyze the medical content and meaning of a urology report.

8. Dive deeper into urology by reviewing the activities at the end of this chapter and online at Medical Terminology Interactive.

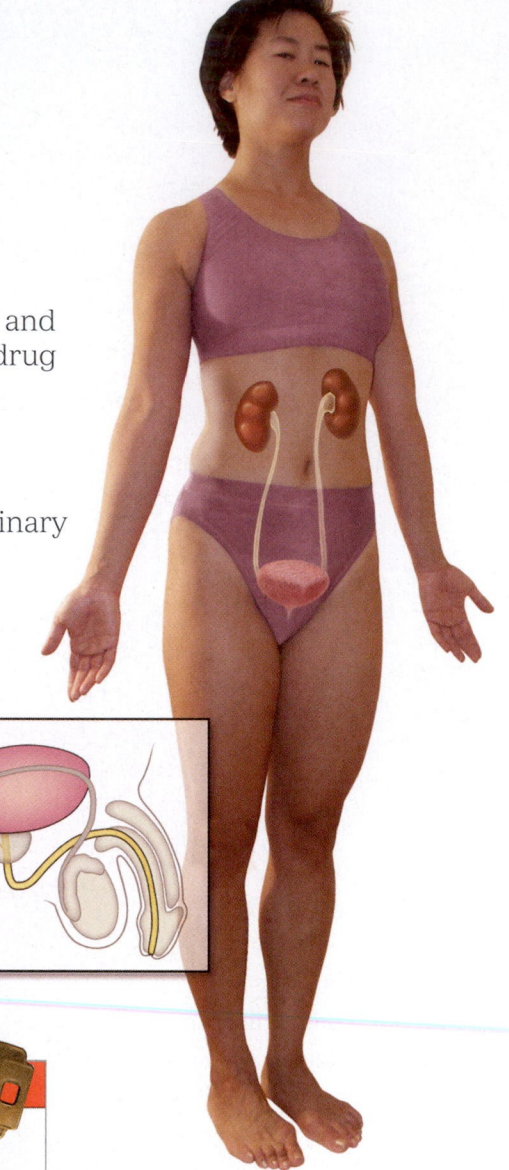

Figure 11-1 ■ **Urinary system.**

The urinary system consists of the kidneys that produce urine, and other structures that transport, store, or excrete urine. In a male, the urinary system continues into the penis (see insert box).

Medical Language Key

To unlock the definition of a medical word, break it into word parts. Define each word part. Put the word part meanings in order, beginning with the suffix, then the prefix (if present), then the combining form(s).

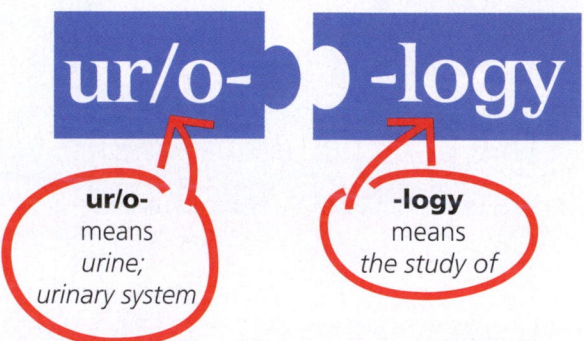

ur/o-
means
*urine;
urinary system*

-logy
means
the study of

	Word Part	Word Part Meaning
Suffix	-logy	*the study of*
Combining Form	ur/o-	*urine; urinary system*

Urology: *The study of the urine and the urinary system (and related structures).*

Anatomy and Physiology

The **urinary system** is a body system that begins with the kidneys. They are located in the **retroperitoneal space,** a small area behind the peritoneum of the abdominal cavity. Other structures of the urinary system are located within the abdominopelvic cavity, and the male urethra is located in the penis (see Figure 11-1 ■). The purpose of the urinary system is to regulate and maintain the composition of the blood and to remove waste products of metabolism from the body by producing, transporting, storing, and excreting urine.

Word Alert

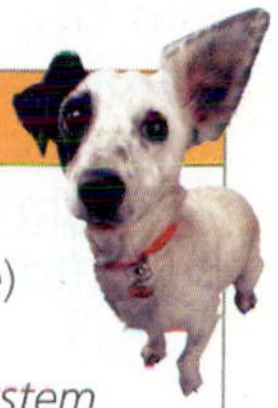

ALTERNATE NAMES

The urinary system is also known as the **urinary tract,** the **genitourinary (GU) system** or genitourinary tract, the **urogenital system** or urogenital tract, and the **excretory system.** Each name highlights a different characteristic of this body system.

1. Genitourinary and urogenital: two systems in close proximity and with shared structures.
2. Tract: a continuing pathway.
3. Excretory: describes the purpose of the system (to excrete urine).

Anatomy of the Urinary System

Kidneys

Each **kidney** is reddish-brown in color and is shaped like (of all things!) a kidney bean. It measures four inches long and two inches wide and weighs less than ½ pound (see Figure 11-2 ■). The upper end of each kidney is

Aorta
Inferior vena cava
Adrenal gland
Rib
Renal vein
Renal artery
Hilum
Retroperitoneal fat
Ureter

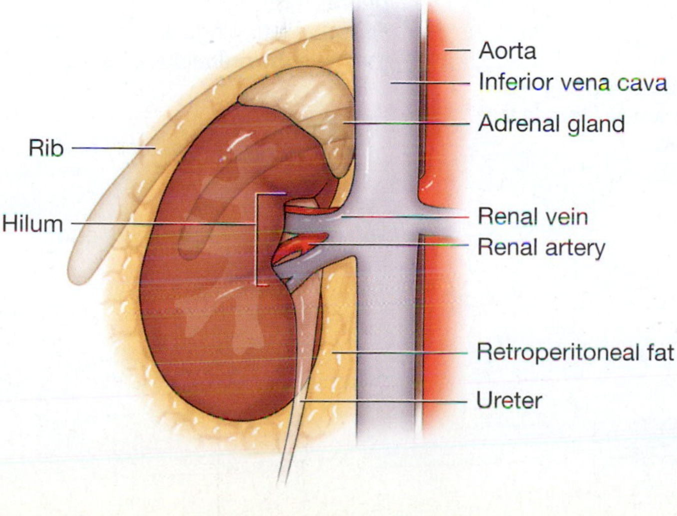

Figure 11-2 ■ Right kidney.
The kidney is shaped like a kidney bean. The adrenal gland of the endocrine system sits on top of the kidney but is not part of the urinary system. Notice the hilum where the renal artery enters and the renal veins and ureter exit the kidney.

positioned under the lower edge of the rib cage in the **flank** area of the back. Each kidney sits within a cushion of fatty tissue in the retroperitoneal space. The **hilum** is an area of indentation on the medial surface of the kidney. The **renal artery** enters there, and the renal vein and ureter exit there.

The adrenal glands sit on top of the kidneys like caps, but they are not part of the urinary system. The adrenal glands are discussed in "Endocrinology," Chapter 14.

A capsule of fibrous connective tissue surrounds the kidney. Just beneath the capsule is the renal **cortex** layer of tissue (see Figure 11-3 ■). Beneath that is the renal **medulla,** which contains triangular-shaped **renal pyramids.** The tip of each renal pyramid connects to the **minor calix,** an area that drains urine. Several minor calices drain into a common area, the **major calix.** The major calices drain into the **renal pelvis,** a large, funnel-shaped cavity that then narrows to become the ureter. Urine flows continuously through the minor calices, into the major calices, into the renal pelvis, and into the ureter.

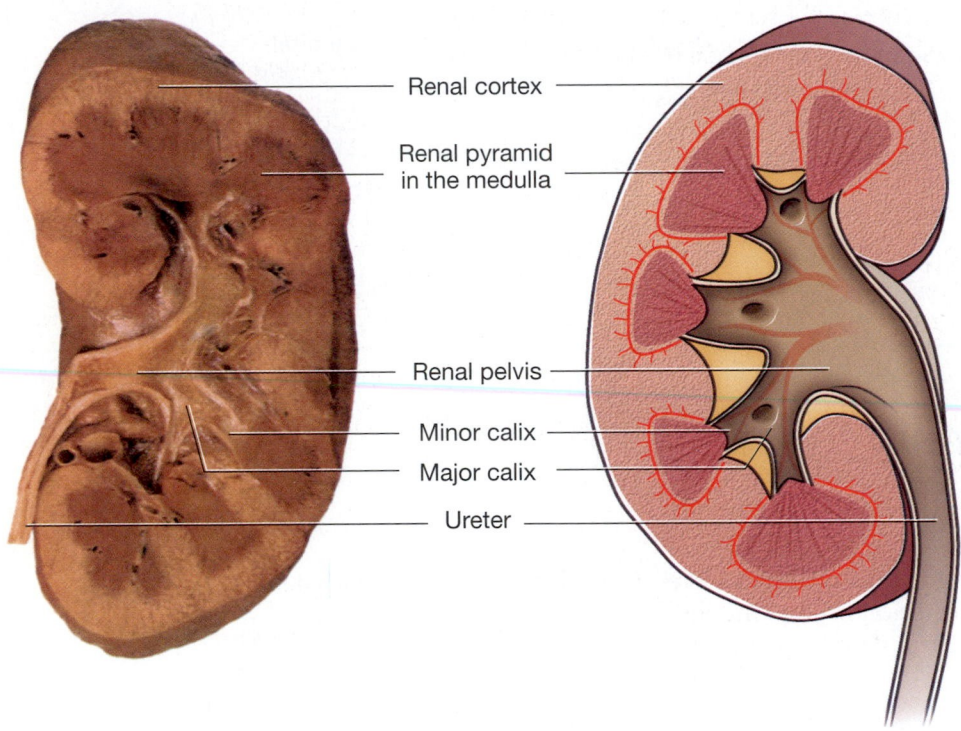

Renal cortex

Renal pyramid in the medulla

Renal pelvis

Minor calix

Major calix

Ureter

Figure 11-3 ■ Cut section of a kidney.
The internal structures of the kidney include the cortex, medulla, renal pyramids, calices, and renal pelvis. The minor and major calices and the pelvis are known as the collecting system because they collect the urine as it is produced. The renal pelvis narrows to become the ureter.

Ureters

Each **ureter** is a 12-inch tube that connects the renal pelvis of the kidney to the bladder (see Figures 11-3, 11-4 ■, 11-5 ■, and 11-6 ■). The ureters connect to the bladder on its posterior side. The **ureteral orifices** are the openings into the bladder. The walls of the ureters are composed of smooth muscle that contracts periodically to propel urine into the bladder, a process known as **peristalsis.**

Bladder

The **bladder** is located in the pelvic cavity and is held in place by ligaments (see Figures 11-4, 11-5, and 11-6). The rounded top of the bladder is the dome or **fundus.** The inside of the bladder is lined with **mucosa,** a mucous membrane. When the bladder is empty, the mucosa collapses into folds or **rugae.** When the bladder is full, smooth muscle in the bladder wall contracts to expel urine. The base of the bladder where it connects to the urethra is the bladder neck. In the bladder neck is a **sphincter,** a muscular ring that opens so that urine can flow into the urethra. The opening and closing of this sphincter is an involuntary reflex that cannot be consciously controlled.

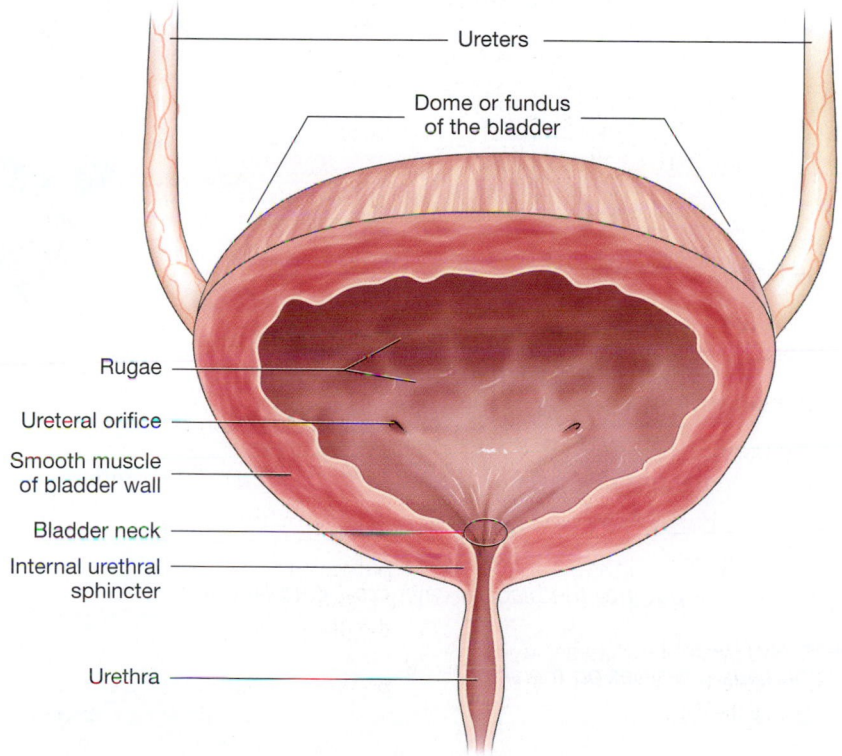

Figure 11-4 ■ Bladder.
The bladder is a hollow cavity that collects and temporarily stores the urine. Rugae are mucous membrane folds in the bladder wall that allow it to expand as it fills.

WORD BUILDING

ureter (YOO-ree-ter) (yoo-REE-ter)

ureteral (yoo-REE-teh-ral)
  ureter/o- *ureter*
  -al *pertaining to*

orifice (OR-ih-fis)

peristalsis (PAIR-ih-STAL-sis)
  peri- *around*
  -stalsis *process of contraction*

bladder (BLAD-er)

vesical (VES-ih-kal)
  vesic/o- *bladder; fluid-filled sac*
  -al *pertaining to*
Vesical is the adjective form for *bladder.* The combining form *cyst/o-* also means *bladder.*

fundus (FUN-dus)

mucosa (myoo-KOH-sah)

mucosal (myoo-KOH-sal)
  mucos/o- *mucous membrane*
  -al *pertaining to*

rugae (ROO-gee)
Ruga is a Latin singular noun. Form the plural by changing *-a* to *-ae.* Because there are so many rugae in the bladder, the singular form is seldom used.

- Ureters
- Dome or fundus of the bladder
- Rugae
- Ureteral orifice
- Smooth muscle of bladder wall
- Bladder neck
- Internal urethral sphincter
- Urethra

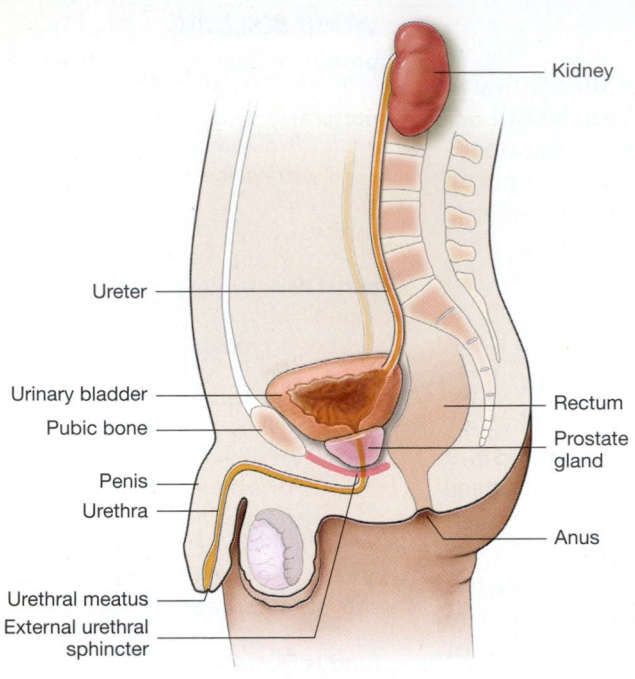

Figure 11-5 ■ **Male urinary system.**
The male urethra is long and travels through the prostate gland and the penis before opening to the outside of the body.

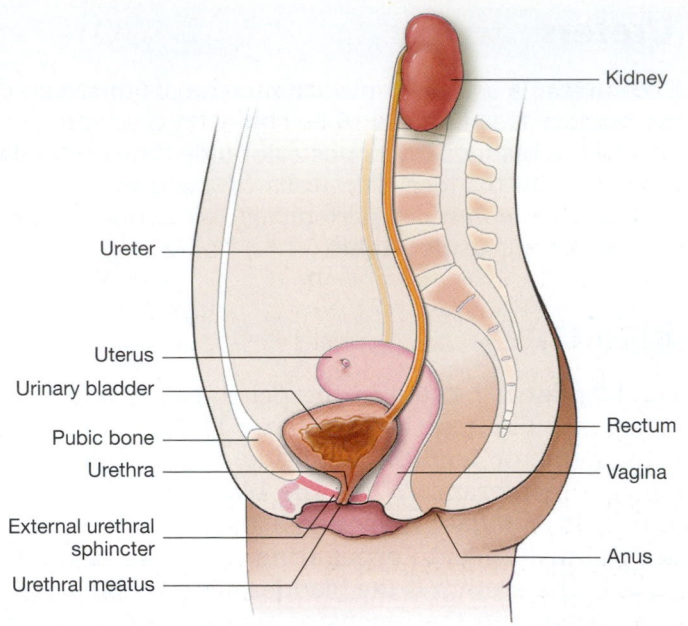

Figure 11-6 ■ **Female urinary system.**
The female urethra is short and straight. Notice how the bladder is beneath the uterus. During pregnancy, the bladder is often compressed by the expanding uterus and fetus inside it.

Word Alert

SOUND-ALIKE WORDS

ureter	(noun)	tube that connects the kidney to the bladder
ureteral	(adjective)	descriptive word for the ureter *Example: The ureteral orifice is the opening of the ureter into the bladder cavity.*
urethra	(noun)	tube that connects the bladder to the outside of the body
urethral	(adjective)	descriptive word for the urethra *Example: The urethra carries urine between the bladder and the outside of the body, and the urethral meatus opens to the outside of the body.*
vesical	(adjective)	descriptive word for the bladder *Example: Intravesical chemotherapy drugs are put into the bladder cavity to treat bladder cancer.*
vesicle	(noun)	small fluid-filled blister on the skin *Example: Herpes zoster virus infection causes vesicles on the skin.*

Urethra

The **urethra** is a tube that carries urine from the bladder to the outside of the body. The **external urethral sphincter** is a muscular ring that can be consciously controlled to release or hold back urine. The **urethral meatus** is where the urethra opens to the outside of the body.

In men, the urethra is 7–8 inches long. As the urethra leaves the bladder, it travels though the center of the **prostate gland,** a spherical gland at the base of the bladder. This part is known as the **prostatic urethra.** The prostate gland is not part of the urinary system; however, enlargement of the prostate gland can affect the urinary system by pressing on and narrowing the urethra. The prostate gland is discussed in "Male Reproductive Medicine," Chapter 12. The external urethral sphincter is located just distal to the prostate gland. The urethra is part of both the urinary and the male reproductive system because it transports both urine and semen. The urethra travels through the length of the **penis** until it reaches the external surface of the body (see Figure 11-5). This part is known as the **penile urethra.** In men, the urethral meatus is located at the tip of the penis. If the male is uncircumcised, the urethral meatus is covered by the foreskin of the penis.

In women, the urethra is much shorter, traveling only 1–2 inches from the bladder to the external surface of the body (see Figure 11-6). The external urethral sphincter is near the distal end of the urethra. The urethral meatus is located just anterior to the external opening of the vagina.

Physiology of the Formation of Urine

The **parenchyma** is the functional or working area of any organ (as opposed to the organ's structural framework). The parenchyma of the kidney is made up of the cortex and the medulla because these areas contain the nephrons. The **nephron,** a microscopic structure, is the functional unit of the kidney and the site of urine production (see Figure 11-7 ■).

The process of urine production begins as the renal artery enters the kidney and divides into smaller arterioles. A single arteriole enters each nephron. The first part of the nephron is the **glomerular capsule** (formerly known as Bowman's capsule). Within this ball-shaped structure, the arteriole divides and forms the **glomerulus,** a network of intertwining capillaries.

The blood flowing through the glomerulus contains waste products from metabolism that are not needed by the body and nutritional substances that are needed by the body. The waste products include

- **urea** (from protein metabolism)
- **creatinine** (from muscle contractions)
- **uric acid** (from purine metabolism to construct cellular DNA and RNA)
- drugs and products of drug metabolism.

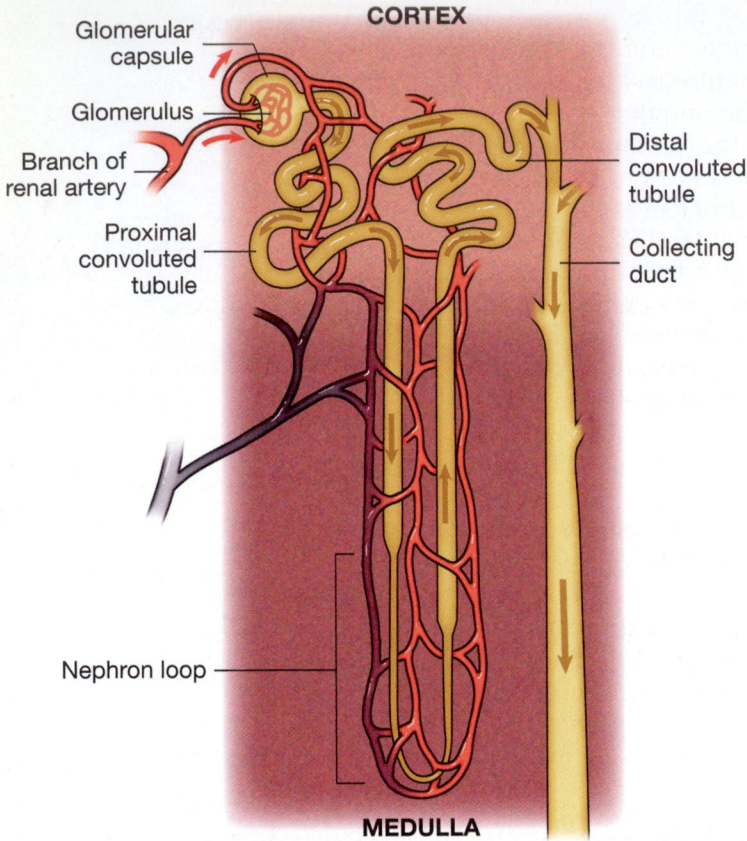

CORTEX

Glomerular capsule

Glomerulus

Branch of renal artery

Proximal convoluted tubule

Distal convoluted tubule

Collecting duct

Nephron loop

MEDULLA

Figure 11-7 ■ Nephron.
The functional unit of the kidney is composed of many smaller structures that filter substances and water out of the blood, help certain substances and some water return to the blood, and send the remaining water and substances as urine to the ureter and bladder.

If these waste products are not excreted in the urine, they quickly reach toxic levels. The nutritional substances include electrolytes, glucose, amino acids, vitamins, and so on. **Electrolytes** are chemicals that have a positive or negative electrical charge and include sodium (Na^+), potassium (K^+), chloride (Cl^-), and bicarbonate (HCO_3^-). Glucose is the simple sugar that the body uses for energy. Amino acids are the building blocks of proteins. These nutritional substances are essential to the health of the body. The job of the nephron is to remove the waste products from the blood but keep the nutritional substances.

The capillaries in the glomerulus have special pores in their walls that are not present in other capillaries in the body. The pressure of the blood pushes the waste products as well as water and nutritional substances through the capillary pores and out into the ball-shaped collecting area of the glomerular capsule. This process is known as **filtration.** Other substances in the blood (red blood cells, white blood cells, platelets, and albumin molecules) are too large to pass through the pores, and so these substances remain in the blood. The capillaries of the glomerulus then combine into a single arteriole that leaves the glomerular capsule and travels along the tubes that make up the rest of the nephron (see Figure 11-7).

The **filtrate** (the solution of waste products, water, and nutritional substances) in the glomerular capsule then flows into the **proximal convoluted**

WORD BUILDING

electrolyte (ee-LEK-troh-lite)
  electr/o- *electricity*
  -lyte *dissolved substance*
Add word parts to make a complete definition of *electrolyte: a dissolved substance (that can conduct) electricity (through a solution).*

filtration (fil-TRAY-shun)
  filtrat/o- *filtering; straining*
  -ion *action; condition*

filtrate (FIL-trayt)
  filtr/o- *filter*
  -ate *composed of; pertaining to*

proximal (PRAWK-sih-mal)
  proxim/o- *near the center or point of origin*
  -al *pertaining to*

convoluted (CON-voh-LOO-ted)

tubule of the nephron. In the proximal convoluted tubule, most of the water and nutritional substances move out of the tubule and return to the blood in a nearby capillary. This process is known as **reabsorption.** However, if, for example, the blood already has a high level of glucose in it (because of just eating a sugary food or because of uncontrolled diabetes mellitus), it cannot reabsorb additional glucose, and so that glucose remains in the proximal convoluted tubule and is excreted in the urine.

The proximal convoluted tubule becomes a U-shaped tubule known as the **nephron loop.** There, more water and electrolytes are reabsorbed. The nephron loop widens to become the distal convoluted tubule. In the **distal convoluted tubule,** more water and electrolytes as well as amino acids and other nutritional substances are reabsorbed. The distal convoluted tubules of many nephrons empty into a common **collecting duct.** Some reabsorption continues to take place in the collecting duct. After that, the fluid that remains is known as **urine.** Urine is produced continuously by the nephrons in the kidneys (see Figure 11-8 ■).

The process of eliminating urine from the body is described in several ways: **urination, micturition, voiding,** or passing water (a layperson's phrase).

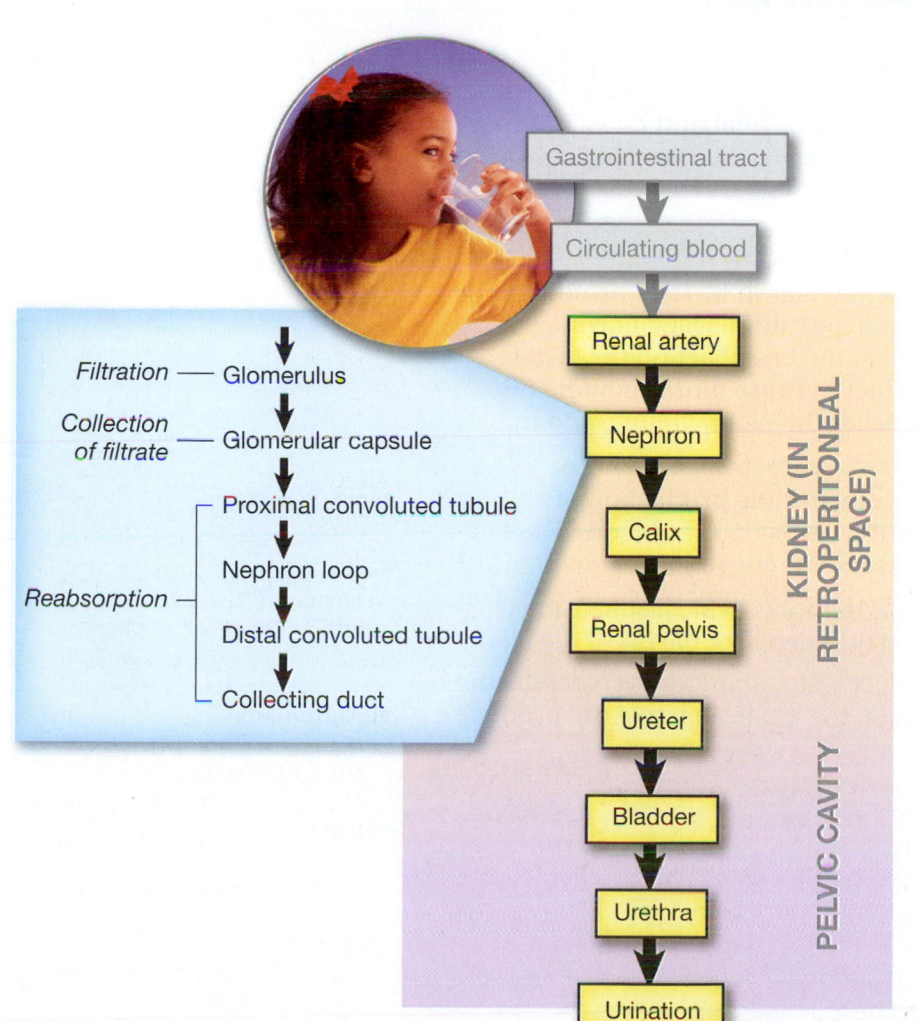

Figure 11-8 ■ **Pathway of urine production and elimination.**

Across the Life Span

Pediatrics. The kidneys of a fetus begin to produce urine by about the 12th week of life. The urine is excreted and becomes part of the amniotic fluid around the fetus. Children ages 1–3 produce about 400–600 cc (about a pint) of urine each day. Children ages 3–8 produce about 600–1000 cc (about a quart) of urine daily.

Adults produce about 1200–1500 cc (1–3 quarts) of urine each day. Each kidney contains more than 1 million individual nephrons. If laid end to end, these nephrons would be 80 miles in length.

Geriatrics. As a person ages, some nephrons deteriorate and die. Because the body does not repair or replace nephrons, the total number of nephrons in the kidneys continues to decline with age, and kidney function also decreases. Poor renal function can significantly prolong the effects of some drugs. Patients with renal disease and older adults are prescribed lower doses of drugs to prevent toxic symptoms due to decreased rates of drug excretion.

Physiology of Other Functions of the Kidneys

The kidneys also help the body to maintain a normal and constant internal environment. *Note:* These functions are separate from that of urine production.

1. If the blood pressure decreases, the kidneys
   - produce concentrated urine with less water in it. The hormone aldosterone (from the adrenal gland) and antidiuretic hormone (from the posterior pituitary gland in the brain) act on the distal convoluted tubule and collecting duct to cause more sodium and water to be reabsorbed. This increases the blood volume and the blood pressure.
   - secrete the enzyme **renin.** Renin stimulates the production of angiotensin, a powerful vasoconstrictor that causes blood vessels to constrict, increasing blood pressure.

2. If the pH of the blood decreases, the kidneys cause bicarbonate (an electrolyte) (HCO_3^-) to be reabsorbed and this increases the pH of the blood.

3. If the number of red blood cells decreases, the kidneys secrete the hormone **erythropoietin** to stimulate the bone marrow to produce more red blood cells.

WORD BUILDING

renin (REE-nin)
  ren/o- *kidney*
  -in *a substance*

erythropoietin
(eh-RITH-roh-POY-eh-tin)
  erythr/o- *red*
  -poietin *a substance that forms*

Vocabulary Review

Anatomy and Physiology

Word or Phrase	Description	Combining Forms
urinary system	Body system that includes the kidneys, ureters, bladder, and urethra. Its function is to produce and excrete urine. It also helps regulate the internal environment of the body by secreting the enzyme renin and the hormone erythropoietin. It is also known as the **urinary tract, genitourinary system** or tract, **urogenital system** or tract, and the **excretory system.**	**urin/o-** *urine; urinary system* **ur/o-** *urine; urinary system* **genit/o-** *genitalia* **excret/o-** *removing from the body*

Kidney

calix	Area at the tip of each renal pyramid. The minor calices take urine to the major calices.	**calic/o-** *calix* **cali/o-** *calix*
cortex	Area of tissue beneath the capsule of the kidney	**cortic/o-** *cortex (outer region)*
flank	Area of the back (between the ribs and the hip bone) that overlies the kidneys	
hilum	Indentation in the medial side of each kidney where the renal artery enters and the renal vein and the ureter exit	**hil/o-** *hilum (indentation in an organ)*
kidney	Organ of the urinary system that produces urine. It is in the **retroperitoneal space,** an area behind the peritoneum of the abdomen.	**ren/o-** *kidney* **nephr/o-** *kidney; nephron* **peritone/o-** *peritoneum*
medulla	Area of tissue beneath the cortex of the kidney. It contains the renal pyramids.	
parenchyma	Functional area of the kidney that is made up of the cortex and medulla and contains the nephrons	
renal pelvis	Large, funnel-shaped cavity within each kidney that collects urine from the major calices and then narrows to become the ureter	**pelv/o-** *pelvis (hip bone; renal pelvis)* **pyel/o-** *renal pelvis*
renal pyramids	Triangular-shaped areas of tissue in the medulla of the kidney	**ren/o-** *kidney*

Nephron

collecting duct	Common passageway that collects fluid from many nephrons. The final step of reabsorption takes place there, and the fluid that remains is urine.	
distal convoluted tubule	Tubule of the nephron that begins at the nephron loop and ends at the collecting duct. Reabsorption takes place there.	**dist/o-** *away from the center or point of origin* **tub/o-** *tube* **tubul/o-** *tube; small tube*
glomerular capsule	Ball-shaped structure that surrounds the glomerulus and collects filtrate. Formerly known as Bowman's capsule.	**glomerul/o-** *glomerulus*
glomerulus	Network of intertwining capillaries within the glomerular capsule in the nephron. Filtration takes place in the glomerulus.	**glomerul/o-** *glomerulus*

Word or Phrase	Description	Combining Forms
nephron	Microscopic functional unit of the kidney	**nephr/o-** *nephron*
nephron loop	Tubule of the nephron that is U-shaped. It begins at the proximal convoluted tubule and ends at the distal convoluted tubule. Reabsorption takes place there. Formerly known as the loop of Henle.	
proximal convoluted tubule	Tubule of the nephron that begins at the glomerular capsule and ends at the nephron loop. Reabsorption takes place there.	**proxim/o-** *near the center or point of origin* **tub/o-** *tube* **tubul/o-** *tube; small tube*

Ureter

Word or Phrase	Description	Combining Forms
peristalsis	Process of smooth muscle contractions that propel urine through the ureter	
ureter	Tube that carries urine from the pelvis of the kidney to the bladder	**ureter/o-** *ureter*
ureteral orifice	Opening at the end of the ureter as it enters the bladder	**ureter/o-** *ureter*

Bladder

Word or Phrase	Description	Combining Forms
bladder	Expandable reservoir for storing urine	**vesic/o-** *bladder; fluid-filled sac* **cyst/o-** *bladder; fluid-filled sac; semisolid cyst*
fundus	Dome-shaped top of the bladder	
mucosa	Mucous membrane lining that is inside the bladder	**mucos/o-** *mucous membrane*
rugae	Folds in the mucosa of the bladder that disappear as the bladder fills with urine	
sphincter	Muscular ring around a tube. The sphincter in the bladder neck is not under conscious control, but the external urethral sphincter is under voluntary, conscious control.	

Urethra

Word or Phrase	Description	Combining Forms
external urethral sphincter	Muscular ring in the urethra. It can be consciously controlled to release or hold back urine.	**urethr/o-** *urethra*
penis	Structure that is part of the male reproductive system. In a man, the inferior part of the urethra passes through the length of the penis, and this is the **penile urethra.**	**pen/o-** *penis*
prostate gland	Gland that is part of the male reproductive system. In a man, the superior part of the urethra passes through the center of the prostate gland, and this is the **prostatic urethra.**	**prostat/o-** *prostate gland*
urethra	Tube that carries urine from the bladder to the outside of the body. In women, it is a short tube but, in men, it goes through the prostate gland and down the length of the penis.	**urethr/o-** *urethra*
urethral meatus	The opening to the outside of the body that is at the end of the urethra	**urethr/o-** *urethra*

Urine Production and Other Kidney Functions

Word or Phrase	Description	Combining Forms
creatinine	Waste product from muscle contractions. It is removed from the blood by the kidneys.	
electrolytes	Substances that have a positive or negative charge and conduct electricity when dissolved in a solution. Excess amounts in the blood are removed by the kidneys. Examples: Sodium, potassium, chloride, bicarbonate	electr/o- *electricity*
erythropoietin	Hormone secreted by the kidneys when the number of red blood cells in the blood decreases. It stimulates the bone marrow to produce more red blood cells.	erythr/o- *red*
filtration	Process in which water, some nutritional substances, and wastes in the blood are all pushed through pores in the capillaries of the glomerulus. The resulting fluid is **filtrate.**	filtrat/o- *filtering; straining* filtr/o- *filter*
reabsorption	Process by which water and nutritional substances in the filtrate move out of the tubule and return to the blood in a nearby capillary	absorpt/o- *absorb; take in*
renin	Enzyme secreted by the kidney when the blood pressure decreases. Renin stimulates the production of angiotensin, a powerful vasoconstrictor.	ren/o- *kidney*
urea	Waste product from protein metabolism. It is removed from the blood by the kidneys.	
uric acid	Waste product from purine metabolism. It is removed from the blood by the kidneys.	
urination	The process of expelling urine from the body. It is also known as **voiding, micturition,** or passing water.	urin/o- *urine; urinary system* micturi/o- *making urine* enur/o- *to urinate*
urine	Water, waste products, and other substances excreted by the kidneys	ur/o- *urine; urinary system*

Labeling Exercise

Match each anatomy word or phrase to its structure and write it in the numbered box for each figure. Be sure to check your spelling. Use the Answer Key at the end of the book to check your answers.

hilum	major calix	minor calix	renal cortex	renal pelvis	renal pyramid	ureter

1.

2.

3.

4.

5.

6.

7.

external urinary sphincter	kidney	penis	prostate gland	ureter	urethra	urethral meatus	urinary bladder

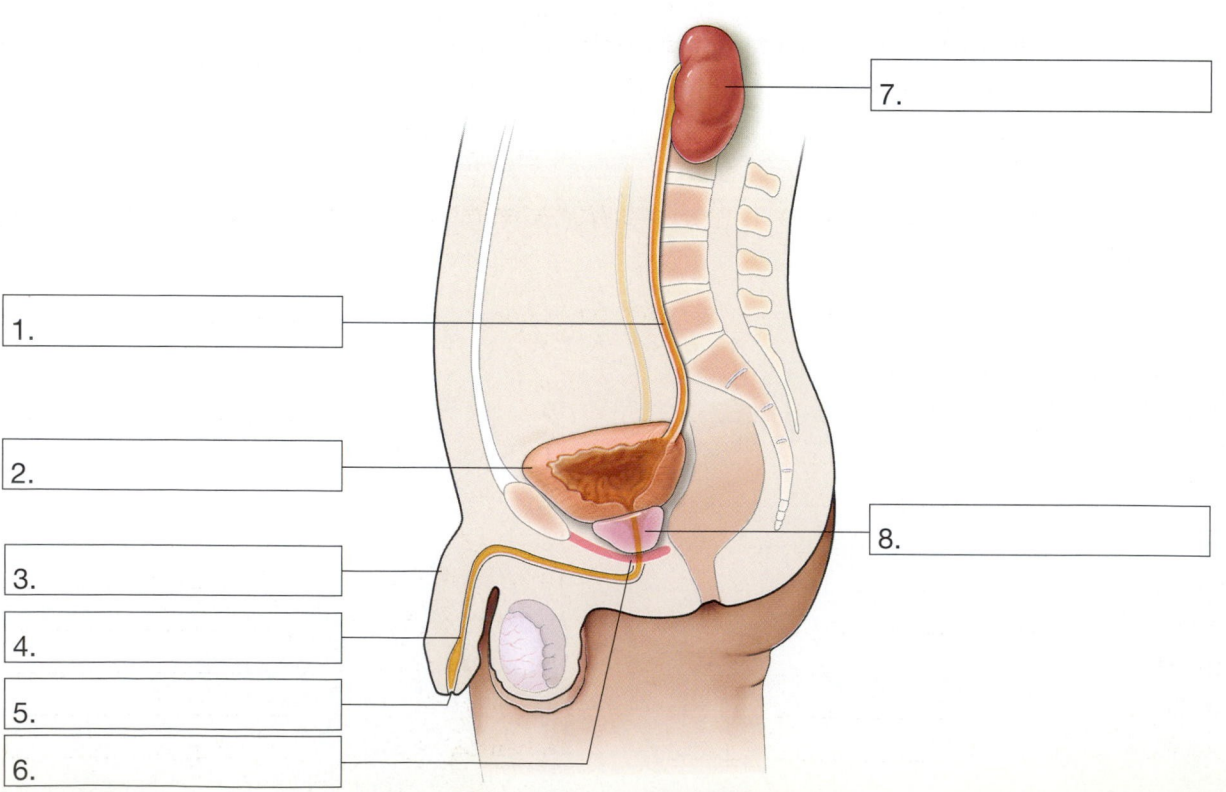

7.

1.

2.

8.

3.

4.

5.

6.

| collecting duct | glomerular capsule | nephron loop | renal artery |
| distal convoluted tubule | glomerulus | proximal convoluted tubule | |

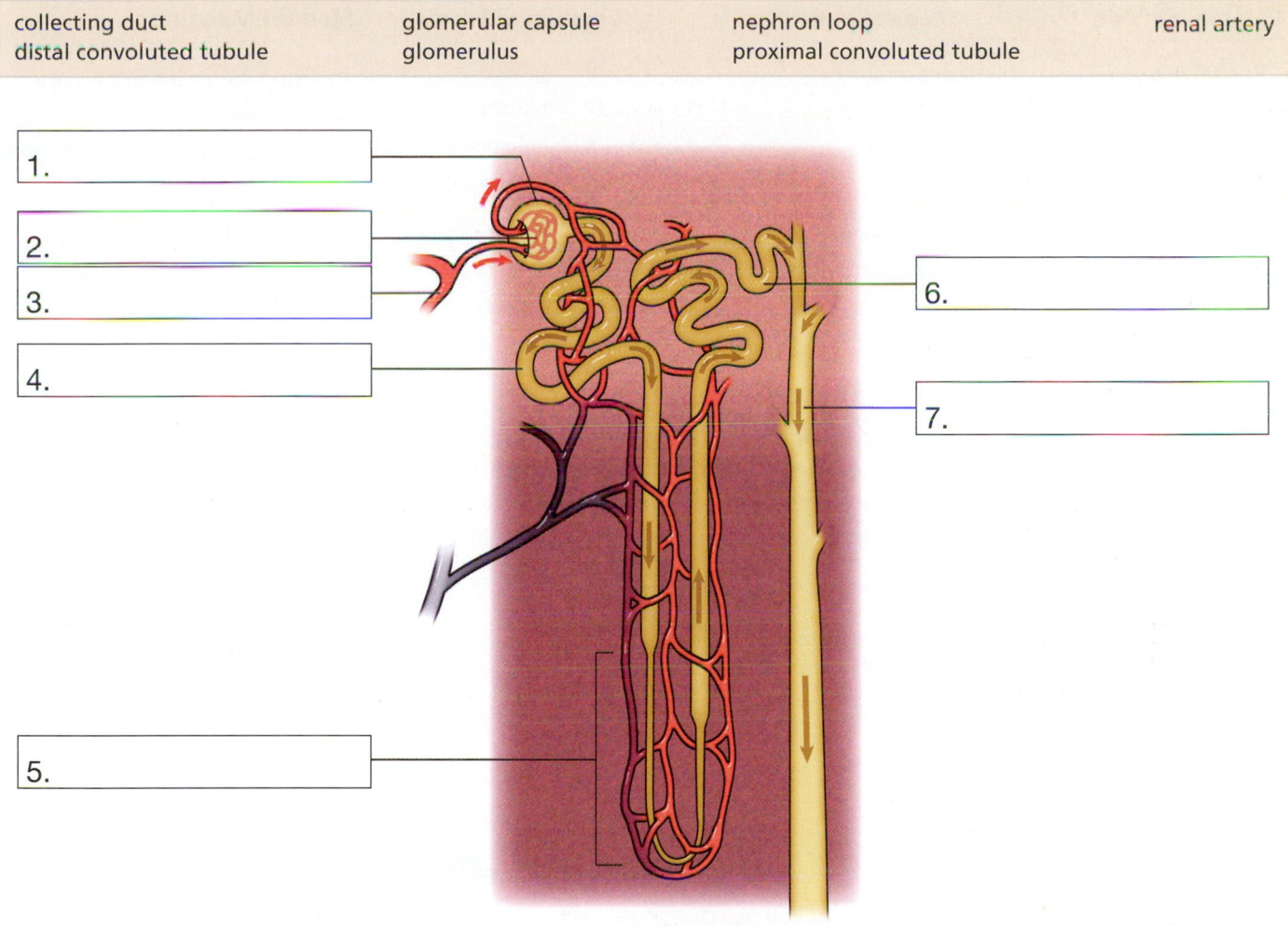

1.

2.

3.

4.

5.

6.

7.

Building Medical Words

Use the Answer Key at the end of the book to check your answers.

Combining Forms Exercise

Before you build urinary words, review these combining forms. Next to each combining form, write its medical meaning. The first one has been done for you.

Combining Form	Medical Meaning	Combining Form	Medical Meaning
1. **absorpt/o-**	absorb; take in	10. excret/o-	
2. calic/o-		11. filtrat/o-	
3. cali/o-		12. filtr/o-	
4. cortic/o-		13. genit/o-	
5. cyst/o-		14. glomerul/o-	
6. dist/o-		15. hil/o-	
7. electr/o-		16. micturi/o-	
8. enur/o-		17. mucos/o-	
9. erythr/o-		18. nephr/o-	

Combining Form	Medical Meaning	Combining Form	Medical Meaning
19. pelv/o-	_____	26. tub/o-	_____
20. pen/o-	_____	27. tubul/o-	_____
21. peritone/o-	_____	28. ureter/o-	_____
22. prostat/o-	_____	29. urethr/o-	_____
23. proxim/o-	_____	30. urin/o-	_____
24. pyel/o-	_____	31. ur/o-	_____
25. ren/o-	_____	32. vesic/o-	_____

Combining Form and Suffix Exercise

Read the definition of the medical word. Look at the combining form that is given. Select the correct suffix from the Suffix List and write it on the blank line. Then build the medical word and write it on the line. (Remember: You may need to remove the combining vowel. Always remove the hyphens and slash.) Be sure to check your spelling. The first one has been done for you.

SUFFIX LIST		
-al (pertaining to)	-eal (pertaining to)	-poietin (a substance that forms)
-ar (pertaining to)	-ic (pertaining to)	-tion (a process; being or having)
-ary (pertaining to)	-ile (pertaining to)	-ule (small thing)
-ate (composed of; pertaining to)	-ory (having the function of)	
-ation (a process; being or having)	-lyte (dissolved substance)	

Definition of the Medical Word	Combining Form	Suffix	Build the Medical Word
1. Pertaining to the mucosa	**mucos/o-** **-al**		mucosal _____

(You think *pertaining to* (-al) + *mucosa* (mucos/o-). You change the order of the word parts to put the suffix last. You write *mucosal*.)

Definition of the Medical Word	Combining Form	Suffix	Build the Medical Word
2. The process of expelling urine from the body	urin/o-	_____	_____
3. Pertaining to the calix	calic/o-	_____	_____
4. Pertaining to the kidney	ren/o-	_____	_____
5. Pertaining to the bladder	vesic/o-	_____	_____
6. Pertaining to the prostate gland	prostat/o-	_____	_____
7. Pertaining to the glomerulus	glomerul/o-	_____	_____
8. Small tube	tub/o-	_____	_____
9. Having the function of removing (waste) from the body	excret/o-	_____	_____
10. Composed of (a substance that has been) filter(ed)	filtr/o-	_____	_____
11. Pertaining to the urine	urin/o-	_____	_____
12. Pertaining to the hilum	hil/o-	_____	_____
13. Pertaining to the ureter	ureter/o-	_____	_____
14. Pertaining to the penis	pen/o-	_____	_____
15. Pertaining to the urethra	urethr/o-	_____	_____
16. Dissolved substance (that can conduct) electricity	electr/o-	_____	_____
17. A process of making urine	micturi/o-	_____	_____
18. A substance (from the kidney) that forms red (blood cells)	erythr/o-	_____	_____

Diseases and Conditions

Kidneys and Ureters

Word or Phrase	Description	Word Building
glomerulonephritis	Complication that develops following an acute infection with streptococcal bacteria or with viruses. The original infection, which is often a strep throat, causes the immune system to produce antibodies. Antibodies combine with the bacteria or viruses to form antigen–antibody complexes that clog the pores of the capillaries of the glomerulus. The kidney becomes inflamed and urine production decreases. Treatment: Antibiotic drugs; corticosteroid drugs to decrease inflammation; renal dialysis, if necessary.	**glomerulonephritis** (gloh-MAIR-yoo-loh-neh-FRY-tis) **glomerul/o-** *glomerulus* **nephr/o-** *kidney; nephron* **-itis** *inflammation of; infection of*
hydronephrosis	Enlargement of the kidney. This is due to the pressure from urine that is backed up in the ureter because of an obstructing stone or stricture. In **caliectasis,** the calices of the kidney are enlarged. In **hydroureter,** only the ureter is enlarged. Treatment: Removal of the stone or stricture.	**hydronephrosis** (HY-droh-neh-FROH-sis) **hydr/o-** *water; fluid* **nephr/o-** *kidney; nephron* **-osis** *condition; abnormal condition; process* **caliectasis** (KAY-lee-EK-tah-sis) **cali/o-** *calix* **-ectasis** *condition of dilation* **hydroureter** (HY-droh-YOO-ree-ter) (HY-droh-yoo-REE-ter) *Hydroureter* is a combination of the combining form *hydro-* (water; fluid) and the word *ureter.*
nephrolithiasis	Kidney stone or **calculus** formation in the urinary system. Kidney stones can vary in size from microscopic (often referred to as sand or gravel) (see Figure 11-9 ■) to large enough to block the ureter or fill the renal pelvis (see Figure 11-10 ■). Kidney stones are composed of magnesium, calcium, or uric acid crystals. **Calculogenesis** or **lithogenesis** is the process of forming stones. **Renal colic** is a spasm of the smooth muscle of the ureter or bladder as the kidney stone's jagged edges scrape the mucosa. This causes severe pain, nausea and vomiting, and hematuria. Many stones reach the bladder and are eliminated from the body with the urine (see Figure 11-19). Stones that do not pass spontaneously can be destroyed by lithotripsy (see Figure 11-25) or removed surgically. Treatment: Analgesic drugs; lithotripsy; surgical procedures of stone basketing or nephrolithotomy.	**nephrolithiasis** (NEF-roh-lih-THY-ah-sis) **nephr/o-** *kidney; nephron* **lith/o-** *stone* **-iasis** *state of; process of* **calculus** (KAL-kyoo-lus) **calculi** (KAL-kyoo-lie) *Calculus* is a Latin singular noun. Form the plural by changing *-us* to *-i.* **calculogenesis** (KAL-kyoo-loh-JEN-eh-sis) **calcul/o-** *stone* **gen/o-** *arising from; produced by* **-esis** *a process* **lithogenesis** (LITH-oh-JEN-eh-sis) **lith/o-** *stone* **gen/o-** *arising from; produced by* **-esis** *a process* **colic** (KAWL-ik) **col/o-** *colon* **-ic** *pertaining to*

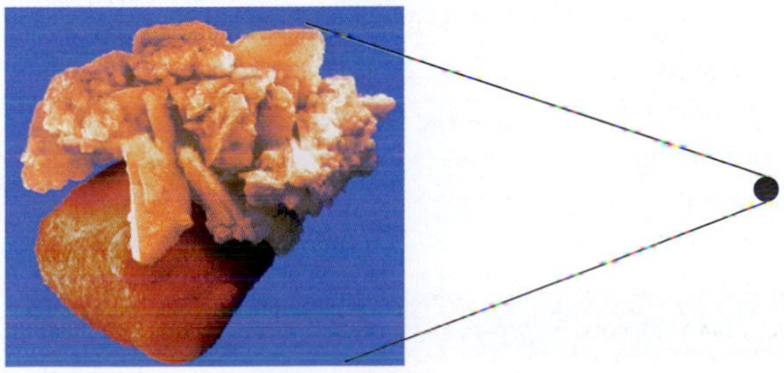

Figure 11-9 ■ Kidney stone.
A kidney stone no bigger than this dot caused hematuria, vomiting, renal colic, and severe pain. Under the microscope, the many sharp, jagged edges of the kidney stone can be seen.

Did You Know?

Egyptian mummies have been found to have kidney stones.

(continued)

Word or Phrase	Description	Word Building
nephrolithiasis (*continued*)	**Figure 11-10 ■ Nephrolithiasis.** These multiple kidney stones in the calices and pelvis of the kidney have become so large that they cannot pass spontaneously. They disrupt the caliceal structure and leave little room in the pelvis for urine.	**Word Alert** **WORDS WITH TWO DIFFERENT MEANINGS** **calculus** A kidney stone / It is also the name of the heel bone. **colic** Spasm of the smooth muscle around the ureters and bladder / Spasm of the smooth muscle around the intestines **pelvis** Funnel-shaped area in the kidney that collects urine / Hip bones (as well as the sacrum and coccyx of the spinal column)
nephropathy	General word for any disease of the kidney. Diabetic nephropathy involves progressive damage to the glomeruli because of diabetes mellitus. The tiny arteries of the glomerulus harden (**glomerulosclerosis**) because of accelerated arteriosclerosis throughout the body. Treatment: Correct the underlying cause; manage the diabetes mellitus.	**nephropathy** (neh-FRAWP-ah thee) **nephr/o-** *kidney; nephron* **-pathy** *disease; suffering* **glomerulosclerosis** (gloh-MAIR-yoo-loh-skleh-ROH-sis) **glomerul/o-** *glomerulus* **scler/o-** *hard; sclera (white of the eye)* **-osis** *condition; abnormal condition; process*
		Select the correct suffix and combining form meanings to get the definition of *glomerulosclerosis: abnormal condition of the glomerulus (becoming) hard.*
nephroptosis	Abnormally low position of a kidney. It sometimes requires surgery, but more often is mentioned as an incidental finding seen on an x-ray.	**nephroptosis** (NEF-rawp-TOH-sis) **nephr/o-** *kidney; nephron* **-ptosis** *state of prolapse; drooping; falling*
nephrotic syndrome	Damage to the pores of the capillaries of the glomerulus. This allows large amounts of albumin (protein) to leak into the urine, decreasing the amount of protein in the blood. This changes the osmotic pressure of the blood and allows fluid to go into the tissues, producing edema in the extremities; fluid also goes into the abdominal cavity, producing **ascites** (a grossly enlarged, fluid-distended abdomen). Treatment: Diuretic drugs to decrease edema; correct the underlying cause.	**nephrotic** (nef-RAWT-ik) **nephr/o-** *kidney; nephron* **-tic** *pertaining to* **ascites** (ah-SY-teez)

Clinical Connections

Dietetics. In the nutritional disease kwashiorkor (protein malnutrition), patients have grossly distended abdomens. The lack of dietary protein causes low blood protein, and fluid moves from the blood into the abdominal cavity. At the same time, their bodies break down muscle tissue to meet the protein needs of the rest of the body. This results in thin extremities (muscle wasting).

Word or Phrase	Description	Word Building

polycystic kidney disease	**Congenital** disease characterized by cysts in the kidney that eventually destroy the nephrons, causing kidney failure (see Figures 11-11 ■ and 11-12). The early stage of this progressive degenerative disease shows few symptoms or signs; often it is not detected until hypertension and already enlarged kidneys are detected upon physical examination. Treatment: Dialysis or kidney transplantation. 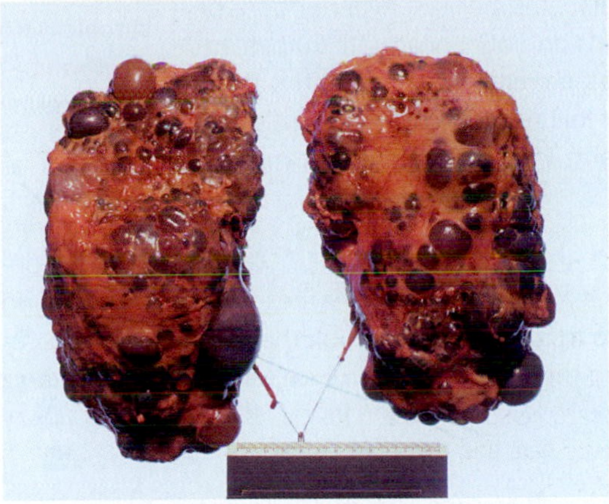
	
	Figure 11-11 ■ Polycystic kidney disease.
	As nonfunctioning cysts replace large numbers of nephrons, the patient's kidney function progressively decreases.
		polycystic (PAWL-ee-SIS-tik)
		  poly- *many; much*
		  cyst/o- *bladder; fluid-filled sac; semisolid cyst*
		  -ic *pertaining to*
		Select the correct combining form meaning to get the definition of *polycystic: pertaining to many semisolid cysts.*
		
		congenital (con-JEN-ih-tal)
		  congenit/o- *present at birth*
		  -al *pertaining to*

pyelonephritis	Inflammation and infection of the pelves of the kidneys. Infection of the kidneys (**nephritis**) also involves the renal pelves. It is caused by a bacterial infection of the bladder that goes up the ureters to the kidneys.	**pyelonephritis** (PY-eh-loh-neh-FRY-tis)
		  pyel/o- *renal pelvis*
		  nephr/o- *kidney; nephron*
		  -itis *inflammation of; infection of*
		
		nephritis (neh-FRY-tis)
		  nephr/o- *kidney; nephron*
		  -itis *inflammation of; infection of*

renal cell cancer	**Cancerous** tumor (**carcinoma**) that arises from tubules in the nephron (see Figure 11-12 ■). **Wilms' tumor** is cancer of the kidney that occurs in children and arises from residual embryonic or fetal tissue; it is also known as a **nephroblastoma.** Treatment: Surgery, radiation therapy, chemotherapy. 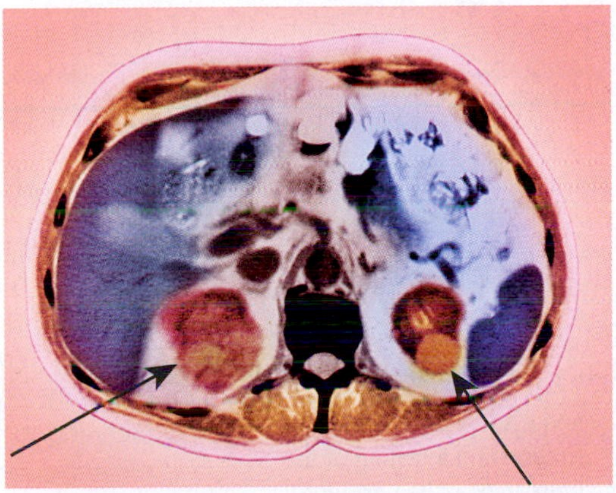
	
	Figure 11-12 ■ CT scan of the kidneys.
	This colorized computerized axial tomography (CT) scan shows the abdominal organs and the kidneys. The bottom center of the image shows the patient's spinal column, and areas around both sides are the patient's ribs. The top of the image is the patient's abdomen. The abdominal organs will seem to you to be in an abnormal, reversed position, unless you understand that a CT scan is read as if you were at the patient's feet and looking up. Therefore, the patient's liver (light and dark blue) lies along the left-hand side of the image. The patient's right kidney (which is on the left-hand side of the image) is enlarged from a cancerous tumor. The patient's left kidney shows two large cysts.
		cancerous (KAN-ser-us)
		  cancer/o- *cancer*
		  -ous *pertaining to*
		
		carcinoma (KAR-sih-NOH-mah)
		  carcin/o- *cancer*
		  -oma *tumor; mass*
		
		Wilms' (WILMZ) **tumor**
		
		nephroblastoma (NEF-roh-blas-TOH-mah)
		  nephr/o- *kidney; nephron*
		  blast/o- *immature; embryonic*
		  -oma *tumor; mass*

Word or Phrase	Description	Word Building
renal failure	Disease in which the kidneys decrease their urine production, and then stop producing urine. **Acute renal failure (ARF)** occurs suddenly and is usually due to trauma, severe blood loss, or overwhelming infection. It is caused by **acute tubular necrosis,** the sudden destruction of large numbers of nephrons and their tubules. **Chronic renal failure (CRF)** begins with renal insufficiency, followed by gradual worsening with progressive damage to the kidneys from diabetes mellitus, hypertension, or glomerulonephritis. Symptoms and signs do not appear until 80 percent of kidney function has been lost. **End-stage renal disease (ESRD)** is the final, irreversible stage of chronic renal failure in which there is little or no remaining kidney function. Treatment: Treat the underlying cause; treat end-stage failure with dialysis.	**acute** (ah-KYOOT) **necrosis** (neh-KROH-sis) **necr/o-** *dead cells, tissue, or body* **-osis** *condition; abnormal condition; process* **chronic** (KRAWN-ik) **chron/o-** *time* **-ic** *pertaining to*
uremia	Excessive amounts of the waste product urea in the blood because of renal failure. The kidneys are unable to remove urea, and it reaches toxic levels in the blood. It is then excreted to a small degree through the sweat glands, making white deposits on the skin that look like ice (uremic frost). Treatment: Dialysis.	**uremia** (yoo-REE-mee-ah) **ur/o-** *urine; urinary system* **-emia** *condition of the blood; substance in the blood*

Bladder

Word or Phrase	Description	Word Building
bladder cancer	Cancerous tumor (carcinoma) of the lining of the bladder, most commonly seen in men over age 60. Hematuria is often the first sign. Treatment: Transurethral resection of the bladder tumor (TURBT), surgical excision of the bladder (cystectomy), radiation therapy, or **intravesical** insertion of chemotherapy drugs through a catheter into the bladder.	**intravesical** (IN-trah-VES-ih-kal) **intra-** *within* **vesic/o-** *bladder; fluid-filled sac* **-al** *pertaining to*
cystitis	Inflammation or infection of the bladder. This is often caused by bacteria in the urethra that ascend into the bladder, particularly in women because of the short length of the urethra. **Interstitial cystitis** is a chronic, progressive infection in which the bladder mucosa becomes extremely irritated and red, with bleeding (see Figure 11-13 ■). **Radiation cystitis** is caused by the irritating effects of radiation therapy given to treat bladder cancer. Treatment: Correct the underlying condition; analgesic drugs and antispasmodic drugs.	**cystitis** (sis-TY-tis) **cyst/o-** *bladder; fluid-filled sac; semisolid cyst* **-itis** *inflammation of; infection of* Select the correct combining form meaning to get the definition of *cystitis: inflammation or infection of the bladder.* **interstitial** (IN-ter-STISH-al) **interstiti/o-** *spaces within tissue* **-al** *pertaining to* **radiation** (RAY-dee-AA-shun) **radi/o-** *radius (forearm bone); x-rays; radiation* **-ation** *a process; being or having* Select the correct combining form meaning to get the definition of *radiation: being or having x-rays or radiation.*

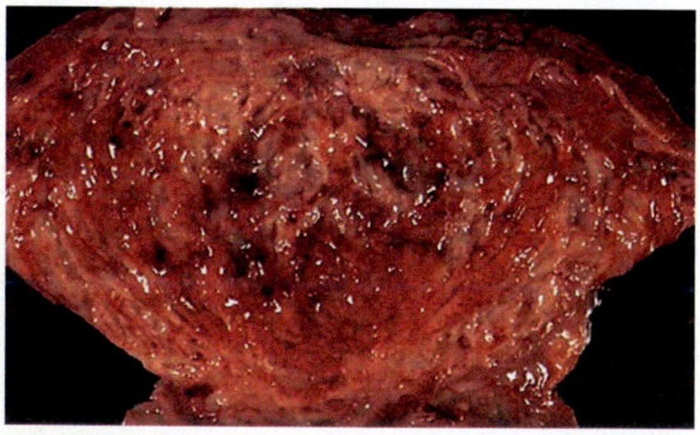

Figure 11-13 ■ Acute cystitis.
This opened bladder from a cadaver shows severe irritation and infection of the mucosa with areas of hemorrhage.

Word or Phrase	Description	Word Building
cystocele	Hernia in which the bladder bulges through a weakness in the muscular wall of the vagina or rectum. This causes retention of the urine that is in the bulge of the hernia. This is also known as a **vesicocele.** Treatment: Surgical repair of the vagina or rectum, if severe.	**cystocele** (SIS-toh-seel) **cyst/o-** *bladder; fluid-filled sac; semisolid cyst* **-cele** *hernia* **vesicocele** (VES-ih-KOH-seel) **vesic/o-** *bladder; fluid-filled sac* **-cele** *hernia*
neurogenic bladder	Urinary retention due to a lack of innervation of the nerves of the bladder. This can be due to a spinal cord injury, spina bifida, multiple sclerosis, or Parkinson's disease. The bladder must be catheterized intermittently because it does not contract to expel urine. Treatment: Catheterization.	**neurogenic** (NYOOR-oh-JEN-ik) **neur/o-** *nerve* **gen/o-** *arising from; produced by* **-ic** *pertaining to*
overactive bladder	Urinary urgency and frequency due to involuntary contractions of the bladder wall as the bladder fills with urine. This sometimes causes incontinence. Treatment: Drugs for overactive bladder.	
urinary retention	Inability to empty the bladder because of an obstruction (enlargement of the prostate gland, kidney stone), nerve damage (neurogenic bladder), or as a side effect of certain types of drugs. Even when the bladder contracts, a large amount of **postvoid residual** urine remains in the bladder. Treatment: Correct the underlying cause.	**retention** (ree-TEN-shun) **retent/o-** *keep; hold back* **-ion** *action; condition* **postvoid** (POST-voyd) *Postvoid* is a combination of the prefix *post-* (after; behind) and the word *void* (urinate).
vesicovaginal fistula	Formation of an abnormal passageway connecting the bladder to the vagina. Urine flows from the bladder into the vagina and leaks continually to the outside of the body. Treatment: Surgical correction.	**vesicovaginal** (VES-ih-koh-VAJ-ih-nal) **vesic/o-** *bladder; fluid-filled sac* **vagin/o-** *vagina* **-al** *pertaining to* **fistula** (FIS-tyoo-lah)

Urethra

Word or Phrase	Description	Word Building
epispadias	Congenital condition in which the female urethral meatus is in an abnormal location near the clitoris, or the male urethral meatus is in an abnormal location on the upper surface of the shaft of the penis rather than at the tip of the glans penis. **Hypospadias** is when the male urethral meatus is in an abnormal location on the underside of the shaft of the penis. Treatment: Surgery (urethroplasty) to reposition the urethral meatus.	**epispadias** (EP-ih-SPAY-dee-as) **epi-** *upon; above* **spad/o-** *tear; opening* **-ias** *condition* **hypospadias** (HY-poh-SPAY-dee-as) **hypo-** *below; deficient* **spad/o-** *tear; opening* **-ias** *condition*
urethritis	Inflammation or infection of the urethra. Gonococcal urethritis is a symptom of the sexually transmitted disease gonorrhea caused by the bacterium *Neisseria gonorrhoeae*. Nongonococcal urethritis is a sexually transmitted disease caused by the bacterium *Chlamydia trachomatis*. Nonspecific urethritis is an inflammation or infection of the urethra from bacteria, chemicals, or trauma; it is not a sexually transmitted disease. Treatment: Antibiotic drugs for an infection.	**urethritis** (YOO-ree-THRY-tis) **urethr/o-** *urethra* **-itis** *inflammation of; infection of*

Urine and Urination

Word or Phrase	Description	Word Building
albuminuria	Presence of albumin in the urine. Albumin is the major protein in the blood, and so this condition is also called **proteinuria.** Normally there is no protein in the urine because albumin molecules are too large to pass through the pores in the capillaries of the glomerulus; but when there is kidney disease, albumin passes through the damaged pores and is excreted in the urine. Albuminuria is an important first sign of kidney disease. It is also present in pregnant women who are developing preeclampsia. Treatment: Correct the underlying cause.	**albuminuria** (AL-byoo-mih-NYOO-ree-ah) **albumin/o-** *albumin* **ur/o-** *urine; urinary system* **-ia** *condition; state; thing* **proteinuria** (PROH-tee-NYOO-ree-ah) **protein/o-** *protein* **ur/o-** *urine; urinary system* **-ia** *condition; state; thing*
anuria	Absence of urine production by the kidneys because of acute or chronic renal failure. Treatment: Diuretic drugs or renal dialysis.	**anuria** (an-YOO-ree-ah) **an-** *without; not* **ur/o-** *urine; urinary system* **-ia** *condition; state; thing*
bacteriuria	Presence of bacteria in the urine. Normally, urine is sterile. Bacteria indicate a urinary tract infection. Treatment: Antibiotic drugs.	**bacteriuria** (BAK-teer-ee-YOO-ree-ah) **bacteri/o-** *bacterium* **ur/o-** *urine; urinary system* **-ia** *condition; state; thing*
dysuria	Difficult or painful urination. It can be due to many factors (kidney stone, cystitis, etc.). Treatment: Correct the underlying cause.	**dysuria** (dis-YOO-ree-ah) **dys-** *painful; difficult; abnormal* **ur/o-** *urine; urinary system* **-ia** *condition; state; thing*
enuresis	Involuntary release of urine in an otherwise normal person who should have already developed bladder control. Nocturnal enuresis is involuntary urination during sleep. Laypersons call this bedwetting. Treatment: Antidiuretic hormone (ADH), a pituitary gland hormone; psychological therapy.	**enuresis** (EN-yoo-REE-sis) **enur/o-** *to urinate* **-esis** *a process* Add words to make a complete definition of *enuresis*: a process *(that causes the patient)* to urinate.
frequency	Urinating often, usually in small amounts. This can be due to a kidney stone, enlargement of the prostate gland, a urinary tract infection, or overactive bladder. Treatment: Correct the underlying cause. Frequency is also normally present during pregnancy when the enlarging uterus limits the capacity of the bladder; however, this is not considered a disease.	
glycosuria	Glucose in the urine. This is an indication of an elevated blood sugar level, as seen in diabetes mellitus. Treatment: Correct the underlying cause.	**glycosuria** (GLY-kohs-YOO-ree-ah) **glycos/o-** *glucose (sugar)* **ur/o-** *urine; urinary system* **-ia** *condition; state; thing*
hematuria	Blood in the urine. This can be gross or frank blood (easily seen with the naked eye), or it can be microscopic blood that can only be detected with laboratory testing. Hematuria can be caused by a kidney stone, cystitis, bladder cancer, and so on. It can also be due to menstrual blood that contaminates a urine specimen. Treatment: Correct the underlying cause.	**hematuria** (HEE-mah-TYOO-ree-ah) **hemat/o-** *blood* **ur/o-** *urine; urinary system* **-ia** *condition; state; thing*

Word or Phrase	Description	Word Building
hesitancy	Inability to initiate a normal stream of urine. There is dribbling, and the urinary stream has a decreased **caliber.** The volume of urine passed is less, and residual urine may remain in the bladder. It can be caused by blockage of the urethra by a kidney stone, a urinary tract infection, or an enlarged prostate gland. Treatment: Correct the underlying cause.	**caliber** (KAL-ih-ber)
hypokalemia	A decreased amount of potassium in the blood. It is usually due to diuretic drugs that cause the kidneys to excrete excessive amounts of urine (and potassium). Treatment: Adjust the dose of the diuretic drug.	**hypokalemia** (HY-poh-kay-LEE-mee-ah) **hypo-** *below; deficient* **kal/i-** *potassium* **-emia** *condition of the blood; substance in the blood*
incontinence	Inability to voluntarily keep urine in the bladder. It can be due to a spinal cord injury, surgery on the prostate gland, unconsciousness, or a mental condition such as dementia. Treatment: Correct the underlying cause.	**incontinence** (in-CON-tih-nens) **in-** *in; within; not* **contin/o-** *hold together* **-ence** *state of* Add words to make a complete definition of *incontinence: state of not (being able) to hold together (all urine in the bladder).*

Across the Life Span

Pediatrics. Incontinence of urine is normal in babies because the nerve connections to the external urethral sphincter do not develop until about 2 years of age—about the time that parents begin toilet training.

Geriatrics. Incontinence can begin as early as middle age. There is relaxation of the muscles of the pelvic floor. When the patient laughs, coughs, or sneezes, increased intra-abdominal pressure causes urine to pass. This is known as **stress incontinence.** Muscle tone can be improved by doing Kegel exercises (the perineum is alternatively tensed and relaxed), or surgery may be needed. In older adults, the bladder has a decreased capacity and does not contract as well, which leaves a postvoid residual of urine with frequency of urination. Dementia often results in incontinence.

Word or Phrase	Description	Word Building
ketonuria	Ketone bodies in the urine. Ketones are waste products produced when fat is metabolized. Ketonuria is seen in patients with diabetes mellitus who metabolize fat for energy because they cannot metabolize glucose. It is also seen in malnourished patients who do not have enough glucose in the blood. Treatment: Correct the underlying cause.	**ketonuria** (KEE-toh-NYOO-ree-ah) **keton/o-** *ketones* **ur/o-** *urine; urinary system* **-ia** *condition; state; thing*
nocturia	Increased frequency and urgency of urination during the night. It can be due to cystitis, an enlarged prostate gland, or decreased capacity of the bladder in older adults. Nocturia is expressed as the number of times the patient voids each night (e.g., nocturia x3). Treatment: Correct the underlying cause.	**nocturia** (nawk-TYOO-ree-ah) **noct/o-** *night* **ur/o-** *urine; urinary system* **-ia** *condition; state; thing*
oliguria	Decreased production of urine due to kidney failure. Dehydration can cause temporary oliguria. Treatment: Correct the underlying cause.	**oliguria** (OL-ih-GYOO-ree-ah) **olig/o-** *scanty; few* **ur/o-** *urine; urinary system* **-ia** *condition; state; thing*

Word or Phrase	Description	Word Building
polyuria	Excessive production of urine due to diabetes mellitus or diabetes insipidus. Treatment: Correct the underlying cause.	**polyuria** (PAWL-ee-YOO-ree-ah) **poly-** *many; much* **ur/o-** *urine; urinary system* **-ia** *condition; state; thing*
pyuria	White blood cells (WBCs) in the urine, indicating a urinary tract infection. Severe pyuria can cause the urine to be cloudy or milky, or the number of white blood cells may be so few that they can be detected only by microscopic examination during a urinalysis. Treatment: Antibiotic drugs.	**pyuria** (py-YOO-ree-ah) **py/o-** *pus* **ur/o-** *urine; urinary system* **-ia** *condition; state; thing*
urgency	Strong urge to urinate and a sense of pressure in the bladder as the bladder contracts repeatedly. It is caused by obstruction from an enlarged prostate gland, a kidney stone, or inflammation from a urinary tract infection. Treatment: Correct the underlying cause.	
urinary tract infection (UTI)	General category of an infection anywhere in the urinary tract. Urinary tract infections are caused by bacteria, most often by *Escherichia coli* (*E. coli*), which is commonly found in the intestines and rectum. Urethritis is when the infection is only in the urethra. Cystitis is when the infection is in the bladder. Pyelonephritis is when the infection is in the kidney. Because of the short length of the urethra in women and its location close to the anus, women are more prone than men to develop urinary tract infections. Catheterization can also introduce bacteria into the urinary tract. Prevention: Patients with frequent urinary tract infections may be told to drink cranberry juice (see Figure 11-14 ■) to make their urine more acidic, as bacteria prefer alkaline, not acidic, urine. Treatment: Antibiotic drugs.	**infection** (in-FEK-shun) **infect/o-** *disease within* **-ion** *action; condition*

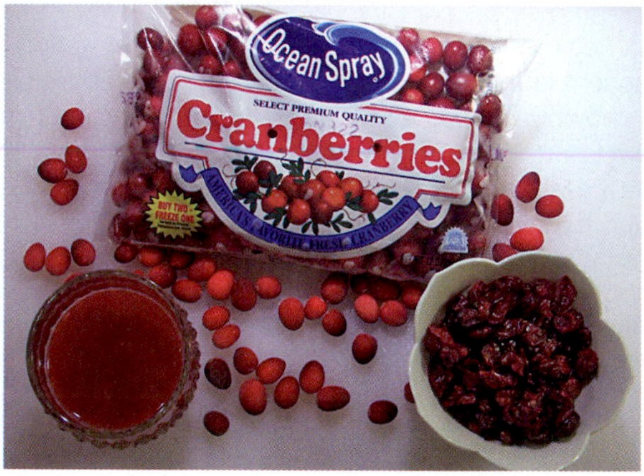

Figure 11-14 ■ **Cranberry juice.**
Patients with urinary tract infections can drink cranberry juice to make their urine more acidic. Bacteria that cause a urinary tract infection multiply rapidly in alkaline urine, but not in acidic urine. Some types of kidney stones form in alkaline urine, but not in acidic urine.

Laboratory and Diagnostic Procedures

Blood Tests

Word or Phrase	Description	Word Building
blood urea nitrogen (BUN)	Measures the amount of urea. It is used to monitor kidney function and the progression of kidney disease or to watch for signs of nephrotoxicity in patients taking aminoglycoside antibiotic drugs.	
creatinine	Measures the amount of creatinine. It is used to monitor kidney function and the progression of kidney disease. Creatinine is measured in conjunction with the BUN to give a comprehensive picture of kidney function.	

Urine Tests

Word or Phrase	Description	Word Building

culture and sensitivity (C&S)	Puts urine onto culture medium in a Petri dish to identify the cause of a urinary tract infection (see Figure 11-15 ■). Microorganisms present in the urine grow into colonies. The specific disease-causing microorganism is identified and tested to determine its sensitivity to various antibiotic drugs.	culture (KUL-chur)
		sensitivity (SEN-sih-TIV-ih-tee)
		  sensitiv/o- affected by; sensitive to
		  -ity state; condition

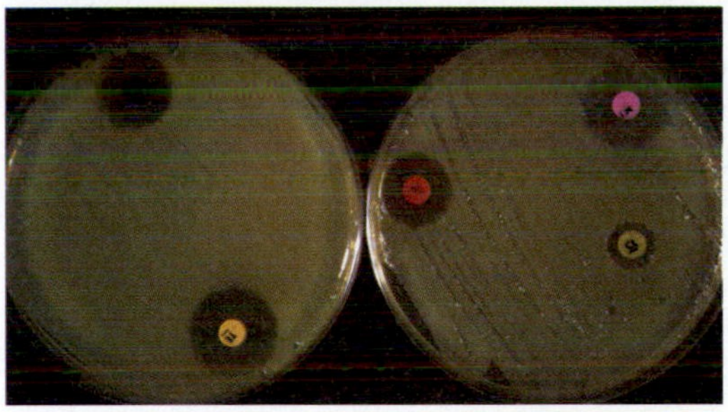

Figure 11-15 ■ Culture and sensitivity testing.
These Petri dishes grew colonies of the bacterium *E. coli*, the most common cause of a urinary tract infection. Antibiotic disks were placed in the Petri dishes. The antibiotic drugs that were most effective against *E. coli* show a large zone of inhibition (clear ring) around the disk where the bacterium could not grow. One of those antibiotic drugs would be prescribed to treat this patient's urinary tract infection.

Word or Phrase	Description	Word Building
drug screening	Performed on a group of employees or athletes to detect any individual who is using illegal, addictive, or performance-enhancing drugs	

leukocyte esterase	Detects esterase, an enzyme associated with leukocytes and a urinary tract infection. This dipstick test gives a quick result so that antibiotic drugs can be started immediately. At the same time, a urine specimen is also sent for C&S.	leukocyte (LOO-koh-site)
		  leuk/o- white
		  -cyte cell
		esterase (ES-ter-ace)

24-hour creatinine clearance	Collects all urine for 24 hours to measure the total amount of creatinine "cleared" (excreted) by the kidneys. The result is compared to the level of creatinine in the blood to determine the level of kidney function.	

Word or Phrase	Description	Word Building
urinalysis (UA)	Describes the characteristics of the urine and detects substances in it. A quick urinalysis can be done with a dipstick test (see Figure 11-16 ■) or the urine specimen can be sent to the laboratory for a full analysis. 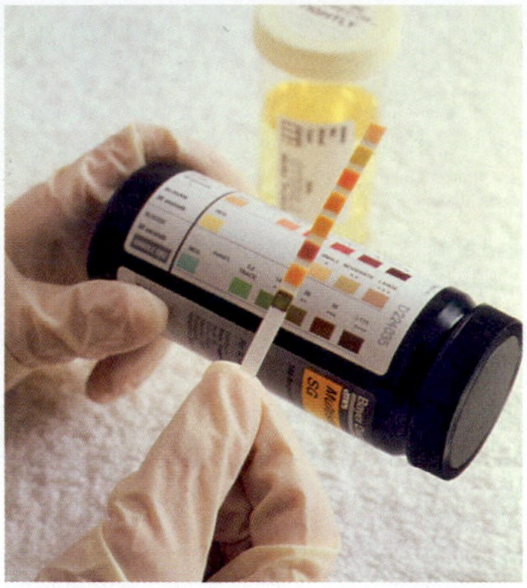 **Figure 11-16 ■ Urine dipstick.** This plastic strip with chemical-impregnated pads can perform several different laboratory tests (pH, protein, glucose, blood, and ketones) with a single dip in a urine specimen. The pads change color over time, and the final color of each pad is compared to a chart on the back of the container that gives a range of colors for each test and the associated test result numbers.	**urinalysis** (yoo-rih-NAL-ih-sis) *Urinalysis* is a combination of the combining form *urin/o-* (urine; urinary system) plus a shortened form of *analysis*.
color	Normal urine is light yellow to amber in color, depending on its concentration. Pink or smoky-colored urine indicates red blood cells from bleeding in the urinary tract. **Turbid** (cloudy or milky) urine indicates white blood cells and a urinary tract infection. The urinary analgesic drug phenazopyridine (Pyridium, Urogesic) turns the urine bright orange.	**turbid** (TUR-bid)
odor	Urine has a faint odor due to the waste products in it. The urine of a patient with uncontrolled diabetes mellitus has a fruity smell because of the glucose in it. When urine stands at room temperature, bacteria from the air grow in it, breaking down the urea into ammonia; this gives old urine its characteristic smell.	

pH	A test of how **acidic** or **alkaline** the urine is. Urine is normally slightly alkaline. Bacteria grow quickly and some types of kidney stones form more readily in alkaline urine.	**pH** (pee-H)
		
		acidic (ah-SID-ik)
		  acid/o- *acid (low pH)*
		  -ic *pertaining to*
		
		alkaline (AL-kah-line)
		  alkal/o- *base (high pH)*
		  -ine *pertaining to*

protein	Protein (or albumin) is not normally found in urine. Its presence (proteinuria or albuminuria) indicates damage to the glomerulus.	**protein** (PROH-teen)
glucose	Glucose is not normally found in urine. Its presence (glycosuria) indicates uncontrolled diabetes mellitus, with excess glucose in the blood "spilling" over into the urine.	**glucose** (GLOO-kohs)
red blood cells (RBCs)	Microscopic examination of urine under high-power magnification to count the number of erythrocytes (red blood cells). Even clear urine can contain **occult (hidden) blood.** This microscopic hematuria is reported as the number of RBCs per high-power field (hpf). If the urine has visible blood, the red blood cell count is reported as "TNTC" (too numerous to count).	**occult** (oh-KULT)

Word or Phrase	Description	Word Building
white blood cells (WBCs)	Microscopic examination of urine under high-power magnification to count the number of leukocytes (white blood cells) to identify a urinary tract infection. If the specimen is milky or cloudy, the white blood cell count is reported as "TNTC."	
ketones	Ketones are not normally found in urine. They are produced when the body cannot use (or does not have enough) glucose and instead metabolizes fat. It is seen in patients with uncontrolled diabetes mellitus, malnutrition, or in marathon runners.	**ketones** (KEE-tohnz)
specific gravity (SG)	Measurement of the concentration of the urine as compared to that of water (specific gravity 1.000). Dilute (not concentrated) urine has a specific gravity of 1.005, while concentrated urine is 1.030. Above 1.030 means the patient is dehydrated. Instruments used to measure specific gravity include a **urinometer** (see Figure 11-17 ■) or a **refractometer**, a handheld instrument that uses light rays that are bent (refracted) by a thin layer of urine spread on glass.	**urinometer** (YOO-rih-NAWM-eh-ter) **urin/o-** *urine; urinary system* **-meter** *instrument used to measure* **refractometer** (REE-frak-TAWM-eh-ter) **refract/o-** *bend; deflect* **-meter** *instrument used to measure*

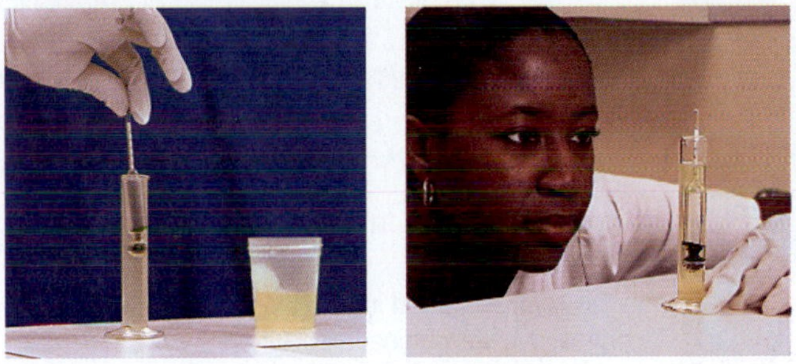

Figure 11-17 ■ Urinometer.
This test tube–like container holds the urine. A calibrated glass weight floats in the urine. The specific gravity is measured where the surface of the urine touches the calibrated scale on the narrowed top of the glass float.

Word or Phrase	Description	Word Building
sediment	There are several types of sediment in the urine. Crystals (calcium oxalate, uric acid, etc.) can become a kidney stone. Casts are protein molecules (**hyaline casts**) or blood (red cell casts) that is molded by the cylindrical shape of the tubules. Epithelial cells are normal in urine sediment because they are shed continuously from the lining of the urinary tract.	**hyaline** (HY-ah-lin) **hyal/o-** *clear, glass-like substance* **-ine** *pertaining to*
other substances	Chemical compounds whose presence helps to diagnose certain disease conditions. Bence Jones protein is seen in multiple myeloma (cancer of the bone marrow). Vanillylmandelic acid (VMA) is seen in pheochromocytoma and neuroblastoma, while 5-HIAA is seen in carcinoid syndrome.	

Radiology and Nuclear Medicine Procedures

Word or Phrase	Description	Word Building

intravenous pyelography (IVP)	Procedure that uses x-rays and radiopaque contrast dye (see Figure 11-18 ■). The dye is injected intravenously and flows through the blood and into the kidneys. It outlines the renal pelves, ureters, bladder, and urethra. It shows any obstruction, blockage, kidney stone, or abnormal anatomy in the urinary tract. It is also known as an **excretory urography**. The x-ray image is known as a **pyelogram** or **urogram**.
	
	Alternatively, **retrograde pyelography** can be done in which a cystoscopy is performed and a catheter is advanced into the ureter and dye is injected. The dye outlines the ureter, as well as the pelvis and calices of the kidney. 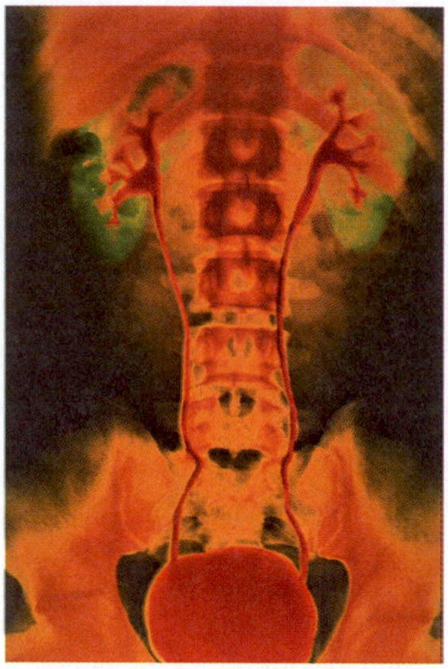
	
	Figure 11-18 ■ Intravenous pyelogram.
	In this color-enhanced image, the contrast dye has outlined structures of the urinary tract from the kidneys to the urethra. This is a normal pyelogram with no evidence of tumor, obstruction, or kidney stone.
		intravenous (IN-trah-VEE-nus)
		  intra- *within*
		  ven/o- *vein*
		  -ous *pertaining to*
		pyelography (PY-eh-LAWG-rah-fee)
		  pyel/o- *renal pelvis*
		  -graphy *process of recording*
		excretory (EKS-kreh-TOH-ree)
		(eks-KREE-toh-ree)
		  excret/o- *removing from the body*
		  -ory *having the function of*
		urography (yoo-RAWG-rah-fee)
		  ur/o- *urine; urinary system*
		  -graphy *process of recording*
		pyelogram (PY-eh-LOH-gram)
		  pyel/o- *renal pelvis*
		  -gram *a record or picture*
		urogram (YOO-roh-gram)
		  ur/o- *urine; urinary system*
		  -gram *a record or picture*
		retrograde (RET-roh-grayd)
		  retro- *behind; backward*
		  -grade *pertaining to going*
		The ending *-grade* contains the combining form *grad/o-* and the single letter suffix *–e*.

kidneys, ureters, bladder (KUB) x-ray	Procedure that uses an x-ray of the kidneys, ureters, and bladder done without contrast dye. It is used to find kidney stones or as a preliminary x-ray (scout film) before performing pyelography.	

nephrotomography	Procedure that uses a computerized axial tomography (CAT) scan and radiopaque contrast dye injected intravenously. It takes x-ray images as multiple "slices" through the kidneys. The images can be examined layer by layer to show the exact location of tumors.	**nephrotomography**
		(NEF-roh-toh-MAWG-rah-fee)
		  nephr/o- *kidney; nephron*
		  tom/o- *cut; slice; layer*
		  -graphy *process of recording*

renal angiography	Procedure that uses x-rays and radiopaque contrast dye. The dye is injected intravenously and flows through the blood into the renal artery. It outlines the renal artery and shows any obstruction or blockage. It is also known as **renal arteriography**. The x-ray image is known as a **renal angiogram** or **renal arteriogram**.	**angiography** (AN-jee-AWG-rah-fee)
		  angi/o- *blood vessel; lymphatic vessel*
		  -graphy *process of recording*
		arteriography
		(ar-TEER-ee-AWG-rah-fee)
		  arteri/o- *artery*
		  -graphy *process of recording*
		angiogram (AN-jee-OH-gram)
		  angi/o- *blood vessel; lymphatic vessel*
		  -gram *a record or picture*
		arteriogram (ar-TEER-ee-oh-gram)
		  arteri/o- *artery*
		  -gram *a record or picture*

Word or Phrase	Description	Word Building
renal scan	Procedure that uses a radioactive isotope injected intravenously. It is taken up by the kidney and emits radioactive particles that are captured by a scanner and made into an image. It is performed after a kidney transplantation to look for signs of organ rejection.	
ultrasonography	Procedure that uses ultra high-frequency sound waves emitted by a transducer or probe to produce an image of the kidneys, ureters, or bladder. The ultrasound image is known as a **sonogram** (see Figure 11-19 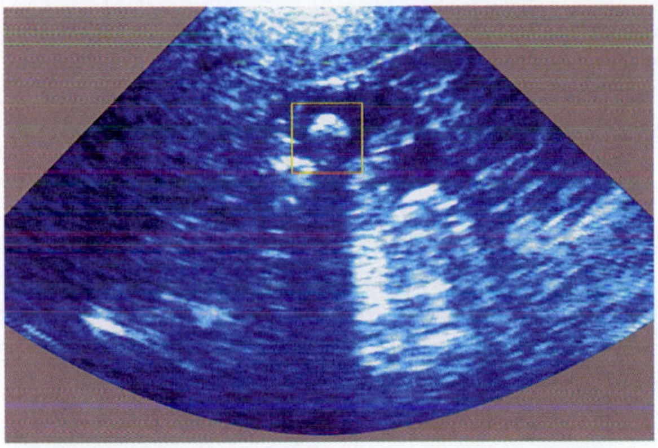 ■). **Figure 11-19 ■ Sonogram.** This ultrasound image shows a kidney stone in the bladder.	**ultrasonography** (UL-trah-soh-NAWG-rah-fee) **ultra-** *beyond; higher* **son/o-** *sound* **-graphy** *process of recording* **sonogram** (SAWN-oh-gram) **son/o-** *sound* **-gram** *a record or picture*

Other Laboratory Tests

cystometry	Procedure that evaluates the function of the nerves to the bladder. A catheter is used to inflate the bladder with liquid (or gas). A **cystometer** attached to the catheter measures the amount of liquid and the pressure in the bladder. The patient indicates when the first urge to urinate occurs. At that time, the cystometer makes a graphic recording known as a **cystometrogram (CMG).**	**cystometry** (sis-TAWM-eh-tree) **cyst/o-** *bladder; fluid-filled sac; semisolid cyst* **-metry** *process of measuring* **cystometer** (sis-TAWM-eh-ter) **cyst/o-** *bladder; fluid-filled sac; semisolid cyst* **-meter** *instrument used to measure* **cystometrogram** (sis-toh-MET-roh-gram) **cyst/o-** *bladder; fluid-filled sac; semisolid cyst* **metr/o-** *measurement* **-gram** *a record or picture*
voiding cystourethrography (VCUG)	Procedure that uses x-rays and radiopaque contrast dye. The dye, which is inserted into the bladder through a cystoscope, outlines the bladder and urethra. The x-ray image, taken while the patient is urinating, is known as a **voiding cystourethrogram.**	**cystourethrography** (sis-toh-yoo-ree-THRAWG-rah-fee) **cyst/o-** *bladder; fluid-filled sac; semisolid cyst* **urethr/o-** *urethra* **-graphy** *process of recording* **cystourethrogram** (sis-toh-yoo-REE-throh-gram) **cyst/o-** *bladder; fluid-filled sac; semisolid cyst* **urethr/o-** *urethra* **-gram** *a record or picture*

Medical and Surgical Procedures

Medical Procedures

Word or Phrase	Description	Word Building

catheterization	Procedure in which a **catheter** (flexible tube) is inserted through the urethra and into the bladder to drain the urine (see Figure 11-20 ■). A straight catheter is inserted each time the bladder becomes full, or it can also be used to obtain a single urine specimen for testing. A **Foley catheter** is an indwelling tube that drains urine continuously. It has an expandable balloon tip that keeps it positioned in the bladder. A **suprapubic catheter** is inserted through the abdominal wall (just above the pubic bone) and into the bladder. It is sometimes inserted after bladder or prostate gland surgery. A **condom catheter** is shaped like a condom (male contraceptive device). It fits snugly over the penis and collects the urine as it leaves the urethra meatus. Foley, suprapubic, and condom catheters are connected to a urine-collecting bag (see Figure 11-22).	**catheterization**
		(KATH-eh-TER-ih-ZAY-shun)
		  catheter/o- *catheter*
		  -ization *process of making, creating, or inserting*
		catheter (KATH-eh-ter)
		Foley (FOH-lee)
		suprapubic (SOO-prah-PYOO-bik)
		  supra- *above*
		  pub/o- *pubis (hip bone)*
		  -ic *pertaining to*
		condom (CON-dom)

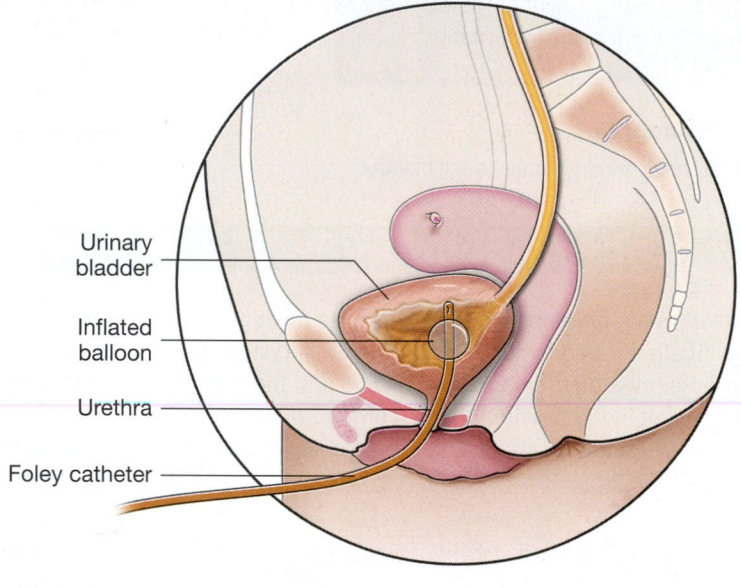

Urinary bladder

Inflated balloon

Urethra

Foley catheter

Figure 11-20 ■ Foley catheter.
The inflated balloon at the tip of the catheter holds the Foley catheter in place in the bladder. The catheter continuously drains urine from the bladder, and the urine is collected in a drainage bag.

Word or Phrase	Description	Word Building
dialysis	Procedure to remove waste products from the blood of a patient in renal failure. There are two types of dialysis: hemodialysis and peritoneal dialysis. **Hemodialysis** uses a fistula or a shunt in the patient's arm (see Figure 11-21 ■). A fistula is created by surgically joining an artery and vein. After surgery, the vein enlarges enough to accommodate two needles, one that removes blood and sends it to the dialysis machine and another that receives purified blood from the dialysis machine and returns it to the body. In a patient whose blood vessels are small, an external shunt (loop of tubing) is used instead to join an artery to the vein. **Peritoneal dialysis** uses a permanent catheter inserted through the abdominal wall. **Dialysate fluid** flows through the catheter and remains in the abdominal cavity for several hours. During that time, the fluid pulls body wastes from the blood. Then the fluid is removed, carrying waste products with it. In **continuous ambulatory peritoneal dialysis (CAPD),** the patient is able to walk around between the three or four daily episodes of dialysis. In **continuous cycling peritoneal dialysis (CCPD),** a machine inserts and removes dialysate fluid several times a night while the patient sleeps. Patients in renal failure continue to undergo dialysis several times a week while waiting for a kidney transplantation.	**dialysis** (dy-AL-ih-sis) **dia-** *complete; completely through* **-lysis** *process of breaking down or destroying* Add words to make a complete definition of *dialysis: the process of breaking down or destroying (wastes) completely through(out the body).* **hemodialysis** (HEE-moh-dy-AL-ih-sis) **hem/o-** *blood* **dia-** *complete; completely through* **-lysis** *process of breaking down or destroying* **peritoneal** (PAIR-ih-toh-NEE-al) **peritone/o-** *peritoneum* **-al** *pertaining to* **dialysate** (dy-AL-ih-sayt) **dia-** *complete; completely through* **lys/o-** *break down; destroy* **-ate** *composed of; pertaining to* **ambulatory** (AM-byoo-lah-TOR-ee) **ambulat/o-** *walking* **-ory** *having the function of*

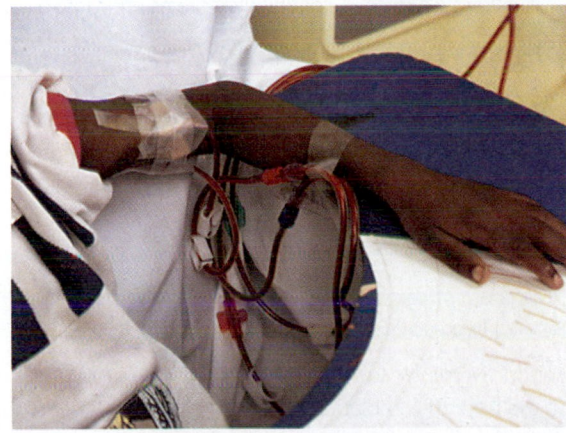
(a)

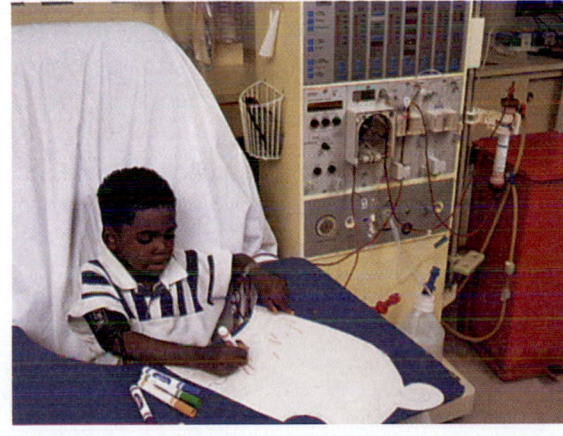
(b)

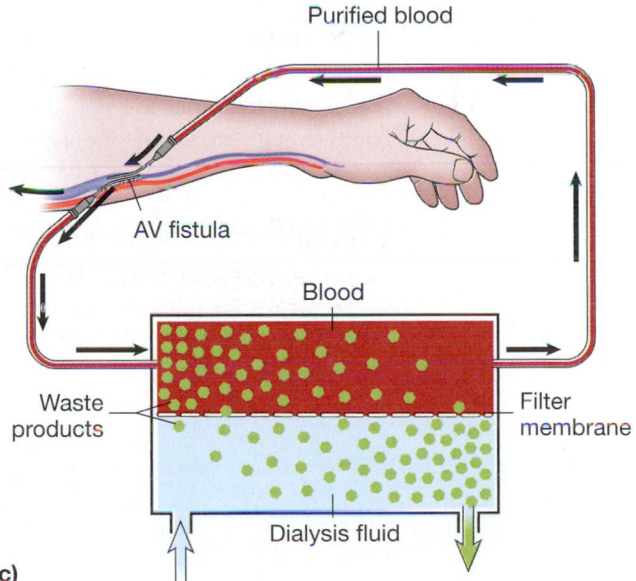
(c)

Figure 11-21 ■ Hemodialysis.

(a) This young patient is undergoing hemodialysis. A shunt was placed in his upper arm where the arteries and veins are larger. It was placed in his left arm because he is right handed. (b) During dialysis he is able to color and read to pass the time while his blood is cleansed of wastes. His blood pressure is checked frequently during dialysis and so the blood pressure cuff is allowed to remain on his right upper arm. (c) The dialysis machine pumps the blood through tubing whose wall is a selectively permeable membrane. Dialysate fluid surrounds the tubing. Wastes and excess amounts of electrolytes and glucose move from an area of higher concentration (in the blood) to an area of lower concentration (dialysate fluid). The blood is pumped back through an arteriovenous (AV) fistula or shunt.

Word or Phrase	Description	Word Building
intake and output (I&O)	Nursing procedure that documents the total amount of fluid intake (oral, nasogastric tube, intravenous line, etc.) and the total amount of fluid output (urine, wound drainage, etc.) (see Figure 11-22 ■). It is used to monitor the body's fluid balance in patients with renal failure, burns, congestive heart failure, large draining wounds, dehydration, overdose of diuretic drugs, etc.	

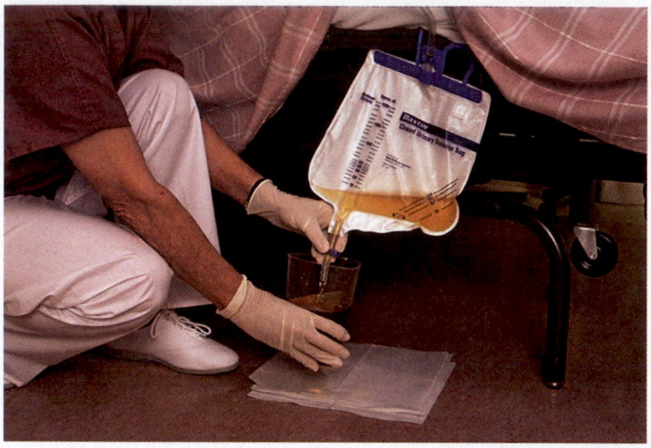

Figure 11-22 ■ **Urine output.**
This nurse is measuring the urine output from a patient who has an indwelling Foley catheter that continuously drains urine into a collecting bag.

Word or Phrase	Description	Word Building
urine specimen	Procedure to obtain a urine specimen for testing. Urine specimens can be tested in the doctor's office with a dipstick (see Figure 11-16). A clean-caught specimen (the urethral meatus is first cleansed) or a catheterized specimen (obtained directly from a catheter) is placed in a sterile container and sent to a laboratory for culture and sensitivity testing.	

Surgical Procedures

Word or Phrase	Description	Word Building
bladder neck suspension	Procedure to correct stress incontinence. A supportive sling of muscle tissue or synthetic material is inserted around the base of the bladder and the urethra to elevate them to a normal position.	**suspension** (sus-PEN-shun) **suspens/o-** *hanging* **-ion** *action; condition*
cystectomy	Procedure to remove the bladder because of bladder cancer. A **radical cystectomy** removes the bladder, surrounding tissues, and lymph nodes.	**cystectomy** (sis-TEK-toh-mee) **cyst/o-** *bladder; fluid-filled sac; semisolid cyst* **-ectomy** *surgical excision* **radical** (RAD-ih-kal) **radic/o-** *all parts including the root* **-al** *pertaining to*

Word or Phrase	Description	Word Building
cystoscopy	Procedure that uses a rigid or flexible **cystoscope** inserted through the urethra in order to examine the bladder (see Figure 11-23 ■). A wide-angle lens and a light allow a full view of the bladder. A video attachment can be used to create a permanent visual record.	**cystoscopy** (sis-TAWS-koh-pee) **cyst/o-** *bladder; fluid-filled sac; semisolid cyst* **-scopy** *process of using an instrument to examine* **cystoscope** (SIS-toh-skohp) **cyst/o-** *bladder; fluid-filled sac; semisolid cyst* **-scope** *instrument used to examine*

Did You Know?

Cystoscopes have been used since the early 1800s. Because this was before the invention of the light bulb, early cystoscopes used a platinum wire that glowed when an electrical current ran through it to illuminate the inside of the bladder.

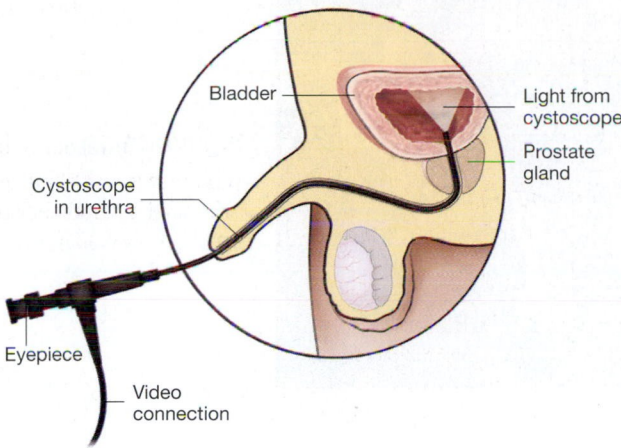

Figure 11-23 ■ Cystoscopy.

The cystoscope is a flexible tube that has a viewing eyepiece and a light to illuminate the inside of the bladder. The cystoscope is inserted through the urethra and into the bladder.

Word or Phrase	Description	Word Building
kidney transplantation	Procedure to remove a severely damaged kidney from a patient with end-stage kidney failure and insert a new kidney from a donor. The patient (the recipient) is matched by blood type and tissue type to the **donor**. The patient's diseased kidney is removed and the donor kidney is sutured in place (see Figure 11-24 ■). Kidney transplantation patients must take immunosuppressant drugs for the rest of their lives to keep their bodies from rejecting their new kidney.	**transplantation** (TRANS-plan-TAY-shun) **transplant/o-** *move something to another place* **-ation** *a process; being or having* **donor** (DOH-nor)

Did You Know?

The first successful kidney transplant occurred in 1954 in the United States between identical twins. It was not until FDA approval of the antirejection immunosuppressant drug cyclosporine in 1984 that transplantation of kidneys from cadavers or unrelated living donors could be performed successfully. In 2009, there were 78,000 patients waiting for kidney transplantations.

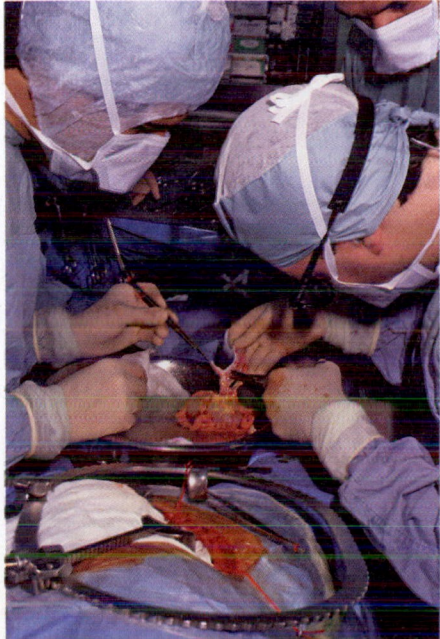

Figure 11-24 ■ Kidney transplantation.

When it was removed, this donor kidney was flushed with a cold solution and kept on ice to preserve it. Now, these surgeons are preparing it for transplantation. The renal artery and vein of the donor kidney will be sutured to the patient's iliac artery and vein in the pelvic cavity. The ureter of the donor kidney will be sutured to the patient's bladder.

Word or Phrase	Description	Word Building

lithotripsy	Procedure that uses sound waves to break up a kidney stone (see Figure 11-25 ■). After an x-ray pinpoints the location of the stone, a **lithotriptor** generates sound waves that break up the stone. Because the sound waves are generated by a source outside the body, the procedure is known as **extracorporeal shock wave lithotripsy (ESWL).** In the surgical procedure **percutaneous ultrasonic lithotripsy,** an endoscope is inserted through the flank skin and into the kidney. A lithotriptor probe is inserted through the endoscope and into the kidney to break up large stones. Sometimes a holmium laser that generates a laser beam is used to break up very hard kidney stones. 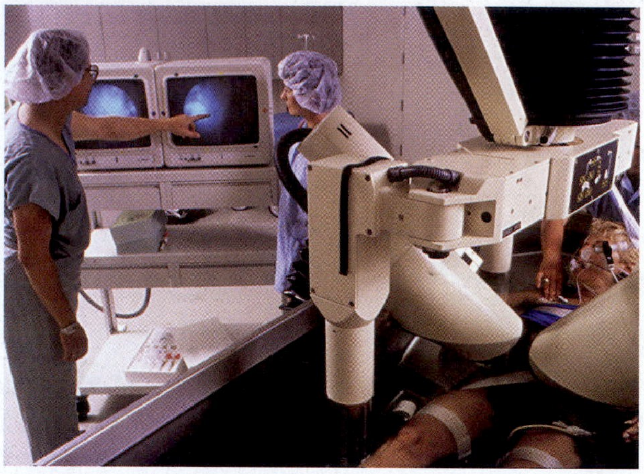
	
	Figure 11-25 ■ Lithotripsy.
	The patient lies on a table or is immersed in a tank of water. The lithotriptor emits sound at a frequency that creates shock waves to break up a kidney stone.
		lithotripsy (LITH-oh-TRIP-see)
		   lith/o- *stone*
		   -tripsy *process of crushing*
		lithotriptor (LITH-oh-TRIP-tor)
		   lith/o- *stone*
		   -triptor *thing that crushes*
		extracorporeal (EKS-trah-kohr-POH-ree-al)
		   extra- *outside of*
		   corpor/o- *body*
		   -eal *pertaining to*
		percutaneous (PER-kyoo-TAY-nee-us)
		   per- *through; throughout*
		   cutane/o- *skin*
		   -ous *pertaining to*
		ultrasonic (UL-trah-SAWN-ik)
		   ultra- *beyond; higher*
		   son/o- *sound*
		   -ic *pertaining to*

nephrectomy	Surgical procedure to remove a diseased or cancerous kidney. Alternatively, a healthy kidney may be removed from a donor so that it can be transplanted into a patient with renal failure.	**nephrectomy** (neh-FREK-toh-mee)
		   nephr/o- *kidney; nephron*
		   -ectomy *surgical excision*

nephrolithotomy	Procedure in which a small incision is made in the skin and an endoscope is inserted in a percutaneous approach into the kidney to remove a kidney stone embedded in the renal pelvis or calices.	**nephrolithotomy**
		(NEF-roh-lih-THAW-toh-mee)
		   nephr/o- *kidney; nephron*
		   lith/o- *stone*
		   -tomy *process of cutting or making an incision*

nephropexy	Procedure to correct a kidney that is in an abnormally low position (nephroptosis) by suturing it back into anatomical position.	**nephropexy** (NEF-roh-PEK-see)
		   nephr/o- *kidney; nephron*
		   -pexy *process of surgically fixing in place*

Word or Phrase	Description	Word Building
renal biopsy	Procedure in which a small piece of kidney is excised for microscopic analysis. This is done to confirm or exclude a diagnosis of cancer or kidney disease.	**biopsy** (BY-awp-see) **bi/o-** *life; living organisms; living tissue* **-opsy** *process of viewing*
stone basketing	Procedure in which a cystoscope is inserted into the bladder. A stone basket (a long-handled instrument with several interwoven wires at its end) is then passed through the cystoscope to snare a kidney stone and remove it.	
transurethral resection of a bladder tumor (TURBT)	Procedure to remove a bladder tumor from inside the bladder. A special cystoscope known as a **resectoscope** is inserted through the urethra into the bladder. It has built-in instruments that resect the bladder tumor, cauterize bleeding blood vessels, and use irrigating fluid to flush pieces of tissue out of the bladder.	**transurethral** (TRANS-yoo-REE-thral) **trans-** *across; through* **urethr/o-** *urethra* **-al** *pertaining to* **resection** (ree-SEK-shun) **resect/o-** *to cut out; remove* **-ion** *action; condition* **resectoscope** (ree-SEK-toh-skohp) **resect/o-** *to cut out; remove* **-scope** *instrument used to examine*
urethroplasty	Procedure that involves plastic surgery to reposition the urethra. It is used to correct congenital hypospadias or epispadias.	**urethroplasty** (yoo-REE-throh-PLAS-tee) **urethr/o-** *urethra* **-plasty** *process of reshaping by surgery*

Drug Categories

These categories of drugs are used to treat urinary diseases and conditions. The most common generic and trade name drugs in each category are listed.

Category	Indication	Examples	Word Building
antibiotic drugs	Used to treat urinary tract infections. These urinary antibiotic drugs have a special affinity for the urinary tract, although other categories of antibiotic drugs are also used to treat urinary tract infections.	nitrofurantoin (Macrobid, Macrodantin), sulfisoxazole (Gantrisin)	**antibiotic** (AN-tee-by-AWT-ik) (AN-tih-by-AWT-ik) **anti-** *against* **bi/o-** *life; living organisms; living tissue* **-tic** *pertaining to*

Clinical Connections			
Pharmacology. Aminoglycoside antibiotic drugs can cause a severe, **nephrotoxic** effect on the kidneys. Patients taking these drugs have their kidney function monitored by periodic BUN and creatinine tests.			**nephrotoxic** (NEF-roh-TAWK-sik) **nephr/o-** *kidney; nephron* **tox/o-** *poison* **-ic** *pertaining to*

Category	Indication	Examples	Word Building
antispasmodic drugs	Relax the smooth muscle in the walls of the ureter, bladder, and urethra. Used to treat spasm from cystitis and overactive bladder.	L-hyoscyamine (Anaspaz, Cystospaz)	**antispasmodic** (AN-tee-spaz-MAWD-ik) **anti-** *against* **spasmod/o-** *spasm* **-ic** *pertaining to*
diuretic drugs	Block sodium from being absorbed from the tubule back into the blood. As the sodium is excreted in the urine, it brings water and potassium with it because of osmotic pressure. This process is known as diuresis. This decreases the volume of blood and is used to treat hypertension, congestive heart failure, and nephrotic syndrome.	furosemide (Lasix), hydrochlorothiazide (HCTZ)	**diuretic** (DY-yoo-RET-ik) **dia-** *complete; completely through* **ur/o-** *urine; urinary system* **-etic** *pertaining to* The *a* in *dia-* is dropped when the word is formed.
drugs for overactive bladder	Block the action of acetylcholine and decrease contractions of the smooth muscle of the bladder	solifenacin (Vesicare), tolterodine (Detrol)	
potassium supplements	Used as a replacement for potassium lost due to diuretic drugs. (Diuretic drugs increase sodium excretion but also potassium excretion because they are both positively charged electrolytes.) The presence of *K* in the drug name refers to the chemical symbol for potassium (K^+).	potassium (Kay Ciel, K-Dur, K-Tab)	
urinary analgesic drugs	Exert a pain-relieving effect on the mucosa of the urinary tract	phenazopyridine (Pyridium, Urogesic)	**analgesic** (AN-al-JEE-zik) **an-** *without; not* **alges/o-** *sensation of pain* **-ic** *pertaining to*

Abbreviations

ARF	acute renal failure	**I&O**	intake and output
BUN	blood urea nitrogen	**IVP**	intravenous pyelography
CAPD	continuous ambulatory peritoneal dialysis	**K, K⁺**	potassium
cath	catheterize or catheterization (slang)	**KUB**	kidneys, ureters, bladder
cc	cubic centimeter (measure of volume)	**mL**	milliliter (measure of volume)
CCPD	continuous cycling peritoneal dialysis	**pH**	potential of hydrogen (acidity or alkalinity)
CRF	chronic renal failure	**RBC**	red blood cell
C&S	culture and sensitivity	**SG**	specific gravity
cysto	cystoscopy (slang)	**sp gr**	
epi	epithelial cell (in the urine specimen) (slang)	**TNTC**	too numerous to count
ESWL	extracorporeal shock wave lithotripsy	**TURBT**	transurethral resection of bladder tumor
ESRD	end-stage renal disease	**UA**	urinalysis
GU	genitourinary gonococcal urethritis	**UTI**	urinary tract infection
		VMA	vanillylmandelic acid
hpf	high-power field	**WBC**	white blood cell

Word Alert

ABBREVIATIONS

Abbreviations are commonly used in all types of medical documents; however, they can mean different things to different people and their meanings can be misinterpreted. Always verify the meaning of an abbreviation.

ARF means *acute renal failure,* but it also means *acute respiratory distress* or *acute rheumatic fever.*

C&S means *culture and sensitivity,* but the sound-alike word *CNS* means *central nervous system.*

CRF means *chronic renal failure,* but it also means *cardiac risk factors.*

GU means *genitourinary,* but it also means *gonococcal urethritis.*

It's Greek to Me!

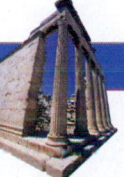

Did you notice that some words have two different combining forms? Combining forms from both Greek and Latin languages remain a part of medical language today.

Word	Greek	Latin	Medical Word Examples
bladder	cyst/o-	vesic/o-	cystitis, vesicovaginal
kidney	nephr/o-	ren/o-	nephritis, renal
kidney stone	lith/o-	calcul/o-	lithotripsy, calculogenesis
make urine	enur/o- urin/o-	mictur/o-	enuresis, micturition urination
renal pelvis	pyel/o-	pelv/o-	pyelonephritis, renal pelvis

CAREER FOCUS

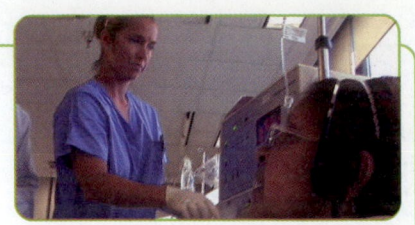

Meet Cindy, a dialysis nurse

"I came into dialysis because my brother actually was on dialysis for a very long time, and it was something I thought would be interesting. The dialysis center let me come in and let me observe for a few hours, and I found that was also very fascinating. I had already been a nurse for over eight years. This dialysis center gave me all the on-the-job training. It was just a whole different field. You really get to know your patients. You do have the time to actually sit down and talk to them. The majority of our patients have hypertension or they have diabetes, so we do a lot of diabetic teaching."

Dialysis nurses are allied health professionals who work in dialysis centers. They specialize in caring for patients with end-stage kidney disease who are receiving dialysis.

    Urologists are physicians who practice in the specialty of urology. They diagnose and treat patients with diseases of the urinary tract. Some urologists further specialize and become **nephrologists** who only treat patients with kidney disease. Physicians can take additional training and become board certified in the subspecialty of pediatric nephrology. Cancerous tumors of the urinary tract are treated medically by an oncologist or surgically by a urologist or a general surgeon.

urologist (yoo-RAWL-oh-jist)
ur/o- *urine; urinary system*
log/o- *word; the study of*
-ist *one who specializes in*

nephrologist (neh-FRAWL-oh-jist)
nephr/o- *kidney; nephron*
log/o- *word; the study of*
-ist *one who specializes in*

myhealthprofessionskit To see Cindy's complete video profile, visit Medical Terminology Interactive at www.myhealthprofessionskit.com. Select this book, log in, and go to the 11th floor of Pearson General Hospital. Enter the Laboratory, and click on the computer screen.

CHAPTER REVIEW EXERCISES

Test your knowledge of the chapter by completing these review exercises. Use the Answer Key at the end of the book to check your answers.

Anatomy and Physiology

Unscramble and Match Exercise

Unscramble the medical word and write the correct spelling of the word on the line, then match each word to its description. The first one has been done for you.

1.	beddrla	_bladder_	_____ Tube from renal pelvis to bladder
2.	deiykns	_____	_____ Proximal and distal convoluted
3.	hulmi	_____	_____ Opening at the end of the ureter or urethra
4.	lbeuut	_____	_____ Contains renal pyramids
5.	eprhstnic	_____	_____ Network of capillaries
6.	gearu	_____	_____ Paired organs shaped like kidney beans
7.	rlelguosum	_____	_____ Ring of muscles around tube
8.	smutea	_____	_____ Tube from bladder to outside the body
9.	aotestrp	_____	_____ Holds urine
10.	rteeur	_____	_____ Male gland around urethra
11.	claxi	_____	_____ Major and minor
12.	ulameld	_____	_____ Indentation in an organ
13.	rthurae	_____	_____ Folds in the bladder mucosa

Sequencing Exercise

Beginning with blood entering the kidney, write each structure of the urinary system in the correct order.

Structures	Correct Order
bladder	1. _____
calix	2. _____
collecting duct	3. _____
distal convoluted tubule	4. _____
glomerular capsule	5. _____
glomerulus	6. _____
nephron loop	7. _____
proximal convoluted tubule	8. _____
renal artery	9. _____
renal pelvis	10. _____
ureter	11. _____
urethra	12. _____
urethral meatus	13. _____

Diseases and Conditions

Matching Exercise

Match each word to its description.

1. anuria
2. dysuria
3. enuresis
4. glycosuria
5. incontinence
6. nocturia
7. oliguria
8. polyuria
9. pyuria
10. retention

_____ Bedwetting
_____ Excessive urine
_____ Difficult urination
_____ Voiding at night
_____ WBCs in the urine
_____ No urine production
_____ Sugar in the urine
_____ Bladder distended with urine
_____ Scanty urine production
_____ Inability to hold urine in the bladder

Antonyms Exercise

For each medical word given, write the antonym (opposite word) on the line.

Medical Word	Antonym		Medical Word	Antonym
1. acute	_____		4. gross blood in the urine	_____
2. polyuria	_____		5. urinary retention	_____
3. epispadias	_____			

Synonyms Exercise

For each medical word given, write the synonym (similar word) on the line.

Medical Term	Synonym		Medical Word	Synonym
1. albuminuria	_____		4. gross blood	_____
2. cystocele	_____		5. nephroblastoma	_____
3. enuresis	_____			

True or False Exercise

Indicate whether each statement is true or false by writing T or F on the line.

1. _____ Wilms' tumor is cancer of the kidney in children.
2. _____ Glomerulonephritis can develop following a strep throat.
3. _____ Albumin and protein are normally found in the urine.
4. _____ Glycosuria is a symptom of renal carcinoma.
5. _____ A spinal cord injury can result in polycystic kidneys.
6. _____ Pyelonephritis is an infection of the renal pelvis and kidney.
7. _____ A vesicovaginal fistula is an abnormal passage between the ureter and vagina.
8. _____ Renal colic is caused by a kidney stone in the intestines.
9. _____ Hydroureter develops because of an obstructing kidney stone.
10. _____ Bacteriuria is a symptom of a urinary tract infection.
11. _____ Calculogenesis is another name for lithogenesis.

Laboratory, Radiology, Surgery, and Drugs

Laboratory Test Exercise

Review the form below for ordering laboratory tests. Find each of the following tests related to urology and put a checkmark next to it.

albumin	creatinine clearance	gonococcus, urethra	urea nitrogen
creatinine	culture, urine	UA (dipstick & microscopic)	uric acid

PANELS AND PROFILES			TESTS	
968T	Lipid Panel	19687W	Bilirubin (Direct)
315F	Electrolyte Panel	265F	HBsAg
10256F	Hepatic Function Panel	51870R	HB Core Antibody
10165F	Basic Metabolic Panel	1012F	Cardio CRP
10231A	Comprehensive Metabolic Panel	23242E	GGT
10306F	Hepatitis Panel, Acute	28852E	Protein, Total
182Aaa	Obstetric Panel	141A	CBC Hemogram
18T	Chem-Screen Panel (Basic)	21105R	hCG, Qualitative, Serum
554T	Chem-Screen Panel (Basic with HDL)	10321A	ANA
7971A	Chem-Screen Panel (Basic with HDL, TIBC)	80185	Cardio CRP with Lipid Profile
TESTS		26F	PT with INR
56713E	Lead, Blood	232Aaa	UA, Dipstick
2782A	Antibody Screen	42A	CBC with Diff
3556F	Iron, TIBC	20867W	HDL Cholesterol
20933E	Cholesterol	31732E	PTT
3084111E	Uric Acid	34F	UA, Dipstick and Microscopic
53348W	Rubella Antibody	20396R	CEA
27771E	Phosphate	45443E	Hematocrit
2111600E	Creatinine	28571E	PSA, Total
29868W	Testosterone, Total	66902E	WBC count
9704F	Creatinine Clearance	20750E	Chloride
19752E	Bilirubin (Total)	7187W	Hemoglobin
30536Rrr	T3, Total	4259T	HIV-1 Antibody
687T	Protein Electrophoresis	45484R	Hemoglobin A1c
3563444R	Digoxin	67868R	Alk Phosphatase
15214R	Glucose, 2-Hour Postprandial	24984R	Iron
30502E	T3, Uptake	28512E	Sodium
7773E	Platelet Count	17426R	ALT
39685R	Dilantin (phenytoin)	**MICROBIOLOGY**	
30494R	Triglycerides	112680E	Group A Beta Strep Culture, Throat
26013E	Magnesium	5827W	Group B Beta Strep Culture, Genitals
15586R	Glucose, Fasting	49932E	Chlamydia, Endocervix/Urethra
30237W	T4, Free	6007W	Culture, Blood
28233E	Potassium	2692E	Culture, Genitals
19208W	AST	2649T	Culture, HSV
30163E	TSH	612A	Culture, Sputum
22764R	Ferritin	6262E	Culture, Throat
20008W	Calcium	6304R	Culture, Urine
54726F	Occult Blood, Stool	50286R	Gonococcus, Endocervix/Urethra
51839W	HAV Antibody, Total	6643E	Gram Stain
430A	Blood Group and Rh Type	**STOOL PATHOGENS**	
28399W	Progesterone	10045F	Culture, Stool
30262E	T4, Total	4475F	Culture, Campylobacter
20289W	Carbon Dioxide	10018T	Culture, Salmonella
1156F	RPR	86140A	E. coli Toxins
30940E	Urea Nitrogen	1099T	Ova and Parasites
17417W	Albumin	**VENIPUNCTURE**	
28423E	Prolactin	63180	Venipuncture

Circle Exercise

Circle the correct word from the choices given.

1. Ultrasonography uses (**radiation, sound waves, x-rays**) to produce an image.

2. To detect the presence of a kidney stone, a/an (**cystometrogram, IVP, KUB**) is performed after contrast dye is injected into a vein.

3. After the diagnosis of renal cell carcinoma was made, a (**biopsy, nephrectomy, nephropexy**) was performed to remove the entire kidney.

4. A (**catheter, cystoscope, shunt**) is a permanent tubing that is surgically inserted in the arm in order to perform hemodialysis.

5. The (**BUN, KUB, UA**) results showed that the urine had TNTC WBC.

6. Urine specific gravity is measured with all of these instruments *except* (**dialysis, refractometer, urinometer**).

7. Intravenous pyelography uses (**a CT scan, contrast dye, sound waves**) to produce an image.

Multiple Choice Exercise

Select the best answer for the question.

1. A culture and sensitivity test on a urine specimen shows the _____.
   a. color and odor of the urine   c. microorganism present and its response to antibiotic drugs
   b. amount of urea and creatinine   d. specific gravity, pH, and sediment

2. Which procedure uses a special solution and machine to remove waste products from the blood?
   a. catheterization   c. lithotripsy
   b. cystoscopy   d. hemodialysis

3. Which drug is used to increase urine output?
   a. diuretic   c. analgesic
   b. antispasmodic   d. antibiotic

Building Medical Words

Review the Combining Forms Exercise and Combining Form and Suffix Exercise that you already completed in the anatomy section on pages 561–562.

Combining Forms Exercise

Before you build urinary words, review these additional combining forms. Next to each combining form, write its medical meaning. The first one has been done for you.

Combining Form	Medical Meaning		Combining Form	Medical Meaning
1. albumin/o-	albumin		12. hyal/o-	
2. ambulat/o-			13. kal/i-	
3. bacteri/o-			14. keton/o-	
4. blast/o-			15. lith/o-	
5. calcul/o-			16. log/o-	
6. catheter/o-			17. neur/o-	
7. chron/o-			18. noct/o-	
8. gen/o-			19. olig/o-	
9. glycos/o-			20. protein/o-	
10. hemat/o-			21. pub/o-	
11. hem/o-			22. py/o-	

Combining Form	Medical Meaning		Combining Form	Medical Meaning
23. retent/o-	_____		27. tom/o-	_____
24. scler/o-	_____		28. tox/o-	_____
25. spad/o-	_____		29. transplant/o-	_____
26. spasmod/o-	_____		30. vagin/o-	_____

Related Combining Forms Exercise

Write the combining forms on the line provided. (Hint: See the It's Greek to Me feature box.)

1. Two combining forms that mean *bladder.* _____
2. Two combining forms that mean *kidney.* _____
3. Two combining forms that mean *kidney stone.* _____
4. Three combining forms that mean *make urine.* _____
5. Two combining forms that mean *renal pelvis.* _____

Combining Form and Suffix Exercise

Read the definition of the medical word. Select the correct suffix from the Suffix List. Select the correct combining form from the Combining Form List. Build the medical word and write it on the line. Be sure to check your spelling. The first one has been done for you.

SUFFIX LIST		COMBINING FORM LIST
-cele (hernia)	-metry (process of measuring)	cali/o- (calix)
-ectasis (condition of dilation)	-pathy (disease; suffering)	catheter/o- (catheter)
-ectomy (surgical excision)	-pexy (process of surgically fixing in place)	cyst/o- (bladder; fluid-filled sac)
-gram (a record or picture)		lith/o- (stone)
-graphy (process of recording)	-ptosis (state of prolapse; drooping; falling)	nephr/o- (kidney; nephron)
-itis (inflammation of; infection of)		pyel/o- (renal pelvis)
-ization (process of making, creating, or inserting)	-scopy (process of using an instrument to examine)	urethr/o- (urethra)
		urin/o- (urine; urinary system)
-meter (instrument used to measure)	-tripsy (process of crushing)	ur/o- (urine; urinary system)

Definition of the Medical Word

1. Inflammation or infection of the urethra
2. State of prolapse or drooping of the kidney
3. Process of recording the renal pelvis (by using contrast dye)
4. Instrument used to measure urine
5. Inflammation or infection of the bladder
6. Condition of dilation of the calix
7. Disease of the kidney
8. Surgical excision of the kidney
9. Process of using an instrument to examine the bladder
10. Hernia of the bladder
11. A record or picture of the urinary system (from contrast dye)
12. Process of inserting a catheter
13. Process of crushing a (kidney) stone (by using sound waves)
14. Process of measuring the bladder
15. Process of surgically fixing in place a kidney

Build the Medical Word

1. urethritis _____
2. _____
3. _____
4. _____
5. _____
6. _____
7. _____
8. _____
9. _____
10. _____
11. _____
12. _____
13. _____
14. _____
15. _____

Prefix Exercise

Read the definition of the medical word. Look at the medical word or partial word that is given (it already contains a combining form and a suffix). Select the correct prefix from the Prefix List and write it on the blank line. Then build the medical word and write it on the line. Be sure to check your spelling. The first one has been done for you.

PREFIX LIST

an- (without; not)	epi- (upon; above)	supra- (above)
anti- (against)	hypo- (below; deficient)	trans- (across; through)
dys- (painful; difficult; abnormal)	poly- (many; much)	

Definition of the Medical Word	Prefix	Word or Partial Word	Build the Medical Word
1. Condition in the blood of below (normal levels of) potassium	hypo-	kalemia	hypokalemia
2. Condition of difficult or painful urine	_____	uria	_____
3. Pertaining to many cysts (in the kidney)	_____	cystic	_____
4. Pertaining to through the urethra	_____	urethral	_____
5. Condition (of being) without urine	_____	uria	_____
6. Pertaining to above the pubic bone	_____	pubic	_____
7. Condition of much urine	_____	uria	_____
8. Pertaining to (a drug that is) against (urinary) spasms	_____	spasmodic	_____
9. Condition upon (the upper surface of the penis having the) opening (for the urethra)	_____	spadias	_____

Multiple Combining Forms and Suffix Exercise

Read the definition of the medical word. Select the correct suffix and combining forms. Then build the medical word and write it on the line. Be sure to check your spelling. The first one has been done for you.

SUFFIX LIST

-al (pertaining to)
-ary (pertaining to)
-esis (a process)
-graphy (process of recording)
-ia (condition; state; thing)
-iasis (state of; process of)
-ic (pertaining to)
-ist (one who specializes in)
-itis (inflammation of; infection of)
-oma (tumor; mass)
-osis (condition; abnormal condition; process)
-tomy (process of cutting or making an incision)

COMBINING FORM LIST

blast/o- (immature; embryonic)	olig/o- (scanty; few)
genit/o- (genitalia)	pyel/o- (renal pelvis)
gen/o- (arising from)	py/o- (pus)
glomerul/o- (glomerulus)	scler/o- (hard)
glycos/o- (glucose; sugar)	tom/o- (cut; slice; layer)
hemat/o- (blood)	tox/o- (poison)
keton/o- (ketones)	vagin/o- (vagina)
lith/o- (stone)	vesic/o- (bladder; fluid-filled sac)
log/o- (the study of)	urin/o- (urine; urinary system)
nephr/o- (kidney; nephron)	ur/o- (urine; urinary system)
noct/o- (night)	

Definition of the Medical Word	Build the Medical Word
1. A process of a stone arising from (the kidney)	lithogenesis
2. Process of cutting or making an incision (into the) kidney (to get) a stone	_____
3. Abnormal condition of the glomerulus of hard(ness)	_____
4. Inflammation or infection of the renal pelvis and kidney	_____
5. Tumor of the kidney (made of) immature, embryonic (cells)	_____
6. Condition of pus in the urine	_____

Definition of the Medical Word

Build the Medical Word

7. State of the kidney (having) stones

_____

8. Pertaining to the genitalia and the urinary system

_____

9. Condition of blood in the urine

_____

10. Process of recording the kidney (as an image of a) cut, slice, or layer

_____

11. Condition of glucose in the urine

_____

12. Pertaining to the bladder and the vagina

_____

13. Condition of scanty urine

_____

14. One who specializes in the study of the kidney

_____

15. Condition of ketones in the urine

_____

16. Pertaining to (a drug affecting the) kidney (as a) poison

_____

17. Condition of (during the) night (making) urine

_____

Abbreviations

Define and Match Exercise

Give the definition for each abbreviation listed below, then match it to its description.

1. BUN   _____   _____ X-ray image of the kidneys after injection of dye

2. cc   _____   _____ Test to determine what is causing a UTI and how to treat it

3. CRF   _____   _____ Long-term decrease in kidney function

4. C&S   _____   _____ Presence of this cell in the urine means infection

5. ESWL   _____   _____ X-ray of the kidneys, ureters, and bladder

6. I&O   _____   _____ Unit of measurement of volume of liquid

7. IVP   _____   _____ Used when there are too many cells to count

8. K   _____   _____ Blood test that measures kidney function

9. KUB   _____   _____ Measures consumption and excretion of fluids

10. TNTC   _____   _____ Includes multiple tests done on one urine specimen

11. UA   _____   _____ An electrolyte

12. WBC   _____   _____ Shock waves that dissolve kidney stones

Applied Skills

Plural Noun and Adjective Spelling Exercise

Read the noun and write the plural and/or adjective form. Be sure to check your spelling. The first one has been done for you.

Singular Noun	Plural Noun	Adjective	Singular Noun	Plural Noun	Adjective
1. cortex	cortices	cortical	6. pelvis	_____	_____
2. glomerulus	_____	_____	7. tubule	_____	_____
3. hilum	_____	_____	8. ureter	_____	_____
4. kidney	_____	_____	9. urethra	_____	_____
5. medulla	_____	_____	10. urine	_____	_____

Medical Report Exercise

This exercise contains an emergency department report. Read the report and answer the questions.

EMERGENCY DEPARTMENT REPORT

PATIENT NAME: NGUYEN, Li

HOSPITAL NUMBER: 082-344-8463

DATE: November 19, 20xx

CHIEF COMPLAINT
This 40-year-old female presented to the emergency department with complaints of abdominal pain, nausea, and vomiting.

HISTORY OF PRESENT ILLNESS
The patient had been seen 3 days earlier in the office of her primary care physician for a complaint of pressure and pain in the urethra. She was given a tentative diagnosis of urinary tract infection. The physician ordered a clean-catch urine specimen, and the patient provided this to a nearby laboratory. The patient was given a prescription for the antibiotic drug Bactrim and the urinary analgesic drug Pyridium. She was told to call the office in 3 days for the result of the urine culture. The patient states that, even though she was on the antibiotic drug, her symptoms worsened over the next 48 hours. She was taking Pyridium regularly, as well as Extra Strength Tylenol, and using a heating pad. She was drinking fluids, including cranberry juice as recommended by her primary care physician to acidify the urine to decrease the growth of bacteria. This evening, when her pain became acute, with pressure in the bladder area, a sense of urgency to urinate, spasm, renal colic, and nausea and vomiting, she presented to the emergency department.

PAST MEDICAL HISTORY
Appendectomy in the remote past. She has a history of kidney stones x2, the last episode being several years ago.

SOCIAL HISTORY
She is married and sexually active in a monogamous relationship. Her husband had a vasectomy several years ago.

PHYSICAL EXAMINATION
Vital signs: Temperature 98.8, pulse 120, respirations 28, blood pressure 140/100; normal blood pressure for her is 116/90. There is tenderness to palpation over the right lumbar and flank areas. There is tenderness to palpation over the suprapubic area. There is no tenderness to palpation elsewhere in the abdomen. Vaginal examination revealed no vaginal discharge or tenderness.

LABORATORY DATA
A catheterized urine specimen was obtained. It showed no bacteria, no gross blood, and no white blood cells. There was, however, microscopic hematuria. A KUB x-ray revealed no abnormalities. A pregnancy test was negative. However, a CT scan revealed a moderately sized kidney stone located in the bladder neck.

DIAGNOSIS
Solitary kidney stone at the bladder neck.

TREATMENT
The patient was given a urine strainer and will strain all urine. She will call to schedule an appointment with a urologist next week so that these multiple episodes of kidney stones can be investigated. If she passes the stone, the patient will bring it to the hospital laboratory for analysis.
In the emergency department, the patient was given pain medication and hydrated with I.V. fluids. When her pain had subsided, she was released. She will follow up as described above.

Alfred J. Strawberry, M.D.

Alfred J. Strawberry, M.D.

AJS:ljs
D: 11/19/xx
T: 11/19/xx

Word Analysis Questions

1. Divide *urologist* into its three word parts and define each word part.

Word Part	Definition

2. Divide *suprapubic* into its three word parts and define each word part.

Word Part	Definition

3. Divide *hematuria* into its three word parts and define each word part.

Word Part	Definition

4. Divide *antibiotic* into its three word parts and define each word part.

Word Part	Definition

5. Define these abbreviations.

   KUB _____

   I.V. _____

6. The phrase "tentative diagnosis of urinary tract infection" could be written with an abbreviation as "tentative diagnosis of a _____."

Fact Finding Questions

1. What type of urine specimen was obtained by the physician's office lab? _____

2. What was the purpose of drinking cranberry juice? _____

3. Define these words.

   renal colic _____

   suprapubic pain _____

4. What type of urine specimen was obtained in the emergency department? _____

5. Why was the patient given a urine strainer? _____

Critical Thinking Questions

1. Why was it important to note that the patient has had an appendectomy? _____

2. Why was it important to note that the patient's husband has had a vasectomy? _____

3. Why were the patient's pulse, respirations, and blood pressure elevated on admission to the emergency department, but not her temperature? _____

4. What did the results of the vaginal examination mean? _____

5. What is the most likely explanation for the microscopic hematuria? _____

On the Job Challenge Exercise

On the job, you will often encounter new medical words. Practice your medical dictionary skills by looking up the medical word in bold and writing its definition on the blank line.

OFFICE CHART NOTE

The patient presented with **strangury** and dysuria. A urinalysis showed both WBCs and RBCs. A diagnosis of cystitis was made, and the patient was given Cipro 250 mg b.i.d. and Pyridium 200 mg q.8h.

Strangury: _____

Hearing Medical Words Exercise

You hear someone speaking the medical words given below. Read each pronunciation and then write the medical word it represents. Be sure to check your spelling. The first one has been done for you.

1. KATH-eh-ter   *catheter* _____
2. KAL-kyoo-lus   _____
3. sis-TY-tis   _____
4. sis-TAWS-koh-pee   _____
5. dis-YOO-ree-ah   _____
6. gloh-MAIR-yoo-loh-neh-FRY-tis   _____
7. HEE-moh-dy-AL-ih-sis   _____
8. LITH-oh-TRIP-see   _____
9. nawk-TYOO-ree-ah   _____
10. PY-eh-loh-neh-FRY-tis   _____

Pronunciation Exercise

Read the medical word that is given. Then review the syllables in the pronunciation. Circle the primary (main) accented syllable. The first one has been done for you.

1. urination (yoo-rih-(nay)-shun)
2. creatinine (kree-at-ih-neen)
3. cystoscopy (sis-taws-koh-pee)
4. excretory (eks-kree-toh-ree)
5. glomerulus (gloh-mair-yoo-lus)
6. hematuria (hee-mah-tyoo-ree-ah)
7. nephrectomy (neh-frek-toh-mee)
8. polyuria (pawl-ee-yoo-ree-ah)
9. pyelonephritis (py-eh-loh-neh-fry-tis)
10. urologist (yoo-rawl-oh-jist)

Multimedia Preview

Immerse yourself in a variety of activities inside Medical Terminology Interactive. Getting there is simple:

1. Click on www.myhealthprofessionskit.com.
2. Select "Medical Terminology" from the choice of disciplines.
3. First-time users must create an account using the scratch-off code on the inside front cover of this book.
4. Find this book and log in using your username and password.
5. Click on Medical Terminology Interactive.
6. Take the elevator to the 11th Floor to begin your virtual exploration of this chapter!

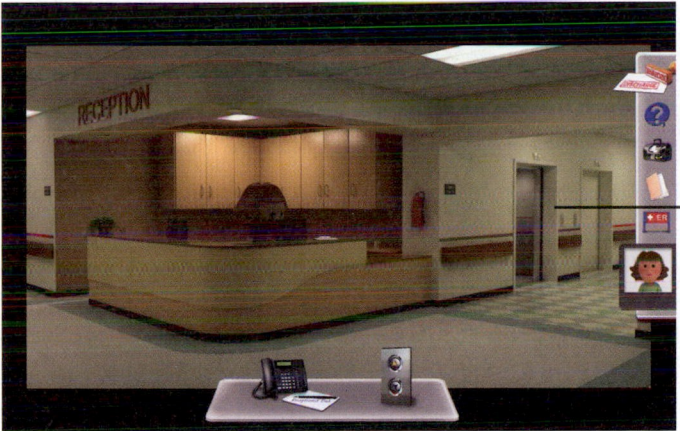 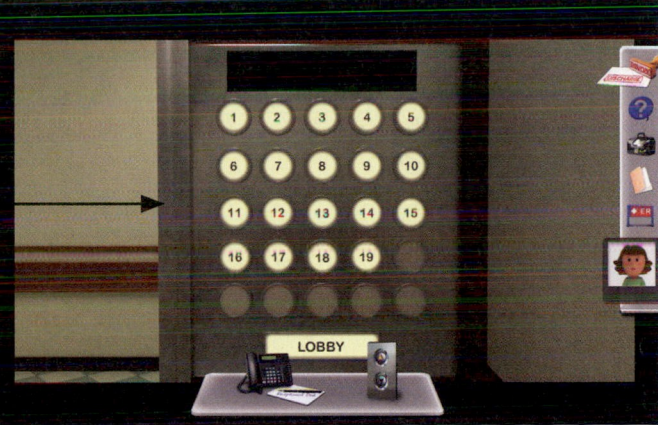

■ **Disease and Other Word Parts Flashcards**
Like the regular word parts flashcards, use customizable flashcards to help you memorize disease names and additional word parts. Print out prepared flashcards or make your own!

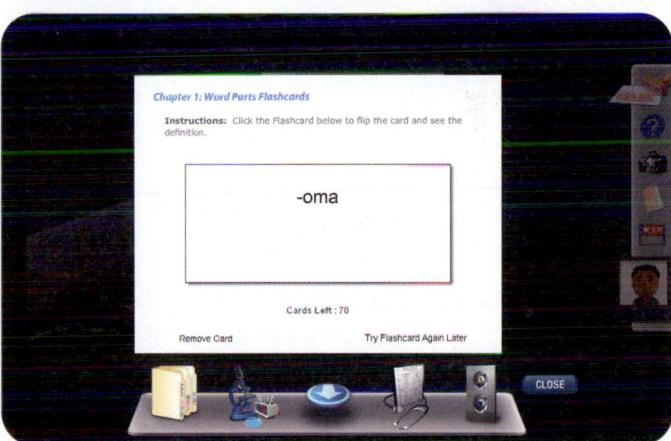

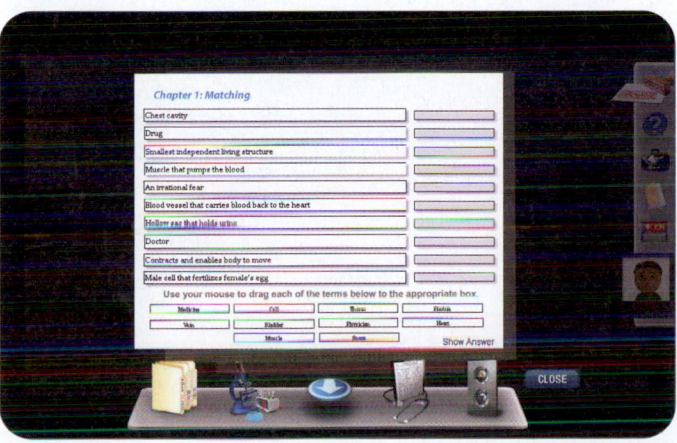

■ **Matching**   Are you a medical terminology matchmaker? See if you can correctly match the term to its corresponding definition. Then check your score to see if all of your choices were matches made in heaven.

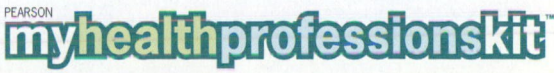

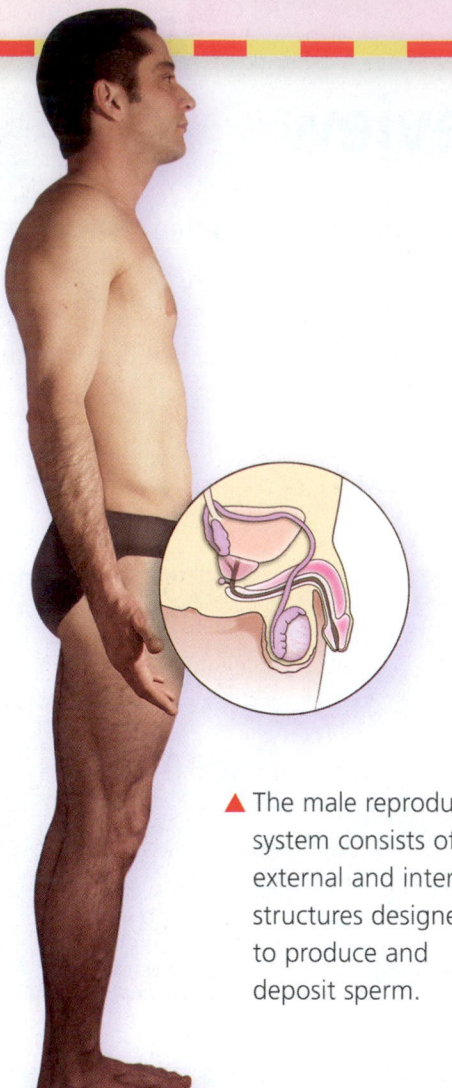

▲ The male reproductive system consists of external and internal structures designed to produce and deposit sperm.

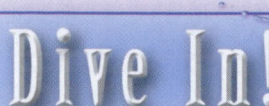

Dive In!

- The sperm of a man is half the size of that of a mouse.
- In the first five years that Viagra was on the market, physicians wrote prescriptions for about one billion tablets.
- Ready to multiply your odds for success? In this chapter we'll explore the language that describes the genitourinary system structures, functions, diseases, and conditions.
- You'll plant the seeds of knowledge once you master the language of male reproduction!

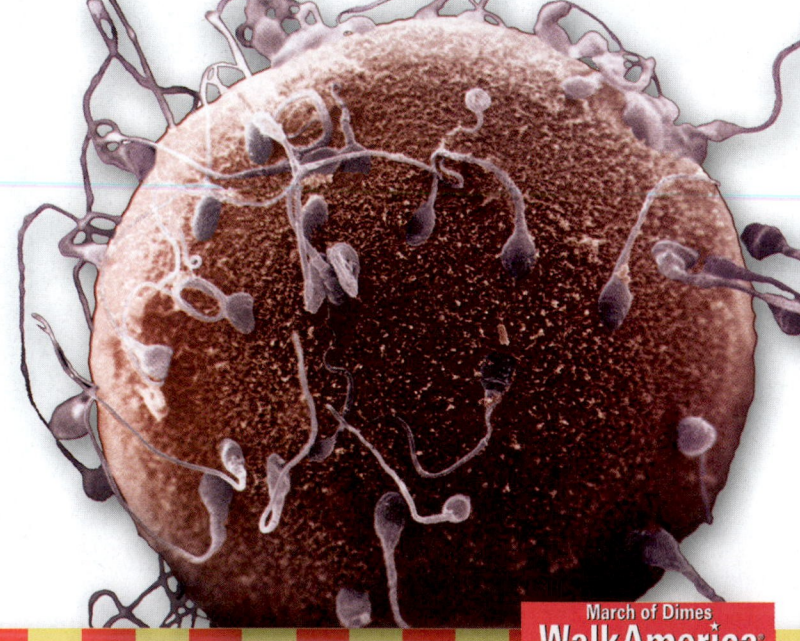

▶ A spermatozoon is nearly 100,000 times smaller than the ovum.

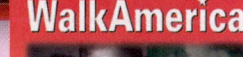
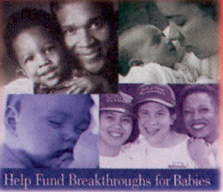
Medicine Through HISTORY

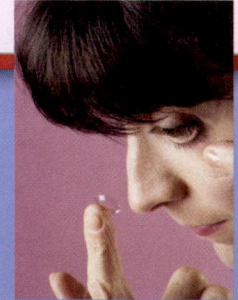

1936

The hard contact lens is invented by an optometrist in New York

1938

The March of Dimes begins to raise money for polio research

12
Male Reproductive Medicine
Male Genitourinary System

Male reproductive (RE-proh-DUK-tive) medicine is the medical specialty that studies the anatomy and physiology of the male genitourinary system and uses diagnostic tests, medical and surgical procedures, and drugs to treat male reproductive diseases.

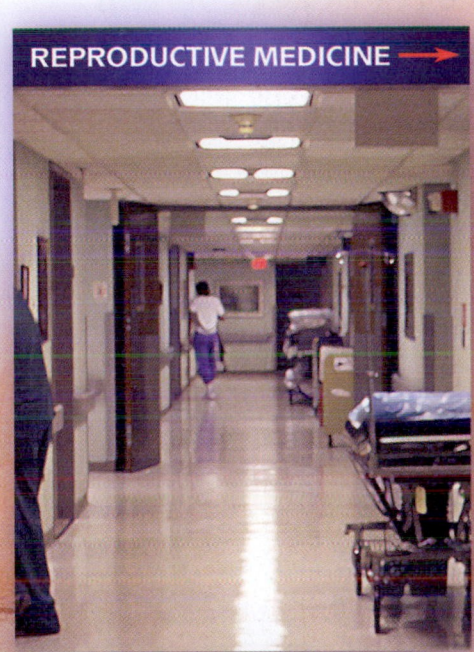

REPRODUCTIVE MEDICINE →

▶ Roosters are male chickens and they showcase their colorful feathers to attract mates for reproduction.

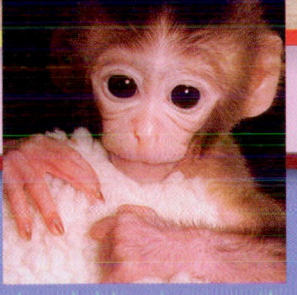

The Rh blood group (first discovered in the Rhesus monkey) is identified by Dr. Karl Landsteiner of Austria

1940

1941

The first commercial batches of the antibiotic drug penicillin (grown from a mold) became available

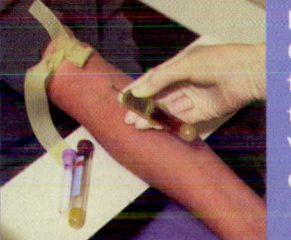

1943

Becton Dickinson Company invents the first vacuum tube, the Vacutainer, for drawing blood

Measure Your Progress: Learning Objectives

After you study this chapter, you should be able to

1. Identify the structures of the male genitourinary system.

2. Describe the processes of spermatogenesis and ejaculation.

3. Describe common male genitourinary diseases and conditions, laboratory and diagnostic procedures, medical and surgical procedures, and drug categories.

4. Give the medical meaning of word parts related to the male genitourinary system.

5. Build male genitourinary words from word parts and divide and define male genitourinary words.

6. Spell and pronounce male genitourinary words.

7. Analyze the medical content and meaning of a male reproductive medicine report.

8. Dive deeper into male reproductive medicine by reviewing the activities at the end of this chapter and online at Medical Terminology Interactive.

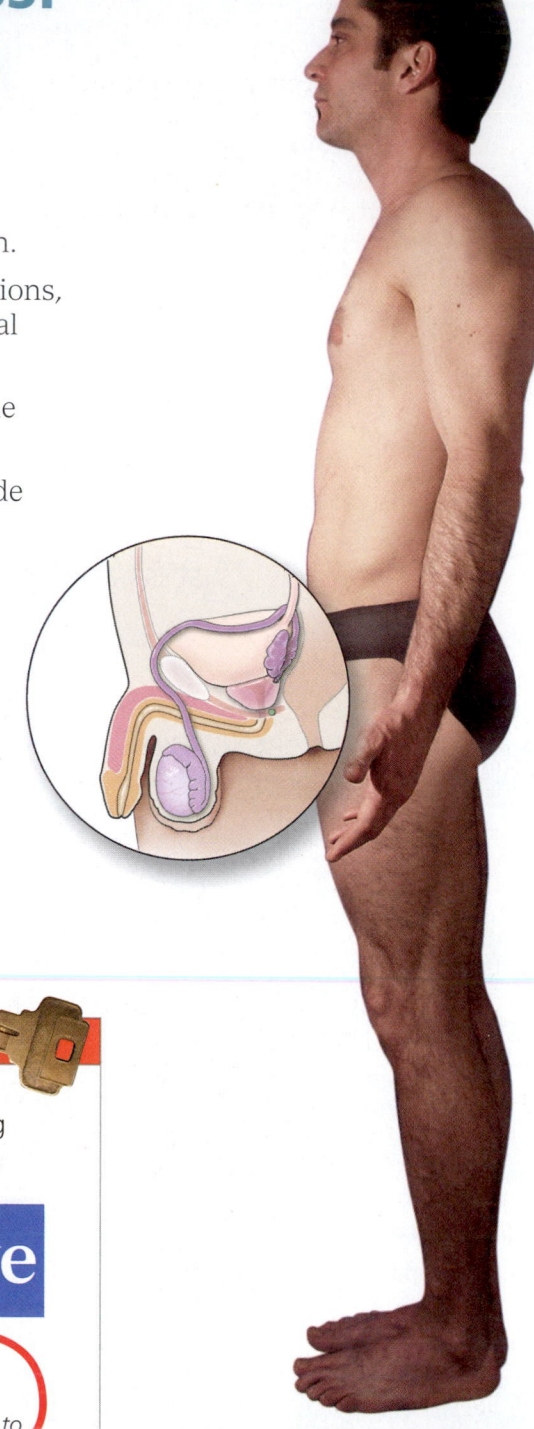

Figure 12-1 ■ Male genitourinary system.

The male genitourinary system is located in the pelvic cavity and outside the body in the area below the pelvic cavity.

Medical Language Key

To unlock the definition of a medical word, break it into word parts. Define each word part. Put the word part meanings in order, beginning with the suffix, then the prefix (if present), then the combining form(s).

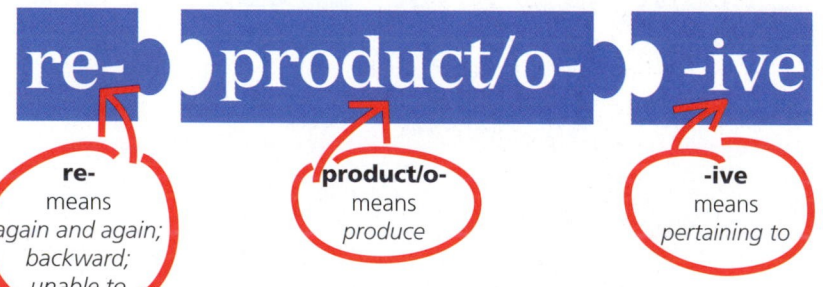

re-
means
again and again;
backward;
unable to

product/o-
means
produce

-ive
means
pertaining to

	Word Part	Word Part Meaning
Suffix	-ive	*pertaining to*
Prefix	re-	*again and again; backward; unable to*
Combining Form	product/o-	*produce*

Reproductive Medicine: (Medical specialty) pertaining to again and again producing (children).

Anatomy and Physiology

The **male genitourinary system** includes both the external and internal genitalia or **genital organs** (see Figure 12-1 ■). The **external genitalia** outside of the body include the scrotum, testes, epididymides, penis, and urethra. The **internal genitalia** within the pelvic cavity include the vas deferens, seminal vesicles, ejaculatory ducts, prostate gland, and bulbourethral glands. The male genitourinary system shares the urethra with the urinary system. The genitourinary system is also known as the **urogenital system** because of the close proximity of these two body systems and their shared structures. The function of the male genitourinary system is to display the male secondary sexual characteristics, produce spermatozoa, and, when appropriate, deposit spermatozoa inside the female.

Anatomy of the Male Genitourinary System

Scrotum

The **scrotum** is a soft pouch of skin behind the penis and in front of the legs (see Figure 12-2 ■). The scrotum is always a few degrees cooler than the core body temperature. This temperature difference is necessary for the proper development of spermatozoa. Muscles in the wall of the scrotum

WORD BUILDING

genitourinary
(JEN-ih-toh-YOO-rih-NAIR-ee)
  genit/o- *genitalia*
  urin/o- *urine; urinary system*
  -ary *pertaining to*

genital (JEN-ih-tal)
  genit/o- *genitalia*
  -al *pertaining to*

genitalia (JEN-ih-TAY-lee-ah)

urogenital (YOO-roh-JEN-ih-tal)
  ur/o- *urine; urinary system*
  genit/o- *genitalia*
  -al *pertaining to*

scrotum (SKROH-tum)

scrotal (SKROH-tal)
  scrot/o- *a bag; scrotum*
  -al *pertaining to*

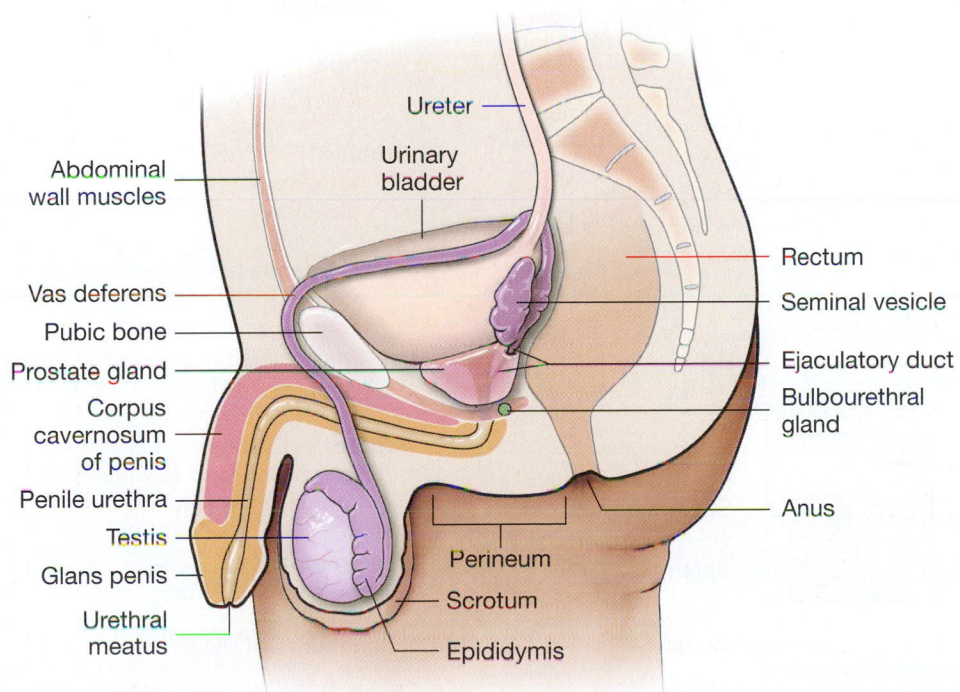

Figure 12-2 ■ External and internal male genitalia.
The internal male genitalia are interconnected with the external male genitalia. The urinary bladder is located near the internal male genitalia. The urethra is shared by the male genitourinary system and the urinary system.

contract or relax to move the scrotum closer to or farther away from the body to adjust to temperature changes in the environment. The **perineum** is the area on the outside of the body between the anus and the scrotum.

Testis and Epididymis

The scrotum contains the **testes** or **testicles.** Each testis is an egg-shaped gland about 2 inches in length (see Figures 12-2 and 12-3 ■). The testes are the **gonads** or sex glands in a male. They function as part of the male genitourinary system and the endocrine system (discussed in "Endocrinology," Chapter 14). (Gonads also include the ovaries, the female sex glands that produce ova, discussed in "Gynecology and Obstetrics," Chapter 13.)

The testes contain the **seminiferous tubules,** tightly coiled tubules that produce **spermatozoa** or **sperm.** Each spermatozoon has a head and a tail or **flagellum** that propels it. The testes are also endocrine glands; their **interstitial cells** (between the seminiferous tubules) secrete the hormone

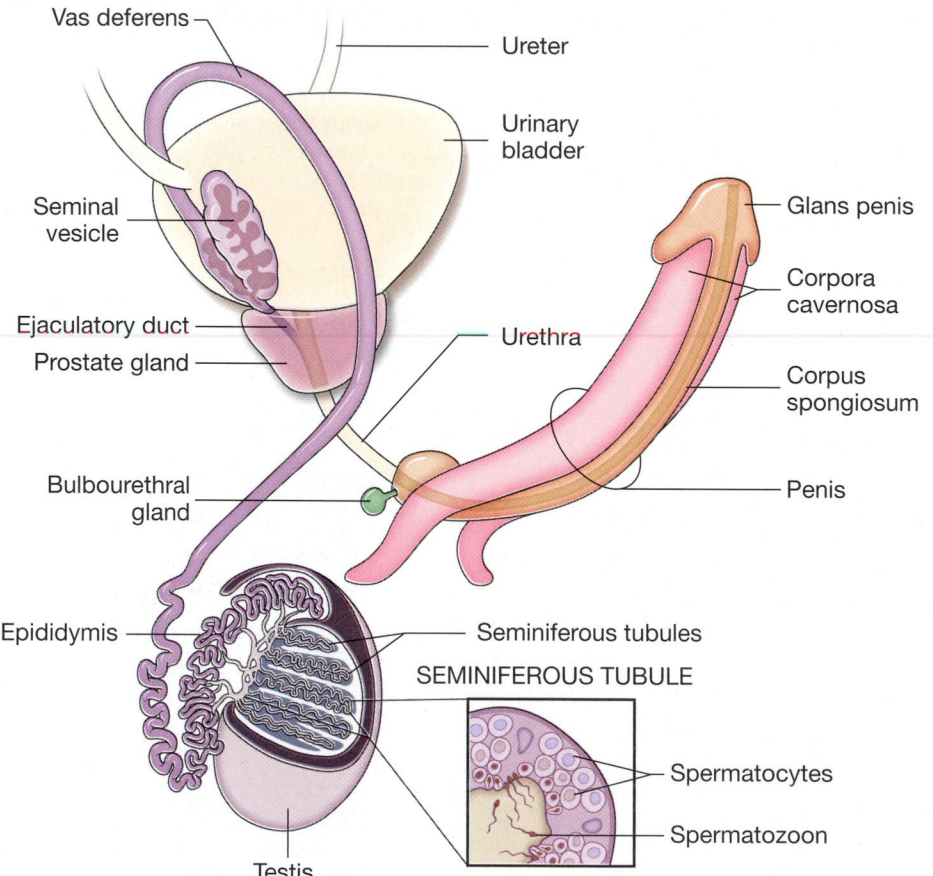

Figure 12-3 ■ Structures of the testis and penis.
The tightly coiled seminiferous tubules and epididymis become the single tubule of the vas deferens. It connects the external genitalia to the internal genitalia. The three columns of erectile tissue in the penis can be seen.

testosterone. **Testosterone** is the most abundant and biologically active of all the male sex hormones; it stimulates spermatozoa to mature. Mature spermatozoa are continuously released into the **lumen** (internal opening) of the seminiferous tubules and carried by fluid into the epididymis. The testes also secrete a small amount of the female hormone estradiol.

The **epididymis** is a long, coiled tube (over 20 feet in length) that is attached to the outer wall of each testis (see Figures 12-2 and 12-3). Within the epididymis, the head of each spermatozoon is given a cap-like layer of enzymes that helps it penetrate and fertilize the ovum of the female. The epididymis also destroys defective spermatozoa. Spermatozoa in the epididymis are mature but not yet moving. The tubules in the inferior section of the epididymis make a U-turn and become a larger, uncoiled duct known as the vas deferens or ductus deferens.

Clinical Connections

Neonatology. Before birth, the fetal testes develop in the pelvic cavity. Each testis has a **spermatic cord** that contains arteries, veins, nerves, and the vas deferens. Two months before birth, a testis and its spermatic cord enter the **inguinal canal,** a passageway that goes through the abdominal muscles, over the pubic bone, through the groin area, and into one side of the scrotum (see Figure 12-4 ■). At some point between birth and 2 years of age, the inguinal canal closes. If it fails to close, a loop of intestine can slip through the inguinal canal and create a bulge in the groin or in the scrotum. This is known as an indirect inguinal hernia.

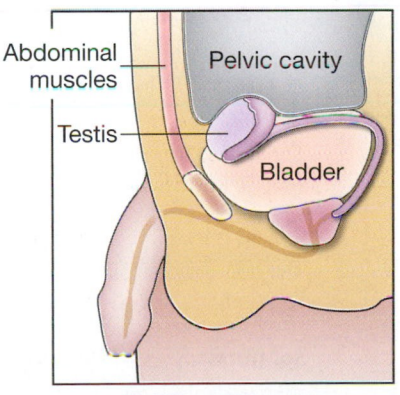
Position of testis in 5-month fetus

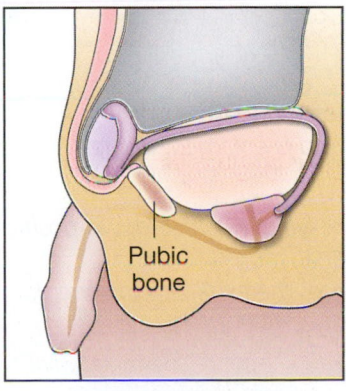
Position of testis in 7-month fetus

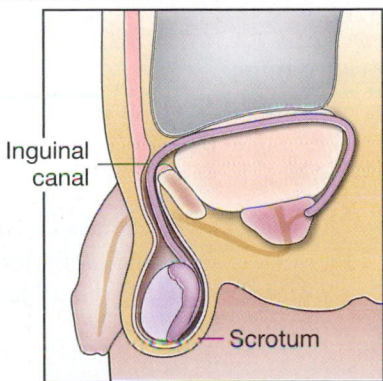
Position of testis in newborn

Figure 12-4 ■ Descent of the testes.
Before birth, the testes and their spermatic cords move from the abdominal cavity, through the inguinal canals, and into the scrotum.

Vas Deferens, Seminal Vesicles, and Ejaculatory Duct

The **vas deferens** (or **ductus deferens**) is a long duct that receives spermatozoa from the epididymis (see Figures 12-2 and 12-3). Spermatozoa can be stored in the vas deferens for several months in an inactive state. The vas deferens travels superiorly through the inguinal canal along with the other structures in the spermatic cord. At the superior end of the inguinal canal, however, the vas deferens continues on alone and goes behind the urinary bladder. There, the vas deferens merges with a seminal vesicle. The **seminal vesicles** are two elongated glands that form a *V* along the posterior wall of the urinary bladder. These glands produce **seminal fluid,** which makes up most of the volume of **semen.** The **ejaculatory duct** is a large collecting duct that holds spermatozoa from each vas deferens and seminal fluid from the seminal vesicles. The ejaculatory duct enters the prostate gland and then joins the prostatic urethra within the prostate gland.

Prostate Gland and Bulbourethral Glands

The **prostate gland** is a round gland at the base of the bladder (see Figures 12-2 and 12-3). It completely surrounds the first part of the urethra (the prostatic urethra). The prostate gland is not part of the urinary system, however. The prostate gland produces **prostatic fluid,** a milky substance that makes up some of the volume of semen. This fluid contains an antibiotic substance that kills bacteria in the woman's vagina, as well as a substance that activates the enzymes in the head of a spermatozoon so that it can penetrate the woman's ovum to fertilize it. Prostatic fluid also contains acid phosphatase, an enzyme that breaks the deposit of semen apart and releases the spermatozoa in the woman's vagina.

The **bulbourethral glands** are small, bulblike glands about the size of peas that are located on either side of the urethra just below the prostate gland (see Figures 12-2 and 12-3). They produce thick mucus that makes up some of the volume of the semen and neutralizes the acidity of any urine remaining in the urethra at the time of ejaculation.

Word Alert

SOUND-ALIKE WORDS

prostate   (noun)   gland that surrounds the urethra in men
Example: When the prostate gland is enlarged, it interferes with urination in men.

prostrate   (adjective)   descriptive word for *lying in a face-down position from humility or exhaustion*
Example: After the marathon race, the exhausted winner lay prostrate on the track.

Penis

The **penis** functions as an organ of the male genitourinary system and the urinary system (see Figures 12-2 and 12-3). The urethra leaves the prostate gland and passes through the length of the penis (penile urethra). The urethral meatus is located at the tip of the **glans penis.** In uncircumcised males, the urethral meatus is covered by the **prepuce** or **foreskin** of the penis. The penis and urethra serve as a passageway for semen (as part of the male genitourinary system) and as a passageway for urine (as part of the urinary system).

Three columns of erectile tissue run the length of the penis. Two of the columns, the **corpora cavernosa,** are located along the upper surface of the penis. The third column, the **corpus spongiosum,** is centered along the underside of the penis. The urethra is located within the corpus spongiosum. These three columns are composed of **erectile tissue** that fills with blood during sexual arousal, causing an **erection** as the penis becomes firm and erect.

Word Alert

SOUND-ALIKE WORDS

gland   (noun)   one of the structures of the endocrine system that secretes hormones into the blood
Example: The anterior pituitary gland in the brain secretes hormones that stimulate the testes at the beginning of puberty.

glans   (noun)   rounded area on top of the shaft of the penis
Example: The glans is covered by the foreskin in uncircumsized males.

Physiology of Spermatogenesis, Sexual Maturity, and Ejaculation

Spermatogenesis

At the onset of **puberty** (or **adolescence**), the anterior pituitary gland in the brain (discussed in "Endocrinology," Chapter 14) begins to secrete hormones to stimulate the testes. **Follicle-stimulating hormone (FSH)**

A Closer Look

Most cells in the body divide by the process of **mitosis,** in which the 46 chromosomes in the nucleus duplicate and then split, creating two identical cells each with 46 chromosomes. However, the production of spermatozoa is different from that of other cells in the body.

During childhood, the seminiferous tubules contain immature **spermatocytes.** These cells are round and each contains 46 chromosomes. First, the 46 chromosomes duplicate by mitosis, and the duplicated chromosomes randomly exchange genetic material. This is how different combinations of genes from the male are passed on to his children. Then the spermatocyte divides two more times and becomes four individual spermatozoon, each with 23 chromosomes; this process is **meiosis.** Spermatozoa (and also ova from the female) are **gametes**, and they have only half of the usual number of chromosomes. Each spermatozoon contains 23 chromosomes. **Spermatogenesis** is the process of producing more spermatozoa.

WORD BUILDING

corpora cavernosa
(KOR-por-ah KAV-er-NOH-sah)
Corpus is a Latin singular noun. Form the plural by changing *-us* to *-ora*.

corpus spongiosum
(KOR-puhs SPUN-jee-OH-sum)

erectile (ee-REK-tile)
　erect/o- *to stand up*
　-ile *pertaining to*

erection (ee-REK-shun)
　erect/o- *to stand up*
　-ion *action; condition*

puberty (PYOO-ber-tee)
　puber/o- *growing up*
　-ty *quality or state*

adolescence (AD-oh-LES-sens)
　adolesc/o- *the beginning of being an adult*
　-ence *state of*

follicle (FAWL-ih-kl)

mitosis (my-TOH-sis)
　mit/o- *threadlike structure*
　-osis *condition; abnormal condition; process*

spermatocyte (SPER-mah-toh-SITE)
　spermat/o- *spermatozoon; sperm*
　-cyte *cell*

meiosis (my-OH-sis)

gamete (GAM-eet)

spermatogenesis
(SPER-mah-toh-JEN-eh-sis)
　spermat/o- *spermatozoon; sperm*
　gen/o- *arising from; produced by*
　-esis *a process*

causes the seminiferous tubules to enlarge. Because these tubules make up 80% of each testis, the testes themselves enlarge significantly during puberty. FSH also stimulates spermatocytes in the testes to begin dividing. **Luteinizing hormone (LH)** stimulates the interstitial cells to begin to secrete testosterone.

WORD BUILDING

luteinizing (LOO-tee-ih-NY-zing)

Sexual Maturity

Also during puberty, testosterone causes the development of the male sexual characteristics: enlargement of the external genitalia; development of large body muscles; deepening of the voice (as the larynx widens); growth of body hair on the face, chest, axillae, and genital area; and development of the sexual drive (see Figure 12-5 ■).

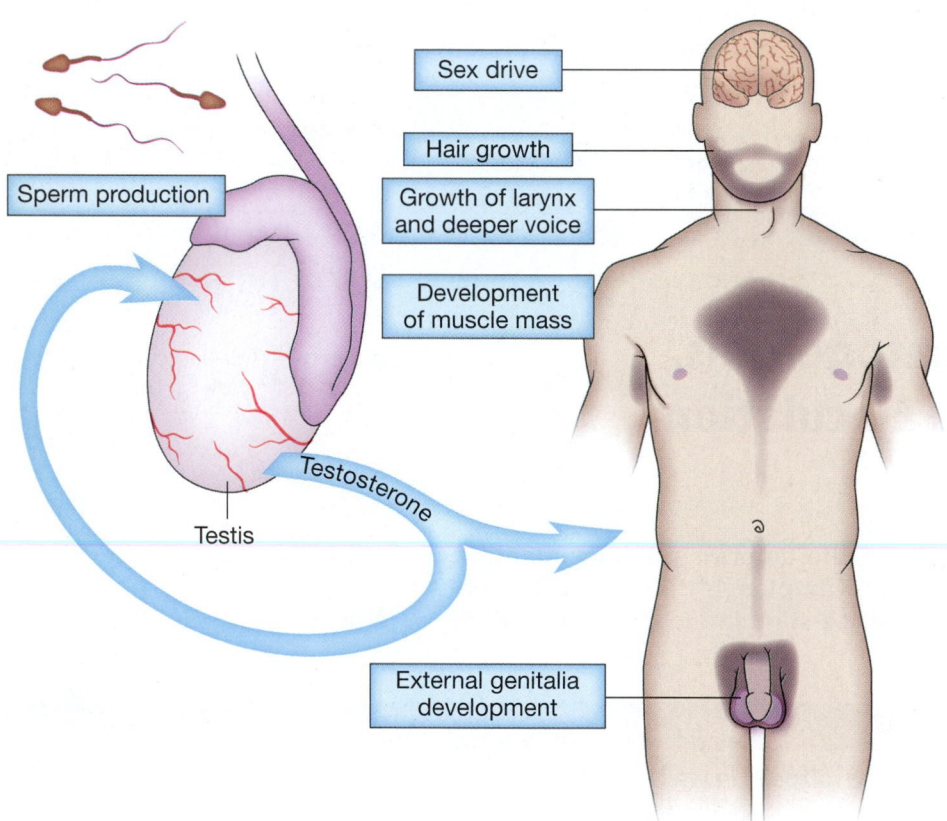

Sex drive

Hair growth

Growth of larynx and deeper voice

Development of muscle mass

Sperm production

Testosterone

Testis

External genitalia development

Figure 12-5 ■ Testosterone.
Testosterone is secreted by interstitial cells between the seminiferous tubules of the testes. Testosterone causes the development of the male sexual characteristics during puberty. It also causes spermatozoa to develop and mature.

Ejaculation

The process of ejaculation begins in response to thoughts or sensations that initiate sexual arousal. Smooth muscle relaxes in the wall of arteries in the penis, and vasodilation increases blood flow within the penis. Veins constrict to keep the corpora cavernosa and the corpus spongiosum distended with blood and produce an erection.

Stimulation from the sympathetic division of the nervous system causes muscles at the base of the penis to contract. Spermatozoa in the vas deferens move into the ejaculatory duct, where they are mixed with fluid from the seminal vesicles. This fluid has a high level of sugar, a source of energy for the spermatozoa. It is at this point that the spermatozoa become active. Then the spermatozoa move into the urethra. The prostate gland contracts, forcing prostatic fluid through ducts into the urethra. As the spermatozoa move through the urethra, they are mixed with mucus from the bulbourethral glands. Semen is a combination of spermatozoa and secretions from the seminal vesicles, prostate gland, and the bulbourethral glands. A series of contractions cause 2–5 mL of semen to be expelled from the penis through the urethral meatus. This process is **ejaculation.** Within this small volume of semen are 100–500 million spermatozoa! Sugar and other nutrients in the semen keep the spermatozoa swimming strongly as they travel through the female cervix, uterus, and uterine tube to fertilize an ovum. The physical union of a male and a female during **sexual intercourse** is known as **coitus.**

WORD BUILDING

ejaculation (ee-JAK-yoo-LAY-shun)
 ejaculat/o- *to expel suddenly*
 -ion *action; condition*

coitus (KOH-ih-tus)
The combining forms *pareun/o-* and *venere/o-* also mean *sexual intercourse.*

Vocabulary Review

Anatomy and Physiology

Word or Phrase	Description	Combining Forms
external genitalia	Scrotum, testes, epididymides, penis, and urethra	**genit/o-** *genitalia*
genital organs	Male internal and external **genitalia**	**genit/o-** *genitalia*
genitourinary system	Two body systems that share some structures: the male genital system and the urinary system. It is also known as the **urogenital system.**	**genit/o-** *genitalia* **urin/o-** *urine; urinary system* **ur/o-** *urine; urinary system*
internal genitalia	Vas deferens, seminal vesicles, ejaculatory ducts, bulbourethral gland, and prostate gland in the pelvic cavity	**genit/o-** *genitalia*

Scrotum, Testis, and Epididymis

epididymis	Long, coiled tube on the outer wall of each testis. It receives spermatozoa from the seminiferous tubules, stores them, and destroys defective spermatozoa.	**didym/o-** *testes (twin structures)*
gonads	The male sex glands (i.e., the testes)	**gon/o-** *seed (ovum or spermatozoon)*
inguinal canal	Passageway in the groin area through which the testes travel as they descend from the abdomen to the scrotum. The open canal should close around the spermatic cord sometime before age 2.	**inguin/o-** *groin*
interstitial cells	Special cells between the seminiferous tubules of the testes. These cells secrete testosterone when stimulated by luteinizing hormone (LH).	**interstiti/o-** *spaces within tissue*
lumen	Central open area throughout the length of a tube or duct (such as the seminiferous tubule, vas deferens, ejaculatory duct, or urethra)	
perineum	Area of skin between the anus and the scrotum	**perine/o-** *perineum*
scrotum	Pouch of skin that holds the two testes	**scrot/o-** *a bag; scrotum*
seminiferous tubules	Tubules within each testis where spermatozoa develop	**semin/i-** *spermatozoon; sperm* **fer/o-** *to bear* **tub/o-** *tube*
spermatic cord	Muscular tube that contains arteries, veins, and nerves for each testis as well as the vas deferens. It passes through the inguinal canal.	**spermat/o-** *spermatozoon; sperm*
spermatozoon	An individual mature sperm. Because it contains 23 chromosomes, it is a gamete. The **flagellum** is the long tail on a spermatozoon that propels it and makes it able to move. It is also known as **sperm.**	**spermat/o-** *spermatozoon; sperm* **sperm/o-** *spermatozoon; sperm*
testes	Egg-shaped gland in each side of the scrotum. It is also known as a **testicle.** It contains interstitial cells that secrete testosterone and seminiferous tubules that produce spermatozoa.	**test/o-** *testis; testicle* **testicul/o-** *testis; testicle* **didym/o-** *testes (twin structures)* **orchi/o-** *testis* **orch/o-** *testis*
testosterone	Most abundant and most biologically active of the male sex hormones secreted by the interstitial cells of the testes. It causes the male sexual characteristics to develop and spermatozoa to mature.	**test/o-** *testis; testicle*

Penis

Word or Phrase	Description	Combining Forms
erection	During sexual arousal, erectile tissue in the penis fills with blood, causing the penis to become firm and erect.	**erect/o-** *to stand up*
penis	Organ of **erectile tissue** that fills with blood during male sexual arousal. The **glans penis** is the rounded area on top of the shaft of the penis. The **corpora cavernosa** are two columns of tissue along the upper surface of the penis. The **corpus spongiosum** is a column of tissue on the underside of the penis. The urethra travels through the corpus spongiosum.	**pen/o-** *penis* **balan/o-** *glans penis* **erect/o-** *to stand up*
prepuce	**Foreskin** of the penis that covers the urethral meatus in an uncircumcised male	

Other Structures

Word or Phrase	Description	Combining Forms
bulbourethral glands	Small, bulblike glands below the prostate gland that secrete mucus into the urethra during ejaculation	**bulb/o-** *like a bulb* **urethr/o-** *urethra*
ejaculatory duct	Duct that collects semen from the vas deferens and the seminal vesicles and empties into the urethra during ejaculation	**ejaculat/o-** *to expel suddenly*
prostate gland	Large, round gland at the base of the bladder. It surrounds the first part of the urethra and produces **prostatic fluid** that becomes part of semen.	**prostat/o-** *prostate gland*
semen	Fluid expelled from the penis during ejaculation. Semen contains spermatozoa, seminal fluid, prostatic fluid, and mucus from the bulbourethral glands.	
seminal vesicles	Glands along the posterior wall of the bladder that secrete **seminal fluid,** a source of energy for the spermatozoa and the main fluid of semen	**semin/o-** *spermatozoon; sperm*
vas deferens	Long tube that receives spermatozoa from the epididymis and carries them to the seminal vesicles. It is also known as the **ductus deferens.**	**vas/o-** *blood vessel; vas deferens*

Spermatogenesis, Sexual Maturity, and Ejaculation

Word or Phrase	Description	Combining Forms
coitus	The physical union of a male and female during **sexual intercourse**	**coit/o-** *sexual intercourse* **pareun/o-** *sexual intercourse* **venere/o-** *sexual intercourse*
ejaculation	Sudden expelling of semen from the penis during sexual arousal of the male	**ejaculat/o-** *to expel suddenly*
follicle-stimulating hormone (FSH)	Hormone secreted by the anterior pituitary gland. It causes the seminiferous tubules of the testes to enlarge during puberty and spermatocytes in the testes to begin dividing.	
gamete	A cell (male spermatozoon or female ovum) that has 23 chromosomes instead of the usual 46 chromosomes like other cells	
luteinizing hormone (LH)	Hormone secreted by the anterior pituitary gland. It causes the interstitial cells of the testes to secrete testosterone.	
meiosis	Process by which a spermatocyte reduces the number of chromosomes in its nucleus to 23, or half the normal number, to create gametes	

Word or Phrase	Description	Combining Forms
mitosis	Process by which most body cells reproduce. The 46 chromosomes in the nucleus duplicate, and then split, creating two identical cells each with 46 chromosomes.	**mit/o-** *threadlike structure*
puberty	Period of time when FSH and LH from the anterior pituitary gland first begin to stimulate the testes. Testosterone causes the male sexual characteristics to develop, and there is a growth spurt. It is also known as **adolescence.**	**puber/o-** *growing up* **adolesc/o-** *the beginning of being an adult*
spermatocyte	Immature spermatozoon in the wall of the seminiferous tubule	**spermat/o-** *spermatozoon; sperm*
spermatogenesis	Process of producing a mature spermatozoon through the processes of mitosis and meiosis	**spermat/o-** *spermatozoon; sperm* **gen/o-** *arising from; produced by*

Labeling Exercise

Match each anatomy word or phrase to its structure and write it in the numbered box. Be sure to check your spelling. Use the Answer Key at the end of the book to check your answers.

bulbourethral gland	epididymis	prostate gland	testis
corpus cavernosum of the penis	glans penis	scrotum	vas deferens
ejaculatory duct	penile urethra	seminal vesicle	

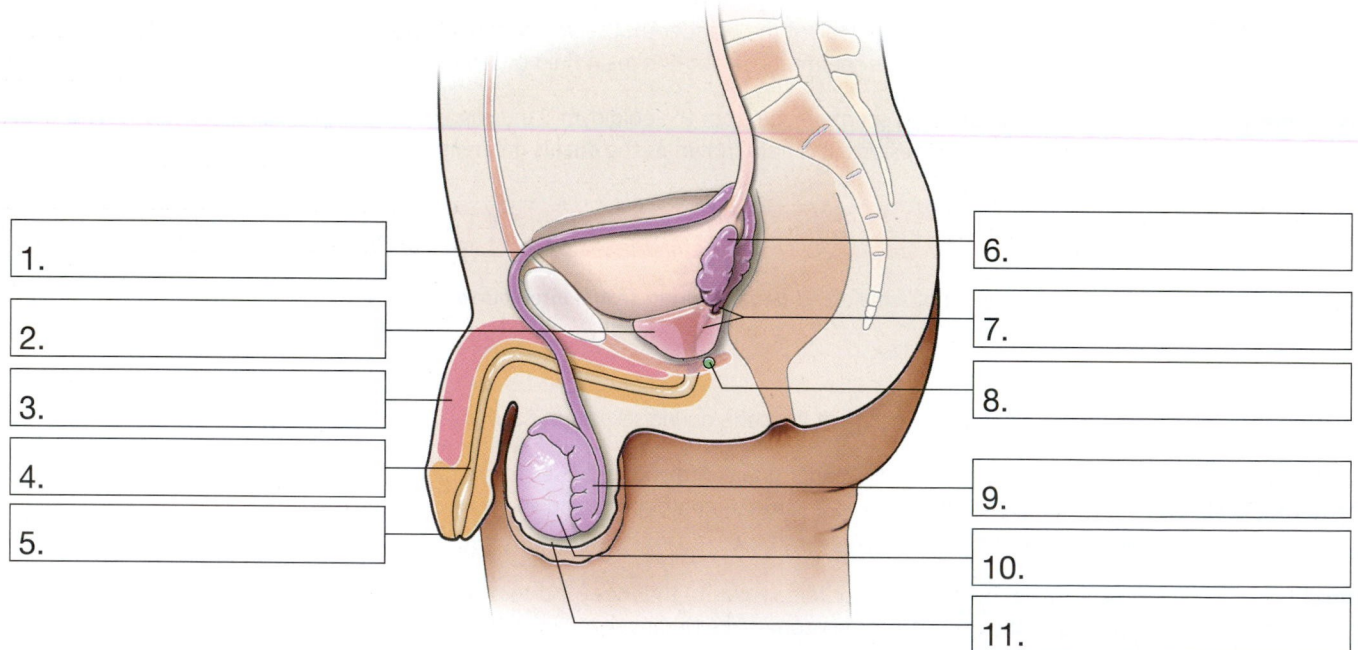

1.

2.

3.

4.

5.

6.

7.

8.

9.

10.

11.

Building Medical Words

Use the Answer Key at the end of the book to check your answers.

Combining Forms Exercise

Before you build male genitourinary words, review these combining forms. Next to each combining form, write its medical meaning. The first one has been done for you.

Combining Form	Medical Meaning	Combining Form	Medical Meaning
1. **adolesc/o-**	the beginning of being an adult	18. pen/o-	
		19. perine/o-	
2. balan/o-		20. product/o-	
3. bulb/o-		21. prostat/o-	
4. coit/o-		22. puber/o-	
5. didym/o-		23. scrot/o-	
6. ejaculat/o-		24. semin/i-	
7. erect/o-		25. semin/o-	
8. fer/o-		26. spermat/o-	
9. genit/o-		27. sperm/o-	
10. gen/o-		28. testicul/o-	
11. gon/o-		29. test/o-	
12. inguin/o-		30. tub/o-	
13. interstiti/o-		31. urethr/o-	
14. mit/o-		32. urin/o-	
15. orchi/o-		33. ur/o-	
16. orch/o-		34. vas/o-	
17. pareun/o-		35. venere/o-	

Combining Form and Suffix Exercise

Read the definition of the medical word. Look at the combining form that is given. Select the correct suffix from the Suffix List and write it on the blank line. Then build the medical word and write it on the line. (Remember: You may need to remove the combining vowel. Always remove the hyphens and slash.) Be sure to check your spelling. The first one has been done for you.

SUFFIX LIST				
-al (pertaining to)	-cyte (cell)	-ic (pertaining to)	-ion (action; condition)	-ty (quality or state)
-ar (pertaining to)	-ence (state of)	-ile (pertaining to)	-ory (having the function of)	-ule (small thing)

Definition of the Medical Word	Combining Form	Suffix	Build the Medical Word
	perine/o- **-al**		
1. Pertaining to the perineum			*perineal*
(You think *pertaining to* (-al) + *the perineum* (perine/o-). You change the order of the word parts to put the suffix last. You write *perineal*.)			
2. Pertaining to the scrotum	scrot/o-	_____	_____
3. State of growing up	puber/o-	_____	_____
4. (Immature) cell (that will become) sperm	spermat/o-	_____	_____
5. Small tube	tub/o-	_____	_____
6. An action (of the penis) standing up	erect/o-	_____	_____
7. State of the beginning of being an adult	adolesc/o-	_____	_____
8. Pertaining to the genitals	genit/o-	_____	_____
9. Pertaining to the testes	testicul/o-	_____	_____
10. Pertaining to the penis	pen/o-	_____	_____
11. Pertaining to the prostate gland	prostat/o-	_____	_____
12. Having the function of expelling (semen) suddenly	ejaculat/o-	_____	_____
13. Pertaining to the groin	inguin/o-	_____	_____

Diseases and Conditions

Testis and Epididymis

Word or Phrase	Description	Word Building
cryptorchism	Failure of one or both of the testicles to descend through the inguinal canal into the scrotum. This causes a low sperm count and male infertility. It is also known as cryptorchidism. Treatment: Testosterone drug; orchiopexy.	**cryptorchism** (krip-TOHR-kiz-em) **crypt/o-** *hidden* **orch/o-** *testis* **-ism** *process; disease from a specific cause*
epididymitis	Inflammation and infection of the epididymis. It is caused by a bacterial urinary tract infection or sexually transmitted diseases such as gonorrhea or chlamydia. Treatment: Antibiotic drugs.	**epididymitis** (EP-ih-DID-ih-MY-tis) **epi-** *upon; above* **didym/o-** *testes (twin structures)* **-itis** *inflammation of; infection of*
infertility	Failure of the woman to conceive after at least 1 year of regular sexual intercourse. If the man is the reason, it can be because of a hormone imbalance of FSH or LH, undescended testicles, a varicocele, genetic abnormalities, damage to the testes from mumps, infection in the testes, too few spermatozoa, or abnormalities of the spermatozoa. Treatment: Correct the underlying cause.	**infertility** (IN-fer-TIL-ih-tee) **in-** *in; within; not* **fertil/o-** *able to conceive a child* **-ity** *state; condition*
oligospermia	Fewer than the normal number of spermatozoa are produced by the testes (see Figure 12-6 ■). This is the most common cause of male infertility. It is caused by a hormone imbalance or an undescended testicle. Treatment: Correct the underlying cause.	**oligospermia** (OH-lih-goh-SPER-mee-ah) **olig/o-** *scanty; few* **sperm/o-** *spermatozoon; sperm* **-ia** *condition; state; thing*

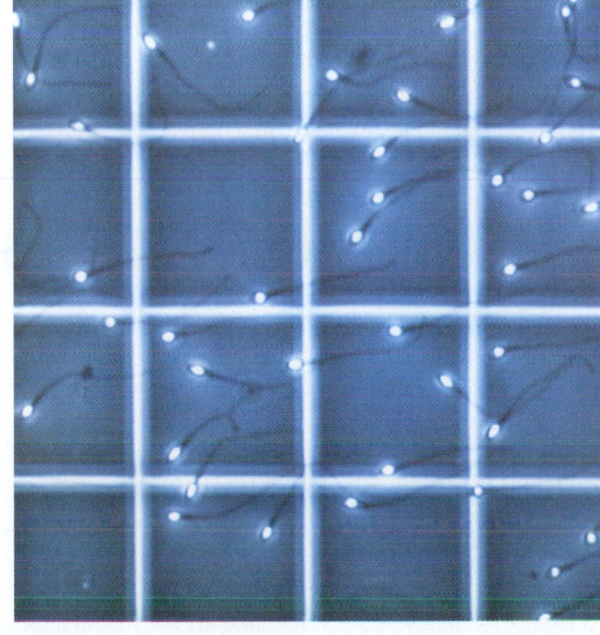
(a)

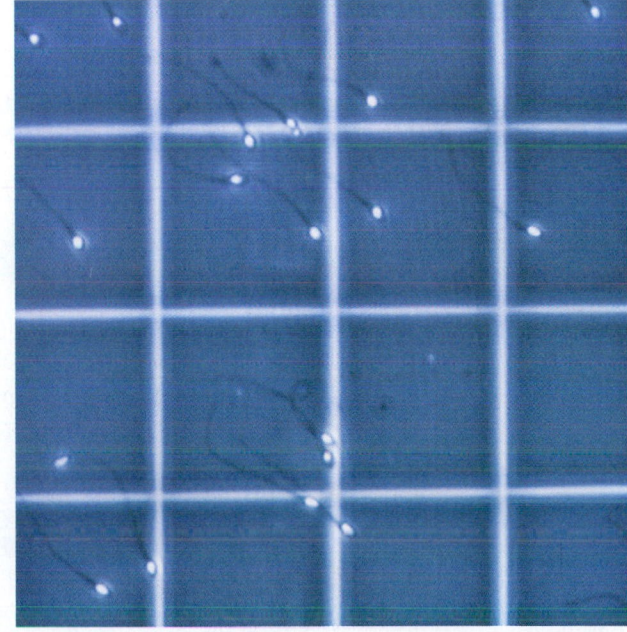
(b)

Figure 12-6 ■ Oligospermia.

(a) A normal number of sperm as seen on a counting grid under the microscope. (b) A decreased number of sperm in a patient with oligospermia.

Word or Phrase	Description	Word Building
orchitis	Inflammation or infection of the testes. It is caused by bacteria, the mumps virus, or trauma. Treatment: Antibiotic drugs for a bacterial infection; an antibiotic drug is not effective against a virus.	**orchitis** (or-KY-tis) **orch/o-** *testis* **-itis** *inflammation of; infection of*
testicular cancer	Cancerous tumor of one of the testes. Almost all of these arise from abnormal spermatocytes, not from other parts of the testes. It is also known as a **seminoma.** Treatment: Chemotherapy drugs and an orchiectomy.	**seminoma** (SEM-ih-NOH-mah) **semin/o-** *spermatozoon; sperm* **-oma** *tumor; mass*
varicocele	Varicose vein in the spermatic cord to the testis. The valves in the vein do not close completely. The vein becomes distended with blood and is painful. A varicocele can cause a low sperm count and infertility. Treatment: Surgical removal of the varicocele.	**varicocele** (VAIR-ih-koh-SEEL) **varic/o-** *varix; varicose vein* **-cele** *hernia*

Prostate Gland

Word or Phrase	Description	Word Building
benign prostatic hypertrophy (BPH)	Benign, gradual enlargement of the prostate gland that normally occurs as a man ages. The enlarged prostate gland compresses the urethra and causes the bladder to retain urine. There is hesitancy and dribbling on urination and a narrowed caliber of the urine stream. Treatment: Drugs to decrease the size of the prostate gland. Surgery: Transurethral resection of the prostate gland (TURP) or an alternate procedure with a laser, microwaves, or radiowaves.	**benign** (bee-NINE) **hypertrophy** (hy-PER-troh-fee) **hyper-** *above; more than normal* **-trophy** *process of development* The ending *–trophy* contains the combining form *troph/o-* and the one-letter suffix *–y.*
cancer of the prostate gland	**Cancerous** tumor of the prostate gland. This **malignancy** is the most common cancer in men. There are few early symptoms or signs because the cancer grows slowly. Later, the cancer makes the prostate feel hard or nodular on digital rectal examination. Treatment: Prostatectomy, radiation therapy, cryosurgery, female hormone drug therapy, or chemotherapy drugs.	**cancerous** (KAN-ser-us) **cancer/o-** *cancer* **-ous** *pertaining to* **malignancy** (mah-LIG-nan-see) **malign/o-** *intentionally causing harm; cancer* **-ancy** *state of*
prostatitis	Acute or chronic bacterial infection of the prostate gland. It is caused by a urinary tract infection or a sexually transmitted disease. Treatment: Antibiotic drug.	**prostatitis** (PRAWS-tah-TY-tis) **prostat/o-** *prostate gland* **-itis** *inflammation of; infection of*

Penis

Word or Phrase	Description	Word Building
balanitis	Inflammation and infection of the glans penis caused by a bacterium, virus, yeast, or fungus. It is often associated with phimosis and inadequate hygiene of the prepuce. Treatment: Antibiotic drug (for a bacterial infection); antifungal drug (for a yeast or fungal infection).	**balanitis** (BAL-ah-NY-tis) **balan/o-** *glans penis* **-itis** *inflammation of; infection of*
chordee	Downward curvature of the penis during an erection. It is caused by a constricting, cordlike band of tissue along the underside of the penis. This is a congenital abnormality that is often associated with hypospadias. Treatment: Surgical correction.	**chordee** (kor-DEE)
dyspareunia	Painful or difficult sexual intercourse or **postcoital** pain. It is caused by a penile or prostatic infection, chordee of the penis, or phimosis. Treatment: Correct the underlying cause.	**dyspareunia** (DIS-pah-ROO-nee-ah) **dys-** *painful; difficult; abnormal* **pareun/o-** *sexual intercourse* **-ia** *condition; state; thing* **postcoital** (post-KOH-ih-tal) **post-** *after; behind* **coit/o-** *sexual intercourse* **-al** *pertaining to*

Word or Phrase	Description	Word Building
erectile dysfunction (ED)	Inability to achieve or sustain an erection of the penis. It can be caused by cardiovascular disease that impedes blood flow into the penis, neurologic disease (such as a spinal cord injury) that impairs sensory stimuli and nerve transmission, a low level of testosterone, the side effects of certain drugs, or psychological factors. It is also known as **impotence.** Treatment: Drugs to stimulate an erection; penile implant.	**erectile** (ee-REK-tile) 　**erect/o-** *to stand up* 　**-ile** *pertaining to* **dysfunction** (dis-FUNK-shun) *Dysfunction* is a combination of the prefix *dys-* (painful; difficult; abnormal) and the word *function.* **impotence** (IM-poh-tens)
phimosis	Congenital condition in which the opening of the foreskin is too small to allow the foreskin to pull back over the glans penis. This traps **smegma** (a white, cheesy discharge of skin cells and oil) and can cause infection. Treatment: Circumcision.	**phimosis** (fih-MOH-sis) 　**phim/o-** *closed tight* 　**-osis** *condition; abnormal condition; process* **smegma** (SMEG-mah)
premature ejaculation	Ejaculation of semen that often occurs with minimal stimulation and before the penis becomes fully erect to penetrate the vagina. This lessens the enjoyment of sexual intercourse and decreases the chance of conception. It can be caused by a hormone imbalance but is more often caused by stress or a psychological reason. Treatment: Correct the underlying cause.	**premature** (pree-mah-CHUR)
priapism	Continuing erection of the penis with pain and tenderness. It is caused by spinal cord injury or a side effect of drugs used to treat erectile dysfunction. Treatment: Correct the underlying cause.	**priapism** (PRY-ah-pizm) 　**priap/o-** *persistent erection* 　**-ism** *process; disease from a specific cause*
sexually transmitted disease (STD)	Contagious disease that is contracted during sexual intercourse with an infected individual (see Table 12-1). A positive test for a sexually transmitted disease means that the patient and all sexual partners need to be treated. Sexually transmitted diseases can also be passed to a fetus (in the uterus or as it travels through the birth canal), causing serious illness, blindness, and even death. It is also known as **venereal disease** (VD). Treatment: Antibiotic drugs or antiviral drugs.	**venereal** (veh-NEER-ee-al) 　**venere/o-** *sexual intercourse* 　**-al** *pertaining to*

Table 12-1   Sexually Transmitted Diseases (STDs)

Physicians are required to report all cases of sexually transmitted diseases to the state health department, which, in turn, reports all cases to the national Centers for Disease Control and Prevention (CDCP).

acquired immunodeficiency syndrome (AIDS)		immunodeficiency
Note: This disease, its history, symptoms, diagnosis, and treatment, are discussed in detail in "Hematology and Immunology," Chapter 6.		(im-myoo-noh-dee-FISH-en-see) 　**immun/o-** *immune response* 　**defici/o-** *lacking; inadequate* 　**-ency** *condition of being*
Pathogen	Human immunodeficiency virus (HIV), a retrovirus	
Symptoms	Men: Fever, night sweats, weight loss, fatigue Women: Same	
Diagnosis	Blood test (ELISA, Western blot, viral RNA load, p24 antigen, CD4 count) or saliva screening test (OraSure)	
Treatment	Oral antiviral drugs taken in combination	
Other	Treatment can only slow the progress of this disease; there is no cure.	

(continued)

Table 12-1   Sexually Transmitted Diseases   (*continued*)

chlamydia		**chlamydia** (klah-MID-ee-ah)
Pathogen	*Chlamydia trachomatis,* a gram-negative coccus (sphere-shaped) bacterium	
Symptoms	Men: Painful urination with burning and itching. Thin, watery discharge from the urethra. Some men have no symptoms. Women: Frequently have no symptoms or a slight vaginal discharge	
Diagnosis	Smear of discharge from urethra (men) or cervix (women) is stained and examined under the microscope	
Treatment	Oral antibiotic drugs	
Other	Most common sexually transmitted disease. It is also known as **nongonococcal urethritis.**	
genital herpes		**herpes** (HER-peez)
Pathogen	Herpes simplex virus (HSV), type 2	
Symptoms	Men: Vesicular lesions (blisters) on the penis, scrotum, perineum, or anus. When the blisters break, they become skin ulcers. There may be flu-like symptoms or no symptoms at all. Women: Same, on the vulva, perineum, anus, or vagina	
Diagnosis	Culture grown from swab of a lesion, polymerase chain reaction test	
Treatment	Topical and oral antiviral drugs shorten the duration of each outbreak	
genital warts (condylomata acuminata) (see Figure 12-7 ■)		**condylomata acuminata** (CON-dih-LOH-mah-tah ah-KOO-mih-NAH-tah)
Pathogen	Human papillomavirus (HPV) Certain strains cause genital warts; other strains cause dysplasia of the cervix, which can lead to cervical cancer in women	
Symptoms	Men: Itching, flesh-colored, irregular lesions that are raised and cauliflower-like Women: Same, with vaginal discharge	
Diagnosis	Visual examination of the skin of the genital area. In women, a Pap smear of the cervix is examined under the microscope.	
Treatment	Topical chemicals or cryosurgery, cautery, or laser to remove warts	
Other	It is also known as **venereal warts.**	

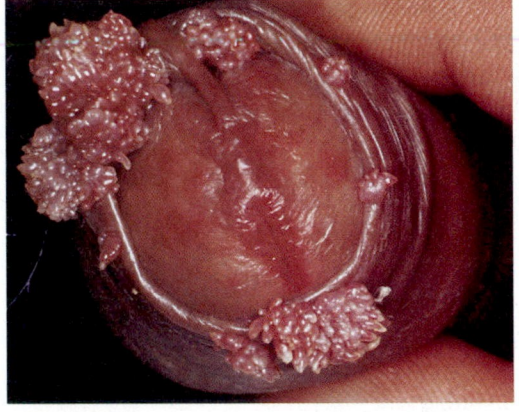 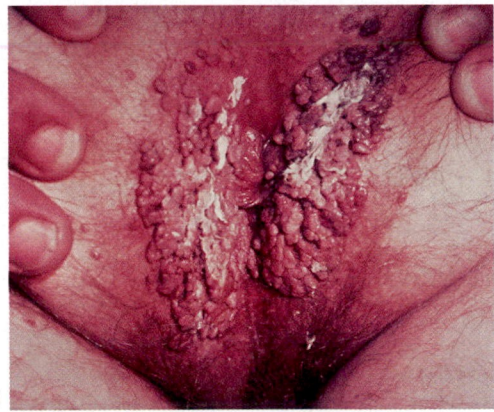

(a)   (b)

Figure 12-7 ■ Genital warts in a male and female.

These raised, irregular, flesh-colored lesions are caused by the human papillomavirus (HPV). Some strains of this virus are associated with cancer of the cervix in women.

Table 12-1   Sexually Transmitted Diseases   (*continued*)

gonorrhea		**gonorrhea** (GAWN-oh-REE-ah)
Pathogen	*Neisseria gonorrhoeae,* a gram-negative diplococcus (double sphere) bacterium. It is also known as **gonococcus (GC).**	**gon/o-** *seed (ovum or spermatozoon)*
Symptoms	Men: Painful urination. Thick yellow discharge from the urethra (gonococcal urethritis). Some men have no symptoms.	**-rrhea** *flow; discharge*
	Women: Painful urination. Thick yellow vaginal discharge. Half of infected women have no symptoms.	
Diagnosis	Gram stain of a smear of the discharge shows characteristic gram-negative intracellular diplococci under the microscope	
	Culture grown from a swab of discharge from the urethra (men) or cervix (women)	
Treatment	Oral antibiotic drug	
Other	Laypersons call this disease *the clap* because of a similar-sounding French word that means *house of prostitution.*	
syphilis		**syphilis** (SIF-ih-lis)
Pathogen	*Treponema pallidum,* a spirochete (spiral) bacterium	**chancre** (SHANG-ker)
Symptoms	Men: Single, painless **chancre** (lesion that ulcerates, forms a crust, and then heals) on the penis. Later, there is fever, rash, and various symptoms that mimic other diseases.	**lues** (LOO-ees)
	Women: Same, with chancre on female genitalia	
Diagnosis	Fluid from a lesion viewed with special illumination under darkfield microscopy shows the spiral bacterium	
	Blood tests for antibodies (RPR, VDRL, FTA-ABS)	
Treatment	Oral antibiotic drug	
Other	It is also known as **lues.**	
trichomoniasis		**trichomoniasis** (TRIK-oh-moh-NY-ah-sis)
Pathogen	*Trichomonas vaginalis,* a protozoan with a flagellum (tail)	
Symptoms	Men: Almost no symptoms	
	Women: Greenish-yellow frothy or bubbly vaginal discharge with a foul odor. Itching of the vulva and vagina.	
Diagnosis	Wet mount preparation of the vaginal discharge examined under the microscope. Culture of the discharge.	
Treatment	Oral antiprotozoal drugs	

Male Breast

Word or Phrase	Description	Word Building
gynecomastia	Enlargement of the male breast. It is caused by an imbalance of testosterone and estradiol because of puberty, aging, surgical removal of the testes, or female hormone drug treatment for prostate cancer. Treatment: Androgen drug. Plastic surgery to decrease breast size.	**gynecomastia** (GY-neh-koh-MAS-tee-ah) **gynec/o-** *female; woman* **mast/o-** *breast; mastoid process* **-ia** *condition; state; thing*

Laboratory and Diagnostic Procedures

Blood Tests

Word or Phrase	Description	Word Building
acid phosphatase	Tests for an enzyme found in the prostate gland. Prostatic acid phosphatase (PAP) only measures acid phosphatase from the prostate gland as opposed to the total acid phosphatase level. Increased levels in the blood indicate cancer of the prostate that has metastasized to the body.	**acid phosphatase** (AS-id FAWS-fah-tays)
hormone testing	Determines the levels of FSH and LH from the anterior pituitary gland and testosterone from the testes. It is used to diagnose infertility problems.	**hormone** (HOR-mohn)
prostate-specific antigen (PSA)	Detects a glycoprotein in cells of the prostate gland. PSA is increased in men with prostate cancer. The higher the level, the more advanced the cancer. The PSA level falls after successful treatment of the cancer.	**antigen** (AN-tih-jen) **anti-** *against* **-gen** *that which produces*
syphilis testing	Blood tests include RPR, VDRL, and FTA-ABS. RPR stands for rapid plasma reagin. VDRL stands for Venereal Disease Research Laboratory. These tests detect an antibody that is produced with syphilis; however, it is also produced with other diseases. FTA-ABS stands for fluorescent treponemal antibody absorption. This test detects the body's specific antibodies against syphilis.	

Semen Tests

Word or Phrase	Description	Word Building
acid phosphatase	There is acid phosphatase in semen. The presence of acid phosphatase in the vagina indicates sexual intercourse has occurred. This test is used in rape investigations.	
DNA analysis	DNA analysis of semen from a crime scene or rape victim can be compared to the samples of known DNA in a criminal database. DNA analysis can also be used to prove paternity (that a particular man is the father of the child being tested).	
semen analysis	Microscopic examination of the spermatozoa (see Figure 12-8 ■). A semen analysis is done as part of a workup for infertility. After not ejaculating for 36 hours, the man gives a semen specimen. A normal **sperm count** is greater than 50 million/mL. The **motility** (forward movement) and **morphology** (normal shape) of the spermatozoa are evaluated. A semen analysis is also done after a vasectomy to verify **aspermia** and a successful sterilization.	**motility** (moh-TIL-ih-tee) **motil/o-** *movement* **-ity** *state; condition* **morphology** (mor-FAWL-oh-jee) **morph/o-** *shape* **-logy** *the study of* **aspermia** (aa-SPER-mee-ah) **a-** *away from; without* **sperm/o-** *spermatozoon; sperm* **-ia** *condition; state; thing*

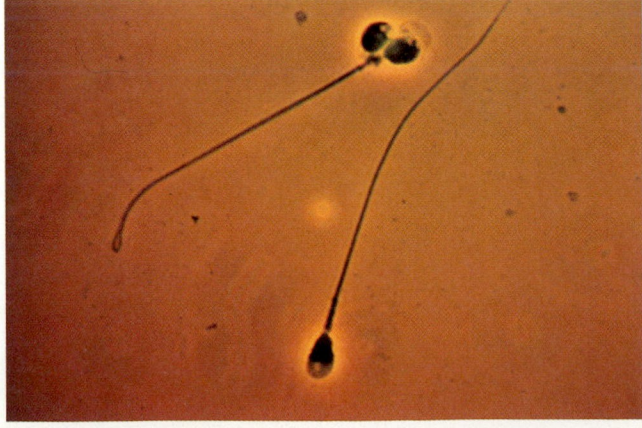

Figure 12-8 ■ Spermatozoa.
The spermatozoon on the right shows normal morphology. Vigorous movement of its flagellum would indicate normal motility. The spermatozoon on the left has an abnormal double head. Abnormal spermatozoa can also have enlarged heads, pin heads, or tails that are kinked, doubled, coiled, or missing. All men produce a few abnormal spermatozoa, but exposure to lead, cigarette smoke, or chemicals can increase this number. Large numbers of abnormal spermatozoa cause male infertility.

Radiologic Tests

Word or Phrase	Description	Word Building
ProstaScint scan	Procedure that uses ProstaScint to detect areas of metastasis from a primary site of prostate cancer. ProstaScint is a combination of a radioactive tracer (indium-111) and a monoclonal antibody that binds to receptors on cancer cells in the prostate gland and elsewhere in the body. The radioactive tracer emits gamma rays that are detected by a gamma scintillation camera and made into an image.	

ultrasonography	Procedure that uses ultra high-frequency sound waves emitted by a transducer or probe to produce an image. Ultrasonography of the testis is used to detect a varicocele or undescended testes. **Transrectal ultrasonography (TRUS)** uses an ultrasound probe inserted into the rectum to obtain an image of the prostate gland or to help guide a needle biopsy of the prostate gland. The **ultrasound** image is a **sonogram.**	**ultrasonography**
		(UL-trah-soh-NAWG-rah-fee)
		  ultra- *beyond; higher*
		  son/o- *sound*
		  -graphy *process of recording*
		
		transrectal (trans-REK-tal)
		  trans- *across; through*
		  rect/o- *rectum*
		  -al *pertaining to*
		
		ultrasound (UL-trah-sound)
		
		sonogram (SAWN-oh-gram)
		  son/o- *sound*
		  -gram *a record or picture*

Medical and Surgical Procedures

Medical Procedures

Word or Phrase	Description	Word Building
digital rectal examination (DRE)	Procedure to palpate the prostate gland. A gloved finger inserted into the rectum is used to feel the prostate gland for signs of tenderness, nodules, hardness, or enlargement. This examination should be done yearly in men over age 40.	**digital** (DIJ-ih-tal) **digit/o-** *digit (finger or toe)* **-al** *pertaining to*
newborn genital examination	The newborn's external genitalia are examined for any sign of abnormal positioning of the urethral meatus (epispadias, hypospadias), ambiguous genitalia, or undescended testicles (see Figure 12-9 ■).	

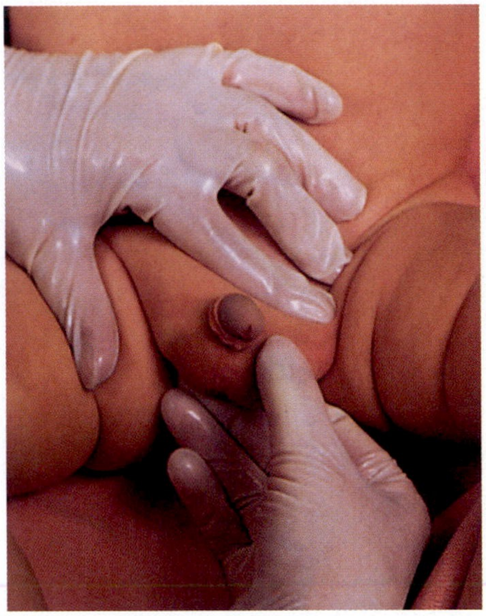

Figure 12-9 ■ Newborn scrotal examination.
The scrotum is palpated during the initial physical assessment of a newborn. Both testes should be descended and present in the scrotum at birth.

Word or Phrase	Description	Word Building
testicular self-examination (TSE)	Palpation of the testes and scrotum to detect lumps, masses, or enlarged lymph nodes. TSE should be done monthly to detect early signs of testicular cancer.	

Surgical Procedures

Word or Phrase	Description	Word Building
biopsy	Procedure to remove tissue from the prostate gland to diagnose prostatic cancer. A large-bore needle is inserted through the rectum or urethra to take a core of prostatic tissue. 　　**Fine-needle aspiration biopsy** of the testis is performed to investigate a low sperm count. A thin needle is inserted and a syringe is used to aspirate tissue. An **incisional biopsy** (open biopsy) is performed when a mass is felt in a testis.	**biopsy** (BY-awp-see) **bi/o-** *life; living organisms; living tissue* **-opsy** *process of viewing* **aspiration** (AS-pih-RAY-shun) **aspir/o-** *to breathe in; to suck in* **-ation** *a process; being or having* **incisional** (in-SIH-shun-al) **incis/o-** *to cut into* **-ion** *action; condition* **-al** *pertaining to*
circumcision	Procedure to remove the prepuce (foreskin). This can be done to correct a tight prepuce and allow better hygiene of the glans penis. The foreskin in newborn babies is often removed because of social customs or religious requirements.	**circumcision** (SER-kum-SIH-shun) **circum-** *around* **cis/o-** *to cut* **-ion** *action; condition*

Word or Phrase	Description	Word Building
orchiectomy	Procedure to remove a testis because of testicular cancer	**orchiectomy** (OR-kee-EK-toh-mee) **orchi/o-** *testis* **-ectomy** *surgical excision*
orchiopexy	Procedure to reposition an undescended testicle and fix it within the scrotum	**orchiopexy** (OR-kee-oh-PEK-see) **orchi/o-** *testis* **-pexy** *process of surgically fixing in place*
penile implant	Procedure to implant an inflatable penile **prosthesis** for patients with erectile dysfunction	**prosthesis** (praws-THEE-sis)
prostatectomy	Procedure to remove the entire prostate gland, along with the lymph nodes, seminal vesicles, and vas deferens because of prostate cancer. A retropubic or a suprapubic surgical approach is used.	**prostatectomy** (PRAWS-tah-TEK-toh-mee) **prostat/o-** *prostate gland* **-ectomy** *surgical excision*
transurethral resection of the prostate (TURP)	Procedure to reduce the size of the prostate gland in patients with benign prostatic hypertrophy. A special cystoscope (a **resectoscope**) is inserted through the urethra. It has built-in cutting instruments and cautery to resect pieces of the prostate gland and cauterize bleeding blood vessels. Chips of prostatic tissue are then irrigated out (see Figure 12-10 ■). TURP has been the most common surgical treatment for a moderately to severely enlarged prostate gland. Other procedures use a	**transurethral** (TRANS-yoo-REE-thral) **trans-** *across; through* **urethr/o-** *urethra* **-al** *pertaining to* **resection** (ree-SEK-shun) **resect/o-** *to cut out and remove* **-ion** *action; condition* **resectoscope** (ree-SEK-toh-skohp) **resect/o-** *to cut out; remove* **-scope** *instrument used to examine*

(continued)

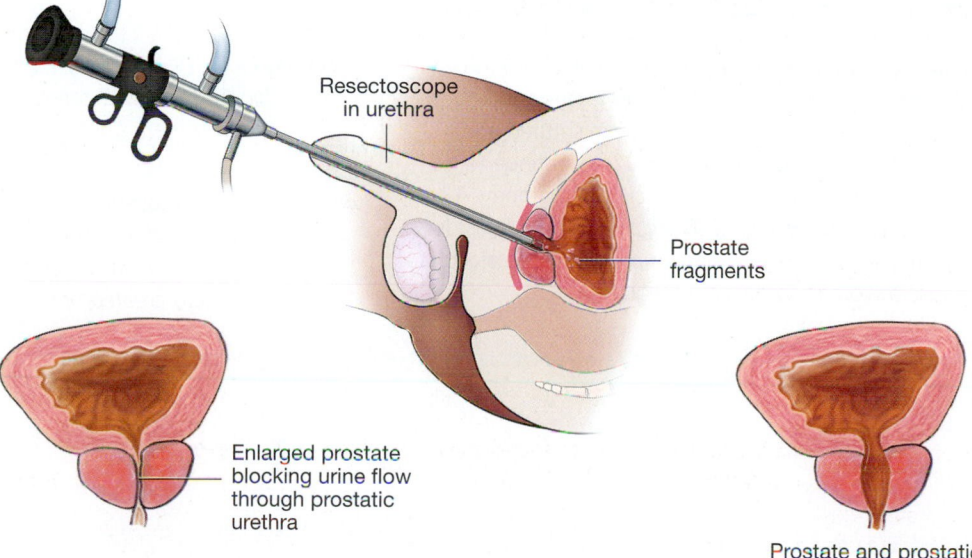

Resectoscope in urethra

Prostate fragments

Enlarged prostate blocking urine flow through prostatic urethra

Prostate and prostatic urethra after TURP

Figure 12-10 ■ Transurethral resection of the prostate (TURP).

This surgical procedure has been the "gold standard" of treatment for benign prostatic hypertrophy for many years.

Word or Phrase	Description	Word Building
transurethral resection of the prostate (*continued*)	laser (see Figure 12-11 ■) to vaporize prostatic tissue. These include **photoselective vaporization of the prostate (PVP)** and **holmium laser ablation of the prostate (HoLAP).** Laser surgery produces the same results as a TURP, but with less bleeding and a shorter recovery time. Minimally invasive procedures for moderate benign prostatic hypertrophy include **transurethral microwave therapy (TUMT),** which uses a microwave antenna on a catheter inserted through the urethra to destroy prostatic tissue with microwaves and heat, and **transurethral needle ablation (TUNA),** which uses a resectoscope to place needles in the prostate gland to destroy prostatic tissue with radio waves and heat.	**ablation** (ah-BLAY-shun) **ablat/o-** *take away; destroy* **-ion** *action; condition*

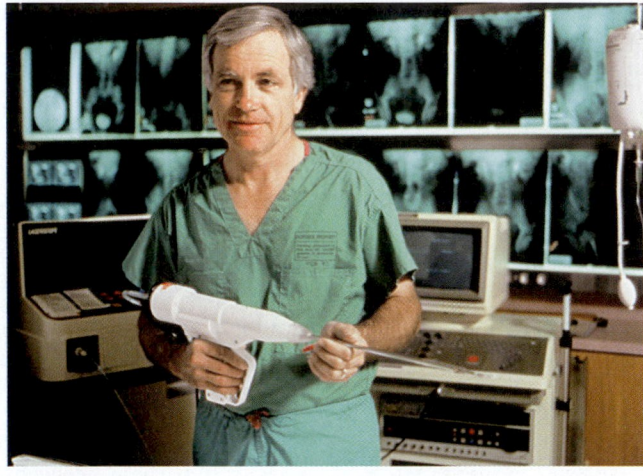

Figure 12-11 ■ Laser for prostate surgery.

This surgeon is showing the handheld laser that is used to perform laser surgery on the prostate gland.

Word or Phrase	Description	Word Building
vasectomy	Procedure in the male to prevent pregnancy in the female. Through a small incision at the base of the scrotum, both vas deferens are divided, a length of each tube is removed, and the cut ends are sutured and crushed or destroyed with electrocautery. Spermatozoa continue to be produced by the testes, but they are absorbed back into the body. A **vasovasostomy** is a reversal of a vasectomy. The cut ends of the vas deferens are rejoined so that spermatozoa are again present in the ejaculate and the male can cause a woman to become pregnant.	**vasectomy** (vah-SEK-toh-mee) **vas/o-** *blood vessel; vas deferens* **-ectomy** *surgical excision* **vasovasostomy** (VAY-soh-vah-SAWS-toh-mee) **vas/o-** *blood vessel; vas deferens* **vas/o-** *blood vessel; vas deferens* **-stomy** *surgically created opening*

Drug Categories

These categories of drugs are used to treat male genitourinary diseases and conditions. The most common generic and trade name drugs in each category are listed.

Category	Indication	Examples	Word Building
androgen drugs	Treat a lack of production of testosterone by the testes because of cryptorchidism, orchiectomy, or decreased levels of LH from the anterior pituitary gland. It is used to treat delayed puberty in boys. *Androgen* refers to testosterone produced by the testes, other testosterone-like hormones, or manufactured testosterone used in drugs.	methyltestosterone (Android, Testred, Virilon), testosterone (Androderm, AndroGel)	**androgen** (AN-droh-jen) **andr/o-** *male* **-gen** *that which produces*
antiviral drugs	Treat viral infections that cause genital herpes and condylomata acuminata. These drugs are applied topically to the affected areas. Oral antiviral drugs are used to treat HIV and AIDS.	Topical: acyclovir (Zovirax), valacyclovir (Valtrex). Oral: zalcitabine (Hivid), zidovudine (Retrovir) for HIV or AIDS	**antiviral** (AN-tee-VY-ral) (AN-tih-VY-ral) **anti-** *against* **vir/o-** *virus* **-al** *pertaining to*
drugs for benign prostatic hypertrophy	Androgen inhibitor drugs inhibit the male hormone dihydrotestosterone, which causes the prostate gland to enlarge. Other drugs relax the smooth muscle in the prostate gland and urethra and allow urine to flow more freely.	Androgen inhibitor drugs: dutasteride (Avodart), finasteride (Proscar). Other drugs: tamsulosin (Flomax), terazosin (Hytrin)	

Did You Know?

Proscar for benign prostatic hypertrophy is also marketed under the trade name Propecia. Propecia comes in a lower dose and is prescribed specifically to treat male-pattern baldness.

Category	Indication	Examples	Word Building
drugs for erectile dysfunction	Promote the release of nitric oxide gas in the tissues and inhibit an enzyme, both of which increases blood flow into the penis to create an erection	sildenafil (Viagra), tadalafil (Cialis), vardenafil (Levitra)	

Abbreviations

AIDS	acquired immunodeficiency syndrome		**LH**	luteinizing hormone
BPH	benign prostatic hypertrophy		**PAP**	prostatic acid phosphatase
CDCP	Centers for Disease Control and Prevention The abbreviation for its older name—Centers for Disease Control (CDC)—is still used.		**PSA**	prostate-specific antigen
			PVP	photoselective vaporization of the prostate
			RPR	rapid plasma reagin (test for syphilis)
DRE	digital rectal examination		**STD**	sexually transmitted disease
ED	erectile dysfunction		**TRUS**	transrectal ultrasound
FSH	follicle-stimulating hormone		**TSE**	testicular self-examination
GC	gonococcus (*Neisseria gonorrhoeae*)		**TUMT**	transurethral microwave therapy
GU	genitourinary		**TUNA**	transurethral needle ablation
HIV	human immunodeficiency virus		**TURP**	transurethral resection of the prostate
HoLAP	holmium laser ablation of the prostate		**VD**	venereal disease
HPV	human papillomavirus		**VDRL**	Venereal Disease Research Laboratory (test for syphilis)
HSV	herpes simplex virus			

Word Alert

ABBREVIATIONS

Abbreviations are commonly used in all types of medical documents; however, they can mean different things to different people and their meanings can be misinterpreted. Always verify the meaning of an abbreviation.

ED means *erectile dysfunction,* but it also means *emergency department.*

PAP means *prostatic acid phosphatase,* but *Pap* is a short form for *Papanicolaou smear.*

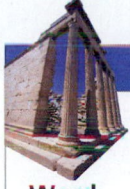

It's Greek to Me!

Did you notice that some words have two different combining forms? Combining forms from both Greek and Latin languages remain a part of medical language today.

Word	Greek	Latin	Medical Word Examples
penis	balan/o-	pen/o-	balanitis, penile
sexual intercourse	pareun/o-	venere/o-	dyspareunia, venereal disease
		coit/o-	postcoital
testis	didym/o-	test/o-	epididymis, testosterone
	orchi/o-	testicul/o-	orchiectomy, testicular
	orch/o-		orchitis

CAREER FOCUS

Meet Mindy, a clinical laboratory scientist and blood bank supervisor

"Clinical laboratory scientist is the newer name, but we know ourselves as medical technologists. In college, I took a microbiology class. I enjoyed it so much that I pursued that as my major. A technologist performs the testing, whether it's hematology, chemistry, blood bank, or microbiology. I have to communicate with the doctors and nurses. I have to have an understanding of medical terminology to be able to communicate clearly with them. When we can interact with the nurses and the doctors to give them the answers they need to care for the patients, that's what's rewarding."

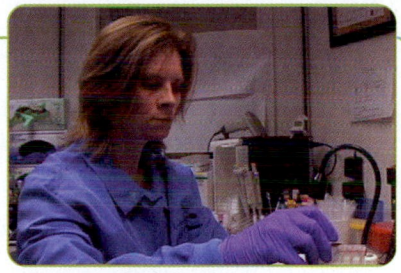

Clinical laboratory scientists are allied health professionals who work in a hospital or a large commercial medical laboratory. They perform all types of laboratory tests on blood, urine, and other body fluids and tissues. They work with microscopes and computerized equipment.

Reproductive medicine physicians treat male (and female) patients who have difficulty conceiving a child because of infertility.

Endocrinologists treat patients with disorders of the endocrine system, including hormonal disorders that affect men, such as infertility. Cancerous tumors of the male genitourinary system are treated medically by an oncologist and surgically by a general surgeon.

clinical (KLIN-ih-kal)
clinic/o- *medicine*
-al *pertaining to*

laboratory (LAB-oh-rah-ᴛᴏʜ-ree)
laborat/o- *workplace; testing place*
-ory *having the function of*

scientist (SY-en-tist)
scient/o- *science; knowledge*
-ist *one who specializes in*

reproductive (REE-proh-DUK-tiv)
re- *again and again; backward; unable to*
product/o- *produce*
-ive *pertaining to*

PEARSON **myhealthprofessionskit**™ To see Mindy's complete video profile, visit Medical Terminology Interactive at www.myhealthprofessionskit.com. Select this book, log in, and go to the 12th floor of Pearson General Hospital. Enter the Laboratory, and click on the computer screen.

CHAPTER REVIEW EXERCISES

Test your knowledge of the chapter by completing these review exercises. Use the Answer Key at the end of the book to check your answers.

Anatomy and Physiology

Fill in the Blank Exercise

Fill in the blank with the correct word from the word list.

ductus deferens	genitals	prepuce	spermatocytes
ejaculatory duct	interstitial	prostate gland	spermatogenesis
epididymis	lumen	sperm	testes
flagellum	perineum	spermatic cord	testosterone

1. Process of making mature sperm _____

2. Internal and external reproductive organs _____

3. Contain the seminiferous tubules that make spermatozoa _____

4. Area between the anus and scrotum _____

5. Opening in the center of a tube or duct _____

6. Synonym for spermatozoa _____

7. Tubule on top of the testis _____

8. Cells that secrete testosterone _____

9. Contains arteries, veins, nerves, and vas deferens _____

10. Immature cells in the seminiferous tubules _____

11. Tail of a sperm _____

12. Hormone that causes the development of male sexual characteristics during puberty _____

13. Also known as the vas deferens _____

14. Vas deferens and seminal vesicles empty into this structure _____

15. Spherical gland at the base of the bladder _____

16. Structure that is still present in an uncircumcised male _____

True or False Exercise

Indicate whether each statement is true or false by writing T or F on the line.

1. _____ The bulbourethral glands are also known as the vas deferens.

2. _____ The external male genitalia are located within the pelvic cavity.

3. _____ Testicles is a synonym for testes.

4. _____ The prostate gland secretes most of the fluid that makes up the volume of an ejaculation.

5. _____ The glans penis is a structure that fills with blood and becomes erect.

6. _____ The flagellum makes a sperm move.

7. _____ The inguinal canal is a passageway from the pelvic cavity to the scrotum.

8. _____ The penis contains erectile tissue.

9. _____ Gametes are cells that are unique because they have a flagellum.

Circle Exercise

Circle the correct word from the choices given.

1. The (**bladder, penis, scrotum**) is a soft sac of skin that holds the testes.
2. The internal male genitalia include all of the following *except* the (**epididymis, prostate gland, vas deferens**).
3. Spermatozoa are produced in the (**scrotum, seminal vesicles, seminiferous tubules**).
4. The spermatic cord contains all of the following *except* (**arteries, ejaculatory duct, vas deferens**).
5. The process by which a cell divides to end up with 23 chromosomes is known as (**meiosis, mitosis, puberty**).

Sequencing Exercise

Beginning with the spermatozoon in the lumen of the seminiferous tubules, use the list of anatomical structures given here to help you arrange the structures in the correct order through which a spermatozoon moves until it leaves the body.

ejaculatory duct	prostatic urethra	urethra in the penis	vas deferens
epididymis	seminiferous tubules	urethral meatus	

1. <u>seminiferous tubules</u> →   2. _____ →   3. _____ →

4. _____ →   5. _____ →   6. _____ →

7. _____

Diseases and Conditions

Matching Exercise

Match each word or phrase to its description.

1. chancre	_____ Caused by *Treponema pallidum*
2. chordee	_____ Failure to conceive
3. condylomata acuminata	_____ Enlargement of the male breasts
4. dyspareunia	_____ Fewer than the normal number of sperm
5. erectile dysfunction	_____ Can be caused by a mumps infection
6. gonorrhea	_____ Painful sexual intercourse
7. gynecomastia	_____ Skin lesion of syphilis
8. herpes simplex virus	_____ Downward curve of the penis during erection
9. infertility	_____ Inability to sustain an erection
10. oligospermia	_____ Genital warts
11. orchitis	_____ Vesicular lesions like blisters on the skin
12. syphilis	_____ Intracellular diplococci under the microscope

Circle Exercise

Circle the correct word from the choices given.

1. Gynecomastia is a disease that affects the (**breasts, penis, scrotum**).
2. Inflammation of the glans penis is known as (**balanitis, gynecomastia, phimosis**).
3. A low number of sperm on a semen analysis is known as (**cryptorchism, oligospermia, varicocele**).
4. Postcoital pain is also known as (**dyspareunia, impotence, venereal disease**).
5. A chancre is seen with the sexually transmitted disease (**genital warts, gonorrhea, syphilis**).

(continued)

6. HIV is a (**bacterium, retrovirus, virus**).

7. All of these diseases can be caused by a sexually transmitted disease *except* (**epididymitis, phimosis, prostatitis**).

8. Postcoital pain occurs after (**ejaculation, sexual intercourse, spermatogenesis**).

9. (**Aspermia, Chordee, Phimosis**) is a congenital condition in which the opening of the foreskin is too small to pull it over the glans penis.

10. AIDS is caused by the (**herpes simplex virus, human immunodeficiency virus, human papillomavirus**).

Laboratory, Radiology, Surgery, and Drugs

Circle Exercise

Circle the correct word from the choices given.

1. The (**acid phosphatase, prostate-specific antigen, sperm count**) is *not* increased in patients with cancer of the prostate.

2. What procedure can be performed by the patient on himself? (**biopsy, circumcision, testicular self-examination**)

3. An (**incisional biopsy, orchiectomy, orchiopexy**) is performed to reposition an undescended testicle.

4. Antibiotic drugs are effective against (**genital warts, gonorrhea, HIV**).

5. A penile implant is used to treat patients with (**aspermia, erectile dysfunction, prostate cancer**).

6. Patients with cancer of the prostate gland are given (**androgen, antibiotic, female hormone**) drugs.

Fill in the Blank Exercise

Fill in the blank with the correct word from the word list.

acid phosphatase	digital rectal exam	resectoscope	varicocelectomy
circumcision	morphology	ultrasonography	vasovasostomy

1. Surgical excision of a varicose vein of the spermatic cord _____

2. Sperm shape that is checked on sperm analysis _____

3. Enzyme found mainly in the prostate gland _____

4. Uses sound waves to create an image _____

5. Should be done yearly for men over age 40 _____

6. Instrument used to perform a TURP _____

7. Procedure to reverse a vasectomy _____

8. Removal of the foreskin of the penis _____

Building Medical Words

Review the Combining Forms Exercise and Combining Form and Suffix Exercise that you already completed in the anatomy section on pages 609–610.

Related Combining Forms Exercise

Write the combining forms on the line provided. (Hint: See the It's Greek to Me feature box.)

1. Two combining forms that mean *penis.* _____

2. Three combining forms that mean *sexual intercourse.* _____

3. Five combining forms that mean *testis.* _____

Combining Forms Exercise

Before you build male genitourinary words, review these additional combining forms. Next to each combining form, write its medical meaning. The first one has been done for you.

Combining Form	Medical Meaning	Combining Form	Medical Meaning
1. aspir/o-	to breathe in; to suck in	14. malign/o-	
2. ablat/o-		15. mast/o-	
3. andr/o-		16. morph/o-	
4. bi/o-		17. motil/o-	
5. cancer/o-		18. olig/o-	
6. cis/o-		19. phim/o-	
7. crypt/o-		20. priap/o-	
8. defici/o-		21. resect/o-	
9. fertil/o-		22. scient/o-	
10. gynec/o-		23. son/o-	
11. immun/o-		24. troph/o-	
12. incis/o-		25. urethr/o-	
13. laborat/o-		26. varic/o-	

Prefix Exercise

Read the definition of the medical word. Look at the medical word or partial word that is given (it already contains a combining form and a suffix). Select the correct prefix from the Prefix List and write it on the blank line. Then build the medical word and write it on the line. Be sure to check your spelling. The first one has been done for you.

PREFIX LIST

a- (away from; without)	in- (in; without; not)	trans- (across; through)
circum- (around)	post- (after; behind)	ultra- (beyond; higher)
dys- (painful; difficult; abnormal)	re- (again and again;	
epi- (upon; above)	backward; unable to)	

Definition of the Medical Word	Prefix	Word or Partial Word	Build the Medical Word
1. Pertaining to through the urethra	trans-	urethral	transurethral
2. Condition of painful or difficult sexual intercourse		pareunia	
3. Process of recording higher (frequency) sound (waves)		sonography	
4. Condition (of being) without spermatozoa		spermia	
5. Action of (going) around (the foreskin) to cut (it off)		cision	
6. Pertaining to again and again producing (children)		productive	
7. Pertaining to after sexual intercourse		coital	
8. Inflammation of (a coiled tube structure that is) upon the testis		didymitis	
9. Condition of not (being) able to conceive a child		fertility	

Combining Form and Suffix Exercise

Read the definition of the medical word. Select the correct suffix from the Suffix List. Select the correct combining form from the Combining Form List. Build the medical word and write it on the line. Be sure to check your spelling. The first one has been done for you.

SUFFIX LIST	COMBINING FORM LIST	
-al (pertaining to)	andr/o- (male)	orch/o- (testis)
-ancy (state of)	balan/o- (glans penis)	phim/o- (closed tight)
-cele (hernia)	bi/o- (life; living tissue)	priap/o- (persistent erection)
-ectomy (surgical excision)	cancer/o- (cancer)	prostat/o- (prostate gland)
-gen (that which produces)	malign/o- (intentionally causing	resect/o- (to cut out; remove)
-ism (process; disease from a specific cause)	harm; cancer)	semin/o- (spermatozoon; sperm)
-itis (inflammation of; infection of)	morph/o- (shape)	varic/o- (varix; varicose vein)
-ity (state; condition)	motil/o- (movement)	vas/o- (blood vessel; vas deferens)
-logy (the study of)	orchi/o- (testis)	venere/o- (sexual intercourse)
-oma (tumor; mass)		
-opsy (process of viewing)		
-osis (condition; abnormal condition; process)		
-ous (pertaining to)		
-pexy (process of surgically fixing in place)		
-scope (instrument used to examine)		

Definition of the Medical Word

1. State of movement (of spermatozoa)

2. Surgical excision of the vas deferens

3. Pertaining to cancer

4. Hernia of a varicose vein (in the spermatic cord)

5. Tumor (of the structure that produces) sperm

6. Inflammation or infection of the testis

7. The study of the shape (of spermatozoa)

8. Surgical excision of the prostate gland

9. Process of surgically fixing in place a testis

10. State of intentionally causing harm (cancer)

11. Inflammation or infection of the glans penis

12. That (a drug) which produces male (characteristics)

13. Process (of removing) and viewing living tissue

14. Instrument used to examine (and then) to cut out and remove (tissue)

15. Pertaining to (any disease transmitted by) sexual intercourse

16. Surgical excision of a testis

17. Inflammation or infection of the prostate gland

18. Disease from a specific cause of a persistent erection

19. Abnormal condition (in which the foreskin opening is) closed tight

Build the Medical Word

1. *motility*
2.
3.
4.
5.
6.
7.
8.
9.
10.
11.
12.
13.
14.
15.
16.
17.
18.
19.

Multiple Combining Forms and Suffix Exercise

Read the definition of the medical word. Select the correct suffix and combining forms. Then build the medical word and write it on the line. Be sure to check your spelling. The first one has been done for you.

SUFFIX LIST	COMBINING FORM LIST	
-ary (pertaining to)	crypt/o- (hidden)	olig/o- (scanty; few)
-ency (condition of being)	defici/o- (lacking; inadequate)	orch/o- (testis)
-esis (a process)	genit/o- (genitalia)	spermat/o- (spermatozoon; sperm)
-ia (condition; state; thing)	gen/o- (arising from; produced by)	sperm/o- (spermatozoon; sperm)
-ism (process; disease from a specific cause)	gynec/o- (female; woman)	urin/o- (urine; urinary system)
-stomy (surgically created opening)	immun/o- (immune response)	vas/o- (blood vessel; vas deferens)
	mast/o- (breast; mastoid process)	

Definition of the Medical Word

Build the Medical Word

1. Condition of being (or having) an immune response (that is) inadequate

   immunodeficiency

2. Pertaining to the genitalia and urinary system

3. Surgically created opening (between one end of the) vas deferens (and the other end of the) vas deferens

4. Condition (of enlargement in which the male's chest resembles the) female breast

5. A process of spermatozoa arising from or produced by (the testis)

6. Disease from a specific cause of hidden testis

7. Condition of few sperm

Abbreviations

Definition Exercise

Write the definition of the following abbreviations.

1. BPH _____

2. ED _____

3. GC _____

4. HSV _____

5. PSA _____

6. STD _____

7. TURP _____

8. VD _____

Applied Skills

Plural Noun and Adjective Spelling Exercise

Fill in the blanks with the correct word form. Be sure to check your spelling. The first one has been done for you.

Singular Noun	Plural Noun	Adjective
1. tubule	<u>tubules</u>	<u>tubular</u>
2. testicle	_____	_____
3. perineum		_____
4. spermatozoon	_____	
5. epididymis	_____	
6. prostate		_____
7. penis		_____

Proofreading and Spelling Exercise

Read the following paragraph. Identify each misspelled medical word and write the correct spelling of it on the line.

The male anatomy is located in the pelvic area. It shares the urethra with the urinary system, and this exits from the glands penis or tip of the penis. The peroneal area is the skin between the anus and skrotum. The testes produce spermatozon if they have descended through the inguinel canal. The epidydimis holds sperm or gameetes. Then sperm travel through the vas deference and ejaculatory duct. The seminole vesicles add fluid, as does the prostrate gland, to make semen.

1. _____		6. _____	
2. _____		7. _____	
3. _____		8. _____	
4. _____		9. _____	
5. _____		10. _____	

English and Medical Word Equivalents Exercise

For each English word or phrase, write its equivalent medical word. Be sure to check your spelling. The first one has been done for you.

English Word	Medical Word	English Word	Medical Word
1. testicular cancer	<u>seminoma</u>	5. undescended testicle	_____
2. pain during intercourse	_____	6. genital warts	_____
3. impotence	_____	7. enlarged prostate	_____
4. sexually transmitted disease	_____		

Dividing Medical Words

Separate these words into their component parts (prefix, combining form, suffix). Note: Some words do not contain all three word parts. The first one has been done for you.

Medical Word	Prefix	Combining Form	Suffix	Medical Word	Prefix	Combining Form	Suffix
1. dyspareunia	<u>dys-</u>	<u>pareun/o-</u>	<u>-ia</u>	5. aspermia	_____	_____	_____
2. venereal	_____	_____	_____	6. priapism	_____	_____	_____
3. circumcision	_____	_____	_____	7. reproductive	_____	_____	_____
4. testicular	_____	_____	_____	8. postcoital	_____	_____	_____

Medical Report Exercise

This exercise contains an operative report. Read the report and answer the questions.

OPERATIVE REPORT

PATIENT: JENKINS, Daniel

MEDICAL RECORD NUMBER: 206-47-5869

DATE OF SURGERY: November 19, 20xx

PREOPERATIVE DIAGNOSES
1. Undescended left testis
2. Left indirect inguinal hernia

POSTOPERATIVE DIAGNOSES
1. Undescended left testis, corrected
2. Left indirect inguinal hernia, repaired

PROCEDURES
1. Left orchiopexy
2. Left inguinal herniorrhaphy

DESCRIPTION OF OPERATIVE PROCEDURE
The patient was placed in the dorsal supine position, and general anesthesia was induced via mask anesthesia. The pubic region and external genitalia were prepped and draped with Betadine antibacterial scrub. A transverse incision was made in the suprapubic skin fold on the left side. It was carried down through subcutaneous tissue and fat. Bleeding was controlled with the electrocautery. The left testis was identified in the operative field and was noted to be lying just within the external inguinal ring. The external oblique fascia was incised with a #15 scalpel and Metzenbaum scissors. The left testis was grasped and freed from its surrounding structures up to the level of the internal inguinal ring. This maneuver freed up the cord so that adequate cord length was obtained. The hernia sac was then opened and dissected up to the level of the inguinal ring, where it was closed with 4-0 Vicryl suture. Then we again turned our attention to the undescended left testis. A scrotal incision was made and a subcutaneous pouch created. The left testis was then brought down into the pouch, and a 3-0 silk suture was placed in the lower pole of the testis, brought out through the scrotal skin, and tied over a cotton pledget to secure the testis in place. A careful search detected no bleeding in the scrotal or groin incisions. The scrotal incision was closed with 5-0 Vicryl. The external oblique fascia was closed with a running 4-0 Vicryl suture. The subcutaneous tissue was closed with 4-0 Vicryl. The skin was closed with a running subcuticular 3-0 Prolene suture, and the child was discharged from the operating room in satisfactory condition.

James R. Bentley, M.D.
_____
James R. Bentley, M.D.

JRB:btg
D: 11/19/xx
T: 11/19/xx

Word Analysis Questions

1. Divide *orchiopexy* into its two word parts and define each word part.

Word Part	Definition
_____	_____
_____	_____

2. An incision in the suprapubic skin fold would be located _____.
   a. below the pubic bone
   b. around the pubic bone
   c. above the pubic bone

Fact Finding Questions

1. In the dorsal supine position, the patient is placed on his (**abdomen, back, side**).

2. In a male, the external genitalia include what five structures?

   _____   _____

   _____   _____

   _____

3. Incisions were made in what two areas? _____   _____

4. The hernia sac was closed with sutures. **True**   **False**

5. *Subcutaneous* means (**around the testis, inside the scrotum, under the skin**).

6. The left testis was not descended. What operative procedure was performed to correct this? _____

Critical Thinking Questions

1. A preoperative diagnosis represents the patient's condition (**before, during, after**) surgery.

2. "The maneuver freed up the cord…" What *cord* does this refer to? **spinal cord**   **spermatic cord**   **umbilical cord**

Hearing Medical Words Exercise

You hear someone speaking the medical words given below. Read each pronunciation and then write the medical word it represents. Be sure to check your spelling. The first one has been done for you.

1. PAIR-ih-NEE-um   *perineum*
2. BAL-ah-NY-tis   _____
3. SHANG-ker   _____
4. DIS-pah-ROO-nee-ah   _____
5. EP-ih-DID-ih-mis   _____
6. GAWN-oh-REE-ah   _____
7. or-KY-tis   _____
8. PRAWS-tah-TEK-toh-mee   _____
9. SEM-ih-NOH-mah   _____
10. SIF-ih-lis   _____

Pronunciation Exercise

Read the medical word that is given. Then review the syllables in the pronunciation. Circle the primary (main) accented syllable. The first one has been done for you.

1. puberty (⟨pyoo⟩-ber-tee)
2. aspermia (aa-sper-mee-ah)
3. ejaculation (ee-jak-yoo-lay-shun)
4. erectile (ee-rek-tile)
5. genitalia (jen-ih-tay-lee-ah)
6. gynecomastia (gy-neh-koh-mas-tee-ah)
7. infertility (in-fer-til-ih-tee)
8. orchiectomy (or-kee-ek-toh-mee)
9. testicular (tes-tik-yoo-lar)
10. venereal (veh-neer-ee-al)

Multimedia Preview

Immerse yourself in a variety of activities inside Medical Terminology Interactive. Getting there is simple:

1. Click on www.myhealthprofessionskit.com.
2. Select "Medical Terminology" from the choice of disciplines.
3. First-time users must create an account using the scratch-off code on the inside front cover of this book.
4. Find this book and log in using your username and password.
5. Click on Medical Terminology Interactive.
6. Take the elevator to the 12th Floor to begin your virtual exploration of this chapter!

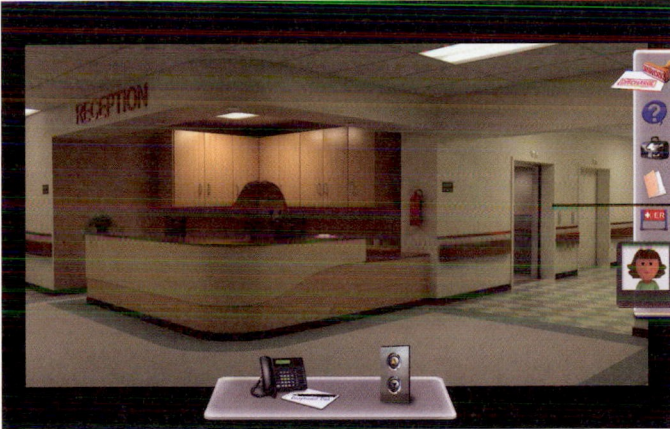 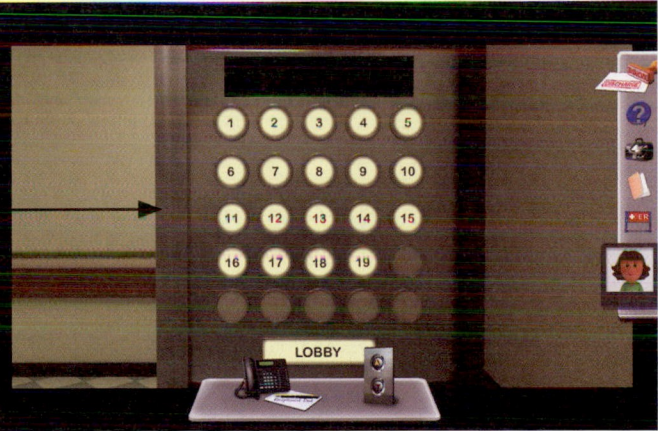

■ **Word Surgery**   Are you ready for the operating room? Use your scalpel to slice each word into its component parts. Then define those parts once they're on your tray. Can you make the cut?

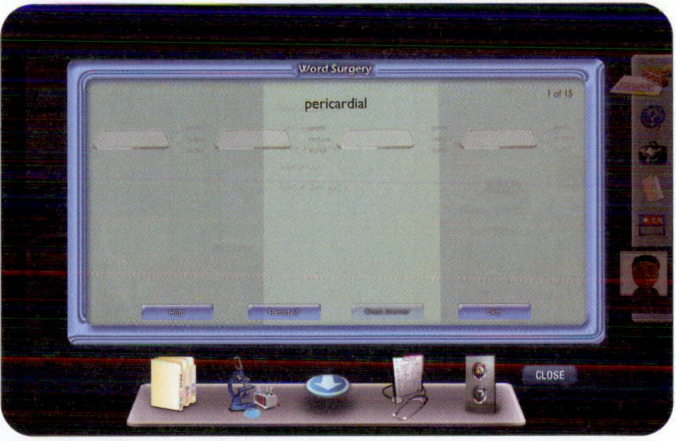

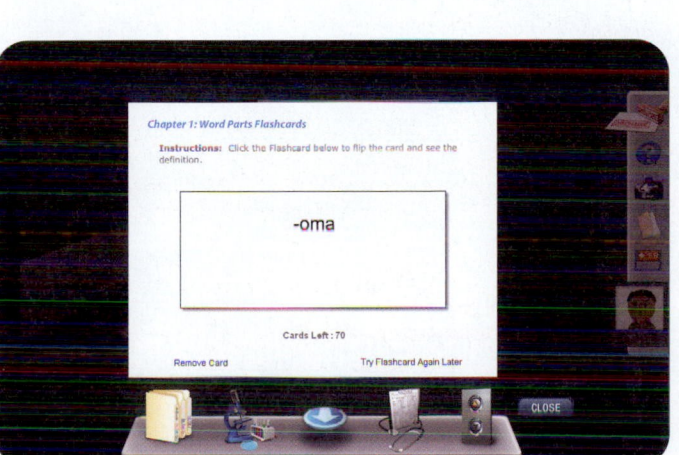

■ **Disease and Other Word Parts Flashcards**
Like the regular word parts flashcards, use customizable flashcards to help you memorize disease names and additional word parts. Print out prepared flashcards or make your own.

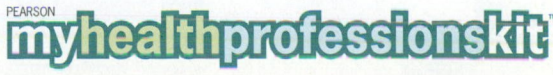

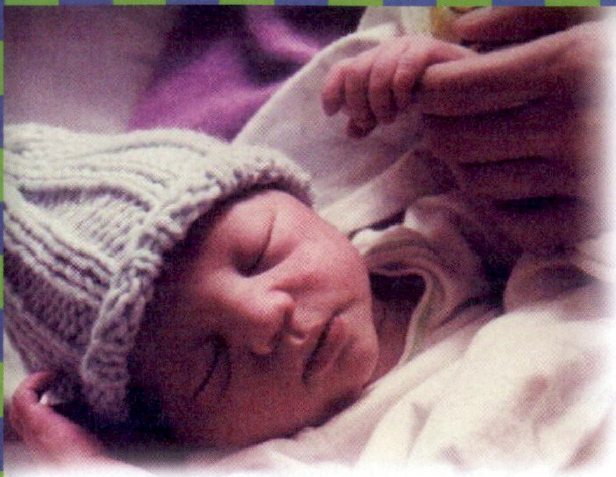

Dive In!

- A baby girl is born with a lifetime supply of eggs in her ovaries.
- At 66 years of age, Adriana Iliescu of Romania was the oldest woman to give birth.
- Are you ready for a chapter that really delivers? Here we'll explore the language that describes the female reproductive system structures, functions, diseases, and conditions.
- You'll have a fertile mind once you master the language of gynecology and obstetrics!

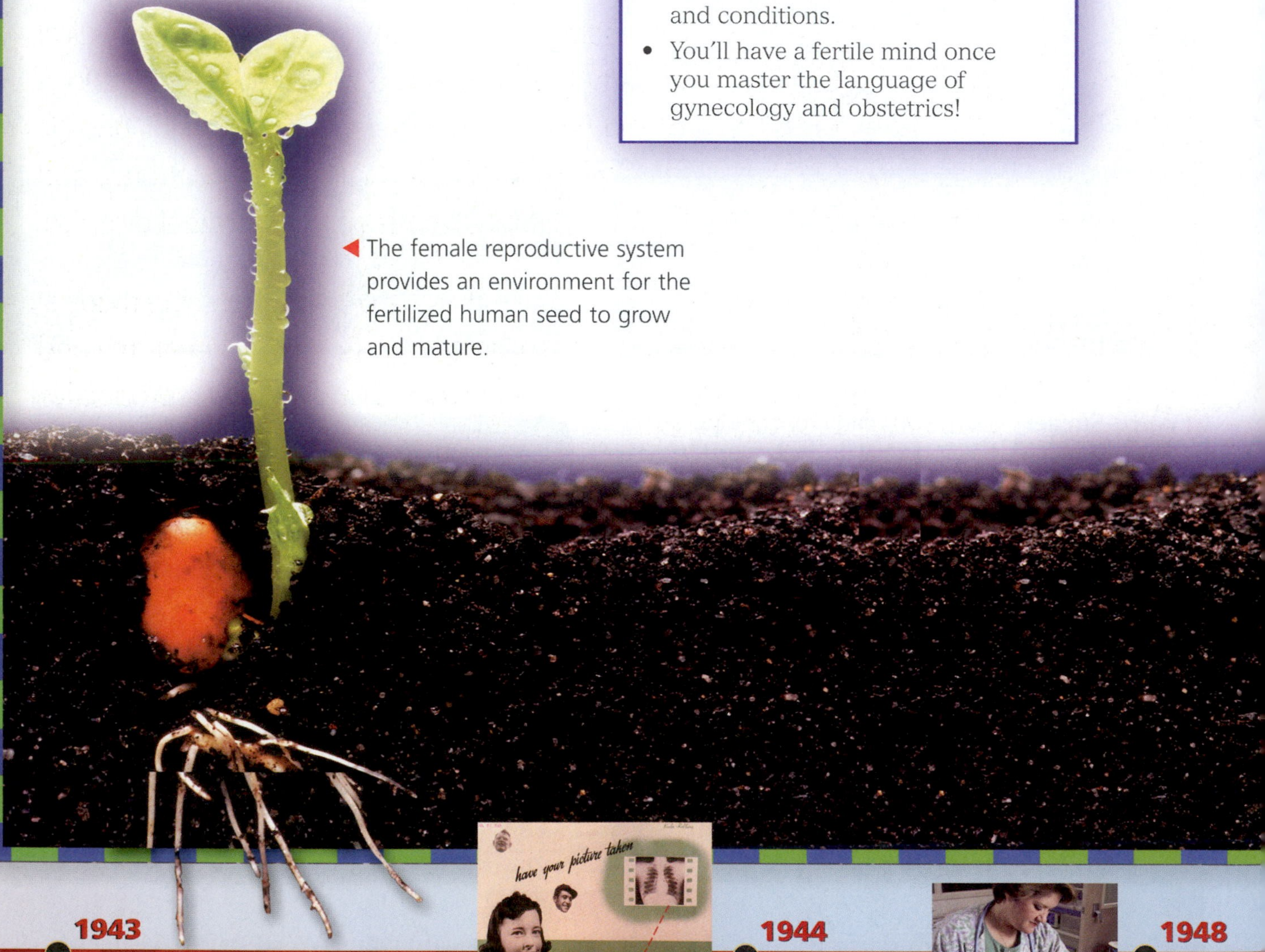

The female reproductive system provides an environment for the fertilized human seed to grow and mature.

Medicine Through HISTORY

1943

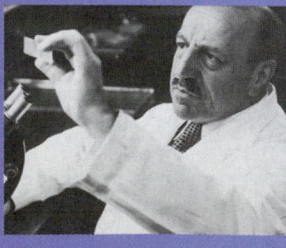

The Pap test for cervical cancer is invented by Dr. George Papanicolaou

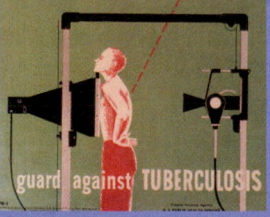

have your picture taken
guard against TUBERCULOSIS

1944

The first drug is developed to treat tuberculosis

Picture Desk, Inc./Kobal Collection

1948

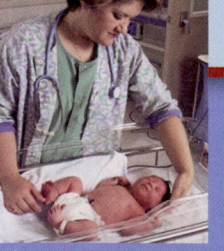

The Apgar score newborn assessment tool is invented by Dr. Virginia Apgar

13
Gynecology and Obstetrics

Female Genital and Reproductive System

Gynecology (GY-neh-KAWL-oh-jee) is the medical specialty that studies the anatomy and physiology of the female genital system and uses diagnostic tests, medical and surgical procedures, and drugs to treat female genital diseases.

Obstetrics (awb-STET-riks) is the medical specialty that studies the anatomy and physiology of the female reproductive system and uses diagnostic tests, medical and surgical procedures, and drugs to monitor normal pregnancy and childbirth and treat diseases.

◀ Like a bird egg, the uterus houses the gestation process.

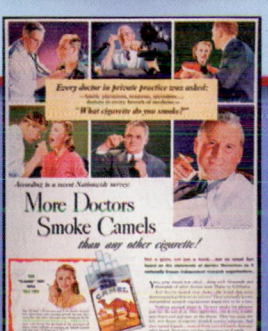

1950

The first scientific research studies are published that link smoking to cancer

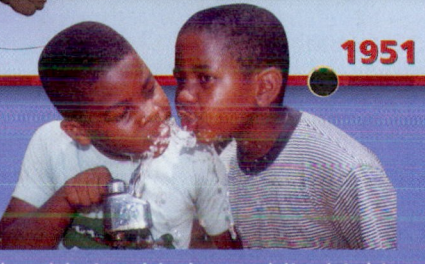

Fluoride is added to public drinking water to prevent dental cavities
©Phil Coale/Silver Image

1951

1951

Prescription drugs are defined by law as those drugs that must be ordered by a physician and dispensed by a pharmacist

Measure Your Progress: Learning Objectives

After you study this chapter, you should be able to

1. Identify the structures of the female genital and reproductive system.
2. Describe the processes of oogenesis, menstruation, conception, and labor and delivery.
3. Describe normal and abnormal findings in the neonate.
4. Describe common female genital and reproductive diseases and conditions, laboratory and diagnostic procedures, medical and surgical procedures, and drug categories.
5. Give the medical meaning of word parts related to the female genital and reproductive system.
6. Build female genital and reproductive words from word parts and divide and define words.
7. Spell and pronounce female genital and reproductive words.
8. Analyze the medical content and meaning of a gynecology report.
9. Dive deeper into gynecology and obstetrics by reviewing the activities at the end of this chapter and online at Medical Terminology Interactive.

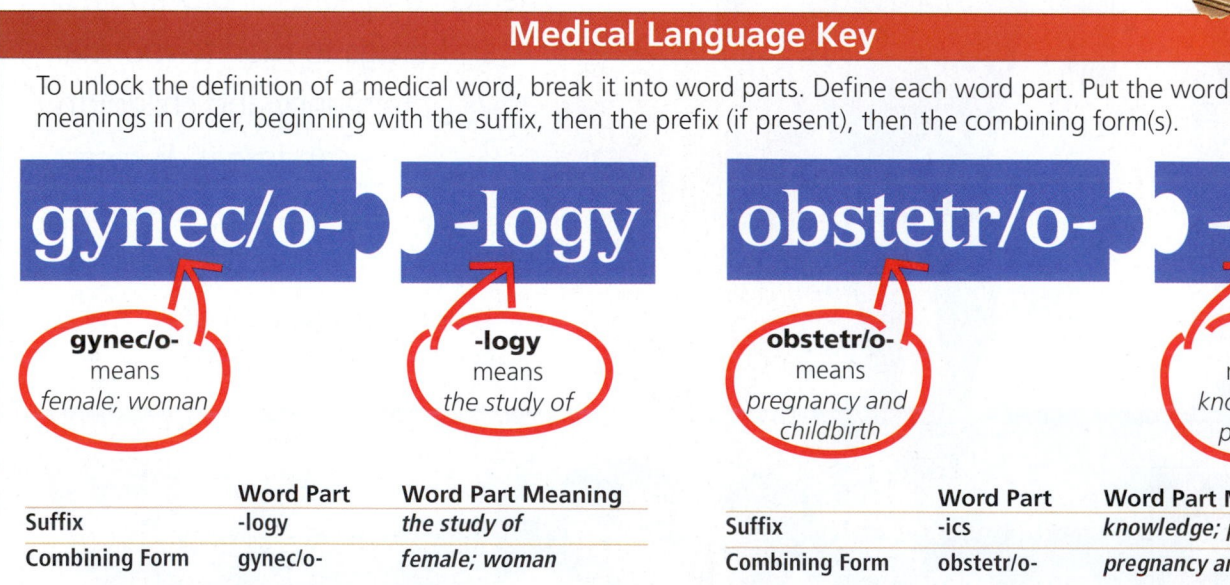

Medical Language Key

To unlock the definition of a medical word, break it into word parts. Define each word part. Put the word part meanings in order, beginning with the suffix, then the prefix (if present), then the combining form(s).

gynec/o- ⬤ -logy

gynec/o- means *female; woman*

-logy means *the study of*

	Word Part	Word Part Meaning
Suffix	-logy	*the study of*
Combining Form	gynec/o-	*female; woman*

Gynecology: The study of females.

obstetr/o- ⬤ -ics

obstetr/o- means *pregnancy and childbirth*

-ics means *knowledge; practice*

	Word Part	Word Part Meaning
Suffix	-ics	*knowledge; practice*
Combining Form	obstetr/o-	*pregnancy and childbirth*

Obstetrics: The knowledge and practice (of treating women during) pregnancy and childbirth.

Anatomy and Physiology

The **female genital and reproductive system** includes both internal and external genitalia or **genital organs** (see Figure 13-1 ■). The **internal genitalia** in the pelvic cavity include the ovaries, uterine tubes, uterus, and vagina. The **external genitalia** include the area of the vulva (the mons pubis, labia majora, labia minora, clitoris, and vaginal introitus). The breasts or mammary glands also play a role in the female reproductive system. The female genital and reproductive system together with the urinary system is known as the

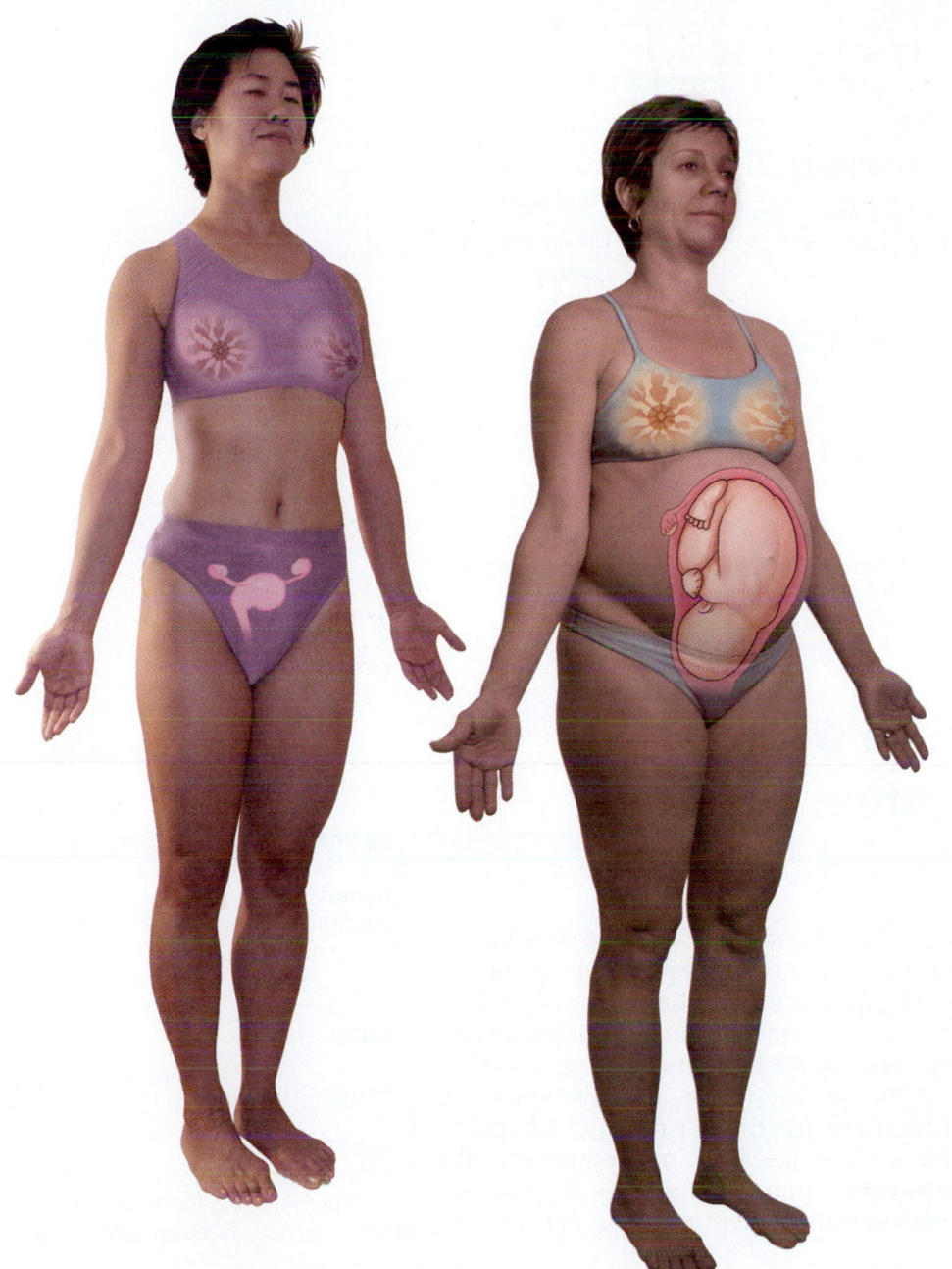

Figure 13-1 ■ Female genital and reproductive system.
The female genital and reproductive system consists of the ovaries, uterine tubes, uterus, and vagina, as well as the external genitalia on the outside of the body. It also includes the breasts. This system undergoes significant changes during pregnancy and childbirth.

genitourinary (GU) system or **urogenital system** because of the close proximity of these two body systems (see Figure 13-2 ■). The function of the female genital and reproductive system is to display the female secondary sexual characteristics, produce ova (eggs), and, when appropriate, conceive and bear children.

WORD BUILDING

genitourinary
(JEN-ih-toh-YOO-rih-NAIR-ee)
 genit/o- *genitalia*
 urin/o- *urine; urinary system*
 -ary *pertaining to*

urogenital (YOO-roh-JEN-ih-tal)
 ur/o- *urine; urinary system*
 genit/o- *genitalia*
 -al *pertaining to*

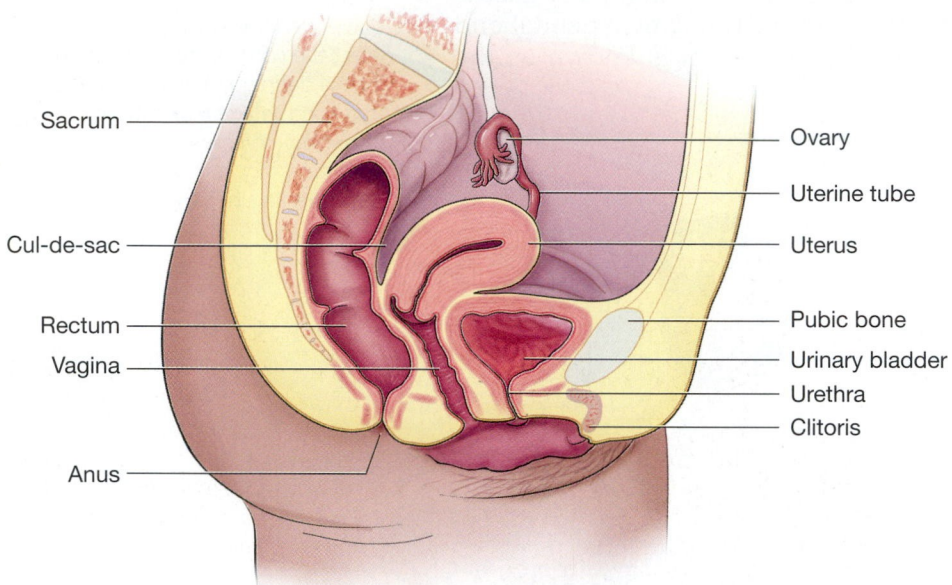

Figure 13-2 ■ Abdominopelvic cavity.
The female genital and reproductive organs in the abdominopelvic cavity lie in close proximity to the organs of the urinary system.

Anatomy of the Female Genital and Reproductive System

Ovaries

An **ovary** is a small egg-shaped gland about 2 inches in length that is near the end of a uterine tube (see Figure 13-3 ■). The ovaries are held in place by the **broad ligament,** a folded sheet of peritoneum that extends to the walls of the pelvic cavity and the **suspensory ligament.** The **ovarian ligament** connects the ovary to the uterus. The ovaries are the **gonads** or sex glands in a female. They function as part of the female genital and reproductive system and the endocrine system (discussed in "Endocrinology," Chapter 14). The ovaries contain **follicles** that rupture, releasing **ova** (eggs) during the menstrual cycle. The ovaries are glands that secrete three hormones (estradiol, progesterone, and testosterone) that affect puberty, menstruation, and pregnancy.

ovary (OH-vah-ree)

ovarian (oh-VAIR-ee-an)
 ovari/o- *ovary*
 -an *pertaining to*
The combining form *oophor/o-* also means *ovary.*

ligament (LIG-ah-ment)

gonad (GOH-nad)
 gon/o- *seed (ovum or spermatozoon)*
 -ad *toward; in the direction of*

follicle (FAWL-ih-kl)

ovum (OH-vum)

ova (OH-vah)
Form the plural by changing *-um* to *-a.* The combining forms *o/o-, ov/i-, ov/o-,* and *ovul/o-* mean *ovum* (egg).

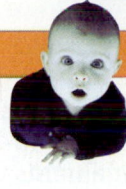

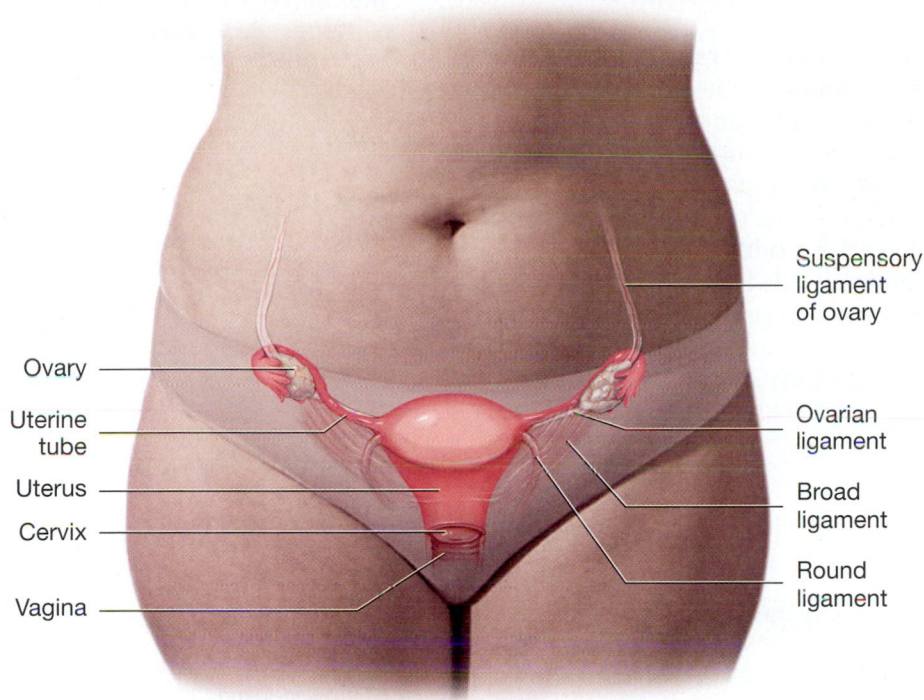

Ovary

Uterine
tube

Uterus

Cervix

Vagina

Suspensory
ligament
of ovary

Ovarian
ligament

Broad
ligament

Round
ligament

Figure 13-3 ■ Ovaries, uterine tubes, and uterus.
The ovaries and uterine tubes lie on either side of the uterus. They are suspended within the abdominopelvic cavity by ligaments. The cervix of the uterus protrudes downward into the vagina.

Uterine Tubes

Each **uterine tube** is about 5 inches in length and is held in place by the broad ligament. The function of the uterine tube is to transport an ovum from the ovary to the uterus. Its medial end is connected to the uterus, but its lateral end is not connected to the ovary (see Figure 13-4). There is an open space (part of the abdominopelvic cavity) between each ovary and its uterine tube. The ovary releases an ovum into this open space. **Fimbriae,** moving, fingerlike projections at the end of the uterine tube, create currents that carry the ovum into the **infundibulum,** the funnel-shaped part of the tube, and then into the **lumen** of the tube. There, the **cilia** (tiny hairs) beat in waves while **peristalsis** (coordinated, wavelike contractions of smooth muscle) propels the ovum toward the uterus. Fluid inside the uterine tube contains nutrients to nourish the ovum on its 3-day journey to the uterus. The uterine tube is also known as the **oviduct.** Collectively, the ovaries and the uterine tubes are known as the **adnexa.**

WORD BUILDING

uterine (YOO-teh-rin) (YOO-teh-rine)
　uter/o- *uterus (womb)*
　-ine *pertaining to*
The combining forms *salping/o-* and *fallopi/o-* also mean *uterine tube.* The uterine tube was formerly known as the fallopian tube.

fimbriae (FIM-bree-ee)
Fimbria is a Latin singular noun. Form the plural by changing *-a* to *-ae.* Because there are so many fimbriae, the singular form is seldom used.

infundibulum (in-fun-DIB-yoo-lum)

lumen (LOO-men)

cilia (SIL-ee-ah)
Cilium is a Latin singular noun. Form the plural by changing *-um* to *-a.*

peristalsis (PAIR-ih-STAL-sis)
　peri- *around*
　stal/o- *contraction*
　-sis *process; condition; abnormal condition*

oviduct (OH-vih-dukt)
　ov/i- *ovum (egg)*
　-duct *duct (tube)*

adnexa (ad-NEK-sah)

adnexal (ad-NEK-sal)
　adnex/o- *accessory connecting parts*
　-al *pertaining to*

Uterus

The **uterus** is an inverted pear-shaped organ about 3 inches in length (see Figure 13-3). The uterus is held in place by the broad ligament, the **round ligaments** at the top of the uterus, and the **uterosacral ligaments** from the uterus to the sacrum of the vertebral column. The **fundus** is the rounded top of the uterus (see Figure 13-4 ■). The **corpus** or body of the uterus is its widest part. The body narrows and becomes the **cervix** (neck of the uterus). Within the uterus is the hollow **intrauterine cavity,** which narrows into the **cervical canal.** The **cervical os** in the center of the cervix is the opening of the cervical canal. The rounded tip of the cervix projects about ½ inch into the vagina.

The wall of the uterus is composed of three layers: perimetrium, myometrium, and endometrium. The **perimetrium** is the outer layer. It is a serous membrane that is part of the peritoneum that lines the abdominopelvic cavity (discussed in "Gastroenterology," Chapter 3). The **myometrium** or uterine muscle contains smooth muscle fibers that are oriented in different directions. This allows the uterus to contract strongly from all sides during labor and the delivery of a baby. The innermost layer, the **endometrium,** lines the intrauterine cavity. It is a mucous membrane that contains glands, and this layer thickens during the menstrual cycle. If an ovum is not fertilized, this lining is shed during menstruation. The superior portion of the uterus is tipped anteriorly and rests on the urinary bladder (see Figure 13-2); this normal position is known as **anteflexion.** The

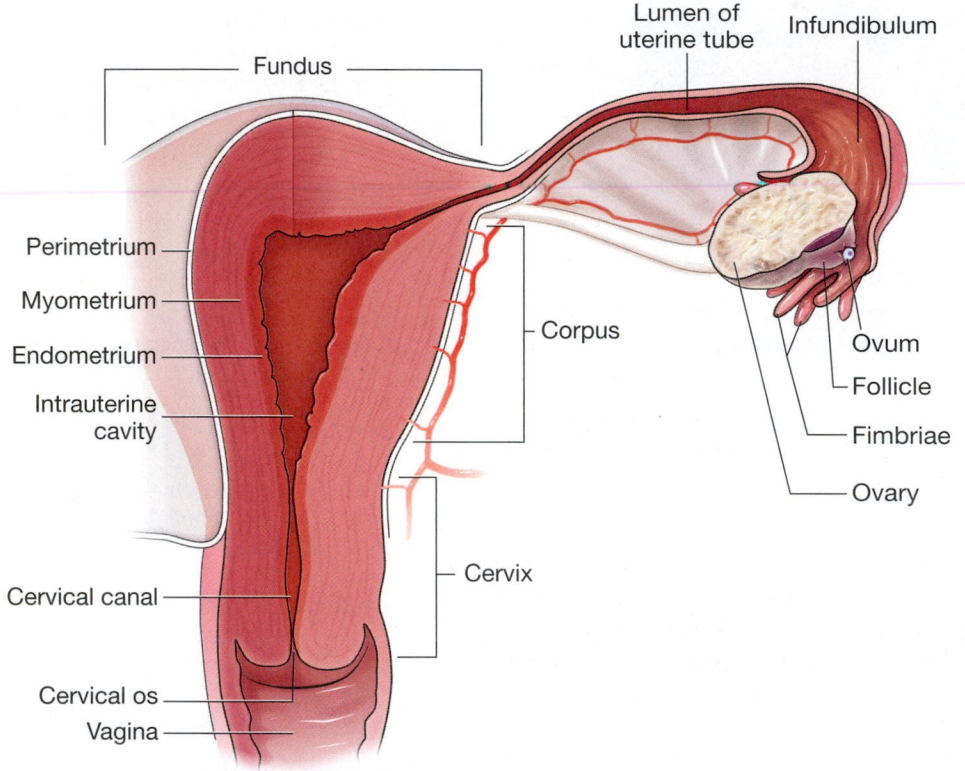

Figure 13-4 ■ Uterus.
The fundus, corpus (body of the uterus), and the cervix are the regions of the uterus. The perimetrium is the outer covering of the uterus. The myometrium is the layer of smooth muscle that makes up the uterine wall. The endometrium is the layer of glands and tissue that lines the intrauterine cavity. The ovary contains a follicle that ruptures and releases an ovum. Movements of the fimbriae draw the ovum into the lumen of the uterine tube that goes to the uterus.

uterus is suspended within the abdominopelvic cavity by the broad ligament and other ligaments that go to the sacrum and to the walls of the pelvic cavity. The broad ligament also creates a small pouch, the **cul-de-sac,** between the uterus and the rectum (see Figure 3-2).

Vagina

The **vagina** is a short, tubelike structure about 3 inches in length (see Figures 13-2 and 13-4). Within the vagina is the open **vaginal canal.** The cervix of the uterus protrudes into the superior end of the vaginal canal. The **fornix** is the area of the vaginal canal that is behind and around the cervix. At the inferior end of the vaginal canal is the **hymen,** an elastic membrane that partially or completely covers the opening, although it is sometimes absent. The hymen, if present, is easily torn by the insertion of a tampon, a vaginal examination, or sexual intercourse. The **vaginal introitus** is the opening to the outside of the body (see Figure 13-5 ■).

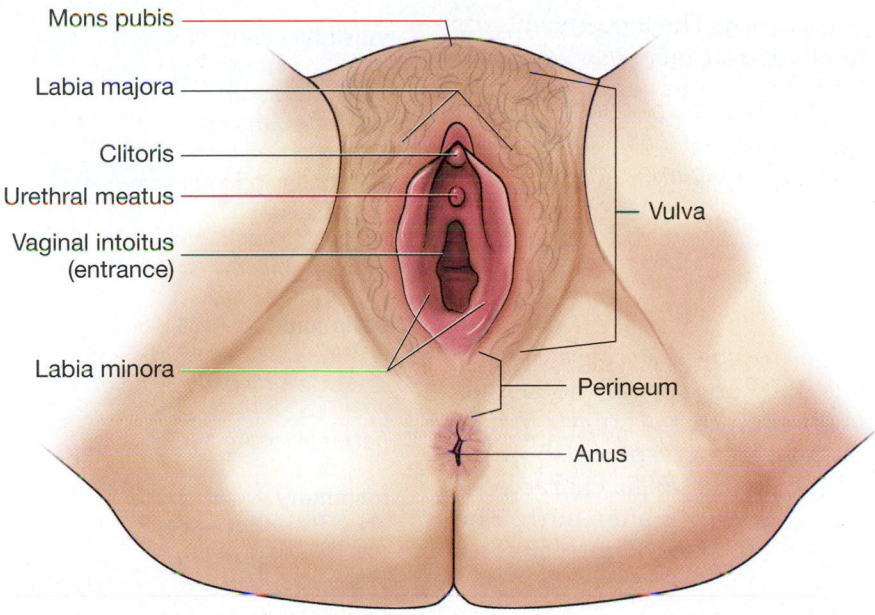

Figure 13-5 ■ External female genitalia.
The labia majora and labia minora protect and partially cover the clitoris, vaginal introitus, and the glands that secrete mucus. The vulva includes all these structures but also includes the mons pubis.

The vagina has three functions. During menstruation, it transports the shed endometrium to the outside of the body. During sexual intercourse, it holds the penis and collects the ejaculate that contains spermatozoa. During birth, it is part of the birth canal that takes the baby to the outside of the mother's body.

External Genitalia

The external genitalia include the labia majora, labia minora, clitoris, vaginal introitus, and glands that produce lubricating secretions (see Figure 13-5). The labia consist of two sets of lip-shaped structures that run anteriorly to posteriorly and partially cover the urethral meatus and vaginal introitus. The thicker, outermost lips, the **labia majora,** are fleshy and covered with pubic

WORD BUILDING

cul-de-sac (KUL-de-sak)
The combining form *culd/o-* means *cul-de-sac.*

vagina (vah-JY-nah)

vaginal (VAJ-ih-nal)
  vagin/o- *vagina*
  -al *pertaining to*
The combining form *colp/o-* also means *vagina.*

fornix (FOR-niks)
The fornix is also known as the vaginal vault.

hymen (HY-men)

introitus (in-TROH-ih-tus)

labia majora
(LAY-bee-ah mah-JOR-ah)

hair on their outer surface. The smooth, thin, inner lips, the **labia minora**, lie beneath the labia majora. The **clitoris** is the organ of sexual response in the female. Its tip is located anterior to the urethral meatus. With sexual stimulation, the clitoris enlarges with blood and becomes firm. The vaginal introitus (entrance to the vagina), is posterior to the urethral meatus. Three sets of glands near the vaginal introitus—**Bartholin's glands,** the **urethral glands,** and **Skene's glands (BUS)**—secrete mucus during sexual arousal. The **vulva** includes all of these structures as well as the **mons pubis** (the rounded, fleshy pad with pubic hair that overlies the pubic bone). The area between the vulva and the anus is the **perineum.**

Word Alert

SOUND-ALIKE WORDS

perineum   (noun)   area between the vulva and the anus
Example: The perineum is an area of skin on the outside of the body.

perimetrium   (noun)   serous membrane on the outside of the uterus
Example: The perimetrium is the outermost layer of the uterus.

peritoneum   (noun)   serous membrane that lines the abdominopelvic cavity
Example: The peritoneum secretes peritoneal fluid that fills the spaces between the intestines and other organs.

Breasts

The breasts or **mammary glands** are located on the chest. Because of their structure of adipose (fatty) tissue and glands, they are part of the integumentary system; and, because of their function, they are part of the female reproductive system. The breasts develop at puberty in response to estradiol secreted by the ovaries. They are one of the female sexual characteristics, and they also provide milk to nourish the newborn after birth. The breasts contain **lactiferous lobules** that produce milk (see Figure 13-6 ■).

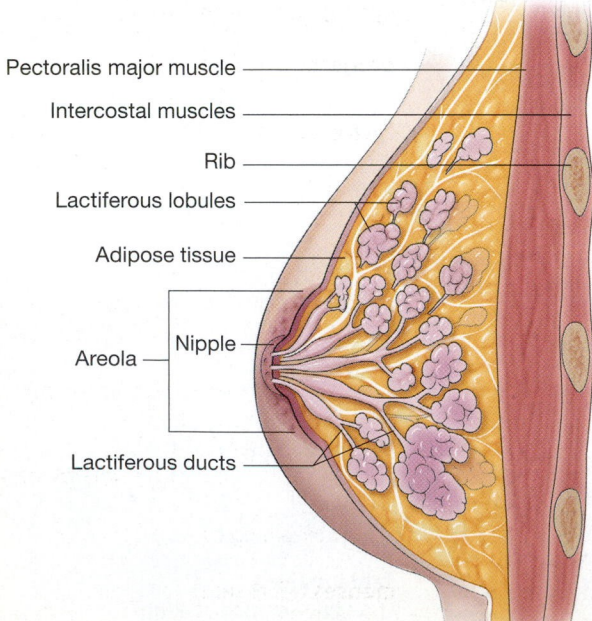

Pectoralis major muscle
Intercostal muscles
Rib
Lactiferous lobules
Adipose tissue
Areola
Nipple
Lactiferous ducts

Figure 13-6 ■ **Breast.**
The breasts or mammary glands develop during puberty, but the lactiferous lobules do not produce milk until after childbirth.

Milk flows through the **lactiferous ducts** to the nipple. The **areola** is the pigmented area around the nipple. The surface of the areola is covered with small, elevated areas that secrete oil to protect the nipple when the baby nurses.

Physiology of Sexual Maturity, Oogenesis, Menstruation, and Conception

Sexual Maturity and Oogenesis

At the onset of puberty (adolescence), the anterior pituitary gland in the brain (discussed in "Endocrinology," Chapter 14) begins to secrete two hormones that stimulate the ovaries.

1. **Follicle-stimulating hormone (FSH).** FSH stimulates a follicle in the ovary to enlarge and produce a mature ovum. **Oogenesis** is the process of forming a mature ovum. Like a spermatozoon, a mature ovum is created by mitosis and meiosis. Like a spermatozoon, the mature ovum is a **gamete.** However, unlike spermatozoa, only a single, large ovum is produced. It contains 23 chromosomes, and the remaining chromosomes are discarded in small packets of cytoplasm known as polar bodies. FSH also stimulates the follicles to secrete estradiol, which causes the development of the female sexual characteristics.

2. **Luteinizing hormone (LH).** LH stimulates a single follicle each month to rupture and release its mature ovum. Then it stimulates the ruptured follicle (corpus luteum) to secrete estradiol and progesterone.

The ovary secretes these three hormones:

1. **Estradiol.** The most abundant and most biologically active of the female hormones. It is secreted by each follicle (and also by the ruptured follicle [corpus luteum] after ovulation). Estradiol causes the development of the female sexual characteristics during puberty: enlargement of the external genitalia, development of the breasts, widening of the pelvis, growth of body hair in the axillary and genital areas, and development of the sexual drive (see Figure 13-7 ■). Estradiol also causes the endometrium (lining of the uterus) to thicken during the menstrual cycle.

2. **Progesterone.** Hormone secreted by a ruptured follicle (corpus luteum) after ovulation. Progesterone also causes the endometrium to thicken.

3. **Testosterone.** A male hormone secreted by cells around the follicle. It plays a role in the female sexual drive.

The Menstrual Cycle

With the onset of puberty, the female begins to ovulate and menstruate. **Menarche** is the beginning of **menstruation,** which occurs with the first **menstrual period** or **menses.**

Each **menstrual cycle,** on average, lasts 28 days and includes four phases: the menstrual phase, the proliferative phase, ovulation, the secretory phase, and the ischemic phase (see Figure 13-8 ■).

WORD BUILDING

areola (ah-REE-oh-lah)

areolae (ah-REE-oh-lee)
Areola is a Latin singular noun. Form the plural by changing -*a* to -*ae*.

areolar (ah-REE-oh-lar)
  areol/o- *small area around the nipple*
  -ar *pertaining to*

oogenesis (OH-oh-JEN-eh-sis)
  o/o- *ovum (egg)*
  gen/o- *arising from; produced by*
  -esis *a process*

gamete (GAM-eet)

luteinizing (LOO-tee-ih-NY-zing)

estradiol (ES-trah-DY-awl)
  estr/a- *female*
  di- *two*
  -ol *chemical substance*
The combining forms *estr/o-* and *gynec/o-* also mean *female.*

progesterone (proh-JES-teh-rohn)

testosterone (tes-TAWS-teh-rohn)

menarche (meh-NAR-kee)
  men/o- *month*
  -arche *a beginning*

menstruation (MEN-stroo-AA-shun)
  menstru/o- *monthly discharge of blood*
  -ation *a process; being or having*

menstrual (MEN-stroo-al)
  menstru/o- *monthly discharge of blood*
  -al *pertaining to*

menses (MEN-seez)

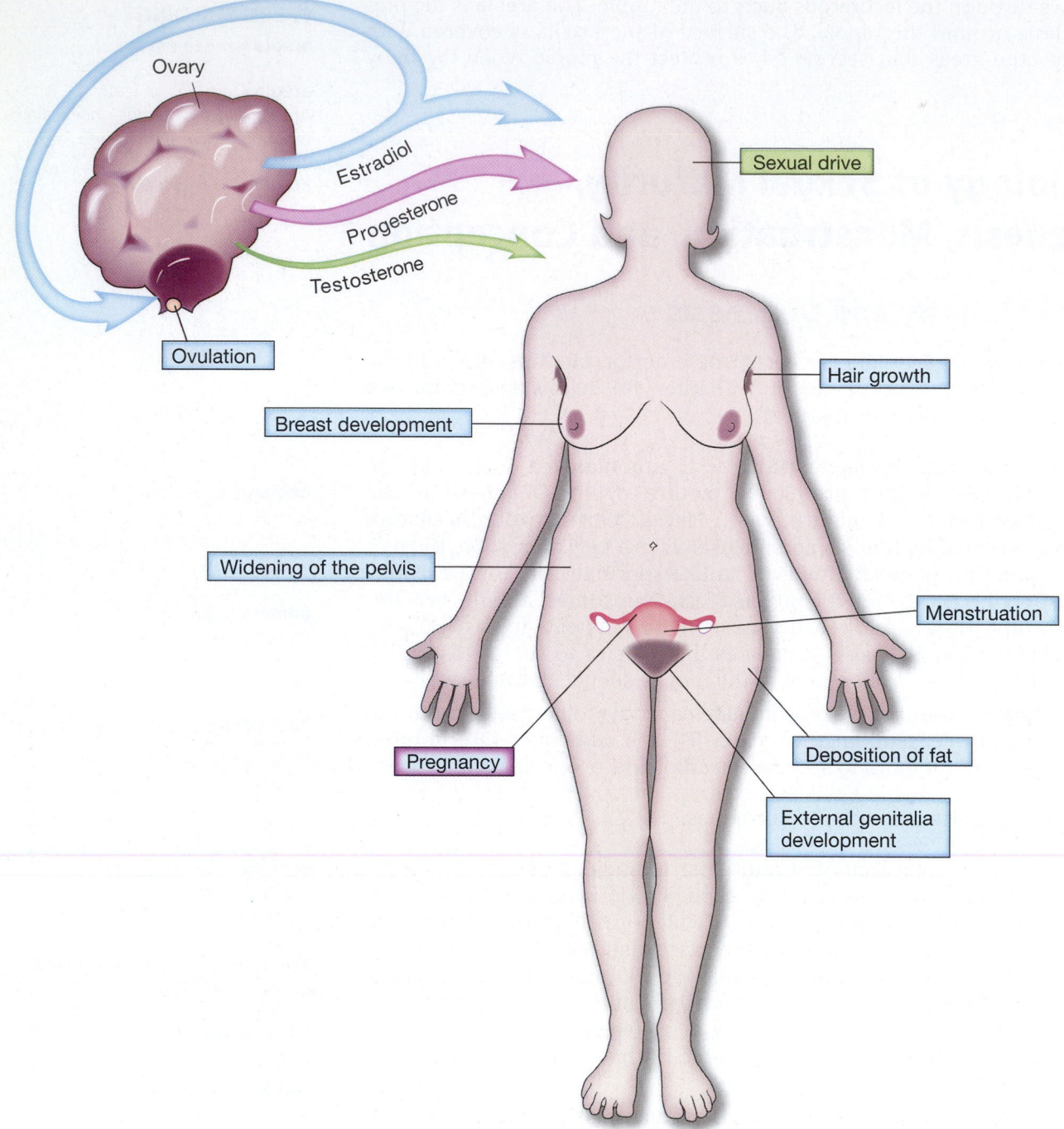

Figure 13-7 ■ **Hormones secreted by the ovaries.**

Estradiol produces the female sexual characteristics during puberty. Estradiol and progesterone stimulate the growth of the endometrium prior to menstruation and also (if an ovum is fertilized) during pregnancy. Testosterone plays a role in the female sexual drive.

THE MENSTRUAL CYCLE

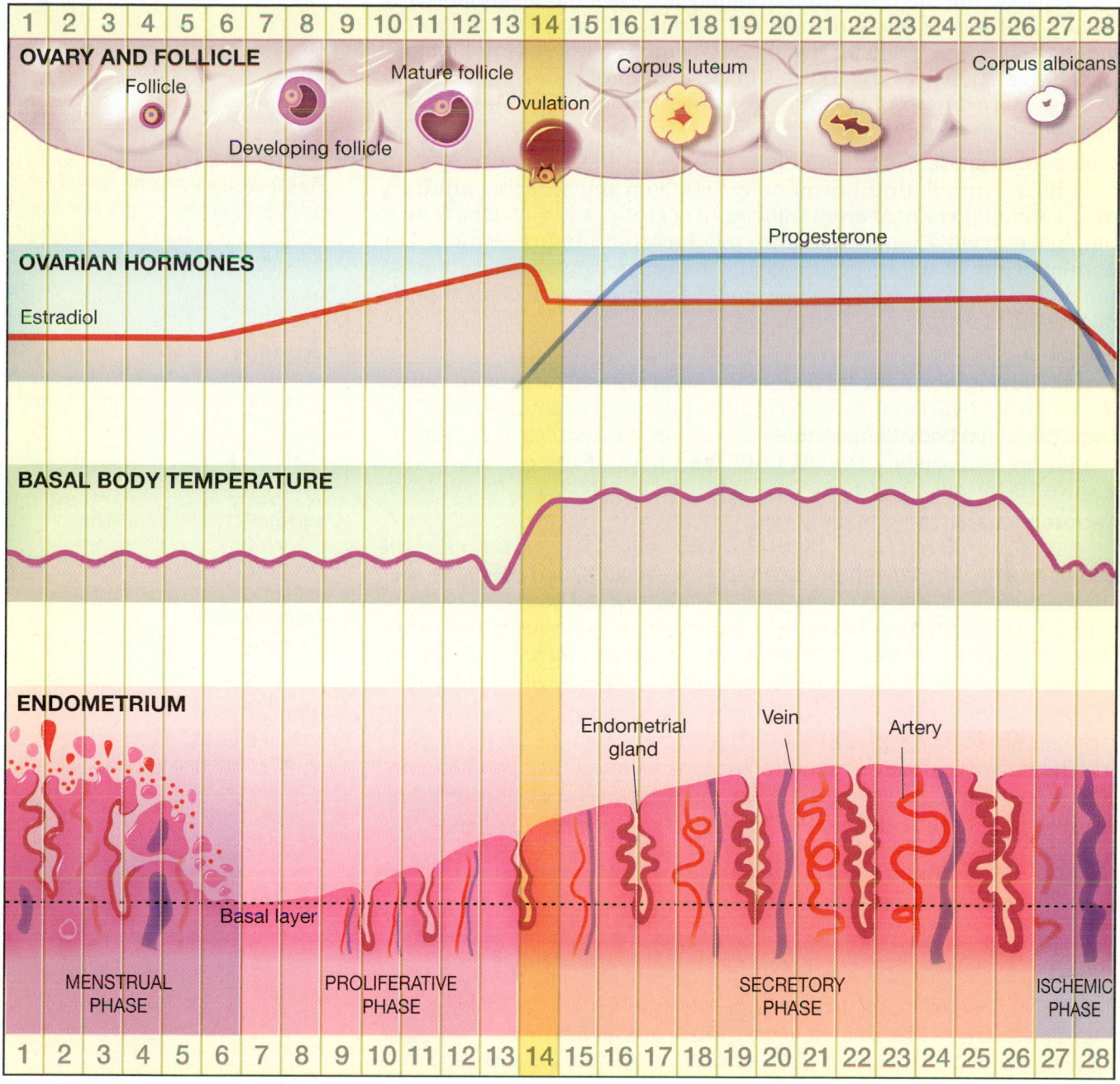

Figure 13-8 ■ Menstrual cycle.

Activities in the ovary are related to those in the uterus during the menstrual cycle. Hormones (estradiol and progesterone) produced by the follicle and then by the corpus luteum cause the endometrium to proliferate. If the ovum is not fertilized, the declining levels of the hormones cause the endometrium to slough off in menstruation.

1. **Menstrual phase** (Days 1–6)

   Menstruation begins. Approximately 30 mL of blood, endometrial tissue, and mucus is shed from the uterus and passes through the vagina. All that remains of the endometrium is a thin layer of glands. At the same time, several follicles in the ovary are enlarging and their ova are maturing in preparation for one of them to be released during ovulation on day 14.

2. **Proliferative phase** (Days 7–13)

   Follicle-stimulating hormone (FSH) from the anterior pituitary gland stimulates the ovarian follicles to secrete estradiol. One follicle becomes greatly enlarged and produces a mature ovum. The endometrium in the uterus becomes thicker because of estradiol. At the end of the proliferative phase, mucus in the cervical canal thins to allow spermatozoa to pass through it.

3. **Ovulation** (Day 14)

   Luteinizing hormone (LH) from the anterior pituitary gland causes the enlarged ovarian follicle to rupture, releasing a mature ovum. The **basal (baseline) body temperature** rises about 0.4 degrees at the time of ovulation and stays elevated until the onset of menstruation (see Figure 13-8).

4. **Secretory phase** (Days 15–26)

   The ruptured ovarian follicle fills with yellow fat and becomes the **corpus luteum.** The corpus luteum secretes estradiol and progesterone. Progesterone causes the endometrial glands of the uterus to enlarge, and the endometrium becomes thicker. Small arteries grow to the innermost edge of the endometrium, ready to nourish a fertilized ovum. The basal body temperature continues to be elevated due to progesterone.

5. **Ischemic phase** (Days 27–28)

   The corpus luteum turns into white scar tissue (corpus albicans) and stops making estradiol and progesterone. The abrupt decrease in these hormones causes the small arteries in the endometrium to contract. This stops the flow of blood and causes ischemia of the tissue. The endometrium begins to slough off, and menstruation (the first phase) begins again.

Did You Know?

In the 1800s, the average age for menarche (the onset of menstruation) was 18 years old. Now the average age for menarche is 12 years old. Researchers point to better health and nutrition in the 1900s as the reason for this trend, but feel that childhood obesity and the presence of estrogen in the environment (from discarded birth control pills) are the reason for the continuing downward trend.

Conception

Of the 100–500 million spermatozoa deposited in the vagina during sexual intercourse, only some are able to reach the ovum in the uterine tube; this occurs 24–48 hours after sexual intercourse. Chemicals secreted by the ovum attract the spermatozoa. A caplike layer of enzymes on the head of each spermatozoon begins to dissolve the layer of cells around the ovum (see Figure 13-9 ■). Many spermatozoa attach to the ovum, but only one penetrates its surface. This is the moment of **fertilization** or **conception.**

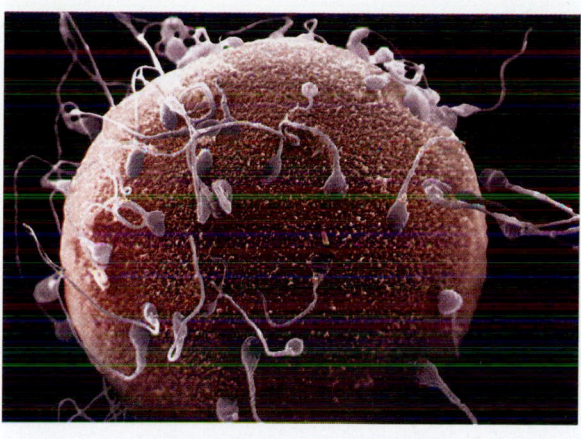

Figure 13-9 ■ An ovum and spermatozoa.

An ovum is nearly 100,000 times larger than a spermatozoon. An ovum and a spermatozoon are gametes that each contain only 23 chromosomes. A fertilized ovum contains 46 chromosomes and is known as a zygote.

After that, the surface of the ovum changes and actually repels the other spermatozoa. When a spermatozoon unites with an ovum, the resulting cell has 46 chromosomes and is known as a **zygote. Pregnancy** begins at the moment of conception.

WORD BUILDING

zygote (ZY-goht)

pregnancy (PREG-nan-see)
   pregn/o- *being with child*
   -ancy *state of*

pregnant (PREG-nant)
   pregn/o- *being with child*
   -ant *pertaining to*

amnion (AM-nee-on)

amniotic (AM-nee-AWT-ik)
   amni/o- *amnion (fetal membrane)*
   -tic *pertaining to*

Clinical Connections

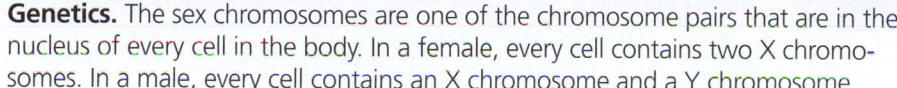

Genetics. The sex chromosomes are one of the chromosome pairs that are in the nucleus of every cell in the body. In a female, every cell contains two X chromosomes. In a male, every cell contains an X chromosome and a Y chromosome.

A spermatozoon contains either the X chromosome or the Y chromosome. The ovum always contains an X chromosome. An X chromosome from the spermatozoon and an X chromosome from the ovum unite to create a female (XX). A Y chromosome from the spermatozoon and an X chromosome from the ovum unite to create a male (XY). **Fraternal twins** occur when the ovary releases two ova that are fertilized by different spermatozoa. Multiple zygotes can develop if the ovary released multiple ova that were all fertilized; this can occur in patients taking ovulation-stimulating drugs for infertility. **Identical twins** occur when one already developing zygote splits to create two separate but identical zygotes.

fraternal (frah-TER-nal)
   fratern/o- *close association or relationship*
   -al *pertaining to*

A zygote immediately begins to divide as it moves through the uterine tube. Within the intrauterine cavity, it sinks into the thick endometrium. At this point, the zygote is a hollow ball with an inner mass of cells and an outer layer.

The inner mass of cells of the zygote becomes the amnion and the embryo. The **amnion** (or bag of waters) is a membrane sac that produces **amniotic fluid.** The developing embryo floats in and is cushioned by the amniotic fluid.

The outer layer of the zygote becomes the **chorion.** It sends fingerlike projections (villi) into the endometrium to absorb nutrients and oxygen. The chorion produces the hormone **human chorionic gonadotropin (HCG).** HCG stimulates the corpus luteum of the ovary to keep producing estradiol and progesterone. This maintains the thickened endometrium to support the developing embryo and prevents menstruation from occurring during the rest of the pregnancy. The chorion becomes the **placenta,** a pancake-like structure about 7 inches in diameter and 1–2 inches thick. By the end of the first trimester of pregnancy, the placenta begins to secrete estradiol and progesterone and takes over the job of the corpus luteum in the ovary. Other

chorion (KOH-ree-on)

chorionic (KOH-ree-ON-ik)
   chorion/o- *chorion (fetal membrane)*
   -ic *pertaining to*

gonadotropin
(GOH-nah-doh-TROH-pin)
   gonad/o- *gonads (ovaries and testes)*
   trop/o- *having an affinity for; stimulating; turning*
   -in *a substance*

placenta (plah-SEN-tah)

placental (plah-SEN-tal)
   placent/o- *placenta*
   -al *pertaining to*

structures in the chorion form the rubbery, flexible **umbilical cord** with its two arteries and one vein that connects the placenta to the fetus. The umbilical cord and placenta bring oxygen, nutrients, and antibodies from the mother to the fetus and remove carbon dioxide and waste products.

After 4 days of development, the zygote is known as an **embryo.** After 8 weeks, it is known as a **fetus** (see Figure 13-10 ■). The fetus, placenta, and all fluids and tissue in the uterus are known as the **products of conception.**

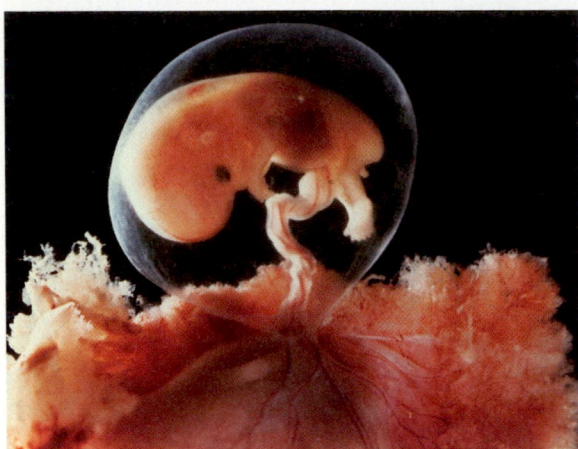

Figure 13-10 ■ Fetus at 9 weeks' gestation.

This fetus, approximately 1 inch in length, is floating in amniotic fluid in the amniotic sac. The beginnings of the eyes, ears, ribs, fingers, and toes are clearly visible. The heart has been beating since the third week of life. The arteries bringing red, oxygenated blood to the fetus are in the umbilical cord.

Gestation is from the moment of conception to the moment of birth. The gestational period is approximately 9 months (38–42 weeks), the average being 40 weeks (see Figure 13-11 ■). Gestation can be divided into three time periods, or trimesters. Each **trimester** is 3 months long. For the fetus, the period of time from conception to birth is the **prenatal period.** For the mother, the period of time from conception to birth is **antepartum.**

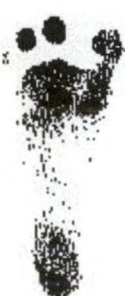

Figure 13-11 ■ Fetal footprint.

This is the actual footprint that appeared on the delivery room record of a fetus who was born prematurely at 23 weeks' gestation.

Did You Know?

The fetus swallows amniotic fluid each day. The fetal kidneys excrete urine into the amniotic fluid. The amniotic fluid contains urea and creatinine (waste products in the urine), skin cells and hair shed by the fetus, and two important substances (lecithin and sphingomyelin) that can be used to determine the maturity of the fetal lungs when the amniotic fluid is tested.

WORD BUILDING

umbilicus (um-BIL-ih-kus)
(UM-bih-LIE-kus)

umbilical (um-BIL-ih-kal)
  umbilic/o- *umbilicus; navel*
  -al *pertaining to*

embryo (EM-bree-oh)

embryonic (EM-bree-ON-ik)
  embryon/o- *embryo; immature form*
  -ic *pertaining to*

fetus (FEE-tus)
Fetus is a Latin singular noun. Its plural form *fetuses* does not follow the regular rule for Latin nouns ending in *-us.*

fetal (FEE-tal)
  fet/o- *fetus*
  -al *pertaining to*

gestation (jes-TAY-shun)
  gestat/o- *from conception to birth*
  -ion *action; condition*

trimester (TRY-mes-ter) (try-MES-ter)

prenatal (pree-NAY-tal)
  pre- *before; in front of*
  nat/o- *birth*
  -al *pertaining to*
The combining form *par/o-* also means *birth.*

antepartum (AN-tee-PAR-tum)
  ante- *forward; before*
  part/o- *childbirth*
  -um *a structure; period of time*

Physiology of Labor and Delivery

As the fetus grows, the uterus expands, taking up space in the mother's abdominal cavity and displacing her abdominal organs. This causes constipation, urinary frequency, and shortness of breath in the mother. During the last trimester of pregnancy, the uterus contracts irregularly to strengthen itself in preparation for childbirth. These are known as **Braxton Hicks contractions** or false labor. Progesterone from the placenta keeps these contractions from becoming labor contractions. The cervical os remains closed (not dilated), and the wall of the cervix remains thick (not effaced). A mucus plug in the cervical os keeps out microorganisms. Late in the pregnancy, the head of the fetus drops into the birth position within the mother's pelvis. This process is known as **engagement.** (It is also known as **lightening** because it eases the mother's shortness of breath.) The fetus usually assumes a head-down position. The head becomes the presenting part (part of the body that will go first through the birth canal). This is a **cephalic presentation.** Any part of the head can be the presenting part, but most commonly it is the top of the head, and this is a **vertex presentation** (see Figure 13-12 ■).

WORD BUILDING

Braxton Hicks (BRAK-ston HIKS)

contraction (con-TRAK-shun)
  contract/o- *pull together*
  -ion *action; condition*

cephalic (seh-FAL-ik)
  cephal/o- *head*
  -ic *pertaining to*

vertex (VER-teks)

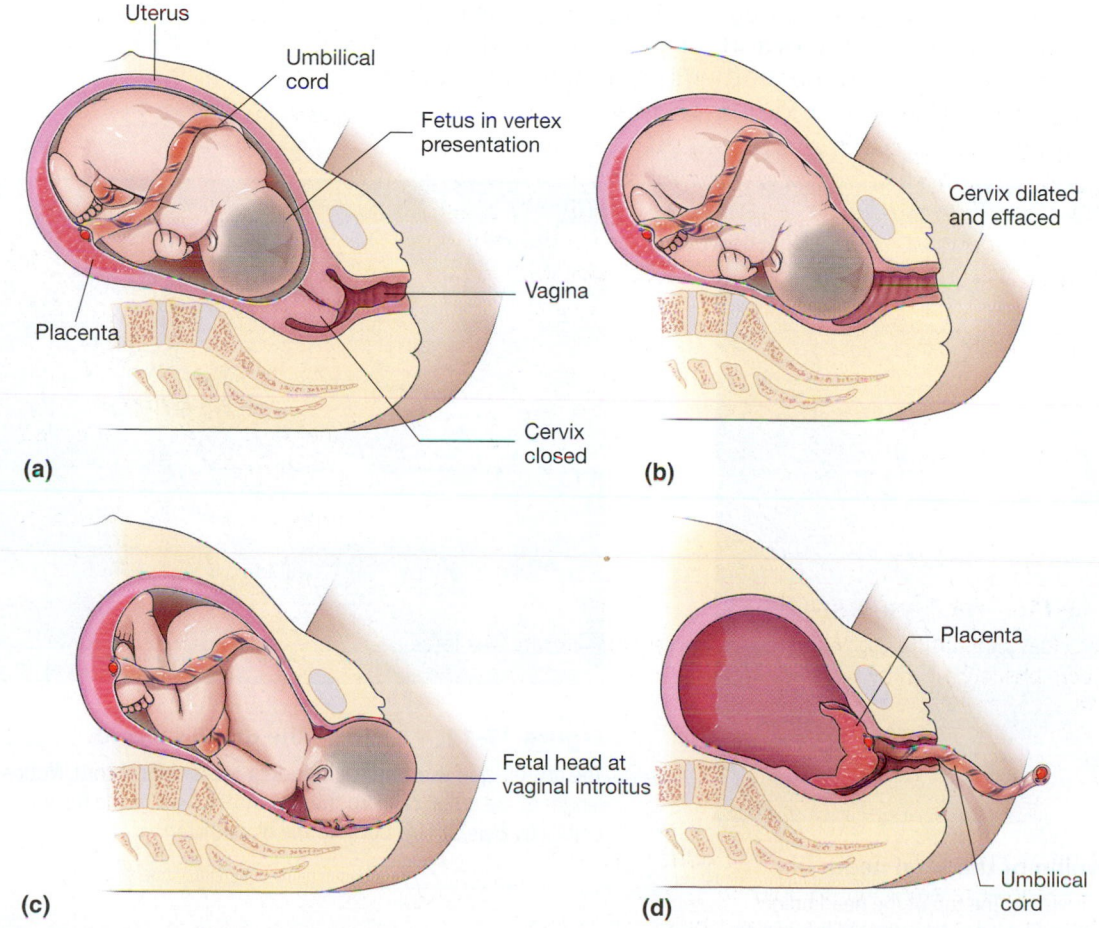

Figure 13-12 ■ Labor and delivery.

(a) This fetus is in a vertex presentation. The cervical os is closed at the beginning of labor. (b) Gradually, the cervix dilates to 10 cm, and its wall thins until it is 100% effaced. (c) The head of the fetus moves through the cervical canal and vagina until the top of the head is visible at the vaginal introitus. (d) After birth, the placenta and umbilical cord are expelled.

Sometime between 38 and 42 weeks' gestation, labor begins. The weight of the fetus presses on the cervix and vagina. This causes the cervix to begin to dilate and stimulates the release of oxytocin from the posterior pituitary gland. The uterus itself also produces oxytoxin. **Oxytocin** causes the uterus to contract regularly. The cervix softens as collagen fibers in its wall break down. This is known as **cervical ripening.**

The process of labor and childbirth is known as **parturition.** It is divided into three stages:

1. **First stage of labor.** Uterine contractions occur about every 30 minutes, increasing in intensity and duration. Cervical **dilation** (widening of the cervical os) progresses from 0 cm to 5 cm, and **effacement** (thinning of the cervical wall) progresses from 0 percent to 50 percent. **Rupture of the membranes (ROM)** occurs, and this releases amniotic fluid. As the uterine contractions intensify, the mother may receive epidural anesthesia to help control the pain. After 8 to 20 hours of labor, the cervix is completely dilated at 10 cm and 100% effaced (see Figure 13-12), and the mother is transferred to the delivery room.

2. **Second stage of labor.** The uterine contractions have brought the head of the fetus into the vagina. The mother is encouraged to push by holding her breath to raise the intra-abdominal pressure. **Crowning** occurs when the top of the head is visible at the vaginal introitus (see Figures 13-12 and 13-13 ■). The head is delivered, and after several more uterine contractions, the shoulders and the rest of the body are delivered. The newborn is placed on the mother's abdomen while the umbilical cord is clamped and cut (see Figure 13-14 ■).

WORD BUILDING

oxytocin (AWK-see-TOH-sin)
  ox/y- *oxygen; quick*
  toc/o- *labor and childbirth*
  -in *a substance*
Select the correct combining form meaning to get the definition of *oxytoxin: a substance (that causes) quick labor and childbirth.*

parturition (PAR-tyoo-RIH-shun)
  parturit/o- *to be in labor*
  -ion *action; condition*

dilation (dy-LAY-shun)
  dilat/o- *dilate; widen*
  -ion *action; condition*

effacement (eh-FAYS-ment)
  efface/o- *do away with; obliterate*
  -ment *action; state*

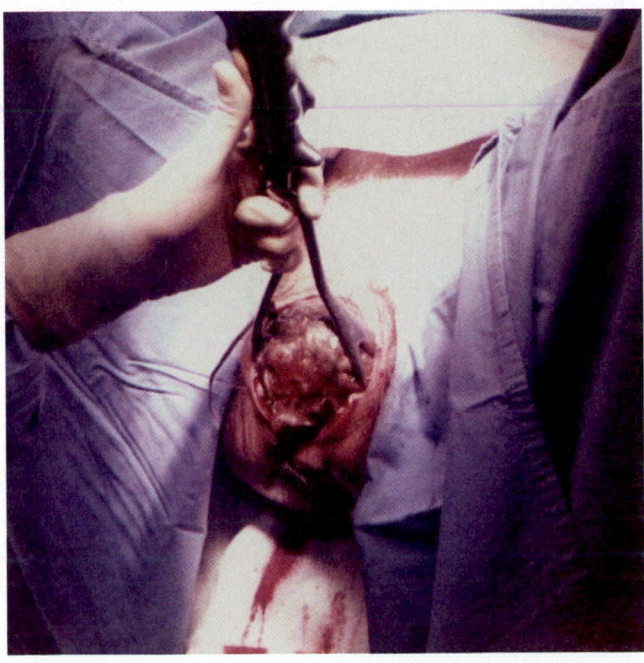

Figure 13-13 ■ **Crowning of the fetal head.**
The hair on the baby's head is visible. The top of the head bulges outwardly with each contraction. The irregular edges of the vagina are from an episiotomy to prevent spontaneous tearing as the baby is born. The obstetrician is using obstetrical forceps to assist in the delivery of the head.

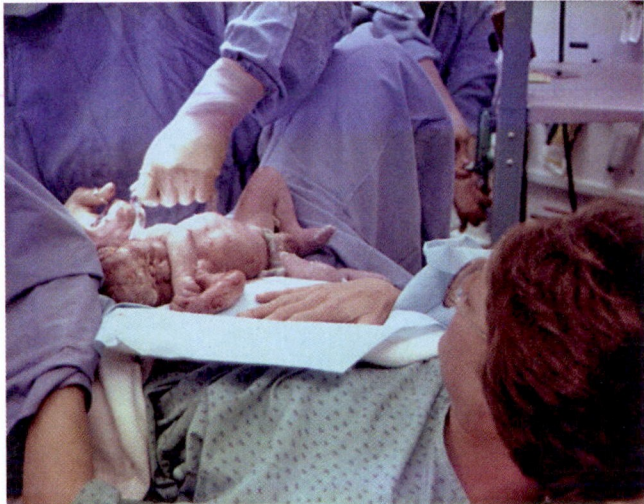

Figure 13-14 ■ **Cutting the umbilical cord.**
The obstetrician uses forceps to clamp the umbilical cord. Notice the length of the umbilical cord from its attachment at the baby's umbilicus, beneath his body, to the obstetrician.

3. **Third stage of labor.** The placenta is delivered about 30 minutes after the birth. The placenta is also known as the afterbirth (see Figure 13-12). Oxytocin causes the uterus to contract to stop blood flow from the raw surfaces where the placenta pulled away. The obstetrician sutures up the episiotomy, if one was performed. The placenta and umbilical cord are sent to pathology for examination. Blood in the umbilical cord is rich in stem cells and can be used for stem cell transplantation (discussed in "Hematology and Immunology," Chapter 6).

For the newborn, the period of time after birth is the **postnatal period.** For the mother, the period of time after birth is **postpartum.** The uterus gradually shrinks in size, a process known as **involution.** Small amounts of blood, tissue, and fluid, known as **lochia,** continue to flow from the uterus for a week until all of the endometrial lining is shed.

Lactation is the production of milk by the breasts when stimulated by the hormone prolactin from the anterior pituitary gland in the brain. After birth, when the newborn cries or sucks, oxytocin secreted by the posterior pituitary gland causes smooth muscles around the lactiferous lobules to contract and expel milk for breastfeeding. This is known as the let-down reflex. The first milk, **colostrum,** is a thick, yellowish fluid. By the third day, the colostrum is replaced by regular breast milk that is thin and white.

Clinical Connections

Immunology (Chapter 6). Colostrum is rich in nutrients and contains maternal antibodies. For the first few days of life, the intestinal tract is more permeable and allows these maternal antibodies to be absorbed into the newborn's blood. Maternal antibodies provide passive immunity to common diseases that the mother has already had. This immunity lasts until the newborn begins to make its own antibodies at about 18 months of age.

WORD BUILDING

postnatal (post-NAY-tal)
  post- *after; behind*
  nat/o- *birth*
  -al *pertaining to*

postpartum (post-PAR-tum)
  post- *after; behind*
  part/o- *childbirth*
  -um *a structure; period of time*

involution (IN-voh-LOO-shun)
  involut/o- *enlarged organ returns to normal size*
  -ion *action; condition*

lochia (LOH-kee-ah)

lactation (lak-TAY-shun)
  lact/o- *milk*
  -ation *a process; being or having*

colostrum (koh-LAWS-trum)

The Newborn

A newborn who is between 38 and 42 weeks' gestation is a **term neonate.** A newborn between 28 and 37 weeks' gestation is **preterm** or **premature,** a reference to the maturity of the internal organs and their ability to function. Because the date of conception is not always known, the gestational age of a newborn is an estimate.

The skin of the newborn is covered with **vernix caseosa,** a thick, white, cheesy substance that protects the skin from amniotic fluid in the uterus (see Figure 13-15 ■). The head can exhibit **molding,** a temporary elongated reshaping of the cranium that occurs as the head passes through the mother's bony pelvis. On the top of the head, the anterior **fontanel** or soft spot is a soft area that bulges when the newborn cries because it is only covered by a layer of fibrous connective tissue, not by bone (see Figure 8-4). There is also a smaller posterior fontanel at the back of the head. The fontanels allow the brain to grow before the bones fuse together. The newborn's face, hands, and feet are often bluish, a temporary condition known as **acrocyanosis.** The first stool is **meconium,** a thick, greenish-black, sticky substance. It contains mucus and bile (from the fetal digestive tract) and skin cells (that were in amniotic fluid swallowed by the fetus).

WORD BUILDING

neonate (NEE-oh-nayt)
  ne/o- *new*
  -nate *thing that is born*

neonatal (NEE-oh-NAY-tal)
  ne/o- *new*
  nat/o- *birth*
  -al *pertaining to*

vernix caseosa
(VER-niks KAY-see-OH-sah)

fontanel (FAWN-tah-NEL)

acrocyanosis (AK-roh-SY-ah-NOH-sis)
  acr/o- *extremity; highest point*
  cyan/o- *blue*
  -osis *condition; abnormal condition; process*

meconium (meh-KOH-nee-um)

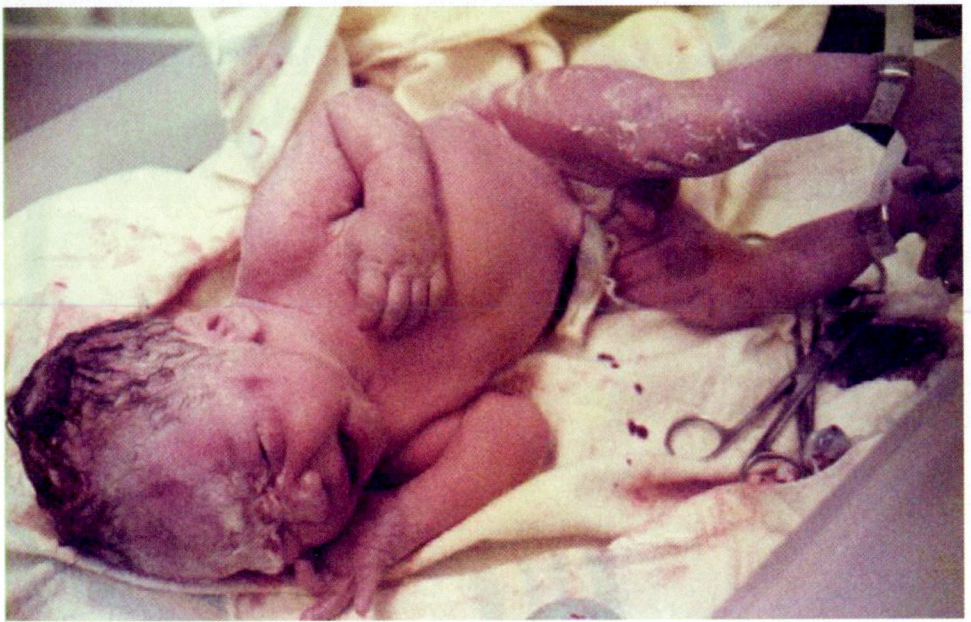

Figure 13-15 ■ Term neonate.
This male newborn is on the warming table in the delivery room. The vernix caseosa has been partially cleaned off of his trunk and arms. His eyes are swollen from the pressure of the birth canal. He is crying vigorously, but his distal extremities still show acrocyanosis (note the bluish color of the right hand and both legs). There is a plastic clamp on the stump of the umbilical cord. There are identification bracelets on both legs.

Vocabulary Review

Female Genital and Reproductive System

Word or Phrase	Description	Combining Forms
external genitalia	Labia majora, labia minora, clitoris, vaginal introitus, Bartholin's glands, urethral glands, and Skene's glands	**genit/o-** *genitalia*
genital organs	External and internal organs and structures of the female genital and reproductive system	**genit/o-** *genitalia*
genitourinary system	Female genital and reproductive system that is in close proximity to the urinary system. It is also known as the **urogenital system.**	**genit/o-** *genitalia* **urin/o-** *urine; urinary system* **ur/o-** *urine; urinary system*
internal genitalia	Ovaries, uterine tubes, uterus, and vagina	**genit/o-** *genitalia*
reproductive system	The other role of the female genital system in conceiving, carrying, and giving birth to a child	**product/o-** *produce*

Ovary and Uterine Tube

Word or Phrase	Description	Combining Forms
adnexa	Accessory organs (the ovaries and uterine tubes) that are connected to the main organ (the uterus)	**adnex/o-** *accessory connecting parts*
follicle	Small area in the ovary that holds an oocyte before puberty and a maturing ovum after puberty. A follicle ruptures at the time of ovulation and becomes the corpus luteum.	
gonads	The ovaries or sex glands in a female	**gon/o-** *seed (ovum or spermatozoon)*
oocyte	Immature egg in the follicle of the fetal ovary	**o/o-** *ovum (egg)*
ovary	Small, egg-shaped gland near the end of the uterine tube. The ovary is held in place by the **broad ligament** and the **suspensory ligament.** The **ovarian ligament** connects the ovary to the uterus. The follicles of the ovary secrete estradiol. The corpus luteum of the ovary secretes estradiol and progesterone. The cells around the follicles secrete testosterone.	**ovari/o-** *ovary* **oophor/o-** *ovary*
ovum	An egg within a follicle in the ovary. A mature ovum is released during ovulation. An ovum is a gamete because it has only 23 chromosomes.	**o/o-** *ovum (egg)* **ov/i-** *ovum (egg)* **ov/o-** *ovum (egg)* **ovul/o-** *ovum (egg)*
uterine tube	Narrow tube that is connected at one end to the uterus. The other end is not directly connected to the ovary. It has a funnel-shaped **infundibulum** and fingerlike **fimbriae** that draw an ovum into the **lumen** (long central opening of the tube). **Cilia** (tiny hairs) inside the uterine tube beat in waves and **peristalsis** (smooth muscle contractions) move the ovum toward the uterus. It is also known as an **oviduct.** Formerly known as the **fallopian tube.**	**uter/o-** *uterus* **stal/o-** *contraction* **ov/i-** *ovum (egg)* **salping/o-** *uterine (fallopian) tube* **fallopi/o-** *uterine (fallopian) tube*

Uterus, Cervix, and Vagina

Word or Phrase	Description	Combining Forms
anteflexion	Normal position of the uterus in which the superior portion is tipped anteriorly on top of the bladder	**flex/o-** *bending*
cervix	Narrow, most inferior part of the uterus. It contains the **cervical canal.** Part of the cervix protrudes into the vagina. The **cervical os** is the small central opening in the cervix.	**cervic/o-** *neck; cervix*
cul-de-sac	Small pouch in the broad ligament that is between the uterus and rectum	**culd/o-** *cul-de-sac*
endometrium	Innermost layer of the uterus that lines the intrauterine cavity. It is a mucous membrane that contains many glands. It thickens and then is shed during the menstrual cycle.	**metri/o-** *uterus (womb)*
myometrium	Smooth muscle layer of the uterine wall. It contracts during menstruation to expel the endometrial lining. It contracts during labor and delivery of the newborn.	**my/o-** *muscle* **metri/o-** *uterus (womb)*
perimetrium	Serous membrane that is the outer layer of the uterus. It is part of the peritoneum that lines the abdominopelvic cavity.	**metri/o-** *uterus (womb)*
uterus	Internal female organ of menstruation and pregnancy. It is also known as the womb. The uterus is held in place by the **broad ligament,** the **round ligaments,** and the **uterosacral ligaments.** The **fundus** is the rounded top of the uterus. The **corpus** is the widest part or body of the uterus. The cervix is the narrow, most inferior part. The hollow **intrauterine cavity** inside the uterus is lined with endometrium.	**uter/o-** *uterus (womb)* **fund/o-** *fundus (part farthest from the opening)* **hyster/o-** *uterus* **metri/o-** *uterus* **metr/o-** *uterus*
vagina	Short tubular structure connected at its superior end to the cervix and at its inferior end to the outside of the body. It contains the **vaginal canal.** The **fornix** is the area of the vaginal canal that is behind and around the cervix. The **hymen** is the elastic membrane that partially or completely covers the inferior end of the vaginal canal. The opening to the outside of the body is the **vaginal introitus.**	**vagin/o-** *vagina* **colp/o-** *vagina*

External Genitalia

Word or Phrase	Description	Combining Forms
BUS	**Bartholin's glands, urethral glands,** and **Skene's glands** are located in or near the vaginal introitus. They secrete mucus during sexual arousal.	**urethr/o-** *urethra*
clitoris	Organ of sexual response in the female that enlarges and becomes engorged with blood	
labia	A pair of fleshy lips covered with pubic hair (the **labia majora**) and a small, thin, inner pair of lips (the **labia minora**) that partially cover the clitoris, urethral meatus, and vaginal introitus	**labi/o-** *lip; labium*
mons pubis	Rounded, fatty pad of tissue covered with pubic hair that lies on top of the pubis (anterior hip bone)	
perineum	Area of skin between the vulva and the anus	**perine/o-** *perineum*
vulva	Area between the inner thighs that includes the external genitalia as well as the mons pubis	**vulv/o-** *vulva* **episi/o-** *vulva*

Breasts

Word or Phrase	Description	Combining Forms
areola	The areola is the pigmented area around the nipple of the breast.	**areol/o-** *small area around the nipple*
lactiferous lobules	Site of milk production in the mammary glands. Prolactin from the anterior pituitary gland stimulates milk production during pregnancy. After birth, oxytocin from the posterior pituitary gland is released when the newborn cries or sucks and this causes the release of milk with the let-down reflex. The milk flows through the **lactiferous ducts** to the nipple.	**lact/i-** *milk* **fer/o-** *to bear* **lact/o-** *milk* **galact/o-** *milk*
mammary glands	The breasts. A female sexual characteristic that develops during puberty. The breasts contain adipose (fatty) tissue and lactiferous lobules. The breasts provide milk to nourish the baby after birth. The nipple is the projecting point of the breast where the lactiferous ducts converge.	**mamm/o-** *breast* **mamm/a-** *breast* **mast/o-** *breast*

Sexual Maturity and Oogenesis

Word or Phrase	Description	Combining Forms
estradiol	Most abundant and biologically active of the female hormones. It is secreted by the follicles of the ovary. During puberty, it causes the development of the female sexual characteristics. It causes the endometrium to thicken during the menstrual cycle. After ovulation, it is secreted by the corpus luteum of the ovary. During pregnancy, it is secreted by the placenta.	**estr/a-** *female* **estr/o-** *female* **gynec/o-** *female*
follicle-stimulating hormone (FSH)	Hormone secreted by the anterior pituitary gland in the brain. It causes a follicle in the ovary to enlarge and produce a mature ovum. FSH also stimulates the follicles to secrete estradiol, which causes the development of the female sexual characteristics.	
gamete	An ovum or spermatozoon. It has 23 chromosomes instead of the usual 46 chromosomes like other cells in the body.	
luteinizing hormone (LH)	Hormone secreted by the anterior pituitary gland in the brain. It causes a follicle to rupture and release a mature ovum.	
oogenesis	Production of a mature ovum from an oocyte through the processes of mitosis and then meiosis	**o/o-** *ovum (egg)* **gen/o-** *arising from; produced by*
progesterone	Hormone secreted by the corpus luteum of the ovary after ovulation. It causes the uterine lining to thicken to prepare for a possible fertilized ovum. During pregnancy, it is secreted by the placenta.	
testosterone	Male hormone secreted by cells around the follicles in the ovary. It plays a role in the female sexual drive.	

Menstruation

Word or Phrase	Description	Combining Forms
corpus luteum	Remnants of a ruptured follicle in the ovary. The corpus luteum is filled with yellow fat and secretes estradiol and progesterone during the menstrual cycle. If the ovum is fertilized, the placenta begins to secrete these hormones, and the corpus luteum becomes white scar tissue.	
ischemic phase	Days 27–28 of the menstrual cycle. The corpus luteum degenerates into white scar tissue (corpus albicans) and stops producing estradiol and progesterone. The endometrium sloughs off, and menstruation begins.	**isch/o-** *keep back; block*
menarche	The first cycle of menstruation at the onset of puberty. This is the first **menstrual period** or **menses.**	**men/o-** *month* **menstru/o-** *monthly discharge of blood*

Word or Phrase	Description	Combining Forms
menstrual cycle	A 28-day cycle that consists of the menstrual phase, proliferative phase, ovulation, secretory phase, and ischemic phase	**menstru/o-** *monthly discharge of blood*
menstrual phase	Days 1–6 of the menstrual cycle. The endometrial lining of the uterus is shed.	**menstru/o-** *monthly discharge of blood*
menstruation	Process in which the endometrium of the uterus is shed each month, causing a flow of blood and tissue through the vagina. Under the influence of estradiol, the endometrium thickens in preparation to receive a fertilized ovum. If the ovum is not fertilized, the endometrium is again shed to begin another menstrual cycle.	**menstru/o-** *monthly discharge of blood*
ovulation	Day 14 of the menstrual cycle. Luteinizing hormone from the anterior pituitary gland causes the ovarian follicle to rupture, releasing the mature ovum. The **basal (baseline) body temperature** rises during ovulation.	**ovul/o-** *ovum (egg)*
proliferative phase	Days 7–13 of the menstrual cycle. A follicle matures in the ovary and the thickness of the endometrium increases.	
secretory phase	Days 15–26 of the menstrual cycle. A ruptured follicle becomes the corpus luteum and secretes estradiol and progesterone. The thickness of the endometrium increases.	**secret/o-** *produce; secrete*
<td colspan="3" align="center">**Conception**</td>
amnion	Membrane sac that produces **amniotic fluid** that surrounds and cushions the developing embryo and fetus. It is also known as the bag of waters.	**amni/o-** *amnion (fetal membrane)*
antepartum	From the mother's standpoint, the period of time from conception until labor and delivery	**part/o-** *childbirth*
chorion	Cells in a zygote that send out fingerlike projections (villi) to penetrate the endometrium to bring nutrients and oxygen to the embryo. It produces human chorionic gonadotropin. It later develops into the placenta.	**chorion/o-** *chorion (fetal membrane)*
embryo	A fertilized ovum (a zygote) is an embryo from 4 days after fertilization through 8 weeks of gestation. Then it becomes a fetus.	**embryon/o-** *embryo; immature form*
fertilization	The act of a spermatozoon uniting with an ovum. It is also known as **conception.**	**fertil/o-** *able to conceive a child* **concept/o-** *to conceive or form*
fetus	An embryo becomes a fetus beginning at 9 weeks of gestation. It is called a fetus until the moment of birth.	**fet/o-** *fetus*
fraternal twins	The ovary releases two ova that are then fertilized at the same time but by different spermatozoa	**fratern/o-** *close association or relationship*
gestation	Period of time from the moment of fertilization of the ovum until birth, approximately 9 months (38–42 weeks)	**gestat/o-** *from conception to birth*
human chorionic gonadotropin (HCG)	Hormone secreted by the chorion of the zygote. It stimulates the corpus luteum of the ovary to keep producing estradiol and progesterone. This maintains the endometrium to support the developing embryo and prevents menstruation for the duration of the pregnancy.	**chorion/o-** *chorion (fetal membrane)* **gonad/o-** *gonads (ovaries and testes)* **trop/o-** *having an affinity for; stimulating; turning*
identical twins	An already developing zygote splits in two. This develops into two separate but identical embryos.	

Word or Phrase	Description	Combining Forms
placenta	Large, pancake-like organ that develops from the chorion. It provides nutrients and oxygen to the developing fetus and removes carbon dioxide and waste products. By the end of the first trimester of pregnancy, it assumes the job of the corpus luteum and secretes estradiol and progesterone to maintain the endometrium during pregnancy. It is also known as the afterbirth.	**placent/o-** *placenta*
pregnancy	State of being with child. It begins at the moment of conception and ends with delivery of the newborn.	**pregn/o-** *being with child*
prenatal period	From the fetus' standpoint, the period of time from conception to birth	**nat/o-** *birth* **par/o-** *birth*
products of conception	The fetus, placenta, and all fluids and tissue in the pregnant uterus	**concept/o-** *to conceive or form*
trimester	A period of 3 months. The time of gestation is divided into three trimesters.	
umbilical cord	Rubbery, flexible cord that connects the placenta to the **umbilicus** (navel) of the fetus. It contains two arteries and one vein.	**umbilic/o-** *umbilicus, (navel)*
zygote	Cell that is the union of a spermatozoon and an ovum. A zygote has 46 chromosomes.	

Labor, Delivery, and Postpartum

Word or Phrase	Description	Combining Forms
Braxton Hicks contractions	Irregular uterine contractions during the last trimester. These strengthen the uterine muscle in preparation for labor. They are also known as false labor.	**contract/o-** *pull together*
cephalic presentation	Position of the fetus in which the head is the presenting part that is first to go through the birth canal. **Vertex presentation** is a type of cephalic presentation in which the top of the head is the presenting part.	**cephal/o-** *head*
cervical ripening	Softening of the cervix as collagen fibers in its wall break down prior to the onset of labor	
colostrum	First milk from the breasts. It is rich in nutrients and contains maternal antibodies to give the newborn passive immunity to common diseases.	
crowning	The top of the fetal head is visible at the vaginal introitus	
dilation	Widening of the cervical os from 0 cm to 10 cm during labor to allow passage of the fetal head	**dilat/o-** *dilate; widen*
effacement	Thinning of the cervical wall, measured as a percentage from 0 percent to 100 percent	**efface/o-** *do away with; obliterate*
engagement	The fetal head drops into position within the mother's pelvis in anticipation of birth. It is also known as **lightening.**	
involution	Process by which the uterus gradually returns to a normal size after childbirth	**involut/o-** *enlarged organ returns to normal size*
lactation	Production of colostrum and then breast milk by the mammary glands after childbirth	**lact/o-** *milk* **lact/i-** *milk* **galact/o-** *milk*

Word or Phrase	Description	Combining Forms
lochia	Small amounts of blood, tissue, and fluid that flow from the uterus after childbirth	
oxytocin	Hormone released by the uterus and by the posterior pituitary gland in the brain. It stimulates the uterus to contract and begin labor. After delivery, it stimulates the uterus to contract to stop hemorrhaging. It stimulates the let-down reflex to get milk flowing for breastfeeding.	**ox/y-** *oxygen; quick* **toc/o-** *labor and childbirth*
parturition	The process of labor and delivery. There are three stages: dilation and effacement of the cervix, delivery of the newborn, delivery of the placenta.	**parturit/o-** *to be in labor*
postnatal period	From the newborn's standpoint, the period of time after birth	**nat/o-** *birth* **par/o-** *birth*
postpartum	From the mother's standpoint, the period of time after delivery	
rupture of the membranes (ROM)	Rupture of the amniotic sac during the first stage of labor, with the release of amniotic fluid that flows out of the vagina	

The Newborn Infant

Word or Phrase	Description	Combining Forms
acrocyanosis	Temporary bluish coloration of the skin of the newborn's face, hands, and feet	**acr/o-** *extremity; highest point* **cyan/o-** *blue*
fontanels	Soft areas on the head between the bones of the cranium in a newborn. In these areas, the brain is only covered with fibrous connective tissue. The largest is the anterior fontanel on the top of the head. There is a smaller posterior fontanel on the back of the head. Fontanels allow the brain to grow before the bones fuse together. They are also known as the soft spots.	
meconium	The first stool passed by a newborn. It is a greenish-black, thick, sticky substance.	
molding	Reshaping of the fetal cranium as it passes through the mother's pelvic bones	
neonate	A newborn from the time of birth until 1 year of age. A **term neonate** is born between 38 and 42 weeks' gestational age. A **preterm** or **premature neonate** is born between 28 to 37 weeks' gestational age. The adjective is **neonatal.**	**ne/o-** *new* **nat/o-** *birth*
vernix caseosa	Thick, white, cheesy substance that covers the skin of the fetus to protect it from amniotic fluid in the uterus	

Labeling Exercise

Match each anatomy word or phrase to its structure and write it in the numbered box for each figure. Be sure to check your spelling. Use the Answer Key at the end of the book to check your answers.

anus	clitoris	labia majora	labia minora	mons pubis	perineum	urethral meatus	vaginal introitus	vulva

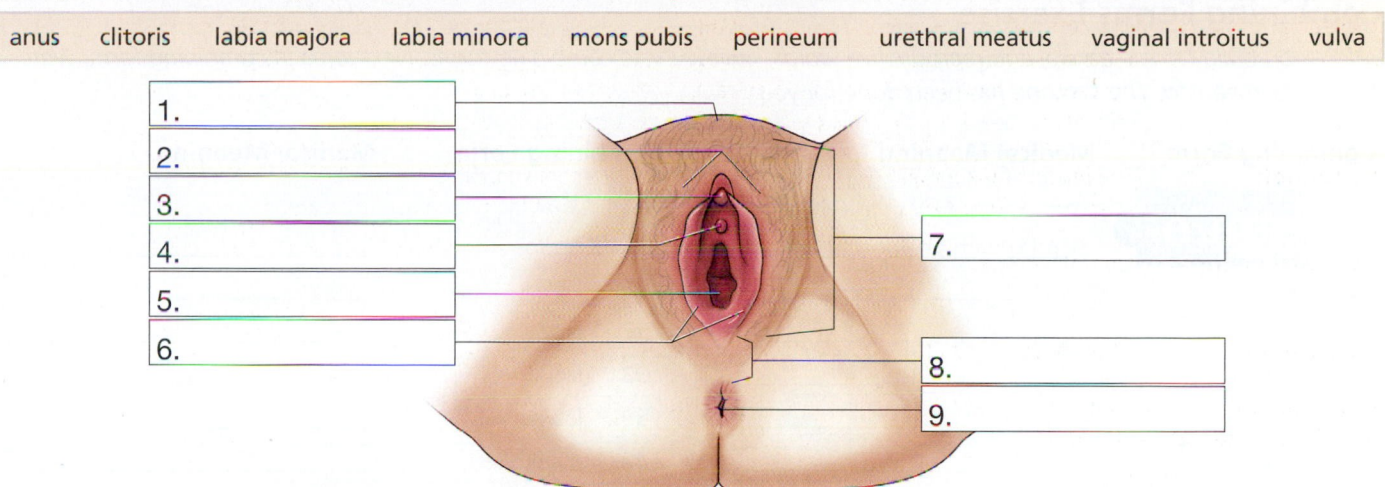

1.
2.
3.
4.
5.
6.
7.
8.
9.

broad ligament	endometrium	intrauterine cavity	ovary	uterine cervix
cervical canal	fimbriae	lumen of uterine tube	ovum	uterine fundus
cervical os	follicle at time of ovulation	myometrium	perimetrium	uterine tube
corpus of uterus	infundibulum	ovarian ligament	round ligament	vagina

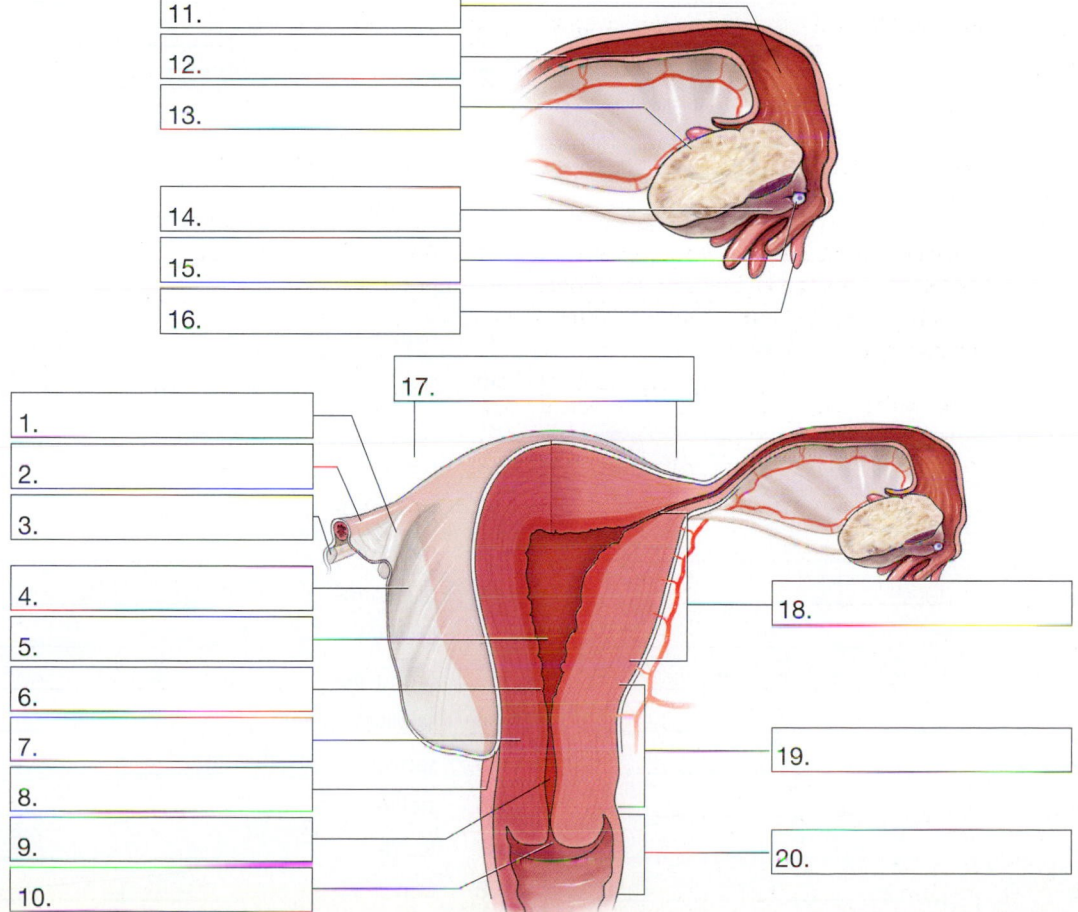

11.
12.
13.
14.
15.
16.
17.

1.
2.
3.
4.
5.
6.
7.
8.
9.
10.

18.
19.
20.

Building Medical Words

Use the Answer Key at the end of the book to check your answers.

Combining Forms Exercise

Before you build female genital and reproductive words, review these combining forms. Next to each combining form, write its medical meaning. The first one has been done for you.

Combining Form	Medical Meaning	Combining Form	Medical Meaning
1. **gon/o-**	seed (ovum or spermatozoon)	35. isch/o-	
2. acr/o-		36. labi/o-	
3. adnex/o-		37. lact/i-	
4. amni/o-		38. lact/o-	
5. areol/o-		39. lob/o-	
6. cephal/o-		40. mamm/a-	
7. cervic/o-		41. mamm/o-	
8. chorion/o-		42. mast/o-	
9. colp/o-		43. men/o-	
10. concept/o-		44. menstru/o-	
11. contract/o-		45. metri/o-	
12. culd/o-		46. metr/o-	
13. cyan/o-		47. my/o-	
14. dilat/o-		48. nat/o-	
15. efface/o-		49. ne/o-	
16. embryon/o-		50. o/o-	
17. episi/o-		51. oophor/o-	
18. estr/a-		52. ovari/o-	
19. estr/o-		53. ov/i-	
20. fallopi/o-		54. ov/o-	
21. fer/o-		55. ovul/o-	
22. fertil/o-		56. ox/y-	
23. fet/o-		57. par/o-	
24. flex/o-		58. part/o-	
25. fratern/o-		59. parturit/o-	
26. fund/o-		60. perine/o-	
27. galact/o-		61. placent/o-	
28. genit/o-		62. pregn/o-	
29. gen/o-		63. product/o-	
30. gestat/o-		64. salping/o-	
31. gonad/o-		65. secret/o-	
32. gynec/o-		66. stal/o-	
33. hyster/o-		67. toc/o-	
34. involut/o-		68. trop/o-	

Combining Form	Medical Meaning		Combining Form	Medical Meaning
69. umbilic/o-	_____		73. uter/o-	_____
70. urethr/o-	_____		74. vagin/o-	_____
71. urin/o-	_____		75. vulv/o-	_____
72. ur/o-	_____			

Combining Form and Suffix Exercise

Read the definition of the medical word. Look at the combining form that is given. Select the correct suffix from the Suffix List and write it on the blank line. Then build the medical word and write it on the line. (Remember: You may need to remove the combining vowel. Always remove the hyphens and slash.) Be sure to check your spelling. The first one has been done for you.

SUFFIX LIST

-al (pertaining to)	-ary (pertaining to)	-ion (action; condition)
-an (pertaining to)	-ation (a process; being or having)	-ization (process of making, creating, or inserting)
-ancy (state of)	-cyte (cell)	
-ant (pertaining to)	-duct (duct; tube)	-ment (action; state)
-ar (pertaining to)	-ic (pertaining to)	-nate (thing that is born)
-arche (a beginning)	-ine (pertaining to)	-tic (pertaining to)

Definition of the Medical Word	Combining Form	Suffix	Build the Medical Word
1. Pertaining to the fundus (of the uterus)	**fund/o-**	**-al**	fundal _____

(You think *pertaining to* (-al) + *the fundus* (fund/o-). You change the order of the word parts to put the suffix last. You write *fundal*.)

Definition of the Medical Word	Combining Form	Suffix	Build the Medical Word
2. Pertaining to the breasts	mamm/o-	_____	_____
3. Pertaining to the uterus	uter/o-	_____	_____
4. Cell (that is an immature) ovum	o/o-	_____	_____
5. Pertaining to the ovary	ovari/o-	_____	_____
6. Pertaining to the areola	areol/o-	_____	_____
7. A process (of having) an ovum (released from the follicle)	ovul/o-	_____	_____
8. A beginning of monthly (periods)	men/o-	_____	_____
9. Pertaining to the cervix	cervic/o-	_____	_____
10. A process (of having) monthly discharge of blood	menstru/o-	_____	_____
11. Pertaining to the amnion	amni/o-	_____	_____
12. A process (of having) milk	lact/o-	_____	_____
13. Pertaining to the accessory connecting parts (the ovary and uterine tube)	adnex/o-	_____	_____
14. Pertaining to the fetus	fet/o-	_____	_____
15. Action to conceive or form	concept/o-	_____	_____
16. Pertaining to being with child	pregn/o-	_____	_____
17. Pertaining to the embryo	embryon/o-	_____	_____
18. Duct (tube that transports) the ovum	ov/i-	_____	_____
19. Pertaining to the vagina	vagin/o-	_____	_____

Definition of the Medical Word	Combining Form	Suffix	Build the Medical Word
20. Pertaining to a lip (structure in the vulvar area)	labi/o-	_____	_____
21. State of being with child	pregn/o-	_____	_____
22. Process of inserting (sperm to be) able to conceive a child	fertil/o-	_____	_____
23. Pertaining to the perineum	perine/o-	_____	_____
24. Thing (baby) that is born new	ne/o-	_____	_____
25. Pertaining to the placenta	placent/o-	_____	_____
26. Action of an enlarged organ (the uterus) returning to normal size	involut/o-	_____	_____
27. Pertaining to the vulva	vulv/o-	_____	_____
28. Action of doing away with or obliterating (the thick wall of the cervix)	efface/o-	_____	_____
29. Condition of conception to birth	gestat/o-	_____	_____

Prefix Exercise

Read the definition of the medical word. Look at the medical word or partial word that is given (it already contains a combining form and a suffix). Select the correct prefix from the Prefix List and write it on the blank line. Then build the medical word and write it on the line. Be sure to check your spelling. The first one has been done for you.

PREFIX LIST		
ante- (forward; before)	peri- (around)	re- (again and again;
endo- (innermost; within)	pre- (before; in front of)	backward; unable to)
intra- (within)	post- (after; behind)	tri- (three)

Definition of the Medical Word	Prefix	Word or Partial Word	Build the Medical Word
1. Pertaining to before the birth	pre-	natal	prenatal
2. Pertaining to within the uterus	_____	uterine	_____
3. Pertaining to again and again producing (children)	_____	productive	_____
4. Condition (of the uterus) of forward bending	_____	flexion	_____
5. A structure (that is) around the uterus	_____	metrium	_____
6. Pertaining to after birth	_____	natal	_____
7. A structure (that is the) innermost (layer) of the uterus	_____	metrium	_____
8. A three-month period (of pregnancy)	_____	mester	_____

Multiple Combining Forms and Suffix Exercise

Read the definition of the medical word. Select the correct suffix and combining forms. Then build the medical word and write it on the line. Be sure to check your spelling. The first one has been done for you.

SUFFIX LIST	COMBINING FORM LIST	
-al (pertaining to)	acr/o- (extremity; highest point)	my/o- (muscle)
-ary (pertaining to)	cyan/o- (blue)	nat/o- (birth)
-esis (a process)	fer/o- (to bear)	ne/o- (new)
-in (a substance)	genit/o- (genitalia)	o/o- (ovum; egg)
-osis (condition; abnormal condition; process)	gen/o- (arising from; produced by)	ox/y- (oxygen; quick)
	lact/i- (milk)	toc/o- (labor and childbirth)
-ous (pertaining to)	metri/o- (uterus; womb)	urin/o- (urine; urinary system)
-um (a structure; period of time)		

Definition of the Medical Word	Combining Form	Combining Form	Suffix	Build the Medical Word
1. Pertaining to milk bear(ing)	**lact/i-**	**fer/o-**	**-ous**	lactiferous
(You think *pertaining to* (-ous) + *milk* (lact/i-) + *bear* (fer/o-). You change the order of the word parts to put the suffix last. You write *lactiferous*.)				
2. Structure of the muscle of the uterus	_____	_____	_____	_____
3. A process of an ovum arising from or produced by (the follicle)	_____	_____	_____	_____
4. Pertaining to a new birth	_____	_____	_____	_____
5. A substance (a hormone that causes) quick labor and childbirth	_____	_____	_____	_____
6. Condition of the extremities (of a newborn being) blue	_____	_____	_____	_____
7. Pertaining to the genital and urinary (system)	_____	_____	_____	_____

Diseases and Conditions

Ovaries and Uterine Tubes

Word or Phrase	Description	Word Building
anovulation	Failure of the ovaries to release a mature ovum at the time of ovulation, although the menstrual cycle is normal. This results in infertility. Anovulation is a normal condition prior to menarche, during pregnancy, and during menopause. Treatment: Hormone drugs to stimulate ovulation.	**anovulation** (AN-aw-vyoo-LAY-shun) **an-** *without; not* **ovul/o-** *ovum (egg)* **-ation** *a process; being or having*
ovarian cancer	**Cancerous** tumor of an ovary. This **malignancy** often does not cause symptoms until it is quite large and has already metastasized. Treatment: Surgical excision and chemotherapy.	**cancerous** (KAN-ser-us) **cancer/o-** *cancer* **-ous** *pertaining to* **malignancy** (mah-LIG-nan-see) **malign/o-** *intentionally causing harm; cancer* **-ancy** *state of*
polycystic ovary syndrome	The ovaries contain multiple cysts (see Figure 13-16 ■). A follicle matures and enlarges, but fails to rupture to release an ovum; it then becomes a cyst. With each menstrual cycle, the cysts enlarge, causing pain. This happens month after month until the ovaries are filled with cysts. This syndrome is associated with amenorrhea or menometrorrhagia, infertility, obesity, and insulin resistance syndrome with the development of type 2 diabetes mellitus. Treatment: Oral contraceptive drug (to correct hormone levels), weight control, oral antidiabetic drug. **Figure 13-16 ■ Polycystic ovary syndrome.** The ovary is filled with both small and large cysts. Some of them contain blood.	**polycystic** (PAWL-ee-SIS-tik) **poly-** *many; much* **cyst/o-** *bladder; fluid-filled sac; semisolid cyst* **-ic** *pertaining to*
salpingitis	Inflammation or infection of the uterine tube that narrows or blocks the lumen of the tube. It is due to endometriosis or pelvic inflammatory disease. With **hydrosalpinx,** inflammation fills the tube with fluid. With **pyosalpinx,** infection fills the tube with pus. Treatment: Treat the underlying cause.	**salpingitis** (SAL-pin-JY-tis) **salping/o-** *uterine (fallopian) tube* **-itis** *inflammation of; infection of* **hydrosalpinx** (HY-droh-SAL-pinks) **hydr/o-** *water; fluid* **-salpinx** *uterine (fallopian) tube* **pyosalpinx** (PY-oh-SAL-pinks) **py/o-** *pus* **-salpinx** *uterine (fallopian) tube*

Uterus

Word or Phrase	Description	Word Building
endometrial cancer	Cancerous tumor of the endometrium of the uterus. The earliest sign is abnormal bleeding. It is also known as **uterine cancer.** Treatment: Hysterectomy; chemotherapy.	

Word or Phrase	Description	Word Building
endometriosis	Endometrial tissue in abnormal places. The endometrium sloughs off during menstruation but is forced upward through the uterine tubes and out into the pelvic cavity because the uterus is in an abnormal, retroflexed position. The endometrial tissue implants itself on the outside of the ovaries and uterus and on the walls of the abdominopelvic cavity. These tissue implants remain alive and sensitive to hormones. Endometrial implants in the uterine tubes cause blockage, scarring, and infertility. Endometriosis on the ovary can form "chocolate cysts" that contain old, dark blood. During each menstrual cycle, the implants in the abdominopelvic cavity thicken and slough off, forming more implants with old blood and tissue debris (see Figure 13-17 ■). They also form adhesions between the internal organs. Endometriosis causes pelvic inflammation, pelvic pain, and pain during sexual intercourse. Treatment: Hormone drugs to suppress the menstrual cycle (to make the implants shrivel up) or laparoscopic surgery to destroy the implants.	**endometriosis** (EN-doh-MEE-tree-OH-sis) **endo-** *innermost; within* **metri/o-** *uterus (womb)* **-osis** *condition; abnormal condition; process*

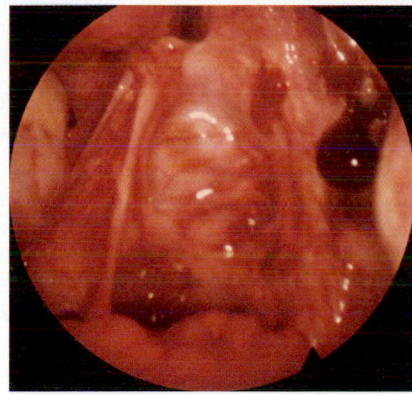

Figure 13-17 ■ Endometriosis.
The cul-de-sac outside of the uterus shows many endometrial implants with evidence of new and old blood.

Word or Phrase	Description	Word Building
leiomyoma	Benign smooth muscle tumor of the myometrium (see Figure 13-18 ■). It can be small or as large as a soccer ball. There is pelvic pain, excessive uterine bleeding, and painful sexual intercourse. Treatment: Uterine artery embolization, myomectomy, or hysterectomy, depending on the size of the tumor.	**leiomyoma** (LIE-oh-my-OH-mah) **lei/o-** *smooth* **my/o-** *muscle* **-oma** *tumor; mass* *Leiomyoma* is a Greek singular noun. Form the plural by changing *-oma* to *-omata*. **leiomyomata** (LIE-oh-my-OH-mah-tah)

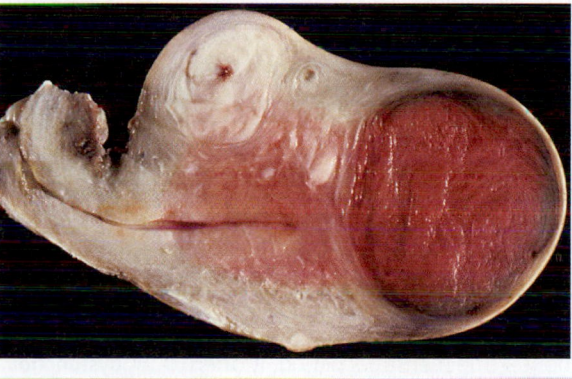

Figure 13-18 ■ Leiomyoma.
This pathology specimen of the cut section of a uterus contains a large, benign, red leiomyoma.

Word or Phrase	Description	Word Building
leiomyosarcoma	Cancerous smooth muscle tumor of the myometrium. Treatment: Hysterectomy and chemotherapy or radiation therapy.	**leiomyosarcoma** (LIE-oh-MY-oh-sar-KOH-mah) **lei/o-** *smooth* **my/o-** *muscle* **sarc/o-** *connective tissue* **-oma** *tumor; mass*

Word or Phrase	Description	Word Building
myometritis	Inflammation or infection of the myometrium. It is associated with pelvic inflammatory disease. **Pyometritis** is an infection of the myometrium that creates pus in the intrauterine cavity. Treatment: Antibiotic drug.	**myometritis** (MY-oh-mee-TRY-tis) **my/o-** *muscle* **metr/o-** *uterus (womb)* **-itis** *inflammation of; infection of* **pyometritis** (PY-oh-mee-TRY-tis) **py/o-** *pus* **metr/o-** *uterus (womb)* **-itis** *inflammation of; infection of*
pelvic inflammatory disease (PID)	Infection of the cervix that ascends to the uterus, uterine tubes, and ovaries. It is often caused by a sexually transmitted disease. There is pelvic pain, fever, and vaginal discharge. If untreated, it can cause scars that block the uterine tubes and infertility. Treatment: Antibiotic drug.	**inflammatory** (in-FLAM-ah-TOR-ee) **inflammat/o-** *redness and warmth* **-ory** *having the function of*
retroflexion of the uterus	Abnormal position in which the entire uterus is bent backward while the cervix is in a normal position. It is associated with the development of endometriosis. It is also known as **retroversion** of the uterus.	**retroflexion** (REH-troh-FLEK-shun) **retro-** *behind; backward* **flex/o-** *bending* **-ion** *action; condition* **retroversion** (REH-troh-VER-shun) **retro-** *behind; backward* **vers/o-** *to travel; to turn* **-ion** *action; condition*
uterine fibroids	Benign fibrous tissue tumor of the myometrium. It can be small or large, and there are usually several. There is pain and prolonged menstrual periods. Treatment: Uterine artery embolization, myomectomy, or hysterectomy, depending on the number and size of the fibroids.	**fibroid** (FY-broyd) **fibr/o-** *fiber* **-oid** *resembling*
uterine prolapse	Descent of the uterus from its normal position. This is caused by stretching of ligaments that support the uterus and weakness in the muscles of the floor of the pelvic cavity. It occurs after childbirth or because of age. The uterus can be so prolapsed that the cervix is visible at the vaginal introitus. Severe prolapse affects urination and bowel movements. It is also known as **uterine descensus.** Treatment: Molded plastic form (a pessary) inserted in the vagina to move the cervix upward; hysterectomy or uterine suspension.	**prolapse** (PROH-laps) **descensus** (dee-SEN-sus)

Menstrual Disorders

Word or Phrase	Description	Word Building
amenorrhea	Absence of monthly menstrual periods. It is caused by a hormone imbalance, thyroid disease, or a tumor of the uterus or ovary. Poor nutrition, stress, chronic disease, intense exercise, or the psychiatric illness of anorexia nervosa can also cause amenorrhea. (*Note:* Amenorrhea is normal before puberty, during pregnancy, and after menopause.) Treatment: Correct the underlying cause.	**amenorrhea** (AH-meh-noh-REE-ah) **a-** *away from; without* **men/o-** *month* **-rrhea** *flow; discharge*
dysfunctional uterine bleeding (DUB)	Sporadic menstrual bleeding without a true menstrual period. It often occurs with anovulation. The endometrium sloughs off from time to time, but never reaches a full thickness because there is no ovulation and no corpus luteum to secrete progesterone. Treatment: Hormone therapy to restore normal menstruation.	**dysfunctional** (dis-FUNK-shun-al) *Dysfunctional* is a combination of the prefix *dys-* (painful; difficult; abnormal), the English word *function* (physiologic working), and the suffix *–al* (pertaining to).

Word or Phrase	Description	Word Building
dysmenorrhea	Painful menstruation. During menstruation, the uterus releases **prostaglandin** to constrict blood vessels in the uterine wall and prevent excessive bleeding. A very high level of prostaglandin causes cramping and temporary ischemia of the myometrium, both of which cause pain. There is also nausea, dizziness, backache, and diarrhea. Pelvic inflammatory disease, endometriosis, or uterine fibroids can also cause dysmenorrhea. Treatment: Nonsteroidal anti-inflammatory drugs to block the production of prostaglandin; correct the underlying cause.	**dysmenorrhea** (DIS-men-oh-REE-ah) **dys-** *painful; difficult; abnormal* **men/o-** *month* **-rrhea** *flow; discharge* **prostaglandin** (PRAWS-tah-GLAN-din)
menopause	Normal cessation of menstrual periods, occurring around middle age. The **perimenopausal period** is the time around menopause when menstrual periods first become irregular and menstrual flow is lighter. Menopause is also known as **climacteric** or the change of life. Treatment: Hormone replacement therapy (HRT) on a short-term basis.	**menopause** (MEN-oh-pawz) **men/o-** *month* **-pause** *cessation* **perimenopausal** (PAIR-ee-MEN-oh-PAW-zal) **peri-** *around* **men/o-** *month* **paus/o-** *cessation* **-al** *pertaining to* **climacteric** (kly-MAK-ter-ik) (KLY-mak-TAIR-ik)

A Closer Look

As a woman ages, the follicles deteriorate and stop secreting estradiol. Ovulation and menstruation cease. Decreased estradiol causes vaginal dryness, vaginal atrophy, and dryness of the skin. The breasts decrease in size. The anterior pituitary gland responds to low estradiol levels in the blood by secreting more follicle-stimulating hormone (FSH). This causes occasional ovulation and menstruation during the perimenopausal period. These bursts of FSH (which often occur at night) produce vasodilation, and the patient experiences hot flashes with perspiration and flushing. Frequent hot flashes throughout the night can cause sleeplessness and fatigue.

Word or Phrase	Description	Word Building
menorrhagia	A menstrual period with excessively heavy flow or a menstrual period that lasts longer than 7 days. It is caused by a hormone imbalance, uterine fibroids, or endometriosis. **Menometrorrhagia** is excessively heavy menstrual flow during menstruation or at other times of the month. **Metrorrhagia** is excessively heavy bleeding at a time other than menstruation. This can be caused by a tubal pregnancy or uterine cancer. Heavy uterine bleeding of any type can cause anemia. Treatment: Hormone therapy or correct the underlying cause.	**menorrhagia** (MEN-oh-RAY-jee-ah) **men/o-** *month* **rrhag/o-** *excessive flow or discharge* **-ia** *condition; state; thing*
oligomenorrhea	A menstrual period with very light flow or infrequent menstrual cycles (longer than 35 days before the next cycle begins) in a woman who previously had normal menstruation. It is caused by a hormone imbalance. Treatment: Hormone therapy.	**oligomenorrhea** (OL-ih-goh-MEN-oh-REE-ah) **olig/o-** *scanty; few* **men/o-** *month* **-rrhea** *flow; discharge*
premenstrual syndrome (PMS)	Breast tenderness, fluid retention, bloating, and mild mood changes (irritability, anger, sadness) a few days before the onset of menstruation. It is caused by high levels of estradiol and progesterone just prior to menstruation. Treatment: Over-the-counter drugs that relieve pain and fluid retention.	**premenstrual** (pree-MEN-stroo-al) **pre-** *before; in front of* **menstru/o-** *monthly discharge of blood* **-al** *pertaining to*

Word or Phrase	Description	Word Building
premenstrual dysphoric disorder (PMDD)	Symptoms of PMS plus feelings of depression, anxiety, tearfulness, mood shifts, difficulty concentrating, sleeping and eating disturbances, and breast, joint, and muscle pain. It is a psychiatric mood disorder caused by an alteration in the levels of the neurotransmitters serotonin and norepinephrine in the brain. Treatment: Antianxiety drugs, antidepressant drugs, and pain reliever drugs.	**dysphoric** (dis-FOR-ik) **dys-** *painful; difficult; abnormal* **phor/o-** *to bear; to carry; range* **-ic** *pertaining to*

Cervix

Word or Phrase	Description	Word Building
cervical cancer	Cancerous tumor of the cervix. If the cancer is still localized, it is **carcinoma *in situ* (CIS).** There is severe dysplasia of the cells as seen on a Pap smear. Later there is ulceration and bleeding. Infection with human papillomavirus (HPV; genital warts, a sexually transmitted disease) predisposes to the development of cervical cancer. Treatment: Conization or hysterectomy.	**carcinoma** (KAR-sih-NOH-mah) **carcin/o-** *cancer* **-oma** *tumor; mass* **in situ** (IN SY-too)
cervical dysplasia	Abnormal growth of squamous cells in the surface layer of the cervix (see Figure 13-19 ■). Cervical dysplasia is seen on an abnormal Pap smear. Severe dysplasia is a precancerous or cancerous condition. Treatment: Treat the underlying infection or cancer. **Figure 13-19 ■ Cervical dysplasia.** A plastic speculum is used to visualize the cervix. The cervix shows a high degree of cervical dysplasia (classified as CIN II on a Pap smear). These areas of redness are abnormal cells that may develop into cancer.	**dysplasia** (dis-PLAY-zee-ah) **dys-** *painful; difficult; abnormal* **plas/o-** *growth; formation* **-ia** *condition; state; thing* Select the correct prefix meaning to get the definition of *dysplasia*: *condition of abnormal growth.*
incompetent cervix	Spontaneous, premature dilation of the cervix during the second trimester of pregnancy. This can result in spontaneous abortion of the fetus. Treatment: Bed rest and placement of a cerclage.	**incompetent** (in-COM-peh-tent)

Vagina and Perineum

Word or Phrase	Description	Word Building
bacterial vaginosis	Bacterial infection of the vagina due to *Gardnerella vaginalis*. There is a white or grayish vaginal discharge that has a fishy odor. This is not a sexually transmitted disease. Treatment: Antibiotic drug.	**vaginosis** (VAJ-ih-NOH-sis) **vagin/o-** *vagina* **-osis** *condition; abnormal condition; process*
candidiasis	Yeast infection of the vagina due to *Candida albicans*. There is vaginal itching and **leukorrhea,** a cheesy, white discharge. Candidiasis can occur after taking an antibiotic drug for a bacterial infection; the drug kills the disease-causing bacteria but also kills the normal bacterial flora of the vagina. Then yeast, which is not affected by the antibiotic drug, multiplies and causes an infection. Treatment: Antiyeast drug applied topically in the vagina.	**candidiasis** (KAN-dih-DY-ah-sis) **candid/o-** *Candida (a yeast)* **-iasis** *state of; process of* **leukorrhea** (LOO-koh-REE-ah) **leuk/o-** *white* **-rrhea** *flow; discharge*
cystocele	Herniation of the bladder into the vagina because of a weakness in the vaginal wall. It is caused by childbirth or age. It can result in urinary retention. Treatment: Colporrhaphy.	**cystocele** (SIS-toh-seel) **cyst/o-** *bladder; fluid-filled sac; semisolid cyst* **-cele** *hernia*
dyspareunia	Painful or difficult sexual intercourse. This can happen when the hymen is across the vaginal introitus or because of infection (of the vagina, cervix, or uterus), pelvic inflammatory disease, endometriosis, or retroflexion of the uterus. Treatment: Correct the underlying cause.	**dyspareunia** (DIS-pah-ROO-nee-ah) **dys-** *painful; difficult; abnormal* **pareun/o-** *sexual intercourse* **-ia** *condition; state; thing*
rectocele	Herniation of the rectum into the vagina because of a weakness in the vaginal wall. It is caused by childbirth or age. It can interfere with bowel movements. Treatment: Colporrhaphy.	**rectocele** (REK-toh-seel) **rect/o-** *rectum* **-cele** *hernia*
vaginitis	Vaginal inflammation or infection. It can be caused by irritation from chemicals in spermicidal jelly or douches. It can also be caused by candidiasis (yeast infection) or a sexually transmitted disease. Treatment: Treat the underlying cause.	**vaginitis** (VAJ-ih-NY-tis) **vagin/o-** *vagina* **-itis** *inflammation of; infection of*

Clinical Connections

Public Health. The first cases of **toxic shock syndrome** were seen in women in 1980. There was a high fever, vomiting, diarrhea, and hypotension (shock). Physicians interviewed patients and family members to discover a common link. All of the patients had used super-absorbent **tampons** during their menstrual period. The super-absorbent tampons held the menstrual blood over an extended period of time until the normally harmless vaginal bacterium *Staphylococcus aureus* multiplied in the old blood and released toxins. Also, the larger size of the tampon created small tears in the vaginal wall that allowed the toxins to enter the blood.	**toxic** (TAWK-sik) **tox/o-** *poison* **-ic** *pertaining to* **tampon** (TAM-pawn)

Breasts

Word or Phrase	Description	Word Building

breast cancer	**Cancerous** tumor, usually an **adenocarcinoma** of the lactiferous lobules of the breast. A lump is detected upon mammography or breast self-examination. There can be swelling in the area, enlarged lymph nodes, and nipple discharge. Advanced breast cancer has **peau d'orange,** dimpling of the breast skin, and nipple retraction (see Figures 13-20 ■ and 13-21 ■). Long-term hormone replacement therapy with an estrogen drug after menopause increases the risk of breast cancer. The genetic mutations BRCA1 or BRCA2 increase the risk of developing breast cancer. Treatment: Lumpectomy or mastectomy, chemotherapy, radiation therapy.	**adenocarcinoma** (AD-eh-noh-KAR-sih-NOH-mah)
		  aden/o- *gland*
		  carcin/o- *cancer*
		  -oma *tumor; mass*
		
		peau d'orange (poh-deh-RAHNJ)

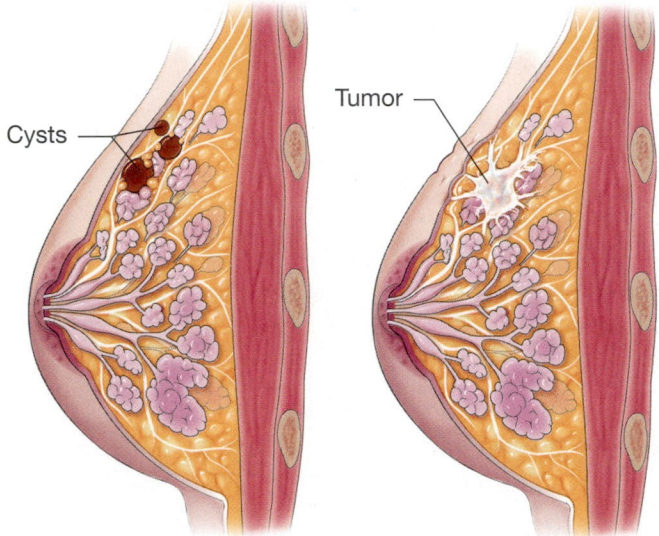

Figure 13-20 ■ Breast with cancer and cysts.
A lump in the breast can be a benign cyst (fibrocystic disease) or it can be cancer. The presence of many cysts can make it difficult to detect a cancerous tumor on mammography.

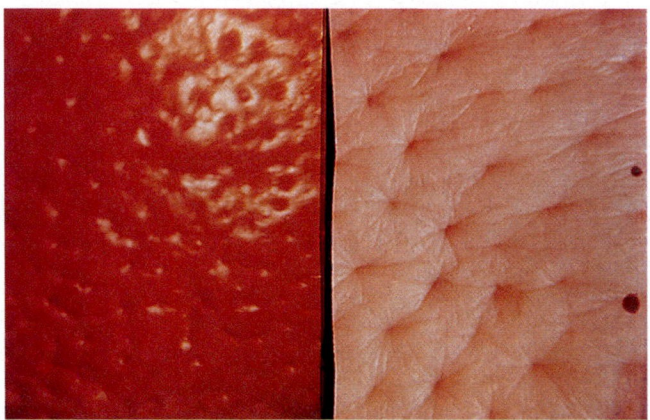

Figure 13-21 ■ Peau d'orange.
As a cancerous tumor spreads, it pulls on structures inside the breast, and this causes the dimpling effect on the skin (right) of peau d'orange, which resembles the pores in the skin of an orange (left).

Word or Phrase	Description	Word Building

failure of lactation	Lack of production of milk in the breasts following pregnancy. It is caused by hyposecretion of prolactin from the anterior pituitary gland. The breasts do not produce milk or produce insufficient milk to breast-feed the baby. Treatment: Switch to bottle feeding.	**lactation** (lak-TAY-shun)
		  lact/o- *milk*
		  -ation *a process; being or having*

fibrocystic disease	Benign condition in which numerous fibrous and fluid-filled cysts form in one or both breasts (see Figure 13-20). The size of the cysts can change in response to hormone levels. The cysts are painful and tender. Severe fibrocystic disease makes it difficult to detect a cancerous tumor on mammography, and so the physician may order an MRI scan instead. Treatment: Hormone therapy. Elimination of certain foods (chocolate, caffeine) from the diet sometimes helps.	**fibrocystic** (FY-broh-SIS-tik)
		  fibr/o- *fiber*
		  cyst/o- *bladder; fluid-filled sac; semisolid cyst*
		  -ic *pertaining to*

galactorrhea	Discharge of milk from the breasts when the patient is not pregnant or breastfeeding. It is caused by an increased level of prolactin from an adenoma (benign tumor) of the anterior pituitary gland. Treatment: Drug to decrease prolactin production or surgery to remove the adenoma from the anterior pituitary gland in the brain.	**galactorrhea** (gah-LAK-toh-REE-ah)
		  galact/o- *milk*
		  -rrhea *flow; discharge*

Pregnancy and Labor and Delivery

Word or Phrase	Description	Word Building
abnormal presentation	Birth position in which the presenting part of the fetus is not the head. In a **breech** presentation, the presenting part is the buttocks, buttocks and feet, or just the feet (see Figure 13-22 ■). If the fetus is in a transverse lie (the fetal vertebral column is perpendicular to the mother's vertebral column), the shoulder or arm is the presenting part. It is also known as **malpresentation** of the fetus (see Figure 13-23 ■). Treatment: Version maneuver to turn the fetus or delivery by cesarean section.	**breech** (BREECH) **malpresentation** (MAL-pree-sen-TAY-shun) The prefix *mal-* means *bad; inadequate.*

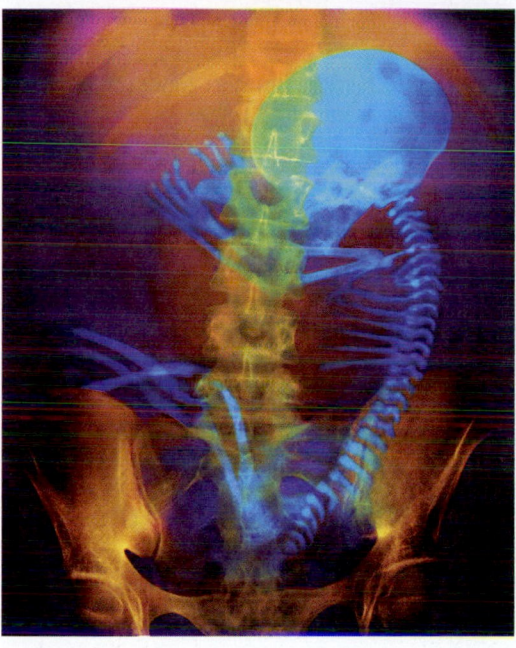

Figure 13-22 ■ Breech position.
This colorized x-ray shows a single fetus in a breech presentation. The fetal spine is on the right-hand side of the image, and the legs are bent.

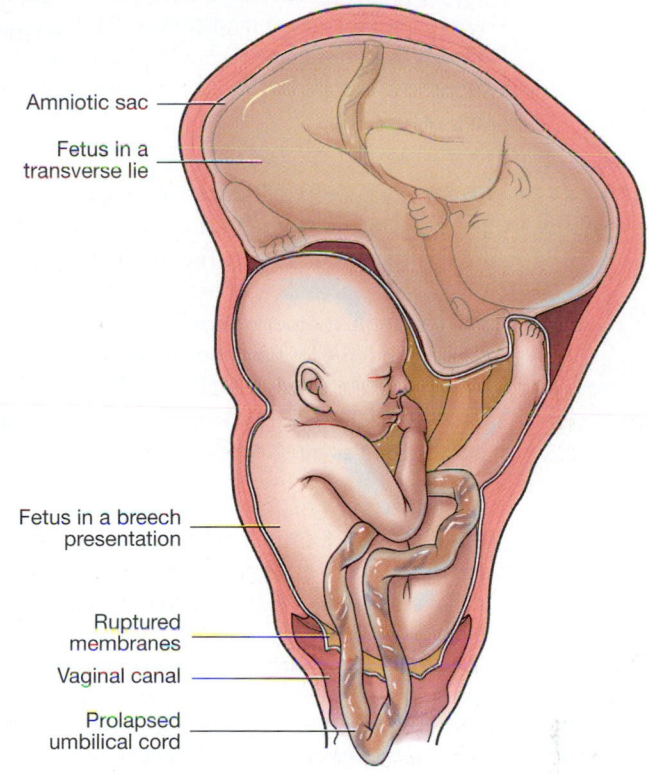

Amniotic sac

Fetus in a transverse lie

Fetus in a breech presentation

Ruptured membranes

Vaginal canal

Prolapsed umbilical cord

Figure 13-23 ■ Malpresentation of fraternal twins.
One twin is in the breech position with the buttocks as the presenting part. The amniotic sac around this fetus has already ruptured, and the umbilical cord has prolapsed into the vaginal canal. The second twin, still in its amniotic sac, is in a transverse lie position.

Word or Phrase	Description	Word Building
abruptio placentae	Complete or partial separation of the placenta from the uterine wall before the third stage of labor. This results in uterine hemorrhage that threatens the life of the mother as well as disruption of blood flow and oxygen through the umbilical cord, which threatens the life of the fetus. Treatment: Emergency cesarean section.	**abruptio placentae** (ab-RUP-shee-oh plah-SEN-tee)

cephalopelvic disproportion (CPD)	The size of the fetal head exceeds the size of the opening in the mother's pelvic bones. Treatment: Cesarean section.	**cephalopelvic** (SEF-ah-loh-PEL-vik)
		   cephal/o- *head*
		   pelv/o- *pelvis (hip bone; renal pelvis)*
		   -ic *pertaining to*
		disproportion (DIS-proh-POR-shun)

Did You Know?

Skeletons of prehistoric women have been discovered that show cephalopelvic disproportion with the skull of the baby still tightly wedged in the mother's pelvic bones.

Word or Phrase	Description	Word Building
dystocia	Any type of difficult or abnormal labor and delivery. Treatment: Correct the underlying cause.	**dystocia** (dis-TOH-see-ah) **dys-** *painful; difficult; abnormal* **toc/o-** *labor and childbirth* **-ia** *condition; state; thing*
ectopic pregnancy	Implantation of a fertilized ovum somewhere other than in the uterus. It can occur in the cervix, ovary, or abdomen, but most commonly occurs in the uterine tube (a **tubal pregnancy**). This occurs more readily if the uterine tube has scar tissue or a blockage in it. The patient has a positive pregnancy test, but there is abdominal tenderness as the uterine tube swells from the developing embryo. The tube can bleed, a condition known as **hemosalpinx.** The tube can suddenly rupture, causing severe blood loss and shock. Treatment: Salpingectomy to remove the embryo and uterine tube.	**ectopic** (ek-TOP-ik) **ectop/o-** *outside of a place* **-ic** *pertaining to* **tubal** (TOO-bal) **tub/o-** *tube* **-al** *pertaining to* **hemosalpinx** (HEE-moh-SAL-pinks) **hem/o-** *blood* **-salpinx** *uterine (fallopian) tube*
gestational diabetes mellitus	Temporary disorder of glucose metabolism that occurs only during pregnancy. Increased levels of estradiol and progesterone block the action of insulin from the pancreas. The function of insulin is to metabolize glucose. A decreased level of insulin leads to a high level of unmetabolized glucose in the mother's blood. Excess glucose crosses the placenta and causes the fetus to grow too rapidly (because its pancreas produces insulin that metabolizes the glucose). Treatment: Dietary management, oral antidiabetic drug during pregnancy. This condition ceases with childbirth, but the mother often develops type 2 diabetes mellitus later in life.	**gestational** (jes-TAY-shun-al) **gestat/o-** *from conception to birth* **-ation** *a process; being or having* **-al** *pertaining to* **diabetes** (DY-ah-BEE-teez) **mellitus** (MEL-ih-tus)
hydatidiform mole	Abnormal union of an ovum and spermatozoon. It produces hundreds of small, fluid-filled sacs but no embryo. The chorion produces HCG, so the patient has early signs of pregnancy. However, the hydatidiform mole grows more rapidly than a normal pregnancy, and the uterus is much larger than expected for the gestational age. Surgery: Removal of the hydatidiform mole or hysterectomy.	**hydatidiform** (HY-dah-TID-ih-form) **hydatidi/o-** *fluid-filled vesicles* **-form** *having the form of* **mole** (MOHL)
mastitis	Inflammation or infection of the breast. It is caused by milk engorgement in the breast or by an infection, usually due to the bacterium *Staphylococcus aureus* from the infant's mouth or the mother's skin. The affected breast is red and swollen, and the mother has a fever. Treatment: Pumping of breast milk. Antibiotic drug to treat the infection.	**mastitis** (mas-TY-tis) **mast/o-** *breast; mastoid process* **-itis** *inflammation of; infection of*
morning sickness	Nausea and vomiting during the first trimester of pregnancy. It is thought to be due to elevated estradiol and progesterone levels. **Hyperemesis gravidarum** is excessive vomiting that causes weakness, dehydration, and fluid and electrolyte imbalance. Treatment: Intravenous fluids for severe hyperemesis gravidarum.	**hyperemesis** (HY-per-EM-eh-sis) **hyper-** *above; more than normal* **-emesis** *condition of vomiting* **gravidarum** (GRAV-ih-DAIR-um)
oligohydramnios	Decreased volume of amniotic fluid. The fetus swallows amniotic fluid but does not excrete a similar volume in its urine because of a congenital abnormality of the fetal kidneys. Treatment: Surgery to the fetus while *in utero* or after birth.	**oligohydramnios** (OL-ih-goh-hy-DRAM-nee-ohs) **olig/o-** *scanty; few* **hydr/o-** *water; fluid* **-amnios** *amniotic fluid* **in utero** (IN YOO-ter-oh)

Word or Phrase	Description	Word Building
placenta previa	Incorrect position of the placenta with its edge partially or completely covering the cervical canal (see Figure 13-24 ■). During labor when the cervix dilates, the connection between the placenta and uterus is disrupted. This causes moderate-to-severe bleeding in the mother and disrupts the flow of blood to the fetus. Treatment: Cesarean section.	**placenta previa** (plah-SEN-tah PREE-vee-ah)

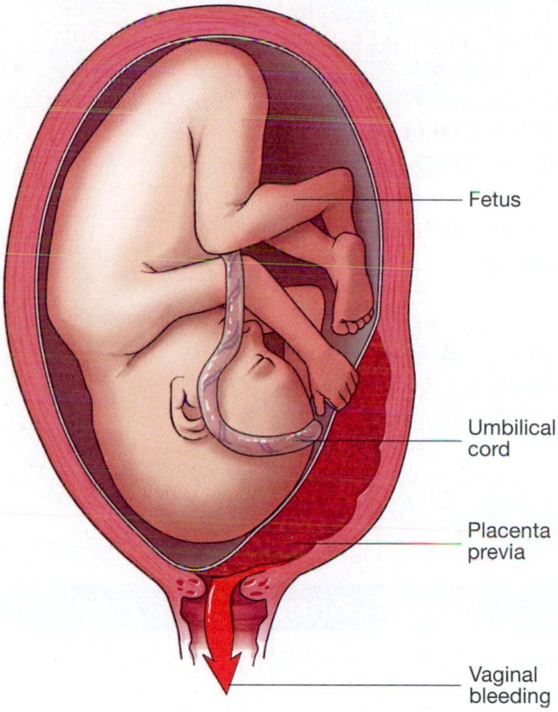

Fetus

Umbilical cord

Placenta previa

Vaginal bleeding

Figure 13-24 ■ Placenta previa.
A low position of the placenta can cause bleeding when the cervix dilates during labor and delivery.

Word or Phrase	Description	Word Building
polyhydramnios	Increased volume of amniotic fluid. It is caused by maternal diabetes mellitus, twin gestation, abnormalities in the fetus. Treatment: Correct the underlying cause.	**polyhydramnios** (PAWL-ee-hy-DRAM-nee-ohs) **poly-** *many; much* **hydr/o-** *water; fluid* **-amnios** *amniotic fluid*
postpartum hemorrhage	Continual bleeding from the site where the placenta separated after delivery. The uterus is boggy and does not become firm. It is caused by hyposecretion of oxytocin from the posterior pituitary gland in the brain. Treatment: Manual massage of the uterus. Intravenous drug therapy with an oxytocin drug.	**hemorrhage** (HEM-oh-rij) **hem/o-** *blood* **-rrhage** *excessive flow or discharge*
preeclampsia	Hypertensive disorder of pregnancy with increased blood pressure, edema, weight gain, and protein in the urine (proteinuria). The nephrons of the kidneys allow large protein molecules from the blood to be lost in the urine. A low level of protein changes the osmotic pressure of the blood and allows fluid to move into the tissues where it collects as edema. Preeclampsia can progress to **eclampsia** in which the patient has seizures. Treatment: Bed rest, antihypertensive and antiseizure drugs.	**preeclampsia** (PREE-ee-KLAMP-see-ah) **pre-** *before; in front of* **eclamps/o-** *a seizure* **-ia** *condition; state; thing* **eclampsia** (ee-KLAMP-see-ah)
premature labor	Regular uterine contractions that occur before the fetus is mature. The cervix can dilate and small amounts of blood or amniotic fluid can leak out. Treatment: Bed rest, tocolytic drug.	
premature rupture of membranes (PROM)	Spontaneous rupture of the amniotic sac and loss of amniotic fluid before labor begins. The mother must deliver or risk the development of infection within 24 hours. Treatment: Induction of labor.	

Word or Phrase	Description	Word Building
prolapsed cord	A loop of umbilical cord becomes caught between the presenting part of the fetus and the birth canal (see Figure 13-23). This occurs if the membranes rupture before the fetal head (or other presenting part) is fully engaged in the mother's pelvis. With each uterine contraction, the umbilical cord is compressed, causing decreased blood flow to the fetus and fetal distress. Treatment: Change the mother's position to move the position of the cord, give oxygen to the mother. Surgery: Cesarean section.	**prolapse** (PROH-laps)

spontaneous abortion (SAB)	Loss of a pregnancy. An early spontaneous abortion usually occurs because of a genetic abnormality or poor implantation of the embryo within the endometrium. A later spontaneous abortion can occur because of preterm labor or an incompetent cervix. In an incomplete abortion, the embryo or fetus is expelled but the placenta and other tissues remain in the uterus. It is also known as a **miscarriage.**	**abortion** (ah-BOR-shun)
		  abort/o- *stop prematurely*
		  -ion *action; condition*

uterine inertia	Weak or uncoordinated contractions during labor. It is caused by (1) decreased levels of oxytocin from the posterior pituitary gland; (2) a uterus that is very distended with multiple fetuses and unable to contract normally; or (3) cephalopelvic disproportion or malpresentation of the fetus. A related condition is **arrest of labor** in which uterine contractions have ceased. It is also known as **failure to progress,** as the cervix does not dilate and efface. Treatment: Intravenous oxytocin drug; cesarean section for cephalopelvic disproportion; version or cesarean section for malpresentation.	**inertia** (in-ER-shah) (in-ER-shee-ah)

Clinical Connections

Psychiatry (Chapter 17). Postpartum depression is a mood disorder with symptoms of mild-to-moderate depression, anxiousness, irritability, tearfulness, and fatigue. It is caused by hormonal changes after birth and by feelings of overwhelming responsibility and fatigue. It was formerly known as **involutional melancholia** because it occurs at the time of involution of the uterus.

Dietetics. A lack of folic acid during pregnancy can cause a neural tube defect in the fetus. Prenatal vitamins for pregnant women and enrichment of cereals and other grain products with added folic acid have greatly decreased the incidence of neural tube defects.

There are many stories about the food cravings of pregnant women: pickles, ice cream, and so forth. Some pregnant women experience **pica,** an unnatural craving for and compulsive eating of substances with no nutritional value, such as clay, chalk, starch, or dirt.

depression (dee-PRESH-un)
  depress/o- *press down*
  -ion *action; condition*

involutional (IN-voh-LOO-shun-al)
  involut/o- *enlarged organ returns to normal size*
  -ion *action; condition*
  -al *pertaining to*

melancholia (MEL-an-KOH-lee-ah)
  melan/o- *black*
  chol/o- *bile; gall*
  -ia *condition; state; thing*

pica (PY-kah) (PEE-kah)

Fetus and Neonate

| apnea | Temporary or permanent cessation of breathing in the newborn after birth. The newborn is said to be **apneic.** The immature central nervous system of a newborn fails to maintain a consistent respiratory rate, and there are occasional long pauses between periods of regular breathing. Treatment: Apnea monitor in the hospital and at home. | **apnea** (AP-nee-ah)
  a- *away from; without*
  -pnea *breathing*
apneic (AP-nee-ik)
  a- *away from; without*
  pne/o- *breathing*
  -ic *pertaining to* |

Word or Phrase	Description	Word Building
fetal distress	Lack of oxygen to the fetus because of decreased blood flow through the placenta or umbilical cord. The fetus has bradycardia and passes meconium because of the stress of a decreased level of oxygen. Treatment: Mother is given oxygen; possible cesarean section.	
growth abnormalities	Many factors affect the growth rate of the embryo and fetus. Maternal illness, malnutrition, and smoking can make the fetus **small for gestational age (SGA)**. This is known as **intrauterine growth retardation (IUGR)**. Diabetes mellitus in the mother can make the fetus **large for gestational age (LGA)**. A fetus within the normal growth range for weight and length is said to be **appropriate for gestational age (AGA)**. Treatment: Correct the underlying cause.	

jaundice	Yellowish discoloration of the skin in a newborn. During gestation, the fetus has extra red blood cells that are no longer needed at birth. Their destruction releases hemoglobin, which is converted into unconjugated bilirubin. The immature newborn liver is not able to conjugate this much bilirubin, and it builds up in the blood (**hyperbilirubinemia**), moves into the tissues, and causes jaundice. The more premature the newborn, the greater the chance of developing jaundice. Treatment: **Phototherapy** with bililights, special fluorescent lights that break down bilirubin in the skin to make it water soluble so it can be excreted by the kidneys.	**jaundice** (JAWN-dis)
		
		hyperbilirubinemia (HY-per-BIL-ih-ROO-bih-NEE-mee-ah)
		  hyper- *above; more than normal*
		  bilirubin/o- *bilirubin*
		  -emia *condition of the blood; substance in the blood*
		
		phototherapy (FOH-toh-THAIR-ah-pee)
		  phot/o- *light*
		  -therapy *treatment*

meconium aspiration	Fetal distress causes the fetus to pass meconium into the amniotic fluid. This can get in the mouth and nose, and, if inhaled with the first breath, it causes severe respiratory distress. Treatment: Suctioning of the newborn's nose and mouth. Use of oxygen and a ventilator after birth.	**aspiration** (AS-pih-RAY-shun)
		  aspir/o- *to breathe in; to suck in*
		  -ation *a process; being or having*

nuchal cord	Umbilical cord is wrapped around the neck of the fetus. A loose nuchal cord can be present without causing a problem. A tight nuchal cord with one or more loops around the neck can impair blood flow to the brain, causing brain damage or fetal death. Treatment: Emergency cesarean section.	**nuchal** (NOO-kal)
		  nuch/o- *neck*
		  -al *pertaining to*

respiratory distress syndrome (RDS)	Difficulty inflating the lungs to breathe because of a lack of surfactant. This occurs mainly in premature newborns. It was previously known as hyaline membrane disease (HMD). Treatment: Surfactant drug given through the endotracheal tube; oxygen and a ventilator.	**respiratory** (RES-pih-rah-TOR-ee) (reh-SPYR-ah-tor-ee)
		  re- *again and again; backward; unable to*
		  spir/o- *breathe; a coil*
		  -atory *pertaining to*

Laboratory and Diagnostic Procedures

Gynecologic Diagnostic Procedures

Word or Phrase	Description	Word Building
acid phosphatase	Enzyme from the prostate gland that is found in the semen. The presence of acid phosphatase in the vagina indicates sexual intercourse and can be used in rape investigations.	**acid phosphatase** (AS-id FAWS-fah-tays)

BRCA1 or BRCA2 gene	Blood test that shows if a patient has inherited the BRCA1 or BRCA2 gene, **genetic** mutations that significantly increase the risk of developing breast or ovarian cancer. BRCA stands for **br**east **ca**ncer.	**gene** (JEEN)
		 genetic (jeh-NET-ik)
		  gene/o- *gene*
		  -tic *pertaining to*

biopsy	Procedure to remove a small piece of tissue for examination to look for abnormal or cancerous cells. A breast biopsy can be done by **fine-needle aspiration** (a very fine needle is inserted into the mass and a syringe is used to aspirate tissue) or by **vacuum-assisted biopsy** (a probe with a cutting device is inserted through the skin and rotated to pull in multiple specimens). For an endometrial biopsy, a speculum is used to visualize the cervix and a dilator expands the cervical os. A pipette or catheter is inserted into the uterus and rotated while suction pulls in tissue. This is used to diagnose abnormal uterine bleeding and uterine cancer. For larger biopsy specimens, a surgical procedure is performed. First mammography or ultrasound is used to identify the location of the mass, and a needle or wire marker is inserted to pinpoint the site. A **stereotactic biopsy** uses three different angles of mammography to precisely locate the mass. For an **incisional biopsy,** an incision is made in the skin overlying the mass and a large part (but not all) of the mass is removed. For an **excisional biopsy,** the entire mass is removed along with a surrounding margin of normal tissue.	**biopsy** (BY-awp-see)
		  bi/o- *life; living organisms; living tissue*
		  -opsy *process of viewing*
		 aspiration (AS-pih-RAY-shun)
		  aspir/o- *to breathe in; to suck in*
		  -ation *a process; being or having*
		 stereotactic (STAIR-ee-oh-TAK-tic)
		  stere/o- *three dimensions*
		  tact/o- *touch*
		  -ic *pertaining to*
		 incisional (in-SIH-shun-al)
		  incis/o- *to cut into*
		  -ion *action; condition*
		  -al *pertaining to*
		 excisional (ek-SIH-shun-al)
		  excis/o- *to cut out*
		  -ion *action; condition*
		  -al *pertaining to*

estrogen receptor assay	**Cytology** test performed on breast tissue that has already been diagnosed as malignant. This test looks for a large number of estrogen receptors on the tumor cell. If present, this means that the tumor requires estrogen (estradiol) in order to grow and that chemotherapy drugs that block estrogen would be effective in treating this cancer.	**receptor** (ree-SEP-tor)
		  recept/o- *receive*
		  -or *person or thing that produces or does*
		 assay (AS-say)
		 cytology (sy-TAWL-oh-jee)
		  cyt/o- *cell*
		  -logy *the study of*

Word or Phrase	Description	Word Building

Pap smear	Screening cytology test used to detect abnormal cells or carcinoma *in situ* (CIS) in the cervix. It is also known as a Pap test. This is an **exfoliative cytology** test because it examines cells that have been scraped off of the cervix. A small plastic or wooden spatula is used to scrape off **ectocervical cells** from the outside wall of the cervix. Then a **cytobrush** is inserted into the cervical os to obtain **endocervical cells** (see Figure 13-25 ■). A cervical broom (Papette®) can obtain both types of cells at the same time and also test for HPV. The cell specimen is transferred to a glass slide and sprayed with a fixative. Alternatively, with **liquid cytology**, the specimen is rinsed in a vial of fixative. This captures all the cells, prevents cell drying, and gives a more accurate result. The slides or vials are sent to the laboratory where the cells are examined under a microscope for abnormalities (see Figure 13-26 ■). The Bethesda System is used to report Pap smear results.	**Pap smear**
		
		 exfoliative (eks-FOH-lee-ah-tiv)
		
		 cytology (sy-TAWL-oh-jee)
		   cyt/o- *cell*
		   -logy *the study of*
		
		 ectocervical (EK-toh-SER-vih-kal)
		   ecto- *outermost; outside*
		   cervic/o- *neck; cervix*
		   -al *pertaining to*
		
		 endocervical (EN-doh-SER-vih-kal)
		   endo- *innermost; within*
		   cervic/o- *neck; cervix*
		   -al *pertaining to*

(continued)

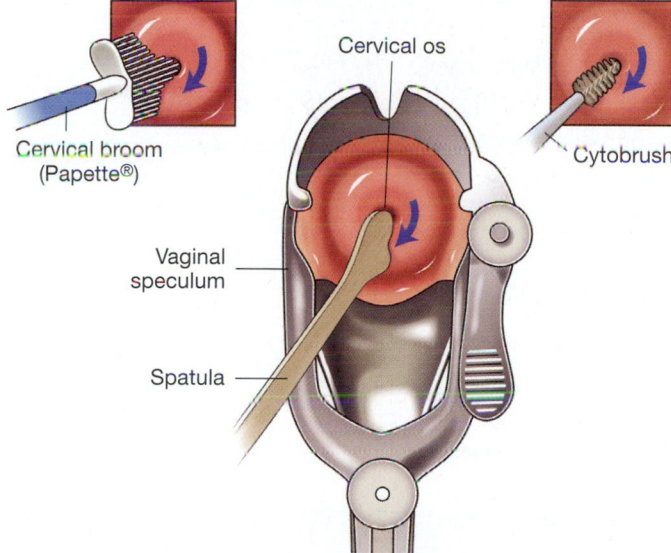
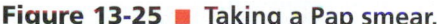

Figure 13-25 ■ Taking a Pap smear.
A metal vaginal speculum is used to move the vaginal walls apart to expose the cervix. Cells from the cervix are obtained using a wooden spatula and a cytobrush or by using a cervical broom (Papette®). A microscope is used to examine the cells and detect cells that are precancerous or cancerous.

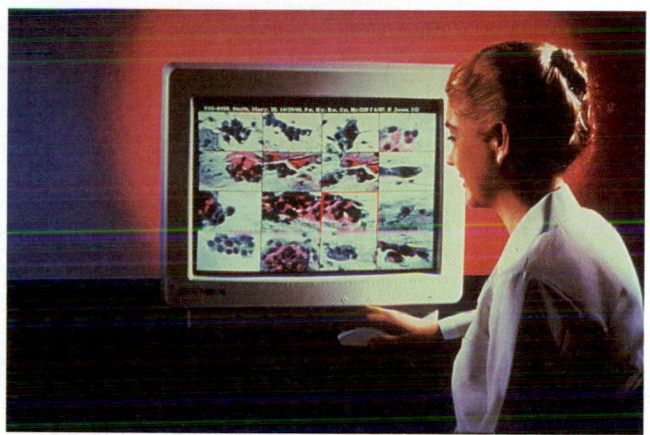

Figure 13-26 ■ Reading a Pap smear.
This pathologist is using a viewing screen and special computer software to review Pap smears to look for evidence of cancer.

Word or Phrase	Description	Word Building
Pap smear (*continued*)	<table><tr><td colspan="2">**A Closer Look**</td></tr></table>	

A Closer Look

PAP SMEAR TERMINOLOGY

(Bethesda System Guidelines)

Specimen Adequacy

- Satisfactory (enough cells were collected; cell quality was sufficient for diagnosis)
- Unsatisfactory (enough cells were not collected; cell quality was poor)

Normal Pap Smear

Findings are reported as:

    Negative for intraepithelial lesion or malignancy. (The presence of infectious organisms [Trichomonas, herpes, HPV] is also reported.)

Abnormal Pap Smear

Findings are reported as one of the following:

ASC-US	Atypical squamous cells of unknown significance
ASC-H	Atypical squamous cells of unknown significance, cannot exclude HSIL
LSIL*	Low-grade squamous intraepithelial lesion
HSIL**	High-grade squamous intraepithelial lesion
SCC	Squamous cell carcinoma

*LSIL includes several levels that are classified as cervical intraepithelial neoplasia (CIN I).
**HSIL includes several levels that are classified as CIN II through III.

Word or Phrase	Description	Word Building
wet mount	Cytology test for yeasts, parasites, or bacteria. A swab of vaginal discharge is sent to the laboratory. The cells are placed on a slide, mixed with saline solution, and examined under a microscope. It is also known as a **wet prep.**	

Infertility Diagnostic Tests

Word or Phrase	Description	Word Building
antisperm antibody test	Test that detects antibodies against sperm in the woman's cervical mucus. Some antibodies attack the tail of the spermatozoon so that it cannot swim; other antibodies prevent the spermatozoon from penetrating the ovum. Men produce antibodies to their own spermatozoa after a vasectomy when the spermatozoa must be absorbed by the body. These antibodies remain even after reversal of the vasectomy.	**antibody** (AN-tee-BAWD-ee) (AN-tih-BAWD-ee) **anti-** *against* **-body** *a structure or thing*
hormone testing	Blood test to determine the levels of FSH and LH from the anterior pituitary gland and estradiol and progesterone from the ovaries. It is used to diagnose menstruation and infertility problems.	

Pregnancy and Neonatal Diagnostic Tests

Word or Phrase	Description	Word Building

amniocentesis	Test of the amniotic fluid. Using ultrasound guidance, a needle is inserted through the abdomen and into the uterus to obtain amniotic fluid (see Figure 13-27 ■). This is done between 15 and 18 weeks' gestation. The following tests are performed.
	
	1. **Chromosome studies** of fetal skin cells can determine the sex of the fetus and identify genetic abnormalities such as Down syndrome.
	2. **Alpha fetoprotein (AFP).** An increased level indicates a neural tube defect (myelomeningocele).
	3. **L/S ratio** (lecithin/sphingomyelin) test for fetal lung maturity. **Lecithin** is a component of surfactant that keeps the alveoli from collapsing with each exhalation. The **sphingomyelin** level is higher when the fetal lungs are immature; when the lungs are mature the lecithin level is higher. 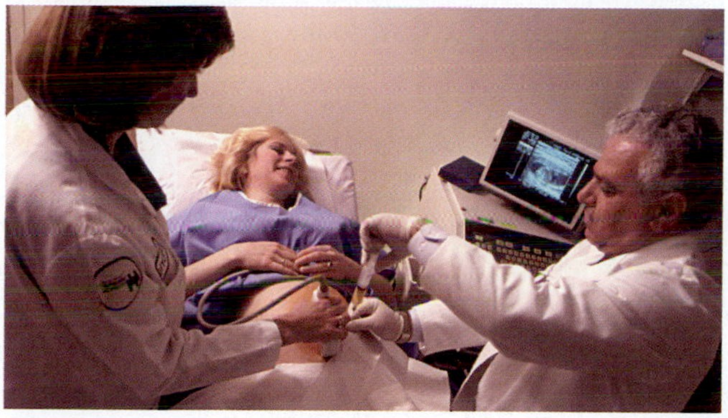
	
	Figure 13-27 ■ Amniocentesis.
	The obstetrician is withdrawing amniotic fluid through a needle inserted into the intrauterine cavity. The position of the needle was verified by ultrasound (as shown on the monitor screen). The technician is holding the ultrasound transducer that is emitting sound waves to produce the image.
		amniocentesis (AM-nee-oh-sen-TEE-sis)
		  amni/o- *amnion (fetal membrane)*
		  -centesis *procedure to puncture*
		
		chromosome (KROH-moh-sohm)
		  chrom/o- *color*
		  -some *a body*
		Add words to make a complete definition of *chromosome: a body (within the nucleus that takes on) color (when stained).*
		
		alpha fetoprotein
		(AL-fah FEE-toh-PROH-teen)
		
		lecithin (LES-ih-thin)
		
		sphingomyelin (SFING-goh-MY-eh-lin)

chorionic villus sampling (CVS)	Genetic test of the chorionic villi of the placenta. A needle is inserted through the abdomen, or a catheter is inserted through the cervix to aspirate placental tissue. This test is performed when a fetal genetic defect is suspected. It can be performed at 12 weeks, which is earlier than an amniocentesis, but it cannot detect neural tube defects in the fetus.	**chorionic** (KOH-ree-ON-ik)
		  chorion/o- *chorion (fetal membrane)*
		  -ic *pertaining to*
		
		villus (VIL-us)
		Villus is a Latin singular noun. Form the plural by changing *–us* to *–i.*

pregnancy test	Blood test to detect human chorionic gonadotropin (HCG) secreted by the fertilized ovum. Serum HCG is positive just 9 days after conception. Home pregnancy tests that detect HCG in the urine are easy to use but are not always accurate. Only a positive blood test (serum beta HCG) is diagnostic of pregnancy. The presence of HCG does not indicate that the pregnancy is normal because HCG is also produced in an ectopic pregnancy and hydatidiform mole.	

Radiologic Procedures

Word or Phrase	Description	Word Building
hystero-salpingography	Procedure in which radiopaque contrast dye is injected through the cervix into the uterus. It coats and outlines the uterus and uterine tubes and shows narrowing, scarring, and blockage. The x-ray image is a **hysterosalpingogram.** This test is done as part of an infertility workup.	**hysterosalpingography** (HIS-ter-oh-SAL-ping-GAWG-rah-fee) **hyster/o-** *uterus (womb)* **salping/o-** *uterine (fallopian) tube* **-graphy** *process of recording* **hysterosalpingogram** (HIS-ter-oh-sal-PING-goh-gram) **hyster/o-** *uterus (womb)* **salping/o-** *uterine (fallopian) tube* **-gram** *a record or picture*
mammography	Procedure that uses x-rays to create an image of the breast. The breast is compressed and slightly flattened (see Figure 13-28 ■). Mammography is used to detect areas of microcalcification, infection, cysts, and tumors, many of which cannot be felt on a breast examination. The x-ray image is a **mammogram.** Xeromammography uses a special plate instead of an x-ray plate, and the image is developed with dry powder rather than liquid chemicals. The image is printed on paper and is a **xeromammogram.** 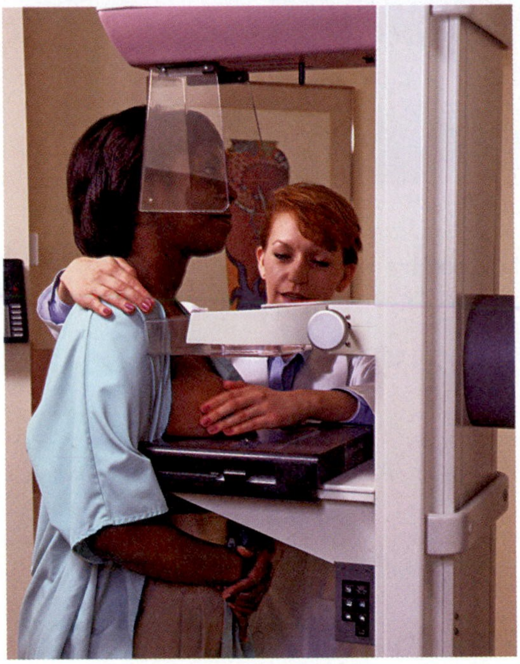 **Figure 13-28 ■ Mammography.** A mammogram is the image obtained when an x-ray beam passes through the breast to an x-ray plate. The breast is compressed because the less distance the x-ray travels the sharper the image that is obtained.	**mammography** (mah-MAWG-rah-fee) **mamm/o-** *breast* **-graphy** *process of recording* **mammogram** (MAM-oh-gram) **mamm/o-** *breast* **-gram** *a picture or record* **xeromammography** (ZEER-oh-mah-MAWG-rah-fee) **xer/o-** *dry* **mamm/o-** *breast* **-graphy** *process of recording* **xeromammogram** (ZEER-oh-MAM-oh-gram) **xer/o-** *dry* **mamm/o-** *breast* **-gram** *a picture or record*

Word or Phrase	Description	Word Building

ultrasonography	Radiologic procedure that uses ultra high-frequency sound waves emitted by a transducer or probe to produce an image on a computer screen. Three-dimensional ultrasonography couples the ultrasound with a position sensor to generate a high-resolution image in three dimensions (see Figure 13-29 ■). The **ultrasound** image is a **sonogram.**
	
	Ultrasonography of the breast or uterus can differentiate between benign, fluid-filled tumors (cysts) and solid tumors that need to be biopsied. A pelvic ultrasound can be used to diagnose a normal pregnancy versus a hydatidiform mole or ectopic pregnancy. In early pregnancy, the beating heart is seen. The image can show multiple fetuses and the sex of the fetus. An ultrasound is done routinely at 16–20 weeks in a normal pregnancy to estimate the gestational age. Serial ultrasounds can be done over time if there is a question of intrauterine growth retardation. The length of the femur, the **biparietal diameter (BPD)** (distance between the two parietal bones of the cranium), and the crown-to-rump length are used to calculate the gestational age of the fetus. The image can show the position of the placenta to diagnose placenta previa. Pelvic ultrasound is used during amniocentesis to locate a large area of amniotic fluid in which to insert the needle (see Figure 13-27). A **transvaginal ultrasound** uses an ultrasound probe inserted into the vagina to determine the thickness of the endometrium in patients with abnormal uterine bleeding.
		ultrasonography
		(UL-trah-soh-NAWG-rah-fee)
		  ultra- *beyond; higher*
		  son/o- *sound*
		  -graphy *process of recording*
		
		ultrasound (UL-trah-sound)
		
		sonogram (SAWN-oh-gram)
		  son/o- *sound*
		  -gram *a record or picture*
		
		biparietal (BY-pah-RY-eh-tal)
		  bi- *two*
		  pariet/o- *wall of a cavity*
		  -al *pertaining to*
		
		transvaginal (trans-VAJ-ih-nal)
		  trans- *across; through*
		  vagin/o- *vagina*
		  -al *pertaining to*

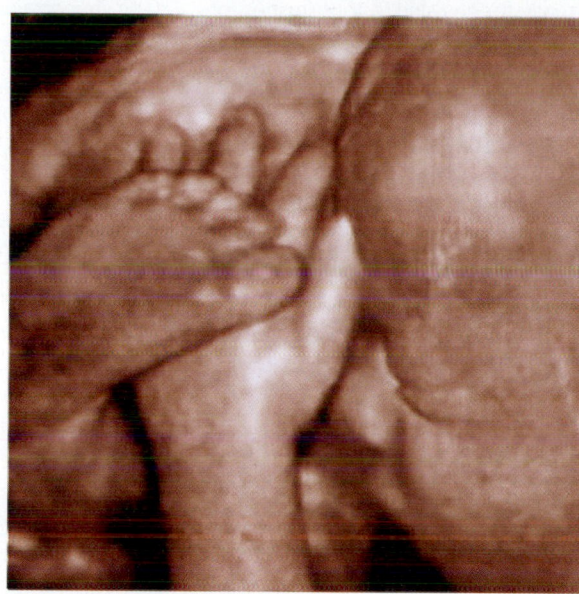

Figure 13-29 ■ Three-dimensional ultrasonography.
Sound waves generated by a transducer bounce off the uterus and are captured to create a computer image. The fine details of the fetus are clearly visible in this type of ultrasound.

Medical and Surgical Procedures

Medical Procedures of the Internal Genitalia

Word or Phrase	Description	Word Building
colposcopy	Procedure that uses a magnifying, lighted scope to visually examine the vagina and cervix	**colposcopy** (kohl-PAWS-koh-pee) **colp/o-** *vagina* **-scopy** *process of using an instrument to examine*
cryosurgery	Procedure to destroy small areas of abnormal tissue on the cervix. Colposcopy is used to visualize the cervical lesions. Then a **cryoprobe** containing extremely cold liquid nitrogen is touched to the areas to freeze and destroy the abnormal tissues.	**cryosurgery** (KRY-oh-SER-jer-ee) **cry/o-** *cold* **surg/o-** *operative procedure* **-ery** *process of* **cryoprobe** (KRY-oh-prohb) **cry/o-** *cold* **-probe** *rodlike instrument*
gynecologic examination	Procedure to physically examine the external and internal genitalia. This is performed with the patient supine in the **dorsal lithotomy position.** The hips and knees are flexed, and the feet are elevated in stirrups. The external genitalia are examined visually for any skin lesions, rashes, or discharge from the vagina. The internal genitalia are examined using a **bimanual examination** (see Figure 13-30 ■). A mass, cystocele, rectocele, or any enlargement of the uterus can be palpated with the gloved hands. Tenderness to palpation can indicate infection or endometriosis. A **speculum** is inserted into the vagina and a Pap smear is performed (see Figure 13-31 ■). The cervix is examined visually for abnormalities.	**gynecologic** (GY-neh-koh-LAW-jik) **gynec/o-** *female; woman* **log/o-** *word; the study of* **-ic** *pertaining to* **dorsal** (DOR-sal) **dors/o-** *back; dorsum* **-al** *pertaining to* **lithotomy** (lih-THAW-toh-mee) **lith/o-** *stone* **-tomy** *process of cutting or making an incision* **speculum** (SPEK-yoo-lum) **bimanual** (by-MAN-yoo-al) **bi-** *two* **manu/o-** *hand* **-al** *pertaining to*

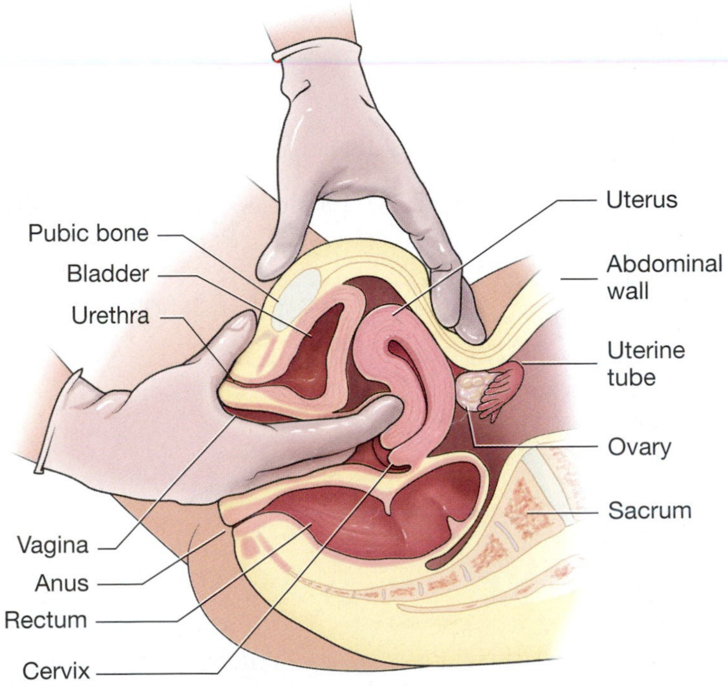

Pubic bone

Bladder

Urethra

Vagina

Anus

Rectum

Cervix

Uterus

Abdominal wall

Uterine tube

Ovary

Sacrum

Figure 13-30 ■ Bimanual examination.

By using both hands, the physician is able to examine the shape of the uterus and detect tenderness and masses.

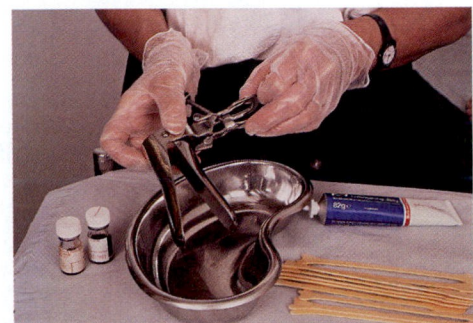

Figure 13-31 ■ Speculum.

A speculum (metal or plastic) has two blades that are pressed together when the speculum is inserted into the vagina and then move apart to separate the walls of the vaginal canal so that the cervix can be seen.

Medical Procedures of the Breast

Word or Phrase	Description	Word Building
breast self-examination (BSE)	Systematic palpation of all areas of the breast and under the arm to detect lumps, masses, or enlarged lymph nodes (see Figure 13-32 ■). BSE should be done monthly to detect early signs of breast cancer. 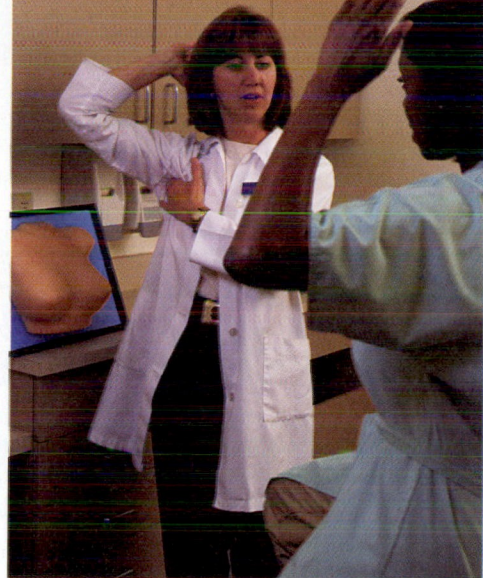 **Figure 13-32 ■ Breast self-examination.** This nurse is instructing the patient on how to perform self-examination of the breasts. All areas of the breasts are palpated in a systematic way. The lymph nodes under the arm are also palpated for any sign of enlargement.	
Tanner staging	System used to describe the development of the female breasts from childhood through puberty. There are five different stages, from Tanner stage 1 (nipple and areola are flat against the chest wall) to Tanner stage 5 (enlargement of the entire breast). The Tanner system is also used to describe the development of the female external genitalia.	

Medical Procedures for Obstetrics

amniotomy	Procedure in which a hook is inserted into the cervical os to rupture the amniotic sac and induce labor	**amniotomy** (AM-nee-AW-toh-mee) **amni/o-** *amnion (fetal membrane)* **-tomy** *process of cutting or making an incision*
Apgar score	Procedure that assigns a score to a newborn at 1 and 5 minutes after birth. Points (0–2) are given for the heart rate, respiratory rate, muscle tone, response to stimulation, and skin color, for a total possible score of 10.	**Apgar** (AP-gar)
assisted delivery	Procedure in which obstetrical forceps or a vacuum extractor is used to facilitate delivery of the head of the fetus (see Figure 13-13)	
epidural anesthesia	Local anesthesia produced by injecting an anesthetic drug into the epidural space between vertebrae in the lower back. This blocks pain and sensation from the abdomen, perineum, and legs and decreases labor pain. Epidural anesthesia is not given until the cervix is already more than 4 cm dilated; otherwise, it can prolong labor.	**epidural** (EP-ih-DOO-ral) **epi-** *upon; above* **dur/o-** *dura mater* **-al** *pertaining to* **anesthesia** (AN-es-THEE-zee-ah) **an-** *without; not* **esthes/o-** *sensation; feeling* **-ia** *condition; state; thing*

Word or Phrase	Description	Word Building
fundal height	The distance in centimeters from the top of the symphysis pubis to the top of the uterine fundus. It is a general indication of fetal growth.	**fundal** (FUN-dal) **fund/o-** *fundus (part farthest from the opening)* **-al** *pertaining to*
induction of labor	Procedure that uses an oxytocin drug to cause labor to begin. This is done when the mother is past her estimated due date or when the health of the mother or fetus necessitates delivery.	**induction** (in-DUK-shun) **induct/o-** *a leading in* **-ion** *action; condition*
Nägele's rule	Procedure used to calculate the patient's estimated date of birth (EDB) or due date. Often the patient does not remember the date of the first day of her last menstrual period (LMP), and so the EDB is just an approximate date. Estimated date of confinement (EDC) is an older phrase that indicated when a woman was to be confined to her home around her due date.	**Nägele** (NAY-gel)
nonstress test (NST)	An external monitor on the mother's abdomen prints out the fetal heart rate. A normal test (reactive test) will show at least two fetal heart rate accelerations associated with fetal movement. A nonreactive test, which is abnormal, is followed by a **biophysical profile (BPP)** that combines a nonstress test with an ultrasound to show fetal movement, fetal heart rate, and amniotic fluid volume.	**biophysical** (BY-oh-FIZ-ih-kal) **bi/o-** *life; living organisms; living tissue* **physic/o-** *body* **-al** *pertaining to*
obstetrical history	Good prenatal care includes documentation of past pregnancies and deliveries. A **nulligravida** is a woman who has never been pregnant and is not pregnant now. A **primigravida** is a woman who is pregnant for the first time. A **multigravida** is a woman who has been pregnant more than once. If she has borne many children, she is said to be **multiparous.** In the past, the obstetrical history was documented as **gravida (G), para (P),** and **abortion (Ab).** A woman who was G3, P3, Ab 0 had been pregnant three times and given birth three times. A woman who had had twins would be G1, P2. The G/TPAL system is used more often now because it provides more details. G Number of times pregnant T Number of term births P Number of premature births A Number of abortions (spontaneous or induced) L Number of living children	**nulligravida** (NUL-ih-GRAV-ih-dah) **null/i-** *none* **-gravida** *pregnancy* **primigravida** (PRY-mih-GRAV-ih-dah) **prim/i-** *first* **-gravida** *pregnancy* **multigravida** (MUL-tih-GRAV-ih-dah) **mult/i-** *many* **-gravida** *pregnancy* **multiparous** (mul-TIP-ah-rus) **mult/i-** *many* **par/o-** *birth* **-ous** *pertaining to* **gravida** (GRAV-ih-dah) **para** (PAIR-ah) **abortion** (ah-BOR-shun) **abort/o-** *stop prematurely* **-ion** *action; condition*
therapeutic abortion (TAB)	Procedure for planned termination of a pregnancy at any time during gestation. All products of conception are removed from the uterus with suction. It is also known as an **elective abortion.**	**therapeutic** (THAIR-ah-PYOO-tik) **therapeut/o-** *treatment* **-ic** *pertaining to* **abortion** (ah-BOR-shun) **abort/o-** *stop prematurely* **-ion** *action; condition* **elective** (ee-LEK-tiv)
version	Procedure to manually correct a breech or other malpresentation prior to delivery. The physician puts his/her hands on the mother's abdominal wall and manipulates the position of the fetus.	**version** (VER-zhun) **vers/o-** *to travel; to turn* **-ion** *action; condition*

A Closer Look

Assisted reproductive technology (ART) uses technology to assist the process of conception. For *in vitro* **fertilization (IVF),** the woman receives ovulation-stimulating drugs. Then mature ova are harvested with a needle inserted into the ovary. Some of the ova are combined with spermatozoa and allowed to grow from 2 to 5 days in a culture medium. Then one fertilized ovum (or more) is placed in the uterus. The newborns were known as test tube babies. For **zygote intrafallopian transfer (ZIFT),** the same procedure is followed but the fertilized ovum (zygote) is grown outside the mother for several days and then is placed in the uterine (fallopian) tube. For **gamete intrafallopian transfer (GIFT),** the ova and spermatozoa (gametes) are collected, but then both are placed in the uterine (fallopian) tube.

When the man has a low sperm count or the woman's cervical mucus contains antibodies against sperm, the man's sperm may be collected, concentrated, and inserted directly into the uterus, a procedure known as **intrauterine insemination.** In men with a very low sperm count, sperm can be taken from the testis or epididymis. Then, under a microscope, a micropipette is used to inject a single sperm into one ovum, a procedure known as **intracytoplasmic sperm injection (ICSI)** (see Figure 13-33 ■)

in vitro (IN VEE-troh)

intrafallopian
(IN-trah-fah-LOH-pee-an)
  intra- *within*
  fallopi/o- *uterine (fallopian) tube*
  -an *pertaining to*

insemination (in-SEM-ih-NAY-shun)
  insemin/o- *plant a seed*
  -ation *a process; being or having*

intracytoplasmic
(IN-trah-SY-toh-PLAS-mik)
  intra- *within*
  cyt/o- *cell*
  plasm/o- *plasma*
  -ic *pertaining to*

injection (in-JEK-shun)
  inject/o- *insert; put in*
  -ion *action; condition*

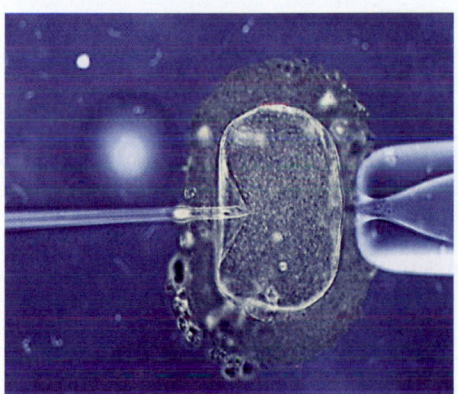

Figure 13-33 ■ Intracytoplasmic sperm injection (ICSI).
A type of assisted reproductive technology. Under the microscope, a micropipette (on the left) is used to penetrate an ovum and insert a single spermatozoon to fertilize it.

Surgical Procedures of the Uterus, Uterine Tubes, and Ovaries

Word or Phrase	Description	Word Building

dilation and curettage (D&C)	Procedure to remove abnormal tissue from inside the uterus. The cervix is dilated with progressively larger dilators inserted into the cervical os. A **tenaculum** (long, scissors-like instrument with two curved, pointed ends) is used to grasp and hold the cervix. Then a **curet** (instrument with a sharp-edged circular or oval ring at one end) is inserted to scrape the endometrium. Alternatively, a vacuum aspirator is inserted to suction out pieces of endometrium. This procedure is performed for abnormal uterine bleeding or suspected uterine cancer. It is also used to perform a therapeutic abortion or remove the products of conception following a spontaneous but incomplete abortion.	**dilation** (dy-LAY-shun)
		   dilat/o- *dilate; widen*
		   -ion *action; condition*
		
		 curettage (kyoo-reh-TAWZH)
		
		 tenaculum (teh-NAK-yoo-lum)
		
		 curet (kyoo-RET)

endometrial ablation	Procedure that uses heat or cold to destroy the endometrium. A laser, hot fluid in a balloon, or an electrode with electrical current is inserted into the uterus. Alternatively, a cryoprobe is inserted to freeze the endometrium. It is used to treat dysfunctional uterine bleeding.	**ablation** (ah-BLAY-shun)
		   ablat/o- *take away; destroy*
		   -ion *action; condition*

Word or Phrase	Description	Word Building
hysterectomy	Procedure to remove the uterus. An **abdominal hysterectomy** is performed with a laparoscope through an abdominal incision. A **vaginal hysterectomy** is performed through the vagina. A total hysterectomy involves removing both the uterus and cervix. A **TAH-BSO** is a total abdominal hysterectomy and bilateral salpingo-oophorectomy (removal of both uterine tubes and ovaries). A hysterectomy is done because of uterine fibroids, endometriosis, uterine prolapse, abnormal uterine bleeding, or uterine or cervical cancer. A radical hysterectomy to treat cancer of the uterus involves removal of the uterus, cervix, upper vagina, and pelvic lymph nodes.	**hysterectomy** (HIS-ter-EK-toh-mee) **hyster/o-** *uterus (womb)* **-ectomy** *surgical excision*
laparoscopy	Procedure to visualize the abdominopelvic cavity, uterus, uterine tubes, and ovaries for diagnosis, biopsy, or surgery. A small incision is made near the umbilicus, and carbon dioxide gas is used to inflate the abdominal cavity. Then a **laparoscope,** a fiberoptic **endoscope,** is inserted through the incision (see Figure 13-34 ■). Grasping and cutting instruments are inserted through other abdominal incisions. Pelvic adhesions, pelvic inflammatory disease, and endometriosis can be treated, and a **laparoscopic** hysterectomy can be done, if needed.	**laparoscopy** (LAP-ah-RAWS-koh-pee) **lapar/o-** *abdomen* **-scopy** *process of using an instrument to examine* **laparoscope** (LAP-ah-ROH-skohp) **lapar/o-** *abdomen* **-scope** *instrument used to examine* **endoscope** (EN-doh-skohp) **endo-** *innermost; within* **-scope** *instrument used to examine* **laparoscopic** (LAP-ah-roh-SKAWP-ik) **lapar/o-** *abdomen* **scop/o-** *examine with an instrument* **ic-** *pertaining to*

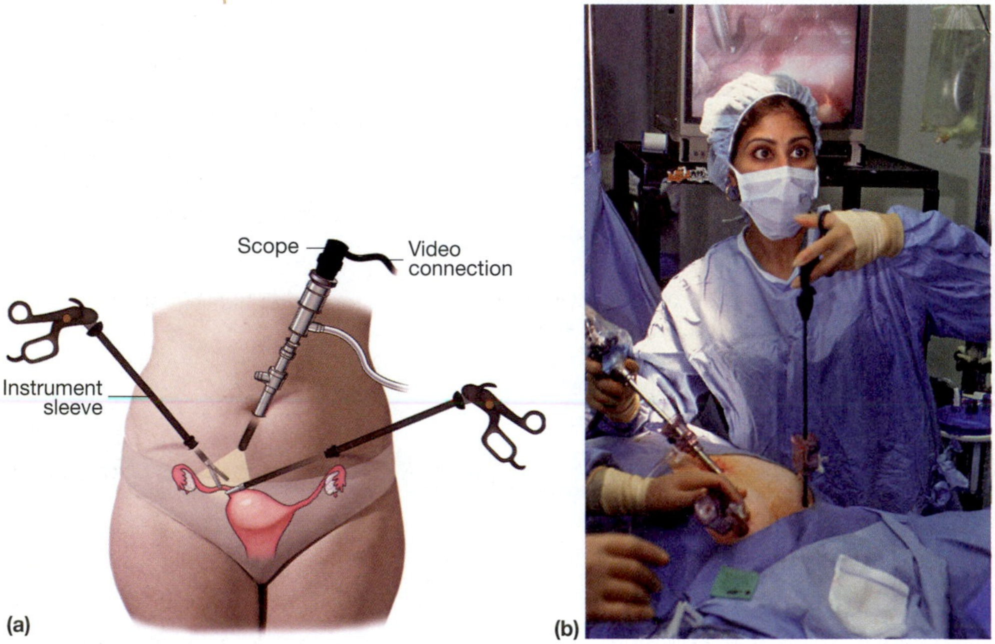

Scope — Video connection

Instrument sleeve

(a)   (b)

Figure 13-34 ■ Laparoscopic surgery.
(a) Small incisions in the abdomen allow visualization of the uterus, uterine tubes, and ovaries with a lighted scope. (b) The image can be seen on screens in the operating room. The surgeon watches the image on the screen as she manipulates the grasping and cutting instruments.

Word or Phrase	Description	Word Building
myomectomy	Procedure to remove leiomyomata or fibroids from the uterus. This procedure can be done vaginally or through a laparoscope in the abdomen.	**myomectomy** (MY-oh-MEK-toh-mee) **my/o-** *muscle* **om/o-** *tumor; mass* **-ectomy** *surgical excision*
oophorectomy	Procedure to remove an ovary because of large ovarian cysts or ovarian cancer. A **bilateral oophorectomy** removes both ovaries.	**oophorectomy** (OH-of-or-EK-toh-mee) **oophor/o-** *ovary* **-ectomy** *surgical excision* **bilateral** (by-LAT-er-al) **bi-** *two* **later/o-** *side* **-al** *pertaining to*

Word or Phrase	Description	Word Building
salpingectomy	Procedure to remove the uterine tube because of ovarian cancer or an ectopic pregnancy in the tube. A bilateral salpingectomy removes both uterine tubes. A **bilateral salpingo-oophorectomy (BSO)** removes both uterine tubes and both ovaries.	**salpingectomy** (SAL-pin-JEK-toh-mee) **salping/o-** *uterine (fallopian) tube* **-ectomy** *surgical excision* **salpingo-oophorectomy** (sal-PING-goh-OH-of-or-EK-toh-mee) **salping/o-** *uterine (fallopian) tube* **oophor/o-** *ovary* **-ectomy** *surgical excision*
tubal ligation	Procedure to prevent pregnancy. A short segment of each uterine tube is removed. The cut ends are sutured and then crushed or cauterized. The woman continues to ovulate, but the ovum cannot travel to the uterus and sperm cannot reach the ovum. It is also known as "getting your tubes tied." A **tubal anastomosis** is a procedure to rejoin the uterine tube segments so that the woman can get pregnant again.	**tubal** (TOO-bal) **tub/o-** *tube* **-al** *pertaining to* **ligation** (ly-GAY-shun) **ligat/o-** *to tie up; to bind* **-ion** *action; condition* **anastomosis** (ah-NAS-toh-MOH-sis) **anastom/o-** *create an opening between two structures* **-osis** *condition; abnormal condition; process*
uterine artery embolization	Procedure used to treat uterine fibroids. A catheter is inserted into the femoral artery in the groin and threaded to the uterine artery. Radiopaque contrast dye is injected to identify the smaller artery that supplies blood to a large fibroid. Tiny particles are injected to block that artery. Without a blood supply, the fibroid shrinks in size.	**embolization** (EM-bol-ih-ZAY-shun) **embol/o-** *embolus (occluding plug)* **-ization** *process of making, creating, or inserting*
uterine suspension	Procedure to suspend and fix the uterus in an anatomically correct position. It is used to correct a retroverted uterus or uterine prolapse. The ligaments holding the uterus are shortened, which pulls the uterus up into a normal position. It is also known as a **hysteropexy.**	**suspension** (sus-PEN-shun) **suspens/o-** *hanging* **-ion** *action; condition* **hysteropexy** (HIS-ter-oh-PEK-see) **hyster/o-** *uterus (womb)* **-pexy** *process of surgically fixing in place*

Surgical Procedures of the Cervix and Vagina

Word or Phrase	Description	Word Building
colporrhaphy	Procedure to suture a weakness in the vaginal wall. This procedure is done to correct a cystocele or a rectocele.	**colporrhaphy** (kohl-POR-ah-fee) **colp/o-** *vagina* **-rrhaphy** *procedure of suturing*
conization	Procedure to remove a large, cone-shaped section of tissue that includes the cervical os and part of the cervical canal. It is used to diagnose a lesion or excise an abnormal area identified by a Pap smear. A laser knife or a loop electrosurgical excision procedure (LEEP) with a hot wire loop is used to burn and cut away the tissue. Alternately, a scalpel (cold knife conization) can be used so that no cells are damaged by heat.	**conization** (KOH-nih-ZAY-shun) **con/o-** *cone* **-ization** *the process of making, creating, or inserting*
culdoscopy	Procedure in which an endoscope is inserted into the vagina and then pushed through the posterior wall of the vagina (in the area of the cul-de-sac behind the cervix) and into the pelvic cavity. This procedure is performed under local anesthesia and leaves no abdominal scars. It is used to examine the cul-de-sac and the external surfaces of the uterus, uterine tubes, and ovaries for signs of endometriosis or adhesions.	**culdoscopy** (kul-DAWS-koh-pee) **culd/o-** *cul-de-sac* **-scopy** *process of using an instrument to examine*

Surgical Procedures of the Breast

Word or Phrase	Description	Word Building
lumpectomy	Procedure to excise a small malignant tumor of the breast. Adjacent normal breast tissue and the axillary lymph nodes are also removed in case any cancerous cells have already spread to them.	**lumpectomy** (lum-PEK-toh-mee) *Lumpectomy* is a combination of the English word *lump* and the suffix *–ectomy* (surgical excision).
mammaplasty	Procedure to change the size, shape, or position of the breast. It is also known as a **mammoplasty**. An **augmentation mammaplasty** enlarges the size of a small breast by inserting a breast **prosthesis** or implant under the skin or chest muscles (see Figure 13-35 ■). A **reduction mammaplasty** reduces the size of a large, **pendulous** breast. The procedure can be performed in conjunction with a **mastopexy** or breast lift to reposition a sagging breast. A **reconstructive mammaplasty** is done to reconstruct a breast after a mastectomy. 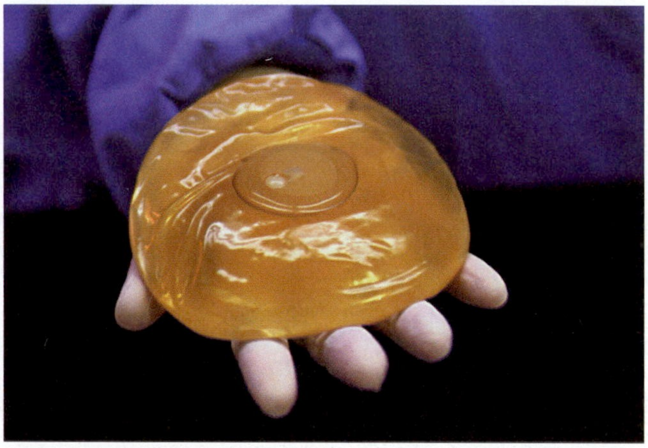 **Figure 13-35 ■ Breast implant.** A breast implant is a soft-walled container filled with silicone gel or saline (salt water). It is placed beneath the skin of the breast or beneath the pectoralis major muscle of the chest.	**mammaplasty** (MAM-ah-PLAS-tee) **mamm/a-** *breast* **-plasty** *process of reshaping by surgery* **mammoplasty** (MAM-oh-plas-tee) **mamm/o-** *breast* **-plasty** *process of reshaping by surgery* **augmentation** (AWG-men-TAY-shun) **augment/o-** *increase in size or degree* **-ation** *a process; being or having* **prosthesis** (praws-THEE-sis) **reduction** (re-DUK-shun) **reduct/o-** *to bring back; decrease* **-ion** *action; condition* **pendulous** (PEN-dyoo-lus) **pendul/o-** *hanging down* **-ous** *pertaining to* **mastopexy** (MAS-toh-PEK-see) **mast/o-** *breast; mastoid process* **-pexy** *process of surgically fixing in place* **reconstructive** (REE-con-STRUK-tiv) **re-** *again and again; backward; unable to* **construct/o-** *to build* **-ive** *pertaining to*
mastectomy	Surgical resection of all or part of the breast to excise a malignant tumor. In a **simple** or **total mastectomy,** the entire breast, the overlying skin, and nipple are removed, but not the chest muscle or axillary lymph nodes. In a **modified radical mastectomy,** an **axillary node dissection** is also performed and some of the axillary lymph nodes are removed. In a **radical mastectomy,** the pectoralis major and minor muscles of the chest wall are also removed; this procedure is performed infrequently. A **prophylactic mastectomy** can be performed to prevent breast cancer from occurring in women who have a strong family history of breast cancer.	**mastectomy** (mas-TEK-toh-mee) **mast/o-** *breast; mastoid process* **-ectomy** *surgical excision* **radical** (RAD-ih-kal) **radic/o-** *all parts including the root* **-al** *pertaining to* **dissection** (dih-SEK-shun) **dissect/o-** *to cut apart* **-ion** *action; condition* **prophylactic** (PROH-fih-LAK-tik) **pro-** *before* **phylact/o-** *guarding; protecting* **-ic** *pertaining to*

Word or Phrase	Description	Word Building
reconstructive breast surgery	Procedure to rebuild a breast after a mastectomy. This can be done at the same time as the mastectomy or in a later operation. A breast prosthesis or a TRAM flap (see Figure 13-36 ■) is used to recreate the fullness of the breast. With a breast prosthesis procedure, a tissue expander (a saline-filled silicone bag) is first inserted to stretch the skin to accommodate a breast prosthesis, which is inserted later. For a **TRAM (transverse rectus abdominis muscle) flap,** an incision is made around a transverse area of the abdomen. Skin, fat, and muscle are excised, except for one end that is left attached to blood vessels (pedicle graft). Alternatively, the latissimus dorsi muscle of the back can be used. Then the flap is tunneled under the skin of the upper abdomen and positioned at the site of the previous mastectomy. Later, a tattoo is done on the skin to create an areola and nipple.	**reconstructive** (REE-con-STRUK-tiv) **re-** *again and again; backward; unable to* **construct/o-** *to build* **-ive** *pertaining to* Select the correct prefix meaning to get the definition of *reconstructive: pertaining to again building (the breast).* **transverse** (trans-VERS) **trans-** *across; through* **-verse** *to travel; to turn*

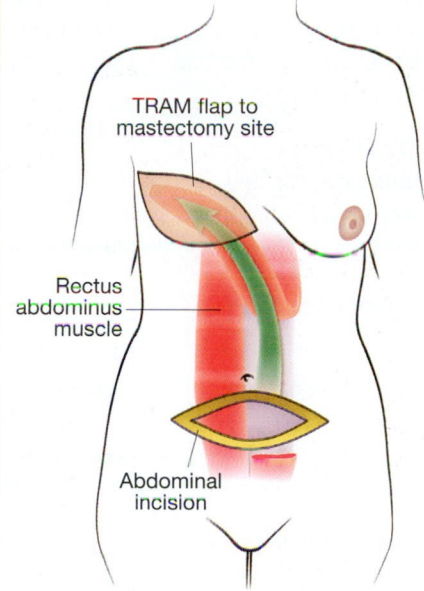

TRAM flap to mastectomy site

Rectus abdominus muscle

Abdominal incision

Figure 13-36 ■ TRAM flap reconstruction.
This reconstructive surgery uses a skin, fat, and muscle flap from the abdomen to reconstruct the breast following a mastectomy. This provides a natural feel to the reconstructed breast and takes the place of a synthetic breast implant.

Surgical Procedures in Obstetrics

cerclage	Procedure to place a purse-string suture around the cervix to prevent it from dilating prematurely. The suture is removed prior to delivery.	**cerclage** (sir-CLAWJ)
cesarean section	Procedure to deliver a fetus. It is done because of cephalopelvic disproportion, failure to progress during labor, the mother being past the due date, or health problems in the mother or fetus. The fetus is delivered through an incision in the abdominal wall and uterus. It is also known as a C section. A vaginal birth after a previous cesarean section is abbreviated as VBAC.	**cesarean** (seh-ZAY-ree-an)
episiotomy	Surgical incision in the posterior edge of the vagina to prevent a spontaneous tear during delivery of the baby's head (see Figure 13-13). Spontaneous vaginal tears usually have ragged tissue edges that are difficult to suture and can extend into the rectum, causing incontinence.	**episiotomy** (eh-PIS-ee-AW-toh-mee) **episi/o-** *vulva* **-tomy** *process of cutting or making an incision*

Drug Categories

These categories of drugs are used to treat female genital and reproductive diseases and conditions. The most common generic and trade name drugs in each category are listed.

Category	Indication	Examples	Word Building
drugs for amenorrhea and abnormal uterine bleeding	Correct lack of hormones	gonadorelin (Lutrepulse), medroxyprogesterone (Provera), progesterone (Crinone)	
drugs for contraception	Suppress the release of FSH and LH from the anterior pituitary gland. Other drugs (not listed here) kill sperm or keep them from reaching the uterus.	Oral contraceptive pill (OCP): Cyclessa, Ortho-Novum, Seasonale Intrauterine device: Mirena Transdermal patch: Ortho Evra Vaginal ring: NuvaRing	**contraception** (CON-trah-SEP-shun) *Contraception* is a combination of the prefix *contra-* (against) and a shortened form of the word *conception*.
drugs for dysmenorrhea	Treat the pain associated with dysmenorrhea. These are nonsteroidal anti-inflammatory drugs (NSAIDs).	ibuprofen (Motrin), mefenamic acid (Ponstel), naproxen (Aleve)	
drugs for endometriosis	Suppress the menstrual cycle for several months and cause endometrial implants in the pelvic cavity to atrophy	goserelein (Zoladex), leuprolide (Lupron Depot)	
drugs for premature labor	Treat premature contractions by relaxing the smooth muscle of the uterine wall. They are known as **tocolytic drugs.**	magnesium sulfate, terbutaline	**tocolytic** (TOH-koh-LIT-ik) **toc/o-** *labor and childbirth* **ly/o-** *break down; destroy* **-tic** *pertaining to*
drugs for premenstrual dysphoric disorder (PMDD)	Treat the depression and anxiety associated with this mood disorder	fluoxetine (Sarafem), paroxetine (Paxil), sertraline (Zoloft)	
drugs for vaginal yeast infections	Topical antifungal drugs used to treat *Candida albicans* infection of the vagina	clotrimazole (Gyne-Lotrimin, Mycelex), miconazole (Monistat 3)	
drugs used to dilate the cervix	Prostaglandin drug applied topically to the cervix to cause dilation and effacement.	dinoprostone (Cervidil, Prepidil)	
drugs used to induce labor	Stimulate the uterus and increase the strength and frequency of contractions of the smooth muscle of the uterine wall	oxytocin (Pitocin)	
hormone replacement therapy (HRT) drugs	Treat the symptoms and consequences of menopause (hot flashes, vaginal dryness, osteoporosis) caused by decreased levels of estradiol. Long-term estrogen use has been associated with an increased risk of breast cancer, endometrial cancer, and thrombophlebitis.	conjugated estrogens (Premarin), estradiol (Climara, Estraderm, Vivelle)	**estrogen** (ES-troh-jen) **estr/o-** *female* **-gen** *that which produces* Estrogen is a drug form of estradiol.

Category	Indication	Examples	Word Building
ovulation-stimulating drugs	Stimulate the anterior pituitary gland to release FSH and LH to cause ovulation. Used to treat infertility. These drugs cause several mature ova to be released at the same time for *in vitro* fertilization.	clomiphene (Clomid), human chorionic gonadotropin (Pregnyl, Profasi)	

Did You Know?

On November 20, 1997, a mother in Iowa gave birth to the world's only surviving set of septuplets. The four boys and three girls were born prematurely at only 30 weeks' gestation. The mother was taking ovulation-stimulating drugs for infertility at the time. On January 26, 2009, a mother in California gave birth to the world's only surviving set of octuplets. With ovulation-stimulating drugs and assisted reproductive technology (ART), the mother had her six previously frozen zygotes implanted in her uterus. Then two zygotes split into identical twins to make a total of eight (six boys and two girls).

Abbreviations

AB, Ab	abortion	**G**	gravida
AFP	alpha fetoprotein	**GIFT**	gamete intrafallopian transfer
AGA	appropriate for gestational age	**G/TPAL**	see *G* and *TPAL*
ART	assisted reproductive technology	**GYN**	gynecology
ASC-H	atypical squamous cells, cannot exclude HSIL	**HCG, hCG**	human chorionic gonadotropin
ASC-US	atypical squamous cells of undetermined significance	**HPV**	human papillomavirus
		HRT	hormone replacement therapy
BBT	basal body temperature	**HSG**	hysterosalpingography
BPD	biparietal diameter (of fetal head)	**HSIL**	high-grade squamous intraepithelial lesion
BPP	biophysical profile	**ICSI**	intracytoplasmic sperm injection
BRCA	breast cancer (gene)	**IUGR**	intrauterine growth retardation
BSE	breast self-examination	**IVF**	*in vitro* fertilization
BSO	bilateral salpingo-oophorectomy	**L&D**	labor and delivery
Bx	biopsy	**LEEP**	loop electrocautery excision procedure
Ca	cancer, carcinoma	**LGA**	large for gestational age
CIN	cervical intraepithelial neoplasia	**LH**	luteinizing hormone
CIS	carcinoma *in situ*	**LMP**	last menstrual period
CNM	certified nurse midwife	**L/S**	lecithin/sphingomyelin (ratio)
CPD	cephalopelvic disproportion	**LSIL**	low-grade squamous intraepithelial lesion
CS	cesarean section ("C-section")	**NB**	newborn
CVS	chorionic villus sampling	**NICU**	neonatal intensive care unit
D&C	dilation and curettage	**NST**	nonstress test
DUB	dysfunctional uterine bleeding	**NSVD**	normal spontaneous vaginal delivery
EDB	estimated date of birth	**OB**	obstetrics
EDC	estimated date of confinement	**OB/GYN**	obstetrics and gynecology
EGA	estimated gestational age	**OCP**	oral contraceptive pill
FHR	fetal heart rate	**P**	para
FSH	follicle-stimulating hormone	**Pap**	Papanicolaou (smear or test)

PID	pelvic inflammatory disease		**TAB**	therapeutic abortion
PMDD	premenstrual dysphoric disorder		**TAH-BSO**	total abdominal hysterectomy and bilateral salpingo-oophorectomy
PMS	premenstrual syndrome			
PROM	premature rupture of membranes		**TPAL**	term newborns, premature newborns, abortions, living children
ROM	rupture of membranes			
SAB	spontaneous abortion		**TRAM**	transverse rectus abdominis muscle (flap)
SCC	squamous cell carcinoma		**TVH**	total vaginal hysterectomy
SGA	small for gestational age		**VBAC**	vaginal birth after cesarean section ("V-back")
STD	sexually transmitted disease		**ZIFT**	zygote intrafallopian transfer

Word Alert

ABBREVIATIONS

Abbreviations are commonly used in all types of medical documents; however, they can mean different things to different people and their meanings can be misinterpreted. Always verify the meaning of an abbreviation.

AI means *artificial insemination,* but it also means *apical impulse, aortic insufficiency,* and *artificial intelligence.*

Ca means *cancer,* but it also means the mineral *calcium.*

D&C means *dilation and curettage,* but it can be confused with *D/C* (*discontinued* or *discharge*).

EDC means *estimated date of confinement,* but it also means *extensor digitorum communis* (a muscle).

G means *gravida,* but it also means *gauge (of a needle).*

P means *para,* but it also means the mineral *phosphorus.*

ROM means *rupture of membranes,* but it also means *range of motion.*

It's Greek to Me!

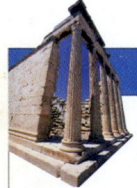

Did you notice that some words have two different combining forms? Combining forms from both Greek and Latin languages remain a part of medical language today.

Word	**Greek**	**Latin**	**Medical Word Examples**
birth	par/o-	nat/o-	multiparous, prenatal
breast	mast/o-	mamm/a-, mamm/o-	mastitis, mammaplasty, mammography
female; woman	gynec/o-	estr/a-, estr/o-	gynecology, estradiol, estrogen
milk	galact/o-	lact/i-, lact/o-	galactorrhea, lactiferous, lactation
ovary	oophor/o-	ovari/o-	oophorectomy, ovarian
ovum	o/o-	ov/i-, ov/o-, ovul/o-	oocyte, oviduct, ovum, ovulation
uterus	hyster/o-	uter/o-	hysterectomy, uterine
	metri/o-, metr/o-		endometriosis, metrorrhagia
vagina	colp/o-	vagin/o-	colposcopy, vaginal
vulva	episi/o-	vulv/o-	episiotomy, vulvar

CAREER FOCUS

Meet Michele, a nurse midwife

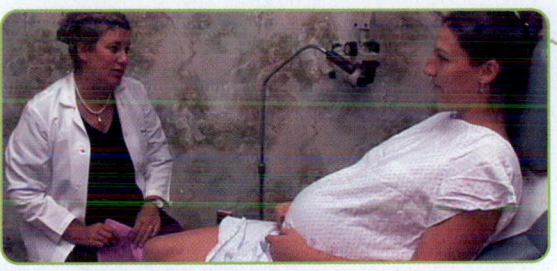

"I think the role of the nurse midwife differs from that of a physician in that you're more holistically focused on the whole person. You look at psychological factors, social factors. You provide more support and more education. I work in an outpatient setting, providing GYN services. I do labor and delivery in the hospital. I have many clients that I'm seeing for their second and third babies. So that's kind of nice to see growing families. It's a very rewarding career because you get to see new families blossoming."

Nurse midwives are allied health professionals who (with the supervision of a physician) manage a patient's prenatal care, delivery, and postpartum care. They are employed in hospitals, obstetrician offices, and birthing centers. They also manage home births.

   Gynecologists are physicians who practice in the medical specialty of gynecology. They diagnose and treat patients with diseases of the female genital and reproductive system. Most gynecologists are also obstetricians who continue to care for their patients during pregnancy and childbirth. **Obstetricians** are physicians who practice in the medical specialty of obstetrics. Obstetricians deliver babies and perform cesarean sections. **Neonatologists** are physicians who practice in the medical specialty of neonatology. They diagnose and treat the fetus during pregnancy and labor and the newborn infant after birth. Most neonatologists work in the neonatal intensive care unit (NICU) in a hospital. **Pediatricians** are physicians who practice in the medical specialty of pediatrics. They diagnose and treat newborns, infants, children, and adolescents. Endocrinologists treat patients with disorders of the endocrine system, including hormonal disorders that affect menstruation. Cancerous tumors of the female genital and reproductive system are treated medically by an oncologist and surgically by a general surgeon.

nurse midwife (NURS MID-wyfe)

gynecologist (GY-neh-KAWL-oh-jist)
  gynec/o- *female; woman*
  log/o- *word; the study of*
  -ist *one who specializes in*

obstetrician (AWB-steh-TRISH-an)
  obstetr/o- *pregnancy and childbirth*
  -ician *a skilled professional or expert*

neonatologist
(NEE-oh-nay-TAWL-oh-jist)
  ne/o- *new*
  nat/o- *birth*
  log/o- *word; the study of*
  -ist *one who specializes in*

pediatrician (PEE-dee-ah-TRISH-an)
  ped/o- *child*
  iatr/o- *physician; medical treatment*
  -ician *a skilled professional or expert*

CHAPTER REVIEW EXERCISES

Test your knowledge of the chapter by completing these review exercises. Use the Answer Key at the end of the book to check your answers.

Anatomy and Physiology

Matching Exercise

Match each word or phrase to its description.

1. breasts
2. cervix
3. ovaries
4. perineum
5. uterine tube
6. uterus
7. vagina
8. vulva

_____ Gonads

_____ Parts of this organ are the fundus and the body

_____ Follicles in these glands rupture to release a mature ovum

_____ Also known as the mammary glands

_____ Area of skin between the vulva and the anus

_____ Has a lumen and a fimbriated end

_____ Has a muscular layer known as the myometrium

_____ Also known as the oviduct

_____ Contains the fornix

_____ The labia are located within this area

_____ The uterine tubes and these are collectively known as the adnexa

_____ The hymen sometimes covers the inferior end of this structure

_____ Contain the lactiferous lobules

_____ Contains an os

_____ Normal position is anteflexion

True or False Exercise

Indicate whether each statement is true or false by writing T or F on the line.

1. _____ A newborn is also known as a neonate.

2. _____ The Bartholin's and Skene's glands secrete mucus during menstruation.

3. _____ The cervical canal is a continuation of the intrauterine cavity.

4. _____ The uterus is suspended within the pelvic cavity only by the broad ligament.

5. _____ The funnel-like widening at the end of the uterine tube is known as the infundibulum.

6. _____ FSH and LH are secreted by the ovary.

7. _____ The onset of menstruation is known as menarche.

8. _____ Ovulation occurs on the first day of the menstrual cycle.

9. _____ Human chorionic gonadotropin is secreted by the vagina.

10. _____ The prenatal period is the period of time before conception.

11. _____ A vertex presentation is the presence of lochia after delivery.

12. _____ Oxytocin causes the uterus to contract.

13. _____ Acrocyanosis is a bluish discoloration of a newborn's face and chest.

Fill in the Blank Exercise

Fill in the blank with the correct word or phrase from the word list.

amnion	false labor	fetus	gestation	presenting part	umbilical cord
embryo	fertilization	gamete	placenta	trimester	zygote
engagement					

1. Fertilized ovum with 46 chromosomes _____

2. Also known as conception _____

3. Part of fetus that will go first through the birth canal _____

4. Cells that become the amniotic sac and fluid _____

5. A spermatozoon or an ovum with 23 chromosomes _____

6. Source of nutrients and oxygen for the fetus _____

7. Connects the placenta to the fetus _____

8. Developmental stage before fetus _____

9. What the embryo is known as after week 8 _____

10. Time from conception to birth _____

11. Equals 3 months' time _____

12. Fetal head drops into position in mother's pelvis _____

13. Also known as Braxton Hicks contractions _____

Sequencing Exercise

Beginning with the fetal head moving into the mother's pelvis, write each event of labor and delivery in the order in which it occurs.

Event	Correct Order
birth of the newborn	1. _____
dilation and effacement	2. _____
crowning	3. _____
engagement	4. _____
involution	5. _____
placenta delivered	6. _____

Matching Exercise

Match each word or phrase to its description.

1. Apgar   _____ Newborn cries and breasts release milk

2. colostrum   _____ Widening of the diameter of the cervical os

3. crowning   _____ Release of amniotic fluid

4. dilation   _____ Time period after birth (for the mother)

5. effacement   _____ Thinning of the cervical wall

6. lactation   _____ Fetal scalp visible at vaginal introitus

7. let-down reflex _____ Production of breast milk after childbirth

8. postpartum   _____ Quick scoring system to assess newborn well-being

9. rupture of membranes _____ First milk from the breast; contains maternal antibodies

Diseases and Conditions

Matching Exercise

Match each word or phrase to its description.

1. breasts
2. breast skin
3. bimanual
4. dorsal lithotomy
5. lymph nodes
6. nipple
7. Tanner stage
8. uterus
9. vaginal speculum

_____ System to describe stages of breast development

_____ Gynecologic exam that uses both hands

_____ Can be pendulous

_____ Instrument that pushes apart the vaginal walls

_____ Axillary ones are enlarged from breast cancer

_____ Standard gynecologic examination position

_____ Where the lactiferous ducts come together

_____ Peau d'orange dimpling associated with cancer

_____ When prolapsed, its cervix can be seen at the vaginal introitus

Circle Exercise

Circle the correct word from the choices given.

1. Galactorrhea is a disease that affects the (**breasts, perineum, vagina**).
2. (**Amenorrhea, Dysmenorrhea, Menometrorrhagia**) is the complete absence of monthly menstrual periods.
3. (**Cervical, Endometrial, Ovarian**) cancer is the most difficult to detect and is often widespread before symptoms become severe.
4. Dyspareunia and dysmenorrhea are symptoms of (**endometriosis, menopause, pregnancy**).
5. A yeast infection in the vagina is known as (**anovulation, candidiasis, hydrosalpinx**).
6. (**Menometrorrhagia, Metrorrhagia, Myometritis**) is an inflammation or infection in the muscular wall of the uterus.
7. An ectopic pregnancy can result in (**eclampsia, hemosalpinx, involution**).
8. Mastitis is a postpartum inflammation of the (**breast, perineum, uterus**).
9. (**Gestational diabetes mellitus, Prolapsed cord, Salpingitis**) cuts off the supply of oxygen to the fetus.
10. Yellowish discoloration of the skin in the neonate is known as (**acrocyanosis, apnea, jaundice**).
11. Pain during sexual intercourse is known as (**abortion, dyspareunia, eclampsia**).

Matching Exercise

Match each word or phrase to its description.

1. candidiasis
2. endometriosis
3. galactorrhea
4. leiomyomata
5. menopause
6. oligomenorrhea
7. pyosalpinx
8. uterine descensus

_____ Yeast infection of the vagina

_____ Discharge of milk from the breast without pregnancy

_____ Climacteric

_____ Prolapse of the uterus

_____ Many smooth muscle tumors of the uterus

_____ Pus in the uterine tube

_____ Scanty menstrual flow

_____ "Chocolate cysts" on the ovary

Laboratory, Radiology, Surgery, and Drugs

True or False Exercise

Indicate whether each statement is true or false by writing T or F on the line.

1. _____ The presence of the BRCA1 gene greatly increases the risk of developing fibrocystic disease of the breast.

2. _____ A fine-needle aspiration biopsy uses a small needle to inject drugs into a cancerous tumor.

3. _____ Dysplasia is an abnormality of the cell that always means it is malignant.

4. _____ The estrogen receptor assay predicts whether estrogen-blocking drugs will be successful in treating a patient's breast cancer.

5. _____ A Pap smear is reported as one of two results, either negative for cancerous cells or positive for cancerous cells.

6. _____ During a LEEP procedure, a cold knife is used to cut away a cone of tissue from the cervix.

7. _____ A lumpectomy is a more extensive procedure than a mastectomy.

8. _____ A hysteropexy is also known as a uterine suspension.

9. _____ Hormone replacement therapy treats the vaginal dryness and hot flashes associated with menopause.

10. _____ Hysterosalpingography can show blockage in the uterine tubes.

Matching Exercise

Match each word or phrase to its description.

1. colposcope   _____ Used to hold the cervix in a fixed position during an examination

2. cryoprobe   _____ Low-power microscope used to examine the cervix

3. curet   _____ X-ray image of the breast

4. incisional biopsy   _____ Only part of a tumor is excised

5. laparoscope   _____ Instrument used to freeze cervical lesions

6. mammogram   _____ Ring instrument with a sharp edge for scraping

7. Pap smear   _____ Uses sound waves to produce an image

8. tenaculum   _____ Drug used to stop premature labor

9. tocolytic   _____ Exfoliative cytology test

10. ultrasound   _____ Fiberoptic endoscope

Multiple Choice Exercise

Circle the choice that best answers the question.

1. Surgical procedure used to suture a weakness in the vaginal wall.
   a. cystocele   c. conization
   b. cryosurgery   d. colporrhaphy

2. A hysterectomy can be performed _____.
   a. through the vagina   c. laparoscopically
   b. through the abdominal wall d. all of the above

3. A breast lift is another name for a/an _____.
   a. augmentation mammoplasty c. reduction mammoplasty
   b. mastopexy   d. mastectomy

4. Drugs used to treat dysmenorrhea include _____.
   a. NSAID drugs   c. antiviral drugs
   b. antibiotic drugs   d. HRT

Building Medical Words

Review the Combining Forms Exercise, Combining Form and Suffix Exercise, Prefix Exercise, and Multiple Combining Forms and Suffix Exercise that you already completed in the anatomy section on pages 660–663.

Combining Forms Exercise

Before you build gynecologic and obstetrical words, review these additional combining forms. Next to each combining form, write its medical meaning. The first one has been done for you.

Combining Form	Medical Meaning	Combining Form	Medical Meaning
1. ablat/o-	take away; destroy	16. manu/o-	
2. abort/o-		17. mult/i-	
3. cancer/o-		18. nuch/o-	
4. cephal/o-		19. null/i-	
5. con/o-		20. obstetr/o-	
6. cry/o-		21. olig/o-	
7. cyst/o-		22. ped/o-	
8. eclamps/o-		23. pelv/o-	
9. ectop/o-		24. plas/o-	
10. hem/o-		25. prim/i-	
11. hydatidi/o-		26. py/o-	
12. hydr/o-		27. rect/o-	
13. lapar/o-		28. rrhag/o-	
14. lei/o-		29. surg/o-	
15. leuk/o-		30. xer/o-	

Related Combining Forms Exercise

Write the combining forms on the line provided. (Hint: See the It's Greek to Me feature box.

1. Two combining forms that mean *birth*. _____
2. Two combining forms that mean *ovary*. _____
3. Two combining forms that mean *vagina*. _____
4. Two combining forms that mean *vulva*. _____
5. Three combining forms that mean *breast*. _____
6. Three combining forms that mean *female; woman*. _____
7. Four combining forms that mean *ovum*. _____
8. Four combining forms that mean *uterus*. _____

Combining Form and Suffix Exercise

Read the definition of the medical word. Select the correct suffix from the Suffix List. Select the correct combining form from the Combining Form List. Build the medical word and write it on the line. Be sure to check your spelling. The first one has been done for you.

SUFFIX LIST

- -al (pertaining to)
- -cele (hernia)
- -centesis (procedure to puncture)
- -ectomy (surgical excision)
- -form (having the form of)
- -graphy (process of recording)
- -gravida (pregnancy)
- -ic (pertaining to)
- -ion (action; condition)

- -itis (inflammation of; infection of)
- -ization (process of making, creating, or inserting)
- -pause (cessation)
- -pexy (process of surgically fixing in place)
- -plasty (process of reshaping by surgery)
- -probe (rodlike instrument)

- -rrhaphy (procedure of suturing)
- -rrhea (flow; discharge)
- -salpinx (uterine tube)
- -scope (instrument used to examine)
- -scopy (process of using an instrument to examine)
- -tomy (process of cutting or making an incision)

COMBINING FORM LIST

- abort/o- (stop prematurely)
- amni/o- (amnion)
- colp/o- (vagina)
- con/o- (cone)
- cry/o- (cold)
- culd/o- (cul-de-sac)
- cyst/o- (bladder)

- ectop/o- (outside of a place)
- episi/o- (vulva)
- galact/o- (milk)
- hem/o- (blood)
- hydatidi/o- (fluid-filled vesicles)
- hyster/o- (uterus; womb)

- lapar/o- (abdomen)
- leuk/o- (white)
- mamm/o- (breast)
- mast/o- (breast)
- men/o- (month)
- nuch/o- (neck)

- oophor/o- (ovary)
- prim/i- (first)
- py/o- (pus)
- rect/o- (rectum)
- salping/o- (uterine tube)
- vagin/o- (vagina)

Definition of the Medical Word	Build the Medical Word
1. Pertaining to the (umbilical cord around the fetus') neck	nuchal
2. Flow of milk (from the breasts when the patient is not pregnant)	
3. Inflammation or infection in the uterine tube	
4. Cessation of a monthly (menstrual period)	
5. Hernia of the bladder (into the vagina)	
6. Process of surgically fixing (back in) place a (sagging) breast	
7. Inflammation or infection of the vagina	
8. Discharge of white (cheesy material from the vagina)	
9. Rodlike instrument (that is) cold (to destroy abnormal tissue on the cervix)	
10. (Woman in a) pregnancy (that is her) first	
11. Instrument used to examine the abdomen	
12. Pertaining to (a fertilized ovum implanting) outside of a place (where it should)	
13. Process of cutting or making an incision into the vulva	
14. Uterine tube (that contains) blood	
15. Inflammation or infection of the breast	
16. Having the form (of a pregnancy but only having) fluid-filled vesicles	
17. Hernia of the rectum (into the vagina)	
18. Surgical excision of the uterine tube	
19. Process of using an instrument to examine the vagina	
20. Procedure to puncture the amnion	

Definition of the Medical Word	**Build the Medical Word**
21. Process of making (and removing) a cone (of tissue from the cervix)	_____
22. Surgical excision of the breast	_____
23. Process of using an instrument to examine the cul-de-sac	_____
24. Uterine tube (that contains) pus	_____
25. Procedure of suturing the vagina	_____
26. Action to stop prematurely (the development of an embryo or fetus)	_____
27. Surgical excision of the uterus	_____
28. Process of recording (an image of) the breast	_____
29. Process of reshaping by surgery the (size, shape, or position) of the breast	_____
30. Surgical excision of the ovary	_____

Prefix Exercise

Read the definition of the medical word. Look at the medical word or partial word that is given (it already contains a combining form and a suffix). Select the correct prefix from the Prefix List and write it on the blank line. Then build the medical word and write it on the line. Be sure to check your spelling. The first one has been done for you.

PREFIX LIST		
an- (without; not)	endo- (innermost; within)	pre- (before; in front of)
bi- (two)	hyper- (above; more than normal)	trans- (across; through)
dys- (painful; difficult; abnormal)	poly- (many; much)	

Definition of the Medical Word	**Prefix**	**Word or Partial Word**	**Build the Medical Word**
1. Condition of an abnormal growth (of squamous cells on the cervix)	*dys-*	plasia	*dysplasia*
2. Pertaining to before (the occurrence of the) monthly discharge of blood	_____	menstrual	_____
3. Pertaining to many semisolid cysts (in the ovary)	_____	cystic	_____
4. Discharge (that is) painful and difficult each month	_____	menorrhea	_____
5. Abnormal condition of the innermost (lining) in the uterus	_____	metriosis	_____
6. Abnormal condition of more than normal vomiting	_____	emesis	_____
7. Pertaining to (using) two hands (to do an examination)	_____	manual	_____
8. Pertaining to through the vagina	_____	vaginal	_____
9. Condition (of a pregnant woman) before (she has a) seizure	_____	eclampsia	_____
10. Condition of painful or difficult sexual intercourse	_____	pareunia	_____
11. Process of being without ovulation	_____	ovulation	_____
12. Condition of painful or difficult labor and childbirth	_____	tocia	_____

Multiple Combining Forms and Suffix Exercise

Read the definition of the medical word. Select the correct suffix and combining forms. Then build the medical word and write it on the line. Be sure to check your spelling. The first one has been done for you.

SUFFIX LIST	COMBINING FORM LIST	
-amnios (amniotic fluid) -ectomy (surgical excision) -ery (process of) -gram (a record or picture) -ia (condition; state; thing) -ic (pertaining to) -itis (inflammation of; infection of) -oma (tumor; mass) -ous (pertaining to) -rrhea (flow; discharge)	cephal/o- (head) cry/o- (cold) hydr/o- (water; fluid) hyster/o- (uterus; womb) lei/o- (smooth) men/o- (month) metr/o- (uterus; womb) mult/i- (many) my/o- muscle	olig/o- (scanty; few) oophor/o- (ovary) par/o- (birth) pelv/o- (pelvis; hip bone) py/o- (pus) rrhag/o- (excessive flow or discharge) salping/o- (uterine tube) surg/o- (operative procedure)

Definition of the Medical Word

Build the Medical Word

1. Inflammation with pus in the uterus — *pyometritis*

2. Tumor of the smooth muscle (in the uterus) — _____

3. Pertaining to the head (of the fetus) and the pelvis (of the mother) — _____

4. (Condition in which the) amniotic fluid is a scanty fluid — _____

5. Pertaining to (a woman who has had) many births — _____

6. A record or picture of the uterus and uterine tubes (using contrast dye) — _____

7. Process of using cold (to destroy tissue during) an operative procedure — _____

8. Surgical excision of the uterine tubes and the ovaries — _____

9. Flow that is scanty for the month(ly menses) — _____

10. Condition of month(ly menses having) excessive flow or discharge — _____

Abbreviations

Matching Exercise

Match each abbreviation to its definition.

1. ASC-US   _____ Due date

2. BSE   _____ Untreated, this can cause adhesions, scarring, and infertility

3. Bx   _____ Uses a loop with electrical current running through it to cut away tissue

4. CIS   _____ Uterus and bilateral uterine tubes and ovaries are surgically removed

5. EDC   _____ Includes physical symptoms of PMS plus mood disorder

6. FSH   _____ Surgical flap to reconstruct breast after mastectomy

7. HRT   _____ Abbreviation for biopsy

8. LEEP   _____ Drug therapy to treat the symptoms of menopause

9. OCP   _____ Oral drug used to prevent pregnancy

10. PID   _____ Cancer still confined to one location

(continued)

11. PMDD   _____ Hormone that makes the follicles produce a mature ovum

12. TAH-BSO   _____ Abnormal Pap smear finding

13. TRAM   _____ Having a vaginal birth after a prior cesarean section

14. VBAC   _____ Important way to detect breast cancer

Applied Skills

Plural Noun and Adjective Spelling Exercise

Read the noun and write the plural and/or adjective forms. Be sure to check your spelling. The first one has been done for you.

Singular Noun	Plural Noun	Adjective
1. areola	areolae	areolar
2. amnion		_____
3. breast	_____	_____
4. cervix		_____
5. fetus	_____	_____
6. ovary	_____	_____
7. ovum	_____	
8. perineum		_____
9. placenta		_____
10. umbilicus		_____
11. uterus		_____
12. vagina		_____

Proofreading and Spelling Exercise

Read the following paragraph. Identify each misspelled medical word and write the correct spelling of it on the line.

A woman may request a gynicologic exam because of pain and dysparunia. When the doctor does a GYN examination, the uteris can be felt, but not the uterin tubes. A pregnant woman's obstetical history notes that she is a primogravida. Her doctor might recommend an amniosentesis and a cecarean section. An older woman might need to have a histerectomy and an ophorectomy.

1. _____   6. _____

2. _____   7. _____

3. _____   8. _____

4. _____   9. _____

5. _____   10. _____

English and Medical Word Equivalents Exercise

For each English word, write its equivalent medical word. Be sure to check your spelling.

English Word	Medical Word
1. breasts	_____
2. afterbirth	_____
3. baby	_____
4. bag of waters	_____
5. false labor	_____
6. getting your tubes tied	_____
7. soft spot (on the newborn's head)	_____
8. womb	_____
9. excessive morning sickness	_____

You Write the Medical Report

You are a healthcare professional interviewing a patient. Listen to the patient's statements and then enter them in the patient's medical record using medical words and phrases. Be sure to check your spelling. The first one has been done for you.

1. The patient says, "I didn't produce any milk with my last pregnancy."

   You write: The patient has a history of <u>failure of lactation.</u>

2. The patient says, "I had my womb taken out, with all my tubes and my ovaries too. That was last year."

   You write: The patient had a _____ and a bilateral _____ last year.

3. The patient says, "I am having itching and a white, cheesy discharge from my vagina because of a yeast infection. I want an antibiotic drug."

   You write: The patient is complaining of _____ coming from the vagina due to an infection with the yeast _____. She was prescribed the topical _____ drug Monistat.

4. The patient says, "I can finally breathe because the baby's head dropped down yesterday. I am due on January 21."

   You write: Based on my examination and the mother's comments, there is _____ of the fetal head in the maternal pelvis. Her _____ [abbreviation] is January 21.

5. The patient says, "I had a workup done last month because I couldn't get pregnant. They said I had an infection in my tubes and that my ovaries had lots of cysts in them. I also had pain when I had sexual intercourse with my husband. They took a scope and looked into my abdomen to check this out, and they said that was because of pieces of the lining of the uterus being in the wrong places."

   You write: The patient had an _____ workup last month. She was found to have _____ and _____ ovary syndrome. She also complained of _____ during sexual intercourse with her husband. She had a _____ to investigate this and was diagnosed as having _____.

6. The patient says, "I started my periods when I was 16. I always have pain with my periods. Recently, my periods have changed and are very light. But I am too young to be in the change of life."

   You write: Patient had _____ at age 16. She reports she has always had _____ with her periods. Recently, she has noticed _____. She is only 30, and so this is probably a hormonal imbalance and not the beginning of _____.

Medical Report Exercise

This exercise contains a History and Physical Examination done in the neonatal intensive care unit. Read the report and answer the questions.

HISTORY AND PHYSICAL EXAMINATION

PATIENT: KAISER, Baby Boy

MEDICAL RECORD NUMBER: 03-7843

DATE OF BIRTH: November 19, 20xx

DATE OF ADMISSION TO NICU: November 19, 20xx

HISTORY
This is a 3360 g, full-term white male infant, who was transferred from the delivery room to the NICU after birth because of respiratory distress. The infant was born to a 34-year-old mother with an EDB of 11/22/xx, and he had an EGA of 40 weeks.

MATERNAL HISTORY
The mother was G2, TPAL 0-0-1-0 with a SAB 2 years ago. The mother had prenatal care beginning in the first trimester of this pregnancy. She took prenatal vitamins. She denied the use of alcohol, smoking, or drugs. A sonogram on 10/10/xx showed a single fetus in breech presentation at 35 weeks' gestation.

LABOR AND DELIVERY HISTORY
The membranes ruptured spontaneously 14 hours prior to the onset of labor. The mother had a temperature of 103.2 degrees prior to delivery and was started on an antibiotic drug. A version of the breech presentation was performed. Labor was induced and lasted 8 hours.

The baby was born via a normal spontaneous vaginal delivery. Apgars were 8 and 8 at 1 and 5 minutes, respectively. There was no evidence of meconium aspiration on visualization of the mouth, pharynx, and vocal cords. The infant was tachypneic despite suctioning and the administration of blow-by oxygen and was brought to the neonatal intensive care unit.

PHYSICAL EXAMINATION
Heart rate 200 beats/minute, respiratory rate 70/minute, temperature 101.2, weight 3360 g, length 54 cm, head circumference 33.5 cm. General: Full-term, AGA male. Alert, active, responsive. Head: Moderate molding present. Fontanels soft. Palate intact. Eyes: Pupils equal and reactive to light. Chest symmetrical. Now pink in room air with only mild tachypnea and mild sternal retractions. Breath sounds equal bilaterally. Clavicles intact. Abdomen: Bowel sounds present. No hepatosplenomegaly. There is a 3-vessel umbilical cord. Genitalia normal. Anus patent. Neurologic: Strong cry, strong suck, normal muscle tone.

IMPRESSION
Term male infant, estimated gestational age of 38.5 weeks, appropriate for gestational age. Rule out pneumonia.

PLAN
Admit to the neonatal intensive care unit. Vital signs q.1h. until stable. Cardiorespiratory monitor. Intravenous fluids of dextrose 10% in water at 80 cc/kg/day. Hold oral feedings for now. Chest x-ray to rule out aspiration pneumonia.

Bonita C. Grant, M.D.
_____
Bonita C. Grant, M.D.

BCG: cgm
D: 11/19/xx
T: 11/19/xx

Word Analysis Questions

1. Give the definitions of these abbreviations.

   a. AGA _____

   b. EDB _____

   c. EGA _____

   d. NICU _____

   e. SAB _____

2. A sonogram showed the fetus at 35 weeks' gestation. If you wanted to use the adjective form of *gestation*, you would say, "The fetus had a _____ age of 35 weeks."

3. Divide *gestational* into its three word parts and define each word part.

Word Part	Definition
_____	_____
_____	_____
_____	_____

4. Divide *prenatal* into its three word parts and define each word part.

Word Part	Definition
_____	_____
_____	_____
_____	_____

5. What is the abbreviation for the medical phrase *normal spontaneous vaginal delivery?* _____

Fact Finding Questions

1. The sonogram (ultrasound) done on 10/10/xx showed what fetal presentation? _____

2. What procedure was performed to correct this presentation? Circle the correct answer.

   Apgar   repeat sonogram   version   vaginal delivery

3. What does the mother's TPAL score of 0-0-1-0 mean? _____

4. What moderate condition of the head was noted on the physical examination? _____

5. The newborn's estimated gestational age was 38.5 weeks. Is this a term newborn?   **Yes   No**

6. Where are the fontanels located? _____

7. What test was ordered to rule out aspiration pneumonia? _____

Critical Thinking Questions

1. Rupture of the membranes many hours prior to delivery can cause infection in the mother and in the newborn. What information is given in the record that tells you that the newborn did develop an infection? _____

2. Circle the correct answer. If there had been meconium-stained amniotic fluid, the newborn experienced **(apnea, fetal distress, premature birth)**.

Dividing Medical Words

Separate these words into their component parts (prefix, combining form, suffix). Note: Some words do not contain all three word parts. The first one has been done for you.

Medical Word	Prefix	Combining Form	Suffix	Medical Word	Prefix	Combining Form	Suffix
1. menstruation	_____	menstru/o-	-ation	6. dysmenorrhea	_____	_____	_____
2. prenatal	_____	_____	_____	7. lactation	_____	_____	_____
3. neonate	_____	_____	_____	8. postpartum	_____	_____	_____
4. anovulation	_____	_____	_____	9. retroversion	_____	_____	_____
5. polycystic	_____	_____	_____	10. cystocele	_____	_____	_____

Hearing Medical Words Exercise

You hear someone speaking the medical words given below. Read each pronunciation and then write the medical word it represents. Be sure to check your spelling. The first one has been done for you.

1. BY-awp-see   biopsy
2. meh-NAR-kee   _____
3. mah-MAWG-rah-fee   _____
4. lak-TAY-shun   _____
5. AM-nee-oh-sen-TEE-sis   _____
6. SIS-toh-seel   _____
7. DIS-pah-ROO-nee-ah   _____
8. eh-PIS-ee-AW-toh-mee   _____

Pronunciation Exercise

Read the medical word that is given. Then review the syllables in the pronunciation. Circle the primary (main) accented syllable. The first one has been done for you.

1. menopause ((men)-oh-pawz)
2. colostrum (koh-laws-trum)
3. mammary (mam-ah-ree)
4. ovarian (oh-vair-ee-an)
5. intrauterine (in-trah-yoo-ter-in)
6. dysmenorrhea (dis-men-oh-ree-ah)
7. vagina (vah-jy-nah)
8. mastectomy (mas-tek-toh-mee)

Multimedia Preview

Immerse yourself in a variety of activities inside Medical Terminology Interactive. Getting there is simple:

1. Click on www.myhealthprofessionskit.com.
2. Select "Medical Terminology" from the choice of disciplines.
3. First-time users must create an account using the scratch-off code on the inside front cover of this book.
4. Find this book and log in using your username and password.
5. Click on Medical Terminology Interactive.
6. Take the elevator to the 13th Floor to begin your virtual exploration of this chapter!

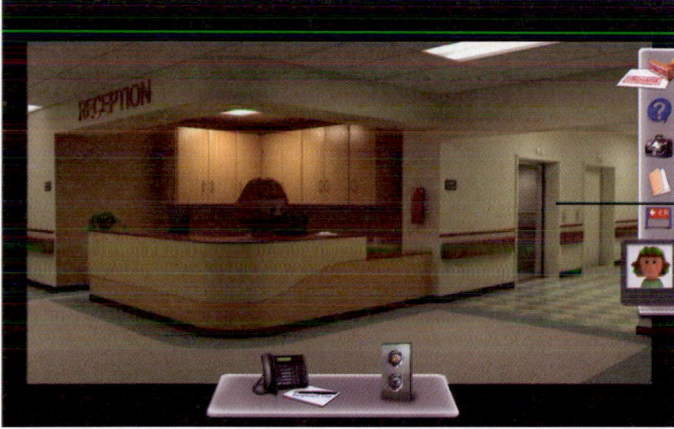 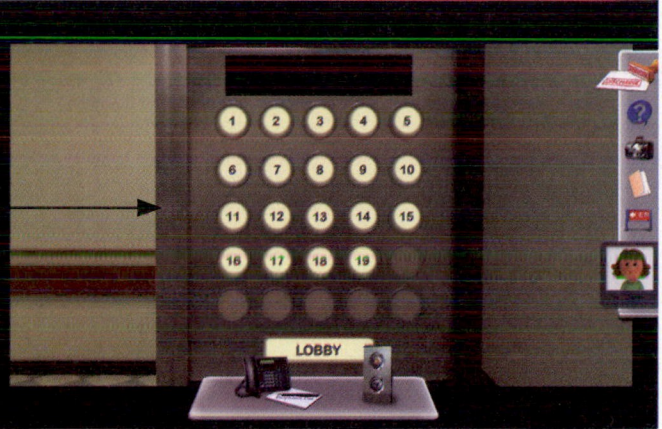

■ **Beat the Clock** Challenge the clock by testing your medical terminology smarts against time. Click here for a game of knowledge, spelling, and speed. Can you correctly answer 20 questions before the final tick?

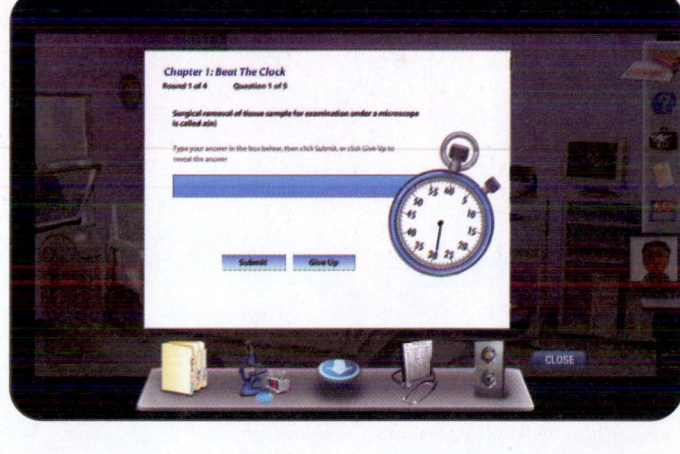

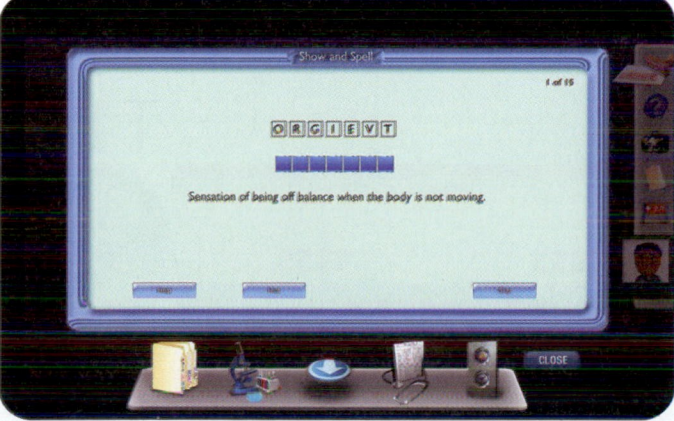

■ **Show and Spell** We're all mixed up, but maybe you can help. Unscramble the letters to form a word that matches the definition provided. When you finish, you'll be dizzy with delight.

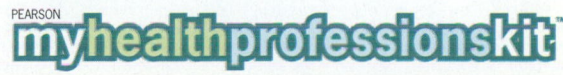

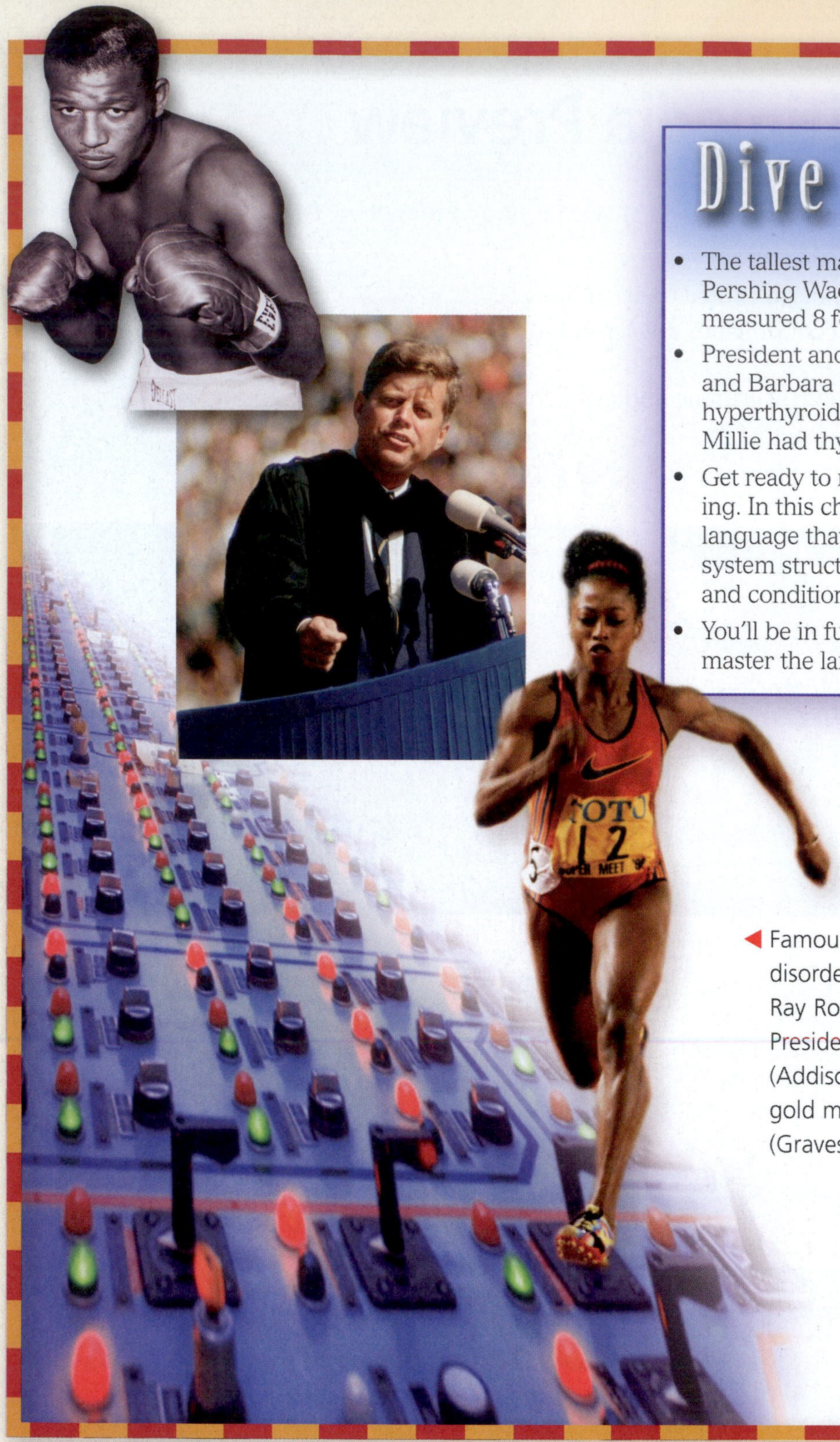

Dive In!

- The tallest man on record was Robert Pershing Wadlow of Illinois, who measured 8 feet, 11.1 inches.

- President and First Lady George and Barbara Bush both had hyperthyroidism. Even their dog Millie had thyroid problems.

- Get ready to regulate your understanding. In this chapter we'll explore the language that describes the endocrine system structures, functions, diseases, and conditions.

- You'll be in full control once you master the language of endocrinology!

◀ Famous sufferers of endocrine disorders: boxing legend Sugar Ray Robinson (diabetes mellitus); President John F. Kennedy (Addison's Disease); Olympic gold medalist Gail Devers (Graves' Disease).

Medicine Through HISTORY

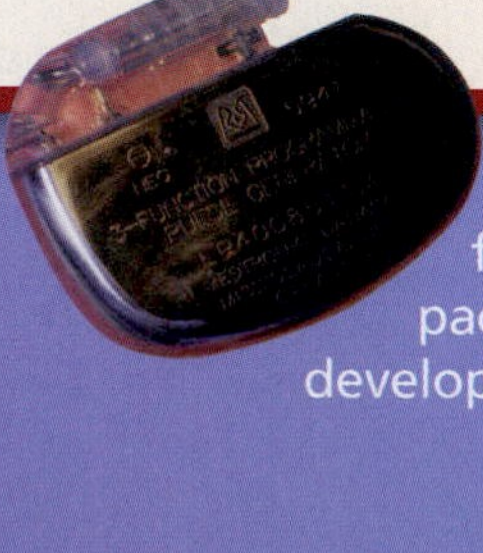

1952
The first cardiac pacemaker is developed

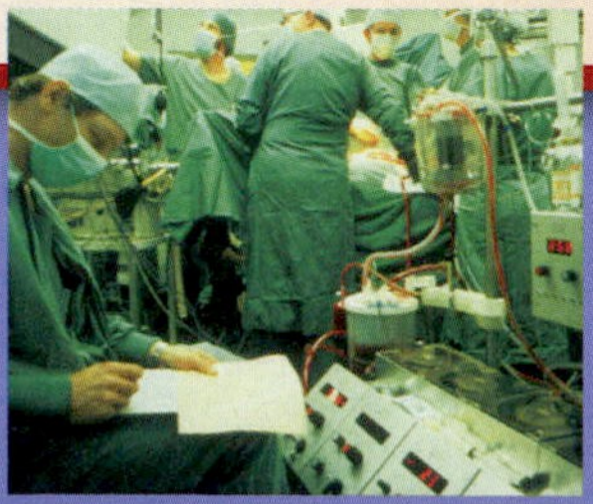

1953
The heart-lung machine for use during open heart surgery is invented by Dr. John Gibbon

1955 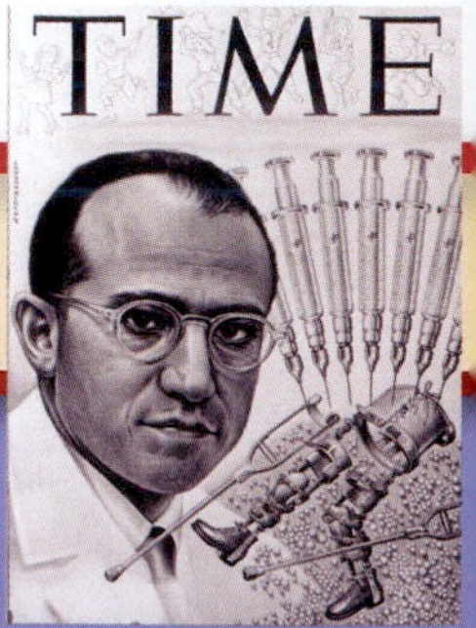
The first polio vaccine (a solution of dead virus) is developed by Dr. Jonas Salk. The oral polio vaccine that uses live, weakened virus is developed by Dr. Albert Sabin in 1961

TIME

14
Endocrinology
Endocrine System

Endocrinology (EN-doh-krin-AWL-oh-jee) is the medical specialty that studies the anatomy and physiology of the endocrine system and uses diagnostic tests, medical and surgical procedures, and drugs to treat endocrine system diseases.

◄ The endocrine system contains organs and glands that secrete hormones to regulate various body functions.

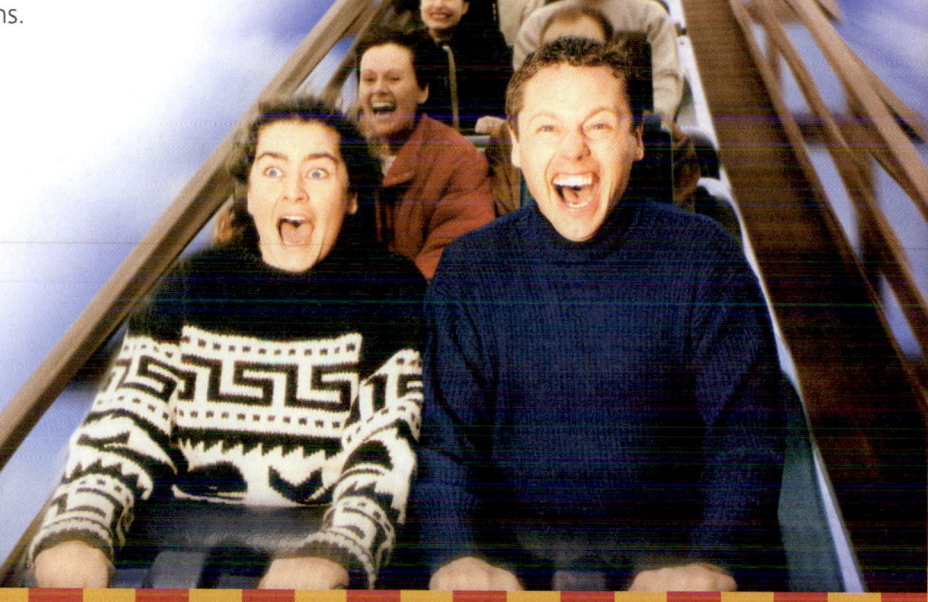

▶ A roller-coaster of hormones is being secreted in the bodies of these riders as they experience fear, stress, joy, and excitement.

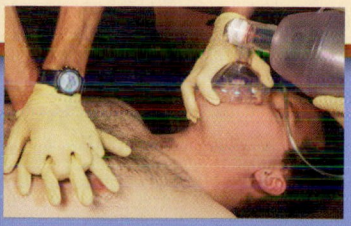

1957

The development of cardiopulmonary resuscitation (CPR) techniques begins with the creation of the ABCs (airway, breathing, circulation)

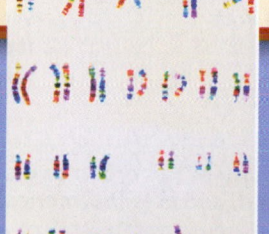

1959

Patients with Down syndrome and mental retardation are found to have an abnormal number of chromosomes

Measure Your Progress: Learning Objectives

After you study this chapter, you should be able to

1. Identify the structures of the endocrine system.

2. Describe the process of hormone response and feedback.

3. Describe common endocrine diseases and conditions, laboratory and diagnostic procedures, medical and surgical procedures, and drug categories.

4. Give the medical meaning of word parts related to the endocrine system.

5. Build endocrine words from word parts and divide and define endocrine words.

6. Spell and pronounce endocrine words.

7. Analyze the medical content and meaning of an endocrinology report.

8. Dive deeper into endocrinology by reviewing the activities at the end of this chapter and online at Medical Terminology Interactive.

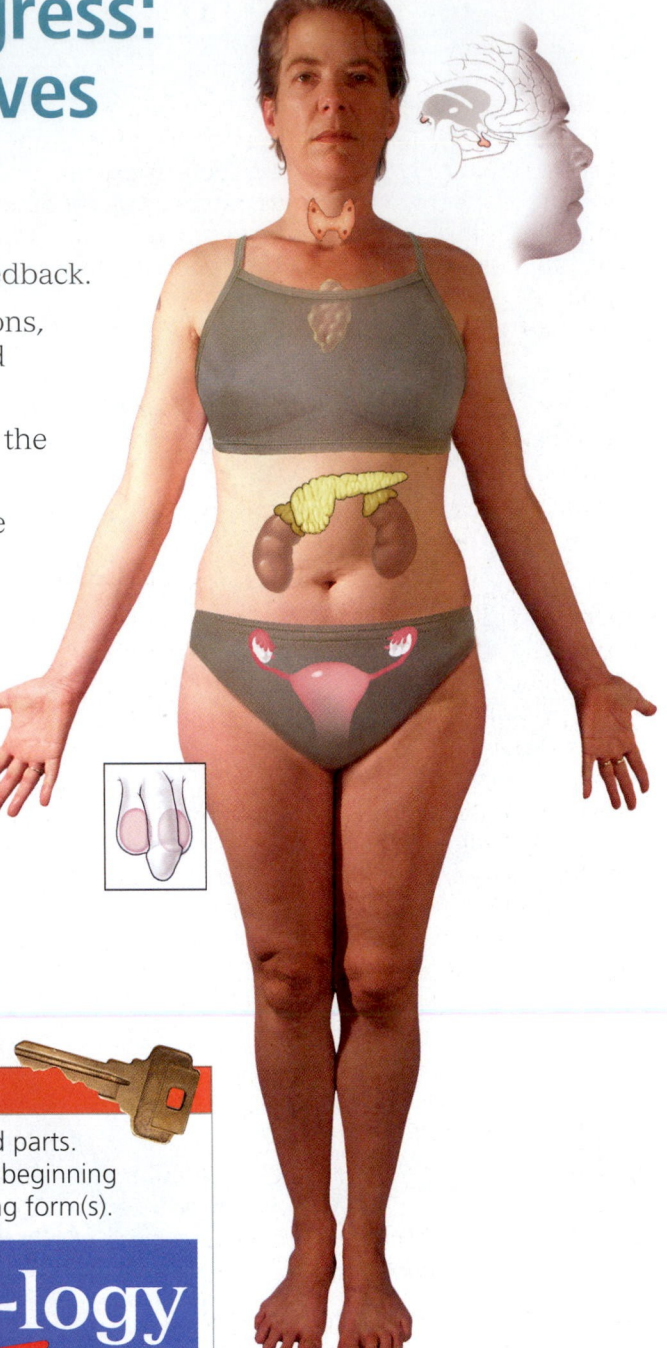

Figure 14-1 ■ **Endocrine system.**
The endocrine system consists of glands that perform very different functions. They are related to each other because they all secrete hormones into the blood.

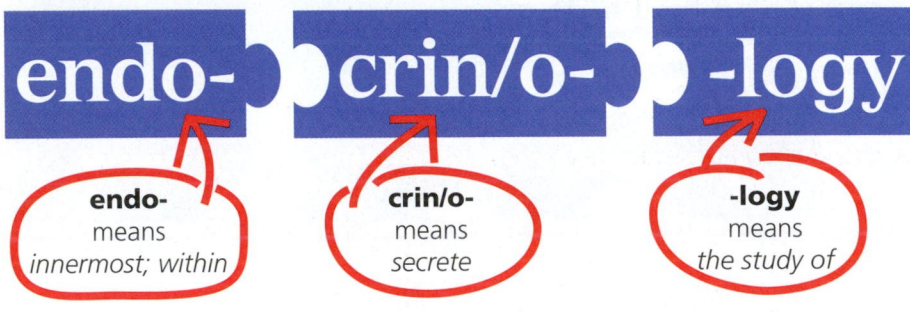

Medical Language Key

To unlock the definition of a medical word, break it into word parts. Define each word part. Put the word part meanings in order, beginning with the suffix, then the prefix (if present), then the combining form(s).

endo- | **crin/o-** | **-logy**

endo-
means
innermost; within

crin/o-
means
secrete

-logy
means
the study of

	Word Part	Word Part Meaning
Suffix	-logy	*the study of*
Prefix	endo-	*innermost; within*
Combining Form	crin/o-	*secrete*

Endocrinology: *The study of (an organ or gland) within (the body that) secretes (hormones).*

Anatomy and Physiology

The **endocrine system** is different from other body systems in that it is made up of **glands** that are in various parts of the body (see Figure 14-1 ■). Endocrine glands produce and secrete hormones into the blood. These glands include the hypothalamus, pituitary gland, pineal gland, thyroid gland, parathyroid glands, thymus, pancreas, adrenal glands, ovaries, and testes. Some, but not all, of these glands are influenced by hormones from the pituitary gland.

However, all endocrine glands are alike in these ways:

1. They secrete substances known as **hormones.**
2. They secrete their hormones directly into the blood and not through ducts.
3. These hormones regulate specific body functions.

One of the functions of the endocrine system is to keep the body in **homeostasis.** This is a state of equilibrium of the internal environment of the body so that all body systems can function optimally. The endocrine system plays a role in homeostasis by regulating body fluids, electrolytes, glucose, cellular metabolism, growth, and the wake–sleep cycle; other body systems regulate other factors of homeostasis.

Some endocrine glands do "double duty" as part of another body system, such as the pituitary gland (nervous system), thymus (immune system), pancreas (digestive system), or ovaries and testes (genital and reproductive system). Because the hypothalamus belongs to the nervous system and the endocrine system and the posterior pituitary gland contains the axons of neurons from the hypothalamus, their shared functions and structures are reflected in the word **neuroendocrine.**

Word Alert

SOUND-ALIKE WORDS

endocrine   (adjective)   descriptive word for glands that secrete hormones directly into the blood
Example: The thyroid gland is one of the glands of the endocrine system.

exocrine   (adjective)   descriptive word for glands that release substances through ducts (not directly into the blood)
Example: The sebaceous glands in the skin are exocrine glands that produce oil.

Anatomy of the Endocrine System

Hypothalamus

The **hypothalamus** is in the center of the brain, on top of the brainstem, and (as its name implies), just below the thalamus. The hypothalamus forms the floor and part of the walls of the third ventricle in the brain, and it has a stalk of blood vessels and nerves that connects it to the pituitary

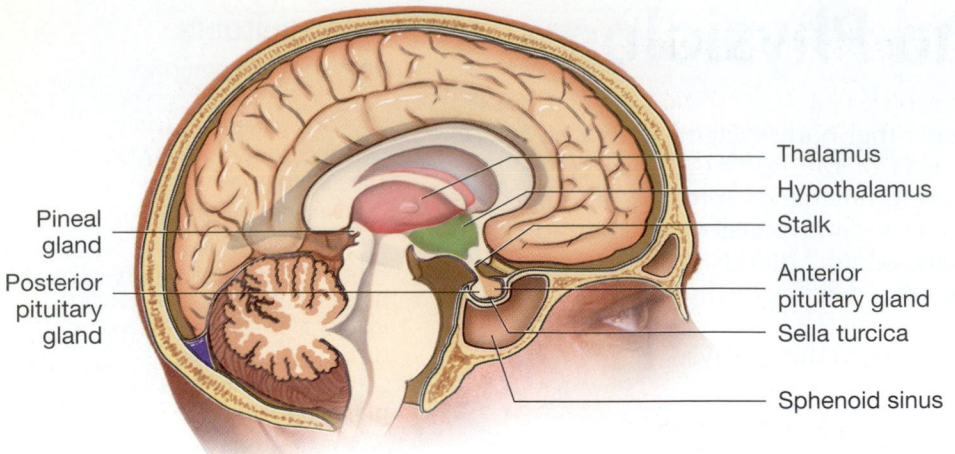

Pineal gland
Posterior pituitary gland
Thalamus
Hypothalamus
Stalk
Anterior pituitary gland
Sella turcica
Sphenoid sinus

Figure 14-2 ■ Endocrine glands in the brain.
The hypothalamus forms the floor and part of the walls of the third ventricle, as well as the stalk of tissue that goes to the pituitary gland. The pituitary gland sits in a bony cup in the sphenoid bone. The pineal gland is located between the two lobes of the thalamus.

gland (see Figure 14-2 ■). The hypothalamus functions as part of both the nervous system (discussed in "Neurology," Chapter 10) and the endocrine system. As an endocrine gland, the hypothalamus secretes substances that stimulate or inhibit the secretion of hormones from the anterior pituitary gland. The hypothalamus also produces two hormones of its own—antidiuretic hormone (ADH) and oxytocin—but these are stored in the posterior pituitary gland. These hormones are secreted when the hypothalamus sends a nerve impulse through the stalk to the posterior pituitary gland.

Pituitary Gland

The **pituitary gland** (**hypophysis**) is within the brain, just above the sphenoid sinus, and it sits in a bony cup (the **sella turcica**) of the sphenoid bone (see Figure 14-2). The pituitary gland is a small, bulb-shaped gland at the end of the stalk from the hypothalamus. Even though it is about the size of a pea and weighs only a fraction of an ounce, the pituitary gland is known as the master gland of the body because the effects of its hormones are felt throughout the body. It has two lobes, each of which contains a different gland: the **anterior pituitary gland** (or **adenohypophysis**) and the **posterior pituitary gland** (or **neurohypophysis**).

Anterior Pituitary Gland   The anterior pituitary gland secretes seven hormones (see Figure 14-3 ■).

1. **Thyroid-stimulating hormone (TSH).** This hormone causes the thyroid gland to grow, and stimulates it to secrete the thyroid hormones T_3 and T_4.

2. **Follicle-stimulating hormone (FSH).** In females, this hormone stimulates follicles in the ovaries to produce mature ova and to secrete the hormone estradiol. In males, it stimulates the seminiferous tubules of the testes to produce spermatozoa.

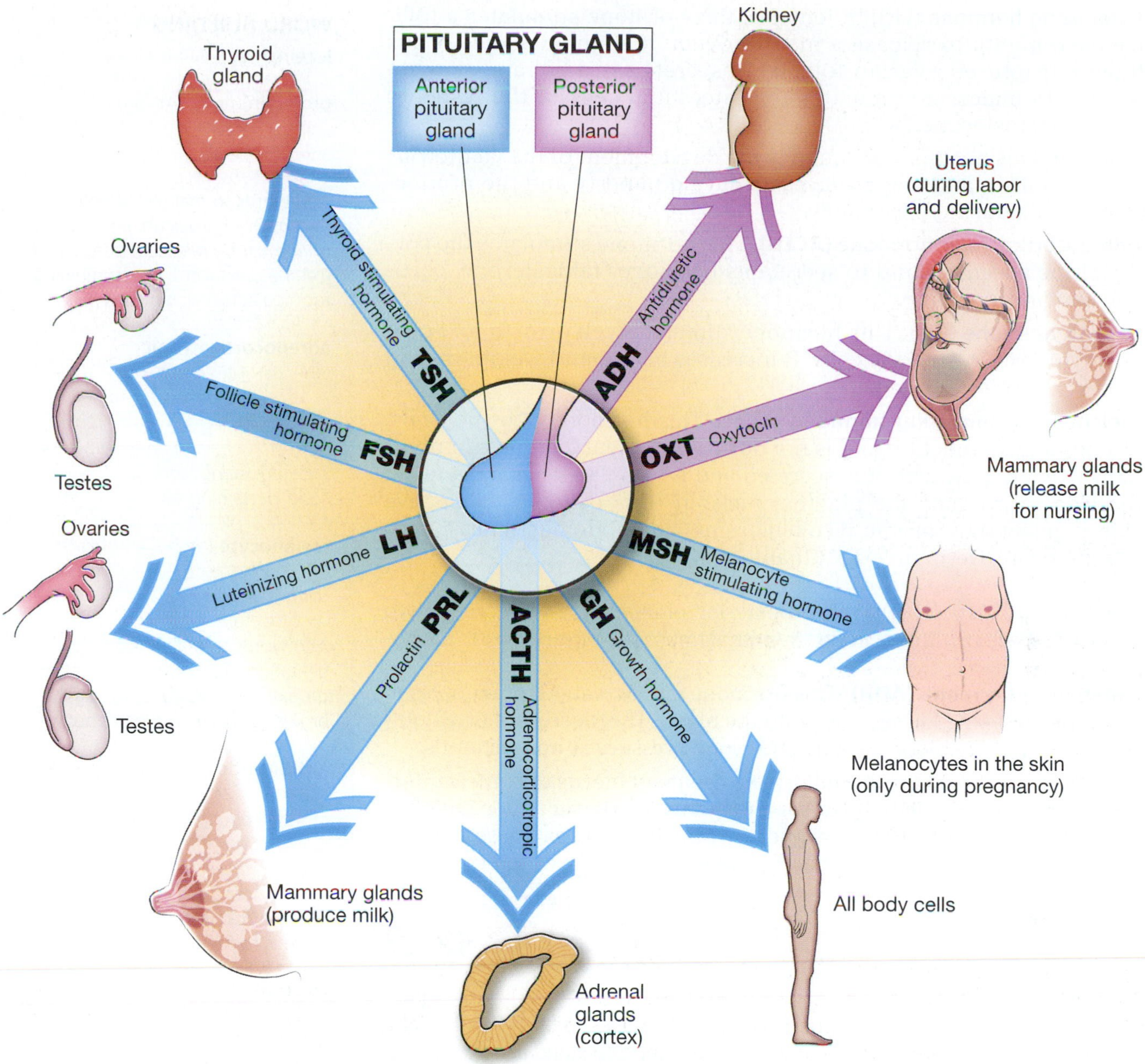

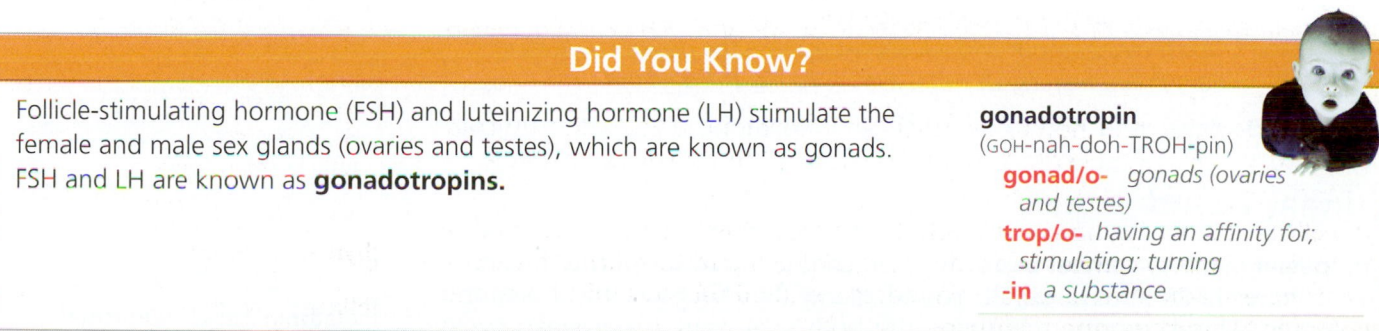

PITUITARY GLAND

Anterior pituitary gland

Posterior pituitary gland

Kidney

Thyroid gland

Ovaries

Testes

Ovaries

Testes

Thyroid stimulating hormone **TSH**

Follicle stimulating hormone **FSH**

Luteinizing hormone **LH**

Prolactin **PRL**

ACTH Adrenocorticotropic hormone

ADH Antidiuretic hormone

OXT Oxytocin

MSH Melanocyte stimulating hormone

GH Growth hormone

Uterus (during labor and delivery)

Mammary glands (release milk for nursing)

Melanocytes in the skin (only during pregnancy)

Mammary glands (produce milk)

Adrenal glands (cortex)

All body cells

Figure 14-3 ■ Hormones of the anterior and posterior pituitary gland.
The anterior pituitary gland produces and secretes seven different hormones. The posterior pituitary gland stores and secretes two hormones that are actually produced by the hypothalamus.

Did You Know?

Follicle-stimulating hormone (FSH) and luteinizing hormone (LH) stimulate the female and male sex glands (ovaries and testes), which are known as gonads. FSH and LH are known as **gonadotropins.**

gonadotropin
(GOH-nah-doh-TROH-pin)
gonad/o- *gonads (ovaries and testes)*
trop/o- *having an affinity for; stimulating; turning*
-in *a substance*

3. **Luteinizing hormone (LH).** In females, this hormone stimulates a follicle each month to release a mature ovum. It stimulates the corpus luteum (ruptured ovarian follicle) to secrete estradiol and progesterone. In males, it stimulates the interstitial cells of the testes to secrete testosterone.

4. **Prolactin.** This hormone stimulates the development of the lactiferous lobules (milk glands) in the breasts during puberty and the production of milk during pregnancy.

5. **Adrenocorticotropic hormone (ACTH).** This hormone stimulates the cortex of the adrenal gland to secrete its hormones (aldosterone, cortisol, and androgens).

6. **Growth hormone (GH).** This hormone stimulates cell growth and protein synthesis in all body cells. It increases height and weight during puberty.

7. **Melanocyte-stimulating hormone (MSH).** This hormone does not have any significant function and is not normally present in adults. In pregnant women, however, it is secreted and it stimulates melanocytes in the skin to produce the pigment melanin. This causes a distinctive skin pigmentation on the face (chloasma) and abdomen (linea nigra) (discussed in "Dermatology," Chapter 7).

Posterior Pituitary Gland   The posterior pituitary gland secretes two hormones that are produced in the hypothalamus (see Figure 14-3).

1. **Antidiuretic hormone (ADH).** This hormone moves water from tubules in the nephron of the kidney back into the blood. This decreases urine output and keeps the blood volume and blood pressure at normal levels.

2. **Oxytocin.** This hormone stimulates the pregnant uterus to contract during labor and childbirth. It causes the uterus to contract after the birth to prevent hemorrhaging. It also causes the breasts to release milk for nursing ("let-down reflex") when the newborn baby cries or sucks.

Word Alert

SOUND-ALIKE WORDS

melanin   (noun)   dark brown or black pigment produced by melanocytes in the skin; melanocyte-stimulating hormone (MSH) and sunlight stimulate the melanocytes to form melanin.
Example: Sunshine increases the level of melanin in the skin, causing it to tan.

melatonin   (noun)   hormone secreted by the pineal gland; it is associated with the wake-sleep cycle.
Example: Daylight and sunshine decrease the melatonin level in the brain, helping us to be awake during the daytime.

Pineal Gland

The **pineal gland** (or **pineal body**) is between the two lobes of the thalamus (see Figure 14-2). It is a small, round gland that secretes the hormone **melatonin.** This hormone maintains the body's 24-hour wake–sleep cycle and regulates the onset and duration of sleep. Increased amounts of melatonin are secreted during the winter.

WORD BUILDING

luteinizing (LOO-tee-ih-NY-zing)

prolactin (proh-LAK-tin)
  pro- *before*
  lact/o- *milk*
  -in *a substance*
Add words to make a complete definition of *prolactin: a substance (that must be released) before milk (can be produced).* The combining form *galact/o-* also means *milk.*

adrenocorticotropic
(ah-DREE-noh-KOR-tih-koh-TROH-pik)
  adren/o- *adrenal gland*
  cortic/o- *cortex (outer region)*
  trop/o- *having an affinity for; stimulating; turning*
  -ic *pertaining to*

melanocyte (meh-LAN-oh-site)
(MEL-ah-NOH-site)
  melan/o- *black*
  -cyte *cell*
Add words to make a complete definition of *melanocyte: a cell (in the skin that produces the dark brown or) black (pigment melanin).*

antidiuretic (AN-tee-DY-yoo-RET-ik)
  anti- *against*
  dia- *complete; completely through*
  ur/o- *urine; urinary system*
  -etic *pertaining to*
The *a* in *dia-* is dropped when the word is formed.

oxytocin (AWK-see-TOH-sin)
  ox/y- *oxygen; quick*
  toc/o- *labor and childbirth*
  -in *a substance*

pineal (PIN-ee-al)

melatonin (MEL-ah-TOH-nin)

Thyroid Gland

The **thyroid gland** has two **lobes** connected by a thin bridge of tissue (the **isthmus**). The thyroid gland is in the neck on either side of the trachea and across its anterior surface (see Figure 14-4 ■). The thyroid gland secretes three hormones.

1. **T_3 (triiodothyronine).** This hormone increases the rate of cellular metabolism.
2. **T_4 (thyroxine).** This hormone is secreted, but then most of it is changed by the liver into T_3.
3. **Calcitonin.** This hormone regulates the amount of calcium in the blood. If the calcium level is too high, calcitonin moves calcium from the blood and deposits it in the bones. Calcitonin has an opposite effect from that of parathyroid hormone secreted by the parathyroid glands.

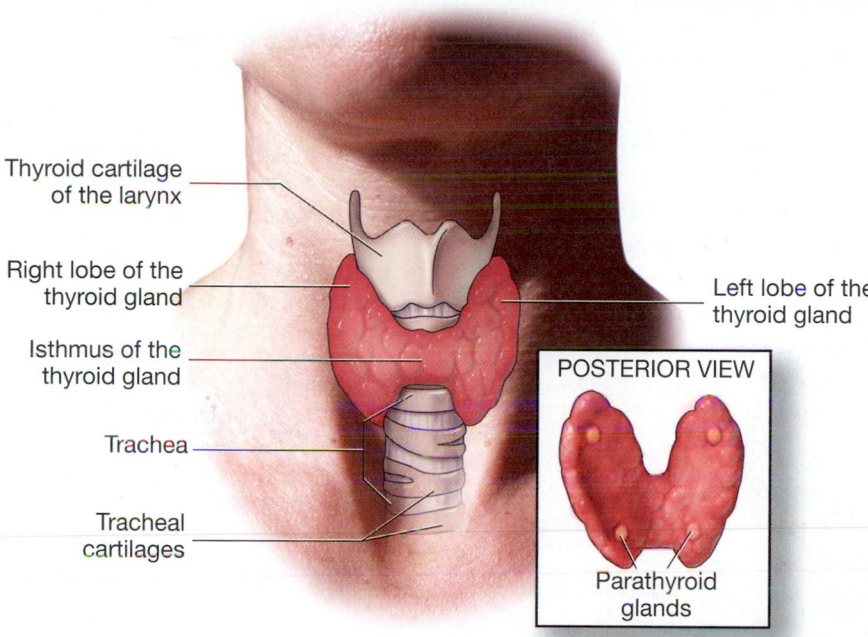

Thyroid cartilage of the larynx

Right lobe of the thyroid gland

Isthmus of the thyroid gland

Trachea

Tracheal cartilages

Left lobe of the thyroid gland

POSTERIOR VIEW

Parathyroid glands

Figure 14-4 ■ Thyroid gland and parathyroid glands.

This anterior view of the thyroid gland shows its two lobes connected by the isthmus, a bridge of tissue. The thyroid cartilage of the larynx mirrors the shield-like shape of the thyroid gland. However, the thyroid cartilage is part of the respiratory system, not the endocrine system. The parathyroid glands are located on the posterior surface of the thyroid gland.

The thyroid gland secretes T_3 and T_4 when stimulated by TSH from the anterior pituitary gland. When the thyroid gland is functioning properly, producing neither too much nor too little of these thyroid hormones, this steady state is known as **euthyroidism.**

Parathyroid Glands

The four **parathyroid glands** are on the posterior surface of the thyroid gland (see Figure 14-4). Each gland is about the size of a grain of rice. The parathyroid glands secrete **parathyroid hormone,** which regulates the amount of calcium in the blood. If the calcium level is too low, parathyroid hormone moves calcium from the bones into the blood. Parathyroid hormone has an opposite effect from that of calcitonin secreted by the thyroid gland.

Thymus Gland

The **thymus gland** is a pink gland with two lobes that is posterior to the sternum, within the mediastinum of the thoracic cavity. During childhood and puberty, the thymus gland is large, but it shrinks during adulthood. The thymus gland functions as part of both the body's immune response (discussed in "Hematology and Immunology," Chapter 6) and the endocrine system. As an endocrine gland, the thymus secretes **thymosins,** which cause immature T lymphocytes in the thymus to develop and mature.

Pancreas

The **pancreas** is a yellow, elongated, triangular gland that is posterior to the stomach (see Figure 14-5 ■). The pancreas functions as part of both the digestive system (discussed in "Gastroenterology," Chapter 3) and the endocrine system. As an endocrine gland, the pancreas secretes three hormones from groups of cells known as **islets of Langerhans.**

1. **Glucagon.** This hormone is secreted by **alpha cells** in the islets of Langerhans. When the blood glucose level is too low, glucagon breaks down **glycogen** (glucose stored in the liver and skeletal muscles) to release **glucose** into the blood.

WORD BUILDING

thymus (THY-mus)

thymic (THY-mik)
   thym/o- *thymus; rage*
   -ic *pertaining to*

thymosin (thy-MOH-sin)

pancreas (PAN-kree-as)

pancreatic (PAN-kree-AT-ik)
   pancreat/o- *pancreas*
   -ic *pertaining to*

islets of Langerhans
(EYE-lets of LAHNG-er-hanz)

glucagon (GLOO-kah-gawn)
   gluc/o- *glucose (sugar)*
   ag/o- *to lead to*
   -on *a substance; structure*

glycogen (GLY-koh-jen)
   glyc/o- *glucose (sugar)*
   -gen *that which produces*

glucose (GLOO-kohs)
   gluc/o- *glucose (sugar)*
   -ose *full of*
The combining form *glycos/o-* also means *glucose (sugar).*

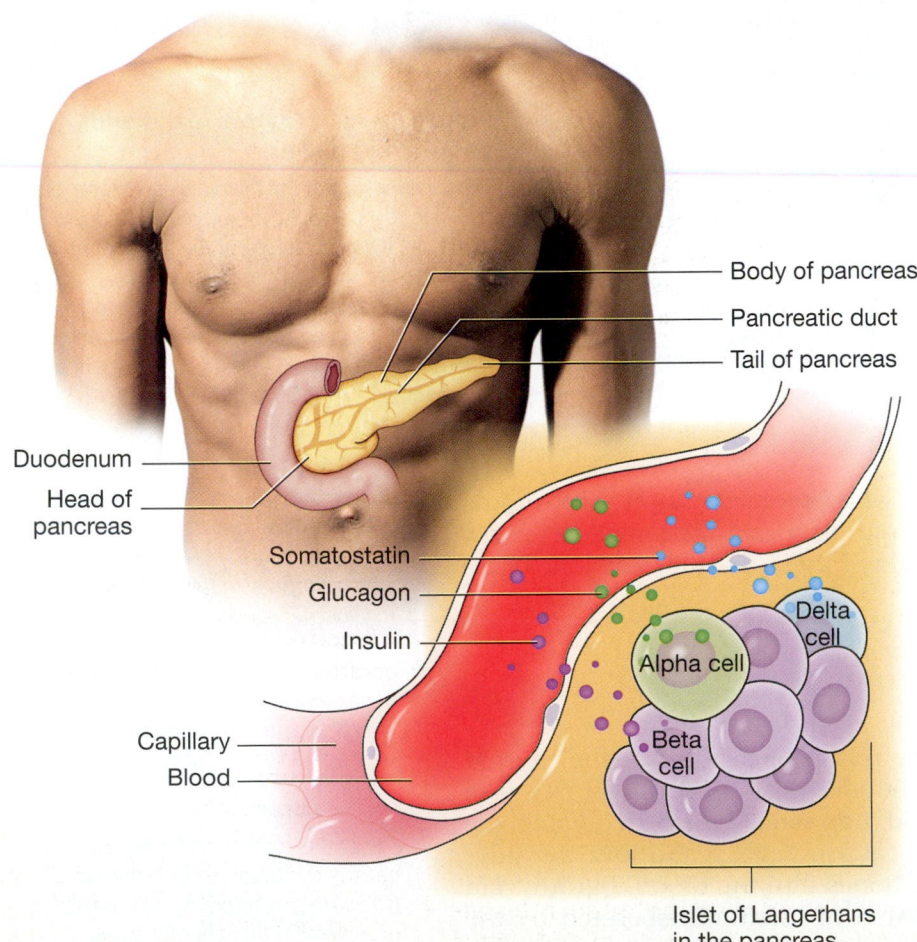

Body of pancreas
Pancreatic duct
Tail of pancreas
Duodenum
Head of pancreas
Somatostatin
Glucagon
Insulin
Delta cell
Alpha cell
Beta cell
Capillary
Blood
Islet of Langerhans in the pancreas

Figure 14-5 ■ **Pancreas.**
The pancreas is composed of small groups (islands) of cells known as the islets of Langerhans. Each islet is located next to a capillary so that the secreted hormones (glucagon, insulin, and somatostatin) can move directly into the blood.

2. **Insulin.** This hormone is secreted by **beta cells** in the islets of Langerhans. Insulin transports glucose to a body cell, binds to an insulin receptor on the cell membrane, and transports glucose into the cell so that it can be metabolized to produce energy.

3. **Somatostatin.** This hormone is secreted by **delta cells** in the islets of Langerhans. Somatostatin prevents glucagon and insulin from being secreted. It also prevents growth hormone (from the anterior pituitary gland) from being secreted.

Adrenal Glands

The **adrenal gland** is draped over the superior end of each kidney (see Figure 14-6 ■). The adrenal gland contains two different glands: an outer layer (cortex) and an inner layer (medulla). Each of these layers functions independently of the other and secretes its own hormones.

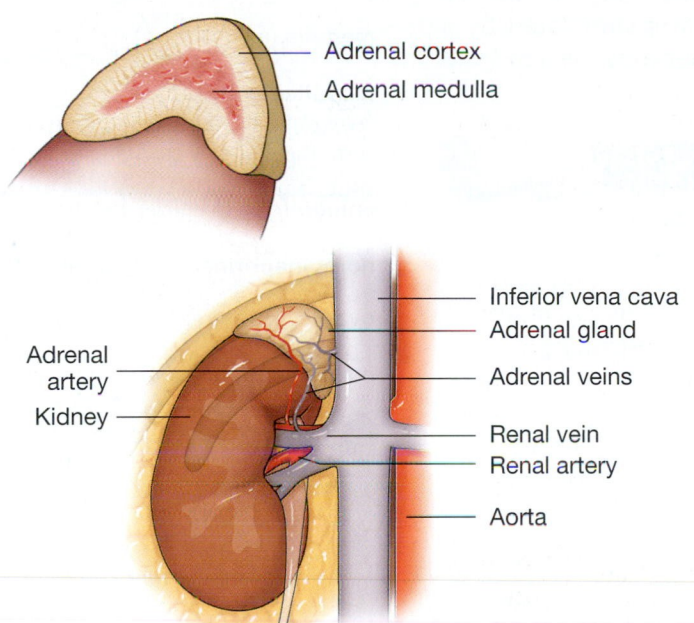

Figure 14-6 ■ Adrenal gland.

The adrenal gland is on top of and next to the kidney, but the adrenal gland is part of the endocrine system while the kidney belongs to the urinary system. The two parts of the adrenal gland, the cortex and the medulla, function as two separate endocrine glands.

Word Alert

SOUND-ALIKE WORDS

aden/o-   (combining form)   a gland
             Example: An adenoma is a benign tumor of a gland.

adren/o-   (combining form)   adrenal gland
              Example: Each adrenal gland sits on top of a kidney.

Adrenal Cortex   The **adrenal cortex** secretes three groups of hormones: mineralocorticoids, glucocorticoids, and androgens. The adrenal cortex secretes these hormones when stimulated by ACTH from the anterior pituitary gland.

1. **Aldosterone.** This hormone is the most abundant and biologically active of the **mineralocorticoid** hormones. The adrenal cortex secretes aldosterone when the blood pressure is low. It moves sodium and water

in tubules in the nephron of the kidney to the blood while allowing potassium to be excreted in the urine. This increases the blood volume and blood pressure.

2. **Cortisol.** This hormone is the most abundant and biologically active of the **glucocorticoid** hormones. It breaks down stored glycogen and increases the amount of glucose in the blood. It decreases the formation of proteins and new tissue, and it also exerts a strong anti-inflammatory effect.

3. **Androgens.** This group of hormones are male sex hormones. The adrenal cortex secretes androgens, but the testes secrete testosterone, the most abundant and biologically active of the androgens. In the blood, some of the androgens are changed to **estrogens** (female sex hormones). (The ovaries secrete estradiol, the most abundant and biologically active of the estrogens.)

Adrenal Medulla The **adrenal medulla** secretes the hormones **epinephrine** and **norepinephrine** into the blood when it is stimulated by a nerve impulse from the sympathetic division of the nervous system (discussed in "Neurology," Chapter 10).

Clinical Connections

Neurology (Chapter 10). When a person experiences danger or anger, the hypothalamus uses the sympathetic nervous system to trigger the release of epinephrine. This prepares the body to either fight or run away from the danger. Epinephrine increases the heart rate, constricts the smooth muscle of the blood vessels to raise the blood pressure, increases the respiratory rate, and dilates the bronchioles to increase air flow into the lungs.

Ovaries

The **ovaries** are small, egg-shaped glands in the pelvic cavity. The ovaries function as part of both the female reproductive system (discussed in "Gynecology and Obstetrics," Chapter 13) and the endocrine system. As an endocrine gland, the follicles of the ovary secrete **estradiol** when stimulated by FSH from the anterior pituitary gland. Estradiol is the most abundant and most biologically active female hormone. The corpus luteum (ruptured ovarian follicle) secretes estradiol and **progesterone** when stimulated by LH from the anterior pituitary gland. The cells around the follicle secrete testosterone (a male sex hormone) when stimulated by LH from the anterior pituitary gland.

Testes

The **testes** or **testicles** are egg-shaped glands in the scrotum, a pouch of skin behind the penis. The testes function as part of both the male genitourinary system (discussed in "Male Reproductive Medicine," Chapter 12) and the endocrine system. As an endocrine gland, the seminiferous tubules of the testes produce spermatozoa when stimulated by FSH from the anterior pituitary gland. Interstitial cells of the testes secrete testosterone when stimulated by LH from the anterior pituitary gland. **Testosterone** is the most abundant and biologically active of all the androgens (male sex hormones).

WORD BUILDING

cortisol (KOR-tih-sawl)

glucocorticoid
(GLOO-koh-KOR-tih-koyd)
  gluc/o- *glucose (sugar)*
  cortic/o- *cortex (outer region)*
  -oid *resembling*

androgen (AN-droh-jen)
  andr/o- *male*
  -gen *that which produces*
The combining form *viril/o-* means *masculine.*

estrogen (ES-troh-jen)
  estr/o- *female*
  -gen *that which produces*

medulla (meh-DUL-ah)

medullae (meh-DUL-ee)
Medulla is a Latin singular noun. Form the plural by changing *-a* to *-ae.*

epinephrine (EP-ih-NEF-rin)

norepinephrine (NOR-ep-ih-NEF-rin)

ovary (OH-vah-ree)

ovarian (oh-VAIR-ee-an)
  ovari/o- *ovary*
  -an *pertaining to*

estradiol (ES-trah-DY-awl)
  estr/a- *female*
  di- *two*
  -ol *chemical substance*

progesterone (proh-JES-ter-ohn)

testis (TES-tis)

testes (TES-teez)
Testis is a Latin singular noun. Form the plural by changing *-is* to *-es.*

testicle (TES-tih-kl)

testicles (TES-tih-kls)
Testicle is a combination of *testis* and the suffix *-cle* (small thing).

testicular (tes-TIK-yoo-lar)
  testicul/o- *testis; testicle*
  -ar *pertaining to*

testosterone (tes-TAWS-teh-rohn)
Testosterone contains the combining forms *test/o-* (testis; testicle) and *steroid/o-* (steroid) and the suffix *-one* (chemical substance).

Physiology of Hormone Response and Feedback

While the nervous system uses neurotransmitters as chemical messengers that travel between two neurons (or a neuron and an organ), the endocrine system uses hormones as chemical messengers. Hormones are secreted into the blood and travel throughout the body. Some neurotransmitters (epinephrine and norepinephrine) are also hormones because they are secreted by a gland and travel in the blood.

As they travel in the blood, hormones come in contact with all tissues, but they only exert an effect on glands or organs that have **receptors** to which they can bind. A hormone is like a key that unlocks receptors on a gland or organ and produces an effect. Other hormones cannot unlock those receptors.

A unique feature of the endocrine system is the "chain reaction" sequence of effects: A hormone released by an endocrine gland can stimulate another endocrine gland to release its hormones and then those hormones stimulate receptors on an organ to produce an effect.

The action of hormones involves **stimulation** or **inhibition.** Some hormones, such as the releasing hormones of the hypothalamus, stimulate an endocrine gland to release its hormones. Other hormones, such as the inhibiting hormones of the hypothalamus, keep an endocrine gland from releasing its hormones.

When two hormones, such as T_3 and T_4, work in conjunction with one another to accomplish an enhanced effect, this is **synergism.** When two hormones, such as calcitonin and parathyroid hormone, exert an opposite effect, this is **antagonism** (see Figure 14-7 ■).

The endocrine system maintains body homeostasis through the use of hormones and a negative feedback mechanism. For example, after the anterior pituitary gland secretes thyroid-stimulating hormone, it then monitors the blood levels of thyroid hormones. If the levels are still low (negative feedback), the anterior pituitary gland secretes more thyroid-stimulating hormone.

WORD BUILDING

receptor (ree-SEP-ter)
recept/o- receive
-**or** person or thing that produces or does

stimulation (STIM-yoo-LAY-shun)
stimul/o- exciting; strengthening
-**ation** a process; being or having

inhibition (IN-hih-BISH-un)
inhibit/o- block; hold back
-**ion** action; condition

synergism (SIN-er-jizm)
syn- together
erg/o- activity; work
-**ism** process; disease from a specific cause

antagonism (an-TAG-on-izm)
antagon/o- oppose or work against
-**ism** process; disease from a specific cause

	HORMONE	ACTION	SOURCE	
BODY METABOLISM	T3 and T4	↑ Increases metabolism	Thyroid	
BLOOD GLUCOSE	Cortisol	↑ Increases blood glucose (stored glycogen converted to glucose)	Adrenal cortex	
	Glucagon	↑ Increases blood glucose	Pancreas	
	Epinephrine	↑ Increases blood glucose	Adrenal medulla	
	Insulin	↓ Decreases blood glucose	Pancreas	
BLOOD CALCIUM	Parathyroid hormone	↑ Increases blood calcium	Parathyroid	
	Calcitonin	↓ Decreases blood calcium	Thyroid	
BLOOD SODIUM	Aldosterone	↑ Increases blood sodium	Adrenal cortex	

Figure 14-7 ■ Effects of hormones.

Hormones from the various endocrine glands affect body metabolism, blood glucose, blood calcium, and blood sodium in complementary or opposite ways.

Vocabulary Review

Anatomy and Physiology

Word or Phrase	Description	Combining Forms
endocrine system	Body system that includes glands that secrete hormones into the blood. These glands include the hypothalamus, pituitary gland, pineal gland, thyroid gland, parathyroid glands, thymus, pancreas, adrenal glands, ovaries, and testes. The endocrine system is also known as the **neuroendocrine system.**	**crin/o-** *secrete* **neur/o-** *nerve*
gland	Structure of the endocrine system that secretes one or more hormones into the blood	**glandul/o-** *gland*
homeostasis	State of equilibrium of the internal environment of the body. The endocrine system plays a role in homeostasis by regulating body fluids, electrolytes, glucose, cellular metabolism, growth, and the wake–sleep cycle.	**home/o-** *same*
hormone	Chemical messenger of the endocrine system that is produced by a gland and secreted into the blood	**hormon/o-** *hormone*

Hypothalamus

hypothalamus	Endocrine gland within the brain just below the thalamus. The hypothalamus secretes substances that stimulate or inhibit the secretion of hormones from the anterior pituitary gland. It also produces antidiuretic hormone (ADH) and oxytocin. These two hormones are stored in the posterior pituitary gland.	**thalam/o-** *thalamus*

Pituitary Gland

adrenocorticotropic hormone (ACTH)	Hormone secreted by the anterior pituitary gland. It stimulates the adrenal cortex to secrete its hormones.	**adren/o-** *adrenal gland* **cortic/o-** *cortex (outer region)* **trop/o-** *having an affinity for; stimulating; turning*
anterior pituitary gland	It secretes thyroid-stimulating hormone (TSH), follicle-stimulating hormone (FSH), luteinizing hormone (LH), prolactin, adrenocorticotropic hormone (ACTH), growth hormone (GH), and melanocyte-stimulating hormone (MSH). It is also known as the **adenohypophysis.**	**pituit/o-** *pituitary gland* **aden/o-** *gland* **hypophys/o-** *pituitary gland*
antidiuretic hormone (ADH)	Hormone produced by the hypothalamus but stored and secreted by the posterior pituitary gland. It moves sodium and water from tubules in the nephron of the kidney into the blood. This decreases urine output and keeps the blood volume and blood pressure normal.	**ur/o-** *urine; urinary system*
follicle-stimulating hormone (FSH)	Hormone secreted by the anterior pituitary gland. In females, it stimulates follicles in the ovary to produce mature ova and to secrete the hormone estradiol. In males, it stimulates the seminiferous tubules of the testes to produce spermatozoa.	**stimul/o-** *exciting; strengthening*
gonadotropins	Category of hormones that stimulates the male and female sex glands (gonads). It includes follicle-stimulating hormone (FSH) and luteinizing hormone (LH).	**gonad/o-** *gonads (ovaries and testes)* **trop/o-** *having an affinity for; stimulating; turning*

Word or Phrase	Description	Combining Forms
growth hormone (GH)	Hormone secreted by the anterior pituitary gland. It stimulates cell growth and protein synthesis in all body cells. It increases height and weight during puberty.	
luteinizing hormone (LH)	Hormone secreted by the anterior pituitary gland. In females, it stimulates a follicle in the ovary to release a mature ovum. It stimulates the corpus luteum (ruptured ovarian follicle) to secrete estradiol and progesterone. In males, it stimulates the interstitial cells of the testes to secrete testosterone.	
melanocyte-stimulating hormone (MSH)	Hormone secreted by the anterior pituitary gland. It is secreted in pregnant women and stimulates melanocytes in the skin to produce melanin. This causes skin pigmentation on the face and abdomen.	**melan/o-** *black*
oxytocin	Hormone produced by the hypothalamus but stored and secreted by the posterior pituitary gland. It stimulates the pregnant uterus to contract during labor and childbirth. It causes the uterus to contract after birth to prevent hemorrhaging. It causes the breasts to release milk for nursing ("let-down reflex") when the baby cries or sucks.	**ox/y-** *oxygen; quick* **toc/o-** *labor and childbirth*
pituitary gland	Endocrine gland in the brain that is connected by a stalk of tissue to the hypothalamus. It sits in the bony cup of the **sella turcica** of the sphenoid bone. It is also known as the **hypophysis.** It is the master gland of the body. It consists of two separate glands: the anterior pituitary gland and the posterior pituitary gland.	**pituit/o-** *pituitary gland* **hypophys/o-** *pituitary gland* **pituitar/o-** *pituitary gland*
posterior pituitary gland	It stores antidiuretic hormone (ADH) and oxytocin produced by the hypothalamus; it secretes these hormones in response to a nerve impulse from the hypothalamus. It is also known as the **neurohypophysis.**	**pituit/o-** *pituitary gland* **neur/o-** *nerve* **hypophys/o-** *pituitary gland*
prolactin	Hormone secreted by the anterior pituitary gland. It stimulates the development of the lactiferous lobules (milk glands) in the breasts during puberty and the production of milk during pregnancy.	**lact/o-** *milk* **galact/o-** *milk*
thyroid-stimulating hormone (TSH)	Hormone secreted by the anterior pituitary gland. It causes the thyroid gland to grow and stimulates it to secrete the thyroid hormones T_3 and T_4.	**thyr/o-** *shield-shaped structure (thyroid gland)* **stimul/o-** *exciting; strengthening*

Pineal Gland

melatonin	Hormone secreted by the pineal gland. It maintains the 24-hour wake–sleep cycle.	
pineal gland	Endocrine gland between the two lobes of the thalamus. It secretes the hormone melatonin. It is also known as the **pineal body.**	

Thyroid Gland

calcitonin	Hormone secreted by the thyroid gland. It regulates the amount of calcium in the blood. If the calcium level is too high, calcitonin moves calcium from the blood and deposits it in the bones.	**calc/i-** *calcium* **ton/o-** *pressure; tone* **calc/o-** *calcium*
euthyroidism	State of normal functioning of the hormones of the thyroid gland	**thyroid/o-** *thyroid gland*
T_3	Hormone secreted by the thyroid gland. It increases the rate of cellular metabolism. It is also known as **triiodothyronine.**	**iod/o-** *iodine* **thyr/o-** *shield-shaped structure (thyroid gland)*

Word or Phrase	Description	Combining Forms
T₄	Hormone secreted by the thyroid gland. Most of it is changed into T_3 by the liver. It is also known as **thyroxine.**	
thyroid gland	Endocrine gland in the neck that secretes the hormones T_3, T_4, and calcitonin. Its two **lobes** and narrow connecting bridge **(isthmus)** have a shieldlike shape.	**thyr/o-** *shield-shaped structure (thyroid gland)*

Parathyroid Glands

parathyroid glands	Four endocrine glands on the posterior surface of the lobes of the thyroid gland. They secrete parathyroid hormone.	**thyr/o-** *shield-shaped structure (thyroid gland)*
parathyroid hormone	Hormone secreted by the parathyroid glands. It regulates the amount of calcium in the blood. If the calcium level is too low, parathyroid hormone moves calcium from the bones to the blood.	**thyr/o-** *shield-shaped structure (thyroid gland)*

Thymus Gland

thymus	Endocrine gland posterior to the sternum and within the mediastinum. It secretes a group of hormones known as **thymosins.** They cause immature T lymphocytes in the thymus to mature.	**thym/o-** *thymus; rage*

Pancreas

glucagon	Hormone secreted by alpha cells in the islets of Langerhans. It breaks down stored glycogen to increase the glucose in the blood.	**gluc/o-** *glucose (sugar)* **ag/o-** *to lead to*
glucose	A simple sugar in foods and also the sugar in the blood (produced when the hormones glucagon or cortisol break down stored glycogen)	**gluc/o-** *glucose (sugar)* **glycos/o-** *glucose (sugar)*
glycogen	Glucose stored in the liver and skeletal muscles. Glycogen is broken down into glucose by the hormone glucagon from the pancreas and by the hormone cortisol from the adrenal cortex.	**glyc/o-** *glucose (sugar)*
insulin	Hormone secreted by beta cells in the islets of Langerhans. It facilitates the transport of glucose into the cells where it is metabolized for energy.	**insul/o-** *island* **insulin/o-** *insulin*
pancreas	Endocrine gland posterior to the stomach. It contains the **islets of Langerhans** (alpha, beta, and delta cells) that secrete the hormones glucagon, insulin, and somatostatin.	**pancreat/o-** *pancreas*
somatostatin	Hormone secreted by delta cells in the islets of Langerhans. It prevents the hormones glucagon and insulin from being secreted by the pancreas. It prevents growth hormone from being secreted by the anterior pituitary gland.	**somat/o-** *body* **stat/o-** *standing still; staying in one place*

Adrenal Glands

adrenal cortex	Outermost layer of the adrenal gland. It secretes three groups of hormones: mineralocorticoids (aldosterone), glucocorticoids (cortisol), and androgens (male sex hormones).	**adren/o-** *adrenal gland* **cortic/o-** *cortex (outer region)*
adrenal glands	Endocrine glands on top of the kidneys. An adrenal gland contains a cortex and a medulla, each of which is a gland that secretes its own hormones.	**adren/o-** *adrenal gland* **adrenal/o-** *adrenal gland* **ren/o-** *kidney*

Word or Phrase	Description	Combining Forms
adrenal medulla	Innermost layer of the adrenal gland. It secretes the hormones epinephrine and norepinephrine when stimulated by a nerve impulse from the sympathetic division of the nervous system.	**adren/o-** *adrenal gland*
aldosterone	Most abundant and biologically active of the mineralocorticoid hormones secreted by the adrenal cortex. The adrenal cortex secretes aldosterone when the blood pressure is low. It moves sodium and water from the tubules in nephrons in the kidney to the blood while allowing potassium to be excreted in the urine.	
androgens	Male sex hormones, such as testosterone from the testes, and other androgens secreted by the adrenal cortex. In the blood, androgens from the adrenal cortex are changed into estrogens.	**andr/o-** *male* **viril/o-** *masculine*
cortisol	Most abundant and biologically active of the glucocorticoid hormones secreted by the adrenal cortex. It breaks down glycogen to increase the level of glucose in the blood. It decreases the formation of proteins and new tissues, and it has an anti-inflammatory effect. The adrenal cortex secretes cortisol when stimulated by ACTH from the anterior pituitary gland.	
epinephrine	Hormone secreted by the adrenal medulla in response to a nerve impulse from the sympathetic division of the nervous system	
estrogens	Female sex hormones, such as estradiol from the ovaries. In the blood, androgens from the adrenal cortex are changed into estrogens.	**estr/o-** *female*
glucocorticoids	Group of hormones secreted by the adrenal cortex. See *cortisol*.	**gluc/o-** *glucose (sugar)* **cortic/o-** *cortex (outer region)*
mineralocorticoids	Group of hormones secreted by the adrenal cortex. See *aldosterone*.	**mineral/o-** *mineral; electrolyte* **cortic/o-** *cortex (outer region)*
norepinephrine	Hormone secreted by the adrenal medulla	

Ovaries

Word or Phrase	Description	Combining Forms
estradiol	Female sex hormone that is the most abundant and biologically active of all the estrogens. Estradiol is secreted by the follicles and corpus luteum of the ovary when stimulated by the follicle-stimulating hormone (FSH) from the anterior pituitary gland.	**estr/a-** *female*
ovaries	Endocrine glands near the uterus; they are also the female sex glands (gonads). Follicle-stimulating hormone (FSH) from the anterior pituitary gland stimulates the follicles of the ovary to secrete estradiol. LH stimulates the corpus luteum (ruptured follicle) to secrete estradiol and progesterone. The cells around the follicles secrete the male hormone testosterone.	**ovari/o-** *ovary*
progesterone	Female sex hormone secreted by the corpus luteum of the ovary when stimulated by luteinizing hormone (LH) from the anterior pituitary gland	

Testes

Word or Phrase	Description	Combining Forms
testes	Endocrine glands on either side of the scrotum; they are also the male sex glands (gonads). They are also known as **testicles.** Follicle-stimulating hormone (FSH) from the anterior pituitary gland stimulates their seminiferous tubules to produce spermatozoa. Luteinzing hormone (LH) from the anterior pituitary gland stimulates their interstitial cells to secrete testosterone.	**test/o-** *testis; testicle* **testicul/o-** *testis; testicle*
testosterone	Male sex hormone that is the most abundant and biologically active of the androgens. Testosterone is secreted by the interstitial cells of the testes when stimulated by luteinizing hormone (LH) from the anterior pituitary gland.	**test/o-** *testis; testicle*

Hormone Response and Feedback

Word or Phrase	Description	Combining Forms
antagonism	Process in which two hormones exert opposite effects	**antagon/o-** *oppose or work against*
inhibition	Action of a hormone to prevent or inhibit an endocrine gland from secreting its hormones	**inhibit/o-** *block; hold back*
receptor	Structure on the cell membrane of an organ or gland where a hormone binds and exerts an effect	**recept/o-** *receive*
stimulation	Action of a hormone that causes an endocrine gland to secrete its hormones	**stimul/o-** *exciting; strengthening*
synergism	Process in which two hormones work together to accomplish an enhanced effect	**erg/o-** *activity; work*

Labeling Exercise

Match each anatomy word or phrase to its structure and write it in the numbered box for each figure. Be sure to check your spelling. Use the Answer Key at the end of the book to check your answers.

adrenal gland	ovary	parathyroid glands	pituitary gland	thymus
hypothalamus	pancreas	pineal body	testis	thyroid gland

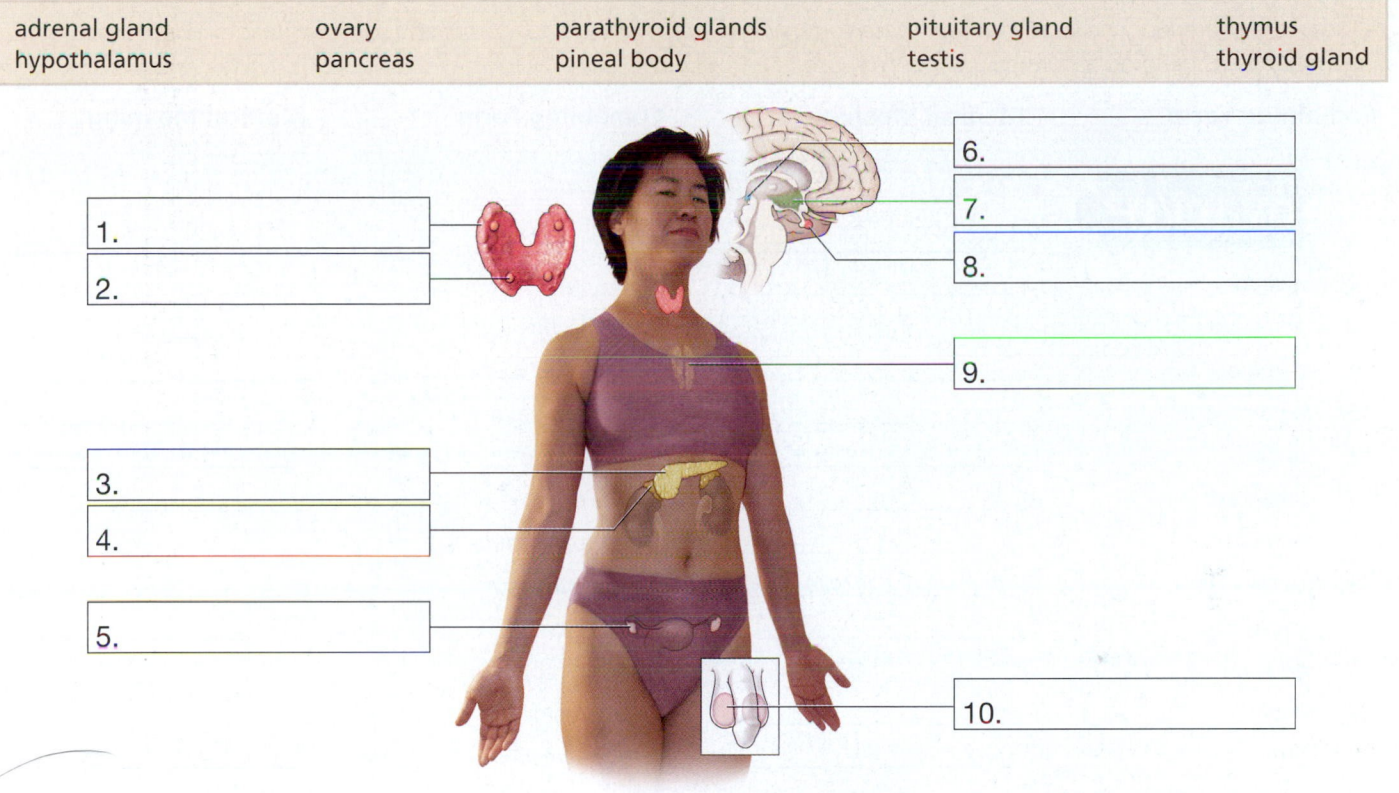

1.
2.
3.
4.
5.
6.
7.
8.
9.
10.

isthmus of thyroid gland	right lobe of the thyroid gland	trachea
left lobe of the thyroid gland	thyroid cartilage of the larynx	tracheal cartilage
parathyroid glands		

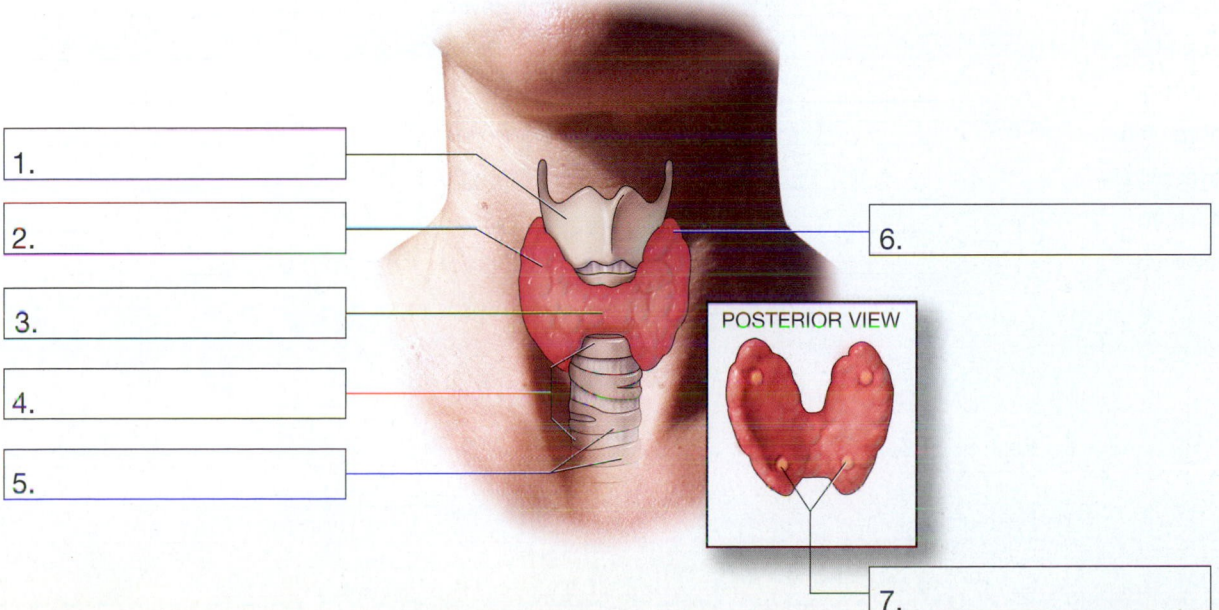

POSTERIOR VIEW

1.
2.
3.
4.
5.
6.
7.

Building Medical Words

Use the Answer Key at the end of the book to check your answers.

Combining Forms Exercise

Before you build endocrine words, review these combining forms. Next to each combining form, write its medical meaning. The first one has been done for you.

Combining Form	Medical Meaning	Combining Form	Medical Meaning
1. **ovari/o-**	ovary	27. insul/o-	
2. aden/o-		28. iod/o-	
3. adrenal/o-		29. lact/o-	
4. adren/o-		30. melan/o-	
5. ag/o-		31. mineral/o-	
6. andr/o-		32. neur/o-	
7. antagon/o-		33. ox/y-	
8. anter/o-		34. pancreat/o-	
9. calc/i-		35. pituitar/o-	
10. calc/o-		36. pituit/o-	
11. cortic/o-		37. recept/o-	
12. crin/o-		38. ren/o-	
13. erg/o-		39. somat/o-	
14. estr/a-		40. stat/o-	
15. estr/o-		41. stimul/o-	
16. galact/o-		42. testicul/o-	
17. glandul/o-		43. test/o-	
18. gluc/o-		44. thalam/o-	
19. glyc/o-		45. thym/o-	
20. glycos/o-		46. thyr/o-	
21. gonad/o-		47. thyroid/o-	
22. home/o-		48. toc/o-	
23. hormon/o-		49. ton/o-	
24. hypophys/o-		50. trop/o-	
25. inhibit/o-		51. ur/o-	
26. insulin/o-		52. viril/o-	

Combining Form and Suffix Exercise

Read the definition of the medical word. Look at the combining form that is given. Select the correct suffix from the Suffix List and write it on the blank line. Then build the medical word and write it on the line. (Remember: You may need to remove the combining vowel. Always remove the hyphens and slash.) Be sure to check your spelling. The first one has been done for you.

SUFFIX LIST		
-al (pertaining to)	-gen (that which produces)	-oid (resembling)
-an (pertaining to)	-ic (pertaining to)	-or (person or thing that produces or does)
-ar (pertaining to)	-ism (process; disease from a	-stasis (condition of staying in one place)
-ation (a process; being or having)	specific cause)	

Definition of the Medical Word	Combining Form	Suffix	Build the Medical Word

thym/o-   -ic

1. Pertaining to the thymus — thymic

   (You think *pertaining to* (-ic) + *the thymus* (thym/o-). You change the order of the word parts to put the suffix last. You write *thymic*.)

2. Pertaining to (substances from endocrine glands) — hormon/o-
3. That which produces male (characteristics) — andr/o-
4. Pertaining to the ovary — ovari/o-
5. Condition of staying in one place (and being the) same — home/o-
6. A process of exciting — stimul/o-
7. (A gland) resembling a shield-shaped structure — thyr/o-
8. Pertaining to the pancreas — pancreat/o-
9. Pertaining to the testicle — testicul/o-
10. Person or thing that produces or receives — recept/o-
11. Process to oppose or work against — antagon/o-

Prefix Exercise

Read the definition of the medical word. Look at the medical word or partial word that is given (it already contains a combining form and a suffix). Select the correct prefix from the Prefix List and write it on the blank line. Then build the medical word and write it on the line. Be sure to check your spelling. The first one has been done for you.

PREFIX LIST		
ad- (toward)	hypo- (below; deficient)	pro- (before)
eu- (normal; good)	para- (beside; apart from; two parts of a pair; abnormal)	syn- (together)

Definition of the Medical Word	Prefix	Word or Partial Word	Build the Medical Word

hypo-   physial

1. Pertaining to something below (the pituitary gland) that grows | | | hypophysial
2. Process of a normal thyroid | | thyroidism |
3. (Structures) resembling two parts of a pair (on the) thyroid gland | | thyroid |
4. Pertaining to (a gland) below the thalamus | | thalamic |
5. A substance (that must be released) before milk (can be produced) | | lactin |
6. Process (of being) together to work | | ergism |
7. Pertaining to (a gland) toward the kidney | | renal |

Diseases and Conditions

Anterior Pituitary Gland: All Hormones

Word or Phase	Description	Word Building
hyperpituitarism	**Hypersecretion** of one or all of the hormones of the anterior pituitary gland. It is caused by a benign tumor (**adenoma**) in the pituitary gland. Treatment: Drug therapy to suppress secretion of the hormone, or surgery to remove the adenoma, or radiation therapy to destroy the adenoma.	**hyperpituitarism** (HY-per-pih-TOO-ih-tah-rizm) **hyper-** *above; more than normal* **pituitar/o-** *pituitary gland* **-ism** *process; disease from a specific cause* **adenoma** (AD-eh-NOH-mah) **aden/o-** *gland* **-oma** *tumor; mass* **adenomata** (AD-eh-NOH-mah-tah) *Adenoma is a Greek noun. Form the plural by changing -oma to -omata.*
hypopituitarism	Hyposecretion of one or more of the hormones of the anterior pituitary gland. It is caused by an injury or a defect in the pituitary gland. **Panhypopituitarism** is hyposecretion of all of the hormones. Treatment: Drug therapy to replace the hormone.	**hypopituitarism** (HY-poh-pih-TOO-ih-tah-rizm) **hypo-** *below; deficient* **pituitar/o-** *pituitary gland* **-ism** *process; disease from a specific cause* **panhypopituitarism** (pan-HY-poh-pih-TOO-eh-tah-rizm) The prefix *pan-* means *all*.

Anterior Pituitary Gland: Prolactin

Word or Phase	Description	Word Building
galactorrhea	Hypersecretion of prolactin. It is caused by an adenoma in the anterior pituitary gland. The high level of prolactin causes the breasts to produce milk, even though the patient is not pregnant. It also inhibits the secretion of FSH and LH and this stops menstruation. Treatment: Drug therapy to suppress secretion of prolactin, or surgery to remove the adenoma, or radiation therapy to destroy the adenoma.	**galactorrhea** (gah-LAK-toh-REE-ah) **galact/o-** *milk* **-rrhea** *flow; discharge*
failure of lactation	Hyposecretion of prolactin. It is caused by a defect in the anterior pituitary gland. The low level of prolactin causes the lactiferous lobules (milk glands) in the breasts not to develop during puberty, and the breasts do not make enough milk for breastfeeding after the baby is born. Treatment: None.	**lactation** (lak-TAY-shun) **lact/o-** *milk* **-ation** *a process; being or having*

Anterior Pituitary Gland: Growth Hormone

Word or Phrase	Description	Word Building
gigantism	Hypersecretion of growth hormone during childhood and puberty (see Figure 14-8 ■). It is caused by an adenoma in the anterior pituitary gland. The high level of growth hormone causes the bones and tissues to grow excessively. Treatment: Drug therapy to suppress secretion of growth hormone, or surgery to remove the adenoma, or radiation therapy to destroy the adenoma.	**gigantism** (jy-GAN-tizm) (JY-gan-tizm) **gigant/o-** *giant* **-ism** *process; disease from a specific cause*

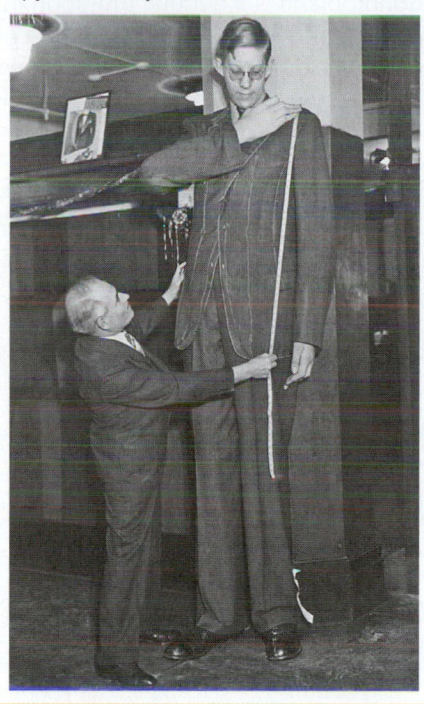

Figure 14-8 ■ Gigantism.
The tallest man who ever lived suffered from gigantism. His name was Robert Wadlow. He was born in 1918 in Illinois and was of average weight and length at birth. By the time he was 18 years old, he was 8'11" and weighed 491 pounds. He wore size 37AA shoes that were over 18" in length. He died in 1940, at the age of 22. The tallest living man now is Bao Xishun, a herdsman in Mongolia, China. He was born in 1951 and is 7'9".

Word or Phrase	Description	Word Building
acromegaly	Hypersecretion of growth hormone during adulthood. It is caused by an adenoma in the anterior pituitary gland. Because the growth plates at the ends of the long bones have already fused, the patient cannot grow taller. So, the high level of growth hormone causes the facial features, jaw, hands, and feet to widen and enlarge (see Figure 14-9 ■). Treatment: Drug therapy to suppress secretion of growth hormone, or surgery to remove the adenoma, or radiation therapy to destroy the adenoma.	**acromegaly** (AK-roh-MEG-ah-lee) **acr/o-** *extremity; highest point* **-megaly** *enlargement*

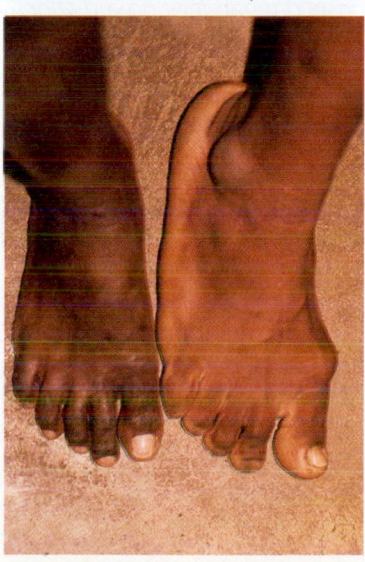

Figure 14-9 ■ Acromegaly.
Increased levels of growth hormone in adulthood cause the face and extremities to widen rather than grow longer. The foot on the left is normal. The foot on the right shows acromegaly with enlargement and widening.

Word or Phrase	Description	Word Building
dwarfism	Hyposecretion of growth hormone during childhood and puberty. It is caused by a defect in the anterior pituitary gland. The low level of growth hormone causes a lack of growth and short stature, but with normal body proportions. Treatment: Drug therapy with growth hormone.	**dwarfism** (DWORF-izm) *Dwarfism* is a combination of the word *dwarf* and the suffix *-ism* (process; disease from a specific cause).

Clinical Connections

Genetics. Dwarfism has many causes. Achondroplasia is a genetic mutation in which cartilage does not convert to bone. This results in a dwarf with small extremities but a normal-sized trunk. Short stature in an otherwise normal person can also be caused by severe malnutrition, very short parents (heredity), or severe kidney or heart disease.

Posterior Pituitary Gland: Antidiuretic Hormone (ADH)

Word or Phrase	Description	Word Building
syndrome of inappropriate ADH (SIADH)	Hypersecretion of antidiuretic hormone (ADH). It is caused by an adenoma in the posterior pituitary gland. (It can also be caused by brain infections, multiple sclerosis, or a stroke.) The high level of ADH causes excessive amounts of water to move into the blood. This dilutes the blood, creates a low level of sodium, and causes headache, weakness, confusion, and eventually coma. Treatment: Restriction of water intake. Surgery to remove the adenoma or radiation therapy to destroy the adenoma.	
diabetes insipidus (DI)	Hyposecretion of antidiuretic hormone (ADH). It is caused by a defect in the posterior pituitary gland. (It can also be caused by a brain infection, head trauma, or heredity.) The low level of ADH causes excessive amounts of water to be excreted in the urine (**polyuria**). There is also weakness (due to water loss and dehydration) and thirst with increased intake of fluids (**polydipsia**). Treatment: Drug therapy with antidiuretic hormone.	**diabetes** (DY-ah-BEE-teez) **insipidus** (in-SIP-ih-dus) **polyuria** (PAWL-ee-YOO-ree-ah) **poly-** *many; much* **ur/o-** *urine; urinary system* **-ia** *condition; state; thing* **polydipsia** (PAWL-ee-DIP-see-ah) **poly-** *many; much* **dips/o-** *thirst* **-ia** *condition; state; thing*

Did You Know?

The Latin word *insipidus* and the English word *insipid* mean *lacking a distinctive appearance or taste*. Patients with diabetes insipidus have tasteless, dilute urine, like water, while the urine of patients with diabetes mellitus is sweet.

Posterior Pituitary Gland: Oxytocin

Word or Phrase	Description	Word Building
	There is no specific disease associated with hypersecretion of oxytocin.	
uterine inertia	Hyposecretion of oxytocin. It is caused by a defect in the posterior pituitary gland. Before birth, the low level of oxytocin causes weak and uncoordinated contractions of the pregnant uterus. This prolongs labor and delays the birth of the baby. After the birth of the baby, the low level of oxytocin causes postpartum hemorrhage (the uterus does not contract, and there is hemorrhaging at the site where the placenta separated from the uterus.) Treatment: Drug therapy with oxytocin hormone.	**uterine** (YOO-ter-in) (YOO-ter-ine) **uter/o-** *uterus (womb)* **-ine** *pertaining to* **inertia** (in-ER-shah) (in-ER-shee-ah) **postpartum** (post-PAR-tum) **post-** *after; behind* **-partum** *childbirth*

Pineal Gland: Melatonin

Word or Phrase	Description	Word Building
	There is no specific disease associated with hyposecretion of melatonin.	
seasonal affective disorder (SAD)	Hypersecretion of melatonin. It is caused by a defect in the pineal gland. The high level of melatonin causes depression, weight gain, and an increased desire for food and sleep. This occurs most often during the winter months when there are fewer hours of bright sunlight. Treatment: Exposure to sunlight or to bright light from a light box. Drug therapy of melatonin and/or antidepressant drugs.	**affective** (ah-FEK-tiv) **affect/o-** *state of mind; mood; to have an influence on* **-ive** *pertaining to*

Thyroid Gland: T$_3$ and T$_4$ Thyroid Hormones

hyperthyroidism	Hypersecretion of T$_3$ and T$_4$ thyroid hormones. It is caused by an adenoma (also known as a nodule) in the thyroid gland. (It can also be caused by hypersecretion of TSH from an adenoma in the anterior pituitary gland.) The high levels of T$_3$ and T$_4$ cause tremors of the hands, tachycardia, palpitations, restlessness, nervousness, diarrhea, insomnia, fatigue, and generalized weight loss. The thyroid gland is enlarged (a goiter) and can be felt on palpation of the neck. The eyes are dry and irritated with slow eyelid closing (lid lag). Hyperthyroidism is also known as **thyrotoxicosis** because of the toxic effect of the high levels of thyroid hormones. The sudden onset of severe hyperthyroidism is known as a **thyroid storm.** The most common type of hyperthyroidism is **Graves' disease.** This is an autoimmune disease in which the body produces antibodies that stimulate TSH receptors on the thyroid gland, and this increases the production of thyroid hormones. The entire thyroid gland becomes enlarged (diffuse toxic goiter), and there is **exophthalmos** (see Figure 14-10 ■). Treatment: Drug therapy to suppress secretion of T$_3$ and T$_4$, or surgery to remove the thyroid gland (thyroidectomy), or radiation therapy to destroy the thyroid gland.	**hyperthyroidism** (HY-per-THY-royd-izm) **hyper-** *above; more than normal* **thyroid/o-** *thyroid gland* **-ism** *process; disease from a specific cause* **thyrotoxicosis** (THY-roh-TAWK-sih-KOH-sis) **thyr/o-** *shield-shaped structure (thyroid gland)* **toxic/o-** *poison; toxin* **-osis** *condition; abnormal condition; process* **Graves' disease** (GRAYVZ) **exophthalmos** (EKS-awf-THAL-mohs) *Exophthalmos* is a combination of the prefix *ex-* (away from; out) and the Greek word *ophthalmos* (eye). *(continued)*

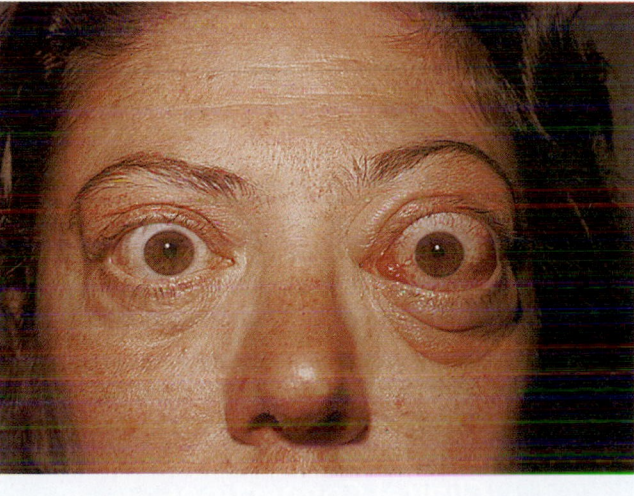

Figure 14-10 ■ Exophthalmos.

Exophthalmos is a well-known sign of hyperthyroidism. Edema behind the eyeballs causes them to bulge and protrude forward, and the large amount of white sclerae makes the eyes appear to be staring.

Word or Phrase	Description	Word Building

hyperthyroidism
(*continued*)

A Closer Look

A goiter is a chronic and progressive enlargement of the thyroid gland (see Figure 14-11 ■). It is also known as **thyromegaly**. A physician can feel this enlargement during a physical examination (see Figure 14-12 ■) even before it becomes visible. A goiter can occur with hyperthyroidism, thyroid cancer, thyroiditis, or hypothyroidism. The causes of goiter include the following:

1. An **adenoma** or nodule growing in the thyroid gland. This is known as an **adenomatous goiter** or **nodular goiter.** If there are many nodules, it is a **multinodular goiter.** An adenoma or nodule usually is benign, but can be cancerous.
2. A cancerous tumor growing in the thyroid gland.
3. Chronic inflammation of the thyroid gland as seen in thyroiditis.
4. A lack of iodine in the soil, water, and diet. This causes the thyroid gland to enlarge to help it capture more iodine. This is known as a **simple goiter,** a **nontoxic goiter,** or an **endemic goiter** (because it occurs in people who live in an area where the soil is poor in iodine). The widespread use of iodized salt has decreased the incidence of this type of goiter.

goiter (GOY-ter)

thyromegaly (THY-roh-MEG-ah-lee)
  thyr/o- *shield-shaped structure (thyroid gland)*
  -megaly *enlargement*

adenoma (AD-eh-NOH-mah)
  aden/o- *gland*
  -oma *tumor; mass*

adenomatous (AD-eh-NOH-mah-tus)
  aden/o- *gland*
  -oma *tumor; mass*
  -tous *pertaining to*

nodular (NAWD-yoo-lar)
  nod/o- *node (knob of tissue)*
  -ular *pertaining to a small thing*

multinodular
(MUL-tee-NAWD-yoo-lar)
  mult/i- *many*
  nodul/o- *small, knobby mass*
  -ar *pertaining to*

nontoxic (non-TAWK-sik)
  non- *not*
  tox/o- *poison*
  -ic *pertaining to*

endemic (en-DEM-ik)
  en- *in; within; inward*
  dem/o- *people; population*
  -ic *pertaining to*

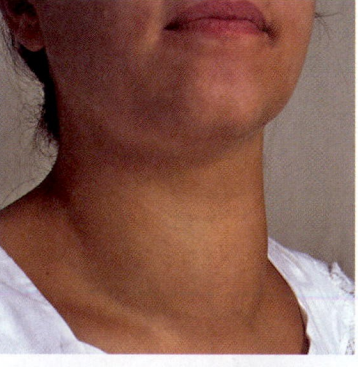

Figure 14-11 ■ Goiter.
A goiter can be a mild, subtle swelling in the neck, or it can enlarge enough to cause difficulty swallowing and breathing.

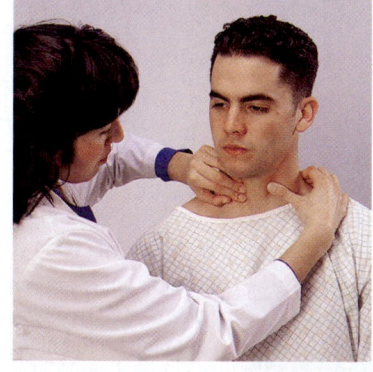

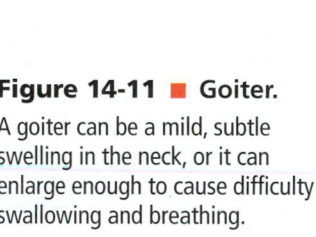

Figure 14-12 ■ Physical examination of the thyroid gland.
The anterior location of the thyroid gland means that even mild enlargement can be detected. This physician is palpating the edges of the patient's thyroid gland to determine its size.

Clinical Connections

Dietetics. The production of T_3 is dependent on adequate amounts of the trace mineral iodine in the diet. The ancient Chinese used seaweed to treat goiter because seaweed contains iodine. Iodine can be obtained from eating seafood, from vegetables grown in soil that contains iodine, and from drinking water that contains iodine. In the Great Lakes and Midwest of the United States, the soil and water are deficient in iodine. This is known as the "goiter belt" because persons living there tend to develop goiter from having too little iodine. Iodine was first added to table salt in 1924, and iodized salt was sold everywhere by 1940.

Word or Phrase	Description	Word Building
hypothyroidism	Hyposecretion of T_3 and T_4 thyroid hormones. It is usually caused by an inadequate amount of iodine in the diet. (It can also be caused by Hashimoto's thyroiditis (see *thyroiditis*), by treatments for hyperthyroidism that remove or destroy the thyroid gland, or by hyposecretion of TSH from the anterior pituitary gland. It can also be caused by a defect in the thyroid gland at birth that causes **congenital hypothyroidism.**) The low levels of T_3 and T_4 cause goiter, fatigue, decreased body temperature, dry hair and skin, constipation, and weight gain. Severe hypothyroidism in adults is characterized by **myxedema** with swelling of the subcutaneous and connective tissues, tingling in the hands and feet because of nerve compression, lack of menstruation, hair loss, an enlarged heart, bradycardia, an enlarged tongue, slow speech, and mental impairment. Untreated congenital hypothyroidism results in mental retardation (**cretinism**). Treatment: Drug therapy with T_3 and T_4 hormones.	**hypothyroidism** (HY-poh-THY-royd-izm) **hypo-** *below; deficient* **thyroid/o-** *thyroid gland* **-ism** *process; disease from a specific cause* **congenital** (con-JEN-ih-tal) **congenit/o-** *present at birth* **-al** *pertaining to* **myxedema** (MIK-seh-DEE-mah) **myx/o-** *mucus-like substance* **-edema** *swelling* **cretinism** (KREE-tin-izm)
thyroid carcinoma	Malignant tumor of the thyroid gland. There is hoarseness, neck pain, and enlargement of the lymph nodes. Treatment: Surgery to remove the thyroid gland (thyroidectomy) or radiation therapy to destroy the thyroid gland.	**carcinoma** (KAR-sih-NOH-mah) **carcin/o-** *cancer* **-oma** *tumor; mass*
thyroiditis	Chronic inflammation and progressive destruction of the thyroid gland. The most common type is **Hashimoto's thyroiditis,** an autoimmune disorder in which the body forms antibodies against the thyroid gland. The thyroid becomes inflamed and enlarged (goiter). Over time, the patient develops hypothyroidism as thyroid tissue is destroyed and replaced by fibrous tissue. Treatment: Drug therapy with T_3 and T_4 hormones.	**thyroiditis** (THY-roy-DY-tis) **thyroid/o-** *thyroid gland* **-itis** *inflammation of; infection of* **Hashimoto** (HAH-shee-MOH-toh)

Parathyroid Glands: Parathyroid Hormone

Word or Phrase	Description	Word Building
hyperpara-thyroidism	Hypersecretion of parathyroid hormone. It is caused by an adenoma in the parathyroid gland. The high level of parathyroid hormone moves calcium from the bones to the blood, and the calcium level in the blood is too high (**hypercalcemia**). The bones become demineralized and prone to fracture. There is also muscle weakness, fatigue, and depression. Excess calcium is excreted in the urine, and this can form kidney stones. Treatment: Surgery to remove the parathyroid glands.	**hyperparathyroidism** (HY-per-PAIR-ah-THY-royd-izm) **hyper-** *above; more than normal* **para-** *beside; apart from; two parts of a pair; abnormal* **thyroid/o-** *thyroid gland* **-ism** *process; disease from a specific cause* **hypercalcemia** (HY-per-kal-SEE-mee-ah) **hyper-** *above; more than normal* **calc/o-** *calcium* **-emia** *condition of the blood; substance in the blood*

Word or Phrase	Description	Word Building
hypopara-thyroidism	Hyposecretion of parathyroid hormone. It is caused by the accidental removal of the parathyroid glands during a thyroidectomy. The low level of parathyroid hormone causes the calcium level in the blood to become very low (**hypocalcemia**). This causes irritability of the nerves, skeletal muscle cramps, or sustained muscle spasm (tetany). Treatment: Drug therapy with parathyroid hormone.	**hypoparathyroidism** (HY-poh-PAIR-ah-THY-royd-izm) **hypo-** *below; deficient* **para-** *beside; apart from; two parts of a pair; abnormal* **thyroid/o-** *thyroid gland* **-ism** *process; disease from a specific cause* **hypocalcemia** (HY-poh-kal-SEE-mee-ah) **hypo-** *below; deficient* **calc/o-** *calcium* **-emia** *condition of the blood; substance in the blood*

Pancreas: Insulin

hyperinsulinism	Hypersecretion of insulin. It is caused by an adenoma in the pancreas. (It also occurs in a newborn baby when the mother has uncontrolled diabetes or gestational diabetes.) The high level of insulin causes **hypoglycemia** (a low level of glucose in the blood). There is shakiness, headache, sweating, dizziness, and even fainting. If left untreated, hypoglycemia can progress to insulin shock and then coma as the blood glucose level becomes too low to support brain activity. Treatment: Supplemental sugar or sugar drink orally or dextrose intravenous fluids. Surgery to remove the adenoma.	**hyperinsulinism** (HY-per-IN-soo-lin-izm) **hyper-** *above; more than normal* **insulin/o-** *insulin* **-ism** *process; disease from a specific cause* **hypoglycemia** (HY-poh-gly-SEE-mee-ah) **hypo-** *below; deficient* **glyc/o-** *glucose (sugar)* **-emia** *condition of the blood; substance in the blood*

Did You Know?

Persons with a normal level of insulin can also become hypoglycemic when they are dieting or fasting. Diabetic patients can become hypoglycemic when they take an oral antidiabetic drug or inject insulin but then skip a meal.

Clinical Connections

Neonatology. The growing embryo of a mother with uncontrolled diabetes or gestational diabetes is used to a high level of glucose in its blood (from the mother via the umbilical cord), and its pancreas constantly secretes large amounts of insulin before birth. After birth, the baby is not drinking much milk, but its pancreas continues to produce large amounts of insulin. Then the baby can suddenly become hypoglycemic and even have seizures or go into a coma.

Word or Phrase	Description	Word Building
insulin resistance syndrome	Hypersecretion of insulin. This occurs when receptors on body cells resist and do not allow insulin to transport glucose into the cell. There is a high level of glucose remaining in the blood (hyperglycemia) and a high level of insulin as the pancreas continues to secrete insulin to try to overcome the resistance. Eventually, the pancreas is unable to produce more insulin, and the patient develops diabetes mellitus. Treatment: Appropriate treatment for the diabetes mellitus. "Your chart says you have IRS . . . It's either a problem with insulin resistance syndrome or the Internal Revenue Service."	**resistance** (ree-ZIS-tans) **resist/o-** *withstand the effect of* **-ance** *state of*

diabetes mellitus (DM)	Hyposecretion of insulin. It is caused by an inability of the beta cells of the pancreas to secrete enough insulin. A person who has diabetes mellitus is a **diabetic.** A brittle diabetic has difficulty controlling the blood glucose level, with frequent swings from hyperglycemia to hypoglycemia.
	        The low level of insulin in the blood results in an increased level of glucose in the blood (**hyperglycemia**). Excess glucose in the blood is excreted in the urine (**glycosuria**). As it is excreted, it holds water to it by osmosis, and this increases the amount of urine (**polyuria**). With excessive urination, the patient becomes thirsty and drinks often (**polydipsia**). The patient also feels hungry and eats often (**polyphagia**) because the glucose in the blood cannot be metabolized by the cells.
	        There are three main types of diabetes mellitus: type 1, type 1.5, and type 2 (see Table 14-1). "Sugar diabetes" is a layperson's phrase for diabetes mellitus. Treatment: Drug therapy with injections of insulin or oral antidiabetic drugs (depending on the type of diabetes mellitus). Diet management, weight control, and exercise.
		diabetes (DY-ah-BEE-teez)
		mellitus (MEL-ih-tus)
		diabetic (DY-ah-BET-ik)
		diabet/o- *diabetes*
		-ic *pertaining to*
		hyperglycemia (HY-per-gly-SEE-mee-ah)
		hyper- *above; more than normal*
		glyc/o- *glucose (sugar)*
		-emia *condition of the blood; substance in the blood*
		glycosuria (GLY-kohs-YOO-ree-ah)
		glycos/o- *glucose (sugar)*
		ur/o- *urine; urinary system*
		-ia *condition; state; thing*
		polyuria (PAWL-ee-YOO-ree-ah)
		poly- *many; much*
		ur/o- *urine; urinary system*
		-ia *condition; state; thing*
		polydipsia (PAWL-ee-DIP-see-ah)
		poly- *many; much*
		dips/o- *thirst*
		-ia *condition; state; thing*
		polyphagia (PAWL-ee-FAY-jee-ah)
		poly- *many; much*
		phag/o- *eating; swallowing*
		-ia *condition; state; thing*

A Closer Look

Gestational diabetes mellitus occurs only during pregnancy. The mother's pancreas is temporarily unable to secrete enough insulin to meet the increased demands from enlarged body tissues. This is because the increased levels of estradiol and progesterone during pregnancy block the action of insulin. This type of diabetes mellitus resolves once the pregnancy is delivered. However, many patients develop type 2 diabetes later in life.

gestational (jes-TAY-shun-al)
gestat/o- *from conception to birth*
-ation *a process; being or having*
-al *pertaining to*

Table 14-1　**Diabetes Mellitus**

Type	Type 1	Type 1.5	Type 2
Other Names	Insulin-dependent diabetes mellitus (IDDM) Juvenile-onset diabetes mellitus	Slow onset Type I Latent autoimmune diabetes in adults (LADA)	Non-insulin-dependent diabetes mellitus (NIDDM) Adult-onset diabetes mellitus (AODM)
Onset	Child, adolescent, young adult	Adult	Adult
Percentage of all diabetics	10%	15%	75%
Amount of insulin	None secreted	Too little secreted	Too little secreted
Autoimmune disease	Yes	Yes	No
Antibodies present	Yes	Yes	No
Insulin resistance	No	No	Yes
Body weight	Normal	Normal	Obese
Associated diseases	None	None	Increased cholesterol and triglyceride blood levels, hypertension, gout
Contributing factors	Heredity, triggered by viral illness	Heredity	Heredity, obesity
Drug therapy	Insulin	Insulin and oral antidiabetic drugs	Oral antidiabetic drugs, occasionally insulin

Word Alert

SOUND-ALIKE WORDS

diabetes insipidus	Caused by hyposecretion of antidiuretic hormone (ADH) from the posterior pituitary gland
diabetes mellitus	Caused by hyposecretion of insulin or resistance to the insulin that is secreted

A Closer Look

Excessive urination (polyuria) is a symptom of both diabetes insipidus and diabetes mellitus, but for different reasons. In diabetes insipidus, a lack of ADH causes excessive production of urine. In diabetes mellitus, excess glucose excreted in the urine holds water to it by osmotic pressure, increasing the volume of urine.

Word or Phrase	Description	Word Building
ketoacidosis	A high level of **ketones** in the blood. This occurs in diabetes mellitus when there is no insulin to metabolize glucose and the body turns to other sources of energy such as fat or protein. Body fat contains the most calories per gram, but fat does not metabolize cleanly and leaves ketones, an acidic byproduct. The patient's breath has a unique "fruity" or "nail polish" odor from the high level of glucose and ketones in the blood. A diabetic coma occurs when a very high level of ketones (which are acidic) lowers the pH of the blood to the point that chemical reactions in the body cannot occur and the patient becomes unconscious. Treatment: Drug therapy with insulin.	**ketoacidosis** (KEE-toh-AS-ih-DOH-sis) **ket/o-** *ketones* **acid/o-** *acid (low pH)* **-osis** *condition; abnormal condition; process* **ketones** (KEE-tohnz)

A Closer Look

Complications of uncontrolled diabetes mellitus affect various organs of the body.

1. **Diabetic neuropathy.** Decreased or abnormal sensation in the extremities because of nerve damage due to demyelination of the nerves.
2. **Diabetic nephropathy.** Degenerative changes, fibrosis, and scarring in the nephrons of the kidneys because of the local effect of high levels of glucose and ketones.
3. **Diabetic retinopathy.** Degenerative changes of the retina of the eye because of the local effect of high levels of glucose and ketones. There is formation of new, abnormally fragile blood vessels that produce frequent hemorrhages.
4. **Atherosclerosis.** Fatty deposits and plaque formation with hardening of the arteries, which is accelerated in diabetes mellitus because of abnormalities in fat metabolism.
5. **Impotence.** Nerve damage and atherosclerosis of the arteries to the penis result in difficulty having an erection.

neuropathy (nyoo-RAWP-ah-thee)
  neur/o- *nerve*
  -pathy *disease; suffering*

nephropathy (neh-FRAWP-ah-thee)
  nephr/o- *kidney; nephron*
  -pathy *disease; suffering*

retinopathy (RET-ih-NAWP-ah-thee)
  retin/o- *retina (of the eye)*
  -pathy *disease; suffering*

Clinical Connections

Podiatry. Diabetic patients are at high risk for developing gangrene of the feet because of atherosclerosis. They are advised to see a podiatrist or physician to have their toenails trimmed. Poor eyesight (from age and diabetic retinopathy) coupled with decreased sensation in the lower extremities (diabetic neuropathy) makes it easy for diabetic patients to cut themselves when trimming their toenails. Small cuts do not heal because of poor blood flow from atherosclerosis. A continuously high level of glucose in the blood suppresses the action of white blood cells that fight infection, and so a small cut can form an ulcer that can progress to gangrene of the foot.

Adrenal Cortex: Aldosterone

hyperaldosteronism	Hypersecretion of aldosterone. It is caused by an adenoma in the adrenal cortex. (It can also be caused by hypersecretion of ACTH from an adenoma in the anterior pituitary gland.) A high level of aldosterone (1) moves large amounts of sodium and water in the nephron of the kidney back to the blood (this causes hypertension) and (2) sends large amounts of potassium to be excreted in the urine (this causes electrolyte imbalance and weakness). Treatment: Surgery to remove the adenoma.	**hyperaldosteronism** (HY-per-al-DAWS-ter-ohn-izm) *Hyperaldosteronism* is a combination of the prefix *hyper-* (above; more than normal), *aldosterone* (with the -e deleted), and the suffix -*ism* (process; disease from a specific cause).

Word or Phrase	Description	Word Building
hypoaldosteronism	Hyposecretion of aldosterone. It is caused by an inherited genetic abnormality of the adrenal cortex. There is dizziness, a low level of sodium in the blood, weakness, and decreased blood pressure. Treatment: Drug therapy: Aldosterone drug.	**hypoaldosteronism** (HY-poh-al-DAWS-ter-ohn-izm)

Adrenal Cortex: Cortisol

Cushing's syndrome	Hypersecretion of cortisol. It is caused by an adenoma in the adrenal cortex. (It can also occur in a patient who takes corticosteroid drugs on a long-term basis.) The high level of cortisol breaks down too much glycogen, causing a high level of glucose in the blood. This results in rapid weight gain, with deposits of fat in the face (moon face) (see Figure 14-13 ■), upper back (buffalo hump), and abdomen. There is a thinning of connective tissue in the skin of the face that allows the blood vessels to show through, giving a reddened appearance to the cheeks. The thinned connective tissue in the skin across the obese abdomen is stretched, causing small hemorrhages and red and purple striae. There is also a wasted appearance of the muscles in the extremities and muscle weakness because of the lack of protein synthesis (see Figure 14-13). (When there is hypersecretion of ACTH because of an adenoma in the anterior pituitary gland, this causes the adrenal cortex to secrete an excess of all of its hormones, including androgens, which produces dark facial hair [hirsutism] and amenorrhea in women. This is known as Cushing's disease.) Treatment: Surgery to remove the adenoma. Discontinue corticosteroid drugs.	**Cushing** (KOOSH-ing) **syndrome** (SIN-drohm) **syn-** *together* **-drome** *a running*

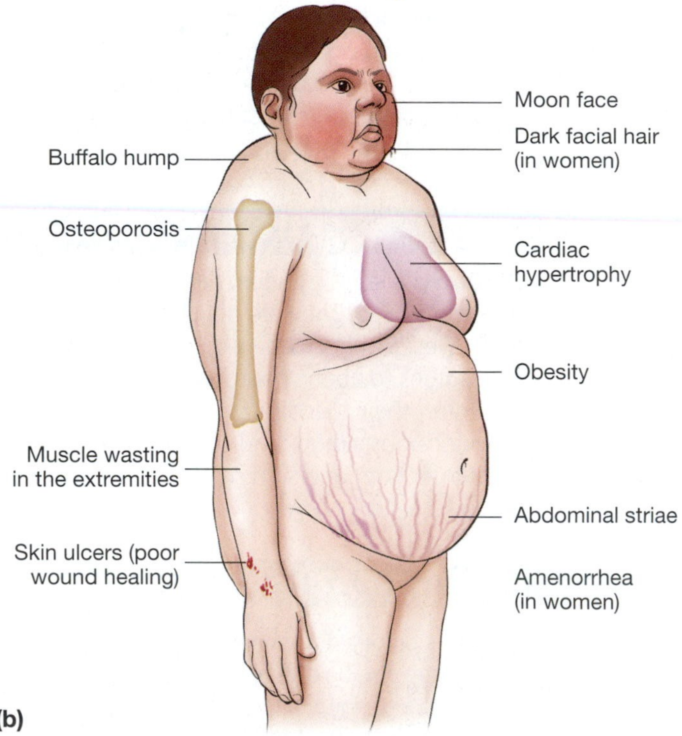

Figure 14-13 ■ Cushing's syndrome.

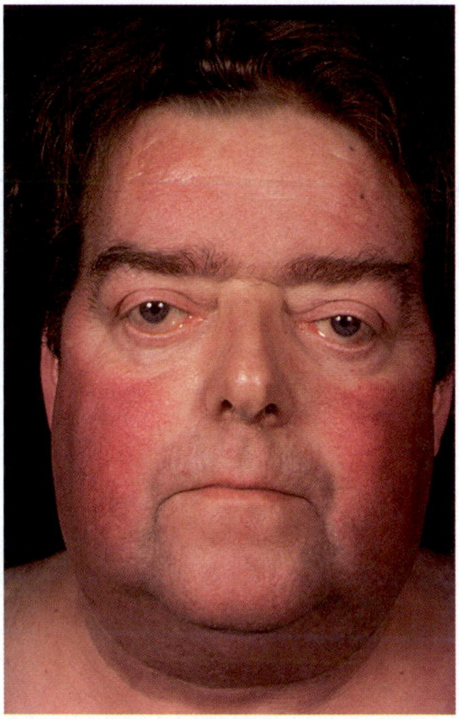

(a) This patient shows the characteristic signs of Cushing's syndrome. Deposits of fat in the cheeks give a moon face appearance. Breakdown of protein in the connective tissues of the skin makes the skin thin, allowing blood vessels to show through and give the cheeks a reddened appearance. (b) The abdomen is obese, while the extremities are thin and there is muscle wasting and weakness. Dark facial hair and amenorrhea occur only with Cushing's disease.

Word or Phrase	Description	Word Building
Addison's disease	Hyposecretion of cortisol. This is an autoimmune disease in which the body produces antibodies that destroy the adrenal cortex. (It can also be caused by hyposecretion of ACTH from the anterior pituitary gland.) There is a low level of blood glucose, fatigue, weight loss, and decreased ability to tolerate stress, disease, or surgery. Patients have an unusual bronzed color to the skin, even in areas not exposed to the sun. Treatment: Drug therapy with corticosteroid drugs.	**Addison** (AD-ih-son)

Adrenal Cortex: Androgens

	There is no specific disease associated with hyposecretion of androgens.	
adrenogenital syndrome	Hypersecretion of androgens. It is caused by an adenoma in the adrenal gland. In girls, the clitorus and labia enlarge and resemble a penis and scrotum. In boys, it causes precocious puberty. In adult females, it causes **virilism** with masculine facial features and body build, **hirsutism** (excessive, dark hair on the forearms and face), and amenorrhea. Treatment: Surgery to remove the adenoma.	**adrenogenital** (ah-DREE-noh-JEN-ih-tal) **adren/o-** adrenal gland **genit/o-** genitalia **-al** pertaining to **virilism** (VIR-ih-lizm) **viril/o-** masculine **-ism** process; disease from a specific cause **hirsutism** (HER-soo-tizm) **hirsut/o-** hairy **-ism** process; disease from a specific cause

Adrenal Medulla: Epinephrine and Norepinephrine

	There is no specific disease associated with hyposecretion of epinephrine and norepinephrine.	
pheochromo-cytoma	Hypersecretion of epinephrine and norepinephrine. It is caused by an adenoma in the adrenal medulla. The high levels of epinephrine and norepinephrine cause heart palpitations, severe sweating, and headaches with severe hypertension that can cause a stroke. Treatment: Surgery to remove the adenoma.	**pheochromocytoma** (FEE-oh-KROH-moh-sy-TOH-mah) **phe/o-** gray **chrom/o-** color **cyt/o-** cell **-oma** tumor; mass Add words to make a complete definition of *pheochromocytoma*: *tumor (with a) gray color to the cells (when viewed under a microscope).*

Ovaries: Estradiol and Progesterone

precocious puberty	Hypersecretion of estradiol. It is caused by an adenoma in the ovary. (It can also be caused by hypersecretion of FSH and LH from an adenoma in the anterior pituitary gland.) The high level of estradiol causes premature development of the breasts and female sexual characteristics, with menstruation and ovulation, in a child. Treatment: Surgery to remove the adenoma.	**precocious** (prih-KOH-shus) **puberty** (PYOO-ber-tee) **puber/o-** growing up **-ty** quality or state
infertility	Hyposecretion of estradiol or an imbalance in the amount of estradiol and progesterone. (It can also be caused by a lack of FSH and LH from the anterior pituitary gland.) There is a lack of ovulation, abnormal menstruation, or a history of miscarriages. Treatment: Drug therapy with female hormone drugs.	**infertility** (IN-fer-TIL-ih-tee) **in-** in; within; not **fertil/o-** able to conceive a child **-ity** state; condition

Word or Phrase	Description	Word Building
menopause	Hyposecretion of estradiol. This is a normal result of the aging process in which the ovaries secrete less and less estradiol. The low level of estradiol causes vaginal dryness, thinning of the hair, and lack of sexual drive. As the hypothalamus senses low estradiol levels, it stimulates the anterior pituitary gland to secrete FSH and LH to stimulate the ovary. This causes hot flashes. Treatment: Drug therapy with female hormone (hormone replacement therapy), but only for a limited time due to the increased risk of breast and endometrial cancer, blood clots, stroke, heart attack, and dementia.	**menopause** (MEN-oh-pawz) **men/o-** *month* **-pause** *cessation*

Testes: Testosterone

Word or Phrase	Description	Word Building
precocious puberty	Hypersecretion of testosterone. It is caused by an adenoma in the testis. (It can also be caused by hypersecretion of FSH and LH from an adenoma in the anterior pituitary gland.) The high level of testosterone causes the premature development of the male sexual characteristics, with development of a beard, deepening of the voice, and sperm production in a child. Treatment: Surgery to remove the adenoma.	**precocious** (prih-KOH-shus) **puberty** (PYOO-ber-tee) **puber/o-** *growing up* **-ty** *quality or state*
gynecomastia	Hyposecretion of testosterone. This is a normal result of the aging process in which the testes secrete less and less testosterone. (It can also be caused by surgical removal of the testes due to cancer.) However, androgens continue to be secreted by the adrenal cortex and converted to estrogens in the blood. The low level of testosterone now in an imbalance with the level of estrogens causes enlargement of the male breasts. Gynecomastia can also be caused by estrogen drug treatment for prostate cancer, by excessive alcohol consumption, or as a side effect of some drugs. Treatment: Drug therapy with androgen drugs. Plastic surgery to decrease the breast size.	**gynecomastia** (GY-neh-koh-MAS-tee-ah) **gynec/o-** *female; woman* **mast/o-** *breast; mastoid process* **-ia** *condition; state; thing*
infertility	Hyposecretion of testosterone. It is caused by failure of one or both of the testes to descend into the scrotum before birth. (It can also be caused by surgical removal of the testes due to cancer. It can also be caused by an imbalance or lack of FSH and LH from the anterior pituitary gland.) The low level of testosterone causes too few spermatozoa to be produced. Treatment: Surgery to bring the testes into the scrotum in a child or drug therapy with an androgen drug.	**infertility** (IN-fer-TIL-ih-tee) **in-** *in; within; not* **fertil/o-** *able to conceive a child* **-ity** *state; condition*

Laboratory and Diagnostic Procedures

Blood Tests

Word or Phase	Description	Word Building
antithyroglobulin antibodies	Detects antibodies against thyroglobulin (precursor hormone to T_3 and T_4) in the thyroid gland. A positive test result indicates Hashimoto's thyroiditis.	**antithyroglobulin** (AN-tee-THY-roh-GLAWB-yoo-lin) **anti-** *against* **thyr/o-** *shield-shaped structure (thyroid gland)* **globul/o-** *shaped like a globe* **-in** *a substance*
calcium	Measures the level of calcium. It is done to determine if the parathyroid gland is secreting a normal amount of parathyroid hormone.	**calcium** (KAL-see-um)

Word or Phrase	Description	Word Building
cortisol level	Measures the level of cortisol. It is done to determine if the adrenal cortex is secreting a normal amount of cortisol. (It also indirectly determines if the anterior pituitary gland is secreting ACTH to stimulate the adrenal cortex to secrete cortisol.) A metabolite of cortisol, **17-hydroxycorticosteroids,** can also be measured in the urine to indirectly measure the level of cortisol in the blood.	**cortisol** (KOR-tih-sawl) **hydroxycorticosteroids** (hy-DRAWK-see-KOR-tih-koh-STAIR-oydz)
fasting blood sugar (FBS)	Measures the level of glucose after the patient has fasted (not eaten) for at least 12 hours. It is used to determine if the pancreas is secreting a normal amount of insulin.	
FSH assay and LH assay	Measures the levels of follicle-stimulating hormone (FSH) and luteinizing hormone (LH). It is done to determine if the anterior pituitary gland is secreting a normal amount of FSH and LH.	**assay** (AS-say)

glucose self-testing	Self-test that measures the level of glucose (blood sugar). Diabetic patients test their own blood glucose level one or more times each day (see Figure 14-14 ■).	**glucose** (GLOO-kohs)
		  gluc/o- *glucose (sugar)*
		  -ose *full of*

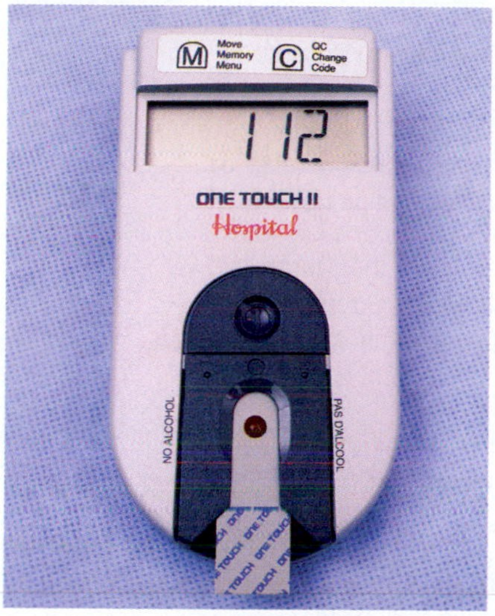

Figure 14-14 ■ Blood glucose monitor.
The patient pricks the fingertip and the drop of blood is placed on a test strip. It is inserted into the blood glucose monitor and the monitor displays the numerical value of the patient's blood glucose level. The blood glucose level is normally between 70 and 150 mg/dL in a person who does not have diabetes mellitus.

Word or Phrase	Description	Word Building

glucose tolerance test (GTT)	Blood and urine tests that measure the level of glucose. It is done to determine if the pancreas is secreting a normal amount of insulin. After the patient has fasted for 12 hours, blood and urine specimens are obtained. Then the patient drinks glucose (in a sugary drink known as **Glucola**) or is given **dextrose** intravenously. Blood and urine specimens are obtained every hour for 4 hours. Normally, the blood glucose returns to normal within one to two hours. High blood and urine levels of glucose indicate diabetes mellitus. It is also known as an **oral glucose tolerance test (OGTT).**	**Glucola** (gloo-KOH-lah)
		dextrose (DEKS-trohs)
		  dextr/o- *right; sugar*
		  -ose *full of*

growth hormone	Measures the level of growth hormone (GH). It is done to determine if the anterior pituitary gland is secreting a normal amount of growth hormone.	
hemoglobin A$_{1C}$ (HbA$_{1C}$)	Measures the A$_{1C}$ fraction of hemoglobin in red blood cells. Hemoglobin A$_{1C}$ binds with glucose. Because red blood cells only live about 12 weeks, the hemoglobin A$_{1C}$ result indicates the average level of blood glucose during the previous 12 weeks. It is used to monitor how well a diabetic patient is controlling the blood glucose level with diet and drugs. It is also known as **glycohemoglobin** or **glycosylated hemoglobin.**	**hemoglobin A$_{1C}$** (HEE-moh-GLOH-bin AA-one-see) **glycohemoglobin** (GLY-koh-HEE-moh-GLOH-bin) **glycosylated** (gly-KOH-sih-lay-ted)

Word or Phrase	Description	Word Building
testosterone	Measures the levels of total testosterone and free testosterone. It is done to determine if the testes are secreting a normal amount of testosterone. (It also indirectly determines if the anterior pituitary gland is secreting luteinizing hormone to stimulate the testes to secrete testosterone.)	
thyroid function tests (TFTs)	Measures the levels of T_3, T_4, and TSH. It is done to determine if the thyroid gland is secreting normal amounts of thyroid hormones. (It also determines if the anterior pituitary gland is secreting enough thyroid-stimulating hormone to stimulate the thyroid to secrete its hormones.) The test uses a radioimmunoassay (RIA) technique in which antibodies labeled with radioactive isotopes combine with thyroid hormones and the amount of radioactivity is measured. Another test value, the free thyroxine index (FTI) or T_7, can be calculated from this.	

Urine Tests

Word or Phrase	Description	Word Building
ADH stimulation test	Measures the concentration of urine. It is done to determine if the posterior pituitary gland is secreting a normal amount of antidiuretic hormone (ADH). The patient does not drink water for 12 hours; then a urine specimen is obtained. Then ADH is given (as the drug vasopressin), the patient drinks water, and another urine specimen is obtained. In a patient with diabetes insipidus, the second urine specimen will be more concentrated because of the ADH (vasopressin). It is also known as the **water deprivation test.**	
estradiol	Measures the level of estradiol. It is done to determine if the ovaries are secreting a normal amount of estradiol. (It also indirectly determines if the anterior pituitary gland is secreting follicle-stimulating hormone to stimulate the ovaries to secrete estradiol.)	
urine dipstick	Measures glucose, ketones, and other substances in the urine. This is a rapid screening test used to evaluate diabetic patients.	
vanillylmandelic acid (VMA)	A 24-hour urine test that measures the levels of epinephrine and norepinephrine. It is done to determine if the adrenal medulla is secreting a normal amount of these hormones. Vanillylmandelic acid (VMA), a byproduct of these hormones, is measured.	**vanillylmandelic acid** (VAN-ih-lil-man-DEL-ik AS-id)

Radiology Tests

Word or Phrase	Description	Word Building

radioactive iodine uptake (RAIU) and thyroid scan	Procedure that combines a radioactive iodine uptake procedure and a thyroid scan. The radioactive iodine uptake demonstrates how well the thyroid gland is able to absorb iodine from the blood. The thyroid scan shows the size and shape of the thyroid gland. Two radioactive tracers are given, orally and intravenously. A normal scan will show uniform distribution of radioactive tracer throughout the thyroid gland. An adenoma appears as a bright ("hot") spot because of its increased uptake of radioactive iodine compared to the rest of the gland. A darker area (a "cold" spot) can either be a cyst or a cancerous tumor of the thyroid gland (neither of which take up iodine) (see Figure 14-15 ■).	**radioactive** (RAY-dee-oh-AK-tiv)
		  radi/o- *radius (forearm bone); x-rays; radiation*
		  act/o- *action*
		  -ive *pertaining to*
		iodine (EYE-oh-dine) (EYE-oh-deen)

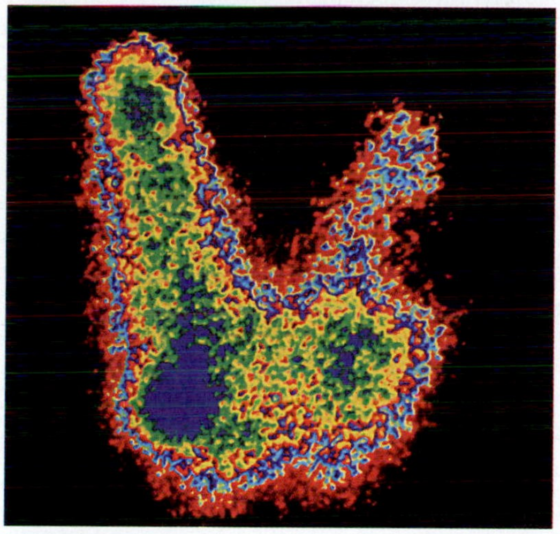

Figure 14-15 ■ Thyroid scan.
This patient's thyroid scan shows a large, dark area in the inferior portion of one lobe. This is a "cold" spot, an area of decreased uptake of radioactive tracer. A "cold" spot can be a cyst or a cancerous tumor.

Medical and Surgical Procedures

Medical Procedures

Word or Phase	Description	Word Building
ADA diet	Special physician-prescribed diet for diabetic patients that follows the guidelines of the American Diabetes Association (ADA). The amounts of carbohydrate and fat are limited. The physician orders the upper limit for the total daily number of calories for a diabetic patient in the hospital. Example: 1200-calorie ADA diet. Rather than using the ADA diet, diabetic patients can just count calories. A dietitian or diabetes educator helps the patient plan a menu that fits lifestyle and food preferences.	

Surgical Procedures

Word or Phrase	Description	Word Building

adrenalectomy	Procedure to remove the adrenal gland because of an adenoma or cancerous tumor.	**adrenalectomy** (ah-DREE-nal-EK-toh-mee)
		  adrenal/o- *adrenal gland*
		  -ectomy *surgical excision*

fine-needle biopsy	Procedure that uses a fine needle to take a small sample of tissue from a thyroid nodule seen on a thyroid scan. The tissue is sent to the laboratory to determine if the nodule is benign or malignant.	**biopsy** (BY-awp-see)
		  bi/o- *life; living organisms; living tissue*
		  -opsy *process of viewing*

Word or Phrase	Description	Word Building
parathyroidectomy	Procedure to remove one or more of the parathyroid glands to control hyperparathyroidism. Also, a parathyroidectomy can occur accidentally when the thyroid gland is surgically removed.	**parathyroidectomy** (PAIR-ah-THY-roy-DEK-toh-mee) **para-** *beside; apart from; two parts of a pair; abnormal* **thyroid/o-** *thyroid gland* **-ectomy** *surgical excision*
thymectomy	Procedure to remove the thymus in patients with myasthenia gravis	**thymectomy** (thy-MEK-toh-mee) **thym/o-** *thymus; rage* **-ectomy** *surgical excision*
thyroidectomy	Procedure to remove the thyroid gland. All of the thyroid gland can be removed or just one part or one lobe (**subtotal thyroidectomy** or **thyroid lobectomy**).	**thyroidectomy** (THY-roy-DEK-toh-mee) **thyroid/o-** *thyroid gland* **-ectomy** *surgical excision*
		lobectomy (loh-BEK-toh-mee) **lob/o-** *lobe of an organ* **-ectomy** *surgical excision*
transsphenoidal hypophysectomy	Procedure to remove an adenoma from the pituitary gland (hypophysis). The pituitary gland is difficult to visualize through an incision in the cranium, so the incision is made through the sphenoid sinus (transsphenoidal).	**transsphenoidal** (TRANS-sfee-NOY-dal) **trans-** *across; through* **sphenoid/o-** *sphenoid bone; sphenoid sinus* **-al** *pertaining to*
		hypophysectomy (HY-pawf-ih-SEK-toh-mee) **hypophys/o-** *pituitary gland* **-ectomy** *surgical excision*

Drug Categories

These categories of drugs are used to treat endocrine diseases and conditions. The most common generic and trade name drugs in each category are listed.

Category	Indication	Examples	Word Building
antidiabetic drugs	Treat type 2 diabetes mellitus by stimulating the pancreas to secrete more insulin or increase the number of insulin receptors. These drugs are given orally. They are not insulin and they are not used to treat patients with type 1 diabetes mellitus.	glyburide (DiaBeta, Micronase), metformin (Glucophage), rosiglitazone (Avandia), sitagliptin (Januvia)	**antidiabetic** (AN-tee-DY-ah-BET-ik) **anti-** *against* **diabet/o-** *diabetes* **-ic** *pertaining to*
antithyroid drugs	Treat hyperthyroidism by inhibiting the production of T_3 and T_4. Radioactive sodium iodide 131 (I-131) is given orally. It is taken up by the thyroid gland and emits low-level beta and gamma radiation that destroys thyroid cells. It has a short half-life and is excreted in the urine, limiting the number of cells that are destroyed. Some functioning thyroid gland tissue can remain.	methimazole (Tapazole), radioactive sodium iodide 131 (I-131)	**antithyroid** (AN-tee-THY-royd) **anti-** *against* **thyr/o-** *shield-shaped structure (thyroid gland)* **-oid** *resembling*

Category	indication	Examples	Word Building
corticosteroid drugs	Mimic the action of hormones from the adrenal cortex. They are used to treat severe inflammation. They are used to treat Addison's disease.	dexamethasone (Decadron), hydrocortisone (Cortef, Solu-Cortef), prednisone (Deltasone, Meticorten)	**corticosteroid** (KOR-tih-koh-STAIR-oyd) **cortic/o-** *cortex (outer region)* **-steroid** *steroid*
growth hormone drugs	Provide growth hormone.	somatrem (Protropin), somatropin (Humatrope, Nutropin)	
insulin	Treats type 1 and type 1.5 diabetes mellitus. It can also be used to treat type 2 diabetes mellitus that cannot be controlled with oral antidiabetic drugs. Insulin must be injected from one to several times each day to control the blood glucose (see Figure 14-16 ■). Insulin is classified according to how quickly it acts (which depends on the size of the insulin crystal) and how many hours its therapeutic effect continues (see Figure 14-17 ■).	Rapid-acting (regular) insulins: Humulin R, insulin aspart (NovoLog), insulin lispro (Humalog), Novolin R, Regular Iletin II. Intermediate-acting (NPH or lente) insulins: Humulin N, Lente Iletin II, Novolin N. Long-acting insulins: insulin detemir (Levemir), insulin glargine (Lantus).	**insulin** (IN-soo-lin)

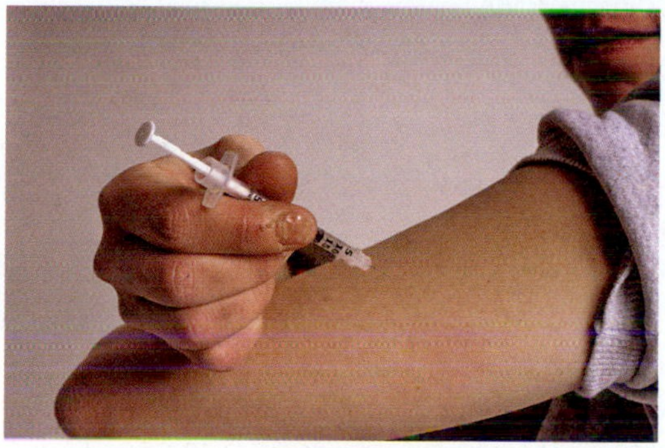

Figure 14-16 ■ Insulin injection.
Insulin is a liquid drug that must be injected subcutaneously into the fat layer beneath the skin. The needle is inserted at an angle so that it does not go into the muscle layer. The back of the arms, abdomen, and many other sites can be used for insulin injections. A new site must be selected for each injection.

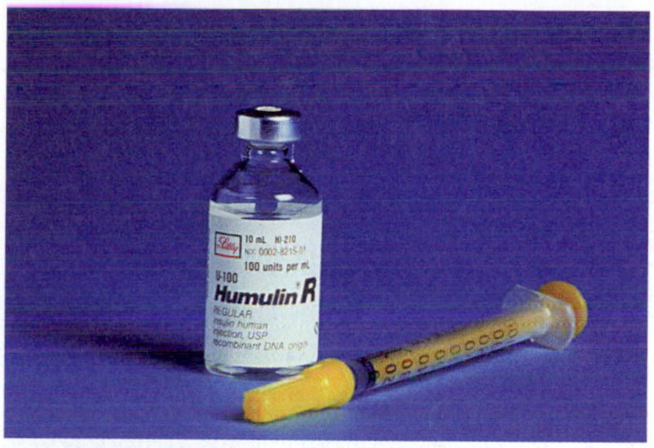

Figure 14-17 ■ Humulin R insulin.
This insulin is a rapid-acting insulin. The R stands for *regular insulin*. Humulin is a trade name for insulin that is manufactured by recombinant DNA technology. In the past, all insulin drugs were produced from ground-up animal pancreas.

Category	indication	Examples	Word Building
thyroid supplement drugs	Treat a lack of thyroid hormones and hypothyroidism	levothyroxine (Levothroid, Synthroid), liothyronine (Cytomel), liotrix (Thyrolar)	

Abbreviations

ACTH	adrenocorticotropic hormone
ADA	American Diabetes Association, American Dietetic Association
ADH	antidiuretic hormone
Ca, Ca⁺⁺	calcium
CDE	certified diabetes educator
DI	diabetes insipidus
DKA	diabetic ketoacidosis
DM	diabetes mellitus
FBS	fasting blood sugar
FSH	follicle-stimulating hormone
FTI	free thyroxine index
GH	growth hormone
GTT	glucose tolerance test
HbA$_{1C}$	hemoglobin A$_{1C}$
IDDM	insulin-dependent diabetes mellitus
IRS	insulin resistance syndrome
K, K⁺	potassium

LADA	latent autoimmune diabetes in adults
LH	luteinizing hormone
MSH	melanocyte-stimulating hormone
Na, Na⁺	sodium
NIDDM	non-insulin-dependent diabetes mellitus
NPH	neutral protamine Hagedorn (type of insulin)
OGTT	oral glucose tolerance test
RAIU	radioactive iodine uptake
RIA	radioimmunoassay
SAD	seasonal affective disorder
SIADH	syndrome of inappropriate ADH
T$_3$	triiodothyronine
T$_4$	thyroxine
T$_7$	free thyroxine index (FTI)
TFTs	thyroid function tests
TSH	thyroid-stimulating hormone
VMA	vanillylmandelic acid

Word Alert

ABBREVIATIONS

Abbreviations are commonly used in all types of medical documents; however, they can mean different things to different people and their meanings can be misinterpreted. Always verify the meaning of an abbreviation.

ADA means *American Diabetes Association,* but it also means *American Dietetic Association.*

Ca means *calcium,* but it also means *cancer.*

GTT means *glucose tolerance test,* but *gtt.* means *drops.*

NPH means *neutral protamine Hagedorn* (insulin), but it also means *normal pressure hydrocephalus.*

It's Greek to Me!

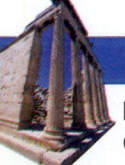

Did you notice that some words have two different combining forms? Combining forms from both Greek and Latin languages remain a part of medical language today.

Word	Greek	Latin	Medical Word Examples
female	gynec/o-	estr/a-, estr/o-	gynecomastia, estradiol, estrogens
male, masculine	andr/o-	viril/o-	androgens, virilism
milk	galact/o-	lact/o-	galactorrhea, lactation
pituitary gland	hypophys/o-	pituitar/o-, pituit/o-	adenohypophysis, hypopituitarism, pituitary

CAREER FOCUS

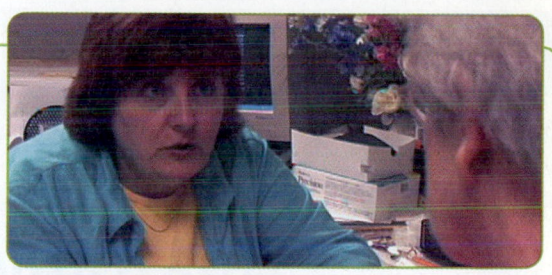

Meet Maureen, a diabetes educator

"I worked in a large city hospital that had a very large diabetic population, and that's how I got interested in the disease. On a typical day we see patients who have had diabetes anywhere from just a few weeks to years. Diabetic education has really changed a lot, because we're really trying to empower the patient. The person lives with diabetes every day, so they should have the tools to take care of their diabetes. The more information they have, the better choices that they're going to make. What we try and do is teach them how—about their food, how to monitor their blood glucose, what their medications are, how to take them properly and consistently, and what to do if their blood glucose is either too high or too low."

Diabetes educators are allied health professionals who counsel and educate patients with diabetes mellitus and their families. They work in hospitals, clinics, and some physicians' offices.

Endocrinologists are physicians who practice in the specialty of endocrinology. They diagnose and treat patients with diseases of the endocrine system. Some endocrinologists specialize and become **diabetologists** who only treat patients with diabetes mellitus. Physicians can take additional training and become board certified in the subspecialties of reproductive endocrinology or pediatric endocrinology. Surgery on the endocrine system is performed by a general surgeon or a neurosurgeon. Cancerous tumors of the endocrine system are treated medically by an oncologist or surgically by a general surgeon or neurosurgeon.

endocrinologist
(EN-doh-krih-NAWL-oh-jist)
  endo- *innermost; within*
  crin/o- *secrete*
  log/o- *word; the study of*
  -ist *one who specializes in*

diabetologist
(DY-ah-beh-TAWL-oh-jist)
  diabet/o- *diabetes*
  log/o- *word; the study of*
  -ist *one who specializes in*

PEARSON myhealthprofessionskit™ To see Maureen's complete video profile, visit Medical Terminology Interactive at www.myhealthprofessionskit.com. Select this book, log in, and go to the 14th floor of Pearson General Hospital. Enter the Laboratory, and click on the computer screen.

CHAPTER REVIEW EXERCISES

Test your knowledge of the chapter by completing these review exercises. Use the Answer Key at the end of the book to check your answers.

Anatomy and Physiology

Location Exercise

Identify the area of the body where each of these endocrine structures is located. The first one has been done for you.

Endocrine Gland or Organ   **Location**

1. hypothalamus   in the center of the brain, on top of the brainstem, below the thalamus

2. pituitary gland   _____

3. pineal gland   _____

4. thyroid gland   _____

5. parathyroid glands   _____

6. thymus   _____

7. pancreas   _____

8. adrenal glands   _____

9. ovaries   _____

10. testes   _____

Unscramble and Match Exercise

Unscramble the letters to spell a hormone. Write its correct spelling on the blank line, then match the hormone with the gland or organ that secretes it. Note: Some glands or organs will have more than one hormone. The first one has been done for you.

1. nnsuiil   insulin_____   _____ anterior pituitary gland
2. daltsoerone   _____   _____ posterior pituitary gland
3. HST   _____   _____ pineal gland
4. cooxtyin   _____   _____ thyroid gland
5. HACT   _____   __1__ pancreas
6. nacggoul   _____   _____ adrenal cortex
7. HAD   _____   _____ adrenal medulla
8. ephpiinener   _____   _____ testes
9. tttesosroeen   _____   _____ ovaries
10. tlcainrop   _____
11. tolmeanin   _____
12. dloiaerst   _____
13. yxhtroien   _____

Circle Exercise

Circle the correct word from the choices given.

1. The (**pineal gland, pancreas, testis**) secretes the male hormone testosterone.

2. The (**ovary, pituitary, thymus**) secretes estradiol and is responsible for sexual characteristics in the female.

3. The (**ovaries, parathyroid glands, testes**) are four small glands located on the thyroid gland.

4. The (**adrenal gland, pancreas, pituitary gland**) contains two areas called the cortex and the medulla.

5. The (**adrenal gland, pituitary gland, thymus**) shrinks in size in adults.

Diseases and Conditions

Matching Exercise

Match each word or phrase to its description.

1. thyromegaly
2. diabetes insipidus
3. myxedema
4. exophthalmos
5. galactorrhea
6. gigantism
7. menopause
8. polydipsia
9. uterine inertia

_____ Bulging, staring eyes

_____ Excessive thirst

_____ Not enough ADH

_____ Hyposecretion of estradiol

_____ Too little oxytocin

_____ Severe hypothyroidism in an adult

_____ Milk secretion from breasts of nonpregnant female

_____ Enlargement of the thyroid gland

_____ Hypersecretion of growth hormone during childhood

True or False Exercise

Indicate whether each statement is true or false by writing T or F on the line.

1. _____ A goiter is also known as thyromegaly.

2. _____ Diabetes insipidus is also known as sugar diabetes.

3. _____ Addison's disease is also known as thyrotoxicosis.

4. _____ Cretinism in a child is caused by a lack of the same hormone as dwarfism in a child.

5. _____ Gestational diabetes only occurs in men.

6. _____ Moon face and buffalo hump are characteristics of Cushing's syndrome.

7. _____ Gynecomastia is the overproduction of milk by the breasts during pregnancy.

Laboratory, Radiology, Surgery, and Drugs

Circle Exercise

Circle the correct word from the choices given.

1. Which disease is associated with the adrenal cortex? (**diabetes, thyroiditis, virilism**)

2. A cold or hot nodule might be seen on a/an (**ACTH stimulation test, fasting blood glucose, thyroid scan**).

3. A large volume of urine could indicate (**diabetes insipidus, precocious puberty, thyroid storm**).

4. HbA_{1C} is also known as (**antithyroglobulin antibodies, FSH, glycosylated hemoglobin**).

5. A person taking Synthroid would have had the (**adrenal gland, ovary, thyroid gland**) surgically removed.

6. All of the following are laboratory tests for diabetes *except* (**calcium, fasting blood glucose, GTT**).

7. Thyroid function tests include all of the following *except* (**estradiol, T_4, TSH**).

Matching Exercise

Match each word or phrase to its description.

1. antidiabetic drugs
2. corticosteroid drugs
3. insulin
4. lobectomy
5. radioactive I-131
6. thymectomy

_____ Surgical treatment for myasthenia gravis

_____ Removes just part of the thyroid gland

_____ Used to treat patients with type 2 diabetes mellitus

_____ Patients with Addison's disease must take these

_____ This drug is given by subcutaneous injection

_____ Emits gamma radiation that destroys the thyroid

Laboratory Test Exercise

Review the form below for ordering laboratory tests. Find each of the following tests related to endocrinology and put a check next to it.

electrolyte panel	potassium	sodium	T_4, total
glucose, fasting	prolactin	T_3, total	TSH
glucose tolerance test (GTT)			

PANELS AND PROFILES			TESTS		
968T		Lipid Panel	19687W		Bilirubin (Direct)
315F		Electrolyte Panel	265F		HBsAg
10256F		Hepatic Function Panel	51870R		HB Core Antibody
10165F		Basic Metabolic Panel	1012F		Cardio CRP
10231A		Comprehensive Metabolic Panel	23242E		GGT
10306F		Hepatitis Panel, Acute	28852E		Protein, Total
182Aaa		Obstetric Panel	141A		CBC Hemogram
18T		Chem-Screen Panel (Basic)	21105R		hCG, Qualitative, Serum
554T		Chem-Screen Panel (Basic with HDL)	10321A		ANA
7971A		Chem-Screen Panel (Basic with HDL, TIBC)	80185		Cardio CRP with Lipid Profile
TESTS			26F		PT with INR
56713E		Lead, Blood	232Aaa		UA, Dipstick
2782A		Antibody Screen	42A		CBC with Diff
3556F		Iron, TIBC	20867W		HDL Cholesterol
20933E		Cholesterol	31732E		PTT
3084111E		Uric Acid	34F		UA, Dipstick and Microscopic
53348W		Rubella Antibody	20396R		CEA
27771E		Phosphate	45443E		Hematocrit
2111600E		Creatinine	28571E		PSA, Total
29868W		Testosterone, Total	66902E		WBC count
9704F		Creatinine Clearance	20750E		Chloride
19752E		Bilirubin (Total)	7187W		Hemoglobin
30536Rrr		T3, Total	4259T		HIV-1 Antibody
687T		Protein Electrophoresis	45484R		Hemoglobin A1c
3563444R		Digoxin	67868R		Alk Phosphatase
15214R		Glucose, 2-Hour Postprandial	24984R		Iron
30502E		T3, Uptake	28512E		Sodium
7773E		Platelet Count	17426R		ALT
39685R		Dilantin (phenytoin)	**MICROBIOLOGY**		
30494R		Triglycerides	112680E		Group A Beta Strep Culture, Throat
26013E		Magnesium	5827W		Group B Beta Strep Culture, Genitals
15586R		Glucose, Fasting	49932E		Chlamydia, Endocervix/Urethra
30237W		T4, Free	6007W		Culture, Blood
28233E		Potassium	2692E		Culture, Genitals
19208W		AST	2649T		Culture, HSV
30163E		TSH	612A		Culture, Sputum
22764R		Ferritin	6262E		Culture, Throat
20008W		Calcium	6304R		Culture, Urine
54726F		Occult Blood, Stool	50286R		Gonococcus, Endocervix/Urethra
51839W		HAV Antibody, Total	6643E		Gram Stain
430A		Blood Group and Rh Type	**STOOL PATHOGENS**		
28399W		Progesterone	10045F		Culture, Stool
30262E		T4, Total	4475F		Culture, Campylobacter
20289W		Carbon Dioxide	10018T		Culture, Salmonella
1156F		RPR	86140A		E. coli Toxins
30940E		Urea Nitrogen	1099T		Ova and Parasites
17417W		Albumin	**VENIPUNCTURE**		
28423E		Prolactin	63180		Venipuncture

Building Medical Words

Review the Combining Forms Exercise, Combining Form and Suffix Exercise, and Prefix Exercise that you already completed in the anatomy section on pages 726–727.

Combining Forms Exercise

Before you build endocrine words, review these additional combining forms. Next to each combining form, write its medical meaning. The first one has been done for you.

Combining Form	Medical Meaning		Combining Form	Medical Meaning
1. acid/o-	acid (low pH)	16.	mast/o-	
2. acr/o-		17.	men/o-	
3. chrom/o-		18.	mult/i-	
4. cyt/o-		19.	myx/o-	
5. dem/o-		20.	nephr/o-	
6. dextr/o-		21.	neur/o-	
7. diabet/o-		22.	nod/o-	
8. dips/o-		23.	nodul/o-	
9. fertil/o-		24.	phag/o-	
10. genit/o-		25.	phe/o-	
11. gestat/o-		26.	retin/o-	
12. gigant/o-		27.	sphenoid/o-	
13. gynec/o-		28.	toxic/o-	
14. hirsut/o-		29.	tox/o-	
15. ket/o-		30.	ur/o-	

Multiple Combining Forms and Suffix Exercise

Read the definition of the medical word. Select the correct suffix and combining forms. Then build the medical word and write it on the line. Be sure to check your spelling. The first one has been done for you.

SUFFIX LIST	COMBINING FORM LIST	
-al (pertaining to)	acid/o- (acid; low pH)	ket/o- (ketones)
-ar (pertaining to)	adren/o- (adrenal gland)	mast/o- (breast; mastoid process)
-ia (condition; state; thing)	chrom/o- (color)	mult/i- (many)
-oma (tumor; mass)	cyt/o- (cell)	nodul/o- (small, knobby mass)
-osis (condition; abnormal condition;	genit/o- (genitalia)	phe/o- (gray)
process)	glycos/o- (glucose; sugar)	ur/o- (urine; urinary system)
	gynec/o- (female; woman)	

Definition of the Medical Word

1. Pertaining to many small, knobby masses

2. Abnormal condition (in which) ketones (cause the blood to become) acid with a low pH

3. Pertaining to the adrenal gland (hormones affecting the) genitalia

4. Tumor (with a) gray color to the cells (when viewed under the microscope) (Hint: Use 3 combining forms.)

5. Condition (in a man of having) a female (appearing) breast

6. Condition of glucose in the urine

Build the Medical Word

1. multinodular

2.

3.

4.

5.

6.

Combining Form and Suffix Exercise

Read the definition of the medical word. Select the correct suffix from the Suffix List. Select the correct combining form from the Combining Form List. Build the medical word and write it on the line. Be sure to check your spelling. The first one has been done for you.

SUFFIX LIST	COMBINING FORM LIST	
-ectomy (surgical excision)	acr/o- (extremity; highest point)	myx/o- (mucus-like substance)
-edema (swelling)	aden/o- (gland)	nod/o- (node)
-ic (pertaining to)	adrenal/o- (adrenal gland)	thym/o- (thymus; rage)
-ism (process; disease from a specific cause)	diabet/o- (diabetes)	thyr/o- (thyroid gland)
-itis (inflammation of; infection of)	galact/o- (milk)	thyroid/o- (thyroid gland)
-megaly (enlargement)	gigant/o- (giant)	tox/o- (poison)
-oma (tumor; mass)	hirsut/o- (hairy)	viril/o- (masculine)
-rrhea (flow; discharge)	hypophys/o- (pituitary gland)	
-ular (pertaining to a small thing)		

Definition of the Medical Word

1. Pertaining to a toxin or poison

2. Pertaining to a nodule

3. Surgical excision of the pituitary gland

4. Inflammation or infection of the thyroid gland

5. Tumor or mass in a gland

6. Surgical excision of the adrenal gland

7. Pertaining to diabetes

8. Enlargement of the thyroid gland

9. Disease from a specific cause of (hypersecretion of androgens causing) hairiness

10. Flow or discharge of milk (from the breast of a nonpregnant female)

11. Swelling (in the subcutaneous and connective tissues) from a mucus-like substance

12. Surgical excision of the thyroid gland

13. Disease from a specific cause (of too much growth hormone that makes a person a) giant

14. Enlargement of the extremities

15. Disease from a specific cause of (too much androgen that makes a female to be) masculine

16. Surgical excision of the thymus

Build the Medical Word

toxic _____

Prefix Exercise

Read the definition of the medical word. Look at the medical word or partial word that is given (it already contains a combining form and suffix). Select the correct prefix from the Prefix List and write it on the blank line. Then build the medical word and write it on the line. Be sure to check your spelling. The first one has been done for you.

PREFIX LIST

anti- (against)	in- (in; within; not)	poly (many; much)
en- (in; within; inward)	para- (beside; apart from; two	trans- (across; through)
hyper- (above; more than normal)	parts of a pair; abnormal)	
hypo- (below; deficient)		

Definition of the Medical Word	Prefix	Word or Partial Word	Build the Medical Word
1. Substance in the blood of more than normal calcium	hyper-	calcemia	hypercalcemia
2. Substance in the blood of deficient glucose	_____	glycemia	_____
3. Condition of not (being) able to conceive a child	_____	fertility	_____
4. Disease from a specific cause of more than normal thyroid gland (hormones)	_____	thyroidism	_____
5. Pertaining to (being present) within a population	_____	demic	_____
6. Condition of much urine	_____	uria	_____
7. Surgical excision of two parts of a pair (of a gland on the) thyroid gland	_____	thyroidectomy	_____
8. Pertaining to (a drug that is) against diabetes	_____	diabetic	_____
9. Substance in the blood of more than normal glucose	_____	glycemia	_____
10. Pertaining to (a surgical approach to the pituitary gland that goes) through the sphenoid bone or sphenoid sinus	_____	sphenoidal	_____

Abbreviations

Abbreviation Exercise

Give the abbreviation for the following definitions.

1. Type 1 diabetes mellitus _____
2. A group of tests that pertain to thyroid gland function _____
3. Blood test that measures glucose level after not eating _____
4. Diabetes with burning of fat and acidic blood _____
5. Organization for diabetes education and information _____
6. Measures the average blood sugar over several months _____
7. Depression related to low levels of light _____
8. Certified instructor who teaches about diabetic diets _____
9. Syndrome in which receptors resist the effect of insulin _____
10. Triiodothyronine _____

Applied Skills

Plural Noun and Adjective Spelling Exercise

Read the noun and write the plural form and/or adjective form. Be sure to check your spelling. The first one has been done for you.

Singular Noun	Plural Noun	Adjective
1. hypophysis		hypophysial
2. adenoma	_____	
3. cortex	_____	_____
4. gland	_____	_____
5. hormone	_____	
6. hypothalamus		_____
7. ovary	_____	_____
8. pancreas		_____
9. testis	_____	_____
10. thymus		_____

Proofreading and Spelling Exercise

Read the following paragraph. Identify each misspelled medical word and write the correct spelling of it on the line.

Endocrineology is the study of glands and hormones. The pitutary gland is the master gland. In diabetes mellitis, there is too much glukose and not enough insulin. A tumor in the adrenal medula is a feochromocytoma. If there is an adenoma in the thyroid gland, then a thyroectomy would be done. Graves' disease is known for exofthalmos and a goiter. An enlarged thyroid gland is thyromegalee. Galactorhea is milk production in a woman who is not pregnant.

1. _____	6. _____
2. _____	7. _____
3. _____	8. _____
4. _____	9. _____
5. _____	10. _____

Medical Report Exercise

This exercise contains a physician's office chart note. Read the report and answer the questions.

CHART NOTE

HISTORY

This is a 54-year-old male who presents with fatigue. He also has headaches. Because of a history of some visual field deficits during his headaches, his ophthalmologist ordered an MRI of the brain. I reviewed the scans and did not see anything but the expected postsurgical changes of the brain. Lab tests show that he does have some residual function of the pituitary gland, so his endocrinologist only placed him on testosterone patches and thyroid hormone replacement (Synthroid). He also has a history of depression, which could explain the fatigue and headache, or they could be due to low thyroid hormone replacement levels.

PHYSICAL EXAMINATION

HEENT: Normal. Lungs: Clear to auscultation. Cardiovascular: Regular rate and rhythm, without murmurs, rubs, or gallops. Abdomen: Nondistended, nontender. Extremities: No edema.

ASSESSMENT

1. Fatigue. Possibly hypothyroidism. Will check T_3, T_4, and TSH levels.
2. Headache, possibly within the context of depression. He is on a rather low dose of an antidepressant drug at this time.
3. Hypopituitarism, after surgical removal of an adenoma.

PLAN

1. Will obtain an FSH, LH, free and total testosterone, and baseline ACTH.
2. Follow up in 1 week.

Edward Allen Selcher, M.D.

Edward Allen Selcher, M.D.

EAS:blg
D: 11/19/xx
T: 11/19/xx

Word Analysis Questions

1. Divide *endocrinologist* into its four word parts and define each word part.

Word Part	Definition
_____	_____
_____	_____
_____	_____
_____	_____

2. Divide *hypopituitarism* into its three word parts and define each word part.

Word Part	Definition
_____	_____
_____	_____
_____	_____

3. What is the abbreviation for *thyroid-stimulating hormone?* _____

Fact Finding Questions

1. Besides the physician who dictated this report, what two physician specialists have also recently seen the patient?

   _____

   _____

2. What two hormones does the patient already take as drugs for hormone replacement therapy?

   _____

   _____

3. What do these abbreviations mean?

   ADH: _____

   FSH: _____

   LH: _____

4. The patient is taking Synthroid for his (**headaches, hypothyroidism, lungs**). Circle the correct answer.

Critical Thinking Questions

1. The patient's fatigue, headache, and visual field defect could be signs of a recurring tumor in the brain. What test has already been done to look for a tumor?

   _____

2. The patient's MRI of the brain showed postsurgical changes, meaning changes that are present because of a surgery that was done. Which endocrine gland was operated on in the past?

   _____

3. Which of the patient's drugs correlates with doing the lab tests for T_3, T_4, and TSH?

   _____

Hearing Medical Words Exercise

You hear someone speaking the medical words given below. Read each pronunciation and then write the medical word it represents. Be sure to check your spelling. The first one has been done for you.

1. DY-ah-BEE-teez   *diabetes*   5. IN-fer-TIL-ih-tee   _____

2. AD-eh-NOH-mah   _____   6. SIN-er-jizm   _____

3. GLAN-dyoo-lar   _____   7. THY-roy-DEK-toh-mee   _____

4. HY-per-gly-SEE-mee-ah   _____

Pronunciation Exercise

Read the medical word that is given. Then review the syllables in the pronunciation. Circle the primary (main) accented syllable. The first one has been done for you.

1. hormone (HOR-mohn)

2. ovarian (oh-vair-ee-an)

3. cortisol (kor-tih-sawl)

4. diabetic (dy-ah-bet-ik)

5. endocrinology (en-doh-krih-nawl-oh-jee)

6. homeostasis (hoh-mee-oh-stay-sis)

7. pituitary (pih-too-eh-tair-ee)

Multimedia Preview

Immerse yourself in a variety of activities inside Medical Terminology Interactive. Getting there is simple:

1. Click on www.myhealthprofessionskit.com.
2. Select "Medical Terminology" from the choice of disciplines.
3. First-time users must create an account using the scratch-off code on the inside front cover of this book.
4. Find this book and log in using your username and password.
5. Click on Medical Terminology Interactive.
6. Take the elevator to the 14th Floor to begin your virtual exploration of this chapter!

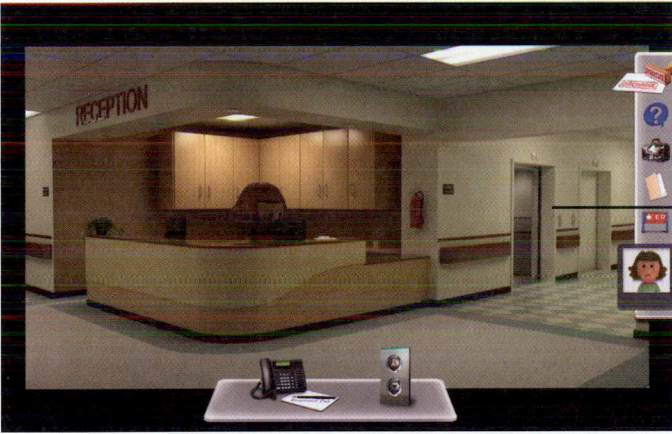 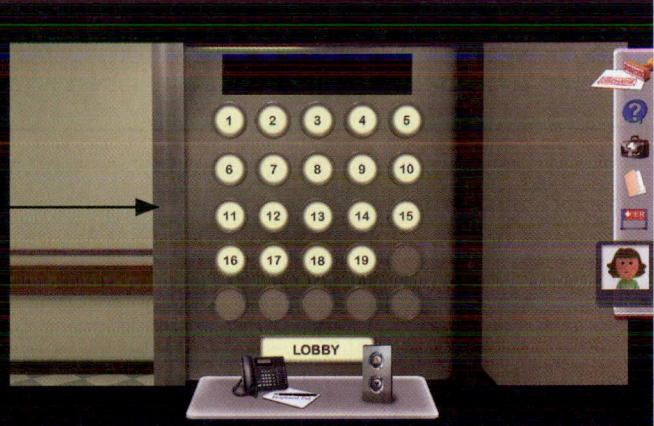

■ **Word Up!**   Catch it while you can! Challenge yourself to match the definition to the corresponding word part as your choices swirl around the screen. See how many you can match up correctly before your time is up!

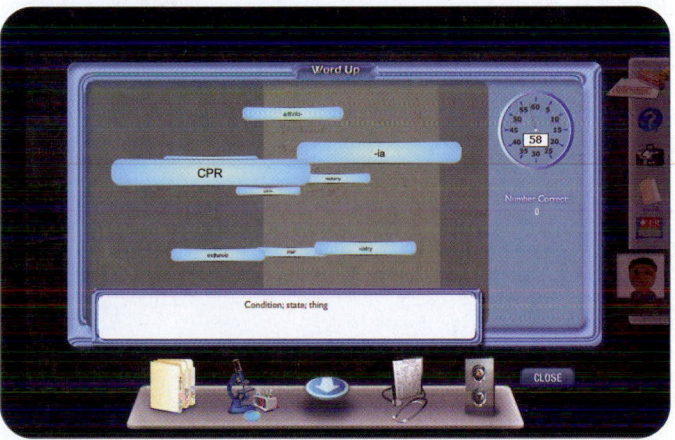

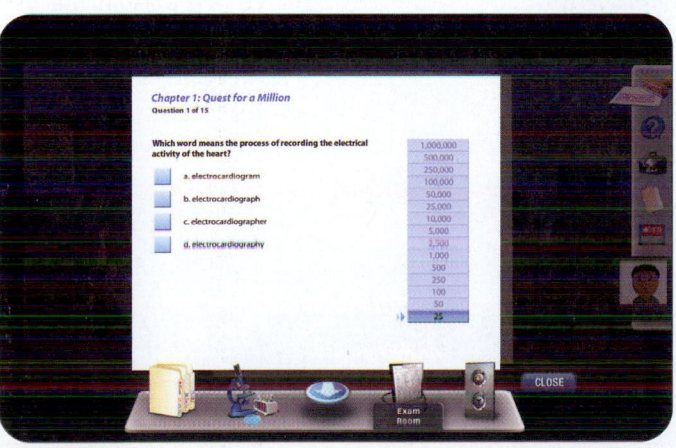

■ **Quest for a Million**   Who wants to win a million points? If it's you, then click on this game to begin your challenge. If you correctly answer 15 questions in a row, then you're a winner. But be very careful, because one wrong response will take you back down to zero.

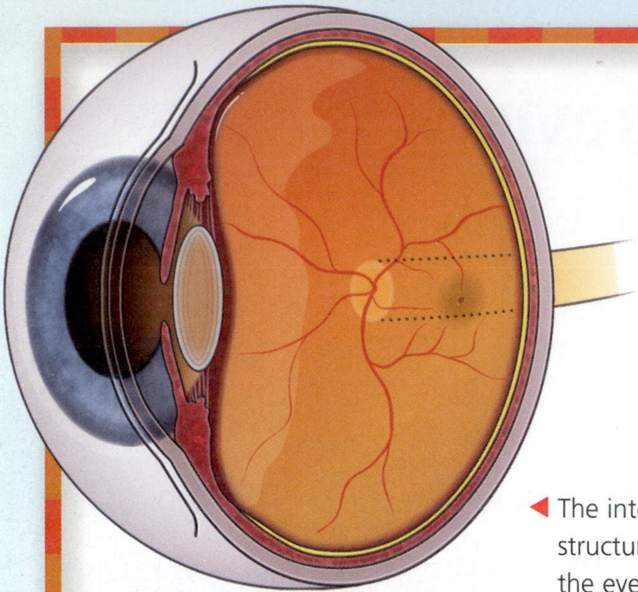

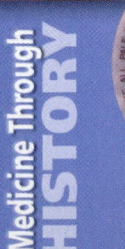

The internal structure of the eye.

Dive In!

- The eyes can distinguish nearly 7 million different shades of color.
- After his retirement, Crayola's most senior crayon maker Emerson Moser revealed that he was actually colorblind.
- Leonardo da Vinci devised the first concept for the contact lens.
- Set your sights on becoming a star pupil. In this chapter we'll explore the language that describes the eye structures, functions, diseases, and conditions.
- You'll be seeing clearly once you master the language of ophthalmology!

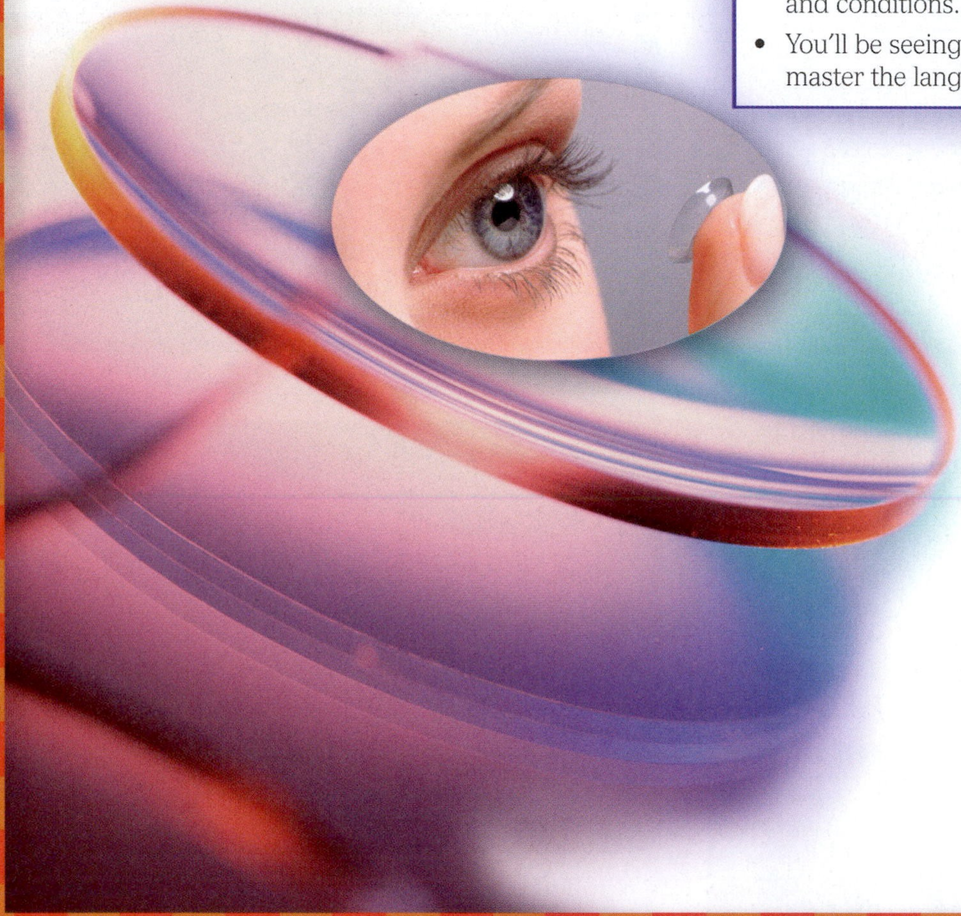

Since the 1940s contact lenses have been used by millions around the world to correct their vision.

Medicine Through HISTORY

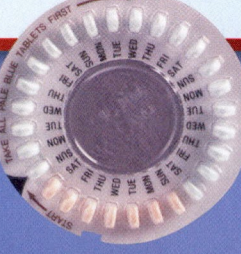

1960

The first oral contraceptive pill is introduced

1961

The first breast silicone implant surgery is performed

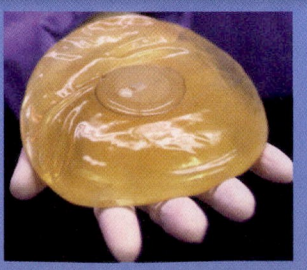

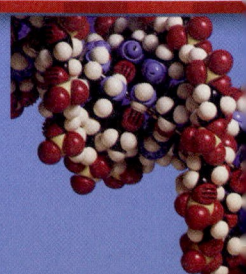

Ophthalmology

Eye

Ophthalmology (AWF-thal-MAWL-oh-jee) is the medical specialty that studies the anatomy and physiology of the eye and uses diagnostic tests, medical and surgical procedures, and drugs to treat eye diseases.

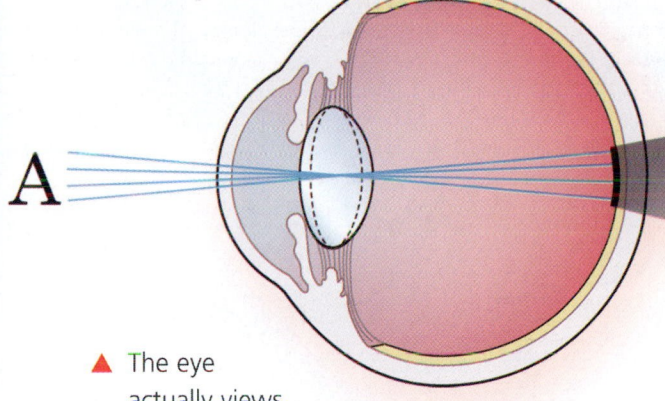

▲ The eye actually views images upside down and backward until the brain turns the image right side up.

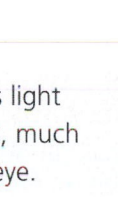

▶ Cameras process light to create images, much like the human eye.

1962

Watson and Crick receive the Nobel Prize for identifying the double-helix structure of DNA in the nucleus of a cell

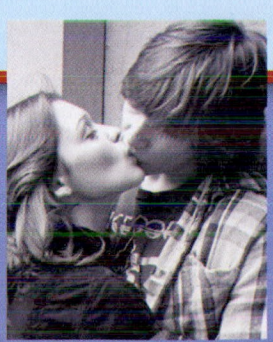

1964

Epstein-Barr virus is discovered to be the cause of "kissing disease" (infectious mononucleosis)

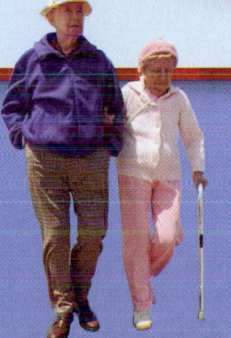

1965

Medicare and Medicaid begin to provide medical coverage for the elderly and the poor

Measure Your Progress: Learning Objectives

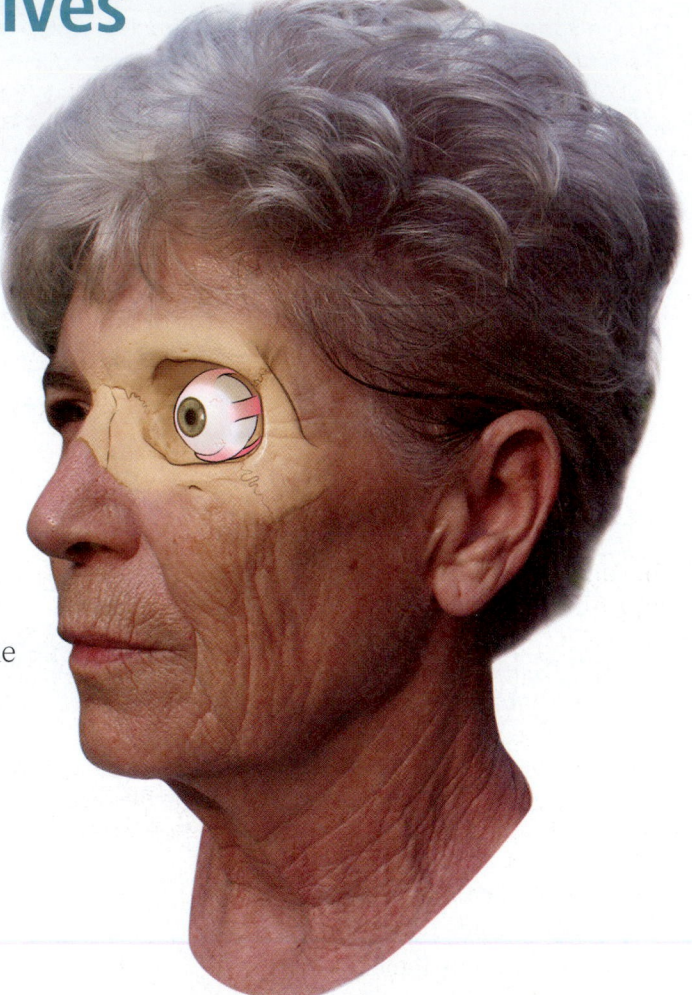

After you study this chapter, you should be able to

1. Identify the structures of the eye.

2. Describe the process of vision.

3. Describe common eye diseases and conditions, laboratory and diagnostic procedures, medical and surgical procedures, and drug categories.

4. Give the medical meaning of word parts related to the eye.

5. Build eye words from word parts and divide and define words related to the eye.

6. Spell and pronounce eye words.

7. Analyze the medical content and meaning of an ophthalmology report.

8. Dive deeper into ophthalmology by reviewing the activities at the end of this chapter and online at Medical Terminology Interactive.

Figure 15-1 ■ Eye.
The eyes consist of two identical but individual organs that sit in bony sockets of the cranium. By nerves, they connect to the structures in the brain to provide the special sense of sight.

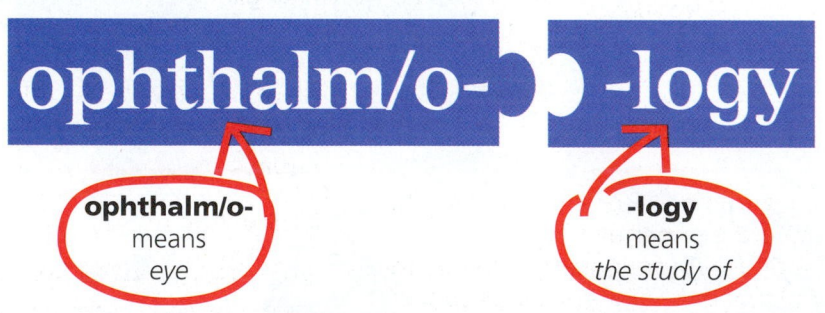

Medical Language Key

To unlock the definition of a medical word, break it into word parts. Define each word part. Put the word part meanings in order, beginning with the suffix, then the prefix (if present), then the combining form(s).

ophthalm/o- ⬡⬡ -logy

ophthalm/o-
means
eye

-logy
means
the study of

	Word Part	Word Part Meaning
Suffix	-logy	*the study of*
Combining Form	ophthalm/o-	*eye*

Ophthalmology: *The study of the eye (and related structures).*

Anatomy and Physiology

The eyes belong to a body system that consists of two identical main organs and many associated structures (see Figure 15-1 ■). Each eye or **optic globe** is located within an **orbit,** a hollow bony socket in the anterior cranium. The walls of the orbit are made up of several different cranial and facial bones (discussed in "Orthopedics," Chapter 8). The bony orbit surrounds all but the anterior surface of the eye. In the posterior wall of the orbit, the optic nerve (cranial nerve II), arteries, and veins come through openings in the bone to reach the eye. Within the bony orbit, a layer of fat cushions and protects the eye. The purpose of the eyes is to provide sensory information that can be interpreted by the visual cortex in the brain to become the sense of sight.

Anatomy of the Eye

Eyelid and Lacrimal Gland

The upper and lower **eyelids** protect the delicate tissues of the eye (see Figure 15-2 ■). The eyelids blink involuntarily to prevent foreign substances from entering the eye. The eyelids also blink many times a minute to spread a layer of tears that keeps the surface of the eye moist. At the edges of the eyelids, sebaceous glands secrete oil that acts as a barrier to keep tears in the eye. The **eyelashes** form a protective barrier that extends outward from the eye to catch foreign substances before they come in contact with the eye. The sebaceous glands and eyelashes are part of the integumentary system (discussed in "Dermatology," Chapter 7).

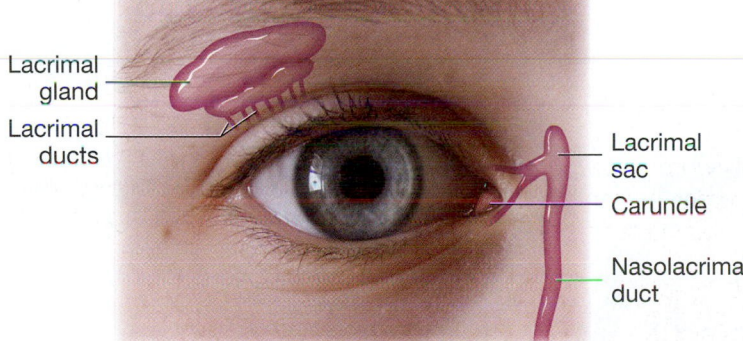

Lacrimal gland
Lacrimal ducts
Lacrimal sac
Caruncle
Nasolacrimal duct

Figure 15-2 ■ Lacrimal glands.
The lacrimal glands secrete tears to lubricate the anterior surface of the eye. Excess tears flow into the lacrimal sac, drain into the nasolacrimal duct, and eventually enter the nose.

The **caruncle** is the red, triangular tissue at the medial corner where the eyelids meet. The **lacrimal gland** is located in the superior-lateral aspect of each eye (see Figure 15-2). The lacrimal glands continuously secrete tears that travel through the **lacrimal ducts.** Large amounts of tears are produced when the eye is irritated or invaded by a foreign substance and during times of emotional distress. Tears contain an antibacterial enzyme to prevent bacterial infections. At the medial aspects of the upper and lower eyelids, two tiny openings drain away excess tears. The tears flow into the **lacrimal sac** and then into the **nasolacrimal duct** to the inside of the nose. That is why when your eyes water, your nose also runs!

Conjunctiva, Sclera, and Cornea

The **conjunctiva** is a delicate, transparent mucous membrane that covers the insides of the eyelids and the anterior surface of the eye (see Figure 15-4). The conjunctiva produces watery, clear mucus that traps any foreign substances on the surface of the eye.

The **sclera** is a tough, fibrous connective tissue that forms a continuous outer layer around the eye. This tissue is white and opaque and, where it can be seen between the eyelids, is known as the white of the eye (see Figures 15-3 ■ and 15-4 ■). The sclera protects the internal structures of the eye and helps maintain the shape of the eye. The sclera is the site of attachment for all of the muscles that move the eye (see Figure 15-9).

WORD BUILDING

conjunctiva (CON-junk-TY-vah)
(con-JUNK-tih-vah)

conjunctivae (CON-junk-TY-vee)
(con-JUNK-tih-vee)
Conjunctiva is a Latin singular noun. Form the plural by changing *-a* to *-ae*.

conjunctival (CON-junk-TY-val)
(con-JUNK-tih-val)
  conjunctiv/o- *conjunctiva*
  -al *pertaining to*

sclera (SKLEER-ah)

sclerae (SKLEER-ee)
Sclera is a Latin singular noun. Form the plural by changing *-a* to *-ae*.

scleral (SKLEER-al)
  scler/o- *hard; sclera (white of the eye)*
  -al *pertaining to*

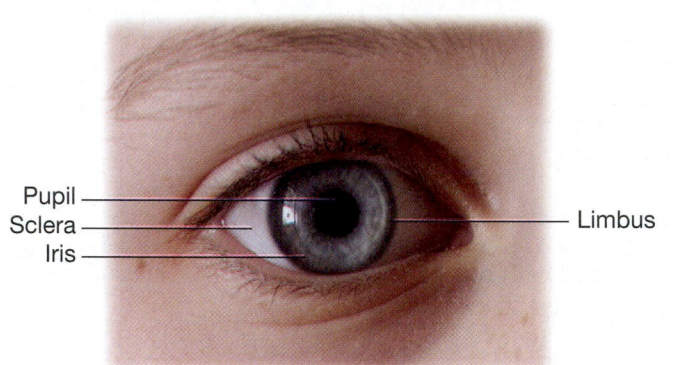

Pupil —
Sclera —
Iris —
— Limbus

Figure 15-3 ■ Anterior surface of the eye.
The anterior surface is the only part of the eye that is visible on the surface of the body. The sclera (white of the eye), iris, pupil, and limbus are part of this area.

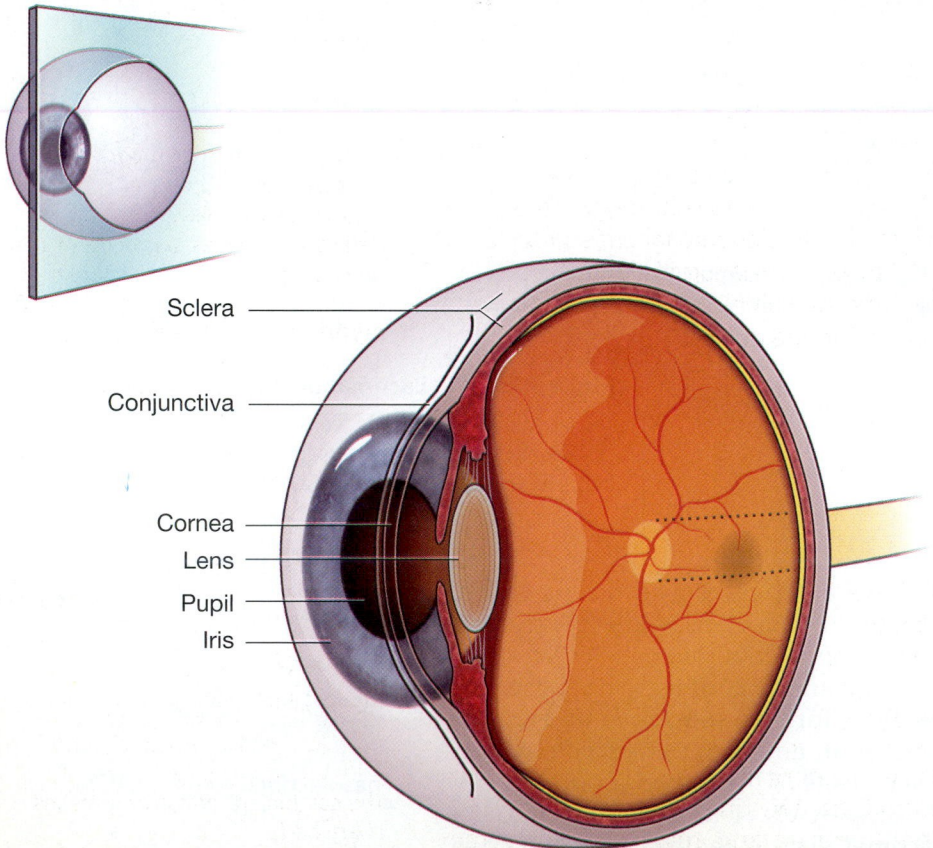

Sclera —
Conjunctiva —
Cornea —
Lens —
Pupil —
Iris —

Figure 15-4 ■ Internal structures at the front of the eye.

The conjunctiva covers the anterior surface of the eye and the inner eyelids. The sclera surrounds the entire eye. On the anterior surface of the eye, the sclera changes into the transparent cornea. The colored iris and the central pupil can be seen through the cornea. The lens of the eye is behind the iris.

Across the anterior part of the eye, the sclera changes into a transparent layer known as the **cornea** (see Figure 15-4). The transitional line between the white sclera and the clear cornea is known as the **limbus** (see Figure 15-3). The cornea allows light to enter the eye. It also bends (refracts) the rays of light. The cornea itself contains no blood vessels. It receives oxygen and nutrients from tears that flow across its surface and from aqueous humor that flows beneath it in the anterior chamber. The cornea does have nerves, however, and is the most sensitive area on the anterior surface of the eye.

Iris and Pupil

The iris and pupil can be seen behind the transparent cornea. The **iris** is a circular structure whose color is determined by genetics. At the center of the iris is the **pupil,** a round opening that allows light rays to enter the eye (see Figure 15-4). The pupil itself appears black because very little light is reflected from the back of the eye. However, if you take a picture with flash photography, this intense light does reflect from the back of the eye, and the photograph shows an eye with a red pupil.

In bright light, muscles in the iris contract to constrict and decrease the diameter of the pupil. This process, which is known as **miosis,** keeps too much light from entering the eye. In dim light, muscles in the iris relax to dilate and increase the diameter of the pupil. This process, which is known as **mydriasis,** allows more light to enter the eye.

Clinical Connections

Genetics. Eye color is a genetically determined trait. In each cell, chromosome 15 contains genes for brown/blue and brown/brown eye colors. Chromosome 19 contains a gene for blue/green eye colors. Each parent contributes combinations of these genes to their baby.

At birth, all babies' eyes appear slate gray to blue in color because of the lack of the brown pigment melanin in the iris. Exposure to light triggers the production of melanin by melanocytes in the iris. Babies who inherit a brown/brown or brown/blue gene have a large number of melanocytes in their iris, and they develop dark brown or light brown eyes. Babies who inherit a blue/blue or blue/green gene have no melanocytes in the iris, and their eyes are blue, hazel, or green.

Choroid and Ciliary Body

The **choroid** is a spongy membrane of blood vessels that is part of the internal structure of the eye (see Figure 15-5 ■). It begins at the outer edge of the iris. It cannot be seen on the anterior surface of the eye because it lies beneath the opaque white sclera. In the posterior cavity, the choroid is the middle layer between the sclera and the retina. The blood vessels of the choroid supply blood to the entire eye.

The **ciliary body** is an extension of the choroid (see Figure 15-5). It attaches to suspensory ligaments that hold the lens in place behind the iris. The ciliary body contains muscles that contract and relax to change the

---

WORD BUILDING

cornea (KOR-nee-ah)

corneae (KOR-nee-ee)
Cornea is a Latin singular noun. Form the plural by changing -*a* to -*ae*.

corneal (KOR-nee-al)
   corne/o- *cornea (of the eye)*
   -al *pertaining to*
The combining form *kerat/o-* also means *cornea.*

limbus (LIM-bus)

iris (EYE-ris)

irides (IHR-ih-deez)
Iris is a Greek singular noun. Form the plural by changing -*is* to *ides.*

iridal (IHR-ih-dal) (EYE-rih-dal)
   irid/o- *iris (colored part of the eye)*
   -al *pertaining to*
The combining form *ir/o-* also means *iris.*

pupil (PYOO-pil)

pupillary (PYOO-pih-LAIR-ee)
   pupill/o- *pupil (of the eye)*
   -ary *pertaining to*
The combining form *cor/o-* also means *pupil.*

miosis (my-OH-sis)
   mi/o- *narrowing*
   -osis *condition; abnormal condition; process*
Add words to make a complete definition of *miosis: a process of narrowing (the size of the pupil).*

mydriasis (mih-DRY-eh-sis)
   mydr/o- *widening*
   -iasis *state of; process of*

choroid (KOH-royd)

choroidal (koh-ROY-dal)
   choroid/o- *choroid (middle layer around the eye)*
   -al *pertaining to*

ciliary (SIL-ee-AIR-ee)
   cili/o- *hairlike structure*
   -ary *pertaining to*
The combining form *cycl/o-* means *ciliary body.*

shape of the lens to focus light rays coming through the pupil. The ciliary body also produces aqueous humor.

The **uvea** or **uveal tract** is a collective word for the iris, choroid, and ciliary body.

WORD BUILDING

uvea (YOO-vee-ah)

uveal (YOO-vee-al)
  uve/o- *uvea (of the eye)*
  -al *pertaining to*

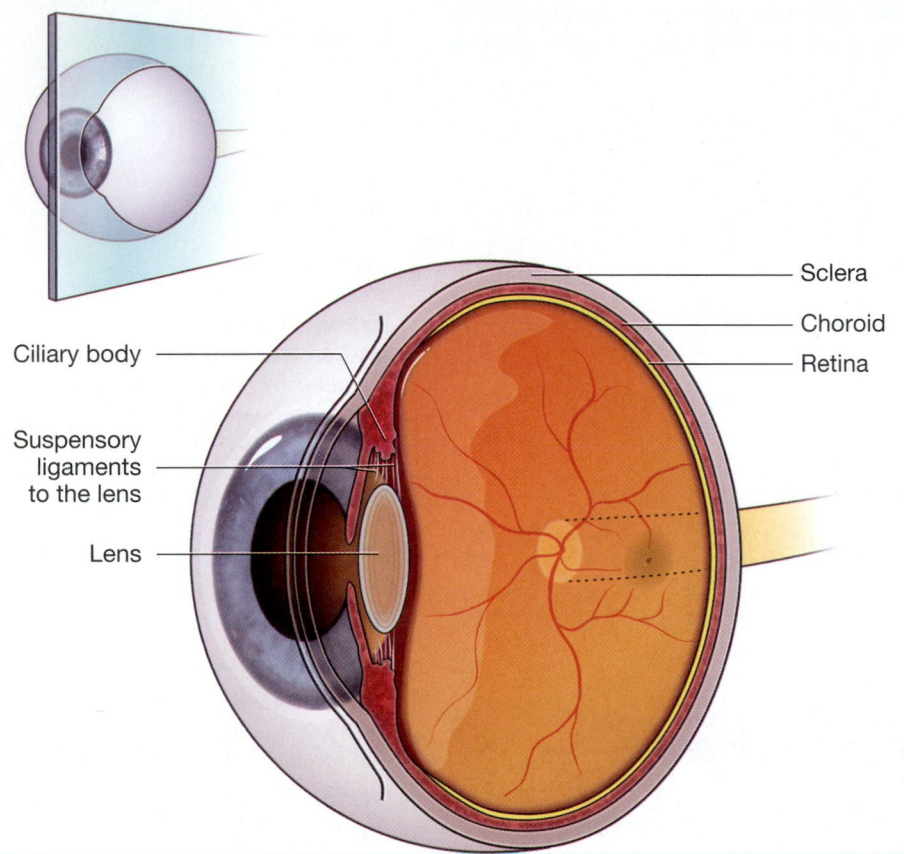

Sclera
Choroid
Retina
Ciliary body
Suspensory ligaments to the lens
Lens

Figure 15-5 ■ **Tissue layers in the eye.**

The sclera (white of the eye) continues around the entire eye. Its tough, fibrous connective tissue helps to maintain the shape of the eye. The choroid contains blood vessels. The ciliary body is an extension of the choroid. The retina lines the curved wall of the posterior cavity.

Lens

The **lens** is a clear, flexible disk behind the pupil. It contains protein molecules arranged in a crystalline structure that makes the lens transparent (see Figure 15-5). The lens is surrounded by the **lens capsule,** a clear membrane. Through the process of **accommodation,** the lens changes shape. The muscles of the ciliary body contract or relax to move the suspensory ligaments to the lens. The lens becomes thicker and more rounded to see objects close by (near vision) or thinner and flatter to see objects at a distance (far vision).

Anterior and Posterior Chambers

The **anterior chamber** is a small space between the cornea and the iris (see Figure 15-6 ■). The **posterior chamber** is a very narrow space posterior to the iris. The iris forms a dividing wall between the anterior and posterior

lens (LENZ)

lenses (LEN-sez)
  lenticul/o- *lens (of the eye)*
  -ar *pertaining to*
The combining forms *lent/o-, phac/o-,* and *phak/o-* also mean *lens.*

capsule (KAP-sool)

capsular (KAP-soo-lar)
  capsul/o- *capsule (enveloping structure)*
  -ar *pertaining to*

accommodation
(ah-KAWM-oh-DAY-shun)
  accommod/o- *to adapt*
  -ation *a process; being or having*

anterior (an-TEER-ee-or)
  anter/o- *before; front part*
  -ior *pertaining to*

posterior (pohs-TEER-ee-or)
  poster/o- *back part*
  -ior *pertaining to*

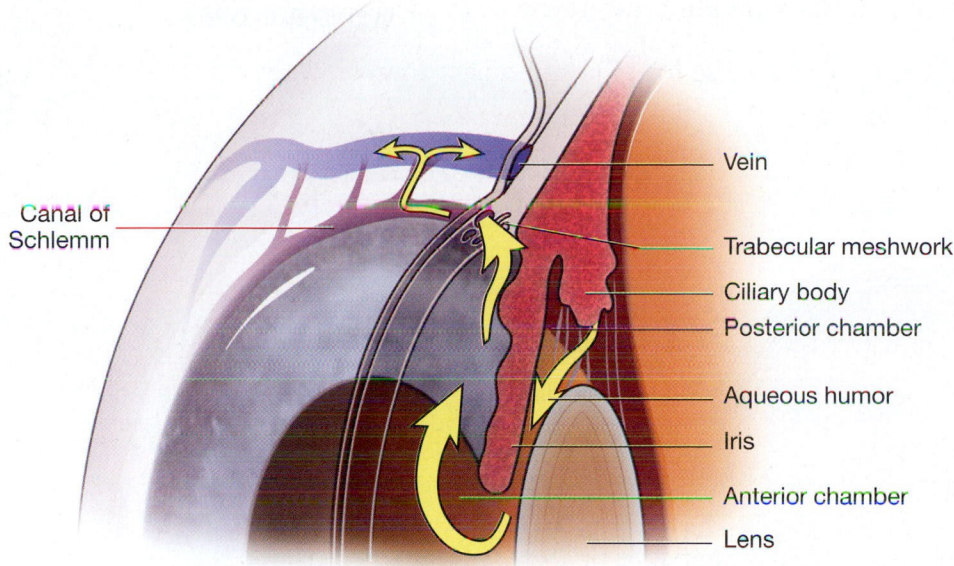

Canal of
Schlemm

Vein

Trabecular meshwork

Ciliary body

Posterior chamber

Aqueous humor

Iris

Anterior chamber

Lens

Figure 15-6 ■ Aqueous humor.
Aqueous humor produced by the ciliary body circulates through the posterior chamber, pupil, and anterior chamber. It drains through the trabecular meshwork.

chambers of the anterior eye. The only opening in this wall is the pupil. The anterior and posterior chambers are both filled with aqueous humor.

Aqueous humor is a clear, watery fluid that is produced continuously by the ciliary body. Aqueous humor carries nutrients and oxygen to the cornea and lens. Aqueous humor circulates through the posterior chamber, through the pupil, and into the anterior chamber. It then drains through the **trabecular meshwork,** interlacing fibers all around the edge of the iris where it meets the cornea and forms an angle. The aqueous humor then drains into the canal of Schlemm, a circular channel around the iris. From there, the aqueous humor is absorbed into veins and taken away by the blood. The rate of production of aqueous humor normally equals the rate of drainage.

Posterior Cavity

The **posterior cavity** is the largest space in the eye. It lies between the lens and the back of the eye (see Figure 15-7 ■). It is filled with **vitreous humor,** a clear, gel-like substance that helps maintain the shape of the eye.

Retina

The **retina** is a thin layer of tissue that lines the curved wall of the posterior cavity (see Figures 15-5, 15-7, and 15-8 ■). The choroid layer lies beneath the retina and provides blood to the retina. **Fundus** is a general word for the retina because it is the area that is farthest from the opening to the eye (the pupil).

There are two distinct landmarks on the retina. The **optic disk** is a bright, yellow-white circle with sharp edges in the area of the retina closest to the nose. This is where the **optic nerve** (cranial nerve II) enters the eye. The

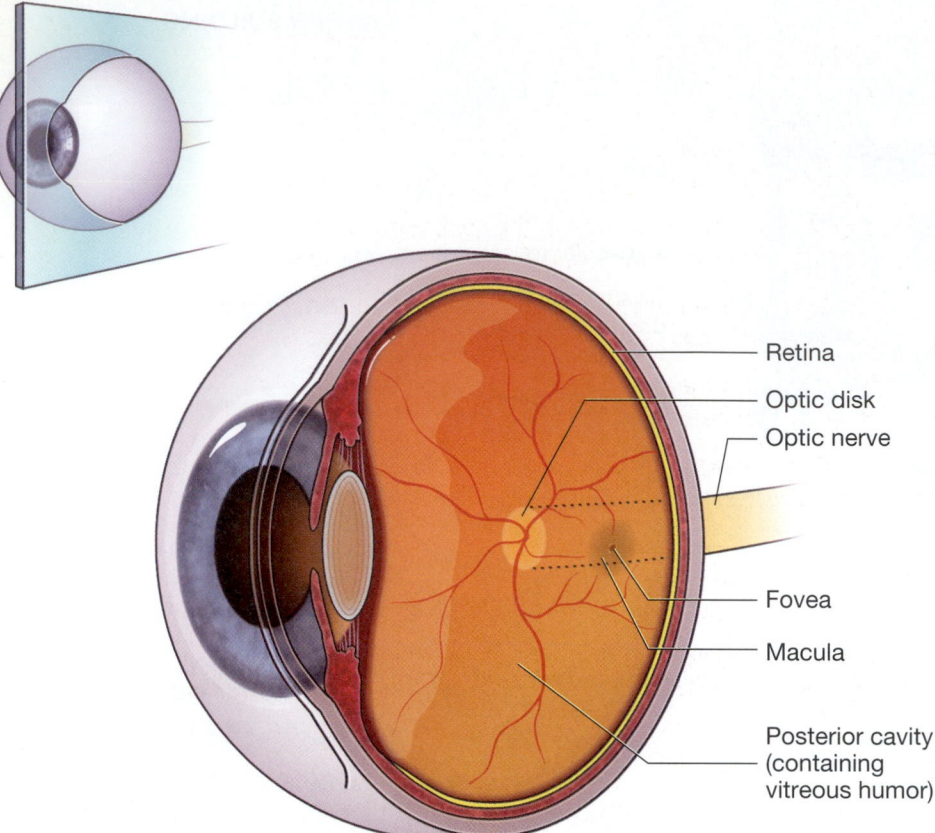

Figure 15-7 ■ **Internal structures at the back of the eye.**

The posterior cavity is filled with vitreous humor. The retina contains the macula (area of sharpest vision) and the optic disk (area where the optic nerve enters).

retinal arteries also enter through the optic disk and spread across the retina, and the retinal veins leave the eye at the optic disk. The optic disk is not stimulated by light or color and cannot receive sensory information. It is known as the **blind spot.** The second landmark is the **macula,** a dark yellow-orange area. The **fovea** is a small depression in the center of the macula. The fovea lies directly opposite the pupil. Light rays entering the pupil fall on the macula, specifically the fovea, which is the area of sharpest vision.

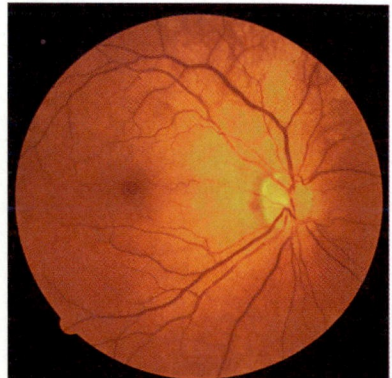
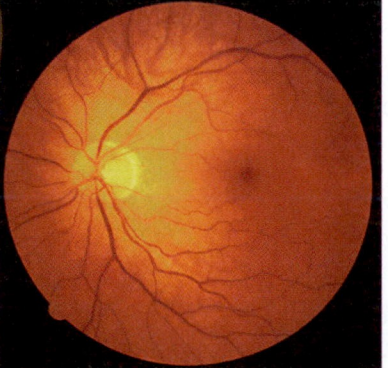

Figure 15-8 ■ **Retinae of both eyes.**

Dilation of the pupil permits visualization of the retina. The structures of the optic disk, retinal blood vessels, and macula can clearly be seen. Note that the size and shape of these structures are not identical in each eye.

WORD BUILDING

macula (MAK-yoo-lah)

maculae (MAK-yoo-lee)
Macula is a Latin singular noun. Form the plural by changing *-a* to *-ae.*

macular (MAK-yoo-lar)
  macul/o- *small area or spot*
  -ar *pertaining to*

fovea (FOH-vee-ah)

foveae (FOH-vee-ee)
Fovea is a Latin singular noun. Form the plural by changing *-a* to *-ae.*

foveal (FOH-vee-al)
  fove/o- *small, depressed area*
  -al *pertaining to*

Word Alert

SOUND-ALIKE WORDS

caruncle   (noun)   red, triangular tissue at the medial corner of the eye
Example: The caruncle became irritated when a foreign substance entered the eye.

carbuncle   (noun)   large abscess on the skin that tunnels through the subcutaneous tissue
Example: A carbuncle contains pus from an infection caused by bacteria on the skin.

macula   (noun)   dark, orange-yellow area with indistinct margins located on the retina
Example: The macula showed degenerative changes.

macule   (noun)   small, flat, pigmented spot on the skin
Example: Sun exposure increases the number of macules (freckles) on the skin.

macular   (adjective)   descriptive word that pertains to the macula of the eye and a macule on the skin
Examples: The patient has macular degeneration of the eye.
The patient has a macular-papular rash on the skin.

miosis   (noun)   decreasing the diameter of the pupil when the muscles of the iris contract
Example: Bright light produces miosis, as the size of the pupil decreases.

mitosis   (noun)   process by which most body cells reproduce
Example: In mitosis, the dividing cell duplicates and then splits into two cells that each have 46 chromosomes.

A Closer Look

The optic nerve (cranial nerve II) is a sensory nerve that carries sensory information from the retina to the optic chiasm. The **oculomotor motor nerve** (cranial nerve III) is a motor nerve that carries motor commands from the midbrain to four of the six extraocular muscles to move the eye, to the eyelids to produce movement, and to the muscles of the iris to contract or relax (to decrease or increase the diameter of the pupil). The trochlear nerve (cranial nerve IV) is a motor nerve that carries motor commands from the midbrain to one extraocular muscle (the superior oblique muscle) to produce movements of the eye. The trigeminal nerve (cranial nerve V) is a sensory nerve that carries sensory information from the skin of the eyelids and eyebrows to the pons in the brainstem. The abducens nerve (cranial nerve VI) is a motor nerve that carries motor commands from the pons to one extraocular muscle (the lateral rectus muscle) to produce movements of the eye. The facial nerve (cranial nerve VII) is a motor nerve that carries motor commands from the pons to the lacrimal glands to produce tears.

oculomotor (AWK-yoo-loh-MOH-tor)
ocul/o- *eye*
-motor *thing that produces movement*

Extraocular Muscles

The **extraocular muscles** control the movements of the eye. Four of these are straight muscles (and have *rectus* in their names). The other two wrap around the eye in a slanted manner (and have *oblique* in their names) (see Figure 15-9 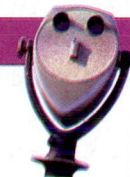). The extraocular muscles are attached to the sclera by tendons. The movement of the extraocular muscles is under voluntary control.

WORD BUILDING

extraocular (EKS-trah-AWK-yoo-lar)
extra- *outside of*
ocul/o- *eye*
-ar *pertaining to*

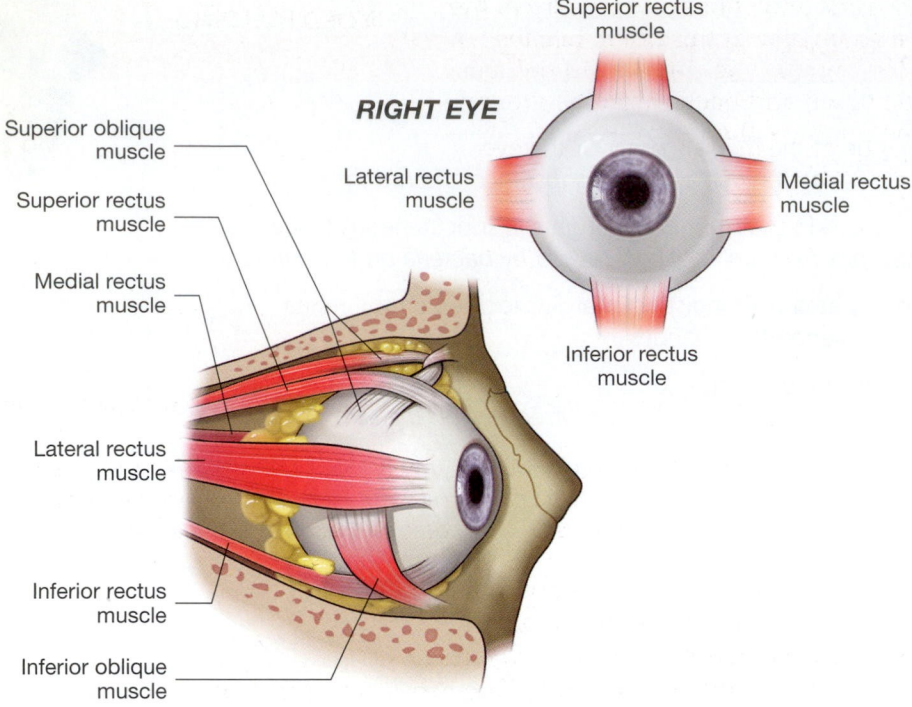

Figure 15-9 ■ Extraocular muscles.
The eye can move in all directions because of six different extraocular muscles attached by tendons to the sclera.

Extraocular Muscles

- **Superior rectus muscle:** Turns the eye superiorly
- **Inferior rectus muscle:** Turns the eye inferiorly
- **Medial rectus muscle:** Turns the eye medially (toward the midline)
- **Lateral rectus muscle:** Turns the eye laterally (away from the midline)
- **Superior oblique muscle:** Turns the eye inferiorly and medially
- **Inferior oblique muscle:** Turns the eye superiorly and laterally

Physiology of Vision

The process of **vision** begins as light rays from an object pass through the cornea, which bends the rays to begin to focus them. The light rays then enter the pupil and pass through the lens. Muscles in the ciliary body contract or relax to change the shape of the lens and focus the light rays. Light rays from objects directly in the line of vision fall on the macula (specifically the fovea), and these objects produce the clearest, sharpest image. Other parts of the retina pick up light rays from objects at the edges of the visual field.

The retina contains special light-sensitive cells known as rods and cones. **Rods** are sensitive in all levels of light and detect black and white, but not color. Rods function in daytime and nighttime vision. It only takes one photon (light particle) to activate a rod, so rods can detect objects in very low light, but they only produce a somewhat grainy black-and-white image of that object.

Cones are only sensitive to color. There are three different types of cones that respond to either red light, green light, or blue light. The cones are concentrated in the macula. It takes many photons to activate a cone, which is why it is difficult to see colors in dim light. Cones produce a sharp color image that is superimposed on the black-and-white image created by the rods.

WORD BUILDING
superior (soo-PEER-ee-or) **super/o-** *above* **-ior** *pertaining to*
inferior (in-FEER-ee-or) **infer/o-** *below* **-ior** *pertaining to*
rectus (REK-tus)
medial (MEE-dee-al) **medi/o-** *middle* **-al** *pertaining to*
lateral (LAT-er-al) **later/o-** *side* **-al** *pertaining to*
oblique (ob-LEEK)
vision (VIH-shun) **vis/o-** *sight; vision* **-ion** *action; condition*

When a person looks at an object, the rods and cones everywhere in the retina respond to the light rays to create an image. At this point, because of the way in which the light rays have been bent by the cornea and the lens, the image of the object is actually upside down and backward when it contacts the retina (see Figure 15-10 ■). The image is then converted to nerve impulses that are transmitted to the optic nerve.

WORD BUILDING

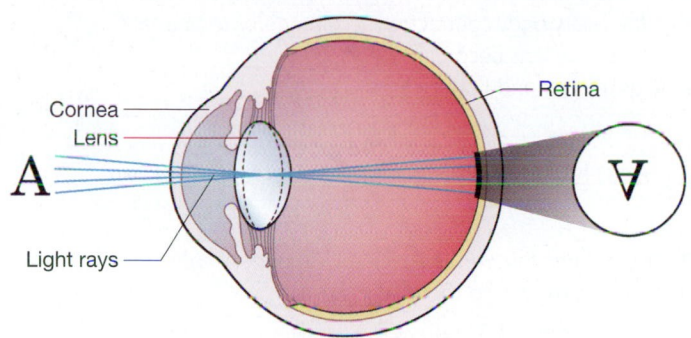

Figure 15-10 ■ **Light rays coming from an object to the retina.**

The cornea and lens focus light rays from an object onto the retina. An object directly in the line of vision produces an image on the macula. This image is sharp and clear, but upside down and backward.

The optic nerve (cranial nerve II) from each eye travels to the **optic chiasm,** a crossing point where parts of one optic nerve cross over to join the optic nerve on the other side, and vice versa. This merges part of the visual field of one eye with part of the visual field of the other eye to create three-dimensional, **stereoscopic vision** with a perception of depth and distance. These combined nerves (now called optic tracts) enter the **thalamus** in the brain. There the sensory information they carry is interpreted by the thalamus and quickly sent to the midbrain. If needed, the midbrain sends out a motor command reflex to blink or move away from something coming toward the eye. The sensory information is also sent to the **visual cortex** in the right and left occipital lobes of the brain (see Figure 15-11 ■). The visual cortex merges the image from each eye to create a single, three-dimensional image and turns that image so that it is right side up and facing in the direction of the original object. Another area in the occipital lobe associates this visual image with long-term visual memories and communicates with the frontal lobe of the brain where decisions are made about the meaning of what was seen and what to do about it.

chiasm (KY-azm)

stereoscopic (STAIR-ee-oh-SKAWP-ik)
  stere/o- *three dimensions*
  scop/o- *examine with an instrument*
  -ic *pertaining to*

thalamus (THAL-ah-mus)

visual (VIH-shoo-al)
  vis/o- *sight; vision*
  -ual *pertaining to*

cortex (KOR-teks)

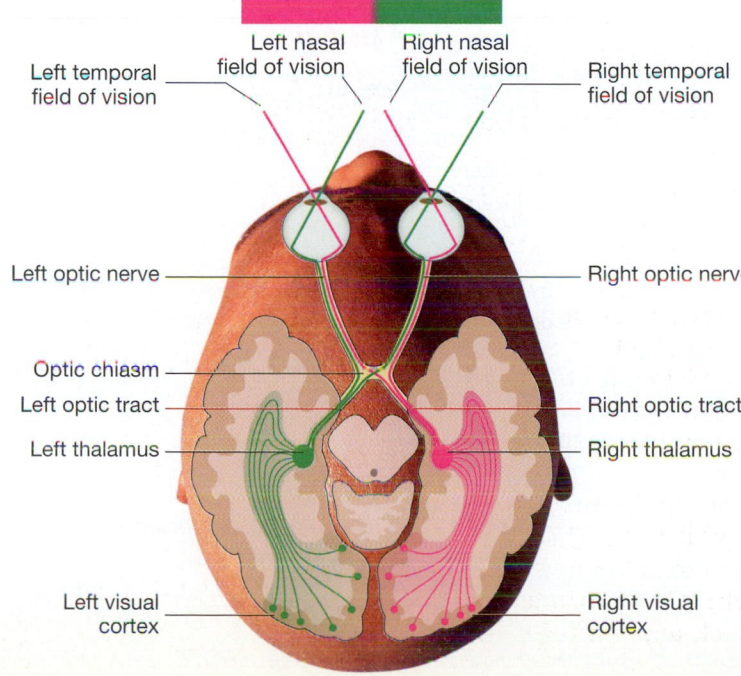

Figure 15-11 ■ **Optic nerve, optic chiasm, thalamus, and visual cortex.**

The image of an object travels as sensory information through the optic nerve (cranial nerve II) to the optic chiasm, through the optic tracts to the thalamus, and then to the visual cortex where it is interpreted.

Vocabulary Review

Anatomy and Physiology

Word or Phrase	Description	Combining Forms
accommodation	Change in the shape of the lens as the muscles of the ciliary body contract or relax to move the suspensory ligaments to the lens. The lens becomes thicker and more rounded to see objects close by or thinner and flatter to see objects at a distance.	**accommod/o-** *to adapt*
anterior chamber	Small space between the cornea and the iris. Aqueous humor circulates through it.	**anter/o-** *before; front part*
aqueous humor	Clear, watery fluid produced by the ciliary body. It circulates through the posterior and anterior chambers and takes nutrients and oxygen to the cornea and lens. It drains through the trabecular meshwork.	**aque/o-** *watery substance*
caruncle	Red, triangular tissue at the medial corner of the eye	
choroid	Spongy membrane of blood vessels that begins at the iris and continues around the eye. In the posterior cavity, it is the middle layer between the sclera and the retina.	**choroid/o-** *choroid (middle layer around the eye)*
ciliary body	Extension of the choroid layer that lies posterior to the iris. It has suspensory ligaments that hold the lens in place. When the ciliary body contracts and relaxes it changes the shape of the lens. It also produces aqueous humor.	**cili/o-** *hairlike structure* **cycl/o-** *ciliary body (of the eye); circle; cycle*
cones	Light-sensitive cells in the retina that detect color. There are three different types of cones that respond to either red light, green light, or blue light.	
conjunctiva	Delicate, transparent mucous membrane that covers the inside of the eyelids and the anterior surface of the eye. It produces clear, watery mucus.	**conjunctiv/o-** *conjunctiva*
cornea	Transparent layer over the anterior part of the eye. This is the same layer that was previously the white sclera. The transitional area where the change occurs is the limbus.	**corne/o-** *cornea (of the eye)* **kerat/o-** *cornea (of the eye); hard, fibrous protein*
extraocular muscles	Six muscles that are attached to the sclera by tendons: **superior rectus muscle, inferior rectus muscle, medial rectus muscle, lateral rectus muscle, superior oblique muscle,** and **inferior oblique muscle.** *Rectus* means *straight,* and *oblique* means *slanted.* They move the eye in all directions. These movements are under voluntary control by the **oculomotor nerve** (cranial nerve III), trochlear nerve (cranial nerve IV), and the abducens nerve (cranial nerve VI).	**ocul/o-** *eye* **super/o-** *above* **infer/o-** *below* **medi/o-** *middle* **later/o-** *side*
eye	Organ that provides sensory information that is interpreted by the brain to become the sense of sight. The eye is also known as the **optic globe.**	**opt/o-** *eye; vision* **ocul/o-** *eye* **ophthalm/o-** *eye*
eyelids	Pair of fleshy structures that blink to keep the surface of the eye moist with tears and prevent foreign substances from entering the eye. They contain the eyelashes and sebaceous glands.	**blephar/o-** *eyelid*
fovea	Small depression in the center of the macula. It is the area of sharpest vision and lies directly opposite the pupil.	**fove/o-** *small, depressed area*

Word or Phrase	Description	Combining Forms
fundus	General word for the retina because it is the area that is farthest from the opening (pupil)	**fund/o-** *fundus (part farthest from the opening)* **fundu/o-** *fundus (part farthest from the opening)*
iris	Circular, colored structure around the pupil. The muscles of the iris contract or relax to decrease or increase the diameter of the pupil. This is under involuntary control by the oculomotor nerve (cranial nerve III). The color of the iris is determined by genetics.	**irid/o-** *iris (colored part of the eye)* **ir/o-** *iris (colored part of the eye)*
lacrimal gland	Gland in the superior-lateral aspect of the eye. It produces and secretes tears through the **lacrimal ducts.** The lacrimal glands produce tears when stimulated by the facial nerve (cranial nerve VII).	**lacrim/o-** *tears* **dacry/o-** *lacrimal sac; tears*
lacrimal sac	Structure that collects tears as they drain from the medial aspect of the eye. It empties into the nasolacrimal duct.	**lacrim/o-** *tears* **dacry/o-** *lacrimal sac; tears*
lens	Clear, flexible disk behind the pupil. It is surrounded by the lens capsule. The muscles of the ciliary body change the lens shape (accommodation) to focus light rays on the retina.	**lenticul/o-** *lens (of the eye)* **lent/o-** *lens (of the eye)* **phac/o-** *lens (of the eye)* **phak/o-** *lens (of the eye)*
lens capsule	Clear membrane that surrounds the lens	**capsul/o-** *capsule (enveloping structure)*
limbus	Border where the white, opaque sclera becomes the transparent cornea over the anterior aspect of the eye	
macula	Dark yellow-orange area with indistinct edges on the retina. It contains the fovea.	**macul/o-** *small area or spot*
miosis	Contraction of the iris muscle to constrict (reduce the size of) the pupil and limit the amount of light entering the eye	**mi/o-** *narrowing*
mydriasis	Relaxation of the iris muscle to dilate (enlarge the size of) the pupil and increase the amount of light entering the eye	**mydr/o-** *widening*
nasolacrimal duct	Structure that carries tears from the lacrimal sac to the inside of the nose	**nas/o-** *nose* **lacrim/o-** *tears*
optic disk	Bright yellow-white circle on the retina where the optic nerve and retinal arteries enter and the retinal veins leave the posterior cavity. It cannot receive sensory information and is known as the blind spot.	**opt/o-** *eye; vision*
optic nerve	Cranial nerve II. It enters the posterior eye at the optic disk. It is a sensory nerve that carries sensory information of visual images from the rods and cones of the retina. At the **optic chiasm** in the brain, parts of each optic nerve cross over to join the optic nerve on the other side. These recombined nerves become the optic tracts that go to the thalamus.	**opt/o-** *eye; vision*
orbit	Bony socket in the cranium that surrounds all but the anterior part of the eye	
posterior cavity	Large space between the lens and the retina. It is filled with vitreous humor.	**poster/o-** *back part* **cav/o-** *hollow space*
posterior chamber	Very narrow space posterior to the iris. Aqueous humor circulates through it.	**poster/o-** *back part*

Word or Phrase	Description	Combining Forms
pupil	Dark, round, central opening in the iris that allows light rays to enter the internal eye. Constriction and dilation of the pupil is under involuntary control through nerve impulses to the muscles of the iris from the oculomotor nerve (cranial nerve III).	**pupill/o-** *pupil (of the eye)* **cor/o-** *pupil (of the eye)*
retina	Layer of tissue that lines the posterior cavity. It contains rods and cones. Landmarks on the retina include the optic disk and the macula.	**retin/o-** *retina (of the eye)*
rods	Light-sensitive cells in the retina. They detect black and white and function in daytime and nighttime vision.	
sclera	White, opaque, tough, fibrous connective tissue that forms the outer layer around most of the eye. It is also known as the white of the eye.	**scler/o-** *hard; sclera (white of the eye)*
stereoscopic vision	Three-dimensional vision with depth and distance perception	**stere/o-** *three dimensions* **scop/o-** *examine with an instrument* **vis/o-** *sight; vision*
thalamus	Relay station in the brain that receives sensory information from the optic tracts and sends it to the midbrain and to the visual cortex in the occipital lobes of the brain	
trabecular meshwork	Interlacing fibers through which the aqueous humor drains. It is all around the iris where the edge of the iris meets the cornea and forms an angle.	**trabecul/o-** *trabecula (mesh)*
uvea	Collective word for the iris, choroid, and ciliary body. It is also known as the **uveal tract.**	**uve/o-** *uvea (of the eye)*
visual cortex	Area in the right and left occipital lobes of the brain that processes vision. It merges the images from each eye to create a single image, then turns the image right side up and facing in the direction of the original object.	**vis/o-** *sight; vision*
vitreous humor	Clear, gel-like substance that fills the posterior cavity of the eye	**vitre/o-** *transparent substance; vitreous humor*

Labeling Exercise

Match each anatomy word or phrase to its structure and write it in the numbered box for each figure. Be sure to check your spelling. Use the Answer Key at the end of the book to check your answers.

caruncle   iris   lacrimal ducts   lacrimal gland   lacrimal sac   limbus   nasolacrimal duct   pupil   sclera

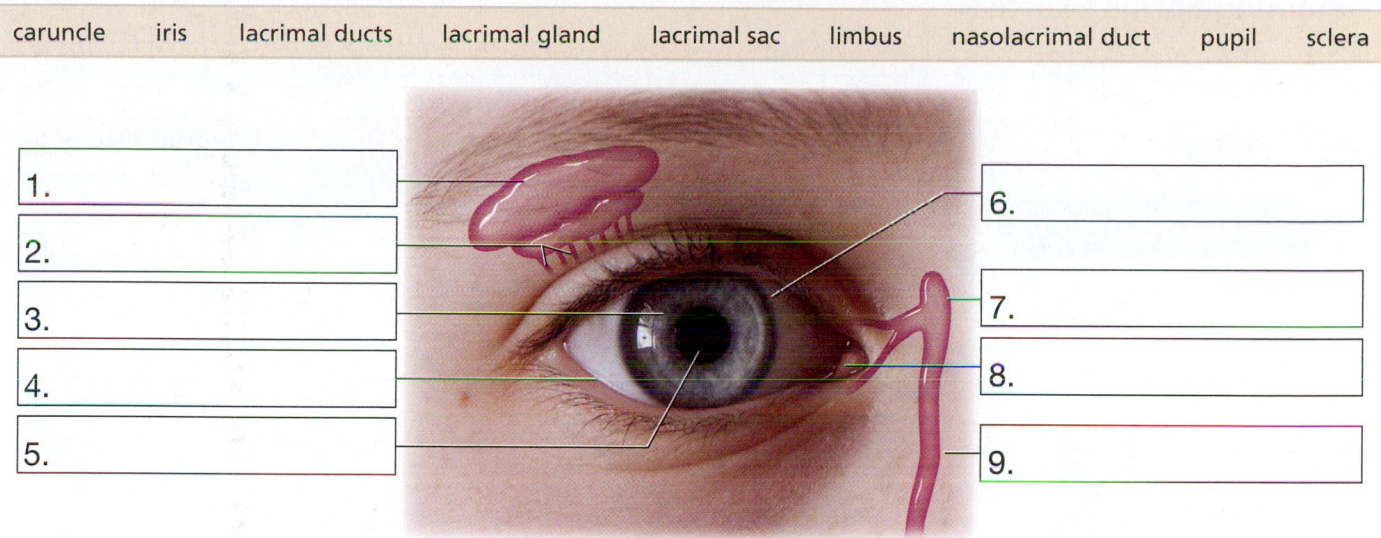

1.

2.

3.

4.

5.

6.

7.

8.

9.

choroid	cornea	lens	optic nerve	retina
ciliary body	fovea	macula	posterior cavity	sclera
conjunctiva	iris	optic disk	pupil	suspensory ligaments

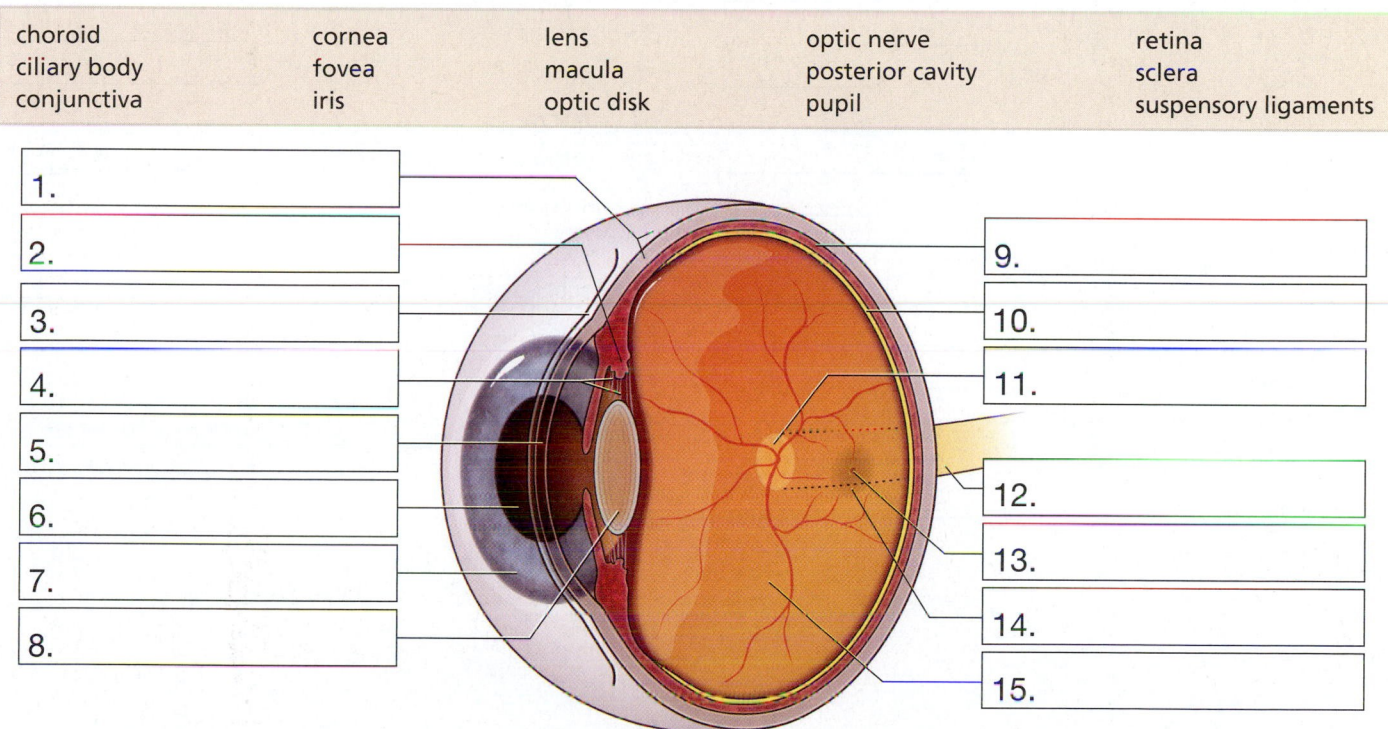

1.

2.

3.

4.

5.

6.

7.

8.

9.

10.

11.

12.

13.

14.

15.

Building Medical Words

Use the Answer Key at the end of the book to check your answers.

Combining Forms Exercise

Before you build eye words, review these combining forms. Next to each combining form, write its medical meaning. The first one has been done for you.

Combining Form	Medical Meaning	Combining Form	Medical Meaning
1. **accommod/o-**	to adapt	24. lent/o-	_____
2. anter/o-	_____	25. macul/o-	_____
3. aque/o-	_____	26. medi/o-	_____
4. blephar/o-	_____	27. mi/o-	_____
5. capsul/o-	_____	28. mydr/o-	_____
6. cav/o-	_____	29. nas/o-	_____
7. choroid/o-	_____	30. ocul/o-	_____
8. cili/o-	_____	31. ophthalm/o-	_____
9. conjunctiv/o-	_____	32. opt/o-	_____
10. corne/o-	_____	33. phac/o-	_____
11. cor/o-	_____	34. phak/o-	_____
12. cycl/o-	_____	35. poster/o-	_____
13. dacry/o-	_____	36. pupill/o-	_____
14. fove/o-	_____	37. retin/o-	_____
15. fund/o-	_____	38. scler/o-	_____
16. fundu/o-	_____	39. scop/o-	_____
17. infer/o-	_____	40. stere/o-	_____
18. irid/o-	_____	41. super/o-	_____
19. ir/o-	_____	42. trabecul/o-	_____
20. kerat/o-	_____	43. uve/o-	_____
21. lacrim/o-	_____	44. vis/o-	_____
22. later/o-	_____	45. vitre/o-	_____
23. lenticul/o-	_____		

Combining Form and Suffix Exercise

Read the definition of the medical word. Look at the combining form that is given. Select the correct suffix from the Suffix List and write it on the blank line. Then build the medical word and write it on the line. (Remember: You may need to remove the combining vowel. Always remove the hyphens and slash.) Be sure to check your spelling. The first one has been done for you.

SUFFIX LIST		
-al (pertaining to)	-iasis (state of; process of)	-osis (condition; abnormal condition; process)
-ar (pertaining to)	-ic (pertaining to)	-ous (pertaining to)
-ary (pertaining to)	-ion (action; condition)	-ual (pertaining to)
-ation (a process; being or having)		

Definition of the Medical Word	Combining Form	Suffix	Build the Medical Word
1. Pertaining to the cornea	**corne/o-**	**-al**	*corneal*

(You think *pertaining to* (-al) + cornea (corne/o-). You change the order of the word parts to put the suffix last. You write *corneal.*)

Definition of the Medical Word	Combining Form	Suffix	Build the Medical Word
2. Pertaining to the retina	retin/o-	_____	_____
3. Pertaining to sight and vision	vis/o-	_____	_____
4. Pertaining to the pupil	pupill/o-	_____	_____
5. Pertaining to the white of the eye	scler/o-	_____	_____
6. Process of widening (of the pupil)	mydr/o-	_____	_____
7. Pertaining to the eye or vision	opt/o-	_____	_____
8. Pertaining to a watery substance (aqueous humor)	aque/o-	_____	_____
9. Pertaining to a small area of spot (on the retina)	macul/o-	_____	_____
10. Pertaining to tears	lacrim/o-	_____	_____
11. Condition of having sight	vis/o-	_____	_____
12. A process of having to adapt (the lens of the eye)	accommod/o-	_____	_____
13. Pertaining to the conjunctiva	conjunctiv/o-	_____	_____
14. Process of narrowing of the pupil	mi/o-	_____	_____

Diseases and Conditions

Eyelid

Word or Phrase	Description	Word Building
blepharitis	Inflammation or infection of the eyelid with redness, crusts, and scales at the bases of the eyelashes. Acute blepharitis is caused by an allergy or infection. Chronic blepharitis is caused by acne rosacea, seborrheic dermatitis, or microscopic mites that live in the sebaceous glands. Treatment: Topical antibiotic or corticosteroid ophthalmic ointment.	**blepharitis** (BLEF-ah-RY-tis) **blephar/o-** *eyelid* **-itis** *inflammation of; infection of*
blepharoptosis	Drooping of the upper eyelid from excessive fat or sagging of the tissues due to age. It can also be from a disease that affects the muscles or nerves (e.g., myasthenia gravis or stroke). Treatment: Blepharoplasty or treat the underlying cause.	**blepharoptosis** (BLEF-ah-rawp-TOH-sis) (BLEF-ah-RAWP-toh-sis) **blephar/o-** *eyelid* **-ptosis** *state of prolapse; drooping; falling*
ectropion	Weakening of connective tissue in the lower eyelid. The lower eyelid turns outward (see Figure 15-12 ■), exposing the conjunctiva and causing dryness and chronic conjunctivitis. Treatment: Artificial tears eye drops or surgical correction.	**ectropion** (ek-TROH-pee-on) **ec-** *out; outward* **trop/o-** *having an affinity for; stimulating; turning* **-ion** *action; condition* Select the correct combining form meaning to get the definition of *ectropion: a condition of outward turning (of the eyelid).*

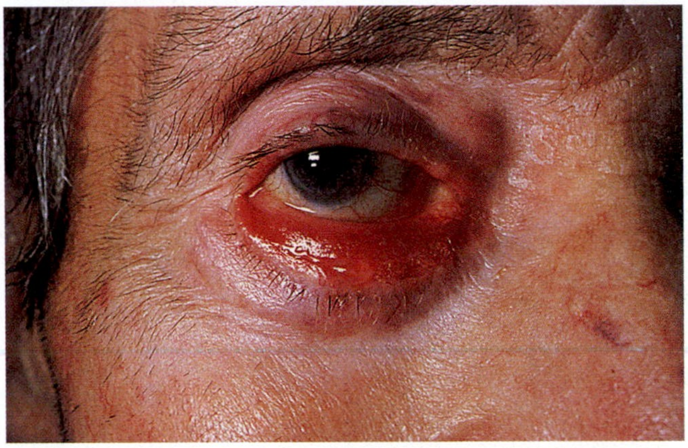

Figure 15-12 ■ Ectropion.

With the eyelid turned outward, the exposed conjunctiva becomes inflamed. Tears spill out, and the surface of the eye is dry and irritated.

Word or Phrase	Description	Word Building
entropion	Weakening of the muscle in the lower eyelid. The lower eyelid turns inward, causing the eyelashes to touch the eye, which results in chronic conjunctivitis and pain. Treatment: Artificial tears eye drops or surgical correction.	**entropion** (en-TROH-pee-on) **en-** *in; within; inward* **trop/o-** *having an affinity for; stimulating; turning* **-ion** *action; condition*
hordeolum	Red, painful swelling or a pimple containing pus on the eyelid. It is caused by a bacterial infection (staphylococcus) in a sebaceous gland. It is also known as a **stye.** Sometimes, when the acute infection subsides, the hordeolum becomes a **chalazion,** a chronically inflamed and granular lump or semisolid cyst. Treatment: Antibiotic drug for a hordeolum; warm compresses or surgical excision for a chalazion.	**hordeolum** (hor-DEE-oh-lum) **chalazion** (kah-LAY-zee-on)

Lacrimal Gland

Word or Phrase	Description	Word Building
dacryocystitis	Bacterial infection of the lacrimal sac. The lacrimal sac is tender and contains pus. Treatment: Oral antibiotic drug.	**dacryocystitis** (DAK-ree-OH-sis-TY-tis) **dacry/o-** *lacrimal sac; tears* **cyst/o-** *bladder; fluid-filled sac; semisolid cyst* **-itis** *inflammation of; infection of*
xerophthalmia	Insufficient production of tears resulting in eye irritation. It is associated with the aging process, an ectropion, or a side effect of certain drugs. It is also known as **dry eyes syndrome.** Treatment: Artificial tears eye drops. Surgery: Insertion of silicone plugs into the opening in the medial aspect of the lower eyelid to keep tears in the eye.	**xerophthalmia** (ZEER-awf-THAL-mee-ah) **xer/o-** *dry* **ophthalm/o-** *eye* **-ia** *condition; state; thing*

Conjunctiva, Sclera, and Cornea

conjunctivitis	Inflamed, reddened, and swollen conjunctiva with dilated blood vessels in the sclera (see Figure 15-13 ■). It is caused by a foreign substance in the eye, a chemical splashed in the eye, allergens or pollution in the air, chlorinated water in swimming pools, mechanical irritation from eyelashes (entropion), or dryness due to a lack of tears. It is also caused by a bacterial or viral infection. Acute contagious bacterial conjunctivitis with mucus discharge is known as **pinkeye.** Treatment: Corticosteroid eye drops for inflammation; topical or oral antibiotic drug for a bacterial infection.	**conjunctivitis** (con-JUNK-tih-VY-tis) **conjunctiv/o-** *conjunctiva* **-itis** *inflammation of; infection of*

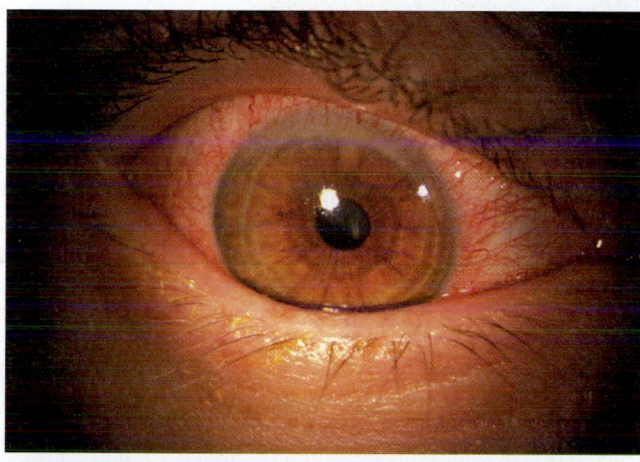

Figure 15-13 ■ Conjunctivitis.
A viral infection has caused the blood vessels in the conjunctiva to become dilated, giving it a reddened, streaky appearance.

Clinical Connections

Neonatology. When a woman with the sexually transmitted disease of gonorrhea gives birth, the eyes of the newborn may become infected from the birth canal. A gonorrheal infection of the eye causes conjunctivitis and can cause blindness. By state law, all newborns are given antibiotic eye drops or eye ointment after birth to prevent blindness caused by gonorrhea. Chlamydia, another organism that causes a sexually transmitted disease of the genital tract, can also cause conjunctivitis in the newborn.

Word or Phrase	Description	Word Building

corneal abrasion	Damage to the most superficial layer of the cornea due to trauma or repetitive irritation, such as a foreign particle under a contact lens. A chronic bacterial infection in an abrasion can cause a **corneal ulcer** with sloughing off of necrotic tissue. This is also known as **ulcerative keratitis**. Treatment: Corticosteroid drugs for inflammation; antibiotic drugs for infection. Surgery: Corneal transplant.	**abrasion** (ah-BRAY-shun)
		  abras/o- *scrape off*
		  -ion *action; condition*
		ulcer (UL-ser)
		ulcerative (UL-ser-AH-tiv)
		  ulcerat/o- *ulcer*
		  -ive *pertaining to*
		keratitis (KAIR-ah-TY-tis)
		  kerat/o- *cornea*
		  -itis *inflammation of; infection of*

exophthalmos	Pronounced outward bulging of the anterior surface of the eye with a startled, staring expression. If just one eye is affected, it often has a tumor behind it. If both eyes are affected, the patient usually has hyperthyroidism (see Figure 14-10). Treatment: Correct the underlying cause.	**exophthalmos** (EKS-awf-THAL-mohs) *Exophthalmos* is a combination of the prefix *ex-* (out; away from) and the Greek word *ophthalmos* (eye).

scleral icterus	Yellow coloration of the conjunctivae, which makes the sclerae also appear yellow. It is caused by **jaundice** due to liver disease (see Figure 15-14 ■). In a patient without jaundice, the sclerae are said to be **anicteric.** Treatment: Correct the underlying cause.
	
		icterus (IK-ter-us)
		icteric (ik-TAIR-ik)
		  icter/o- *jaundice*
		  -ic *pertaining to*
		jaundice (JAWN-dis)
		anicteric (AN-ik-TAIR-ik)
		  an- *without; not*
		  icter/o- *jaundice*
		  -ic *pertaining to*

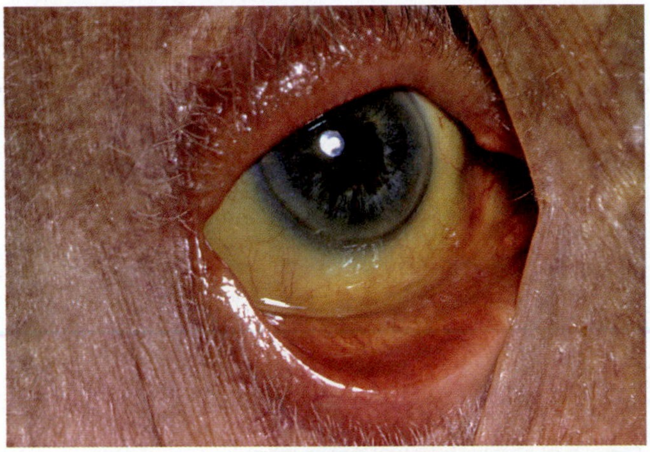

Figure 15-14 ■ Scleral icterus.
This patient's eye has a yellow discoloration. This is due to a high level of bilirubin in the blood that his diseased liver is unable to conjugate.

Iris, Pupil, and Anterior Chamber

Word or Phrase	Description	Word Building

anisocoria	Unequal sizes of the pupils. It is caused by glaucoma, head trauma, stroke, or a tumor that damages the cranial nerve that controls the muscle of the iris (and the size of the pupil). Treatment: Correct the underlying cause.	**anisocoria** (an-EYE-soh-KOH-ree-ah)
		  anis/o- *unequal*
		  cor/o- *pupil (of the eye)*
		  -ia *condition; state; thing*

glaucoma	Increased **intraocular pressure (IOP)** because aqueous humor cannot circulate freely. In open-angle glaucoma, the angle where the edges of the iris and cornea meet is normal and open, but the trabecular meshwork is blocked. Open-angle glaucoma is painless but destroys peripheral vision, leaving the patient with tunnel vision. In closed-angle glaucoma, the angle itself is too narrow and blocks the flow of aqueous humor. Closed-angle glaucoma causes severe pain, blurred vision, and photophobia. Glaucoma can progress to blindness. Treatment: Glaucoma drug to lower intraocular pressure. Surgery: Laser trabeculoplasty.	**glaucoma** (glaw-KOH-mah)
		  glauc/o- *silver gray*
		  oma- *tumor; mass*
		intraocular (IN-trah-AWK-yoo-lar)
		  intra- *within*
		  ocul/o- *eye*
		  -ar *pertaining to*

Word or Phrase	Description	Word Building
hyphema	Blood in the anterior chamber. It is caused by trauma or increased intraocular pressure. Treatment: Topical corticosteroid eye drops or oral corticosteroid drugs; treat underlying glaucoma.	**hyphema** (hy-FEE-mah)
photophobia	Abnormal sensitivity to bright light. It can be associated with inflammation from diseases of the eye or it can be due to increased intracranial pressure or meningitis in the brain. Treatment: Correct the underlying cause.	**photophobia** (FOH-toh-FOH-bee-ah) **phot/o-** *light* **phob/o-** *fear; avoidance* **-ia** *condition; state; thing*
uveitis	Inflammation or infection of the uveal tract. It can be caused by infection in the eye, infection in another part of the body, an allergy, trauma, or an autoimmune disorder. **Iritis** affects the iris. **Choroiditis** affects the choroid membrane. Treatment: Oral corticosteroid or antibiotic drug.	**uveitis** (YOO-vee-EYE-tis) **uve/o-** *uvea (of the eye)* **-itis** *inflammation of; infection of* **iritis** (eye-RY-tis) **ir/o-** *iris (colored part of the eye)* **-itis** *inflammation of; infection of* **choroiditis** (KOH-roy-DY-tis) **choroid/o-** *choroid (middle layer around the eye)* **-itis** *inflammation of; infection of*

Lens

Word or Phrase	Description	Word Building
aphakia	Condition in which the lens of the eye has been surgically removed. In most patients, an artificial intraocular lens is put into the eye during the cataract surgery. Some cataract patients are not good candidates for an artificial intraocular lens. Their cataract is removed, but they wear special cataract eyeglasses, and they remain aphakic.	**aphakia** (ah-FAY-kee-ah) **a-** *away from; without* **phak/o-** *lens (of the eye)* **-ia** *condition; state; thing*
cataract	Clouding of the lens (see Figure 15-15 ■). Protein molecules in the lens begin to clump together. It is caused by aging, sun exposure, eye trauma, smoking, and some drugs. The vision is dull and blurry with faded colors and a yellowish tint around lights. Congenital cataracts are present at birth. Treatment: Cataract surgery (see Figure 15-27).	**cataract** (KAT-ah-rakt)

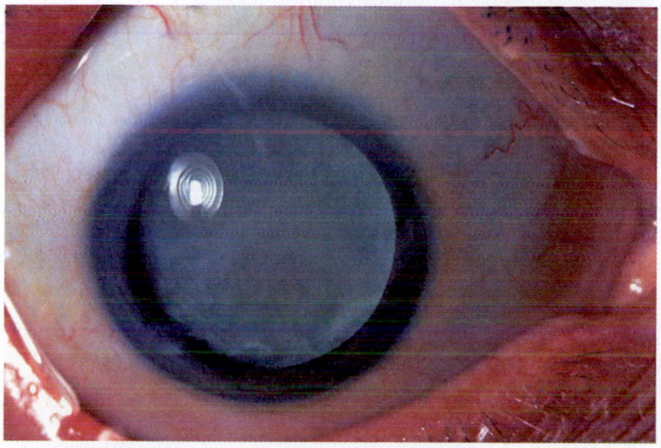

Figure 15-15 ■ Cataract.
As a cataract develops, the lens gradually becomes cloudy and opaque. The vision is blurred and colors appear faded and yellowed.

Word or Phrase	Description	Word Building
presbyopia	Loss of flexibility of the lens with blurry near vision and loss of accommodation. It is caused by aging. Treatment: Corrective eyeglasses.	**presbyopia** (PREZ-bee-OH-pee-ah) **presby/o-** *old age* **-opia** *condition of vision*

Posterior Cavity and Retina

Word or Phrase	Description	Word Building
color blindness	Genetic condition in which the cones (usually the green or red cones) are absent or do not contain enough visual pigment to respond to the light from colored objects. Treatment: None.	

diabetic retinopathy	Chronic, progressive condition of the retina in which a large number of new, fragile blood vessels form (**neovascularization**) in patients with uncontrolled diabetes mellitus (see Figure 15-16 ■). These vessels leak, forming exudates (dried fluid deposits) on the retina. They also rupture easily, causing intraocular hemorrhage. Treatment: Management of diabetes mellitus; surgery with laser photocoagulation (see Figure 15-28).	**diabetic** (DY-ah-BET-ik)
		   diabet/o- *diabetes*
		   -ic *pertaining to*
		retinopathy (RET-ih-NAWP-ah-thee)
		   retin/o- *retina*
		   -pathy *disease; suffering*
		neovascularization
		(NEE-oh-VAS-kyoo-LAR-ih-ZAY-shun)
		   ne/o- *new*
		   vascul/o- *blood vessel*
		   -ization *process of making, creating, or inserting*

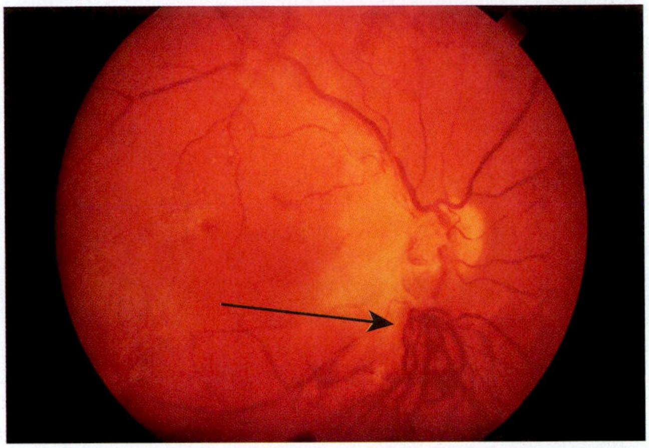

Figure 15-16 ■ Diabetic retinopathy.
This patient's retina shows advanced diabetic retinopathy with neovascularization, the formation of many new, fragile blood vessels (at the bottom of the image).

Word or Phrase	Description	Word Building
floaters and flashers	Floaters are clumps, dots, or strings of collagen molecules that form in the vitreous humor because of aging. Flashers are brief bursts of bright light that occur when the vitreous humor pulls on the retina. Treatment: None.	

macular degeneration	Chronic, progressive loss of central vision as the macula degenerates. In older patients, this is known as age-related macular degeneration (ARMD). In dry macular degeneration (the most common type), the macula deteriorates. In wet macular degeneration, abnormal blood vessels grow under the macula. They are fragile and leak, causing the macula to lift away from the retina. Treatment for wet macular degeneration: Photodynamic therapy to destroy abnormal blood vessels.	**macular** (MAK-yoo-lar)
		   macul/o- *small area or spot*
		   -ar *pertaining to*
		degeneration (DEE-jen-er-AA-shun)
		   de- *reversal of; without*
		   gener/o- *production; creation*
		   -ation *a process; being or having*

night blindness	Marked decrease in visual acuity at night or in dim light. This occurs with aging or when the diet does not contain enough vitamin A. Treatment: Dietary supplement, if needed.	

papilledema	Inflammation and edema of the optic disk. It is caused by increased intracranial pressure from a brain tumor or head trauma. It is also known as a **choked disk.** Treatment: Correct the underlying cause.	**papilledema** (PAP-il-ah-DEE-mah)
		   papill/o- *elevated structure*
		   -edema *swelling*

Word or Phrase	Description	Word Building
retinal detachment	Separation of the retina from the choroid layer beneath it (see Figure 15-17 ■). This can be caused by head trauma. It can occur gradually during aging as the vitreous humor changes from a gel to a watery consistency that flows into tears in the retina and separates the two layers. In diabetic patients, hemorrhage of the fragile retinal blood vessels can separate the layers. Treatment: Retinopexy with cryotherapy or laser photocoagulation.	**detachment** (dee-TACH-ment)

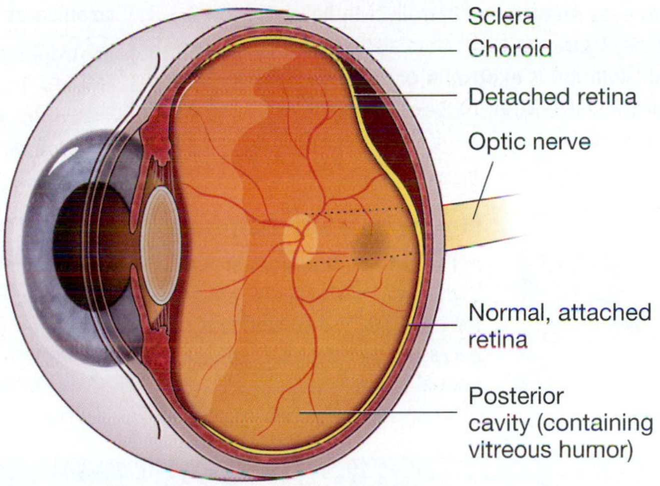

Sclera
Choroid
Detached retina
Optic nerve
Normal, attached retina
Posterior cavity (containing vitreous humor)

Figure 15-17 ■ Retinal detachment.
A gradual partial detachment of the retina is painless. The only symptoms are a sudden increase in the number of floaters and brief flashes of light in the visual field. If untreated, however, it can lead to a complete detachment of the retina.

Word or Phrase	Description	Word Building
retinitis pigmentosa (RP)	Inherited abnormality linked to 70 different genes. The retina has abnormal deposits of pigmentation behind the rods and cones, causing loss of color vision or night vision and loss of central or peripheral vision. It can progress to blindness. Treatment: None.	**retinitis pigmentosa** (RET-ih-NY-tis PIG-men-TOH-sah) **retin/o-** *retina* **-itis** *inflammation of; infection of*
retinoblastoma	Cancerous tumor of the retina in children, arising from abnormal embryonic retinal cells. Treatment: Chemotherapy, radiation therapy, and surgical excision.	**retinoblastoma** (RET-ih-NOH-blas-TOH-mah) **retin/o-** *retina (of the eye)* **blast/o-** *immature; embryonic* **-oma** *tumor; mass*
retinopathy of prematurity	Developing retinal tissue is replaced with fibrous tissue because of using a high level of oxygen therapy in premature babies with immature lungs. It is also known as **retrolental fibroplasia.** Treatment: Laser photocoagulation.	**retinopathy** (RET-ih-NAWP-ah-thee) **retin/o-** *retina (of the eye)* **-pathy** *disease; suffering* **prematurity** (PREE-mah-TYOOR-ih-tee) **pre-** *before; in front of* **matur/o-** *mature* **-ity** *state; condition* **retrolental** (REH-troh-LEN-tal) **retro-** *behind; backward* **lent/o-** *lens (of the eye)* **-al** *pertaining to* **fibroplasias** (FY-broh-PLAY-zee-ah) **fibr/o-** *fiber* **plas/o-** *growth; formation* **-ia** *condition; state; thing*

Extraocular Muscles

Word or Phrase	Description	Word Building
nystagmus	Involuntary rhythmic motions of the eye, particularly when looking to the side. Each back-and-forth motion is known as a "beat." Nystagmus can be caused by multiple sclerosis or Meniere's disease. Treatment: Correct the underlying cause.	nystagmus (nis-TAG-mus)
strabismus	Deviation of one or both eyes medially or laterally. Medial deviation is **esotropia** or **cross-eye** (see Figure 15-18 ■). It is also known as convergent strabismus. Lateral deviation is **exotropia** or **wall-eye.** Treatment: Surgical repositioning of the extraocular muscles, which is done during early childhood. **Figure 15-18 ■ Esotropia.** In this type of strabismus, one or both eyes deviate medially toward the nose. Surgical correction is necessary for the patient to develop normal vision.	strabismus (strah-BIZ-mus) esotropia (ES-oh-TROH-pee-ah) **es/o-** *inward* **trop/o-** *having an affinity for; stimulating; turning* **-ia** *condition; state; thing* exotropia (EKS-oh-TROH-pee-ah) **ex/o-** *away from; external; outward* **trop/o-** *having an affinity for; stimulating; turning* **-ia** *condition; state; thing*

Refractive Disorders of the Eyes

Word or Phrase	Description	Word Building
astigmatism	Surface of the cornea is curved more steeply in one area, so there is no single point of focus. The patient's vision is blurry both near and at a distance. Treatment: Corrective lenses or surgery.	astigmatism (ah-STIG-mah-tizm) **a-** *away from; without* **stigmat/o-** *point; mark* **-ism** *process; disease from a specific cause*
hyperopia	**Farsightedness.** Light rays from a distant object focus correctly on the retina, creating a sharp image. However, light rays from a near object come into focus posterior to the retina, creating a blurred image (see Figure 15-19 ■). **HYPEROPIA (Farsightedness)** Cornea Lens Light rays Far object Position of retina in normal eye Near object **Figure 15-19 ■ Hyperopia.** There is an abnormally short distance between the cornea and the retina. The patient can see things clearly in the distance (farsightedness), but close things are blurry.	hyperopia (HY-per-OH-pee-ah) **hyper-** *above; more than normal* **-opia** *condition of vision* Add words to make a complete definition of *hyperopia: condition of vision (that is sharp at a) more than normal (distance).*

Word or Phrase	Description	Word Building
myopia	**Nearsightedness.** Light rays from a near object focus correctly on the retina, creating a sharp image. However, light rays from a distant object come into focus anterior to the retina, creating a blurred image (see Figure 15-20 ■).	**myopia** (my-OH-pee-ah) **myop/o-** *near* **-opia** *condition of vision* The duplicated letters *op* are deleted when the combining form is joined to the suffix.

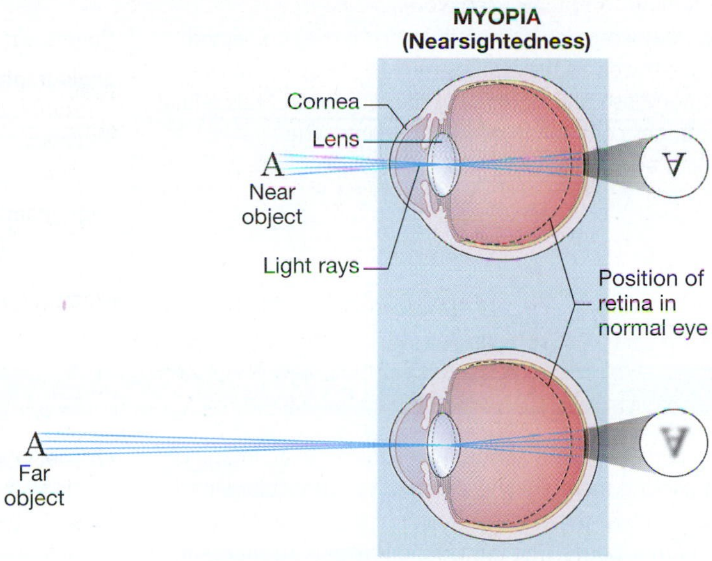

MYOPIA
(Nearsightedness)

Cornea
Lens
A
Near object
Light rays
Position of retina in normal eye
A
Far object

Figure 15-20 ■ Myopia.

There is an abnormally long distance between the cornea and the retina. The patient can see things clearly that are close (nearsightedness), but things in the distance are blurry.

Conditions of the Visual Cortex in the Brain

amblyopia	To prevent double vision, the brain ignores the visual image from an eye with strabismus (the most common cause) or from an eye in which the vision is unfocused or cloudy. This is also known as **lazy eye.** Amblyopia may continue even after the strabismus or other defect is surgically corrected. Treatment: The normal eye is patched until the brain accepts the visual image from the other eye.	**amblyopia** (AM-blee-OH-pee-ah) **ambly/o-** *dimness* **-opia** *condition of vision* Add words to make a complete definition of *amblyopia: condition of vision (with suppression and) dimness (in one eye).*
blindness	Condition of complete or partial loss of vision. It is caused by trauma, eye diseases, or defects in the structure of the eye, optic nerve, or visual cortex in the brain. A patient whose best visual acuity is 20/200 even with corrective lenses is legally blind. Treatment: Correct the underlying cause.	
diplopia	Two visual fields are seen rather than one fused image. It can be caused by ambylopia, by a tumor or trauma that increases intracranial pressure, or by multiple sclerosis that affects nerve conduction to the visual cortex. Treatment: Correct the underlying cause.	**diplopia** (dih-PLOH-pee-ah) **dipl/o-** *double* **-opia** *condition of vision*
scotoma	Temporary or permanent visual field defect in one or both eyes. The defect varies in size and can be patchy or solid, stationary or moving. This is caused by glaucoma, diabetic retinopathy, or macular degeneration when various parts of the retina or optic nerve are destroyed. Also, a hemorrhage (stroke), tumor, or trauma in the occipital lobe on one side of the brain can cause a scotoma in the opposite visual field. **Hemianopia** is loss of one half of the visual field (right or left, top or bottom). Prior to a migraine headache, a patient may see a scintillating scotoma, a moving line of brilliantly flashing bars of light in the visual field. This is also known as hemianopsia. Treatment: Correct the underlying cause.	**scotoma** (skoh-TOH-mah) **scotomata** (skoh-TOH-mah-tah) **scot/o-** *darkness* **-oma** *tumor; mass* **hemianopia** (HEM-ee-ah-NOH-pee-ah) **hemi-** *one half* **an-** *without; not* **-opia** *condition of vision*

Laboratory and Diagnostic Procedures

Diagnostic Procedures

Word or Phrase	Description	Word Building
fluorescein angiography	Procedure in which fluorescein (an orange fluorescent dye) is injected intravenously. The dye travels to the retinal artery in the eye. It glows fluorescent green upon flash photography of the retina. It reveals retinal leaking and hemorrhages common in diabetic patients. The photographic image is an **angiogram.**	**fluorescein** (floo-RES-een) **angiography** (AN-jee-AWG-rah-fee) **angi/o-** *blood vessel; lymphatic vessel* **-graphy** *process of recording* **angiogram** (AN-jee-oh-gram) **angi/o-** *blood vessel; lymphatic vessel* **-gram** *a record or picture*

Radiologic Tests

ultrasonography	Procedure that uses high-frequency sound waves to create an image of the eye. A-scan ultrasound measures the eye prior to intraocular lens insertion. B-scan creates a two-dimensional image of the inside of the eye to show tumors or hemorrhages. The ultrasound image is a **sonogram.**	**ultrasonography** (UL-trah-soh-NAWG-rah-fee) **ultra-** *beyond; higher* **son/o-** *sound* **-graphy** *process of recording* **sonogram** (SAWN-oh-gram) **son/o-** *sound* **-gram** *a record or picture*

Medical and Surgical Procedures

Medical Procedures

Word or Phrase	Description	Word Building
accommodation	Procedure to test the ability of the muscles in the ciliary body to contract and flex the lens as demonstrated on near and distance visual acuity tests	**accommodation** (ah-KAWM-oh-DAY-shun) **accommod/o-** *to adapt* **-ation** *a process; being or having*
color blindness testing	Procedure to determine if a patient has a defect in the red, green, or blue cones in the retina. Each successive color plate requires a higher discrimination of color perception. Color plates that contain numbers are used to test adults (see Figure 15-21 ■), while color plates that contain circles, squares, or animals are used to test children.	

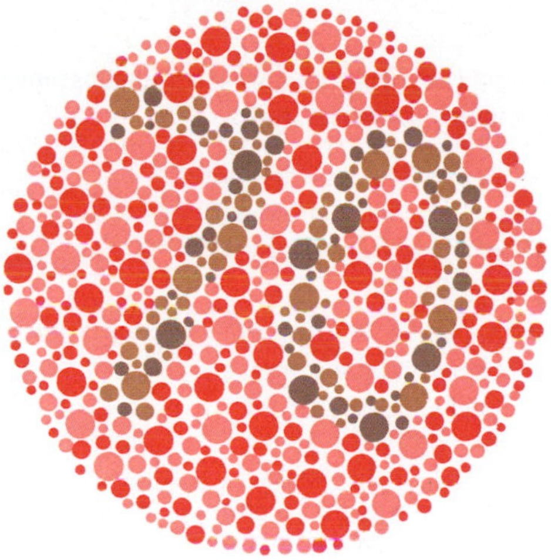

Figure 15-21 ■ **Ishihara color plate for testing color blindness.**
A patient with green color blindness would not be able to distinguish the *70* printed in green.

Word or Phrase	Description	Word Building
convergence	Procedure to test the function of the medial rectus muscles and the ability of both eyes to turn medially. The physician holds up an index finger and moves it progressively closer to the patient's nose. The maximum convergence is called the near point.	**convergence** (con-VER-jens) **converg/o-** *coming together* **-ence** *state of*
dilated funduscopy	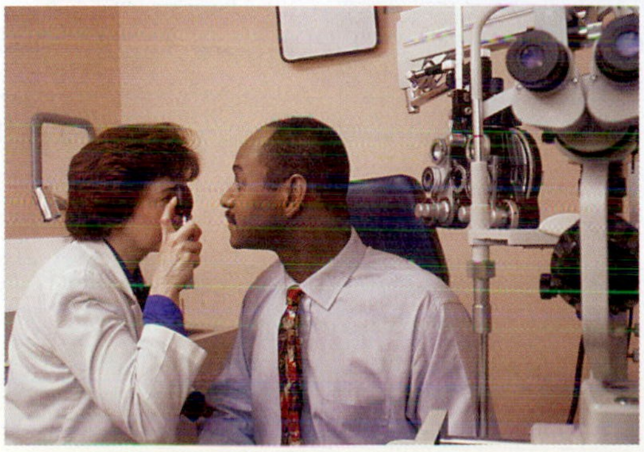 Procedure to examine the posterior cavity. Eye drops are used to dilate the pupil (mydriasis) and to temporarily keep the pupil in a dilated position (**cycloplegia**). An **ophthalmoscope**, a handheld instrument with a light and changeable lenses of different strengths, is used to examine the retina from all angles (see Figure 15-22 ■). Alternatively, the patient can be placed in a darkened room to dilate the pupils. A strobe light creates a sudden flash to illuminate the retina while a Polaroid® picture is taken. This method is able to show about 30% of the retina. Any abnormalities of the retina must be further examined with a dilated funduscopic exam.	**funduscopy** (fun-DUHS-koh-pee) **fundu/o-** *fundus (part farthest from the opening)* **-scopy** *process of using an instrument to examine* **cycloplegia** (SY-kloh-PLEE-jee-ah) **cycl/o-** *ciliary body (of the eye); circle; cycle* **pleg/o-** *paralysis* **-ia** *condition; state; thing* **ophthalmoscope** (awf-THAL-moh-skohp) **ophthalm/o-** *eye* **-scope** *instrument used to examine*

Figure 15-22 ■ **Ophthalmoscope.**
The ophthalmologist selects and dials in a lens on the ophthalmoscope to see a sharp image of the inside of the patient's eye. The lens that she selects corrects the visual defects of her eyes as well as those of the patient.

Word or Phrase	Description	Word Building
eye patching	Procedure in which the eye is covered with a soft bandage and a hard outer shield after eye trauma or eye surgery. Also, a normal eye can be patched to treat amblyopia.	
fluorescein staining	Procedure in which a fluorescein (an orange fluorescent dye) strip or drops are applied topically to the cornea to detect corneal abrasions and ulcers. As a light is used to examine the eye, any corneal abrasions or ulcers glow fluorescent green.	**fluorescein** (floo-RES-een)
gaze testing	Procedure to test the extraocular muscles. The patient's eyes follow the physician's finger from side to side and up and down. **Conjugate gaze** is when both eyes move together as a unit. This is documented in the patient's record as EOMI (extraocular movements intact). **Dysconjugate gaze** is when the eyes do not move together.	**conjugate** (CON-joo-gayt) **conjug/o-** *joined together* **-ate** *composed of; pertaining to* **dysconjugate** (dis-CON-joo-gayt) **dys-** *painful; difficult; abnormal* **conjug/o-** *joined together* **-ate** *composed of; pertaining to*
gonioscopy	Procedure to test for glaucoma. It uses a slit lamp (see Figure 15-25) with a special lens to illuminate and magnify the tiny trabecular mesh-work to look for signs of blockage.	**gonioscopy** (GOH-nee-AWS-koh-pee) **goni/o-** *angle* **-scopy** *process of using an instrument to examine*
peripheral vision	Procedure to test visual acuity at the edges of the visual field. The patient looks straight ahead while the physician moves an object toward the edge of the visual field (from the top, bottom, and both sides). The patient indicates when the object is first seen. Alternatively, a computer projects dots onto a screen with a grid and the patient looks straight ahead and indicates when a dot is seen off to the side.	**peripheral** (peh-RIF-eh-ral) **peripher/o-** *outer aspects* **-al** *pertaining to*
phorometry	Procedure to select the strength of lens that corrects the patient's refractive error to give 20/20 vision. The specifications of that lens are written as a prescription that is duplicated in eyeglasses or contact lenses. A **phorometer** (see Figure 15-23 ■) holds lenses of successive strengths that are dialed into place as the patient looks through the lens at a Snellen chart. Each eye is tested separately.	**phorometry** (foh-RAWM-eh-tree) **phor/o-** *to bear; to carry; range* **-metry** *process of measuring* **phorometer** (foh-RAWM-eh-ter) **phor/o-** *to bear; to carry; range* **-meter** *instrument used to measure*

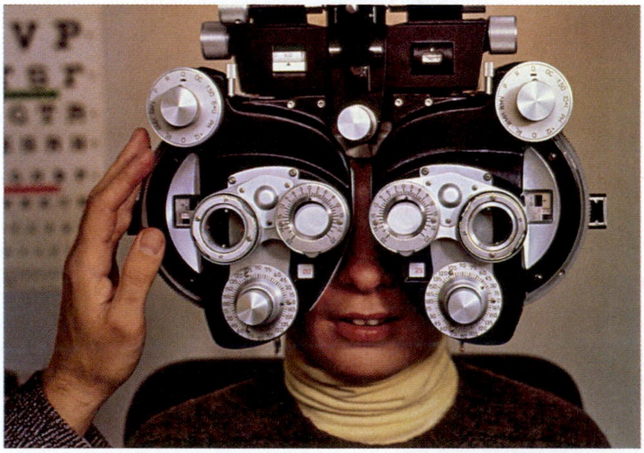

Figure 15-23 ■ Phorometer.
This instrument helps the ophthalmologist select the most accurate corrective lens for the patient.

Word or Phrase	Description	Word Building
pupillary response	Procedure to test that the pupils constrict briskly and equally in response to a bright light (see Figure 15-24 ■). This is documented in the patient's record as *PERRL* (pupils equal, round, and reactive to light). 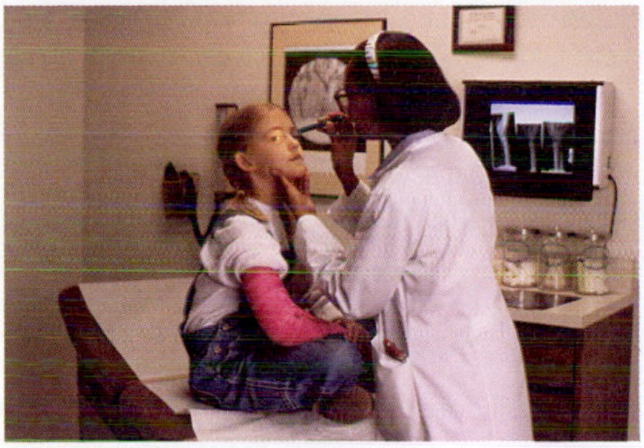 **Figure 15-24 ■ Pupillary response.** This physician is using a penlight to check the response of the pupils. This girl suffered a broken arm and a mild concussion. A sluggish or unequal pupillary response to light could indicate bleeding or edema in her brain.	
slit-lamp examination	Procedure to look for abnormalities of the cornea, anterior chamber, iris, or lens. The slit lamp combines a low-power microscope with a high-intensity blue light beam whose width can be adjusted down to a slit (see Figure 15-25 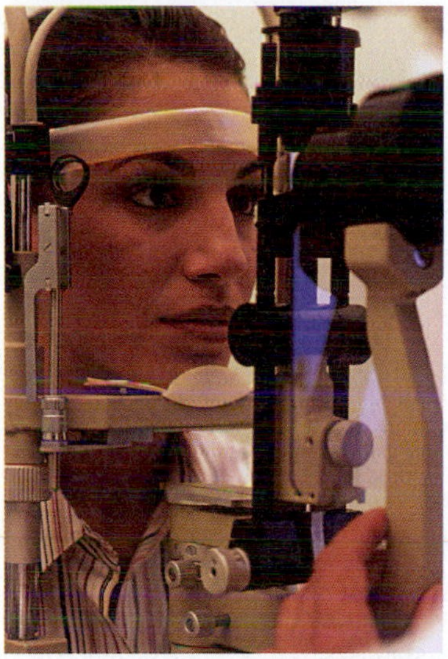 ■). **Figure 15-25 ■ Slit lamp examination.** The patient's chin and forehead are in a fixed position as the slit lamp moves around to magnify, illuminate, and view the eye from different angles.	
tonometry	Procedure to detect increased intraocular pressure and glaucoma. The small, flat disk of the **tonometer** is pressed against the cornea to record intraocular pressure. Alternatively, **air-puff tonometry** emits a short burst of air and measures the pressure of the air rebounding from the cornea without touching the patient's eye.	**tonometry** (toh-NAWM-eh-tree) **ton/o-** *pressure; tone* **-metry** *process of measuring* **tonometer** (toh-NAWM-eh-ter) **ton/o-** *pressure; tone* **-meter** *instrument used to measure*

Word or Phrase	Description	Word Building
visual acuity testing	Procedure to test near and distance visual acuity. Each eye is tested separately. A card with typed sentences of decreasing print size is held at a preset distance of 16 inches to test the near vision. The Snellen chart is used to test distance vision from 20 feet away (see Figure 15-26 ■). As an alternative, the Tumbling E chart has capital *E*s facing in various directions, and the patient indicates which way the legs of the *E* are pointing. Children or patients who are illiterate are tested with charts that use pictures. For a patient with severe vision problems, visual acuity can be measured as the ability to count how many fingers the ophthalmologist holds up or by the ability to perceive light.	**visual** (VIH-shoo-al) **vis/o-** *sight; vision* **-ual** *pertaining to* **acuity** (ah-KYOO-ih-tee) **acu/o-** *needle; sharpness* **-ity** *state; condition*

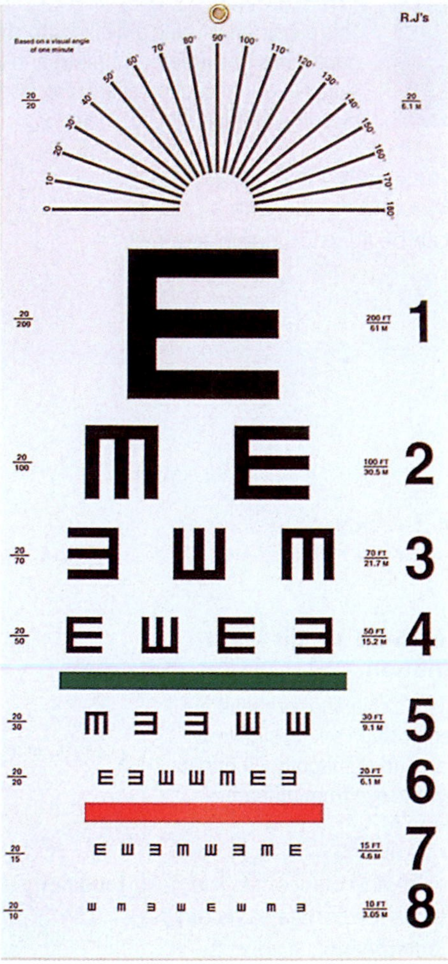

Figure 15-26 ■ **Snellen chart.**
Each line on the chart corresponds to a visual acuity rating. The reference line for this test is 20/20. The first number stands for 20 feet, the distance between the patient and the chart. The second number stands for 20 feet, the distance at which a person with normal vision could see that line. If a patient stands 20 feet from the chart but can only see the top large E (a visual acuity of 20/200), that means he/she can only see the line at 20 feet that a person with normal vision could see from 200 feet away.

Surgical Procedures

blepharoplasty	Plastic surgery procedure on the eyelids to remove fat and sagging skin. It is often done in conjunction with a facelift. It is also done to correct an ectropion or entropion.	**blepharoplasty** (BLEF-ah-roh-PLAS-tee) **blephar/o-** *eyelid* **-plasty** *process of reshaping by surgery*
capsulotomy	Procedure that is only done during cataract extraction when the remaining posterior lens capsule is cloudy or wrinkled. A laser is used to make an opening in the capsule to restore normal vision.	**capsulotomy** (KAP-soo-LAW-toh-mee) **capsul/o-** *capsule (enveloping structure)* **-tomy** *process of cutting or making an incision*

Word or Phrase	Description	Word Building
cataract extraction	Procedure to remove a lens affected by a cataract. Preoperatively, a laser is used to measure the length of the eye and the curvature of the cornea so that a customized intraocular lens (IOL) can be created before the surgery. During an **extracapsular cataract extraction (ECCE),** an incision is made in the sclera, the central part of the lens is removed, the posterior lens capsule is left in place, and the IOL is inserted. During **phacoemulsification,** a small, self-sealing (stitchless) incision is made in the cornea. An ultrasonic probe is inserted and sound waves are used to break up the lens (see Figure 15-27 ■). The pieces are removed with irrigation and aspiration, and the IOL is inserted. The IOL folds to pass through the incision and then unfolds inside the capsule. During an **intracapsular cataract extraction (ICCE),** both lens and lens capsule are completely removed; this operation is performed less often. 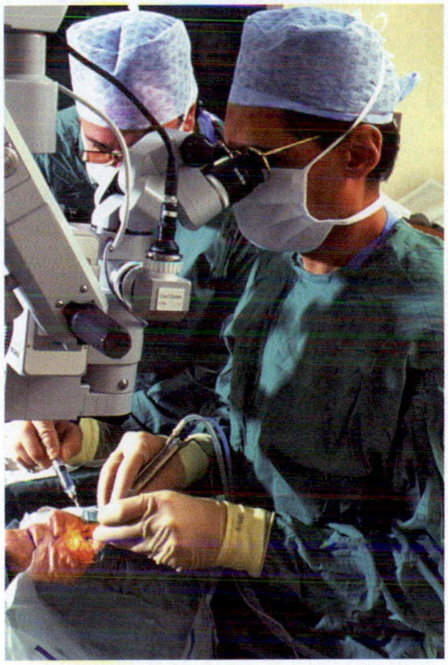 **Figure 15-27 ■ Phacoemulsification.** The surgeon looks through an operating microscope that magnifies the small structures of the eye. He inserts a phacoemulsification probe that emits sound waves to break up the lens.	**extracapsular** (EKS-trah-KAP-soo-lar) **extra-** *outside of* **capsul/o-** *capsule (enveloping structure)* **-ar** *pertaining to* **extraction** (ek-STRAK-shun) **ex-** *out; away from* **tract/o-** *pulling* **-ion** *action; condition* **phacoemulsification** (FAY-koh-ee-MUL-sih-fih-KAY-shun) **phac/o-** *lens (of the eye)* **emulsific/o-** *particles suspended in a solution* **-ation** *a process; being or having* **intracapsular** (IN-trah-KAP-soo-lar) **intra-** *within* **capsul/o-** *capsule (enveloping structure)* **-ar** *pertaining to*
corneal transplantation	Procedure to replace a damaged or diseased cornea. The cornea is removed with a trephine (a round cookie-cutter instrument with a sharp edge). Then a donor cornea is sutured in place with zig-zag sutures. Donor corneas are obtained from people who have died of illness or accident and willed their organs to others.	**transplantation** (TRANS-plan-TAY-shun) **transplant/o-** *move something to another place* **-ation** *a process; being or having*
enucleation	Procedure to remove the eye from the bony orbit because of trauma or a tumor.	**enucleation** (EE-noo-klee-AA-shun) **enucle/o-** *to remove the main part* **-ation** *a process; being or having*
hyperopia surgery	Procedure to correct farsightedness. It uses heat to shrink tissues around the edge of the cornea to produce a greater curvature in the cornea that corrects the refractive error. **Conductive keratoplasty (CK)** uses radiowaves delivered by a probe as thin as a hair to spots around the edge of the cornea. **Laser thermal keratoplasty (LTK)** uses a laser to simultaneously place spots in two concentric circles around the cornea.	**conductive** (con-DUK-tiv) **conduct/o-** *carrying; conveying* **-ive** *pertaining to* **keratoplasty** (KAIR-ah-toh-PLAS-tee) **kerat/o-** *cornea (of the eye); hard, fibrous protein* **-plasty** *process of reshaping by surgery* **laser** (LAY-zer)

Word or Phrase	Description	Word Building
laser photocoagulation	Procedure to seal leaking or hemorrhaging retinal blood vessels in patients with diabetic retinopathy. It is also done to reattach a detached retina. Light from the laser creates heat that coagulates the tissues (see Figure 15-28 ■). If the vitreous humor contains blood, the light from the laser cannot reach the retina, and a **vitrectomy** must be done first to remove the vitreous humor and replace it with a clear man-made fluid. 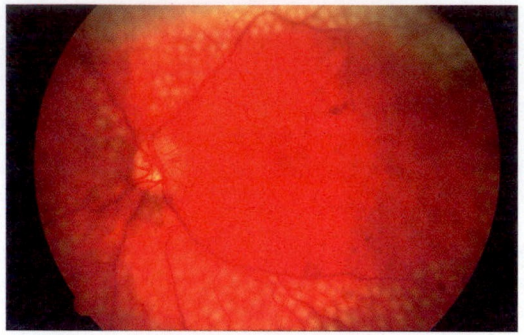 **Figure 15-28 ■ Laser photocoagulation.** This procedure treats leaking or hemorrhaging blood vessels associated with diabetic retinopathy. Here, the laser has been used in multiple small spots around the optic disk to coagulate the tissues.	**photocoagulation** (FOH-toh-koh-AG-yoo-LAY-shun) **phot/o-** *light* **coagul/o-** *clotting* **-ation** *a process; being or having* **vitrectomy** (vih-TREK-toh-mee) **vitre/o-** *transparent substance; vitreous humor* **-ectomy** *surgical excision*
myopia surgery	Procedure to correct nearsightedness. A three-dimensional corneal map is created preoperatively and programmed into the laser. In **laser-assisted *in situ* keratomileusis (LASIK),** a **microkeratome** creates a very thin flap on the surface of the cornea (see Figure 15-29 ■). The flap is peeled back, and a cold laser that cuts tissue without heating it is used to reshape the underlying cornea. The surface flap is then positioned back in place. In **photorefractive keratectomy (PRK),** the cold laser reshapes the curvature of the cornea without the creation of a corneal surface flap. 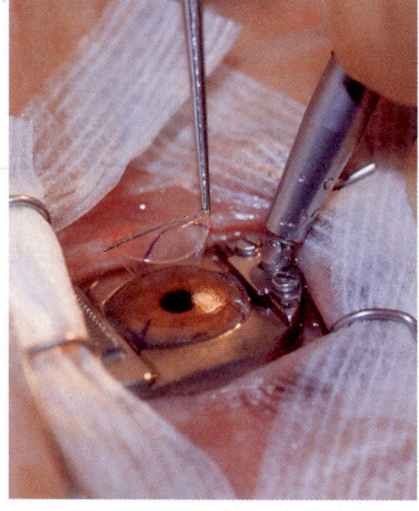 **Figure 15-29 ■ Keratomileusis.** During LASIK surgery, a keratomileusis is done in which a thin flap of cornea is lifted up. Then the laser is used to reshape the cornea, and the corneal flap is positioned back in place.	**in situ** (in SY-too) **keratomileusis** (KER-ah-TOH-my-LOO-sis) **kerat/o-** *cornea (of the eye); hard, fibrous protein* **-mileusis** *process of carving* **microkeratome** (MY-kroh-KAIR-ah-tohm) **micr/o-** *one millionth; small* **kerat/o-** *cornea (of the eye); hard, fibrous protein* **-tome** *instrument used to cut; area with distinct edges* **photorefractive** (FOH-toh-ree-FRAK-tiv) **phot/o-** *light* **refract/o-** *bend; deflect* **-ive** *pertaining to* **keratectomy** (KAIR-ah-TEK-toh-mee) **kerat/o-** *cornea (of the eye); hard, fibrous protein* **-ectomy** *surgical excision*
retinopexy	Procedure to reattach a detached retina. **Cryotherapy** is used to freeze the tissue and fix all three layers (sclera, choroid, retina) together. Alternatively, laser photocoagulation can be done to heat spots on the retina to coagulate and seal them to the layers beneath.	**retinopexy** (RET-ih-noh-PEK-see) **retin/o-** *retina (of the eye)* **-pexy** *process of surgically fixing in place* **cryotherapy** (KRY-oh-THAIR-ah-pee) **cry/o-** *cold* **-therapy** *treatment*

Word or Phrase	Description	Word Building
strabismus surgery	Procedure to correct esotropia or exotropia. During a **resection,** the extraocular muscle on one side is shortened. During a **recession,** the extraocular muscle on the other side is lengthened and reattached.	**resection** (ree-SEK-shun) **resect/o-** *to cut out; remove* **-ion** *action; condition* **recession** (ree-SEH-shun) **recess/o-** *to move back* **-ion** *action; condition*
trabeculoplasty	Procedure to treat open-angle glaucoma. A laser is used to create small holes in half of the trabecular meshwork to increase the flow of aqueous humor. The procedure is usually effective for 5 years, at which time another trabeculoplasty can be performed on the untreated half of the trabecular meshwork.	**trabeculoplasty** (trah-BEK-yoo-loh-PLAS-tee) **trabecul/o-** *trabecula (mesh)* **-plasty** *process of reshaping by surgery*

Drug Categories

These categories of drugs are used to treat eye diseases and conditions. The most common generic and trade name drugs in each category are listed. Note: All drugs used topically in the eye are specially formulated from a solution that is physiologically similar to the fluids of the eye so as not to damage the delicate tissues of the eye.

Category	Indication	Examples	Word Building
antibiotic drugs	Treat bacterial infections of the eye. Antibiotic drugs are not effective against viral infections of the eye.	gentamicin (Garamycin, Genoptic), ofloxacin (Ocuflox)	**antibiotic** (AN-tee-by-AWT-ik) (AN-tih-by-AWT-ik) **anti-** *against* **bi/o-** *life; living organisms; living tissue* **-tic** *pertaining to*
antiviral drugs	Treat viral infections of the eye, specifically herpes simplex virus	trifluridine (Viroptic)	**antiviral** (AN-tee-VY-ral) (AN-tih-VY-ral) **anti-** *against* **vir/o-** *virus* **-al** *pertaining to*
corticosteroid drugs	Treat severe inflammation in the eye	dexamethasone (Maxidex), prednisolone (Pred Forte)	**corticosteroid** (KOR-tih-koh-STAIR-oyd) **cortic/o-** *cortex (outer region)* **-steroid** *steroid*
drugs for glaucoma	Act by decreasing the amount of aqueous humor or by constricting the pupil to open up the angle between the iris and the cornea	betaxolol (Betoptic), carteolol (Ocupress), dorzolamide (Trusopt), pilocarpine (Pilocar), timolol (Timoptic)	
mydriatic drugs	Dilate the pupil to prepare the eye for an internal examination	cyclopentolate (Cyclogyl), tropicamide (Mydriacyl)	**mydriatic** (MIH-dree-AT-ik) **mydr/o-** *widening* **-iatic** *pertaining to a state or process*

Abbreviations

ARMD	age-related macular degeneration	**OS, O.S.***	left eye (Latin, *oculus sinister*)
CK	conductive keratoplasty	**OU, O.U.***	each eye (Latin, *oculus uterque*), both eyes (Latin, *oculus unitas*)
ECCE	extracapsular cataract extraction		
EOM	extraocular movements; extraocular muscles	**PD**	prism diopter
EOMI	extraocular muscles intact	**PDT**	photodynamic therapy
HEENT	head, eyes, ears, nose, and throat	**PERRL**	pupils equal, round, and reactive to light
ICCE	intracapsular cataract extraction	**PERRLA**	pupils equal, round, and reactive to light and accommodation
IOL	intraocular lens		
IOP	intraocular pressure	**PRK**	photorefractive keratectomy
LASIK	laser-assisted *in situ* keratomileusis	**ROP**	retinopathy of prematurity
LTK	laser thermal keratoplasty	**RP**	retinitis pigmentosa
OD, O.D.*	right eye (Latin, *oculus dexter*)	**VF**	visual field
O.D.	Doctor of Optometry		

* According to the Joint Commission on Accreditation of Healthcare Organizations (JCAHO) and the Institute for Safe Medication Practices (ISMP), these abbreviations should not be used. However, because they are still used by some healthcare providers, they are included here.

Word Alert

ABBREVIATIONS

Abbreviations are commonly used in all types of medical documents; however, they can mean different things to different people and their meanings can be misinterpreted. Always verify the meaning of an abbreviation.

O.D. means *right eye* or *Doctor of Optometry,* but it also means *overdose.*

LASIK means *laser assisted* in situ *keratomileusis,* but it can be mistaken for *Lasix,* the trade name of a diuretic drug.

It's Greek to Me!

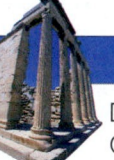

Did you notice that some words have two different combining forms? Combining forms from both Greek and Latin languages remain a part of medical language today.

Word	Greek	Latin	Medical Word Examples
cornea	kerat/o-	corne/o-	keratoplasty, corneal
eye	ophthalm/o-	ocul/o-	ophthalmology, ocular
lens	phac/o-, phak/o-	lent/o-	phacoemulsification, aphakia, retrolental
		lenticul/o-	lenticular
pupil	cor/o-	pupill/o-	anisocoria, pupillary
sight, vision	opt/o-	vis/o-	optic, visual

CAREER FOCUS

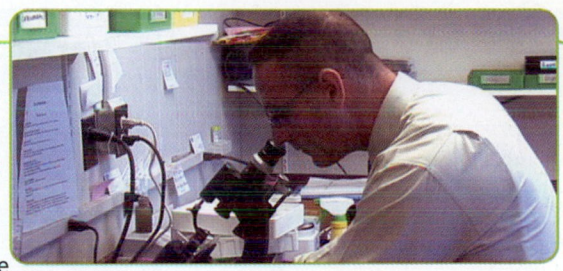

Meet Paul, an optician

"I pick up where the optometrist or ophthalmologist leaves off, by looking at the prescription and suggesting to the patient the selection of frame styles or lens styles. Either we have the lenses here in stock, or we'll order them from a servicing lab that actually manufactures the lens. We use a lensometer to read the prescription of the lens, and we have to make sure we place the optical center of the lens in front of the patient's pupil. This is a fairly busy practice. From 8:00 A.M. to closing, patients come in to purchase new eyewear or have their old eyewear repaired. I've been dealing with the public all my life. When you dispense a pair of glasses to someone and it puts a new light on everything, it's gratifying; it really is."

Opticians are allied health professionals who use automated equipment to cut, grind, and finish lenses to exact specifications based on a written prescription from an optometrist or ophthalmologist. They also prepare contact lenses and instruct the patient in their care and handling. Opticians work in optical stores or in the office of an optometrist or ophthalmologist.

    Optometrists are doctors of **optometry** (O.D.) who have graduated from a school of optometry. They diagnose and treat patients with vision problems and diseases of the eyes. They write prescriptions for eyeglasses and contact lenses. They can administer and prescribe ophthalmic drugs. Optometrists do not perform eye surgery.

    Ophthalmologists are physicians (M.D.) who practice in the medical specialty of ophthalmology. They do all of the things an optometrist does, but they are also able to perform surgery on the eye. Cancerous tumors of the eye are treated medically by an oncologist or surgically by an ophthalmologist.

optician (op-TISH-un)
  opt/o- *eye; vision*
  -ician *skilled professional or expert*

optometrist (op-TAWM-eh-trist)
  opt/o- *eye; vision*
  metr/o- *measurement*
  -ist *one who specializes in*

optometry (op-TAWM-eh-tree)
  opt/o- *eye; vision*
  -metry *process of measuring*

ophthalmologist (AWF-thal-MAWL-oh-jist)
  ophthalm/o- *eye*
  log/o- *word; the study of*
  -ist *one who specializes in*

myhealthprofessionskit To see Paul's complete video profile, visit Medical Terminology Interactive at www.myhealthprofessionskit.com. Select this book, log in, and go to the 15th floor of Pearson General Hospital. Enter the Laboratory, and click on the computer screen.

CHAPTER REVIEW EXERCISES

Test your knowledge of the chapter by completing these review exercises. Use the Answer Key at the end of the book to check your answers.

Anatomy and Physiology

Matching Exercise

Match each word or phrase to its description.

1. ciliary body
2. conjunctiva
3. fovea
4. limbus
5. mydriasis
6. optic chiasm
7. orbit
8. superior rectus muscle
9. suspensory ligaments
10. trabecular meshwork
11. uveal tract
12. visual cortex

_____ Turns the eye upward

_____ Center of the macula

_____ Support the lens

_____ Includes the iris, choroid, and ciliary body

_____ Increases the diameter of the pupil

_____ Bony socket that holds the eye

_____ Filters aqueous humor

_____ Edge of the cornea where it becomes the white sclera

_____ Area in the occipital lobe that processes visual images

_____ Produces aqueous humor

_____ Mucous membrane on the inside of the eyelid

_____ Where the optic nerves cross

Circle Exercise

Circle the correct word from the choices given.

1. The (**iris, limbus, orbit**) is the colored, circular structure around the pupil.
2. The red, triangular tissue at the medial corner of the eye is the (**caruncle, lacrimal gland, trabecular meshwork**).
3. The (**cornea, iris, sclera**) is the tough, fibrous, white outer covering of the eye.
4. The blind spot on the retina corresponds to the (**fundus, macula, optic disk**).
5. Color vision comes from cells known as (**cones, rods, visual cortices**).
6. Cranial nerve (**II, III, IV, V**) is the optic nerve for vision.

True or False Exercise

Indicate whether each statement is true or false by writing T or F on the line.

1. _____ The nasolacrimal duct carries vitreous humor.
2. _____ The sclera is the clear part of the cornea.
3. _____ Eye color is a genetically determined trait.
4. _____ Muscles in the iris contract or relax to constrict or dilate the pupil.
5. _____ At birth, all babies' eyes appear gray-blue.
6. _____ Vitreous humor is a clear, watery fluid.
7. _____ Stereoscopic vision is three-dimensional vision.

Sequencing Exercise

Beginning with the light rays from an object, sequence the structures of the eye in the correct order as the light passes through them.

conjunctiva	fovea of the retina	optic nerve	vitreous humor
cornea	lens	pupil	

1. light rays from an object _____

2. _____

3. _____

4. _____

5. _____

6. _____

7. _____

8. _____

Diseases and Conditions

Circle Exercise

Circle the correct word from the choices given.

1. Involuntary beats of the eye when looking to the side are called (**diplopia, nystagmus, strabismus**).

2. A patient with exophthalmos often has (**blindness, glaucoma, hyperthyroidism**).

3. Increased intraocular pressure is caused by (**conjunctivitis, glaucoma, presbyopia**).

4. Clumps of vitreous humor cause (**color blindness, floaters, strabismus**).

5. Farsightedness is (**astigmatism, hyperopia, myopia**).

Matching Exercise

Match each word or phrase to its description.

1. anisocoria   _____ Malignant eye tumor in children

2. blepharitis   _____ A type of strabismus

3. cataract   _____ Blurry, opaque lens

4. exotropia   _____ Visual field defect

5. macular degeneration _____ Nearsightedness

6. myopia   _____ Unequal pupils

7. retinoblastoma   _____ Inflammation or infection of the eyelid

8. scotoma   _____ Loss of central vision

Laboratory, Radiology, Surgery, and Drugs

True or False Exercise

Indicate whether each statement is true or false by writing T or F on the line.

1. _____ Gonioscopy is used to visualize the trabecular meshwork.

2. _____ A blepharoplasty removes fat and sagging skin from the eyelid.

3. _____ LASIK and PRK are used to surgically correct nearsightedness.

4. _____ Corticosteroid drugs are used to dilate the pupil before an eye exam.

Fill in the Blank Exercise

Fill in the blank with the correct word from the word list.

accommodation	Ishihara	phacoemulsification	Snellen
angiogram	ophthalmoscope	phorometer	tonometry
convergence	penlight	photocoagulation	trabeculoplasty
conjugate gaze	peripheral vision	retinopexy	

1. What can be seen at the edge of the visual field _____

2. Instrument used to do a funduscopic examination _____

3. Testing how well the lens can change shape to focus _____

4. Testing how well the eyes move together as a unit _____

5. Instrument used to check the pupillary response _____

6. Testing how well both eyes focus on a near point _____

7. Test for glaucoma to measure intraocular pressure _____

8. Surgical procedure that uses a laser to seal leaking retinal blood vessels _____

9. Surgical procedure to treat a detached retina _____

10. Instrument that holds lenses of successive strengths to find the best correction for vision _____

11. Test that uses fluorescein to outline the retinal blood vessels _____

12. Color blindness test _____

13. Surgical procedure to treat glaucoma _____

14. Test for visual acuity at a distance _____

15. Breaking up the lens during cataract surgery _____

Building Medical Words

Review the Combining Forms Exercise and Combining Form and Suffix Exercise that you already completed in the anatomy section on pages 774–775.

Combining Forms Exercise

Before you build eye words, review these additional combining forms. Next to each combining form, write its medical meaning. The first one has been done for you.

Combining Form	Medical Meaning	Combining Form	Medical Meaning
1. ambly/o-	dimness	12. es/o-	_____
2. anis/o-	_____	13. ex/o-	_____
3. blast/o-	_____	14. goni/o-	_____
4. coagul/o-	_____	15. icter/o-	_____
5. conjug/o-	_____	16. metr/o-	_____
6. converg/o-	_____	17. micr/o-	_____
7. cry/o-	_____	18. myop/o-	_____
8. cyst/o-	_____	19. ne/o-	_____
9. dipl/o-	_____	20. papill/o-	_____
10. emulsific/o-	_____	21. phob/o-	_____
11. enucle/o-	_____	22. phor/o-	_____

(continued)

Combining Form	Medical Meaning	Combining Form	Medical Meaning
23. phot/o-	_____	27. ton/o-	_____
24. pleg/o-	_____	28. trop/o-	_____
25. presby/o-	_____	29. vascul/o-	_____
26. scot/o-	_____	30. xer/o-	_____

Related Combining Forms Exercise

Write the combining forms on the line provided. (Hint: See the It's Greek to Me feature box.)

1. Two combining forms that mean *cornea.* _____

2. Two combining forms that mean *eye.* _____

3. Two combining forms that mean *pupil.* _____

4. Two combining forms that mean *sight or vision.* _____

5. Four combining forms that mean *lens.* _____

Combining Form and Suffix Exercise

Read the definition of the medical word. Select the correct suffix from the Suffix List. Select the correct combining form from the Combining Form List. Build the medical word and write it on the line. Be sure to check your spelling. The first one has been done for you.

SUFFIX LIST	COMBINING FORM LIST	
-ation (a process; being or having)	blephar/o- (eyelid)	goni/o- (angle)
-ectomy (surgical excision)	conjunctiv/o- (conjunctiva)	ir/o- (iris)
-ence (state of)	converg/o- (coming together)	kerat/o- (cornea)
-itis (inflammation of; infection of)	cry/o- (cold)	presby/o- (old age)
-meter (instrument used to measure)	dipl/o- (double)	retin/o- (retina)
-mileusis (process of carving)	enucle/o- (to remove the main part)	ton/o- (pressure; tone)
-opia (condition of vision)	fundu/o- (fundus; part farthest from	trabecul/o- (trabecula; mesh)
-pathy (disease; suffering)	the opening)	
-pexy (process of surgically fixing in place)		
-plasty (process of reshaping by surgery)		
-ptosis (state of prolapse; drooping)		
-scopy (process of using an instrument to examine)		
-therapy (treatment)		

Definition of the Medical Word   **Build the Medical Word**

1. Inflammation or infection of the conjunctiva   *conjunctivitis* _____

2. Disease of the retina   _____

3. Inflammation or infection of the eyelid   _____

4. Condition of the vision (being) double   _____

5. Condition of vision in old age   _____

6. Process of reshaping by surgery on the trabecula   _____

7. Process of using an instrument to examine the angle (and the trabecular meshwork)   _____

8. Inflammation or infection of the iris   _____

9. State of prolapse or drooping of the eyelid   _____

10. Surgical excision of the cornea   _____

11. State (of the eyes) coming together (as an object moves closer)   _____

12. A process to remove the main part (of the eye)   _____

(continued)

Definition of the Medical Word   **Build the Medical Word**

13. Treatment (that uses) cold (to freeze tissues)   _____

14. Instrument used to measure the pressure (in the eye) _____

15. Process of using an instrument to examine the part (of the eye) that
    is farthest from the opening (the pupil)   _____

16. Process of surgically fixing in place the retina   _____

17. Process of reshaping by surgery on the eyelid   _____

18. Process of carving the cornea   _____

Prefix Exercise

Read the definition of the medical word. Look at the medical word or partial word that is given (it already contains a combining form and a suffix). Select the correct prefix from the Prefix List and write it on the blank line. Then build the medical word and write it on the line. Be sure to check your spelling. The first one has been done for you.

PREFIX LIST

a- (away from; without)	ec- (out; outward)	hemi- (one half)
an- (without; not)	en- (in; within; inward)	intra- (within)
dys- (painful; difficult; abnormal)	extra- (outside of)	retro- (behind; backward)

Definition of the Medical Word	Prefix	Word or Partial Word	Build the Medical Word
1. Condition of inward turning (of the eyelid)	en-	tropion	entropion
2. Condition (of being) without the lens	_____	phakia	_____
3. Pertaining to outside of the capsule (that envelops the lens)	_____	capsular	_____
4. Pertaining to abnormal joined together (movements of the eyes)	_____	conjugate	_____
5. Pertaining to (being) without jaundice (of the eye)	_____	icteric	_____
6. Pertaining to within the eye	_____	ocular	_____
7. Condition of vision of one half (of the visual field) not (being there)	_____	anopia	_____
8. Pertaining to behind the lens	_____	lental	_____
9. Condition of outward turning (of the eyelid)	_____	tropion	_____

Multiple Combining Forms and Suffix Exercise

Read the definition of the medical word. Select the correct suffix and combining forms. Then build the medical word and write it on the line. Be sure to check your spelling. The first one has been done for you.

SUFFIX LIST	COMBINING FORM LIST	
-ation (a process; being or having)	anis/o- (unequal)	metr/o- (measurement)
-ia (condition; state; thing)	blast/o- (immature; embryonic)	ophthalm/o- (eye)
-ist (one who specializes in)	coagul/o- (clotting)	opt/o- (eye; vision)
-itis (inflammation of; infection of)	cor/o- (pupil)	phac/o- (lens)
-oma (tumor; mass)	cycl/o- (ciliary body)	phob/o- (fear; avoidance)
-tome (instrument used to cut)	cyst/o- (fluid-filled sac)	phot/o- (light)
	dacry/o- (tears)	pleg/o- (paralysis)
	emulsific/o- (particles suspended in a solution)	retin/o- (retina)
	es/o- (inward)	trop/o- (having an affinity for; stimulating; turning)
	kerat/o- (cornea)	xer/o- (dry)
	micr/o- (small)	

Definition of the Medical Word

1. Condition (of one of the pupils looking) inward and turning
2. Condition of unequal pupils
3. Instrument used to cut a small area on the cornea
4. Condition of light avoidance
5. Tumor of the retina (composed of) embryonic cells
6. A process (that uses) light (to cause) clotting
7. State (in which the) ciliary body has paralysis (and is kept dilated)
8. Inflammation or infection of (the structure of) tears (that is a) fluid-filled sac
9. A process (in which) the lens (becomes) particles suspended in a solution
10. Condition of dry eyes
11. One who specializes in vision measurement

Build the Medical Word

1. *esotropia*
2. _____
3. _____
4. _____
5. _____
6. _____
7. _____
8. _____
9. _____
10. _____
11. _____

Abbreviations

Matching Exercise

Match each abbreviation to its definition.

1. IOL	_____ Eye muscles that move the eye are intact
2. IOP	_____ Premature babies get this eye disease
3. LASIK	_____ Lens placed within the eye after cataract surgery
4. O.S.	_____ Pupils equal and react normally
5. OU	_____ Surgery for nearsightedness
6. ROP	_____ Glaucoma occurs with this
7. EOMI	_____ Left eye
8. PERRL	_____ Both eyes

Applied Skills

Medical Report Exercise

This exercise contains a Consultation Report from a specialist physician. Read the report and answer the questions.

CONSULTATION REPORT

PATIENT NAME: BROWN, Rubeetha

PATIENT NUMBER: 04-7223

DATE OF CONSULTATION: November 19, 20xx

HISTORY OF PRESENT ILLNESS
This 54-year-old, African American female comes in today as a referral from her primary care physician. She is complaining of bloodshot eyes, headaches, large floaters in her visual field, and blurred vision at close range.

PAST HISTORY
She has had myopia since childhood (onset at age 12). She was diagnosed by a neurologist as having migraines with an aura of scintillating scotomas followed by a temporary visual field defect of hemianopia, "like a gray curtain" coming down. She denies a history of hyperthyroidism, although she has been tested for this on several occasions. She denies hypertension, heart disease, or diabetes. She has some mild osteoarthritis, particularly in her right knee. Past surgeries include a tonsillectomy and an appendectomy in the remote past.

SOCIAL HISTORY
She is married and has 2 children, both living away from home. She works in the member services department of an HMO and does paperwork and computer work all day.

PHYSICAL EXAMINATION
The conjunctivae are infected, and the sclerae are anicteric. There is a soft, movable mass in the margin of the right upper eyelid. The patient states that this was from a trauma and has remained unchanged for many years. This is not a chalazion, just scar tissue. There is a moderate amount of crusted exudate on the eyelids. There is mild exophthalmos bilaterally. PERRL. Extraocular movements intact. Dilating drops were instilled in each eye, and a funduscopy was performed. There is evidence of a developing cataract in the right eye. The retinae bilaterally were normal. There was no suggestion of macular degeneration, and the cup-to-disk ratio was normal. There were no microaneurysms or hemorrhages. There were small clumps of vitreous humor visible in the posterior cavity.

VISUAL TESTING
Distance vision without glasses was 20/200 in both eyes. Peripheral vision was normal. Depth perception was normal. Tonometry showed normal intraocular pressures in both eyes.

DIAGNOSES
1. Eye strain and new-onset presbyopia.
2. Severe myopia. Wears corrective lenses for distance vision.
3. Stage I cataract, O.D.
4. Blepharitis.
5. Vitreous floaters. The patient was advised that although these are annoying and appear large, they are actually small and benign and are the result of the aging process.

PLAN
1. The patient has been given a prescription for new eyeglasses. These will be bifocal lenses to correct her myopia and her new-onset presbyopia.
2. The patient was asked to gently cleanse the eyelids and apply bacitracin ophthalmic ointment b.i.d.

(continued)

3. The patient has been advised of her increased risk of developing glaucoma given her age and race and was advised to have an annual eye examination with tonometry. Follow up in 1 year to evaluate the status of her cataract and do a glaucoma check.

Lauren J. Spiner, M.D.

Lauren J. Spiner, M.D.

LJS: jtr
D: 11/19/xx
T: 11/19/xx

Word Analysis Questions

1. A funduscopy was performed. If you wanted to use the adjective form of funduscopy, you would say, "The patient had a _____ examination performed."

2. Divide *intraocular* into its three word parts and define each word part.

Word Part   **Definition**

_____   _____

_____   _____

_____   _____

3. Divide *anicteric* into its three word parts and define each word part.

Word Part   **Definition**

_____   _____

_____   _____

_____   _____

Fact Finding Questions

1. What part of the eye does a funduscopy examine? _____

2. What eye condition has the patient had since childhood? _____

3. What two visual symptoms does the patient have before the onset of a migraine? _____ _____

4. The mass on the patient's eyelid is a chalazion.   **True   False**

5. What is the meaning of PERRL? _____

6. What abbreviation tells you that the patient's cataract was in the right eye? _____

Critical Thinking Questions

1. The physical finding of crusted exudates on the eyelids corresponds to which diagnosis?

2. Examination of which part of the eye tells you that the patient does not have liver disease?

3. The normal tonometry results ruled out what disease?

4. Why have physicians in the past tested the patient for hyperthyroidism?

Proofreading and Spelling Exercise

Read the following paragraph. Identify each misspelled medical word and write the correct spelling of it on the line.

The eye works with the vizual cortex of the brain for the sense of sight. The aquous humor is clear in the anterior chamber. The layers of the eye are the conjintiva, cornea, and sklera. The retina has the macular where the best vision is. Drops in the eyes cause midriasis so the eyes can be examined. It is not good to have a catarakt or an entropion or blepharotosis. To diagnose eye diseases, a dilated fundoscopic exam is done. The study of the eye is known as ofthalmology.

1. _____   6. _____
2. _____   7. _____
3. _____   8. _____
4. _____   9. _____
5. _____   10. _____

Hearing Medical Words Exercise

You hear someone speaking the medical words given below. Read each pronunciation and then write the medical word it represents. Be sure to check your spelling. The first one has been done for you.

1. AM-blee-OH-pee-ah   *amblyopia*_____
2. KAT-ah-rakt   _____
3. SY-kloh-PLEE-jee-ah   _____
4. my-OH-pee-ah   _____
5. AWF-thal-MAWL-oh-jist   _____
6. op-TISH-un   _____
7. PREZ-bee-OH-pee-ah   _____
8. strah-BIZ-mus   _____
9. toh-NAWM-eh-ter   _____
10. VIT-ree-us HYOO-mor   _____

Pronunciation Exercise

Read the medical word that is given. Then review the syllables in the pronunciation. Circle the primary (main) accented syllable. The first one has been done for you.

1. conjunctiva (con-junk-ty-vah)
2. aphakia (ah-fay-kee-ah)
3. conjunctivitis (con-junk-tih-vy-tis)
4. diplopia (dih-ploh-pee-ah)
5. glaucoma (glaw-koh-mah)
6. macular (mak-yoo-lar)
7. optometrist (op-tawm-eh-trist)
8. phacoemulsification (fay-koh-ee-mul-sih-fih-kay-shun)
9. retinopexy (ret-ih-noh-pek-see)
10. strabismus (strah-biz-mus)

Multimedia Preview

Immerse yourself in a variety of activities inside Medical Terminology Interactive. Getting there is simple:

1. Click on www.myhealthprofessionskit.com.
2. Select "Medical Terminology" from the choice of disciplines.
3. First-time users must create an account using the scratch-off code on the inside front cover of this book.
4. Find this book and log in using your username and password.
5. Click on Medical Terminology Interactive.
6. Take the elevator to the 15th Floor to begin your virtual exploration of this chapter!

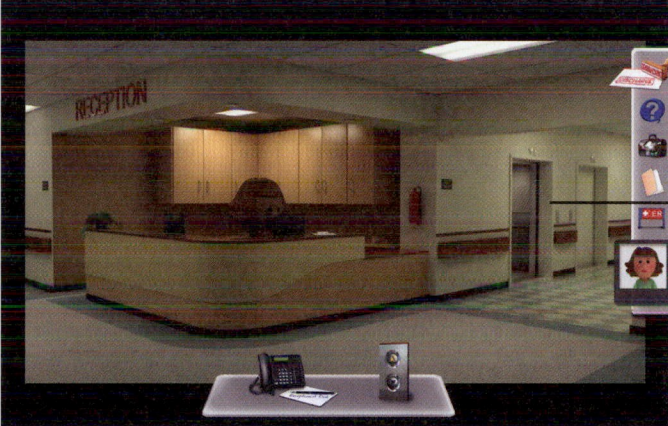 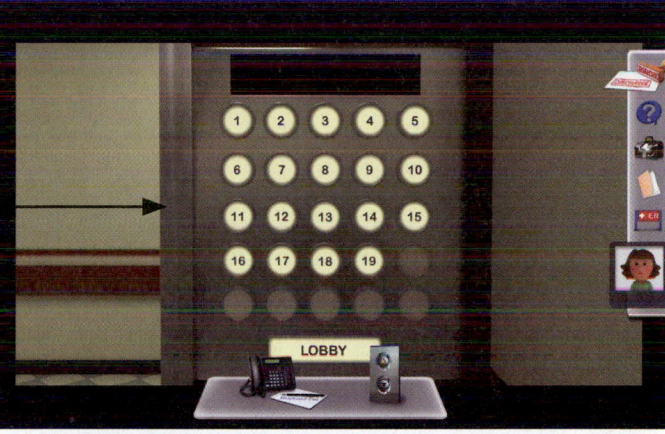

■ **Body Rhythms**   Sing along and learn! We've created a series of original music videos that correspond to each body system. They might not make it to MTV but they'll help you remember basic anatomy and give you a fun study break at the same time.

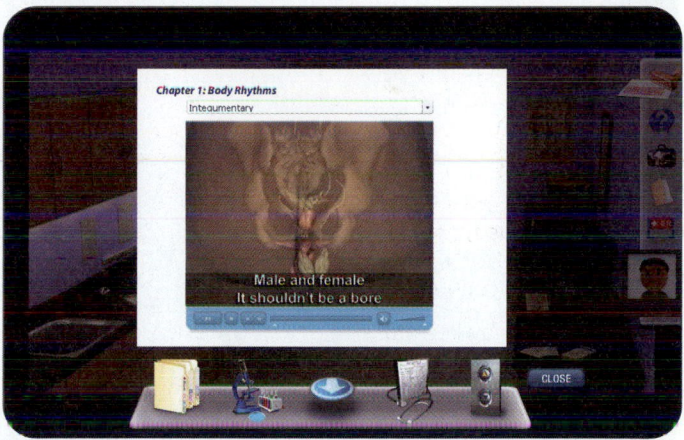

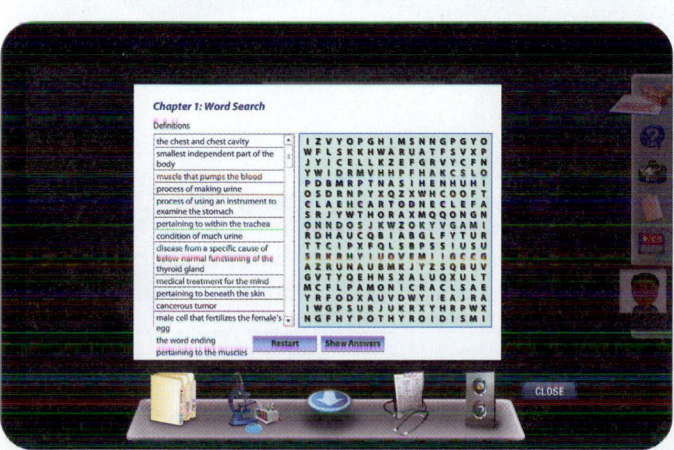

■ **Word Search**   Secret terms are hidden throughout the grid and we simply provide you with clues. Your task is to figure out what terms to find, and then to seek them out. Grab a magnifying glass and your thinking cap. You'll need both!

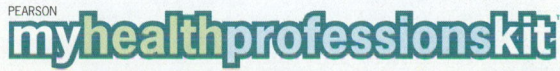

Dive In!

- While our eyes remain the same size from birth, our ears and nose never stop growing.
- Humans can tell the difference between about 10,000 odors.
- This may be tough to swallow, but listen carefully. In this chapter we'll explore the language that describes the structures, functions, diseases, and conditions of the ears, nose, and throat.
- You'll sniff out the truth once you master the language of otolaryngology!

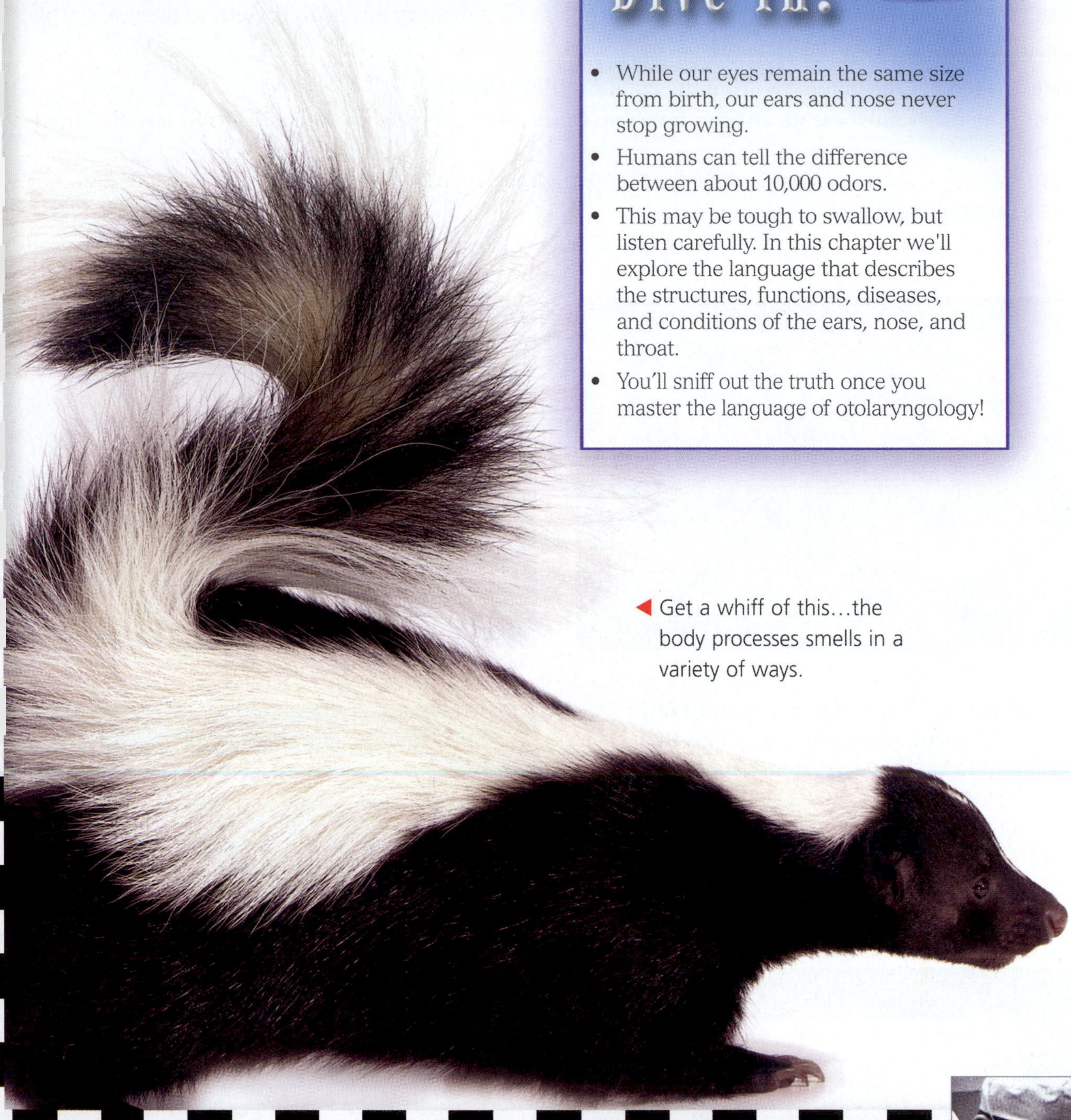

Get a whiff of this…the body processes smells in a variety of ways.

Medicine Through HISTORY

1965

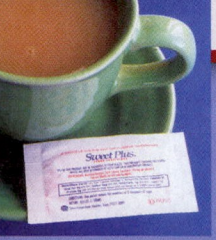

The artificial sweetener aspartame is developed

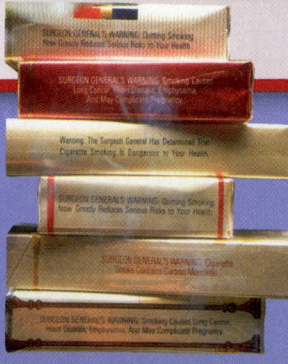

1965

Congress requires a warning label on cigarette packages to say that smoking is hazardous to your health

1967

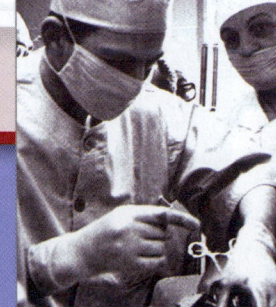

Dr. Christian Barnard performs the first heart transplant operation

Structure Your Progress
Learning Objectives

16

Otolaryngology

Ears, Nose, and Throat

Otolaryngology (OH-toh-LAIR-ing-GAWL-oh-jee) is the medical specialty that studies the anatomy and physiology of the ears, nose, mouth, and throat (ENT) and uses diagnostic tests, medical and surgical procedures, and drugs to treat ENT diseases.

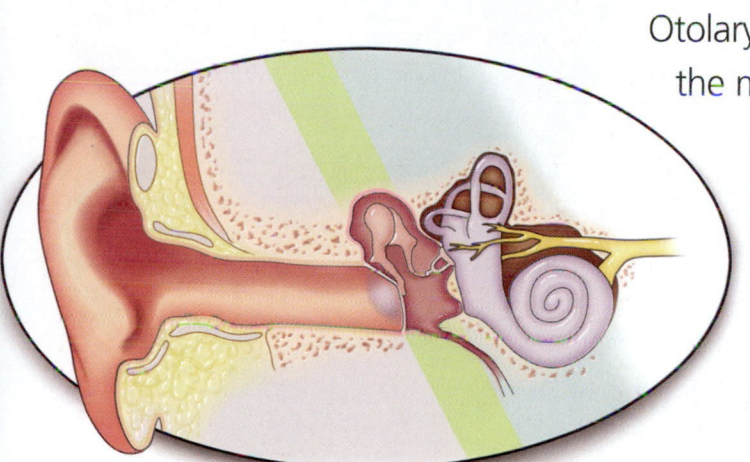

▲ The external, middle, and inner ear form an intricate system to process hearing and enable balance.

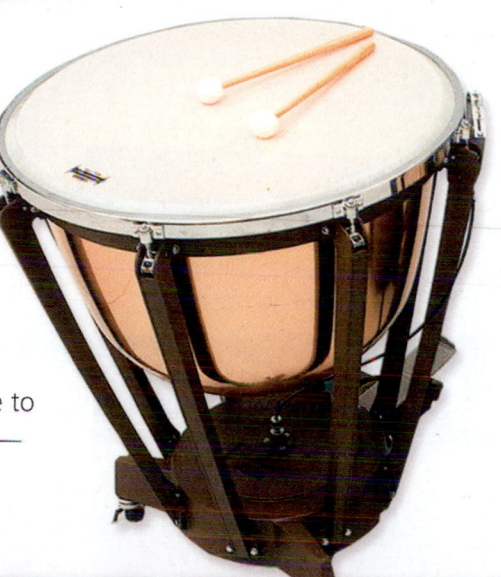
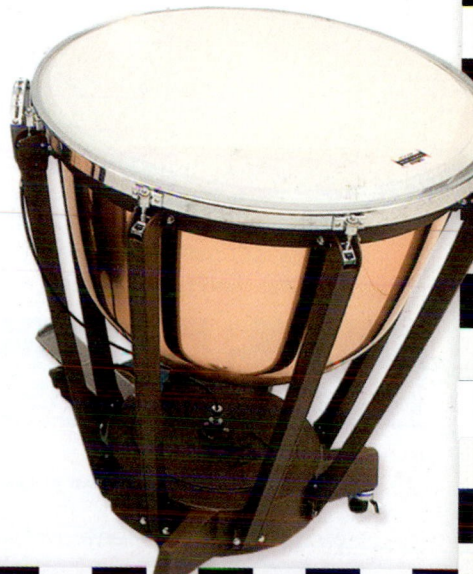

▶ Thin yet rigid; sensitive to pressure and vibration—eardrums work like musical drums

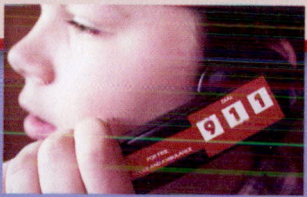

1968

AT&T announces a new national emergency telephone number: 911

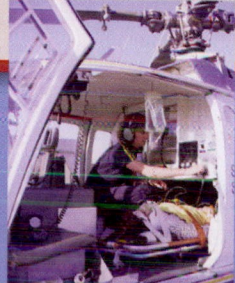

1969

The first Shock Trauma Unit is established at the University of Maryland

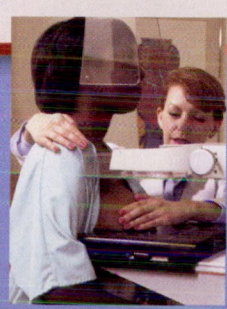

1969

The first mammography of the breast is performed

Measure Your Progress: Learning Objectives

After you study this chapter, you should be able to

1. Identify the structures of the ears, nose, and throat (ENT) system.

2. Describe the process of hearing.

3. Describe common ENT diseases and conditions, laboratory and diagnostic procedures, medical and surgical procedures, and drug categories.

4. Give the medical meaning of word parts related to the ENT system.

5. Build ENT words from word parts and divide and define ENT words.

6. Spell and pronounce ENT words.

7. Analyze the medical content and meaning of an otolaryngology report.

8. Dive deeper into otolaryngology by reviewing the activities at the end of this chapter and online at Medical Terminology Interactive.

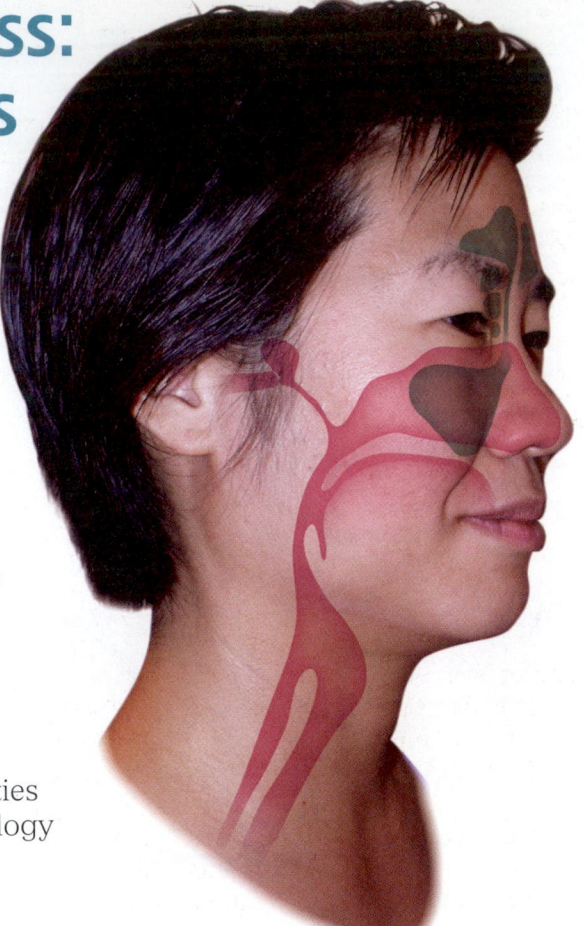

Figure 16-1 ■ **Ears, nose, and throat (ENT) system.**

The ENT system consists of many different structures located in the head and neck. Each of these individual structures is interrelated and connected to one another.

Medical Language Key

To unlock the definition of a medical word, break it into word parts. Define each word part. Put the word part meanings in order, beginning with the suffix, then the prefix (if present), then the combining form(s).

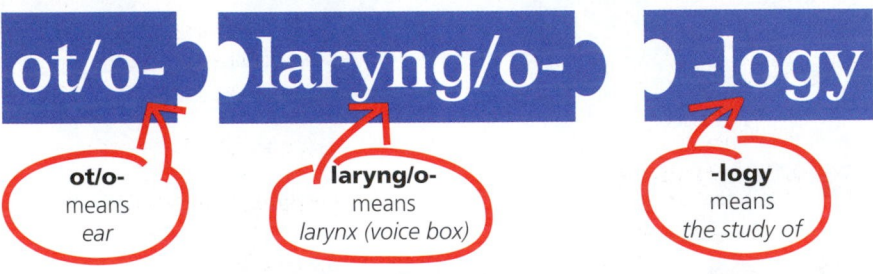

ot/o-
means
ear

laryng/o-
means
larynx (voice box)

-logy
means
the study of

	Word Part	Word Part Meaning
Suffix	-logy	*the study of*
Combining Form	ot/o-	*ear*
Combining Form	laryng/o-	*larynx (voice box)*

Otolaryngology: *The study of the ears, (nose, throat), larynx, (and related structures).*

Although the word *otolaryngology* does not contain combining forms for the nose, mouth, throat, or neck, it is understood that these structures are included in this medical specialty. The word *otorhinolaryngology* does include the combining form *rhin/o-* for nose.

Anatomy and Physiology

The **ears, nose, and throat (ENT) system** is a compact body system that is contained entirely in the head and neck (see Figure 16-1 ■). The head contains the external and internal structures of the ears, nose, and mouth, and the internal structures of the sinuses. The neck contains the internal structures of the pharynx and larynx. The ENT system has several functions. It shares some structures with the gastrointestinal system and the respiratory system, and it serves as a passageway for both food and air. The ENT system also contains lymphoid tissue that functions as part of the immune response. The body's senses of hearing and smell are also part of the ENT system. The structures of the ENT system (along with those of the respiratory system) are used to generate speech.

Anatomy of the ENT System

External Ear

The external ear is the **auricle** or **pinna** (see Figure 16-2 ■). The **helix** is the outer rim of tissue and cartilage that forms a *C* and ends at the earlobe. The **external auditory meatus** is the opening that leads into the **external auditory canal (EAC)**. The **tragus** is the triangular cartilage anterior to the meatus. The canal has glands that secrete **cerumen,** a waxy, sticky substance that traps dirt and has an antibiotic action against microorganisms that enter the canal. At the end of the canal is the **tympanic membrane (TM)** or **eardrum,** a thin membrane that divides the external ear from the middle ear (see Figure 16-3 ■).

Just behind the external ear is the **mastoid process,** a bony projection of the temporal bone of the cranium. The mastoid process is not a solid bone; it contains tiny cavities filled with air. The tendon of the sternocleidomastoid muscle in the neck attaches to the mastoid process.

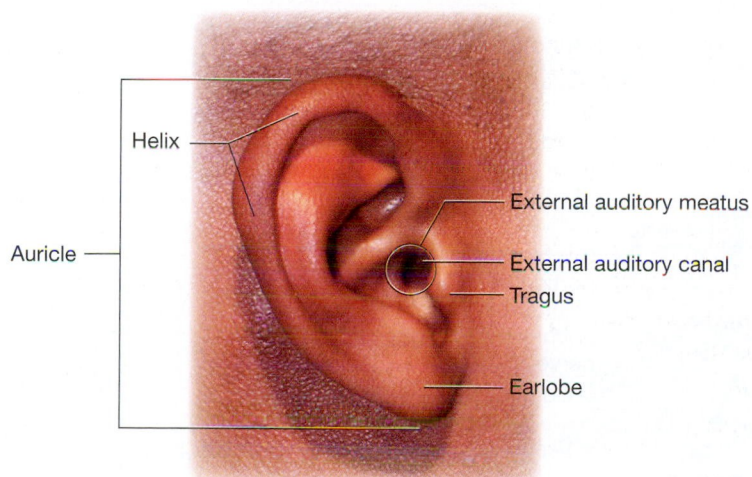

Figure 16-2 ■ **External ear.**
The external ear is composed of several types and shapes of tissue and cartilage. The external ear also includes the external auditory canal that travels into the temporal bone of the cranium.

Labels: Helix, Auricle, External auditory meatus, External auditory canal, Tragus, Earlobe

---

WORD BUILDING

auricle (AW-rih-kl)
  aur/i- *ear*
  -cle *small thing*

auricular (aw-RIK-yoo-lar)
  auricul/o- *ear*
  -ar *pertaining to*

otic (OH-tik)
  ot/o- *ear*
  -ic *pertaining to*
Both *auricular* and *otic* are adjectives that mean *ear*.

pinna (PIN-ah)

pinnae (PIN-ee)
Pinna is a Latin singular noun. Form the plural by changing *-a* to *-ae*.

helix (HEE-liks)

external (eks-TER-nal)
  extern/o- *outside*
  -al *pertaining to*

auditory (AW-dih-TOH-ree)
  audit/o- *the sense of hearing*
  -ory *having the function of*
The combining forms *acous/o-* and *audi/o-* also mean *the sense of hearing*.

meatus (mee-AA-tus)

meati (mee-AA-tie)
Meatus is a Latin singular noun. Form the plural by changing *-us* to *-i*.

tragus (TRAY-gus)

tragi (TRAY-jeye)
Tragus is a Latin singular noun. Form the plural by changing *-us* to *-i*.

cerumen (seh-ROO-men)

tympanic (tim-PAN-ik)
  tympan/o- *tympanic membrane (eardrum)*
  -ic *pertaining to*
The combining form *myring/o-* also means *tympanic membrane (eardrum)*.

mastoid (MAS-toyd)
  mast/o- *breast; mastoid process*
  -oid *resembling*
The combining form *mastoid/o-* also means *mastoid process*.

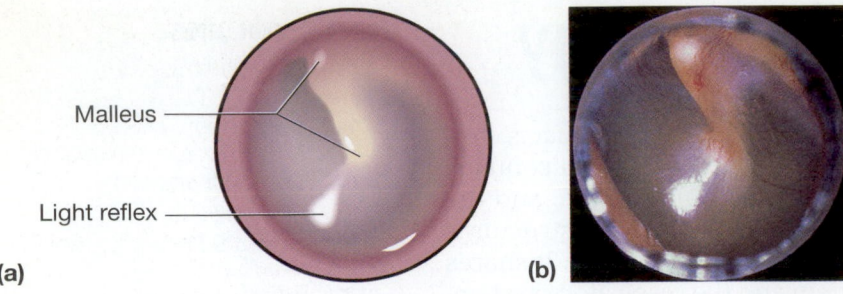

(a) **(b)**

Figure 16-3 ■ **Tympanic membrane.**

A normal tympanic membrane has a gray, pearly color and is so thin that the malleus can be seen behind it. A shiny, reflective strip (reflected light from an otoscope) is seen, which is known as the light reflex.

Middle Ear

The middle ear is a hollow area inside the temporal bone of the cranium (see Figure 16-4 ■). The middle ear contains three tiny bones: the **malleus, incus,** and **stapes,** collectively known as the **ossicles.** These bones are connected to each other by tiny ligaments to form the **ossicular chain.** The first bone, the malleus, is shaped like and also known as the **hammer.** It is connected to the tympanic membrane. Because the tympanic membrane is nearly transparent, the malleus can be seen through it. The second bone, the incus, is shaped like and also known as the **anvil.** The third bone, the stapes, is shaped like and also known as the **stirrup.** The stapes fits into an opening in the temporal bone known as the **oval window.** The **round window,** another opening in the temporal bone, is covered by a membrane. The middle ear is connected to the nasopharynx by the **eustachian tube.** The eustachian tube allows air pressure in the middle ear to equalize with air pressure in the nose and throat and outside the body.

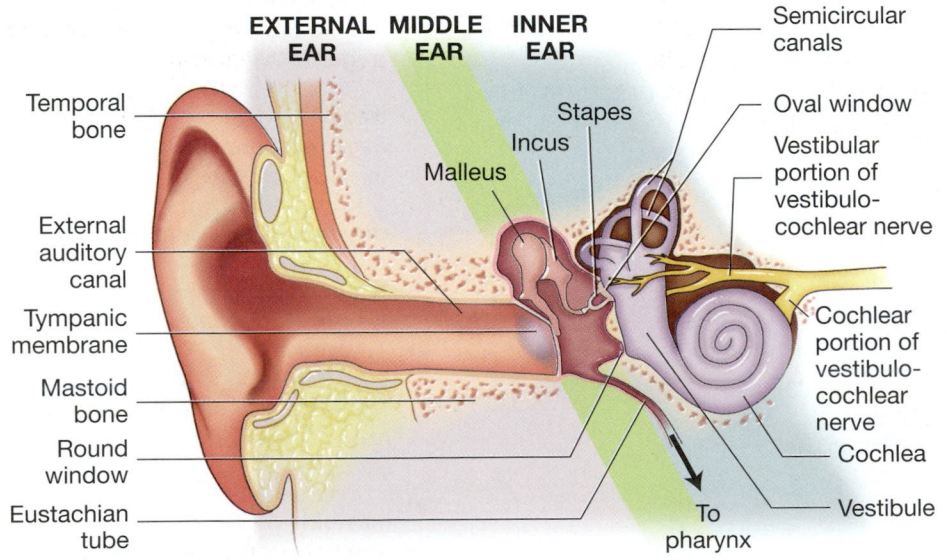

Figure 16-4 ■ **Structures of the middle ear and inner ear.**

Notice the shapes of the malleus, incus, and stapes in the middle ear. Do they look like a hammer, anvil, and stirrup to you? The structures of the inner ear send information about balance and hearing to the brain via the vestibulocochlear nerve.

WORD BUILDING

malleus (MAL-ee-us)

mallei (MAL-ee-eye)
Malleus is a Latin singular noun. Form the plural by changing *-us* to *-i*.

mallear (MAL-ee-ar)
   malle/o- *malleus (hammer-shaped bone)*
   -ar *pertaining to*

incus (ING-kus)

incudes (in-KYOO-deez)

incudal (IN-kyoo-dal)
   incud/o- *incus (anvil-shaped bone)*
   -al *pertaining to*

stapes (STAY-peez)

stapedes (STAY-pee-deez)

stapedial (stay-PEE-dee-al)
   staped/o- *stapes (stirrup-shaped bone)*
   -ial *pertaining to*

ossicle (AWS-ih-kl)
   ossic/o- *bone*
   -cle *small thing*

ossicular (aw-SIK-yoo-lar)
   ossicul/o- *ossicle (little bone)*
   -ar *pertaining to*

eustachian (yoo-STAY-shun)

Word Alert

SOUND-ALIKE WORDS

malleus   (noun)   first bone of the middle ear
Example: An infection in the middle ear caused scar tissue around the malleus and affected the patient's hearing.

malleolus   (noun)   bony projections on the tibia and fibula of the lower leg near the ankle
Example: The lateral malleolus is a bony projection from the distal end of the fibula.

Inner Ear

The temporal bone of the cranium divides the middle ear from the inner ear, with only the round window and oval window connecting the two cavities. The inner ear cavity contains three fluid-filled structures: the vestibule, the semicircular canals, and the cochlea (see Figure 16-4). The **vestibule** is the entrance to the inner ear. One end of the vestibule becomes the three **semicircular canals.** Each of these canals is oriented in a different plane: horizontally, vertically, and obliquely. When you tilt your head forward, backward, or to the side, the semicircular canals send information to the brain about the position of your head and this helps you keep your balance. The other end of the vestibule becomes the coiled **cochlea.** The cochlea sends information to the brain about the frequency and intensity of the sound waves entering the ear. All of the structures of the inner ear are collectively known as the **labyrinth.**

External Nose and Mouth

The external nose is supported by the nasal bone, which forms the bridge of the nose and the **dorsum** (see Figure 16-5 ■). At the nasal tip, the nasal bone becomes cartilage. The **nares** are the external openings or nostrils. The flared cartilage on each side of the nostril is a nasal **ala.**

The lips, cheeks, and chin are supported by the maxilla (upper jawbone) and mandible (lower jawbone). The **nasolabial fold** is the crease in the cheek that goes from the nose to the lip at the corner of the mouth. The **philtrum** is the vertical groove above the upper lip. The chin is also known as the **mentum.**

WORD BUILDING

vestibule (VES-tih-byool)

vestibular (ves-TIB-yoo-lar)
  vestibul/o- *vestibule (entrance)*
  -ar *pertaining to*

semicircular (SEM-ee-SIR-kyoo-lar)
  semi- *half; partly*
  circul/o- *circle*
  -ar *pertaining to*

cochlea (KOHK-lee-ah)

cochleae (KOHK-lee-ee)
Cochlea is a Latin singular noun. Form the plural by changing -a to -ae.

cochlear (KOHK-lee-ar)
  cochle/o- *cochlea (of the inner ear)*
  -ar *pertaining to*

labyrinth (LAB-ih-rinth)
The combining form *labyrinth/o-* means *labyrinth.*

dorsum (DOR-sum)

dorsal (DOR-sal)
  dors/o- *back; dorsum*
  -al *pertaining to*

naris (NAY-ris)

nares (NAY-reez)

ala (AA-lah)

alae (AA-lee)
Ala is a Latin singular noun. Form the plural by changing -a to -ae.

nasolabial (NAY-zoh-LAY-bee-al)
  nas/o- *nose*
  labi/o- *lip; labium*
  -al *pertaining to*
The combining form *cheil/o-* also means *lip.*

philtrum (FIL-trum)

mentum (MEN-tum)
The combining form *ment/o-* means *chin.*

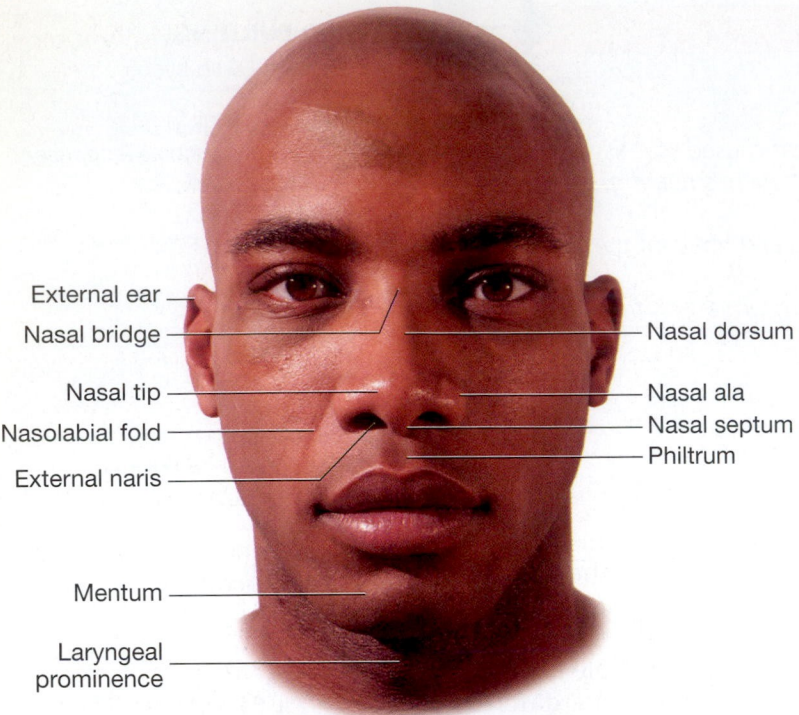

External ear
Nasal bridge
Nasal tip
Nasolabial fold
External naris
Mentum
Laryngeal prominence
Nasal dorsum
Nasal ala
Nasal septum
Philtrum

Figure 16-5 ■ External nose, mouth, and neck.
The external nose is supported by the nasal bone, which transitions to cartilage at the tip of the nose. The tissues of the lips, mouth, and chin are supported by the maxilla and mandible bones. The laryngeal prominence in the neck is composed of cartilage.

Sinuses

A **sinus** is a hollow cavity within a bone that is lined with a mucous membrane. There are four pairs of sinuses, each located within the cranial bone for which they are named (see Figures 16-6 ■ and 16-7 ■). The **frontal sinuses** are within the frontal bone, just above each eyebrow. The **maxillary sinuses,** the largest of the sinuses, are within the maxilla on either side of the nose. The **ethmoid sinuses,** which are groups of small air cells rather than a hollow cavity, are within the ethmoid bone, between the nose and the eyes. The **sphenoid sinuses** are within the sphenoid bone, posterior to the eye and near the pituitary gland of the brain. As a group, these sinuses are also known as the **paranasal sinuses.**

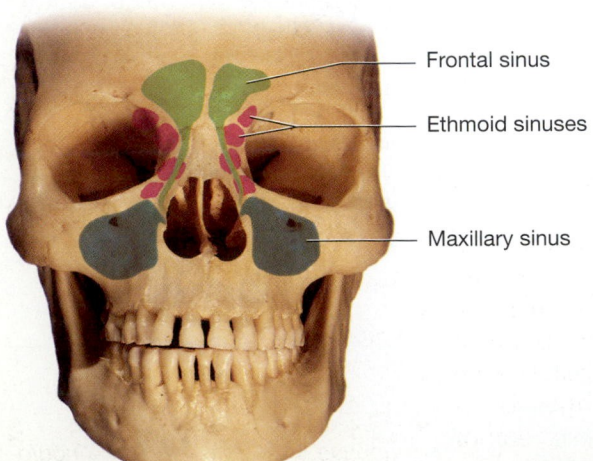

Frontal sinus
Ethmoid sinuses
Maxillary sinus

Figure 16-6 ■ Sinuses.
The sinuses are hollow cavities lined with mucosa within the frontal, maxillary, ethmoid, and sphenoid bones of the cranium and face.

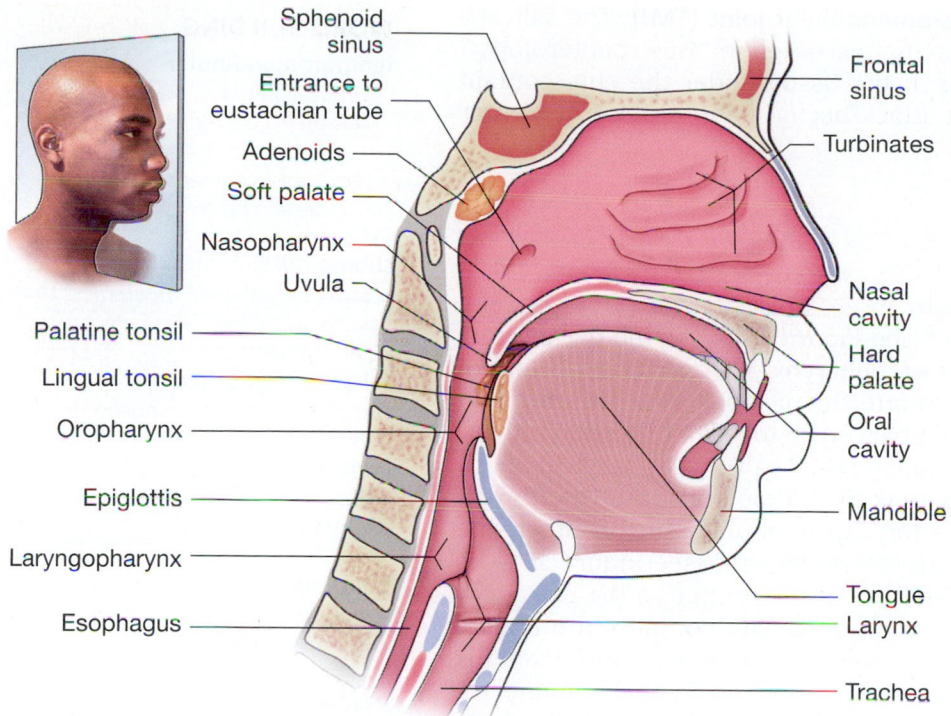

Figure 16-7 ■ **Structures of the internal nose, mouth, and throat.**
This midsagittal section of the head and neck shows the turbinates in the nasal cavity, the structures of the oral cavity, the tonsils and adenoids, and the three parts of the pharynx. Note how anatomically close the pharynx is to the bones of the spinal column.

Nasal Cavity

The **nasal septum** is a vertical wall of cartilage that divides the nasal cavity into right and left sides. In the posterior nasal cavity, this cartilage becomes the ethmoid bone of the cranium. The **nasal cavity** inside the nose is formed by the ethmoid bone of the cranium and by the maxilla of the upper jaw. Along the walls of the nasal cavity are three long, bony projections—the **superior, middle,** and **inferior turbinates.** These are also known as the **nasal conchae.** They are covered with **mucosa,** a mucous membrane that continuously produces **mucus.** They divide and slow down inhaled air and give it warmth and moisture.

Oral Cavity

The **oral cavity** or mouth contains the tongue, hard palate, soft palate, uvula, and teeth (see Figure 16-7). The oral cavity is lined with **oral mucosa** (mucous membrane); it is known as **buccal mucosa** in the cheek area. The **hard palate** or roof of the mouth divides the oral cavity from the nasal cavity. The hard palate is made up of three different cranial bones: the maxilla at the front of the mouth, then the palatine bone, and the vomer bone at the back of the mouth. The posterior hard palate transitions to the tissue of the **soft palate** and the **uvula,** the fleshy hanging part of the soft palate. The mandible forms the floor of the mouth, and the base of the **tongue** is attached to it. Each end of the mandible is attached to the temporal bone of

WORD BUILDING

nasal (NAY-zal)
  nas/o- *nose*
  -al *pertaining to*
Nasal is the adjective form for *nose.* The combining form *rhin/o-* also means *nose.*

septum (SEP-tum)

septal (SEP-tal)
  sept/o- *septum (dividing wall)*
  -al *pertaining to*

cavity (KAV-ih-tee)
  cav/o- *hollow space*
  -ity *state; condition*

superior (soo-PEER-ee-or)
  super/o- *above*
  -ior *pertaining to*

inferior (in-FEER-ee-or)
  infer/o- *below*
  -ior *pertaining to*

turbinate (TER-bih-nayt)
  turbin/o- *scroll-like structure; turbinate*
  -ate *composed of; pertaining to …*

concha (CON-kah)

conchae (CON-kee)
Concha is a Latin singular noun. Form the plural by changing –a to –ae.

mucosa (myoo-KOH-sah)

mucosal (myoo-KOH-sal)
  mucos/o- *mucous membrane*
  -al *pertaining to*

mucus (MYOO-kus)

oral (OR-al)
  or/o- *mouth*
  -al *pertaining to*
Oral is the adjective form for *mouth.*

buccal (BUK-al)
  bucc/o- *cheek*
  -al *pertaining to*

palate (PAL-at)

uvula (YOO-vyoo-lah)

glossal (GLAWS-al)
  gloss/o- *tongue*
  -al *pertaining to*
Glossal is the adjective form for *tongue.* The combining form *lingu/o-* also means *tongue.*

the cranium at the moveable **temporomandibular joint (TMJ)**. The salivary glands secrete saliva into the oral cavity (discussed in "Gastroenterology," Chapter 3). **Submental lymph nodes** in the tissue under the chin contain lymphocytes and macrophages that attack bacteria and viruses that enter the body through the oral cavity.

Pharynx

The **pharynx** or throat is divided into three areas: the nasopharynx, the oropharynx, and the laryngopharynx (see Figure 16-7). As the nasal cavity continues posteriorly, it becomes the **nasopharynx** or uppermost portion of the throat. The eustachian tubes open into the nasopharynx. The roof and walls of the nasopharynx contain the pharyngeal tonsil, a collection of lymphoid tissue commonly known as the **adenoids**. As the nasopharynx continues inferiorly, it becomes the **oropharynx** or middle portion of the throat. The oropharynx contains the **palatine tonsils,** lymphoid tissue on either side of the throat where the soft palate arches downward (see Figure 16-8 ■). The **laryngopharynx** extends from the base of the tongue to the entrances to the esophagus and larynx. The laryngopharynx contains the **lingual tonsils** on either side of the base of the tongue. The tonsils and adenoids are part of the lymphatic system, and they function in the immune response. They contain lymphocytes and macrophages that attack bacteria and viruses in the tissues around the oral cavity.

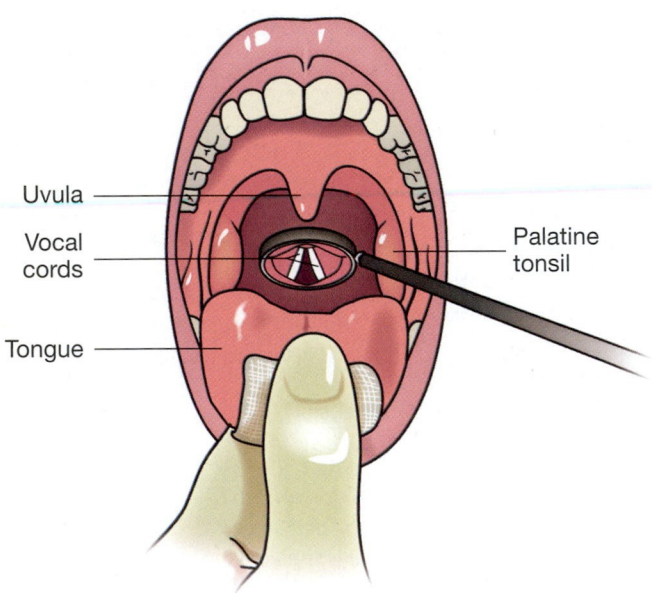

Uvula

Vocal cords

Tongue

Palatine tonsil

Figure 16-8 ■ **Pharynx.**

The pharynx can be examined by holding the tongue with a piece of gauze and pulling it forward. The palatine tonsils can be seen on either side of the oropharynx. A laryngeal mirror can visualize the vocal cords in the larynx. The image of the vocal cords as reflected in the mirror is upside down when compared to the actual position of the vocal cords. The laryngeal mirror can be turned upward to examine the nasopharynx.

Larynx

At its inferior end, the pharynx ends and merges into the larynx that leads to the trachea and the esophagus that leads to the stomach. The **larynx** or voice box is a short, triangular structure. It is surrounded by two thick rings of cartilage that can be clearly seen at the front of the neck as the **laryngeal prominence** (Adam's apple) (see Figure 16-5). At the superior end of the larynx is the **epiglottis**, a lidlike structure (see Figure 16-7). In the middle of the larynx is the **glottis**, a V-shaped structure of cartilage, ligaments, and the **vocal cords** (see Figure 16-8). When you swallow, the larynx moves superiorly and closes against the epiglottis to keep food from entering the lungs. Otherwise, the larynx remains open during breathing, speaking, or singing to allow air to pass over the vocal cords.

The vocal cords relax or tighten to lower or raise the pitch. Men have a large larynx and long vocal cords that vibrate at a slow frequency and produce a lower-pitched voice. Women have shorter vocal cords and a higher-pitched voice. The volume of air from the lungs affects how loud or soft the voice is. The sound of the voice also resonates in the sinuses, adding fullness.

Did You Know?

During speech, exhaled air from the lungs causes the vocal cords to vibrate in a wavelike fashion up to 100 times per second. These vibrations produce sound waves. As the sound waves travel from the vocal cords, they are shaped by the soft palate, tongue, and lips into spoken words.

WORD BUILDING

larynx (LAIR-ingks)

laryngeal (lah-RIN-jee-al)
  laryng/o- *larynx (voice box)*
  -eal *pertaining to*

epiglottis (EP-ih-GLAWT-is)
  epi- *upon; above*
  glott/o- *glottis (of the larynx)*
  -ic *pertaining to*

glottis (GLAWT-is)

vocal (VOH-kal)
  voc/o- *voice*
  -al *pertaining to*

Physiology of the Sense of Hearing

The external ear captures sound waves. They travel down the external auditory canal to the tympanic membrane (see Figure 16-9 ■). There, the sound waves are converted to mechanical motion as they cause the tympanic membrane to move inward and outward. As the tympanic membrane moves, it moves the malleus, the incus, and then the stapes of the middle ear. The stapes transmits this mechanical motion to the oval window. This causes the fluid-filled vestibule to vibrate. This vibration is transmitted to the cochlea. (When the vibration has traveled through the cochlea, it comes back to the vestibule where it causes the round window to bulge. The round window acts as a safety valve in the otherwise rigid bony walls around the inner ear.) Down the length of the coiled cochlea, tiny hair cells detect the loudness (intensity) and pitch (frequency) of the sound. The loudness of the sound correlates to the degree to which the hair cells are distorted. The various frequencies in the sound correlate to the location in the cochlea of the stimulated hairs. The hair cells then send this sensory information as nerve impulses through the cochlear branch of the **vestibulocochlear nerve** (cranial nerve VIII) to the medulla oblongata in the brainstem. From there, the impulses are relayed to the **auditory cortex** in each temporal lobe of the brain.

WORD BUILDING

vestibulocochlear
(ves-TIB-yoo-loh-KOH-klee-ar)
 vestibul/o- *vestibule (entrance)*
 cochle/o- *cochlea (of the inner ear)*
 -ar *pertaining to*

auditory (AW-dih-TOH-ree)
 audit/o- *the sense of hearing*
 -ory *having the function of*
The combining forms *audi/o-* and *acous/o-* also mean *the sense of hearing.*

cortex (KOR-teks)

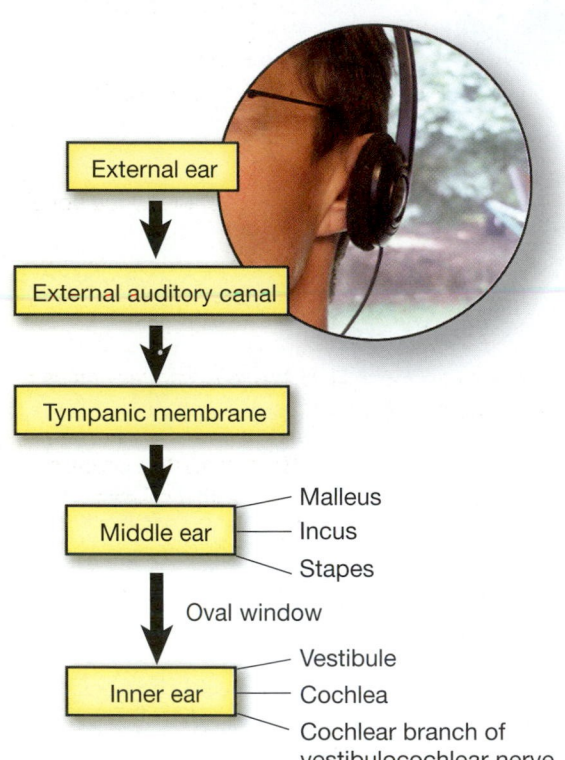

External ear

External auditory canal

Tympanic membrane

Middle ear — Malleus
— Incus
— Stapes

Oval window

Inner ear — Vestibule
— Cochlea
— Cochlear branch of vestibulocochlear nerve

Figure 16-9 ■ The sense of hearing.
Sound travels as sound waves through the external ear canal. Then it is converted to mechanical motion in the middle ear. In the inner ear, it is converted to nerve impulses that travel through the cochlear branch of the vestibulocochlear nerve (cranial nerve VIII).

Vocabulary Review

Ears		
Word or Phrase	**Description**	**Combining Forms**
auditory cortex	Area in each temporal lobe of the brain where sensory information from the ears is interpreted for the sense of hearing	**audit/o-** *the sense of hearing* **audi/o-** *the sense of hearing* **acous/o-** *hearing; sound*
auricle	The visible external ear. It is also known as the **pinna.**	**aur/i-** *ear* **auricul/o-** *ear* **ot/o-** *ear*
cerumen	Sticky wax secreted by glands in the external auditory canal. It traps dirt.	
cochlea	Coiled structure of the inner ear associated with the sense of hearing. It relays sensory information to the brain via the cochlear branch of the vestibulocochlear nerve.	**cochle/o-** *cochlea (of the inner ear)*
eustachian tube	Tube that connects the middle ear to the nasopharynx and equalizes the air pressure between the middle ear and the throat	
external auditory canal	Passageway from the external ear to the middle ear. It contains glands that secrete cerumen.	**extern/o-** *outside* **audit/o-** *the sense of hearing*
external auditory meatus	Opening at the entrance to the external auditory canal	**extern/o-** *outside* **audit/o-** *the sense of hearing*
helix	Rim of tissue and cartilage that forms the C shape of the external ear	
incus	Second bone of the middle ear. It is attached to the malleus on one end and the stapes on the other end. It is also known as the **anvil.**	**incud/o-** *incus (anvil-shaped bone)*
labyrinth	All of the structures of the inner ear	**labyrinth/o-** *labyrinth (of the inner ear)*
malleus	First bone of the middle ear. It is attached to the tympanic membrane on one end and to the incus on the other end. It is also known as the **hammer.**	**malle/o-** *malleus (hammer-shaped bone)*
mastoid process	Bony projection of the temporal bone behind the ear	**mast/o-** *breast; mastoid process* **mastoid/o-** *mastoid process*
ossicles	The three tiny bones of the middle ear: malleus, incus, and stapes. They are also known as the **ossicular chain.**	**ossicul/o-** *ossicle (little bone)* **ossic/o-** *bone*
oval window	Opening in the temporal bone between the middle ear and the vestibule of the inner ear. The opening is covered by the end of the stapes.	
round window	Opening in the temporal bone between the middle ear and the vestibule of the inner ear. The opening is covered with a membrane.	
semicircular canals	Three separate but intertwined canals in the inner ear that are oriented in different planes (horizontally, vertically, obliquely). They help the body keep its balance. They relay sensory information to the brain via the vestibular branch of the vestibulocochlear nerve.	**circul/o-** *circle*
stapes	Third bone of the middle ear. It is attached to the incus on one end and to the oval window on the other end. It is also known as the **stirrup.**	**staped/o-** *stapes (stirrup-shaped bone)*

Word or Phrase	Description	Combining Forms
tragus	Triangular cartilage anterior to the external auditory meatus of the ear	
tympanic membrane	Membrane that divides the external ear from the middle ear. It is also known as the **eardrum.**	**tympan/o-** *tympanic membrane (eardrum)* **myring/o-** *tympanic membrane (eardrum)*
vestibule	Structure at the entrance to the inner ear. It is filled with fluid and is in contact with the oval window and round window. The ends of the vestibule become the semicircular canals and the cochlea.	**vestibul/o-** *vestibule (entrance)*
vestibulocochlear nerve	Cranial nerve VIII that conducts sensory impulses from the semicircular canals and the cochlea to the medulla oblongata of the brainstem	**vestibul/o-** *vestibule (entrance)* **cochle/o-** *cochlea (of the inner ear)*

Sinuses

Word or Phrase	Description	Combining Forms
ethmoid sinuses	Groups of small air cells in the ethmoid bone between the nose and the eyes	**ethm/o-** *sieve*
frontal sinuses	Sinuses above each eyebrow in the frontal bone of the cranium	**front/o-** *front*
maxillary sinuses	Largest of the sinuses. They are on either side of the nose in the maxilla (upper jaw)	**maxill/o-** *maxilla (upper jaw)*
sinus	Hollow cavity within a cranial or facial bone. It is lined with mucosa. The **paranasal sinuses** include all of the sinuses.	**sinus/o-** *sinus* **nas/o-** *nose*
sphenoid sinuses	Sinuses in the sphenoid bone posterior to the nasal cavity and near the pituitary gland of the brain	**sphen/o-** *wedge shape*

Nose and Nasal Cavity

Word or Phrase	Description	Combining Forms
ala	Flared cartilage on each side of the nostril	
mucosa	Mucous membrane lining the nasal cavity that warms and moisturizes the incoming air. It also produces **mucus** to trap foreign particles.	**mucos/o-** *mucous membrane*
naris	One nostril, the opening into the nasal cavity	
nasal cavity	Hollow area inside the nose that is formed by the ethmoid and maxillary bones. It is lined with mucosa.	**nas/o-** *nose* **cav/o-** *hollow space* **rhin/o-** *nose*
nasal dorsum	Vertical ridge in the middle of the external nose. It is supported by the nasal bone.	**dors/o-** *back; dorsum*
nasal septum	Wall of cartilage and bone that divides the nasal cavity into right and left sides	**sept/o-** *septum (dividing wall)*
turbinates	Three long projections of bone (**superior, middle, and inferior turbinates**) covered with mucosa, that jut into the nasal cavity. They break up and give moisture to the air as it enters the nose. They are also known as the **nasal conchae.**	**turbin/o-** *scroll-like structure; turbinate* **super/o-** *above* **infer/o-** *below*

Mouth and Oral Cavity

Word or Phrase	Description	Combining Forms
hard palate	Bone that divides the nasal cavity from the oral cavity. It is made up of the maxilla, palatine, and vomer bones. It is also known as the roof of the mouth.	**palat/o-** *palate*
mentum	The chin. The most anterior part of the mandible (lower jaw).	**ment/o-** *mind; chin*
mucosa	Mucous membrane that produces **mucus.** The **oral mucosa** lines the oral cavity. The **buccal mucosa** lines the cheek area of the oral cavity.	**mucos/o-** *mucous membrane* **or/o-** *mouth* **bucc/o-** *cheek*
nasolabial fold	Skin crease in the cheek from the nose to the lip at the corner of the mouth	**nas/o-** *nose* **labi/o-** *lip; labrum* **cheil/o-** *lip*
oral cavity	Hollow area inside of the mouth that contains the tongue, teeth, hard and soft palates, and uvula. It is lined with oral mucosa.	**or/o-** *mouth*
philtrum	Vertical grooves in the skin of the upper lip	
soft palate	Soft tissue extension of the hard palate at the back of the throat. It ends with the **uvula.**	**palat/o-** *palate*
submental lymph nodes	Lymph nodes in the tissues beneath the chin	**ment/o-** *mind; chin*
temporo-mandibular joint	Moveable joint where ligaments attach each end of the mandible (lower jaw) to the temporal bones of the cranium	**tempor/o-** *temple (side of the head)* **mandibul/o-** *mandible (lower jaw)*
tongue	Large muscle in the oral cavity that is attached to the mandible	**gloss/o-** *tongue* **lingu/o-** *tongue*

Pharynx

Word or Phrase	Description	Combining Forms
adenoids	Lymphoid tissue in the nasopharynx. They are also known as the **pharyngeal tonsils.**	**aden/o-** *gland* **adenoid/o-** *adenoids* **pharyng/o-** *pharynx (throat)* **tonsill/o-** *tonsil*
laryngopharynx	Most inferior part of the throat. It extends from the base of the tongue to the larynx and the entrance to the esophagus.	**laryng/o-** *larynx (voice box)* **pharyng/o-** *pharynx (throat)*
lingual tonsils	Lymphoid tissue located on both sides of the base of the tongue in the laryngopharynx	**lingu/o-** *tongue* **tonsill/o-** *tonsil*
nasopharynx	Uppermost portion of the throat where the posterior nares unite. The nasopharynx contains the openings for the eustachian tubes and the adenoids.	**nas/o-** *nose* **pharyng/o-** *pharynx (throat)*
oropharynx	Middle portion of the throat that lies posterior to the oral cavity. It extends from the soft palate to the epiglottis. It contains the palatine tonsils.	**or/o-** *mouth* **pharyng/o-** *pharynx (throat)*
palatine tonsils	Lymphoid tissue in the oropharynx on either side of the throat where the soft palate arches downward	**palat/o-** *palate* **tonsill/o-** *tonsil*
pharynx	The throat. It is composed of the nasopharynx, oropharynx, and laryngopharynx.	**pharyng/o-** *pharynx (throat)*

Larynx

Word or Phrase	Description	Combining Forms
epiglottis	Lidlike structure that covers the top of the larynx during swallowing	**glott/o-** *glottis (of the larynx)*
glottis	V-shaped structure in the larynx. It contains cartilage, ligaments, and the vocal cords.	**glott/o-** *glottis (of the larynx)*
larynx	Triangular structure in the anterior neck (visible as the **laryngeal prominence** or Adam's apple). It contains the glottis.	**laryng/o-** *larynx (voice box)*
vocal cords	Connective tissue bands in the glottis that vibrate and produce sounds during speaking and singing	**voc/o-** *voice*

Labeling Exercise

Match each anatomy word or phrase to its structure and write it in the numbered box for each figure. Be sure to check your spelling. Use the Answer Key at the end of the book to check your answers.

cochlea	incus	round window	tympanic membrane
cochlear branch of	malleus	semicircular canals	vestibular branch of
vestibulocochlear nerve	mastoid bone	stapes	vestibulocochlear nerve
eustachian tube	oval window	temporal bone	vestibule
external auditory canal			

1.

2.

3.

4.

5.

6.

7.

8.

9.

10.

11.

12.

13.

14.

15.

adenoids
entrance to eustachian tube
epiglottis
esophagus
frontal sinus
hard palate

laryngopharynx
larynx
lingual tonsil
mandible
nasal cavity

nasopharynx
oral cavity
oropharynx
palatine tonsil
soft palate

sphenoid sinus
tongue
trachea
turbinates or conchae
uvula

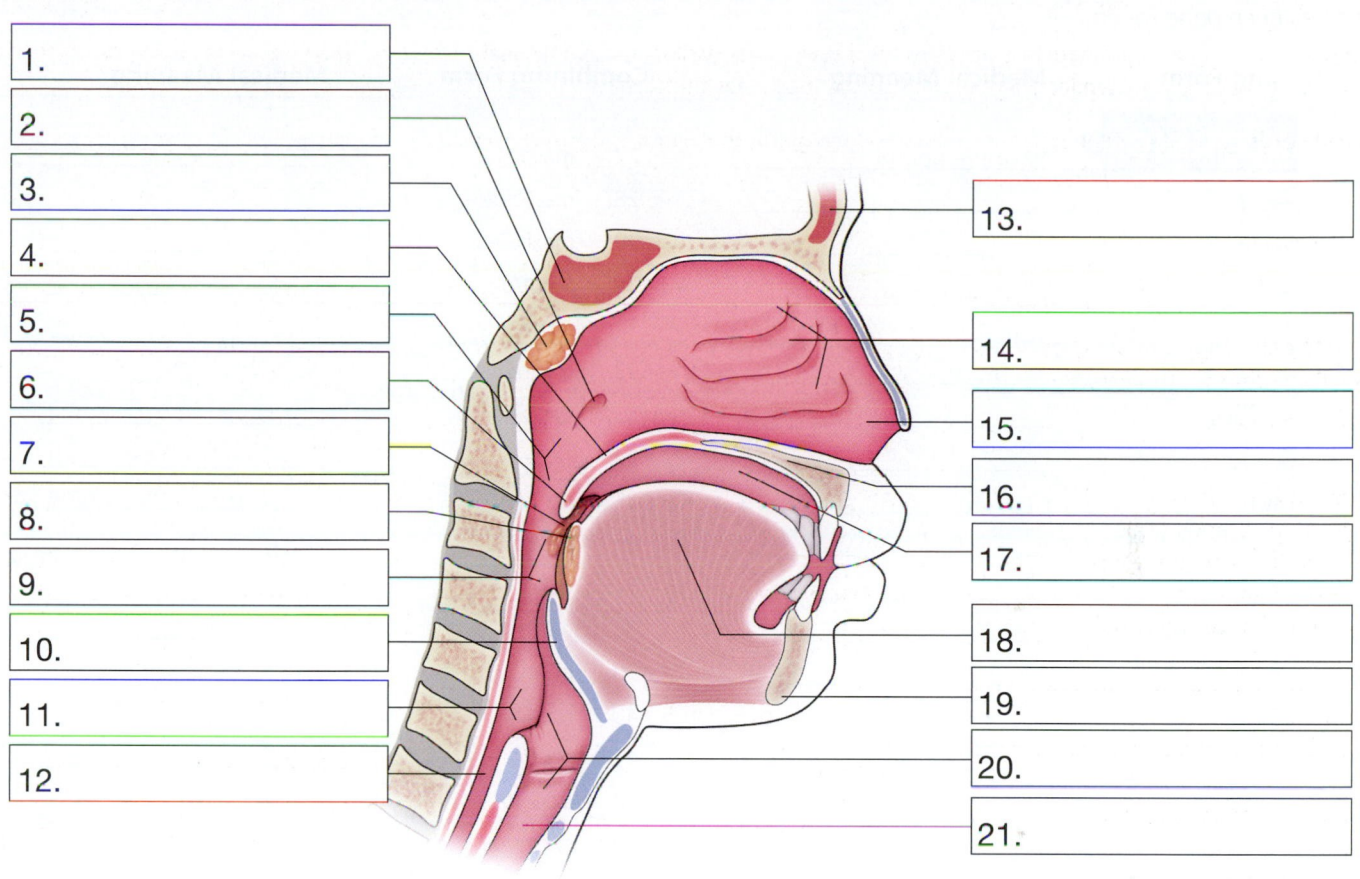

1. _____

2. _____

3. _____

4. _____

5. _____

6. _____

7. _____

8. _____

9. _____

10. _____

11. _____

12. _____

13. _____

14. _____

15. _____

16. _____

17. _____

18. _____

19. _____

20. _____

21. _____

Building Medical Words

Use the Answer Key at the end of the book to check your answers.

Combining Forms Exercise

Before you build ENT words, review these combining forms. Next to each combining form, write its medical meaning. The first one has been done for you.

Combining Form	Medical Meaning	Combining Form	Medical Meaning
1. **acous/o-**	hearing; sound	27. mast/o-	
2. aden/o-		28. mastoid/o-	
3. adenoid/o-		29. maxill/o-	
4. audi/o-		30. ment/o-	
5. audit/o-		31. mucos/o-	
6. aur/i-		32. myring/o-	
7. auricul/o-		33. nas/o-	
8. bucc/o-		34. or/o-	
9. cav/o-		35. ossic/o-	
10. cheil/o-		36. ossicul/o-	
11. circul/o-		37. ot/o-	
12. cochle/o-		38. palat/o-	
13. dors/o-		39. pharyng/o-	
14. ethm/o-		40. rhin/o-	
15. extern/o-		41. sept/o-	
16. front/o-		42. sinus/o-	
17. gloss/o-		43. sphen/o-	
18. glott/o-		44. staped/o-	
19. incud/o-		45. super/o-	
20. infer/o-		46. tempor/o-	
21. labi/o-		47. tonsill/o-	
22. labyrinth/o-		48. turbin/o-	
23. laryng/o-		49. tympan/o-	
24. lingu/o-		50. vestibul/o-	
25. malle/o-		51. voc/o-	
26. mandibul/o-			

Combining Form and Suffix Exercise

Read the definition of the medical word. Look at the combining form that is given. Select the correct suffix from the Suffix List and write it on the blank line. Then build the medical word and write it on the line. (Remember: You may need to remove the combining vowel. Always remove the hyphens and slash.) Be sure to check your spelling. The first one has been done for you.

SUFFIX LIST

-al (pertaining to)	-eal (pertaining to)	-oid (resembling)
-ar (pertaining to)	-ial (pertaining to)	-ory (having the function of)
-ate (composed of; pertaining to)	-ic (pertaining to)	-pharynx (pharynx; throat)
-cle (small thing)		

Definition of the Medical Word	Combining Form	Suffix	Build the Medical Word
1. Pertaining to the palate	**palat/o-**	**-al**	*palatal*
(You think *pertaining to* (-al) + *the palate* (palat/o-). You change the order of the word parts to put the suffix last. You write *palatal*.)			
2. Pertaining to the nose	nas/o-		
3. Having the function of the sense of hearing	audit/o-		
4. Pertaining to the eardrum	tympan/o-		
5. Pertaining to the septum	sept/o-		
6. Composed of a scroll-like structure	turbin/o-		
7. Pertaining to a tonsil	tonsill/o-		
8. Pertaining to the cheek	bucc/o-		
9. Pertaining to the stirrup-shaped bone (in the middle ear)	staped/o-		
10. (Sinus that is) resembling a sieve	ethm/o-		
11. Pertaining to the throat	pharyng/o-		
12. Pertaining to the tongue	gloss/o-		
13. (The part of the) throat (nearest to the) nose	nas/o-		
14. (Lymph structure that is) resembling a gland	aden/o-		
15. Pertaining to the tongue	lingu/o-		
16. Pertaining to the mucous membrane	mucos/o-		
17. Pertaining to the ear	auricul/o-		
18. Pertaining to the mouth	or/o-		
19. Pertaining to (a chain of) little bones (in the middle ear)	ossicul/o-		
20. Small thing (that is the) ear	aur/i-		
21. (Bony process behind the ear) resembling a breast	mast/o-		
22. Pertaining to the voice box	laryng/o-		

Diseases and Conditions

Ears		
Word or Phrase	**Description**	**Word Building**
acoustic neuroma	Benign (not cancerous) tumor of the vestibulocochlear nerve. Depending on the location of the tumor, it can cause pain, dizziness, or hearing loss. Treatment: Surgical excision.	**acoustic** (ah-KOOS-tik) **acous/o-** *hearing; sound* **-tic** *pertaining to* **neuroma** (nyoo-ROH-mah) **neur/o-** *nerve* **-oma** *tumor; mass*
cerumen impaction	Cerumen (earwax), epithelial cells, and hair form a mass that occludes the external auditory canal. It occurs most commonly in older adults because of dry skin, thick cerumen, growth of hair in the external auditory canal and/or the presence of a hearing aid. Treatment: Removal with forceps (see Figure 16-10 ■) or ear drops to soften and wash away cerumen.	**impaction** (im-PAK-shun) **impact/o-** *wedged in* **-ion** *action; condition*

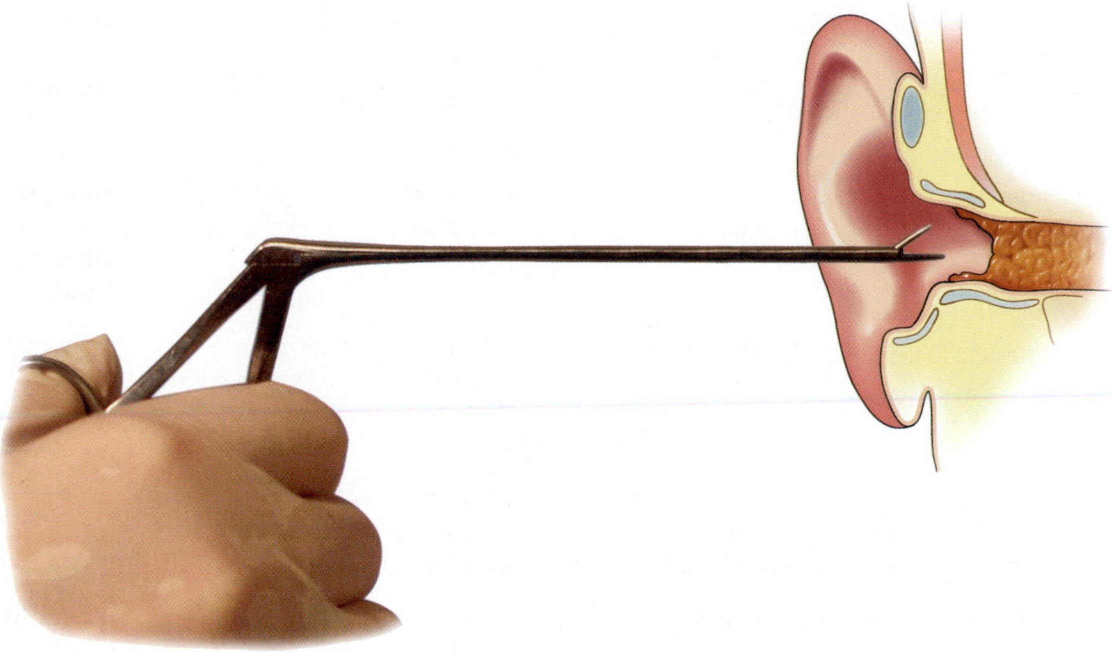

Figure 16-10 ■ Cerumen impaction.
Alligator forceps are used to enter the external auditory canal and remove impacted cerumen or a foreign body. Alligator forceps are so-named because the shape resembles the long nose and open, biting jaws of an alligator.

cholesteatoma	Benign, slow-growing tumor in the middle ear. It contains cholesterol deposits and epithelial cells. It can eventually destroy the bones of the middle ear and extend into the air cells within the mastoid process. The underlying cause usually is chronic otitis media. Treatment: Surgical excision.	**cholesteatoma** (koh-LES-tee-ah-TOH-mah) *Cholesteatoma* is a combination of the word *cholesterol*, the Greek word *stear* (animal fat), and the suffix *-oma* (tumor; mass).

Word or Phrase	Description	Word Building

hearing loss	Progressive, permanent decline in the ability to hear sounds in one or both ears. A foreign body or infection in the external auditory canal, perforation of the tympanic membrane, fluid behind the tympanic membrane, or degeneration of the ossicles of the middle ear keep sound waves from reaching the inner ear. These are types of **conductive hearing loss.** Otosclerosis is also a form of conductive hearing loss (see description in this section). Other causes of hearing loss include disease of the cochlea, damage to the inner ear from excessive noise, or changes due to aging that hinder the production or sending of sensory impulses to the vestibulocochlear nerve. These are types of **sensorineural hearing loss.** A combination of both conductive and sensorineural hearing loss is a **mixed hearing loss. Low-frequency hearing loss** is the inability to hear low-pitched sounds. **High-frequency hearing loss** is the inability to hear high-pitched sounds. Patients with a hearing loss are said to be **hearing impaired** or hard of hearing. **Presbycusis** is bilateral hearing loss due to aging. Total deafness is known as **anakusis.** Deaf-mutism is deafness coupled with the inability to speak. Treatment: Correct the underlying cause; hearing aid; in some cases a cochlear implant may be needed.	**conductive** (con-DUK-tiv)
		   conduct/o- *carrying; conveying*
		   -ive *pertaining to*
		
		sensorineural
		(SEN-soh-ree-NYOOR-al)
		   sensor/i- *sensory*
		   neur/o- *nerve*
		   -al *pertaining to*
		
		presbycusis (PREZ-bee-KOO-sis)
		   presby/o- *old age*
		   -acusis *abnormal condition of hearing*
		Delete the *a* on *–acusis* before joining the word parts.
		
		anakusis (AN-ah-KOO-sis)

Did You Know?
Tone deafness is not a type of hearing loss. It is the inability to identify musical notes and sing in tune with them.

Word or Phrase	Description	Word Building
hemotympanum	Blood in the middle ear behind the tympanic membrane. It can be caused by infection or trauma. Treatment: None usually needed. Treat any infection.	**hemotympanum** (HEE-moh-TIM-pah-num) The combining form *hem/o-* means *blood.*

labyrinthitis	Bacterial or viral infection of the semicircular canals, causing severe vertigo. Treatment: Antibiotic drug for a bacterial infection. Viruses are not sensitive to antibiotic drugs.	**labyrinthitis** (LAB-ih-rin-THY-tis)
		   labyrinth/o- *labyrinth (of the inner ear)*
		   -itis *inflammation of; infection of*

Meniere's disease	Edema of the semicircular canals with destruction of the cochlea, causing tinnitus, vertigo, and hearing loss. It can be caused by head trauma or middle ear infections. Treatment: Correct the underlying cause.	**Meniere's** (MEN-eh-AIRZ)
motion sickness	There is **dysequilibrium** with headache, dizziness, nausea, and vomiting. It is caused by riding in a car, boat, or airplane. Treatment: Drug to treat motion sickness.	**dysequilibrium** (DIS-ee-kwih-LIB-ree-um)

otitis externa	Bacterial infection of the external auditory canal. There is throbbing earache pain (**otalgia**) with a swollen, red canal and serous or purulent drainage. It is caused by a foreign body in the ear or by the patient scratching or probing inside the ear. It is also seen in swimmers whose ear canals are rubbed by ear plugs or softened by exposure to water. It is also known as **swimmer's ear.** Treatment: Correct the underlying cause; topical or oral antibiotic drug.	**otitis externa** (oh-TY-tis eks-TER-nah)
		   ot/o- *ear*
		   -itis *inflammation of; infection of*
		
		otalgia (oh-TAL-jee-ah)
		   ot/o- *ear*
		   alg/o- *pain*
		   -ia *condition; state; thing*

Word or Phrase	Description	Word Building
otitis media	Acute or chronic bacterial infection of the middle ear. There is **myringitis** (redness and inflammation of the tympanic membrane), otalgia, a feeling of pressure, and bulging of the tympanic membrane. There can be an **effusion** (a collection of fluid behind the tympanic membrane that creates an air-fluid level) (see Figure 16-11 ■). This fluid can be **serous** (clear) or **suppurative** (with pus). In children, the effusion can be so thick that it is called **glue ear**. Chronic otitis media can cause a perforation of the tympanic membrane (see Figure 16-12 ■). Otitis media is common in young children because the short eustachian tube is in a nearly horizontal position that allows bacteria to enter from the nasopharynx. If otitis media is left untreated, the tympanic membrane can rupture or the bones of the middle ear can degenerate, resulting in permanent hearing loss. The mastoid process of the temporal bone can also become infected (**mastoiditis**). Treatment: Antibiotic drug; surgery to insert tubes to drain the middle ear.	**otitis media** (oh-TY-tis MEE-dee-ah) **ot/o-** *ear* **-itis** *inflammation of; infection of* **myringitis** (MIR-in-JY-tis) **myring/o-** *tympanic membrane (eardrum)* **-itis** *inflammation of; infection of* **effusion** (ee-FYOO-shun) **effus/o-** *a pouring out* **-ion** *action; condition* **serous** (SEER-us) **ser/o-** *serum of the blood; serumlike fluid* **-ous** *pertaining to* **suppurative** (SUP-uh-RAH-tiv) **suppur/o-** *pus formation* **-ative** *pertaining to* **mastoiditis** (MAS-toy-DY-tis) **mastoid/o-** *mastoid process* **-itis** *inflammation of; infection of*

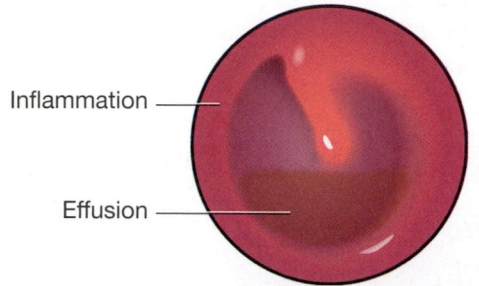

Inflammation

Effusion

Figure 16-11 ■ Myringitis.

The tympanic membrane is red and inflamed. There is dullness with no light reflex. There is a loss of normal landmarks (visibility of the malleus), and the entire tympanic membrane bulges out into the external auditory canal. Fluid from an effusion in the middle ear creates an air-fluid level that can be seen through the tympanic membrane.

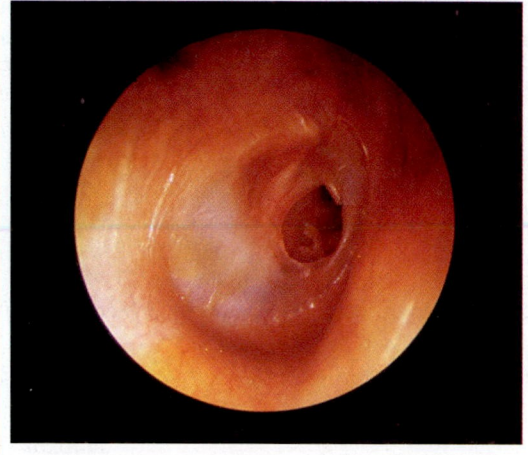

Figure 16-12 ■ Perforated tympanic membrane.

This child's tympanic membrane shows pus and debris in the middle ear with a perforation caused by chronic otitis media.

Word Alert

SOUND-ALIKE WORDS

mastoiditis	(noun)	infection of the air cells in the bone of the mastoid process *Example: The middle ear infection progressed to become mastoiditis.*
mastitis	(noun)	infection of the mammary glands of the breast *Example: Mastitis can develop in nursing mothers.*

otorrhea	Drainage of serous fluid or pus from the ear. It can be caused by otitis externa or otitis media (with a ruptured tympanic membrane). It can also be caused by a fracture of the temporal bone of the cranium with leakage of cerebrospinal fluid through the ear. Treatment: Correct the underlying cause.	**otorrhea** (OH-toh-REE-ah) **ot/o-** *ear* **-rrhea** *flow; discharge*

Word or Phrase	Description	Word Building
otosclerosis	Abnormal deposit of bone in the inner ear, particularly between the stapes and the oval window. The stapes becomes immoveable, causing conductive hearing loss. Certain families have a genetic predisposition to develop otosclerosis. Treatment: Hearing aid, stapedectomy.	**otosclerosis** (OH-toh-skleh-ROH-sis) **ot/o-** *ear* **scler/o-** *hard; sclera (white of the eye)* **-osis** *condition; abnormal condition; process*
ruptured tympanic membrane	Tear in the tympanic membrane due to excessive pressure or infection. In pilots and deep sea divers, unequal air pressure in the middle ear compared to the surrounding air or water pressure can rupture the tympanic membrane. Treatment: Tympanoplasty.	
tinnitus	Sounds (buzzing, ringing, hissing, or roaring) that are heard constantly or intermittently in one or both ears, even in a quiet environment. It is caused by repeated exposure to excessive noise and is associated with hearing loss. It can also be related to the overuse of aspirin. Treatment: Soft background noise (hum of a fan or a device that generates "white noise") to mask tinnitus and allow the patient to sleep.	**tinnitus** (TIN-ih-tus) (tih-NY-tus)
vertigo	Sensation of motion when the body is not moving. It is caused by an upper respiratory infection, middle ear or inner ear infection, head trauma, degenerative changes of the semicircular canals, or Meniere's disease. Treatment: Correct the underlying cause.	**vertigo** (VER-tih-goh)

Sinuses, Nose and Nasal Cavity

Word or Phrase	Description	Word Building
allergic rhinitis	Allergic symptoms in the nose. In response to an inhaled antigen (pollen, dust, animal dander, mold), the immune system produces histamine. This causes nasal stuffiness, sneezing, **rhinorrhea** (clear mucus discharge from the nose), hypertrophy (enlargement) of the turbinates in the nose with red, edematous, and boggy mucous membranes, and **postnasal drip (PND).** When this occurs in spring or fall and coincides with the blooming of certain trees and plants (grasses, maple trees, roses, goldenrod), it is known as **seasonal allergy** or **hay fever.** Treatment: Antihistamine drugs, decongestant drugs, corticosteroid drugs.	**allergic** (ah-LER-jik) **allerg/o-** *allergy* **-ic** *pertaining to* **rhinitis** (ry-NY-tis) **rhin/o-** *nose* **-itis** *inflammation of; infection of* **rhinorrhea** (RY-noh-REE-ah) **rhin/o-** *nose* **-rrhea** *flow; discharge* **postnasal** (post-NAY-zal) **post-** *after; behind* **nas/o-** *nose* **-al** *pertaining to*
anosmia	The temporary or permanent loss of the sense of smell. It is most often caused by head trauma.	**anosmia** (an-AWZ-mee-ah) **an-** *without; not* **osm/o-** *the sense of smell* **-ia** *condition; state; thing*
epistaxis	Sudden, sometimes severe bleeding from the nose. It is due to irritation or dryness of the nasal mucosa and the rupture of a small artery or it can be caused by trauma to the nose. It is also known as a **nosebleed.** Treatment: Topical cautery with heat or chemicals to stop severe bleeding.	**epistaxis** (EP-ih-STAK-sis)
polyp	Benign growth of the mucous membrane in the nose or sinuses. A single polyp may grow large enough to limit the flow of air, or there may be several polyps. Treatment: Polypectomy.	**polyp** (PAWL-ip)

Word or Phrase	Description	Word Building
rhinophyma	Redness and hypertrophy (enlargement) of the nose with small-to-large, irregular lumps. It is caused by the increased number of sebaceous glands associated with acne rosacea of the skin (discussed in "Dermatology," Chapter 7). Treatment: Topical drugs for acne rosacea.	**rhinophyma** (RY-noh-FY-mah) **rhin/o-** *nose* **-phyma** *tumor; growth*
septal deviation	Lateral displacement of the nasal septum, significantly narrowing one nasal airway. This can be a congenital condition or it can be caused by trauma to the nose. Treatment: Surgical correction (septoplasty).	
sinusitis	Acute or chronic bacterial infection in one or all of the sinus cavities (see Figure 16-13 ■). There is headache, pain in the forehead or cheekbones over the sinus, postnasal drainage, fatigue, and fever. **Pansinusitis** involves all the sinuses or all of the sinuses on one side of the face. Treatment: Antibiotic drug; sinus surgery.	**sinusitis** (SY-nyoo-SY-tis) **sinus/o-** *sinus* **-itis** *inflammation of; infection of* **pansinusitis** (PAN-sy-nyoo-SY-tis) **pan-** *all* **sinus/o-** *sinus* **-itis** *inflammation of; infection of*

Nasal septum

Mild sinusitis

Sinusitis with severe mucosal swelling

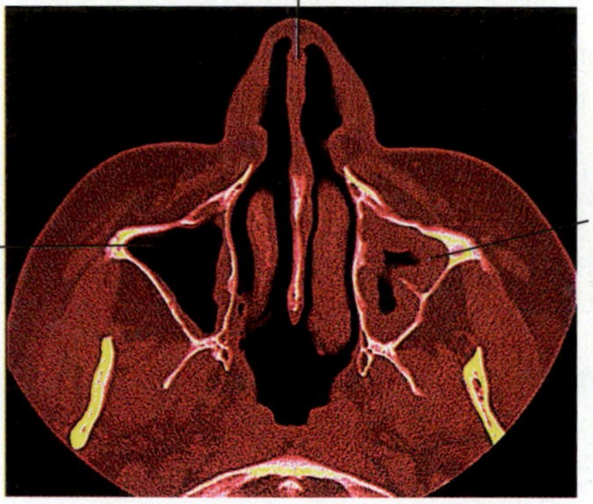

Figure 16-13 ■ Sinusitis.
This CT scan of the head shows the nose at the top of the image with the nasal septum. One of the maxillary sinuses shows sinusitis with severe swelling and thickening of the mucous membrane within the cavity. The other maxillary sinus shows minimal mucosal swelling and is a relatively open cavity.

Word or Phrase	Description	Word Building
upper respiratory infection (URI)	Bacterial or viral infection of the nose that can spread to the throat and ears. The nose is a part of the respiratory system as well as the ENT system. It is also known as a **common cold** or **head cold.** Treatment: Antibiotic drug for a bacterial infection.	

Mouth, Oral Cavity, Pharynx, and Neck

Word or Phrase	Description	Word Building
cancer of the mouth and neck	**Malignant** tumor (**carcinoma**) of squamous epithelial cells in the oral cavity (lips, tongue, gums, cheeks), throat, or larynx. Smoking and using smokeless chewing tobacco can cause this. Treatment: Surgical excision.	**malignant** (mah-LIG-nant) **malign/o-** *intentionally causing harm; cancer* **-ant** *pertaining to* **carcinoma** (KAR-sih-NOH-mah) **carcin/o-** *cancer* **-oma** *tumor; mass*
cervical lymphadenopathy	Enlargement of the lymph nodes in the neck. It is caused by infection, cancer, or the spread of a cancerous tumor from another site. Treatment: Correct the underlying cause.	**cervical** (SER-vih-kal) **cervic/o-** *neck; cervix* **-al** *pertaining to* **lymphadenopathy** (lim-FAD-eh-NAWP-ah-thee) **lymph/o-** *lymph; lymphatic system* **aden/o-** *gland* **-pathy** *disease; suffering*

Word or Phrase	Description	Word Building

cleft lip and palate	Congenital deformity in which the lip or the bones of the right and left maxilla fail to join in the center before birth. The resulting cleft in the skin and bone can be **unilateral** or **bilateral** (see Figure 16-14 ■). The cleft can also extend into the soft palate. The child has difficulty speaking and eating. Treatment: Surgical correction.	**cleft** (KLEFT)
		
		 unilateral (YOO-nih-LAT-eh-ral)
		   uni- *single; not paired*
		   later/o- *side*
		   -al *pertaining to*
		
		 bilateral (by-LAT-eh-ral)
		   bi- *two*
		   later/o- *side*
		   -al *pertaining to*

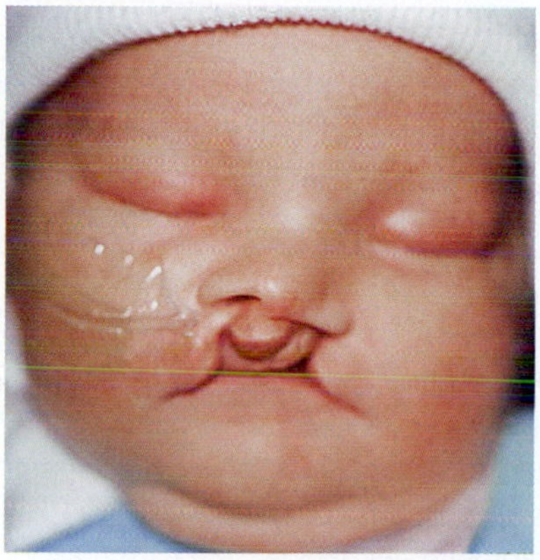

Figure 16-14 ■ Cleft lip and palate.
This infant has a bilateral cleft lip and palate. He has difficulty feeding from the breast or bottle because milk flows into the nasal cavity where it could be inhaled into the lungs. Note the feeding tube inserted in the right nostril and taped to the cheek; it goes to the stomach.

Word or Phrase	Description	Word Building
cold sores	Recurring, painful clusters of blisters on the lips or nose. They are caused by infection with **herpes simplex virus** type 1. After the initial infection, the virus remains dormant in a nerve until triggers of stress, sunlight, illness, or menstruation cause it to erupt again. These are also known as **fever blisters.** Treatment: Topical antiviral drug. *Note:* Herpes simplex type 2 causes genital herpes, a sexually transmitted disease (discussed in "Male Reproductive Medicine," Chapter 12).	**herpes simplex** (HER-peez SIM-pleks)

glossitis	Inflammation of the tongue. It is caused by irritation from spicy or hot food, a food allergy, an infection, or vitamin B deficiency. Treatment: Correct the underlying cause.	**glossitis** (glaw-SY-tis)
		   gloss/o- *tongue*
		   -itis *inflammation of; infection of*

leukoplakia	Benign, thickened, white patch on the mucous membrane of the mouth (see Figure 16-15 ■). It is caused by chronic irritation from tobacco use; it can become cancerous. It is also caused by irritation from an infection with the Epstein-Barr virus, seen in AIDS patients. Treatment: Correct the underlying cause.	**leukoplakia** (LOO-koh-PLAY-kee-ah)
		   leuk/o- *white*
		   plak/o- *plaque*
		   -ia *condition; state; thing*

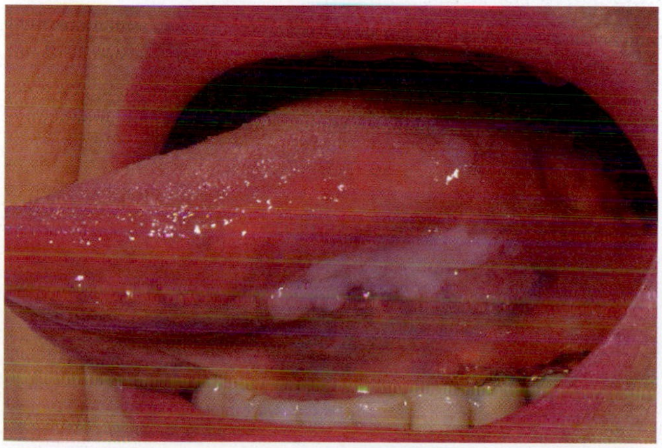

Figure 16-15 ■ Leukoplakia.
Leukoplakia is a precancerous condition. This leukoplakia is under the tongue, but it can occur anywhere in the mouth.

Word or Phrase	Description	Word Building
pharyngitis	Bacterial or viral infection of the throat. When it is caused by the bacterium group A beta-hemolytic **streptococcus,** it is known as **strep throat.** It is important to diagnose strep throat and treat it with an antibiotic drug so that it does not cause the complication of rheumatic heart disease. Treatment: Antibiotic drug.	**pharyngitis** (FAIR-in-JY-tis) **pharyng/o-** *pharynx (throat)* **-itis** *inflammation of; infection of* **streptococcus** (STREP-toh-KAWK-us) **strept/o-** *curved* **-coccus** *spherical bacterium*
temporo-mandibular joint (TMJ) syndrome	Dysfunction of the temporomandibular joint. There is clicking, pain, muscle spasm, and difficulty opening the jaw. It is caused by clenching or grinding the teeth (often during sleep) or by misalignment of the teeth. Treatment: Dental bite guard worn at night, correction of misaligned teeth.	**temporomandibular** (TEM-poh-ROH-man-DIB-yoo-lar) **tempor/o-** *temple (side of the head)* **mandibul/o-** *mandible (lower jaw)* **-ar** *pertaining to*
thrush	Oral infection caused by the yeast *Candida albicans.* It coats the tongue and oral mucosa (see Figure 16-16 ■). Thrush is common in infants, but is also seen in immunocompromised patients with AIDS because their immune system cannot control its growth. It also occurs after a course of antibiotic drugs kills bacteria in the mouth, allowing overgrowth of *Candida albicans.* It is also known as **oral candidiasis.** Treatment: Oral antiyeast drug.	**candidiasis** (KAN-dih-DY-ah-sis) **candid/o-** *Candida (a yeast)* **-iasis** *state of; process of*

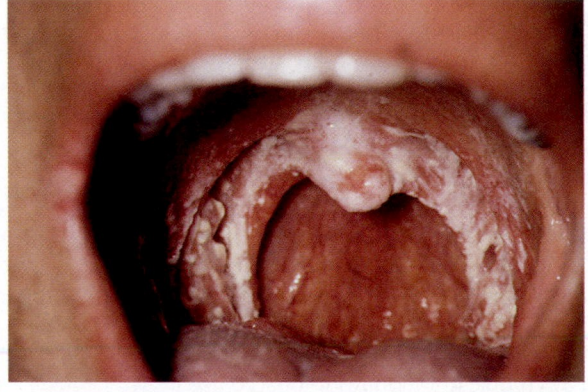

Figure 16-16 ■ Thrush.
The warm, moist environment of the mouth encourages the growth of this yeastlike fungus. It forms a thick white coating that resembles curdled milk, but cannot be wiped away. This 25-year-old man with AIDS has thrush (oral candidiasis) of the soft palate and oropharynx. This is an opportunistic infection that takes advantage of the patient's weakened immune system.

Word or Phrase	Description	Word Building
tonsillitis	Acute or chronic bacterial infection of the pharynx and palatine tonsils (see Figure 16-17 ■). There is a sore throat and difficulty swallowing, with mouth breathing and snoring. The tonsils hypertrophy (enlarge), and the tonsillar crypts contain pus and debris. The adenoids may also hypertrophy and block the eustachian tubes. Treatment: Antibiotic drug, tonsillectomy.	**tonsillitis** (TAWN-sih-LY-tis) **tonsill/o-** *tonsil* **-itis** *inflammation of; infection of*

(continued)

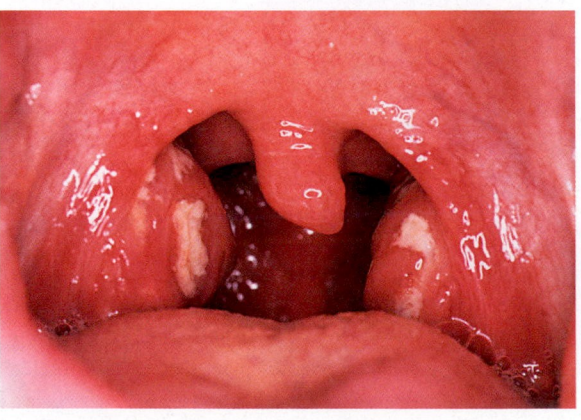

Figure 16-17 ■ Tonsillitis.
This patient has an acute inflammation, infection, and hypertrophy of the palatine tonsils. There are also some areas of white pus from this bacterial infection. The uvula and posterior oropharynx are also inflamed.

Word or Phrase	Description	Word Building
tonsillitis *(continued)*		

<table>
<tr><td colspan="3" align="center">**Word Alert**</td></tr>
<tr><td colspan="3">**MEDICAL WORD SPELLING**</td></tr>
<tr><td>**tonsil**</td><td>the lymph tissue in the throat</td><td>spelled with one *l*</td></tr>
<tr><td>**tonsillitis**</td><td>an inflammation or infection of the tonsils</td><td>spelled with two *l*'s</td></tr>
<tr><td>**tonsillectomy**</td><td>surgical excision of the tonsils</td><td>spelled with two *l*'s</td></tr>
</table>

Larynx

Word or Phrase	Description	Word Building
laryngitis	Hoarseness or complete loss of the voice, difficulty swallowing, and a cough due to swelling and inflammation of the larynx. It is caused by a bacterial or viral infection. Treatment: Antibiotic drug for a bacterial infection.	**laryngitis** (LAIR-in-JY-tis) **laryng/o-** *larynx (voice box)* **-itis** *inflammation of; infection of*
vocal cord nodule or polyp	A nodule is a small, benign, fibrous growth on the surface of the vocal cord. A polyp is a larger, soft growth that contains blood vessels (see Figure 16-18 ■). A nodule or polyp is caused by strain from constant talking or singing or by chronic irritation from smoking or allergies. There is hoarseness and a change in the quality of the voice. Treatment: Voice rest, surgical excision. 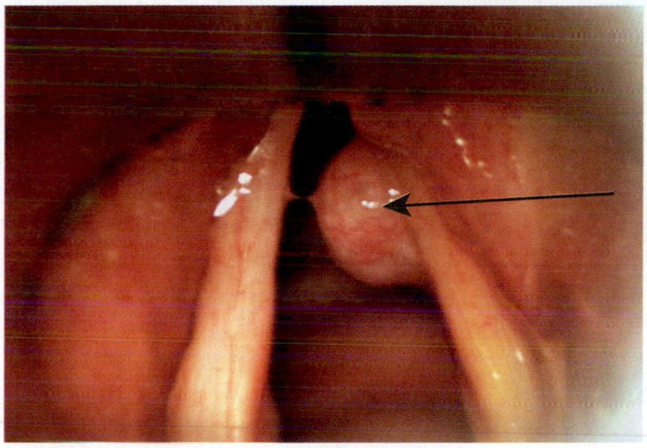 **Figure 16-18 ■ Vocal cord polyp.** This fleshy polyp has a broad base. It is growing on the left vocal cord.	**nodule** (NAWD-yool) **polyp** (PAWL-ip)

Laboratory and Diagnostic Procedures

Hearing Tests

Word or Phrase	Description	Word Building
audiometry	Measures hearing acuity and documents hearing loss (see Figure 16-19 ■). The patient puts on headphones that are connected to an **audiometer,** which produces a series of pure tones, each at a different frequency (high or low pitch) and varying in intensity (loud or soft). The frequency of a tone is measured in **hertz (Hz).** The intensity of a tone is measured in **decibels (dB).** The patient presses a button to signal when the tone is heard. The result, printed on graph paper, is an **audiogram.** In **speech audiometry,** the patient hears spoken words and sentences. If he/she can repeat 50% of the words correctly, then this is the threshold of hearing ability for speech sounds. Both pure tone audiometry and speech audiometry are used to determine whether a patient needs a hearing aid.	**audiometry** (AW-dee-AWM-eh-tree) *audi/o-* the sense of hearing *-metry* process of measuring **audiometer** (AW-dee-AWM-eh-ter) *audi/o-* the sense of hearing *-meter* instrument used to measure **audiogram** (AW-dee-oh-gram) *audi/o-* the sense of hearing *-gram* a record or picture

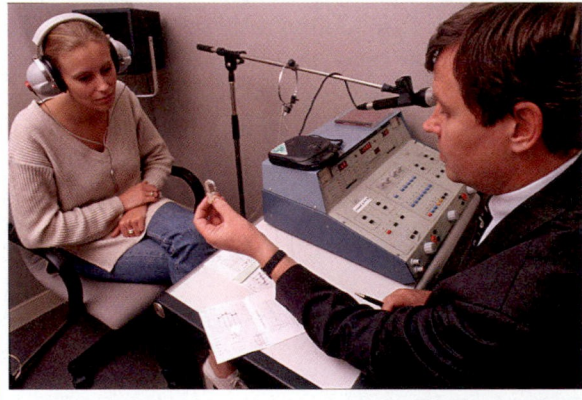

Figure 16-19 ■ Audiometry.
This patient is undergoing audiometry. The headphones cover both ears to keep out outside noises. The hearing in each ear is tested separately, and the patient raises her hand when she hears a sound.

Word or Phrase	Description	Word Building
brainstem auditory evoked response (BAER)	Analyzes the brain's response to sounds. The patient listens as an audiometer produces a series of clicks. An electroencephalography (EEG) is performed at the same time. A lesion or tumor in the auditory cortex of the brain or on the vestibulocochlear nerve will produce an abnormal BAER. It is also known as an **auditory brainstem response (ABR).**	
Rinne and Weber hearing tests	The Rinne tuning fork test evaluates bone conduction versus air conduction of sound in one ear at a time (see Figure 16-20 ■). A vibrating tuning fork is placed against the mastoid process behind one ear to test the bone conduction of sound. Then it is placed next to (but not touching) the same ear. If the sound is louder when the tuning fork is next to the ear, then hearing in that ear is normal and the test is said to be positive (because air conduction normally is greater than bone conduction). If the sound is louder when the tuning fork touches the mastoid process, then the patient has a conductive hearing loss.	**Rinne** (RIN-eh) **Weber** (VAH-ber)

(continued)

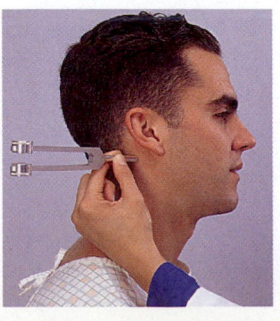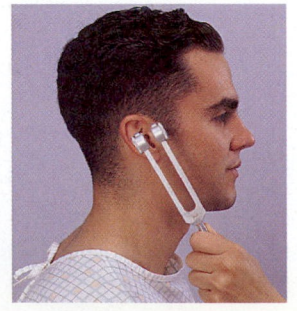

Figure 16-20 ■ Rinne test.
This hearing test uses a vibrating tuning fork to compare bone conduction of sound to air conduction of sound for the same ear.

Word or Phrase	Description	Word Building
Rinne and Weber hearing tests (*continued*)	The Weber tuning fork test evaluates bone conduction of sound in both ears at the same time. The vibrating tuning fork is placed against the center of the forehead or on top of the head. The sound should be heard equally in both ears.	
tympanometry	Measures the ability of the tympanic membrane and the bones of the middle ear to move back and forth. Air pressure (rather than sound vibration) is applied to the external auditory canal. If infection or disease has fixed the middle ear bones, then the tympanic membrane will move very little. This resistance to movement is called **impedance.** The result, printed on graph paper, is called a **tympanogram.**	**tympanometry** (TIM-pah-NAWM-eh-tree) **tympan/o-** *tympanic membrane (eardrum)* **-metry** *process of measuring* **impedance** (im-PEE-dans) **tympanogram** (tim-PAN-oh-gram) **tympan/o-** *tympanic membrane (eardrum)* **-gram** *a record or picture*

Did You Know?

The ear can hear sounds with a frequency as low as 20 Hz or as high as 20,000 Hz. In contrast, a dog can hear from 20 Hz to 45,000 Hz, and a porpoise can hear from 75 Hz to 150,000 Hz. A tuning fork of 256 Hz is used to test the hearing. This frequency corresponds to middle C on the piano.

Laboratory and Radiologic Tests

Word or Phrase	Description	Word Building
culture and sensitivity (C&S)	Laboratory test in which a swab of mucus or pus from the nose, tonsils, or throat (see Figure 16-21 ■) is placed onto culture medium in a Petri dish to identify the cause of an infection. Microorganisms in the mucus or pus grow into colonies, and the specific disease-causing microorganism is identified and tested to determine its sensitivity to various antibiotic drugs.	**culture** (KUL-chur) **sensitivity** (SEN-sih-TIV-ih-tee) **sensitiv/o-** *affected by; sensitive to* **-ity** *state; condition*

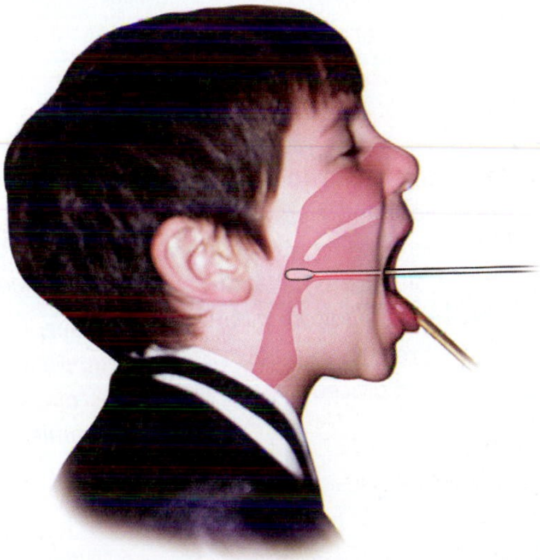

Figure 16-21 ■ Throat swab.
This child is having a swab taken of the oropharynx. The material on the swab will be sent to the laboratory for a culture and sensitivity test.

Word or Phrase	Description	Word Building
rapid strep test	Test kit for strep throat. If it detects beta-hemolytic group A streptococcus, a purplish-pink line appears. Unlike a standard culture and sensitivity test, the result of a rapid strep test is available within the hour so that the physician can immediately prescribe an antibiotic drug.	
RAST	Blood test that measures the amount of IgE produced when the blood is mixed with a specific antigen. It shows which of many allergens the patient is allergic to and how severe the allergy is. RAST stands for radioallergosorbent test.	

Word or Phrase	Description	Word Building
sinus series	Plain x-rays are taken from various angles to show all of the sinuses and confirm or rule out a diagnosis of sinusitis. Sinusitis shows as cloudy, opacified sinuses with thickened mucous membranes. Sometimes an air-fluid level can be seen within the sinus. Often a CT scan is done instead of a plain x-ray to show additional detail (see Figure 16-13).	

Medical and Surgical Procedures

Medical Procedures

Word or Phrase	Description	Word Building
nose, sinus, mouth, and throat examinations	A nasal **speculum** is used to widen the nostril, while a penlight lights the nasal cavity. The frontal and maxillary sinuses are examined for tenderness by pressing with the fingertips on the forehead and cheekbones. A tongue depressor, penlight, and a laryngeal mirror are used to examine the mouth and throat. *That's all you want me to say . . . Ah?*	**speculum** (SPEK-yoo-lum)

otoscopy	Procedure to examine the external auditory canal and tympanic membrane (see Figure 16-22 ■). An **otoscope** provides light and magnification. To assess the mobility of the tympanic membrane, some otoscopes have a rubber bulb that is squeezed to force air into the external auditory canal. The otoscope is pressed against the external auditory meatus to form an air-tight seal, and then the bulb is squeezed. A normal tympanic membrane moves in and out in response to this procedure.	**otoscopy** (oh-TAWS-koh-pee)
		  ot/o- *ear*
		  -scopy *process of using an instrument to examine*
		
		otoscope (OH-toh-skohp)
		  ot/o- *ear*
		  -scope *instrument used to examine*

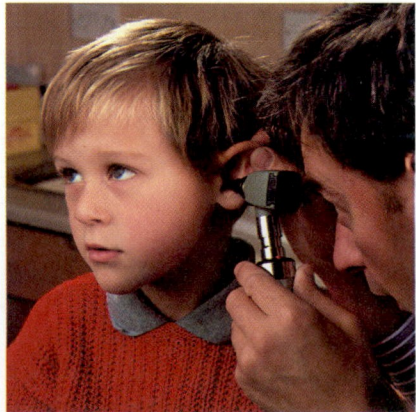

Figure 16-22 ■ Otoscopy.

The physician is using an otoscope to examine this patient's left external auditory canal and tympanic membrane. Before each use, a disposable black plastic tip (speculum) is placed over the part of the otoscope that enters the ear. For patients from 3 years old to adult, the physician gently pulls the helix backward and upward to straighten the external auditory canal and visualize the tympanic membrane. In infants younger than 3, the helix is pulled backward and downward to straighten the external auditory canal.

Word or Phrase	Description	Word Building
Romberg's sign	Procedure to assess equilibrium. The patient stands with the feet together and the eyes closed. Swaying or falling to one side indicates a loss of balance and an inner ear disorder.	**Romberg** (RAWM-berg)

Surgical Procedures

Word or Phrase	Description	Word Building
cheiloplasty	Procedure to repair the lip, usually because of a laceration. A cheiloplasty can be part of a larger surgical procedure to repair a cleft lip and palate.	**cheiloplasty** (KY-loh-PLAS-tee) **cheil/o-** *lip* **-plasty** *process of reshaping by surgery*
cochlear implant	Surgical procedure to insert a small, battery-powered implant beneath the skin behind the ear. Wires from the implant are placed through the round window and into the cochlea of the inner ear. When the implant "hears" a sound, it sends an electrical impulse to stimulate the cochlear portion of the vestibulocochlear nerve.	
endoscopic sinus surgery	Surgical procedure that uses an **endoscope** (a flexible, fiberoptic scope with a magnifying lens and a light source) to examine the nose, sinuses, or throat. **Endoscopy** is used to remove tissue and fluid or perform a biopsy.	**endoscopic** (EN-doh-SKAWP-ik) **endo-** *innermost; within* **scop/o-** *examine with an instrument* **-ic** *pertaining to* **endoscope** (EN-doh-skohp) **endo-** *innermost; within* **-scope** *instrument used to examine* **endoscopy** (en-DAWS-koh-pee) **endo-** *innermost; within* **-scopy** *process of using an instrument to examine*
mastoidectomy	Procedure to remove part of the mastoid process of the temporal bone because of infection	**mastoidectomy** (MAS-toy-DEK-toh-mee) **mastoid/o-** *mastoid process* **-ectomy** *surgical excision*

Word or Phrase	Description	Word Building
myringotomy	Procedure that uses a **myringotome** to make an incision in the tympanic membrane to drain fluid from the middle ear. For chronic middle ear infections, a ventilating tube can also be inserted through the incision to form a permanent opening into the middle ear (see Figure 16-23 ■). This procedure is a **tympanostomy**.	**myringotomy** (MEER-ing-GAW-toh-mee) **myring/o-** *tympanic membrane (eardrum)* **-tomy** *process of cutting or making an incision* **myringotome** (mih-RING-goh-tohm) **myring/o-** *tympanic membrane (eardrum)* **-tome** *instrument used to cut; area with distinct edges* **tympanostomy** (TIM-pan-AWS-toh-mee) **tympan/o-** *tympanic membrane (eardrum)* **-stomy** *surgically created opening*

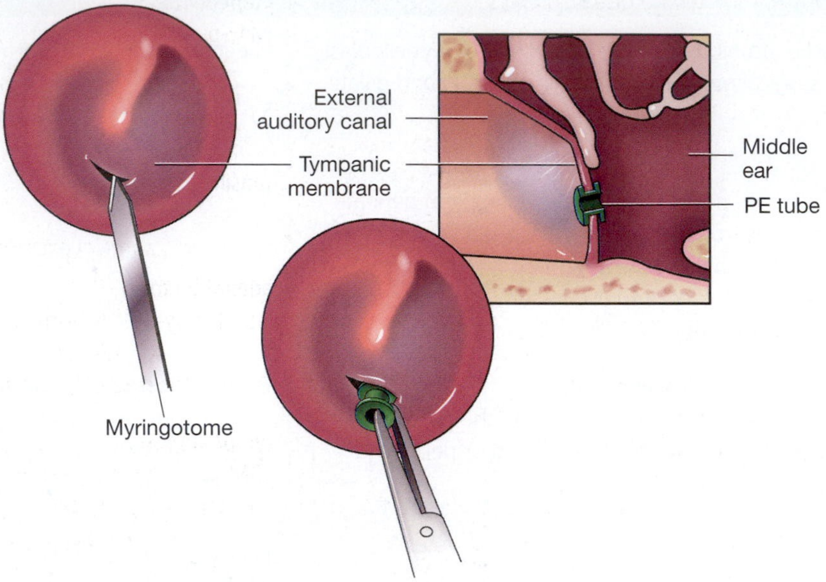

Figure 16-23 ■ Myringotomy and tympanostomy.
A myringotome is used to make an incision in the tympanic membrane. Then a small ventilating tube (tympanostomy tube) is inserted through the incision. This is also known as a PE tube or pressure-equalizing tube.

Word or Phrase	Description	Word Building
otoplasty	Procedure that uses plastic surgery to correct deformities of the external ear. When it corrects protruding ears, it is known as an **ear pinning**.	**otoplasty** (OH-toh-PLAS-tee) **ot/o-** *ear* **-plasty** *process of reshaping by surgery*
polypectomy	Procedure to remove polyps from the nasal cavity, sinuses, or vocal cords	**polypectomy** (PAWL-ih-PEK-toh-mee) **polyp/o-** *polyp* **-ectomy** *surgical excision*
radical neck dissection	Procedure to treat extensive cancer of the mouth and neck. Parts of the jaw bone, tongue (partial **glossectomy**), lymph nodes, and muscles of the neck are removed. The larynx can also be removed (**laryngectomy**).	**radical** (RAD-ih-kal) **radic/o-** *all parts including the root* **-al** *pertaining to* **dissection** (dy-SEK-shun) **dissect/o-** *to cut apart* **-ion** *action; condition* **glossectomy** (glaw-SEK-toh-mee) **gloss/o-** *tongue* **-ectomy** *surgical excision* **laryngectomy** (LAIR-in-JEK-toh-mee) **laryng/o-** *larynx (voice box)* **-ectomy** *surgical excision*
rhinoplasty	Procedure that uses plastic surgery to change the size or shape of the nose	**rhinoplasty** (RY-noh-PLAS-tee) **rhin/o-** *nose* **-plasty** *process of reshaping by surgery*

Word or Phrase	Description	Word Building
septoplasty	Procedure to correct a deviated septum	**septoplasty** (SEP-toh-PLAS-tee) **sept/o-** *septum (dividing wall)* **-plasty** *process of reshaping by surgery*
stapedectomy	Procedure for otosclerosis to remove the diseased part of the stapes and replace it with a prosthetic device	**stapedectomy** (STAY-pee-DEK-toh-mee) **staped/o-** *stapes (stirrup-shaped bone)* **-ectomy** *surgical excision*
tonsillectomy and adenoidectomy (T&A)	Procedure to remove the tonsils and adenoids in patients with chronic tonsillitis and hypertrophy of the tonsils and adenoids	**tonsillectomy** (TAWN-sih-LEK-toh-mee) **tonsill/o-** *tonsil* **-ectomy** *surgical excision* **adenoidectomy** (AD-eh-noy-DEK-toh-mee) **adenoid/o-** *adenoids* **-ectomy** *surgical excision*
tympanoplasty	Procedure to reconstruct a ruptured tympanic membrane	**tympanoplasty** (TIM-pah-noh-PLAS-tee) (TIM-pah-noh-PLAS-tee) **tympan/o-** *tympanic membrane (eardrum)* **-plasty** *process of reshaping by surgery*

Drug Categories

These categories of drugs are used to treat ENT diseases and conditions. The most common generic and trade name drugs in each category are listed.

Category	Indication	Examples	Word Building
antibiotic drugs	Treat bacterial infections of the ears, nose, sinuses, or throat. Antibiotic drugs are not effecttive against viral infections.	amoxicillin (Amoxil), Bactrim, ofloxacin (Floxin Otic), Septra	**antibiotic** (AN-tee-by-AWT-ik) (AN-tih-by-AWT-ik) **anti-** *against* **bi/o-** *life; living organisms; living tissue* **-tic** *pertaining to*
antihistamine drugs	Block the effect of histamine released during an allergic reaction. Histamine causes symptoms of runny, itchy nose and swollen mucous membranes.	cetirizine (Zyrtec), diphenhydramine (Benadryl), fexofenadine (Allegra), loratadine (Claritin, Tavist)	**antihistamine** (AN-tee-HIS-tah-meen)
antitussive drugs	Suppress the cough center in the brain. Some of these drugs contain a narcotic drug.	dextromethorphan (Robitussin CoughGels, Vicks 44), hydrocodone (Hycodan)	**antitussive** (AN-tee-TUS-iv) **anti-** *against* **tuss/o-** *cough* **-ive** *pertaining to*

Category	Indication	Examples	Word Building
antiyeast drugs	Treat yeast infections (oral candidiasis, thrush) of the mouth caused by *Candida albicans*. Solution is swished around the oral cavity and then swallowed.	nystatin (Mycostatin, Nilstat)	**antiyeast** (AN-tee-YEEST)
corticosteroid drugs	Treat inflammation of the ears, nose, or mouth. Topical nose drops, ear drops, or oral drug.	beclomethasone (Beconase), flunisolide (Nasalide), fluticasone (Flonase)	**corticosteroid** (KOR-tih-koh-STAIR-oyd) **cortic/o-** *cortex (outer region)* **-steroid** *steroid*
decongestant drugs	Constrict blood vessels and decrease swelling of the mucous membranes of the nose and sinuses due to colds and allergies. Topical nasal sprays or oral drugs.	oxymetazoline (Afrin 12-hour, Duration), pseudoephedrine (Dimetapp, Drixoral, Sudafed)	**decongestant** (DEE-con-JES-tant) **de-** *reversal of; without* **congest/o-** *accumulation of fluid* **-ant** *pertaining to*
drugs used to treat vertigo and motion sickness	Decrease the sensitivity of the inner ear to motion and keep nerve impulses from the inner ear from reaching the vomiting center in the brain	dimenhydrinate (Dramamine), meclizine (Antivert), scopolamine (Transderm-Scop)	

Clinical Connections

Pharmacology. Aminoglycoside antibiotic drugs are known to damage the cochlea. This drug effect is known as **ototoxicity.** Patients taking aminoglycoside drugs need to have audiometry done periodically to monitor their hearing.

ototoxicity (OH-toh-tawk-SIS-ih-tee)
ot/o- *ear*
toxic/o- *poison; toxin*
-ity *state; condition*

Abbreviations

ABR	auditory brainstem response
AD, A.D.*	right ear (Latin, *auris dextra*)
AS, A.S.*	left ear (Latin, *auris sinister*)
AU, A.U.*	each ear (Latin, *auris uterque*); both ears (Latin, *auris unitas*)
BAER	brainstem auditory evoked response
BOM	bilateral otitis media
C&S	culture and sensitivity
dB, db	decibel
EAC	external auditory canal
ENT	ears, nose, and throat

HEENT	head, eyes, ears, nose, and throat
Hz	hertz
PE	pressure-equalizing (tube)
PND	postnasal drip (or drainage)
RAST	radioallergosorbent test
SOM	serous otitis media
T&A	tonsillectomy and adenoidectomy
TM	tympanic membrane
TMJ	temporomandibular joint
URI	upper respiratory infection

*According to the Joint Commission on Accreditation of Healthcare Organizations (JCAHO) and the Institute for Safe Medication Practices (ISMP), these abbreviations should not be used. However, because they are still used by some healthcare providers, they are included here.

Word Alert

ABBREVIATIONS

Abbreviations are commonly used in all types of medical documents; however, they can mean different things to different people and their meanings can be misinterpreted. Always verify the meaning of an abbreviation.

C&S means *culture and sensitivity*, but the sound-alike abbreviation *CNS* means *central nervous system*.

PND means *postnasal drip*, but it also means *paroxysmal nocturnal dyspnea*.

TM means *tympanic membrane*, but *TMJ* means *temporomandibular joint*.

It's Greek to Me!

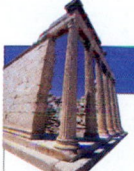

Did you notice that some words have two different combining forms? Combining forms from both Greek and Latin languages remain a part of medical language today.

Word	Greek	Latin	Medical Word Examples
ear	ot/o-	aur/i-, auricul/o-	otic, auricle, auricular
eardrum	tympan/o-	myring/o-	tympanic membrane, myringotomy
hearing	acous/o-	audi/o-, audit/o-	acoustic neuroma, audiogram, auditory canal
lip	cheil/o-	labi/o-	cheiloplasty, nasolabial
nose	rhin/o-	nas/o-	rhinoplasty, nasal
tongue	gloss/o-	lingu/o-	glossectomy, lingual

CAREER FOCUS

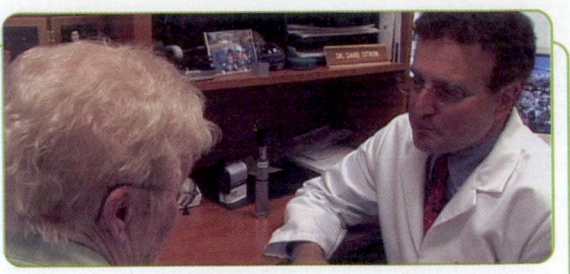

Meet David, an audiologist

"Audiology is very exciting, not just because of all the changes in technology that have occurred, but also the fact that the profession is growing. One very large change is in the area of newborn hearing screening. Now we can screen babies right at birth. There are technologically advanced hearing aids. All of them are programmable by computer; we can individualize each person's hearing profile by programming the hearing aid to meet their specific needs. We tend to see a lot of people who have balance problems because one area of audiology deals with assessing and treating dizziness and vertigo. All audiologists need to have a doctoral degree and the reason for that is because of all the things we do—our scope of practice has grown so much."

Audiologists are allied health professionals who perform hearing tests, diagnose hearing loss, and determine how patients can best use their remaining hearing. They also make and fit hearing aids. Audiologists work in schools, hospitals, physicians' offices, and their own private offices.

Otolaryngologists or **otorhinolaryngologists** are physicians who practice in the medical specialty of otolaryngology. They diagnose and treat patients with diseases of the ears, nose, or throat. They are also known as ENT specialists. When otolaryngologists perform surgery, they are known as head and neck surgeons or **oral and maxillofacial surgeons**. Physicians can take additional training and become board certified in the subspecialties of pediatric otolaryngology, plastic surgery of the head and neck, or allergy and immunology. Malignancies of the ears, nose, and throat are treated medically by an oncologist or surgically by a head and neck surgeon or oral surgeon.

audiologist (AW-dee-AWL-oh-jist)
audi/o- *the sense of hearing*
log/o- *word; the study of*
-ist *one who specializes in*

otolaryngologist
(OH-toh-LAIR-ing-GAWL-oh-jist)
ot/o- *ear*
laryng/o- *larynx (voice box)*
log/o- *word; the study of*
-ist *one who specializes in*

otorhinolaryngologist
(OH-toh-RY-noh-LAIR-ing-GAWL-oh-jist)
ot/o- *ear*
rhin/o- *nose*
laryng/o- *larynx (voice box)*
log/o- *word; the study of*
-ist *one who specializes in*

maxillofacial (MAK-sil-oh-FAY-shal)
maxill/o- *maxilla (upper jaw)*
faci/o- *face*
-al *pertaining to*

PEARSON myhealthprofessionskit™ To see David's complete video profile, visit Medical Terminology Interactive at www.myhealthprofessionskit.com. Select this book, log in, and go to the 16th floor of Pearson General Hospital. Enter the Laboratory, and click on the computer screen.

CHAPTER REVIEW EXERCISES

Test your knowledge of the chapter by completing these review exercises. Use the Answer Key at the end of the book to check your answers.

Anatomy and Physiology

Matching Exercise

Match each word or phrase to its location. Note: Some locations have more than one correct answer.

1. adenoids
2. nasal alae
3. cochlea
4. conchae
5. helix
6. incus
7. malleus
8. nares
9. nasal septum
10. nasopharynx
11. ossicles
12. pinna
13. semicircular canals
14. stapes
15. tonsils
16. tragus
17. turbinates
18. vestibule

_____ External ear
_____ Middle ear
_____ Inner ear
_____ External nose
_____ Nasal cavity
_____ Throat

True or False Exercise

Indicate whether each statement is true or false by writing T or F on the line.

1. _____ The semicircular canals help the body keep its balance.
2. _____ The eustachian tube connects the nasal cavity to the inner ear.
3. _____ The sinuses in the cheek on either side of the nose are the maxillary sinuses.
4. _____ The chin is also known as the mentum.
5. _____ The lingual tonsils are located on either side of the base of the tongue.
6. _____ The pinna is another name for the tragus.
7. _____ The ossicular chain is located in the semicircular canals of the inner ear.
8. _____ The tympanic membrane divides the external auditory canal from the middle ear.

Sequencing Exercise

Beginning where sound enters the external ear, write each structure of the ENT system in the correct order.

| auditory cortex of the brain | external auditory canal | malleus | stapes | vestibule |
| cochlea | incus | oval window | tympanic membrane | vestibulocochlear nerve |

1. external auditory canal →
2. _____ →
3. _____ →
4. _____ →
5. _____ →
6. _____ →
7. _____ →
8. _____ →
9. _____ →
10. _____ →

Diseases and Conditions

True or False Exercise

Indicate whether each statement is true or false by writing T or F on the line.

1. _____ Misalignment of the mandible can cause a vocal cord nodule.

2. _____ Hemotympanum can be caused by pressure, trauma, or acoustic neuroma.

3. _____ Sensorineural hearing loss is caused by a problem in the inner ear.

4. _____ Untreated middle ear infections can progress to otitis externa.

5. _____ The palatine tonsils are also called the adenoids.

6. _____ A benign growth of the mucous membranes of the nose is known as epistaxis.

7. _____ Rhinorrhea is serous drainage from the middle ear.

8. _____ Buzzing or ringing sounds in the ear are known as tinnitus.

Matching Exercise

Match each word or phrase to its description.

1. anosmia   _____ Loss of sense of smell

2. cold sores   _____ Ringing or buzzing in the ears

3. epistaxis   _____ Mouth infection with *Candida albicans*

4. hemotympanum   _____ Describes a fluid that contains pus

5. otitis externa   _____ Blood in the middle ear behind the eardrum

6. otosclerosis   _____ Bleeding from the nose

7. suppurative   _____ Swimmer's ear

8. thrush   _____ Caused by herpes simplex virus type 1

9. tinnitus   _____ Dizziness

10. vertigo   _____ Abnormal bone forms and hardens the stapes and oval window

Laboratory, Radiology, Surgery, and Drugs

Fill in the Blank Exercise

Fill in the blank with the correct word from the word list.

| antihistamine | audiometry | cochlear implant | culture | rhinoplasty |
| antitussive | cheiloplasty | CT scan | otoscopy | Rinne test |

1. Uses a vibrating tuning fork _____

2. Drug used to suppress coughing _____

3. Radiology procedure to view the sinuses _____

4. Plastic surgery on the nose _____

5. Growing microorganism on a medium in a Petri dish _____

6. Procedure to view inside the ear with a lighted instrument _____

7. Drug used to treat allergies _____

8. Test that measures hearing _____

9. Placed in the inner ear to correct total deafness _____

10. Plastic surgery to repair the lip _____

Building Medical Words

Review the Combining Forms Exercise and Combining Form and Suffix Exercise that you already completed in the anatomy section on pages 820–821.

Combining Forms Exercise

Before you build ENT words, review these additional combining forms. Next to each combining form, write its medical meaning. The first one has been done for you.

Combining Form	Medical Meaning	Combining Form	Medical Meaning
1. alg/o-	pain	11. osm/o-	
2. allerg/o-		12. plak/o-	
3. congest/o-		13. polyp/o-	
4. effus/o-		14. presby/o-	
5. hem/o-		15. scler/o-	
6. later/o-		16. scop/o-	
7. leuk/o-		17. sensor/i-	
8. log/o-		18. ser/o-	
9. lymph/o-		19. suppur/o-	
10. neur/o-		20. tuss/o-	

Related Combining Forms Exercise

Write the combining forms on the line provided. (Hint: See the It's Greek to Me feature box.)

1. Three combining forms that mean *ear*. _____

2. Two combining forms that mean *eardrum*. _____

3. Two combining forms that mean *lip*. _____

4. Two combining forms that mean *nose*. _____

5. Two combining forms that mean *tongue*. _____

6. Three combining forms that mean *hearing*. _____

Combining Form and Suffix Exercise

Read the definition of the medical word. Select the correct suffix from the Suffix List. Select the correct combining form from the Combining Form List. Build the medical word and write it on the line. Be sure to check your spelling. The first one has been done for you.

SUFFIX LIST

-ative (pertaining to)
-ectomy (surgical excision)
-ic (pertaining to)
-itis (inflammation of; infection of)
-ive (pertaining to)
-gram (a record or picture)
-metry (process of measuring)

-oma (tumor; mass)
-ous (pertaining to)
-phyma (tumor; growth)
-plasty (process of reshaping by surgery)
-rrhea (flow; discharge)
-scope (instrument used to examine)

-scopy (process of using an instrument to examine)
-stomy (surgically created opening)
-tic (pertaining to)
-tome (instrument used to cut)
-tomy (process of cutting or making an incision)

COMBINING FORM LIST

acous/o- (hearing; sound)
allerg/o- (allergy)
audi/o- (the sense of hearing)
cheil/o- (lip)
gloss/o- (tongue)

labyrinth/o- (labyrinth of the inner ear)
laryng/o- (larynx; voice box)
myring/o- (tympanic membrane; eardrum)
neur/o- (nerve)

ot/o- (ear)
pharyng/o- (pharynx; throat)
polyp/o- (polyp)
rhin/o- (nose)
sept/o- (septum; dividing wall)

ser/o- (serumlike fluid)
suppur/o- (pus formation)
tonsill/o- (tonsil)
tympan/o- (tympanic membrane; eardrum)

Definition of the Medical Word

1. Pertaining to hearing and sound
2. Tumor of the nerve
3. Inflammation or infection of the labyrinth
4. Pertaining to a serum-like fluid
5. Flow or discharge from the nose
6. Process of measuring the tympanic membrane
7. Inflammation or infection of the tonsils
8. Instrument used to examine the ear
9. Tumor or growth of the nose
10. Inflammation or infection of the ear
11. Pertaining to pus formation
12. Surgical excision of the larynx (voice box)
13. Process of reshaping by surgery (on the nasal) septum
14. Surgical excision of a polyp
15. Instrument used to cut the tympanic membrane
16. Inflammation or infection of the pharynx
17. Flow or discharge from the ear
18. Inflammation or infection of the tongue
19. Process of reshaping by surgery (on the) lip
20. Process of cutting or making an incision in the tympanic membrane
21. Surgical excision of the tongue
22. A record or picture of the sense of hearing
23. Inflammation or infection of the larynx
24. Process of using an instrument to examine the ear
25. Process of reshaping by surgery (on the) nose

Build the Medical Word

1. acoustic

Definition of the Medical Word

26. Surgical excision of the tonsils

27. Inflammation or infection of the nose

28. Surgically created opening in the tympanic membrane

29. Pertaining to an allergy

30. Process of reshaping by surgery (on the) ear

Build the Medical Word

_____

_____

_____

_____

_____

Prefix Exercise

Read the definition of the medical word. Look at the medical word or partial word that is given (it already contains a combining form and a suffix). Select the correct prefix from the Prefix List and write it on the blank line. Then build the medical word and write it on the line. Be sure to check your spelling. The first one has been done for you.

PREFIX LIST			
an- (without; not)	bi- (two)	endo- (innermost; within)	post- (after; behind)
anti- (against)	de- (reversal of; without)	pan- (all)	

Definition of the Medical Word	Prefix	Word or Partial Word	Build the Medical Word
1. Pertaining to two sides	bi-	lateral	bilateral
2. Pertaining to (a drug that is) against a cough	_____	tussive	_____
3. Pertaining to (drainage that is) behind the nose	_____	nasal	_____
4. Condition (of being) without the sense of smell	_____	osmia	_____
5. Pertaining to (a drug that does a) reversal of an accumulation of fluid	_____	congestant	_____
6. Pertaining to the innermost parts within (a hollow space) to examine with an instrument	_____	scopic	_____
7. Inflammation or infection of all of the sinuses	_____	sinusitis	_____

Multiple Combining Forms and Suffix Exercise

Read the definition of the medical word. Select the correct suffix and combining forms. Then build the medical word and write it on the line. Be sure to check your spelling. The first one has been done for you.

SUFFIX LIST	COMBINING FORM LIST	
-al (pertaining to)	aden/o- (gland)	neur/o- (nerve)
-ar (pertaining to)	alg/o- (pain)	ot/o- (ear)
-ia (condition; state; thing)	audi/o- (the sense of hearing)	plak/o- (plaque)
-ist (one who specializes in)	laryng/o- (larynx; voice box)	rhin/o- (nose)
-osis (condition; abnormal condition; process)	leuk/o- (white)	scler/o- (hard)
-pathy (disease; suffering)	log/o- (word; the study of)	sensor/i- (sensory)
	lymph/o- (lymph; lymphatic system)	tempor/o- (temple; side of
	mandibul/o- (mandible; lower jaw)	the head)

Definition of the Medical Word

1. Pertaining to a sensory nerve

2. Condition of ear pain

3. Disease of the lymph gland

4. Condition of white plaque (in the mouth)

5. Abnormal condition (in the) ear (of) hardness (of the bones)

Build the Medical Word

sensorineural

_____

_____

_____

_____

(continued)

Definition of the Medical Word	Build the Medical Word
6. Pertaining to the temple and the mandible (joint)	_____
7. One who specializes in the ear, nose, and larynx study of	_____
8. One who specializes in the sense of hearing study of	_____

Applied Skills

Medical Report Exercise

This exercise contains a physician office chart note. Read the report and answer the questions that follow.

OFFICE NOTE

PATIENT NAME: ARQUETTE, Geanne

RECORD NUMBER: 144-26-9842

DATE OF VISIT: November 19, 20xx

HISTORY
This 22-year-old mother of 2 children had a slight fever, a sore throat, and a head cold that developed over a few days after both children had similar symptoms. She states that both children are in day care and many children at the day care center have been ill. A few days later, she also had the acute onset of severe pain and pressure over her right cheekbone and right forehead, but this subsided somewhat more recently. She continued to go to work but, within the last few days, has been experiencing increasing severe fatigue, is slightly dizzy at times, and has some pain in her ears.

PHYSICAL EXAMINATION
On physical examination today, she has only a slightly increased temperature. She has slight pain on palpation of her forehead and cheekbone areas bilaterally. In both ears the TMs are red and bulging outward.

ASSESSMENT
1. Bilateral acute otitis media.
2. Previously acute but now subacute sinusitis.

PLAN
Amoxicillin 500 mg PO b.i.d. × 10 days. She is to call if she has any exacerbation of her symptoms.

Irene S. Klinitski, M.D.
_____
Irene S. Klinitski, M.D.

ISK: mtt
D: 11/19/xx
T: 11/19/xx

Word Analysis Questions

1. Divide *sinusitis* into its two word parts and define each word part.

Word Part	**Definition**
_____	_____
_____	_____

(continued)

2. Divide *bilateral* into its three word parts and define each word part.

Word Part   **Definition**

_____   _____

_____   _____

_____   _____

3. What does the abbreviation *TMs* stand for? _____

Fact Finding Questions

1. Which of the patient's symptoms began with an acute onset? _____

2. What technique was used to do the physical examination of the sinuses? _____

3. What disease is now subacute? _____

4. What drug was prescribed for the patient? _____

Critical Thinking Questions

1. Which of the four headings in this report gives the physician's diagnosis? _____

2. Which sinuses are located beneath the forehead and cheekbones? _____ _____

3. In Diagnosis #1, what abbreviation could be used instead of saying *both ears* or *bilaterally*? _____

4. Describe what symptoms or signs would be considered an exacerbation that might lead the patient to call the office, as instructed.

_____

English and Medical Word Equivalents Exercise

For each English word, write its equivalent medical word. Be sure to check your spelling. The first one has been done for you.

English Word	**Medical Word**	**English Word**	**Medical Word**
1. ear canal	external auditory canal	9. voice box, Adam's apple	_____
2. eardrum	_____	10. hay fever, seasonal allergies	_____
3. earwax	_____	11. common cold, head cold	_____
4. hammer-shaped bone	_____	12. total deafness	_____
5. anvil-shaped bone	_____	13. nosebleed	_____
6. stirrup-shaped bone	_____	14. earache	_____
7. nostril	_____	15. sore throat	_____
8. throat	_____	16. ringing in the ears	_____

On the Job Challenge Exercise

On the job, you will encounter new medical words. Practice your medical dictionary skills by looking up the medical word in bold. Write the definition on the line provided.

OFFICE CHART NOTE (EXCERPT)

DIAGNOSIS: **Rhinitis medicamentosa**, secondary to constant use of Afrin decongestant nasal spray. The patient is to take prednisone 20 mg every day for 5 days to decrease the chronic inflammation. She will refrain from using Afrin spray. She will return in 3 weeks for a full evaluation of her allergies.

---

rhinitis medicamentosa: _____

Hearing Medical Words Exercise

You hear someone speaking the medical words given below. Read each pronunciation and then write the medical word it represents. Be sure to check your spelling. The first one has been done for you.

1. AD-eh-noydz   <u>adenoids</u>
2. AW-dee-AWL-oh-jist   _____
3. KY-loh-PLAS-tee   _____
4. koh-LES-tee-ah-TOH-mah   _____
5. EP-ih-STAK-sis   _____
6. yoo-STAY-shun TOOB   _____
7. LAIR-in-JY-tis   _____
8. MEER-ing-GAW-toh-mee   _____
9. SY-nyoo-SY-tis   _____
10. TAWN-sih-lar   _____

Pronunciation Exercise

Read the medical word that is given. Then review the syllables in the pronunciation. Circle the primary (main) accented syllable. The first one has been done for you.

1. mucosa (myoo-(koh)-sah)
2. audiogram (aw-dee-oh-gram)
3. auricular (aw-rik-yoo-lar)
4. cerumen (seh-roo-men)
5. hemotympanum (hee-moh-tim-pah-num)
6. laryngeal (lah-rin-jee-al)
7. otalgia (oh-tal-jee-ah)
8. postnasal (post-nay-zal)
9. temporomandibular (tem-poh-roh-man-dib-yoo-lar)
10. tonsillar (tawn-sih-lar)

Abbreviations

Matching Exercise

Match each abbreviation to its definition.

1. AD   _____ Tonsillectomy and adenoidectomy
2. BOM   _____ Temporomandibular joint
3. C&S   _____ Postnasal drip
4. ENT   _____ Bilateral otitis media
5. PND   _____ Ears, nose, and throat
6. T&A   _____ Right ear
7. TMJ   _____ Culture and sensitivity

Multimedia Preview

Immerse yourself in a variety of activities inside Medical Terminology Interactive. Getting there is simple:

1. Click on www.myhealthprofessionskit.com.
2. Select "Medical Terminology" from the choice of disciplines.
3. First-time users must create an account using the scratch-off code on the inside front cover of this book.
4. Find this book and log in using your username and password.
5. Click on Medical Terminology Interactive.
6. Take the elevator to the 16th Floor to begin your virtual exploration of this chapter!

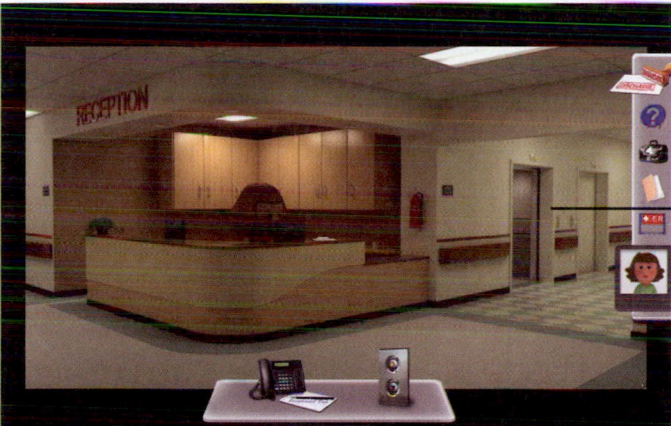 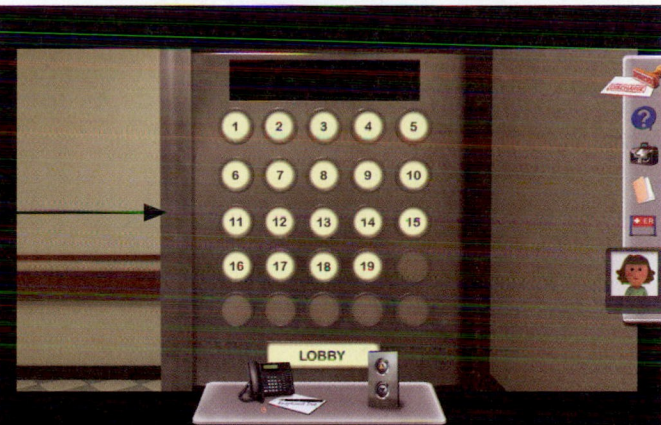

■ **Crossword**   Here is where learning and fun intersect! Simply use the clues to complete the puzzle grid. Whether you're a crossword wizard or only a novice, this activity will reinforce your understanding of key terms and concepts.

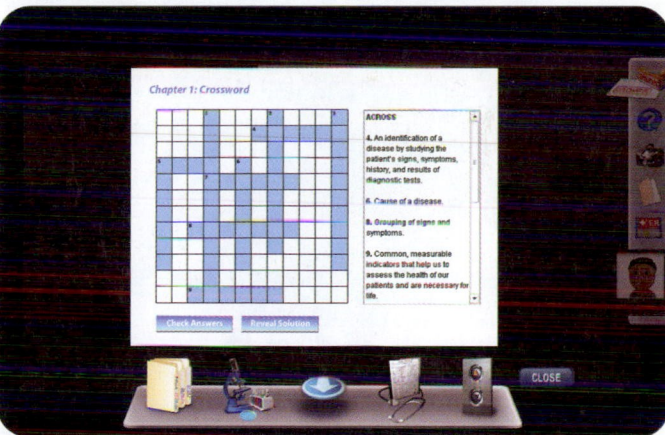

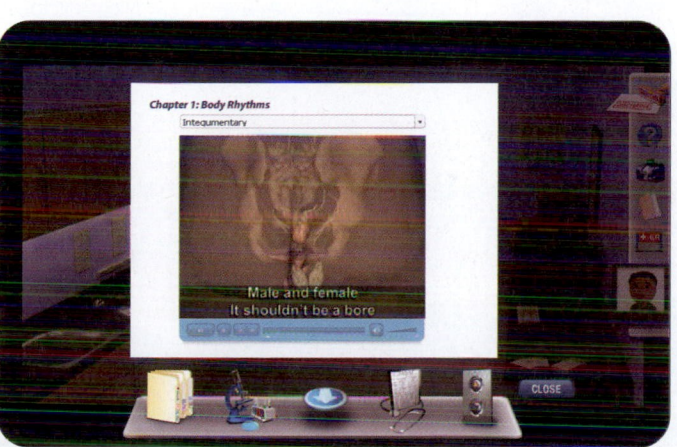

■ **Body Rhythms**   Sing along and learn! We've created a series of original music videos that correspond to each body system. They might not make it to MTV but they'll help you remember basic anatomy and give you a fun study break at the same time.

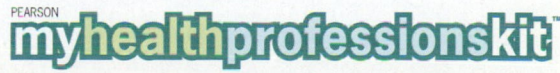

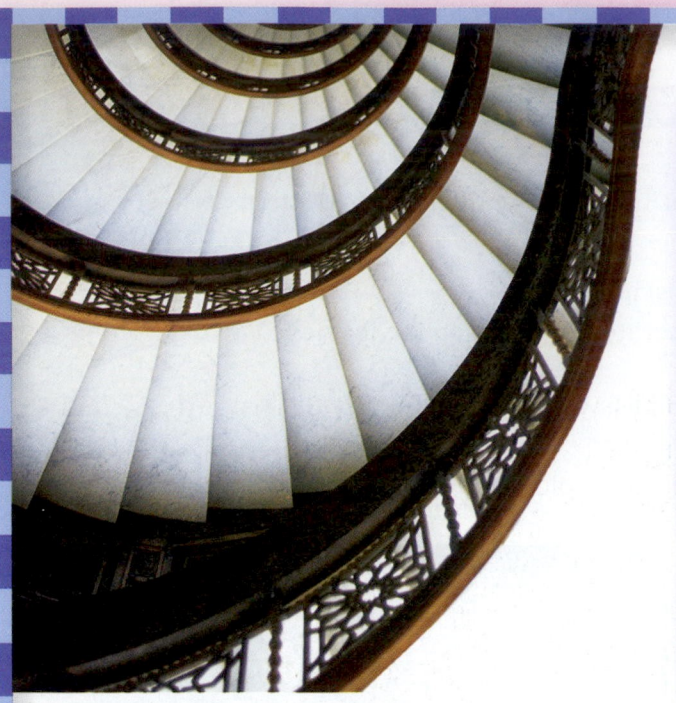

- On average, people fear spiders more than they do death.

- A few famous people who have had depressive mood disorders: Ludwig von Beethoven, Abraham Lincoln, Marilyn Monroe, John Lennon, Kurt Cobain

- Don't panic. It's time to get in the mood. In this chapter we'll explore the language that describes the structures, functions, diseases, and conditions that pertain to psychiatry.

- You'll be on your best behavior once you master the language of the mind!

Mania

Depression

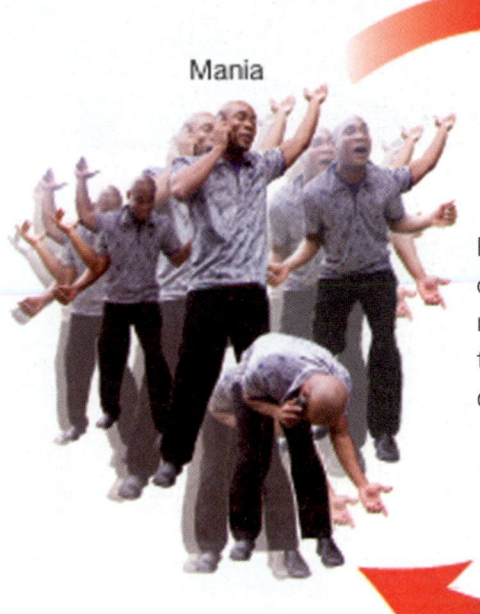

Bipolar disorder is characterized by chronic mood swings between the extremes of depression and mania.

1969

The antianxiety drug Valium becomes the number one prescription drug in the United States with 30 million tablets manufactured each day

1971

The computerized axial tomography (CAT) scan, a radiologic procedure that takes pictures of the body in slices, is introduced

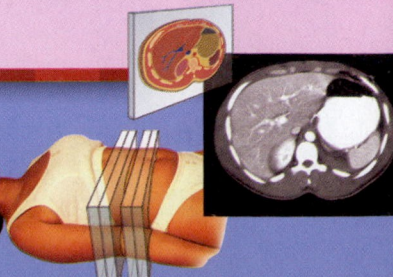

17
Psychiatry

Psychiatry (sy-KY-ah-tree) is the medical specialty that studies the anatomy and physiology of the brain and the functioning of the mind and uses diagnostic tests, medical and psychiatric procedures, and drugs to treat psychiatric diseases.

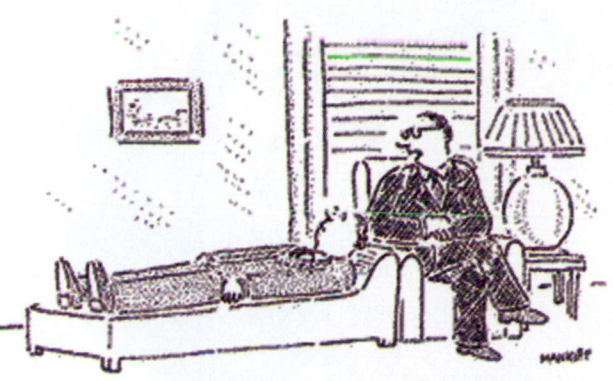

"Wow! You need professional help."

© The New Yorker Collection, 1996, Robert Mankoff from cartoonbank.com. All Rights Reserved.

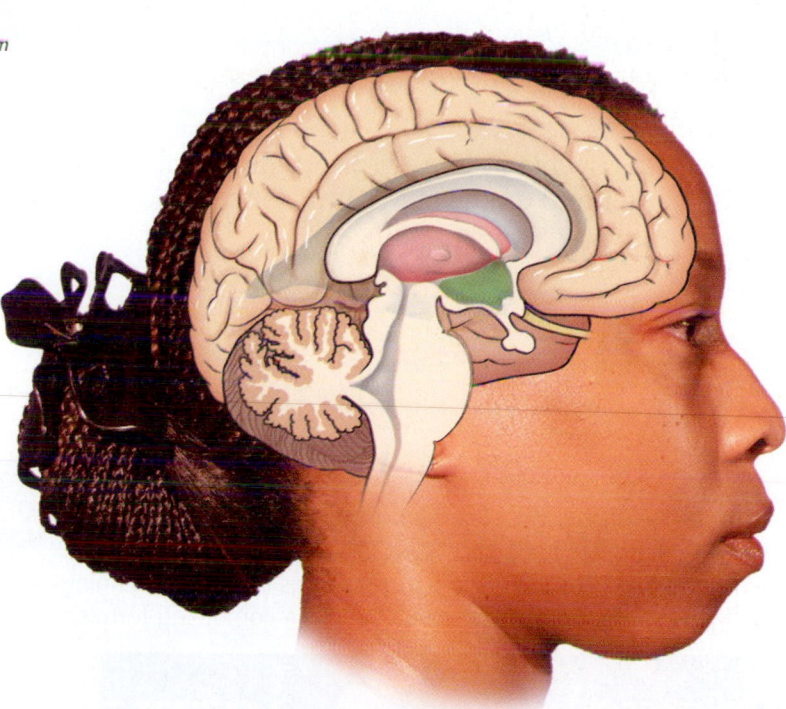

▶ The limbic system processes memories and controls emotion, mood, motivation, and behavior.

1977

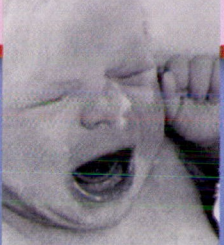

The first whole-body scanner using magnetic resonance imaging (MRI) technology is constructed

1978

Louise Brown becomes the first baby to be conceived by *in vitro* fertilization techniques. She was nicknamed the "test tube baby"

1979

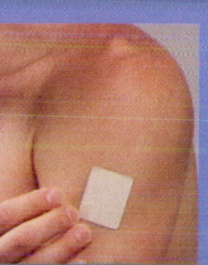

Ciba-Geigy introduces the first transdermal patch drug delivery system

Measure Your Progress: Learning Objectives

After you study this chapter, you should be able to

1. Identify the structures of the brain that are related to psychiatry.

2. Describe the process of an emotional response.

3. Describe common psychiatric diseases and conditions, laboratory and diagnostic procedures, medical and psychiatric procedures and therapies, and drug categories.

4. Give the medical meaning of word parts related to psychiatry.

5. Build psychiatric words from word parts and divide and define psychiatric words.

6. Spell and pronounce psychiatric words.

7. Analyze the medical content and meaning of a psychiatric report.

8. Dive deeper into psychiatry by reviewing the activities at the end of this chapter and online at Medical Terminology Interactive.

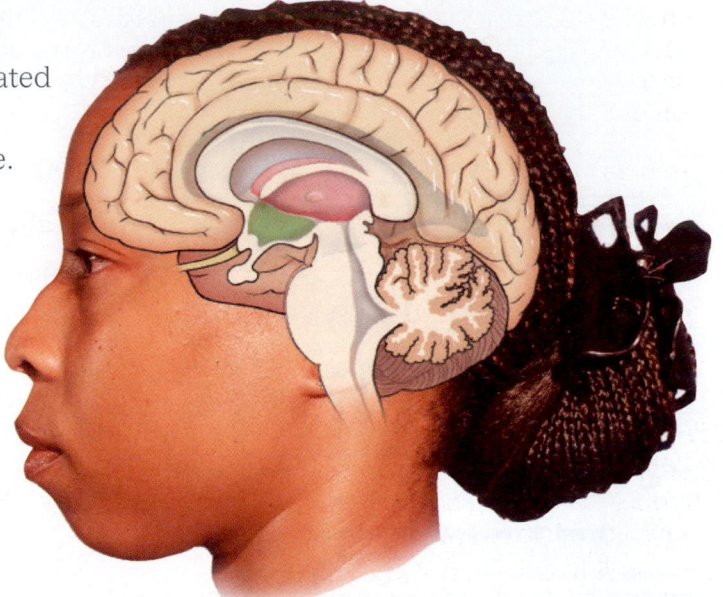

Figure 17-1 ■ The mind.
The mind is a complex interaction between specific anatomical structures of the brain, the mental functions of reasoning, learning, memory, and conscious and subconscious emotions, drives, and desires.

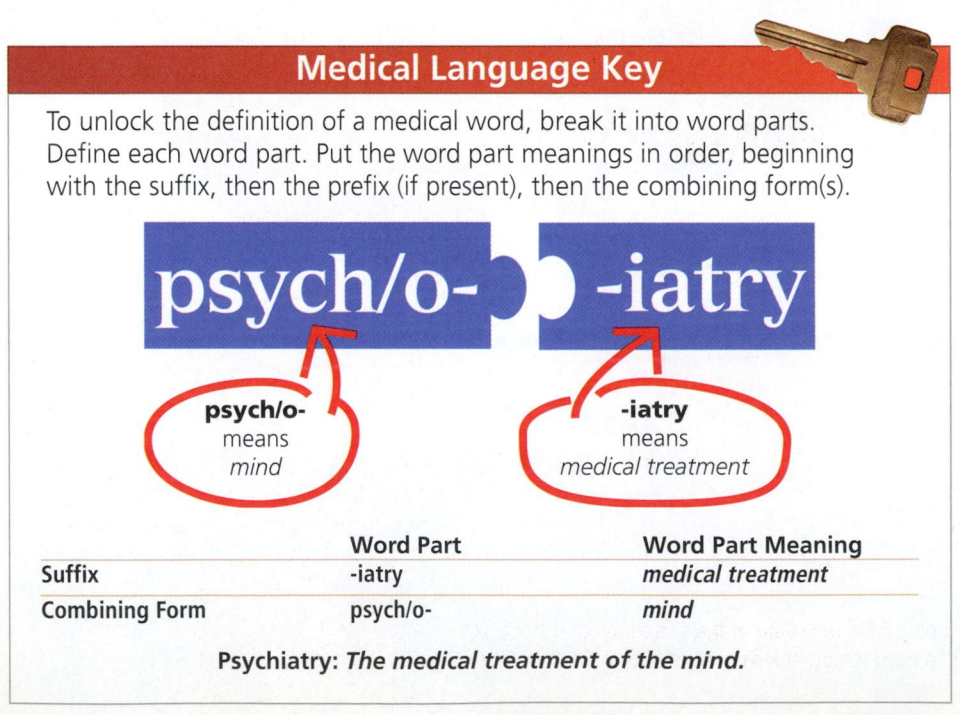

Medical Language Key

To unlock the definition of a medical word, break it into word parts. Define each word part. Put the word part meanings in order, beginning with the suffix, then the prefix (if present), then the combining form(s).

psych/o- ⊃⊂ -iatry

psych/o- means *mind*

-iatry means *medical treatment*

	Word Part	Word Part Meaning
Suffix	-iatry	*medical treatment*
Combining Form	psych/o-	*mind*

Psychiatry: *The medical treatment of the mind.*

Anatomy and Physiology

The structures that pertain to psychiatry are located in the brain (see Figure 17-1 ■). Psychiatry is concerned with physical symptoms and signs as well as behaviors that are the result of thoughts and emotions (for example, a rapid heart rate and agitated behavior due to anger; crying and suicide attempts due to depression; hyperventilation, chest pains, and an anxious facial expression due to fear).

Anatomy Related to Psychiatry

Limbic Lobe and Limbic System

The **limbic lobe** in the brain is along the medial edges of the right and left cerebral hemispheres (just superior to the corpus callosum that is a bridge between the two hemispheres). The limbic lobe includes some of each lobe in the cerebrum, plus a long extension of tissue into the temporal lobe. The limbic lobe is also known as the **cingulate gyrus** because it is in the form of a curved, encircling layer.

The **limbic system** consists of the limbic lobe, thalamus, hypothalamus, and several other smaller structures (see Figure 17-2 ■). The limbic system links the unconscious mind to the conscious mind. The limbic system processes memories and controls emotion, mood, memory, motivation, and behavior.

limbic (LIM-bik)
  limb/o- *edge; border*
  -ic *pertaining to*

cingulate (SIN-gyoo-layt)
  cingul/o- *structure that surrounds*
  -ate *composed of; pertaining to*

gyrus (JY-rus)

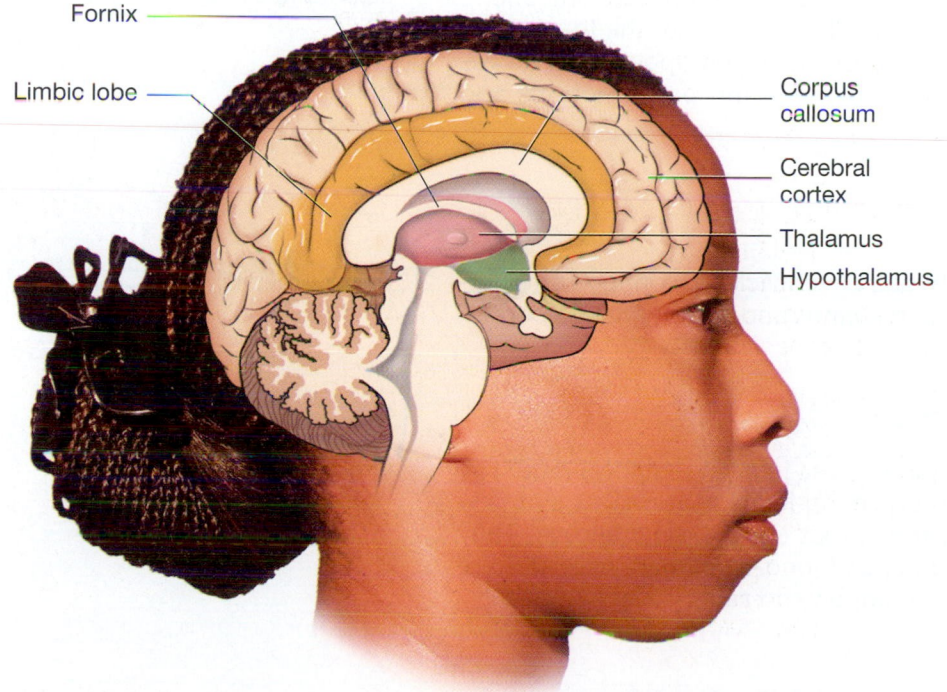

Figure 17-2 ■ **Limbic system.**
This midsagittal section of the brain shows the limbic lobe and some of the structures of the limbic system. The hippocampus and amygdaloid body in each temporal lobe are not visible on this view.

Thalamus

The **thalamus** is in the center of the cerebrum and forms the walls of the third ventricle. The thalamus is part of the nervous system (discussed in "Neurology," Chapter 10). It acts as a relay station, receiving sensory information from the five senses (sight, hearing, taste, smell, and touch) and relaying it to the midbrain (which sends out a motor command if immediate action is needed). The thalamus also relays sensory information to the cerebrum where it is analyzed and compared with memories.

thalamus (THAL-ah-mus)

Hypothalamus

The **hypothalamus,** located below the thalamus, forms the floor and part of the walls of the third ventricle. The hypothalamus is part of the nervous system and the endocrine system (discussed in "Neurology," Chapter 10 and "Endocrinology," Chapter 14). The hypothalamus controls emotions of pleasure, excitement, fear, anger, sexual arousal, and bodily responses to these emotions. The hypothalamus also contains the feeding center and satiety center and regulates the sex drive and sexual behavior. (This behavior is also regulated by the male and female sex hormones and by conscious thought processes from the cerebral cortex.) During times of fear or anger, the hypothalamus sends nerve impulses to the sympathetic division of the nervous system to trigger the "fight or flight" response to danger. The hypothalamus also is active in the learning process and helps short-term memories become permanent long-term memories.

hypothalamus (HY-poh-THAL-ah-mus)

Hippocampus

The **hippocampus** is an elongated, curving structure with two heads, one of which is located in each temporal lobe. The two tails of the hippocampus join as the fornix in the center of the brain. The hippocampus stores long-term memories and helps compare present and past emotions and experiences.

hippocampus (HIP-oh-KAM-pus)

Fornix

The **fornix** is along the floor of each lateral ventricle. It connects the hippocampus in each temporal lobe to the thalamus and to amygdaloid bodies.

fornix (FOR-niks)

Amygdaloid Bodies

The **amygdaloid body** is an almond-shaped area in each temporal lobe. The amygdaloid bodies are involved in interpreting facial expressions and new social situations and identifying situations that could be dangerous. They integrate sensory information, thoughts, and long-term memories and are most active during the emotions of fear, anger, and rage.

amygdaloid (ah-MIG-dah-loyd)
amygdal/o- *almond shape*
-oid *resembling*

Physiology of Emotion and Behavior

A current thought, sensory information from one of the five senses, a recalled memory, or a combination of all three can trigger an emotion. An **emotion** is an intense state of feelings. An intense emotion connected with

emotion (ee-MOH-shun)
emot/o- *moving; stirring up*
-ion *action; condition*

a particular situation causes that situation to imprint deeply in long-term memory. That situation, when later called to mind, brings with it those same intense emotions.

An emotional thought produces an outward display on the face (the person's **affect**) (see Figure 17-3 ■), changes in behavior, and physical symptoms and signs in the body. A person's emotional state of mind may reflect many emotions at the same time (fear, guilt, and anger), but the prevailing, predominant emotion is known as the person's **mood.**

WORD BUILDING

affect (AF-ekt)
_____

affective (ah-FEK-tiv)
  affect/o- *state of mind; mood; to have an influence on*
  -ive *pertaining to*
_____

mood (MOOD)
_____

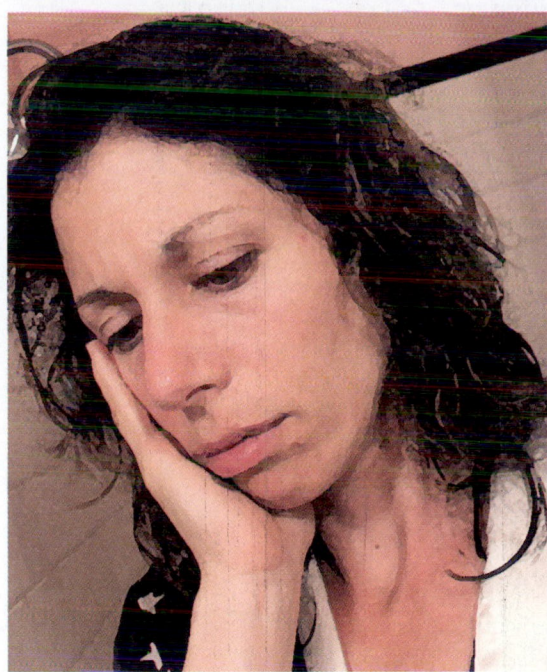

Figure 17-3 ■ Affect.
This woman's affect or facial expression reflects sadness and depression. Emotions are inward thoughts that produce an outward display through facial expressions, body position, and behavior.

Emotions are normal forms of expression, but extremely intense, long-lasting, inappropriate, or absent emotions are signs of mental illness. Injury to the brain or changes in the levels of various neurotransmitters in the brain can produce abnormal emotions and behaviors.

The frontal lobe is the site of reasoning, judgment, planning, organizing, personality, creativity, and recent memories of all of those things. The frontal lobe exerts conscious control over alertness, concentration, and emotions. The frontal lobe also analyzes situations, predicts future events, and weighs the benefits or consequences of actions taken. Injury to the frontal lobe can produce these psychiatric symptoms: flat (unchanging) affect, disinterest in life, inability to concentrate, inappropriate laughing or crying, inappropriate social or sexual behavior, indifference to the consequences of behavior, inability to plan or modify behavior, inability to abide by or create rules to govern behavior, inability to keep commitments, impulsiveness, or an absence of goal-directed behavior.

Injury to the hypothalamus can cause overeating and obesity, disinterest in eating, insomnia, or excessive sleepiness.

Hyperstimulation of the amygdaloid bodies can cause violent, aggressive behavior. Injury to or degeneration of the amygdaloid bodies can cause a loss of the emotions of anger and fear. The patient may recognize a person's face but cannot say if that person is a friend or an enemy. The patient is also unaware of dangerous situations.

Injury to or degeneration of the hippocampus in the temporal lobe can cause the loss of all long-term memory. A patient with Alzheimer's disease with degeneration of those areas may be unable to recognize his/her own face in the mirror.

Neurotransmitters are chemicals that relay messages from one neuron to the next. Neurotransmitters play an important role in emotion and behavior. Increased, decreased, or unbalanced levels of neurotransmitters can cause abnormal emotions and behaviors. Here are some of the most common neurotransmitters:

1. **Norepinephrine.** Neurotransmitter of the sympathetic division of the nervous system. It controls involuntary processes such as the heart rate, respiratory rate, and blood pressure when the body is active or exercising. An increased level of norepinephrine causes aggression, infatuation, and mania. A decreased level causes depression.

2. **Epinephrine.** Neurotransmitter of the sympathetic division of the nervous system. During stress, anxiety, fear, or anger, epinephrine from the adrenal medulla prepares the body for "fight or flight." An increased level of epinephrine causes anxiety, social phobia, performance phobia, and panic attacks.

3. **Dopamine.** Neurotransmitter in the brain. Cocaine, narcotic drugs, and alcohol increase the amount of dopamine, and this causes the euphoria and excitement ("high") craved by addicts. An increased level of dopamine also causes infatuation. A decreased level causes schizophrenia and depression. The combination of an increased level of dopamine in the limbic system and a decreased level of dopamine in the frontal lobe causes paranoia.

4. **Serotonin.** Neurotransmitter in the brain and spinal cord. A decreased level of serotonin causes depression. The combination of a decreased level of serotonin and an increased level of norepinephrine causes violent behavior.

5. **GABA.** Inhibitory neurotransmitter in the brain. A decreased level causes anxiety. GABA stands for gamma-aminobutyric acid.

WORD BUILDING

neurotransmitter
(NYOOR-oh-trans-MIT-er)
 neur/o- *nerve*
 transmitt/o- *to send across or through*
 -er *person or thing that produces or does*

norepinephrine (NOR-ep-ih-NEF-rin)

epinephrine (EP-ih-NEF-rin)

dopamine (DOH-pah-meen)

serotonin (SAIR-oh-TOH-nin)

Vocabulary Review

Anatomy and Physiology

Word or Phrase	Description	Combining Forms
affect	Outward display on the face of inward thoughts and emotions	**affect/o-** *state of mind; mood; to have an influence on*
amygdaloid body	Almond-shaped area within each temporal lobe. It interprets facial expressions and new social situations to identify danger. It combines visual images with long-term memory and is active in the emotions of fear, anger, and rage.	**amygdal/o-** *almond shape*
dopamine	Neurotransmitter in the brain	
emotion	Intense state of feelings	**emot/o-** *moving; stirring up*
epinephrine	Neurotransmitter of the sympathetic division of the nervous system. It is a hormone secreted into the blood by the adrenal medulla to prepare the body for "fight or flight."	
fornix	Connects the hippocampus to the thalamus and amygdaloid bodies	
GABA	Inhibitory neurotransmitter in the brain	
hippocampus	Irregular, curved area within each temporal lobe. It stores long-term memories and helps compare past and present emotions and experiences.	
hypothalamus	Controls emotions (pleasure, excitement, fear, anger, sexual arousal) and bodily responses to emotions. It regulates the sex drive. It contains the feeding and satiety centers. It functions as part of the "fight or flight" response of the sympathetic division of the nervous system. The hypothalamus helps short-term memories become long-term memories.	
limbic lobe	Curved, encircling area of the brain that includes the medial edges of the two cerebral hemispheres and extends into the temporal lobes. It is also known as the **cingulate gyrus.**	**limb/o-** *edge; border* **cingul/o-** *structure that surrounds*
limbic system	Related structures in the brain that control emotion, mood, memory, motivation, and behavior and link the conscious to the unconscious mind. The limbic system consists of the limbic lobe, thalamus, hypothalamus, hippocampus, amygdaloid bodies, and fornix.	**limb/o-** *edge; border*
mood	Prevailing, predominant emotion affecting a person's state of mind	
neurotransmitter	Chemicals that relay messages from one neuron to another	**neur/o-** *nerve* **transmitt/o-** *to send across or through*
norepinephrine	Neurotransmitter of the sympathetic division of the nervous system and in the brain. It controls involuntary processes such as the heart rate, respiratory rate, and blood pressure when the body is active or exercising.	
serotonin	Neurotransmitter in the brain and spinal cord	
thalamus	Relay station that receives sensory information from the senses and relays it to the midbrain (for immediate action in the face of danger) and to the cerebrum (for analysis and comparison with memories)	

Building Medical Words

Use the Answer Key at the end of the book to check your answers.

Combining Forms Exercise

Before you build psychiatric words, review these combining forms. Next to each combining form, write its medical meaning. The first one has been done for you.

Combining Form	Medical Meaning	Combining Form	Medical Meaning
1. **amygdal/o-**	almond shape	5. limb/o-	_____
2. affect/o-	_____	6. neur/o-	_____
3. cingul/o-	_____	7. transmitt/o-	_____
4. emot/o-	_____		

Combining Form and Suffix Exercise

Read the definition of the medical word. Look at the combining form that is given. Select the correct suffix from the Suffix List and write it on the blank line. Then build the medical word and write it on the line. (Remember: You may need to remove the combining vowel. Always remove the hyphens and slash.) Be sure to check your spelling. The first one has been done for you.

SUFFIX LIST			
-ic (pertaining to)	-ion (action; condition)	-ive (pertaining to)	-oid (resembling)

Definition of the Medical Word	Combining Form	Suffix	Build the Medical Word
1. (Structure) resembling an almond shape	**amygdal/o-**	**-oid**	amygdaloid
(You think *resembling* (-oid) + *almond shape* (amygdal/o-). You change the order of the word parts to put the suffix last. You write *amygdaloid*.)			
2. Pertaining to the edge or border	limb/o-	_____	_____
3. Condition or action of stirring up	emot/o-	_____	_____
4. Pertaining to state of mind or mood	affect/o-	_____	_____

Mental Disorders and Conditions

Anxiety Disorders

Anxiety disorders are characterized by the predominant emotion of anxiety, with uneasiness, uncertainty, dread, worry, apprehension, or fear. Bodily symptoms and signs include inability to think clearly, dizziness, dry mouth, chest tightness, palpitations, upset stomach, diarrhea, fine tremor, sweaty palms, inability to relax, heightened startle reflex, fatigue, and irritability. Anxiety itself is an appropriate response to danger, but anxiety disorders are not associated with a specific dangerous situation, person, or thing. Treatment: Antianxiety drugs, antidepressant drugs, psychotherapy, group therapy.

Word or Phrase	Description	Word Building
generalized anxiety disorder	Dwelling on issues that involve "What if . . ." and predicting or fearing that the worst will happen to self, family, or friends	**anxiety** (ang-ZY-eh-tee) **anxi/o-** *fear; worry* **-ety** *condition; state*
obsessive–compulsive disorder	Constant, persistent, uncontrollable thoughts (**obsessions**) that occupy the mind, cause anxiety, and compel the patient to perform excessive, repetitive, or meaningless activities (**compulsions**) for fear of what might happen if these are not done (see Figure 17-4 ■). These activities include washing and cleaning; checking work again and again; checking doors and locks; ordering, labeling, and arranging belongings in a particular sequence; hoarding useless collections of things with an inability to discard things; and repetitive thinking, counting, praying, or making mental lists. These activities consume a significant portion of each day.	**obsession** (awb-SEH-shun) **obsess/o-** *besieged by thoughts* **-ion** *action; condition* **obsessive** (awb-SEH-siv) **obsess/o-** *besieged by thoughts* **-ive** *pertaining to* **compulsion** (com-PAWL-shun) **compuls/o-** *drive or compel* **-ion** *action; condition* **compulsive** (com-PAWL-siv) **compuls/o-** *drive or compel* **-ive** *pertaining to*

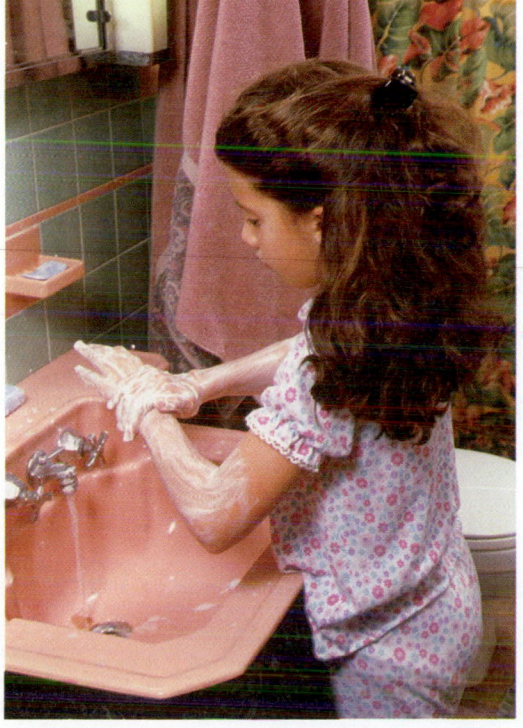

Figure 17-4 ■ **Obsessive–compulsive disorder.**
Washing the hands is a good habit of personal cleanliness. However, when handwashing is excessive and constant to the point that the hands become reddened and raw, and yet the patient cannot stop, then it becomes obsessive–compulsive behavior.

panic disorder	Sudden attack of severe, overwhelming anxiety without an identifiable cause. Patients often feel that they are choking or dying of a heart attack.	**panic** (PAN-ik)

Word or Phrase	Description	Word Building
phobia	Intense, unreasonable fear of a specific thing or situation or even the thought of it (see Table 17-1 and Figure 17-5 ■). Phobias occur when the unconscious mind avoids a real, ongoing conflict by projecting the anxiety onto an unrelated situation or object. Avoidance of the phobia can severely restrict the normal activities of daily life.	**phobia** (FOH-bee-ah) **phob/o-** *fear; avoidance* **-ia** *condition; state; thing* **phobic** (FOH-bik) **phob/o-** *fear; avoidance* **-ic** *pertaining to*

(continued)

Table 17-1   Common Phobias

Phobia	Description	Word Building
acrophobia	Fear of heights	**acrophobia** (AK-roh-FOH-bee-ah) **acr/o-** *extremity; highest point* **phob/o-** *fear; avoidance* **-ia** *condition; state; thing*
agoraphobia	Fear of crowds or public places	**agoraphobia** (AG-or-ah-FOH-bee-ah) **agor/a-** *open area or space* **phob/o-** *fear; avoidance* **-ia** *condition; state; thing*
arachnophobia	Fear of spiders	**arachnophobia** (ah-RAK-noh-FOH-bee-ah) **arachn/o-** *spider; spider web* **phob/o-** *fear; avoidance* **-ia** *condition; state; thing*
claustrophobia	Fear of closed-in spaces	**claustrophobia** (KLAW-stroh-FOH-bee-ah) **claustr/o-** *enclosed space* **phob/o-** *fear; avoidance* **-ia** *condition; state; thing*
microphobia	Fear of germs	**microphobia** (MY-kroh-FOH-bee-ah) **micr/o-** *one millionth; small* **phob/o-** *fear; avoidance* **-ia** *condition; state; thing*
ophidiophobia	Fear of snakes	**ophidiophobia** (oh-FID-ee-oh-FOH-bee-ah) **ophidi/o-** *snake* **phob/o-** *fear; avoidance* **-ia** *condition; state; thing*
social phobia	Fear of being embarrassed or humiliated in front of others, fear of being in a public place, or fear of being the center of attention	**social** (SOH-shal) **soci/o-** *human beings; community* **-al** *pertaining to*
thanatophobia	Fear of death	**thanatophobia** (THAN-ah-toh-FOH-bee-ah) **thanat/o-** *death* **phob/o-** *fear; avoidance* **-ia** *condition; state; thing*
xenophobia	Fear of strangers	**xenophobia** (ZEN-oh-FOH-bee-ah) **xen/o-** *foreign* **phob/o-** *fear; avoidance* **-ia** *condition; state; thing*

Word or Phrase	Description	Word Building

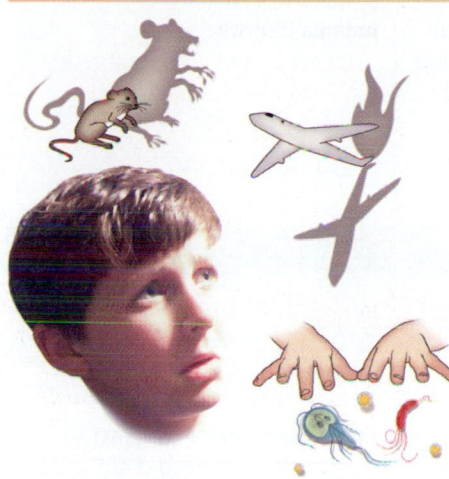

Figure 17-5 ■ Phobias.

Phobias are intense, exaggerated fears of a specific thing or situation.

| **posttraumatic stress disorder (PTSD)** | Continuing, disabling reaction to an excessively traumatic situation or event, such as a war, terrorist attack, torture, rape, kidnapping, natural disaster (e.g., earthquake, flood), explosion, or fire. The patient feels helpless, has a numbed emotional response with disinterest in people and current events, and relives the trauma of the event over and over. Also, there may be chronic anxiety, insomnia, irritability, or occasional violent outbursts. In the past, this was known as combat fatigue or shell shock. | **posttraumatic** (POST-trah-MAT-ik)
post- *after; behind*
traumat/o- *injury*
-ic *pertaining to* |

Eating Disorders

Eating disorders are characterized by abnormal eating patterns, distorted body image, fear, guilt, and depression. The majority of patients are young women. Treatment: Antidepressant drugs, psychotherapy, family therapy.

| **anorexia nervosa** | Extreme, chronic fear of being fat and an obsession to become thinner. The patient decreases food intake to the point of starvation (see Figure 17-6 ■). The patient denies being too thin, denies abnormal eating habits, and tries to keep this a secret from family and friends by making excuses for not eating and wearing clothes that conceal the extreme weight loss. | **anorexia nervosa** (AN-oh-REK-see-ah ner-VOH-sah)
an- *without; not*
orex/o- *appetite*
-ia *condition; state; thing*
Anorexia (discussed in "Gastroenterology," Chapter 3) is a simple loss of appetite due to illness. It is not a psychiatric disorder. |

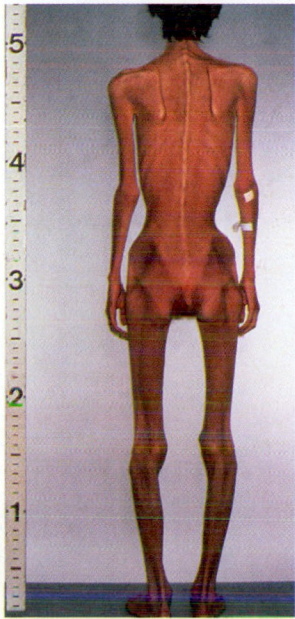

Figure 17-6 ■ Anorexia nervosa.

This patient has long-standing anorexia nervosa. All of the subcutaneous fat on the body is gone because of chronic decreased food intake to the point of starvation. This patient would still deny being too thin and would, in fact, appear to herself as being fat if she looked in a mirror.

Word or Phrase	Description	Word Building
bulimia	Patients gorge themselves on excessive amounts of food (binge eating) and then, for fear of gaining weight, they rid (purge) themselves of food by using laxative drugs or self-induced vomiting. Long-term vomiting wears away tooth enamel, causes inflammation and ulcers in the esophagus, and can lead to death from a low level of potassium in the blood.	**bulimia** (buh-LIM-ee-ah)

Substance-Related Disorders

Substance-related disorders are characterized by the frequent or constant use and abuse of drugs or chemicals to achieve a desired physical or emotional effect (a "high," sedation, or hallucinations). The drugs may be prescription drugs, over-the-counter drugs, tobacco, alcohol, chemicals, or illegal street drugs. After a brief period of use, patients experience **dependence** (the need for the substance in order to prevent withdrawal symptoms). Later, patients exhibit **tolerance** (decreasing effect even with increasing amounts of the substance). Much of the patient's life may center on drug-seeking behavior. Patients are aware of the serious medical conditions related to the use of the substance, but they choose to ignore this and continue to use the substance. **Addiction** is a state of complete physical and psychological dependence on a substance. Treatment: Psychotherapy, group therapy, family therapy, support groups, aversion therapy, medical support for withdrawal symptoms.

The following substances and drugs are often abused:

- Alcohol (beer, wine, liquor, ETOH, rubbing alcohol, wood alcohol)
- Amphetamines (central nervous system stimulant drugs, diet pills, speed)
- Cannabis (marijuana, hashish)
- Cocaine
- **Hallucinogens** (LSD, PCP)
- Inhalants (fumes from paint, paint thinner, cleaning fluid, lighter fluid, liquid glue, correction fluid, felt-tipped markers, or gasoline; aerosol propellant from spray cans)
- Nicotine (cigarettes, cigars, chewing tobacco)
- Opioids (narcotic drugs such as morphine, codeine, Demerol, OxyContin; the street drug heroin)
- Sedatives and antianxiety drugs (barbiturate drugs, sleeping pills, Valium)

dependence (dee-PEN-dens)
depend/o- *to hang onto*
-ence *state of*

tolerance (TAWL-er-ans)
toler/o- *to become accustomed to*
-ance *state of*

addiction (ah-DIK-shun)
addict/o- *surrender to; be controlled by*
-ion *action; condition*

hallucinogen (hah-LOO-sih-noh-jen)
hallucin/o- *imagined perception*
-gen *that which produces*

Affective or Mood Disorders

Mood disorders are characterized by chronic, persistent (longer than 6 months) depression or mood swings alternating between depression and mania. Normal feelings of sadness that diminish over time are considered appropriate and not categorized as a mood disorder. Mood disorders are also known as **affective disorders** because the mood can be seen in the patient's affect (facial expression and body movements). The word *affective* contains the combining form *affect/o-* (state of mind; mood; to have an influence on) and the suffix *-ive* (pertaining to). Treatment: Psychotherapy, antidepressant drugs, drugs for mania.

Word or Phrase	Description	Word Building

bipolar disorder	Chronic mood swings between **mania** and depression (see Figure 17-7 ■). Patients with mania are hyperactive, with limitless energy and extreme happiness (**euphoria**). They have feelings of power and mastery, need little sleep, and are intensely interested in and talk about one thing after another (flight of ideas), making and then quickly discarding plans. Gradually, their thoughts get out of control; they are unable to concentrate and show increasingly poor judgment and recklessness. After an episode of mania, the patient swings abruptly into severe depression. This is also known as **manic-depressive disorder.**	**bipolar** (by-POH-lar)
		  bi- *two*
		  pol/o- *pole*
		  -ar *pertaining to*
		
		mania (MAY-nee-ah)
		  man/o- *thin; frenzy*
		  -ia *condition; state; thing*
		
		euphoria (yoo-FOR-ee-ah)
		  eu- *normal; good*
		  phor/o- *to bear; to carry; range*
		  -ia *condition; state; thing*
		
		manic (MAN-ik)
		
		depressive (dee-PRES-iv)
		  depress/o- *press down*
		  -ive *pertaining to*

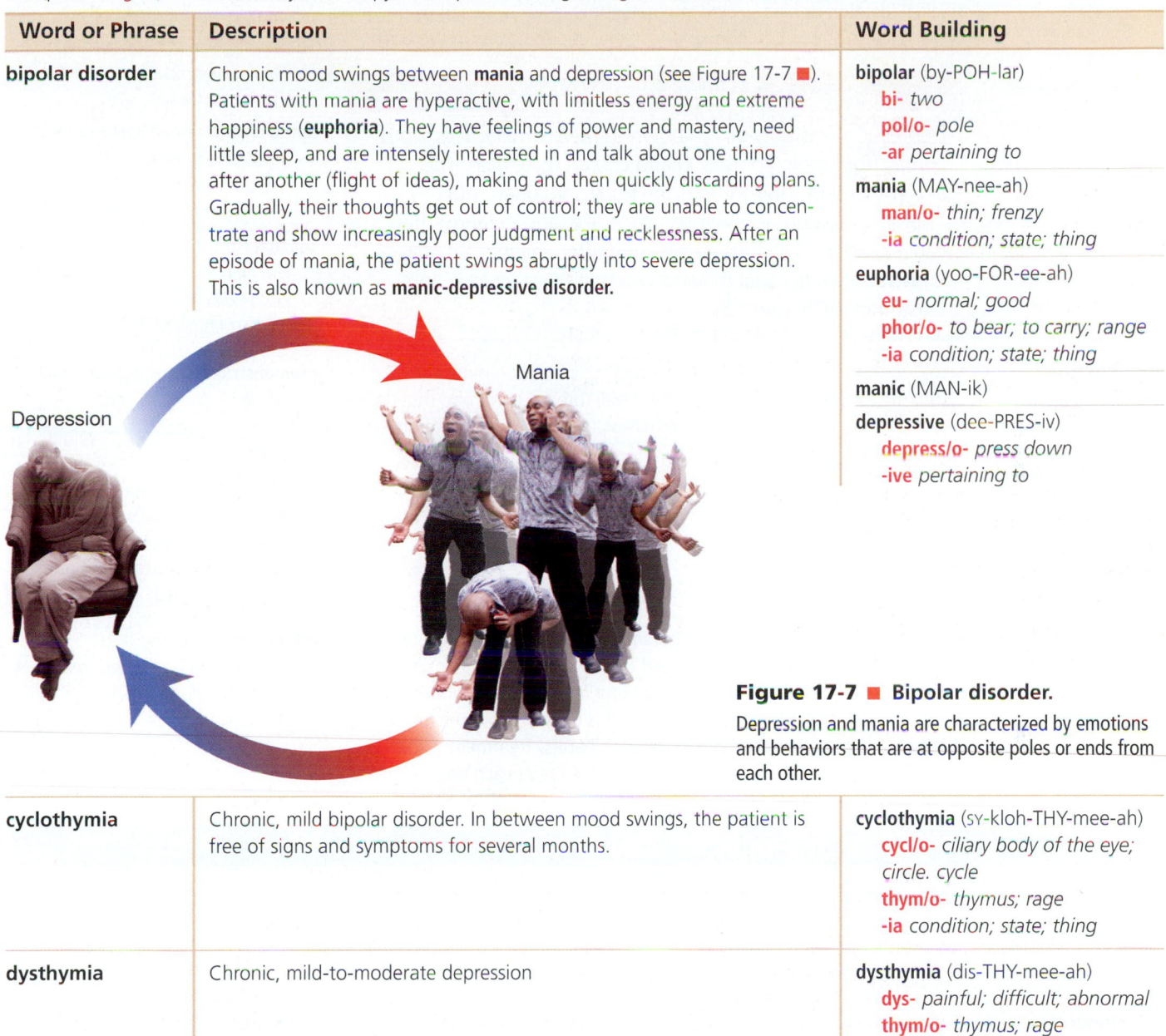

Depression

Mania

Figure 17-7 ■ Bipolar disorder.
Depression and mania are characterized by emotions and behaviors that are at opposite poles or ends from each other.

Word or Phrase	Description	Word Building

cyclothymia	Chronic, mild bipolar disorder. In between mood swings, the patient is free of signs and symptoms for several months.	**cyclothymia** (sy-kloh-THY-mee-ah)
		  cycl/o- *ciliary body of the eye; circle. cycle*
		  thym/o- *thymus; rage*
		  -ia *condition; state; thing*

dysthymia	Chronic, mild-to-moderate depression	**dysthymia** (dis-THY-mee-ah)
		  dys- *painful; difficult; abnormal*
		  thym/o- *thymus; rage*
		  -ia *condition; state; thing*

Word or Phrase	Description	Word Building
major depression	Chronic, severe symptoms of depression with **apathy** (indifference), hopelessness, helplessness, worthlessness, crying, insomnia, lack of pleasure in any activity (**anhedonia**), increased or decreased appetite, inability to make decisions or concentrate, fatigue, and slowed movements. During psychiatric interviews, depressed patients are asked if they have current **suicidal ideation** or past suicide attempts. Depression is caused by decreased levels of norepinephrine, dopamine, and serotonin in the brain.	**depression** (dee-PRESH-un) **depress/o-** *press down* **-ion** *action; condition* **apathy** (AP-ah-thee) **a-** *away from; without* **-pathy** *disease; suffering* The ending –*pathy* contains the combining form *path/o-* and the one-letter suffix –*y*. **anhedonia** (AN-hee-DOH-nee-ah) **an-** *without; not* **hedon/o-** *pleasure* **-ia** *condition; state; thing* **suicidal** (soo-ih-SY-dal) **su/i-** *self* **cid/o-** *killing* **-al** *pertaining to*

Did You Know?

Depression was previously known as *melancholia.* This word comes from *melan/o-* (black) and *chol/e-* (bile; gall). The ancient Greeks thought that the body contained four "humors" (blood, yellow bile, black bile, and phlegm) that caused different moods. Depression after childbirth is still known as involutional melancholia (see "Gynecology and Obstetrics," Chapter 13).

Word or Phrase	Description	Word Building
premenstrual dysphoric disorder (PMDD)	Occurs before the onset of the menstrual cycle and combines the symptoms of premenstrual syndrome (PMS) (breast, joint, and muscle pains) with depression, anxiety, tearfulness, difficulty concentrating, and sleeping and eating disturbances	**premenstrual** (pree-MEN-stroo-al) **pre-** *before; in front of* **menstru/o-** *monthly discharge of blood* **-al** *pertaining to* **dysphoric** (dis-FOR-ik) **dys-** *painful; difficult; abnormal* **phor/o-** *to bear; to carry; range* **-ic** *pertaining to*
seasonal affective disorder (SAD)	Caused by hypersecretion of melatonin from the pineal gland in the brain. Melatonin is normally produced during the night. The longer nights and decreased hours of sunshine during the winter months increase the production of melatonin, and this causes symptoms of depression, weight gain, and altered sleeping habits. Treatment: Exposure to sunlight or the use of a light box for several hours each day.	**affective** (ah-FEK-tiv) **affect/o-** *state of mind; mood; to have an influence on* **-ive** *pertaining to*

Psychosis

Psychoses are characterized by a loss of touch with reality and a disintegration of the thought processes. There is a change in affect and behavior, with inability to communicate effectively or maintain life activities. Schizophrenia is the most common form of psychosis. *Psychosis* (sy-KOH-sis) contains the combining form *psych/o-* (mind) and the suffix *-osis* (condition; abnormal condition; process). Treatment: Antipsychotic drugs, psychotherapy.

Word or Phrase	Description	Word Building
delusional disorder	Continued false beliefs (delusions) concerning events of everyday life. These beliefs are fixed and unchanging despite the efforts of others to persuade or evidence showing otherwise. Common delusions: other people or even strangers are in love with you, your husband or wife is unfaithful, or you have the powers of a god or are a famous person (delusions of grandeur). A patient with **paranoia** or delusions of persecution believes that other people are tying to hurt him/her; the patient is **paranoid.**	**delusional** (dee-LOO-shun-al) **delus/o-** *false belief* **-ion** *action; condition* **-al** *pertaining to* **paranoia** (PAIR-ah-NOY-ah)

Word or Phrase	Description	Word Building

schizophrenia	The most common type of psychosis. There is a chronic loss of touch with reality in most or all aspects of life with bizarre behavior and breakdown of thought processes. The patient is **schizophrenic.** Patients have **hallucinations** (false impressions of vision, smell, sound, taste, or touch). The most common is an auditory hallucination of a voice telling them to do certain things. Patients have delusions of persecution and delusions that others are controlling their thoughts or that they can use their thoughts to control events. Some patients' thoughts are so chaotic that their spoken words are completely meaningless, and they may use **neologisms** (new or made-up words that have no meaning). Patients' emotions and affect are inappropriate and do not correspond to what they are saying. Some patients are rigid and in a stupor (**catatonia**) or their extremities stay fixed in whatever position they are placed (**catalepsy**) (see Figure 17-8 ■), while others have childish, silly behavior (**hebephrenia**). Many patients have their first episode as young adults following a stressful event. Others develop symptoms more slowly over time.	**schizophrenia** (SKIZ-oh-FREE-nee-ah) (SKIT-soh-FREE-nee-ah)
		  schiz/o- *split*
		  phren/o- *diaphragm; mind*
		  -ia *condition; state; thing*
		Select the correct combining form meaning to get the definition of *schizophrenia: condition of a split mind.*
		
		hallucination (hah-LOO-sih-NAY-shun)
		  hallucin/o- *imagined perception*
		  -ation *a process; being or having*
		
		neologism (nee-AWL-oh-jizm)
		  ne/o- *new*
		  log/o- *word; the study of*
		  -ism *process; disease from a specific cause*
		
		catatonia (KAT-ah-TOH-nee-ah)
		  cata- *down*
		  ton/o- *pressure; tone*
		  -ia *condition; state; thing*
		
		catalepsy (KAT-ah-LEP-see)
		  cata- *down*
		  -lepsy *seizure*
		
		hebephrenia (HEE-bah-FREE-nee-ah) (HEB-eh-FREE-nee-ah)
		  hebe/o- *youth*
		  phren/o- *diaphragm; mind*
		  -ia *condition; state; thing*

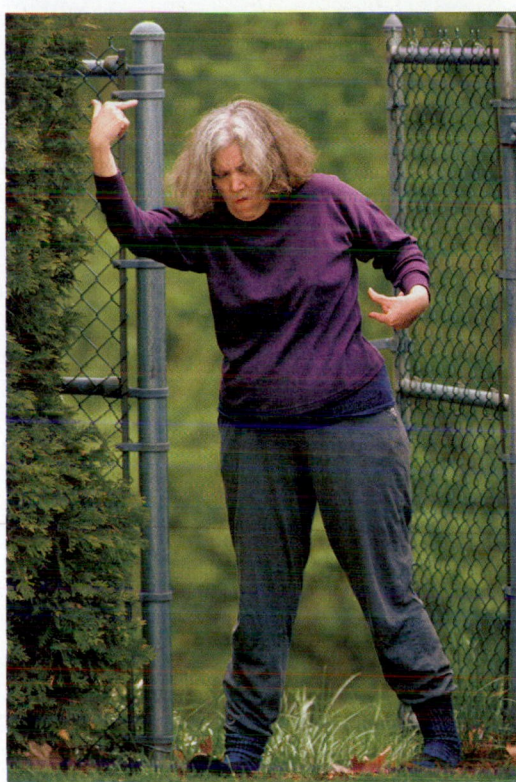

Figure 17-8 ■ Catalepsy.
This patient is showing the unusual fixed position of the extremities that is a common feature of catalepsy. It is associated with catatonic schizophrenia, Parkinson's disease, epilepsy, or can be caused by antipsychotic drugs used to treat schizophrenia.

Did You Know?

Insanity comes from two Latin words meaning *not sound.*

Literature has long depicted an insane person as a lunatic who is influenced by the phases of the moon, with the most severe symptoms during a full moon. *Lunatic* comes from the Latin word *lun/o-* (moon).

Childhood Disorders

Childhood disorders include any behavioral abnormality having to do with feeding, eating, elimination, learning, or motor skills—all major developmental areas during childhood. Treatment: Drugs for ADHD, psychotherapy, group therapy, family therapy.

Word or Phrase	Description	Word Building
attention-deficit hyperactivity disorder (ADHD)	Distractability, short attention span, inability to follow directions, restlessness, hyperactivity, emotional lability, and impulsiveness. It may be caused by mild brain damage at birth, genetic factors, or other abnormalities. It is five times more common in boys than in girls. Most children outgrow the symptoms by late childhood. In the past, it was known as minimal brain dysfunction and attention deficit disorder.	
autism	Inability to communicate or form significant relationships with others, and a lack of interest in doing so. Patients may be of normal intelligence or mentally retarded. The patient may not speak or may have abnormal speech with **echolalia** (automatically repeating what someone else has said). The patient avoids physical contact and eye contact, but is fascinated by objects. There are ritualistic, repetitive behaviors.	**autism** (AW-tizm) **aut/o-** *self* **-ism** *process; disease from a specific cause* **echolalia** (EK-oh-LAY-lee-ah) **ech/o-** *echo (sound wave)* **-lalia** *abnormal condition of speech*
encopresis	Repeated passage of stool into the clothing in a child older than age 5 who does not have a gastrointestinal illness, mental retardation, or a physical disability	**encopresis** (EN-koh-PREE-sis) **en-** *in; within; inward* **copr/o-** *feces; stool* **-esis** *a process*
oppositional defiant disorder	Persistent, aggressive behavior (fighting, arguing, provoking, annoying), defiance of and refusal to obey rules, disrespect for authority figures, with anger, stubbornness, and touchiness. **Conduct disorder** is a more severe form in which the patient physically and sexually assaults others, destroys property, steals, sets fires, or runs away from home.	**oppositional** (AWP-ih-ZIH-shun-al) **oppos/o-** *forceful resistance* **-ition** *condition of having* **-al** *pertaining to*
reactive attachment disorder	Inability to emotionally bond and form intimate relationships with others because of severe abuse or neglect of the patient's basic needs before age 2 when trust is established. There is a lack of trust, watchful wariness, poor eye contact, lack of empathy, inability to show genuine affection, and a lack of a conscience. The patient is difficult to comfort and resists physical contact such as being held, but can show inappropriate friendliness to strangers.	**reactive** (ree-AK-tiv) **react/o-** *reverse movement* **-ive** *pertaining to*
Tourette's syndrome	Frequent, spontaneous, involuntary muscle tics (eye blinking, throat clearing, arm thrusting), vocal tics (grunts, barks), or comments that are socially inappropriate, vulgar, obscene (**coprolalia**), or racist. The patient can only temporarily suppress these tics. The patient also can have echolalia, obsessive–compulsive disorder, and hyperactivity.	**Tourette** (TOOR-et) **coprolalia** (KAWP-roh-LAY-lee-ah) **copr/o-** *feces; stool* **-lalia** *abnormal condition of speech*

Sexual and Gender Identity Disorders

Sexual and gender identity disorders are characterized as accepting or not accepting one's own sexual gender or abnormalities of focusing sexual attention on an object or a person other than a consenting adult. Gender refers to the ways persons act and feel about themselves as a boy/man or girl/woman. Treatment: aversion therapy, cognitive-behavior therapy, group therapy, psychotherapy.

Word or Phrase	Description	Word Building
exhibitionism	Obtaining power, control, and sexual arousal by exposing the genital area in public areas to strangers and seeing their reactions. The patient is an **exhibitionist.**	**exhibitionism** (EK-sih-BIH-shun-izm) **exhibit/o-** *showing* **-ion** *action; condition* **-ism** *process; disease from a specific cause*
fetishism	Obtaining sexual arousal from objects rather than a person. Patients devote a great deal of time to obtaining and using the object (a fetish), which, for men, often includes women's clothing.	**fetishism** (FET-ish-izm)
masochism	Obtaining sexual arousal through abuse, pain, humiliation, or bondage that is done deliberately by another person. The patient is a **masochist.**	**masochism** (MAS-oh-kizm)
pedophilia	Obtaining power, control, and sexual arousal through contact or sexual acts with preadolescent children. The patient is a **pedophile.**	**pedophilia** (PEE-doh-FIL-ee-ah) **ped/o-** *child* **phil/o-** *attraction to; fondness for* **-ia** *condition; state; thing* **pedophile** (PEE-doh-file) **ped/o-** *child* **-phile** *person who is attracted to or is fond of*
rape	Obtaining power, control, and sexual arousal through forced sexual intercourse with a nonconsenting adult. Statutory rape is sexual intercourse with a minor (defined by most states as a person under the age of 18). The patient is a **rapist. Incest** is rape of a child by a parent or relative.	**rape** (RAYP) **rapist** (RAY-pist) **rap/o-** *to seize and drag away* **-ist** *one who specializes in*
sadism	Obtaining power, control, and sexual arousal by deliberately causing abuse, pain, humiliation, or bondage to another person. The patient is a **sadist.**	**sadism** (SAY-dizm) (SAD-izm)
transsexualism	Living or wanting to live as a member of the opposite gender. A **transsexual** believes that he or she has been assigned (by anatomy, parents, or society) a different gender identity and desires to change his or her outward appearance to match what is already felt in the mind as being the true personal identity. Treatment: drug therapy with hormones; a sex reassignment operation.	**transsexualism** (tranz-SEK-shoo-ah-lizm) **trans-** *across; through* **sex/o-** *sex* **-ual** *pertaining to* **-ism** *process; disease from a specific cause*

Word or Phrase	Description	Word Building
transvestism	Wearing clothes (one piece or full outfits) designed or intended for the opposite sex. The person is a **transvestite.** Some are transsexuals (see previous entry) while others do it for sexual arousal.	**transvestism** (trans-VES-tizm) **trans-** *across; through* **vest/o-** *to dress* **-ism** *process; disease from a specific cause*
voyeurism	Obtaining power, control, and sexual arousal by secretively viewing other people who are naked or having sexual relations. The elements of risk and danger as well as knowingly violating another's privacy are part of the experience. The patient is a **voyeur.**	**voyeurism** (VOY-yer-izm)

Cognitive Disorders

Cognitive disorders are characterized by a temporary or permanent impairment of thinking and memory. Treatment: Supportive care, drugs to slow memory loss or improve cognitive function, or psychotherapy.

amnesia	Partial or total loss of long-term memory due to trauma or disease of the hippocampus. The patient is said to be **amnestic.** In **retrograde amnesia,** the patient cannot remember events that occurred before the onset of amnesia. In **anterograde amnesia,** the patient cannot remember events that occurred after the onset of amnesia. In **global amnesia,** all memories (past and present) are lost.	**amnesia** (am-NEE-zee-ah) **amnes/o-** *forgetfulness* **-ia** *condition; state; thing* **amnestic** (am-NES-tik) **amnes/o-** *forgetfulness* **-tic** *pertaining to* **retrograde** (RET-roh-grayd) **retro-** *behind; backward* **-grade** *pertaining to going* **anterograde** (AN-ter-oh-grayd) **anter/o-** *before; front part* **-grade** *pertaining to going* **global** (GLOH-bal) **glob/o-** *shaped like a globe; comprehensive* **-al** *pertaining to*
delirium	Acute confusion, disorientation, and agitation due to toxic levels of body chemicals, drugs, or alcohol in the blood that affect the brain. These acute signs slowly subside as toxic levels of drugs or alcohol in the blood decrease. **Delirium tremens (DT)** is caused by withdrawal symptoms from alcoholic intoxication and includes restlessness, tremors of the hands, hallucinations, sweating, and increased heart rate.	**delirium** (deh-LEER-ee-um) (dee-LEER-ee-um) **delirium tremens** (dee-LEER-ee-um TREM-enz)
dementia	Gradual but progressive deterioration of **cognitive function** due to old age or a neurologic disease. Alzheimer's disease is the most common type of dementia. There is a gradual decline in mental abilities, with forgetfulness, inability to learn new things, inability to perform daily activities, and difficulty making decisions. It can also include personality changes, anxiety, irritability, poor judgment, impulsiveness, hostility, combativeness, depression, and delusions.	**dementia** (dee-MEN-shee-ah) **de-** *reversal of; without* **ment/o-** *mind; chin* **-ia** *condition; state; thing* **cognitive** (KAWG-nih-tiv) **cognit/o-** *thinking* **-ive** *pertaining to*

Impulse Control Disorders

Impulse control disorders are characterized by strong, persistent thoughts (impulses) that occupy the mind and cause tension as the patient decides whether or not to act on them. When the act is performed, the patient feels relief or even pleasure. Treatment: Psychotherapy, counseling with anger management, family therapy.

Word or Phrase	Description	Word Building
intermittent explosive disorder	Sudden, explosively violent, unprovoked attacks of rage that are out of proportion to the stress experienced. Patients always blame their anger on others or on circumstances. There is assault and battery, which is often associated with domestic violence (spousal abuse, child abuse). During psychiatric interviews, patients are asked if they have any **homicidal ideation** about actually killing someone.	**homicidal** (HOH-mih-SY-dal) **hom/i-** *man* **cid/o-** *killing* **-al** *pertaining to* **ideation** (EYE-dee-AA-shun)
kleptomania	Overwhelming impulse to steal things that have little or no value. These things are not stolen out of anger or revenge, and the patient sometimes even secretively returns them. Unlike shoplifting, the patient does not steal in order to obtain something without paying for it. The patient is a **kleptomaniac.**	**kleptomania** (KLEP-toh-MAY-nee-ah) **klept/o-** *to steal* **-mania** *condition of frenzy*
pathological gambling	Constant gambling that interferes with normal life and work activities and creates severe financial problems. Patients lie about how much money they have lost and often place bigger bets to win back lost money.	**pathological** (PATH-oh-LAWJ-ih-kal) **path/o-** *disease; suffering* **log/o-** *word; the study of* **-ical** *pertaining to*
pyromania	Deliberately setting fires for the pleasure of watching the fire and the people sent to fight the fire. Fires are not set to take revenge, conceal a crime, or collect insurance money. The patient is a **pyromaniac.**	**pyromania** (PY-roh-MAY-nee-ah) **pyr/o-** *fire; burning* **-mania** *condition of frenzy*
trichotillomania	Repetitive pulling out hair from the head	**trichotillomania** (TRIK-oh-TIL-oh-MAY-nee-ah) **trich/o-** *hair* **till/o-** *pull out* **-mania** *condition of frenzy*

Personality Disorders

Personality disorders are characterized by a disturbance of one or more aspects of the personality (which is the combination of thoughts, beliefs, emotions, and behaviors that are unique to each person). Patients with personality disorders experience difficulty in interpersonal relationships (marriage, work, social). They are unable to adapt their rigid views, they fail to meet the needs of others, and they have a tendency to blame others for their own failures. Treatment: Psychotherapy, group therapy, family therapy.

antisocial personality	Disregard for the written and unwritten rules and standards of conduct (laws, morals, ethics) of society. Patients lie, steal, and manipulate, showing no empathy for others or guilt or remorse for their actions. There is also fighting, failure to attend school (truancy), vandalism, sexual promiscuity, excessive drinking, the use of illegal drugs, and criminal acts. These patients were previously known as **sociopaths** or **psychopaths.**	**antisocial** (AN-tee-SOH-shal) **anti-** *against* **soci/o-** *human beings; community* **-al** *pertaining to* **personality** (PER-son-AL-ih-tee) **person/o-** *person* **-al** *pertaining to* **-ity** *state; condition*
avoidant personality	Avoidance of social contact because of excessive shyness and extreme fear and sensitivity to criticism or rejection	

Word or Phrase	Description	Word Building
borderline personality	Inability to sustain a stable relationship. Patients fear abandonment and panic when they are alone, rushing into intense, but self-destructive relationships. They tend to see things in black and white—all good or all bad with no middle ground. They are hypersensitive, with strong emotions that can easily change. They have poor tolerance to stress and often overreact.	
dependent personality	Expects and wants to be told what to do and what to think. Patients are passive, have difficulty making decisions, and want others to take care of them and the details of their lives.	**dependent** (dee-PEN-dent) **depend/o-** *to hang onto* **-ent** *pertaining to*
narcissistic personality	Exaggerated sense of self-worth and importance. Patients feel superior to others and believe they are entitled to be the center of attention and to receive compliments, admiration, and affection. They are angry, demanding, and manipulative if others receive more than they do. Their demand to be noticed can be emotional, dramatic, and done for its effect (**histrionic**).	**narcissism** (NAWR-sih-sizm) **histrionic** (HIS-tree-AW-nik)
obsessive–compulsive personality	Inflexible and perfectionistic. Patients feel that everything must be accounted for and in its place, nothing can be left to chance, and they are unwilling to compromise. Patients feel that there is always one best way to do everything and they expect others to act accordingly. Patients keep lists and schedules and are concerned about productivity, but may be so consumed by minor details that they sometimes cannot get the job done. These patients do not have obsessive–compulsive disorder (which was discussed previously).	

Factitious Disorders

Factitious disorders are characterized by physical and/or psychological symptoms that are consciously made up (fabricated) by the patient, and that the patient knows are not true. Patients pretend to be sick (often with symptoms that are difficult to evaluate) or even make themselves sick because of a desire to be cared for. They are intelligent and knowledgeable about medicine, but they are experienced, expert liars who often fool physicians.

Word or Phrase	Description	Word Building
malingering	Exhibiting **factitious** medical or psychiatric symptoms in order to get a tangible reward, such as narcotic drugs or disability payments. Patients are aware that they are lying and know exactly what they want to achieve from their deceptions.	**malingering** (mah-LING-ger-ing) **factitious** (fak-TISH-us) **factiti/o-** *artificial; made up* **-ous** *pertaining to*
Munchausen syndrome	Exhibiting factitious medical or psychiatric symptoms. Patients are aware that they are lying, but are unaware that their motivation is the desire for assistance, attention, compassion, pity, and being excused from the normal expectations of life. Patients are not concerned about the cost of multiple tests, treatments, or surgeries and, in fact, desire to have them.	**Munchausen** (moon-CHOW-zen)
Munchausen by proxy	A person creates illness in another person in order to enjoy the attention that the sick person gets while simultaneously enjoying attention for being the sacrificing, loving caregiver. This can occur in the mother–child relationship and is a form of child abuse. The mother makes up a medical history, induces physical symptoms with drugs, or contaminates specimens for laboratory tests to prolong the child's state of sickness.	**proxy** (PRAWK-see)

Dissociative Disorders

Dissociative disorders are characterized by a breakdown between the conscious mind and the person's identity, personality, and memory. This breakdown is precipitated by a traumatic event or by continuing trauma during childhood. Treatment: Psychotherapy.

Word or Phrase	Description	Word Building
depersonalization	Loss of connection (**dissociative process**) between personal thoughts and a sense of self and the environment. Patients feel as if they are in a dream or watching a movie of themselves, and things seem unreal and strange.	**depersonalization** (dee-PER-son-al-ih-ZAY-shun) **dissociative** (dih-SOH-see-ah-tiv) **dis-** *away from* **soci/o-** *human beings; community* **-ative** *pertaining to*
fugue	Impulsive flight from one's life and familiar surroundings after a traumatic event. The patient begins a new life in a new location and functions normally but is unable to remember anything of the past.	**fugue** (FYOOG)
identity disorder	Loss of connection between the normally integrated functions of conscious thought, perception of the environment, identity, and memory. This loss of connection is done to bury traumatic memories. Two or more distinct personalities are present, each with its own identity and history (made up of parts of the original personality). Each personality is capable of independent thoughts and actions and may be unaware of the other personalities. In the past, this was known as **multiple personality disorder** or **split personality.**	

Somatoform Disorders

Somatoform disorders are characterized by excessive physical complaints that are dramatic but do not fit any medical disease. Diagnostic tests are negative. There is pain in various places in the body with anxiety. Patients have poor insight into their problem and may have experienced trauma prior to the onset of symptoms. Treatment: Psychotherapy, antianxiety drugs.

Word or Phrase	Description	Word Building
body dysmorphic disorder	The patient is continually concerned with minor defects in appearance of the body, particularly of the face, and demands frequent plastic surgery	**dysmorphic** (dis-MOR-fik) **dys-** *painful; difficult; abnormal* **morph/o-** *shape* **-ic** *pertaining to*
conversion disorder	**Somatoform** (neurologic, sensory, or motor) deficits that occur without any physical basis. There may be sudden blindness, deafness, paralysis, or the inability to speak. This begins with **repression** of overwhelming anxiety or internal conflict, which then undergoes a **conversion** to physical symptoms.	**conversion** (con-VER-shun) **con-** *with* **vers/o-** *to travel; to turn* **-ion** *action; condition* **somatoform** (soh-MAT-oh-form) **somat/o-** *body* **-form** *having the form of* **repression** (ree-PRESH-un) **repress/o-** *press back* **-ion** *action; condition*
hypochondriasis	Preoccupation with and misinterpretation of minor body sensations with the fear that these indicate disease. Patients are convinced they have a serious illness and make frequent trips to the doctor despite medical evidence and reassurance to the contrary. The patient is known as a **hypochondriac.**	**hypochondriasis** (HY-poh-con-DRY-ah-sis) **hypo-** *below; deficient* **chondr/o-** *cartilage* **-iasis** *state of; process of*

Laboratory and Diagnostic Procedures

Blood and Urine Tests

Word or Phrase	Description	Word Building
drug level	Blood test to determine the level of an antipsychotic drug in patients who are noncompliant with taking their medicines.	
urine test for drugs	Urine test to detect illegal drugs	

Radiologic Procedures

CT scan or MRI scan	Procedure used to document loss of brain tissue or structural abnormalities of the brain that might be related to a psychiatric illness	
PET scan	Procedure that shows areas of abnormal metabolism in the brain related to dementia and Alzheimer's disease	

Psychiatric Procedures and Tests

Beck Depression Inventory (BDI)	Screening tool that is filled out by the patient to assess the degree of depression. Each item offers four answers that show progressively more depressed emotions: I do not feel sad (0 points), I feel sad (1 point), I am sad all the time (2 points), and I am so sad I can't stand it (3 points). The patient selects the statement that most closely matches his/her feelings.	
Holmes Social Readjustment Rating Scale	Assigns point values to various **stressors** (negative and positive life events) to measure the amount of stress in a patient's life: death of spouse (100 points), divorce (73 points), death of family member (63 points), personal illness (53 points), marriage (50 points), retirement (45 points), pregnancy (40 points), change in finances (38 points), change in jobs (36 points), change in schools (25 points), vacation (13 points), and Christmas (12 points)	**stressor** (STRES-or) **stress/o-** *disturbing stimulus* **-or** *person or thing that produces or does*
intelligence testing	Intelligence tests are administered if the patient is suspected of having any degree of mental impairment or retardation	
psychiatric diagnosis	Diagnosis of any mental or psychiatric illnesses. It is stated in a specific way that involves five axes or aspects, as required by the American Psychiatric Association's publication *Diagnostic and Statistical Manual of Mental Disorders,* fourth edition (DSM-IV) (see Table 17-2).	**psychiatric** (sy-kee-AT-rik) **psych/o-** *mind* **iatr/o-** *physician; medical treatment* **-ic** *pertaining to*

Table 17-2   Psychiatric Diagnosis Format

Axis I	Any psychiatric disorders (except personality disorders and mental retardation)
Axis II	Personality disorders and mental retardation
Axis III	Medical symptoms, signs, and diseases (based on the physical examination, neurologic examination, and mental status examination)
Axis IV	Psychosocial and environmental problems (includes problems with marriage, family, neighbors, community, school, work, housing, finances, health care, police, or the courts)
Axis V	Global Assessment of Functioning (GAF), ranging from 1 to 100 points. A person who is able to manage life's problems, functions in all areas of life, and exhibits no symptoms or signs of mental disorder scores between 91 and 100. Patients with moderate psychiatric disorders or moderate difficulty functioning in social, work, and school situations score between 51 and 60. Patients in constant, severe danger of hurting themselves or others score below 10.

Word or Phrase	Description	Word Building
psychiatric interview	Provides insights into the patient's mental illness. It can be done in a psychiatrist's office or clinic or during admission to an acute care hospital or psychiatric hospital. The patient (or other person if the patient is unable to answer) is asked why he/she came for care, who brought him/her for care, what stressors are going on in his/her life, and about any previous psychiatric illness. The interviewer notes the patient's general appearance and behavior and listens to the patient's answers to analyze speech, content of thoughts, abstract reasoning, insight, and judgment.	
Rorschach test	A set of cards with abstract shapes on them. Patients are asked to describe what the shape of the inkblot represents to them. It is also known as the **inkblot test.**	**Rorschach** (ROHR-shahk)
Thematic Apperception Test (TAT)	Assesses personality, emotions, attitudes, motivation, and conflicts. The patient is shown 31 different pictures of social or interpersonal situations. The patient describes what is happening in the picture or what the theme of the picture is.	**apperception** (AP-er-SEP-shun) **appercept/o-** *fully perceived* **-ion** *action; condition*

Psychiatric Therapies

Word or Phrase	Description	Word Building
art therapy	Uses drawing or creating other types of art while talking with an art therapist. Art therapy relieves stress, allows patients to express their thoughts and emotions safely, and helps them gain insight into their problems. Art therapy helps small children express something they saw or something that was done to them that they cannot describe in words.	**therapy** (THAIR-ah-pee) **therapeutic** (THAIR-ah-PYOO-tik) **therapeut/o-** *therapy; treatment* **-ic** *pertaining to*
aversion therapy	The patient thinks about a desired, but destructive, behavior and this is coupled with a mild electrical shock or a bad smell (such as ammonia). This is a form of conditioning that creates an aversion to doing that behavior. This therapy is used to treat drug and cigarette addiction and sexual identity issues.	**aversion** (ah-VER-shun) **a-** *away from; without* **vers/o-** *to travel; to turn* **-ion** *action; condition*
cognitive-behavioral therapy (CBT)	Based on the premise that beliefs and attitudes (not people or events) cause undesirable or destructive emotions, and that thought patterns and behaviors are learned and can be unlearned. Patients are taught to use guided imagery and self-counseling to produce desirable emotions and behavior. This therapy is used to treat anxiety, panic attacks, phobias, depression, eating disorders, and other behaviors.	**cognitive** (KAWG-nih-tiv) **cognit/o-** *thinking* **-ive** *pertaining to* **behavioral** (bee-HAY-vyer-al) **behav/o-** *activity; manner of acting* **-ior** *pertaining to* **-al** *pertaining to*
detoxication	Observation and medical treatment for a patient with alcoholism undergoing withdrawal. Drugs are given, as needed, to minimize withdrawal symptoms and prevent seizures. This therapy is also known as **detoxification.**	**detoxication** (dee-TAWKS-ih-KAY-shun) **de-** *reversal of; without* **toxic/o-** *poison; toxin* **-ation** *a process; being or having*
electroconvulsive therapy (ECT)	Uses an electrical current and electrodes on the head to produce seizures (convulsions). Patients are given sedative and muscle relaxant drugs to make them unconscious and relaxed. The seizure lasts about 1 minute and the patient awakens within 1 hour. It is used to treat severe depression and schizophrenia. ECT relieves symptoms more quickly than antidepressant drugs (that can take up to a month to become effective). It is also known as **electroshock therapy.**	**electroconvulsive** (ee-LEK-troh-con-VUL-siv) **electr/o-** *electricity* **convuls/o-** *seizure* **-ive** *pertaining to*
family therapy	Involves the entire family, not just the patient. The focus is on relationships and conflicts between family members (what they say to each other, how they say it, and how they act toward each other). The family often labels one family member as the troublemaker, while others can do no wrong. Unless corrected, these fixed roles keep the family members from adopting more appropriate behaviors.	

Word or Phrase	Description	Word Building
group therapy	Provides simultaneous therapy to several patients who have a similar mental illness (such as anxiety, depression, or being a victim of sexual abuse) (see Figure 17-9 ■). Group members share experiences and insights and provide feedback and emotional support to each other.	

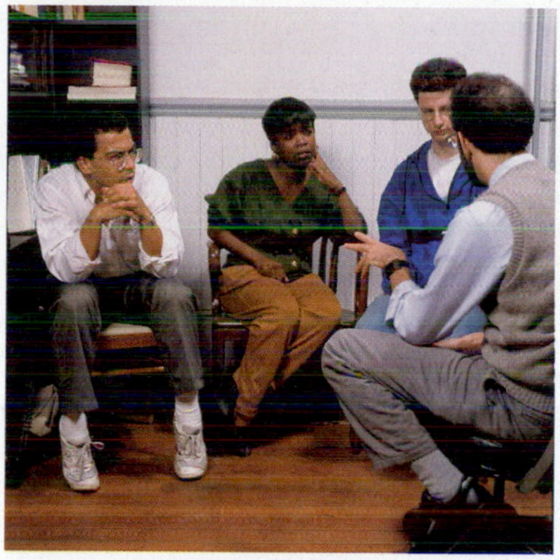

Figure 17-9 ■ Group therapy.
This psychologist is conducting a group therapy session. Group members support or challenge each other while gaining insight into their own problems.

Word or Phrase	Description	Word Building
hypnosis	Places the patient in a sleeplike trance (the patient is still able to remember who they are and what is happening). The therapist makes suggestions that are incorporated in the patient's subconscious mind and later acted upon consciously to some degree. It is used to treat anxiety and phobias and to help patients stop smoking or lose weight. It is also known as **hypnotherapy.**	**hypnosis** (hip-NOH-sis) **hypn/o-** *sleep* **-osis** *condition; abnormal condition; process* **hypnotherapy** (HIP-noh-THAIR-ah-pee) **hypn/o-** *sleep* **-therapy** *treatment*
play therapy	Uses toys and other objects (often dolls) to help young children express emotions and reenact traumatic or abusive events (on a small scale they can control). It is used to treat social withdrawal, anxiety, depression, aggression, and ADHD.	
psychoanalysis	Based on the idea of a conscious and subconscious mind. It was developed by Sigmund Freud to analyze a patient's thoughts and behavior by using interpretation of dreams and hypnosis.	**psychoanalysis** (SY-koh-ah-NAL-ih-sis) **psych/o-** *mind* **analy/o-** *to separate* **-osis** *condition; abnormal condition; process*
psychotherapy	Any therapy (except drug therapy and electroconvulsive therapy) that uses verbal or nonverbal communication between a patient or a group of patients and a psychologist or psychiatrist to treat a mental disorder	**psychotherapy** (SY-koh-THAIR-ah-pee) **psych/o-** *mind* **-therapy** *treatment*
systematic desensitization	Technique in which a patient imagines 10 different scenarios involving a specific phobia (e.g., fear of spiders). Each scenario is associated with progressively greater anxiety. The patient practices relaxation techniques before and after visualizing the first scenario. When the first scenario no longer causes anxiety, the patient moves on to the second, and so forth, until that phobia no longer causes anxiety.	**desensitization** (dee-SEN-sih-tih-ZAY-shun) **de-** *reversal of; without* **sensit/o-** *affected by; sensitive to* **-ization** *process of making, creating, or inserting*
therapeutic milieu	Stable, structured, and safe emotional and physical environment that provides ongoing therapy of various types for a psychiatric patient	**milieu** (meel-YOO)

Drug Categories

These categories of drugs are used to treat psychiatric disorders and conditions. The most common generic and trade name drugs in each category are listed.

Category	Indication	Examples	Word Building
antianxiety drugs	Treat anxiety and neurosis. They are also known as **anxiolytic drugs** and **minor tranquilizers.**	alprazolam (Xanax), chlordiazepoxide (Librium), diazepam (Valium)	**antianxiety** (AN-tee-ang-ZY-eh-tee) **anti-** *against* **anxi/o-** *fear; worry* **-ety** *condition; state* **anxiolytic** (ANG-zee-oh-LIT-ik) **anxi/o-** *fear; worry* **ly/o-** *break down; destroy* **-tic** *pertaining to* **tranquilizer** (TRANG-kwih-LY-zer) **tranquil/o-** *calm* **-izer** *thing that affects in a particular way*
antidepressant drugs	Treat depression by prolonging the action of norepinephrine or serotonin. Categories include tricyclic, tetracyclic, monoamine oxidase inhibitors (MAOIs), selective serotonin reuptake inhibitors (SSRIs), and serotonin and norepinephrine reuptake inhibitors (SNRIs).	bupropion (Wellbutrin), doxepin (Sinequan), duloxetine (Cymbalta), mirtazapine (Remeron), paroxetine (Paxil), sertraline (Zoloft)	**antidepressant** (AN-tee-dee-PRES-ant) **anti-** *against* **depress/o-** *press down* **-ant** *pertaining to*
antipsychotic drugs	Treat psychosis, paranoia, and schizophrenia by blocking dopamine receptors in the limbic system. They are also known as **major tranquilizers.**	aripiprazole (Abilify), chlorpromazine (Thorazine), haloperidol (Haldol), risperidone (Risperdal)	**antipsychotic** (AN-tee-sy-KAWT-ik) **anti-** *against* **psych/o-** *mind* **-tic** *pertaining to*

Did You Know?

Valium comes from the Latin word *valere,* which means *to be healthy.* The plant valerian has been known since the time of Hippocrates to calm the nerves.

Clinical Connections

Pharmacology. Many schizophrenic patients do not continue to take their prescribed antipsychotic drug because of **tardive dyskinesia,** a severe side effect that develops later in the treatment. It causes involuntary, repetitive movements of the face (grimacing, lip smacking, chewing, eye blinking, sticking out the tongue) and movements of the arms and legs (rocking back and forth, marching in place).

tardive (TAR-dive) **tard/o-** *late; slow* **-ive** *pertaining to*

dyskinesia (DIS-kih-NEE-zee-ah) **dys-** *painful; difficult; abnormal* **kines/o-** *movement* **-ia** *condition; state; thing*

Category	Indication	Examples	Word Building
drugs for alcoholism	Inhibit an enzyme that metabolizes the breakdown products of alcohol. Patients on this drug who drink alcohol experience headache, dizziness, nausea, and even heart arrhythmias. This unpleasant reaction is a detriment to drinking alcohol.	disulfiram (Antabuse)	
drugs for bipolar disorder	Lessen the severity of mood swings between the two emotional poles of mania and depression. These include antipsychotic drugs and anticonvulsant drugs.	lamotrigine (Lamictal), levetiracetam (Keppra), lithium (Lithobid)	

Abbreviations

ADD	attention deficit disorder	**OCD**	obsessive–compulsive disorder
ADHD	attention-deficit hyperactivity disorder	**OD**	overdose
BDI	Beck Depression Inventory	**PCP**	phencyclidine (angel dust, a street drug)
CBT	cognitive-behavioral therapy	**PMDD**	premenstrual dysphoric disorder
CNS	central nervous system	**PTSD**	posttraumatic stress disorder
DT	delirium tremens	**Psy**	psychiatry, psychology
ECT	electroconvulsive therapy	**Psych**	psychiatry, psychology
ETOH	ethyl alcohol (liquor)	**SAD**	seasonal affective disorder
LSD	lysergic acid diethylamide (a street drug)	**SSRI**	selective serotonin reuptake inhibitor (drug)
MAO	monoamine oxidase (inhibitor drug)	**TAT**	Thematic Apperception Test

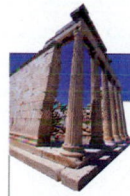

It's Greek to Me!

Did you notice that some words have two different combining forms? Combining forms from both Greek and Latin languages remain a part of medical language today.

Word	Greek	Latin	Medical Word Examples
mind	phren/o-	ment/o-	schizophrenia, mental, dementia
	psych/o-		psychotherapy
self	aut/o-	su/i-	autism, suicide

CAREER FOCUS

Meet Patricia, a social worker

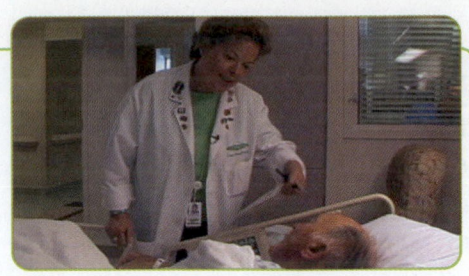

"There are all kinds of jobs you can do when you're a social worker. You can work in nursing homes. You can work in rehab centers. You can work on your own and do private counseling with people who've just gotten a terminal diagnosis. You can work with children. You can work in schools. One of the reasons why I love it is because you never know what you're going to be doing in a day. I'm assigned to a pulmonologist. Each day we go over his case list, and we prioritize who needs to be seen first, who needs home care, who needs nursing home placement, who needs help with prescriptions, who needs somebody to just go in and talk to them. I see my role as helping patients who are in an unfamiliar environment. It's not the best time of their lives. I use medical terminology all day long, especially when calling in the clinical information to the insurance companies."

Social workers are allied health professionals who obtain medical, housing, financial, or other community services and support for patients or clients. Social workers work in the department of human services in government offices, clinics, nursing homes, hospitals, and in psychiatric hospitals.

Psychologists are mental health practitioners who have a doctoral degree (Ph.D.) in **psychology.** They work in psychiatric hospitals, outpatient clinics, and school systems. They administer psychological and intelligence tests and act as therapists for various types of counseling and psychotherapy sessions (family, group, marriage). They are not physicians and cannot prescribe drug therapy.

Psychiatrists are physicians who practice in the mental health specialty of psychiatry. They diagnose and treat patients with mental illness. Physicians can take additional training and become board certified in the subspecialties of child and adolescent psychiatry, geriatric psychiatry, psychosomatic medicine, addiction psychiatry, or forensic psychiatry.

social (SOH-shal)
  soci/o- *human beings; community*
  -al *pertaining to*

psychologist (sy-KAWL-oh-jist)
  psych/o- *mind*
  log/o- *word; the study of*
  -ist *one who specializes in*

psychology (sy-KAWL-oh-jee)
  psych/o- *mind*
  -logy *the study of*

psychiatrist (sy-KY-ah-trist)
  psych/o- *mind*
  iatr/o- *physician; medical treatment*
  -ist *one who specializes in*

myhealthprofessionskit™ To see Patricia's complete video profile, visit Medical Terminology Interactive at www.myhealthprofessionskit.com. Select this book, log in, and go to the 17th floor of Pearson General Hospital. Enter the Laboratory, and click on the computer screen.

CHAPTER REVIEW EXERCISES

Test your knowledge of the chapter by completing these review exercises. Use the Answer Key at the end of the book to check your answers.

Anatomy and Physiology

Matching Exercise

Match each word or phrase to its description. Some structures may have more than one correct description.

1. amygdaloid bodies
2. adrenal medulla
3. hippocampus
4. hypothalamus
5. thalamus
6. frontal lobe

_____ Analyzes situations and weighs consequences and benefits

_____ Contains the satiety and feeding centers

_____ Almond-shaped structures

_____ Relay station that sends sensory information to the brain

_____ Interprets facial expressions and new social situations

_____ Secretes epinephrine for "fight or flight"

_____ Stores long-term memories

_____ Most active with the emotions of fear, anger, and rage

True or False Exercise

Indicate whether each statement is true or false by writing T or F on the line.

1. _____ The hippocampus is the entire anatomical system of the brain that deals with emotions.
2. _____ The limbic lobe is also known as the cingulate gyrus.
3. _____ The hippocampus stores short- and long-term memory.
4. _____ An emotion is an intense state of feeling.
5. _____ The outward expression on a person's face of the inward emotions is known as the mood.
6. _____ Neurotransmitters are chemicals that relay messages from one neuron to the next.
7. _____ Injury to the frontal lobe can produce a flat affect and inability to concentrate.

Matching Exercise

Match each word or phrase to its description. Some words may be used more than once.

1. dopamine
2. epinephrine
3. GABA
4. norepinephrine
5. serotonin

_____ Decreased levels associated with depression

_____ Decreased levels associated with anxiety

_____ Increased levels associated with anxiety, panic attacks, and social phobias

_____ Decreased levels associated with schizophrenia

_____ "Fight or flight" reaction

_____ Increased levels associated with infatuation

Mental Disorders and Conditions

Circle Exercise

Circle the correct word from the choices given.

1. (**Delirium, Panic, Rage**) is a sudden attack of overwhelming anxiety.
2. (**Avoidance, Bulimia, Delusion**) is bingeing on food and then vomiting.
3. (**Delirium, Delirium tremens, Schizophrenia**) is part of the symptoms of withdrawal from alcohol intoxication.
4. Retrograde amnesia causes the patient to forget events that happened (**after, before, during**) a traumatic event.
5. Autistic children can show (**echolalia, encopresis, euphoria**) in their speech.
6. Affective disorders are also known as (**depression, emotions, mood disorders**).
7. Hopelessness, helplessness, and worthlessness are symptoms of (**apathy, depression, withdrawal**).
8. Manic-depressive disorder is also known as (**bipolar disorder, intermittent explosive disorder, sadism**).
9. Making another person sick so that you can get attention is a sign of (**autism, Munchausen by proxy, psychosis**).
10. Doing something for its emotional and dramatic effect is being (**autistic, histrionic, obsessive**).

Matching Exercise

Match each word or phrase to its description.

1. addiction
2. anhedonia
3. conversion disorder
4. dysthymia
5. fugue
6. generalized anxiety disorder
7. identity disorder
8. kleptomania
9. malingering
10. narcissism
11. obsessive–compulsive disorder
12. panic attack
13. schizophrenia
14. sociopath
15. transvestism

_____ Constantly worried about "What if …"

_____ Condition of feeling superior to others and deserving of attention

_____ Physical and psychological dependence on a substance

_____ Performs excessive, repetitive, meaningless activities

_____ Forgetting one's old life and beginning a new life elsewhere

_____ Sudden, severe, overwhelming anxiety

_____ Most common psychosis

_____ Stealing things of no value

_____ Mild, chronic depression

_____ Lack of pleasure in any activity

_____ Sudden blindness or paralysis because of repressed internal conflict

_____ Multiple personality disorder

_____ Pretending to be in pain in order to get narcotic drugs

_____ Dressing as someone of the opposite sex

_____ Antisocial personality prone to violence and criminal acts

True or False Exercise

Indicate whether each statement is true or false by writing T *or* F *on the line.*

1. _____ A mental disorder is the same as a mental illness.
2. _____ Tardive dyskinesia is characterized by vulgar or socially inappropriate comments.
3. _____ Anorexia is the brief name for anorexia nervosa.
4. _____ A hypochondriac fears that every minor body sensation indicates a disease.
5. _____ Childish, silly behavior in schizophrenic patients is known as autism.
6. _____ Obsessive–compulsive disorder is the mildest form of bipolar disorder.
7. _____ Neologisms are made-up words whose meanings are known only to the patient.
8. _____ A fetish is an object used to produce sexual arousal.

Matching Exercise

Match each word or phrase to its description.

1. acrophobia	_____ Fear of closed-in spaces
2. agoraphobia	_____ Fear of strangers
3. arachnophobia	_____ Fear of germs
4. claustrophobia	_____ Fear of death
5. microphobia	_____ Fear of spiders
6. ophidiophobia	_____ Fear of crowds or public places
7. thanatophobia	_____ Fear of heights
8. xenophobia	_____ Fear of snakes

Diagnostic Procedures, Therapies, and Drugs

True or False Exercise

Indicate whether each statement is true or false by writing *T* or *F* on the line.

1. _____ The Rorschach test is another name for the inkblot test.

2. _____ MAOIs and SSRIs are types of drugs used to treat alcoholism.

3. _____ A PET scan looks at abnormal metabolism in the brain of a patient with dementia.

4. _____ Even positive life events are associated with levels of stress.

5. _____ The *Diagnostic and Statistical Manual of Mental Disorders* is published by the American Medical Association.

6. _____ An axis is a way of expressing the severity of a patient's depression.

7. _____ Detoxication is an appropriate therapy for a patient with psychosis.

8. _____ A dysfunctional family often labels one family member as the troublemaker.

9. _____ Hypnosis is also known as hypnotherapy.

10. _____ Tardive dyskinesia can be a severe side effect of antipsychotic drugs.

Matching Exercise

Match each word or phrase to its description.

1. aversion therapy	_____ Stable, structured, safe environment for therapy
2. cognitive-behavioral therapy	_____ All family members receive therapy
3. family therapy	_____ Thoughts can be changed
4. group therapy	_____ Uses toys and dolls to reenact trauma
5. play therapy	_____ Members support each other in therapy
6. psychoanalysis	_____ Uses noxious substances such as ammonia
7. therapeutic milieu	_____ Based on the work of Freud

Building Medical Words

Review the Combining Forms Exercise and Combining Form and Suffix Exercise that you already completed in the anatomy section on page 856.

Combining Forms Exercise

Before you build psychiatric words, review these additional combining forms. Next to each combining form, write its medical meaning. The first one has been done for you.

Combining Form	Medical Meaning	Combining Form	Medical Meaning
1. acr/o-	_extremity; highest point_	26. morph/o-	
2. addict/o-		27. ne/o-	
3. agor/a-		28. obsess/o-	
4. amnes/o-		29. ophidi/o-	
5. anxi/o-		30. ped/o-	
6. arachn/o-		31. phil/o-	
7. aut/o-		32. phob/o-	
8. cid/o-		33. phren/o-	
9. claustr/o-		34. pol/o-	
10. cognit/o-		35. psych/o-	
11. compuls/o-		36. pyr/o-	
12. copr/o-		37. rap/o-	
13. delus/o-		38. schiz/o-	
14. depress/o-		39. sex/o-	
15. factiti/o-		40. soci/o-	
16. hallucin/o-		41. somat/o-	
17. hedon/o-		42. stress/o-	
18. hom/i-		43. su/i-	
19. hypn/o-		44. thanat/o-	
20. iatr/o-		45. therapeut/o-	
21. klept/o-		46. till/o-	
22. log/o-		47. tranquil/o-	
23. man/o-		48. traumat/o-	
24. ment/o-		49. trich/o-	
25. micr/o-		50. xen/o-	

Combining Form and Suffix Exercise

Read the definition of the medical word. Select the correct suffix from the Suffix List. Select the correct combining form from the Combining Form List. Build the medical word and write it on the line. Be sure to check your spelling. The first one has been done for you.

SUFFIX LIST

-al (pertaining to)
-ety (condition; state)
-gen (that which produces)
-ic (pertaining to)
-ion (action; condition)
-ism (process; disease from a specific cause)

-ist (one who specializes in)
-ive (pertaining to)
-lalia (abnormal condition of speech)
-mania (condition of frenzy)
-or (person or thing that produces or does)

-osis (condition; abnormal condition; process)
-ous (pertaining to)
-phile (person who is attracted to or is fond of)
-therapy (treatment)

COMBINING FORM LIST

addict/o- (surrender to; be controlled by)
affect/o- (state of mind; mood)
anxi/o- (fear; worry)
aut/o- (self)
cognit/o- (thinking)

compuls/o- (drive or compel)
copr/o- (feces; stool)
delus/o- (false belief)
factiti/o- (artificial; made up)
hallucin/o- (imagined perception)
hypn/o- (sleep)

klept/o- (to steal)
obsess/o- (besieged by thoughts)
ped/o- (child)
psych/o- (mind)
pyr/o- (fire; burning)

rap/o- (to seize and drag away)
soci/o- (human beings; community)
stress/o- (disturbing stimulus)
therapeut/o- (therapy; treatment)

Definition of the Medical Word

		Build the Medical Word
1.	Action or condition that drives or compels	compulsion
2.	Person or thing that produces a disturbing stimulus	
3.	Condition of (a trance that resembles) sleep	
4.	Pertaining to human beings and community	
5.	Pertaining to thinking	
6.	Condition of (having a) false belief	
7.	That which produces an imagined perception	
8.	Condition of surrender to or being controlled by (something)	
9.	Treatment for the mind	
10.	Person who is attracted to or is fond of a child	
11.	Pertaining to (a medical condition that is) made up	
12.	Abnormal condition of speech (about) feces and stools	
13.	Disease from a specific cause of the self (being unable to form relationships with others)	
14.	Condition of fear and worry	
15.	Condition (of being) besieged by (uncontrollable) thoughts	
16.	Condition of frenzy (of setting) fires and burning	
17.	Pertaining to the state of mind or mood	
18.	One who specializes in (an action) to seize and drag away (a person for forced sexual intercourse)	
19.	Pertaining to (a therapy or) treatment	
20.	Condition of a frenzy to steal	

Prefix Exercise

Read the definition of the medical word. Look at the medical word or partial word that is given (it already contains a combining form and a suffix). Select the correct prefix from the Prefix List and write it on the blank line. Then build the medical word and write it on the line. Be sure to check your spelling. The first one has been done for you.

PREFIX LIST			
an- (without; not)	bi- (two)	dys- (painful; difficult; abnormal)	post- (after; behind)
anti- (against)	de- (reversal of; without)		trans- (across; through)

Definition of the Medical Word	Prefix	Word or Partial Word	Build the Medical Word
1. Pertaining to abnormal (over concern about the body's) shape	*dys-*	morphic	*dysmorphic*
2. A state (of being) without a mind	_____	mentia	_____
3. Pertaining to after an injury	_____	traumatic	_____
4. Pertaining to two poles (of emotion)	_____	polar	_____
5. Condition (of being) without pleasure	_____	hedonia	_____
6. Pertaining to (being) against human beings or community	_____	social	_____
7. Process of a specific disease (of going) across (to a different sexual identity) to dress	_____	vestism	_____

Multiple Combining Forms and Suffix Exercise

Read the definition of the medical word. Select the correct suffix and combining forms. Then build the medical word and write it on the line. Be sure to check your spelling. The first one has been done for you.

SUFFIX LIST	COMBINING FORM LIST	
-al (pertaining to)	acr/o- (extremity; highest point)	ophidi/o- (snake)
-ia (condition; state; thing)	agor/a- (open area or space)	phob/o- (fear; avoidance)
-ic (pertaining to)	arachn/o- (spider; spider web)	phren/o- (diaphragm; mind)
-ism (process; disease from a specific cause)	cid/o- (killing)	psych/o- (mind)
	claustr/o- (enclosed space)	schiz/o- (split)
-mania (condition of frenzy)	hom/i- (man)	su/i- (self)
	iatr/o- (physician; medical treatment)	thanat/o- (death)
	log/o- (word; the study of)	till/o- (pull out)
	micr/o- (small)	trich/o- (hair)
	ne/o- (new)	xen/o- (foreign)

Definition of the Medical Word   Build the Medical Word

1. Condition of a small (thing like a germ causing) fear   *microphobia*

2. Condition of the highest point (height causing) fear   _____

3. Condition of an enclosed space (causing) fear   _____

4. Condition (of having) a split mind   _____

5. Pertaining to self killing   _____

6. Condition of an open area or space (causing) fear   _____

7. Condition of a spider (causing) fear   _____

8. Condition of frenzy (in which) the hair is pulled out (from a person's own head)   _____

9. Pertaining to the mind (being helped) by a physician or medical treatment   _____

(continued)

Definition of the Medical Word

10. Process (of the patient creating) a new (but meaningless) word
11. Condition of a snake (causing) fear
12. Condition of death (causing) fear
13. Pertaining to (someone taking) a man and killing (him)
14. Condition of (something) foreign (or strange causing) fear

Build the Medical Word

_____

_____

_____

_____

_____

Abbreviations

Matching Exercise

Match each abbreviation to its definition.

1. ADHD   _____ Illegal, hallucinogenic drug
2. BDI   _____ Ethyl alcohol
3. ECT   _____ Administration of electricity to cause convulsions
4. ETOH   _____ Characterized by distractibility and hyperactivity
5. LSD   _____ Occurs during the winter months
6. OCD   _____ Mood disorder during premenstrual time
7. PMDD   _____ Characterized by meaningless rituals
8. PTSD   _____ Happens after war, terrorist attacks, or kidnapping
9. SAD   _____ Test to assess the extent of depression

Applied Skills

Proofreading and Spelling Exercise

Read the following paragraph. Identify each misspelled medical word and write the correct spelling of it on the line.

Pyschiatry is the study of the mind, as is psychology. Our inner emotions are expressed as our outward effect. The neurotransmitters dopamin and seratonin are associated with depression. Mild depression is known as disthymia. Suiside attempts are not uncommon in depressed patients, but homocidal ideation is usually expressed by patients who are schizofrenic or have an antisocial personalty. Psychotic patients have strong feelings of paranoya and suspect others are trying to kill them. Patients who always need to be the center of attention are narcistic. Narcotics are drugs and inhaled fumes are substances of abuse and adiction. A theraputic milyoo is a safe, secure environment for therapy.

1. _____   8. _____
2. _____   9. _____
3. _____   10. _____
4. _____   11. _____
5. _____   12. _____
6. _____   13. _____
7. _____   14. _____

Medical Report Exercise

This exercise contains a letter from a psychiatrist to the patient's primary care physician. Read the letter and answer the questions.

Daniel P. Bentley, M.D.
Psychiatric Associates
North Ridge Professional Building, Suite 702
Spring Garden, PA 17103
(717)-643-xxxx

Joseph Gildron, M.D., and Associates, Inc.
Centennial Medical Building, Suite 201
2859 Bonnie Brae Road
Ebensberg, PA 15890

Re: HARDISH, Janine

Dear Dr. Gildron:

Thank you for referring your patient, Mrs. Janine Hardish, to me for psychiatric evaluation.

The patient is a 39-year-old, divorced Caucasian female. She lives in a single-family dwelling with her 2 children. In the past, she has worked part time as a nurses' aide, but is not currently working because of feeling weak, dizzy, and tired. She states that she also feels depressed and hopeless. She claims that she has crying episodes every other day and difficulty sleeping at night.

She presents as a well-groomed lady whose clothes are neat, clean, and in good condition. Her hair is combed and her nails are clean and well manicured. Her affect is moderately bright, and she is alert and oriented to time, person, and place. She is able to answer questions easily, logically, and with a moderate amount of detail. Her thought content is well organized without evidence of flight of ideas or loose associations. Her fund of knowledge appears to be adequate. She is able to count backwards from 100 and to do serial 7s. Her memory for recent and remote events is intact. She was able to name the last 5 presidents. She is able to think of 18 words that begin with the letter "f" in 45 seconds (an above-normal result). However, she states that she feels that her memory is impaired.

She denies delusions or hallucinations. She denies feelings of being persecuted or plotted against. She denies suicidal or homicidal ideation.

She has little contact with her ex-husband, even though they were just divorced. She is experiencing some difficulty with her finances at this time; her husband does send child support payments, but she is not currently working. Her oldest son is experiencing difficulties in his schoolwork and recently was pulled over by the police and given a ticket for speeding.

She has been taking Cymbalta 20 mg P.O. at bedtime, as prescribed by you; however, she has also obtained a prescription for a tricyclic antidepressant drug from another physician and is taking this as well as Ambien for sleep.

It is my opinion that this patient is able to care for her own personal needs, is mentally intact, and has little difficulty relating to others.

DIAGNOSIS

Axis I   Factitious disorder, not otherwise specified.

Axis II   None.

Axis III   Normal mental status and psychiatric evaluation. A complete physical and neurologic examination was not performed. No known documented physical illness.

(continued)

Axis IV   Moderate degree of psychosocial stressors.

Axis V   GAF score is not computed because of factitious disorder.

Thank you for your referral of this patient.

Sincerely,

Daniel P. Bentley, M.D.

Daniel P. Bentley, M.D.

DPB:jbt
D: 11/19/20xx
T: 11/19/20xx

Word Analysis Questions

1. Divide *psychosocial* into its three word parts and define each word part.

    Word Part   **Definition**

    _____   _____

    _____   _____

    _____   _____

2. Divide *factitious* into its two word parts and define each word part.

    Word Part   **Definition**

    _____   _____

    _____   _____

3. Divide *homicidal* into its three word parts and define each word part.

    Word Part   **Definition**

    _____   _____

    _____   _____

    _____   _____

4. A patient who has entertained ideas of suicide is said to be _____ (adjective).

Fact Finding Questions

1. Define *factitious disorder.* _____

2. Name three psychosocial stressors that the patient is currently experiencing.

    a. _____

    b. _____

    c. _____

3. What evidence of drug-seeking behavior is mentioned in this report? _____

Critical Thinking Questions

1. Flight of ideas is associated with which of these diseases? **bipolar disorder**   **gender identity issues**   **suicide**

2. How are delusions different from hallucinations? _____

3. Feelings of being persecuted or plotted against can be labeled as what mental illness? _____

Hearing Medical Words Exercise

You hear someone speaking the medical words given below. Read each pronunciation and then write the medical word it represents. Be sure to check your spelling. The first one has been done for you.

1. ah-DIK-shun   *addiction*
2. ang-ZY-eh-tee   _____
3. dee-LOO-shun   _____
4. dee-TAWK-sih-fih-KAY-shun   _____
5. yoo-FOR-ee-ah   _____
6. KLEP-toh-MAY-nee-ah   _____
7. meel-YOO   _____
8. PAIR-ah-NOY-ah   _____
9. sy-KY-ah-trist   _____
10. SKIT-soh-FREN-ik   _____

Pronunciation Exercise

Read the medical word that is given. Then review the syllables in the pronunciation. Circle the primary (main) accented syllable. The first one has been done for you.

1. panic (pan-ik)
2. cognitive (kawg-nih-tiv)
3. delirium (deh-leer-ee-um)
4. hallucination (hah-loo-sih-nay-shun)
5. hypnosis (hip-noh-sis)
6. phobia (foh-bee-ah)
7. psychiatry (sy-ky-ah-tree)
8. therapeutic (thair-ah-pyoo-tik)

Multimedia Preview

Immerse yourself in a variety of activities inside Medical Terminology Interactive. Getting there is simple:

1. Click on www.myhealthprofessionskit.com.
2. Select "Medical Terminology" from the choice of disciplines.
3. First-time users must create an account using the scratch-off code on the inside front cover of this book.
4. Find this book and log in using your username and password.
5. Click on Medical Terminology Interactive.
6. Take the elevator to the 17th Floor to begin your virtual exploration of this chapter!

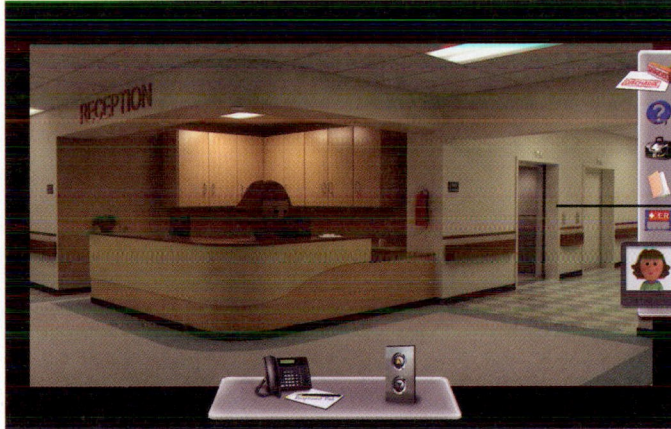
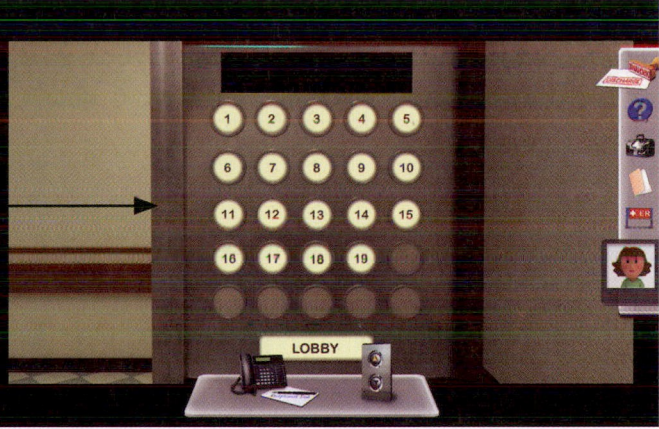

■ **Strikeout** Click on the alphabet tiles to fill in the empty squares in the word or phrase to complete the sentence. This game quizzes your vocabulary and spelling. But choose your letters carefully because three strikes and you're out!

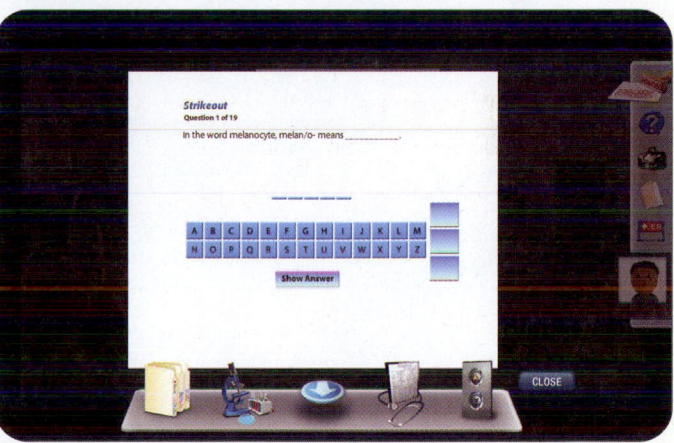

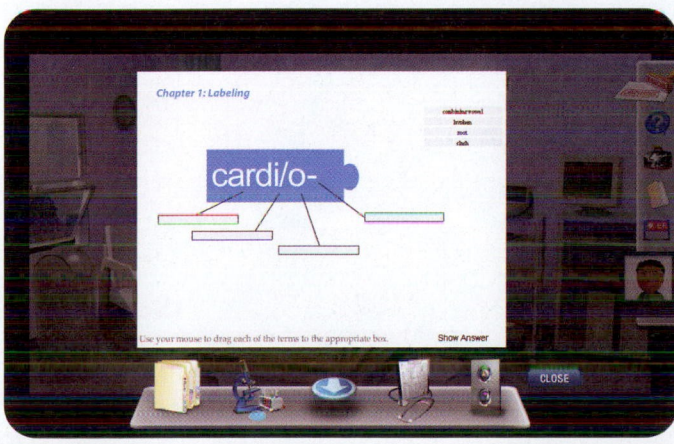

■ **Labeling Exercise** A picture is worth a thousand words . . . only if it's labeled correctly. To review anatomy, click and drag the terms that correlate to a figure from this chapter. All correct labels will lock into place beside the picture.

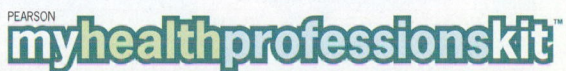

PEARSON
myhealthprofessionskit™

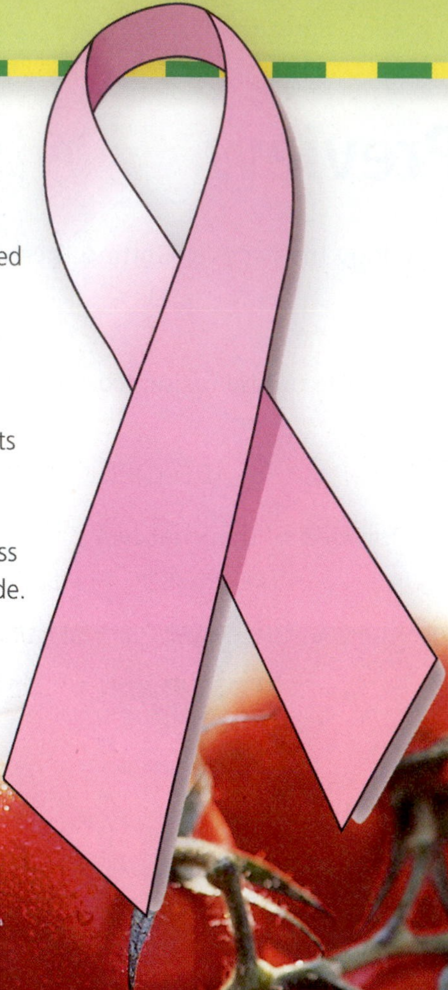

▶ Introduced in 1991, this pink ribbon symbol represents breast cancer awareness worldwide.

Dive In!

- One in two men and one in three women will develop cancer.
- Skin cancer is the most common but lung cancer is the most deadly.
- Cancer mortality rates have declined every year since 1990.
- Two-thirds of cancer deaths can be prevented by healthy lifestyle choices.
- In this chapter we'll explore the language of cancer. Once you master the language of oncology you'll be able to communicate about this serious, but often treatable disease.

Medicine Through HISTORY

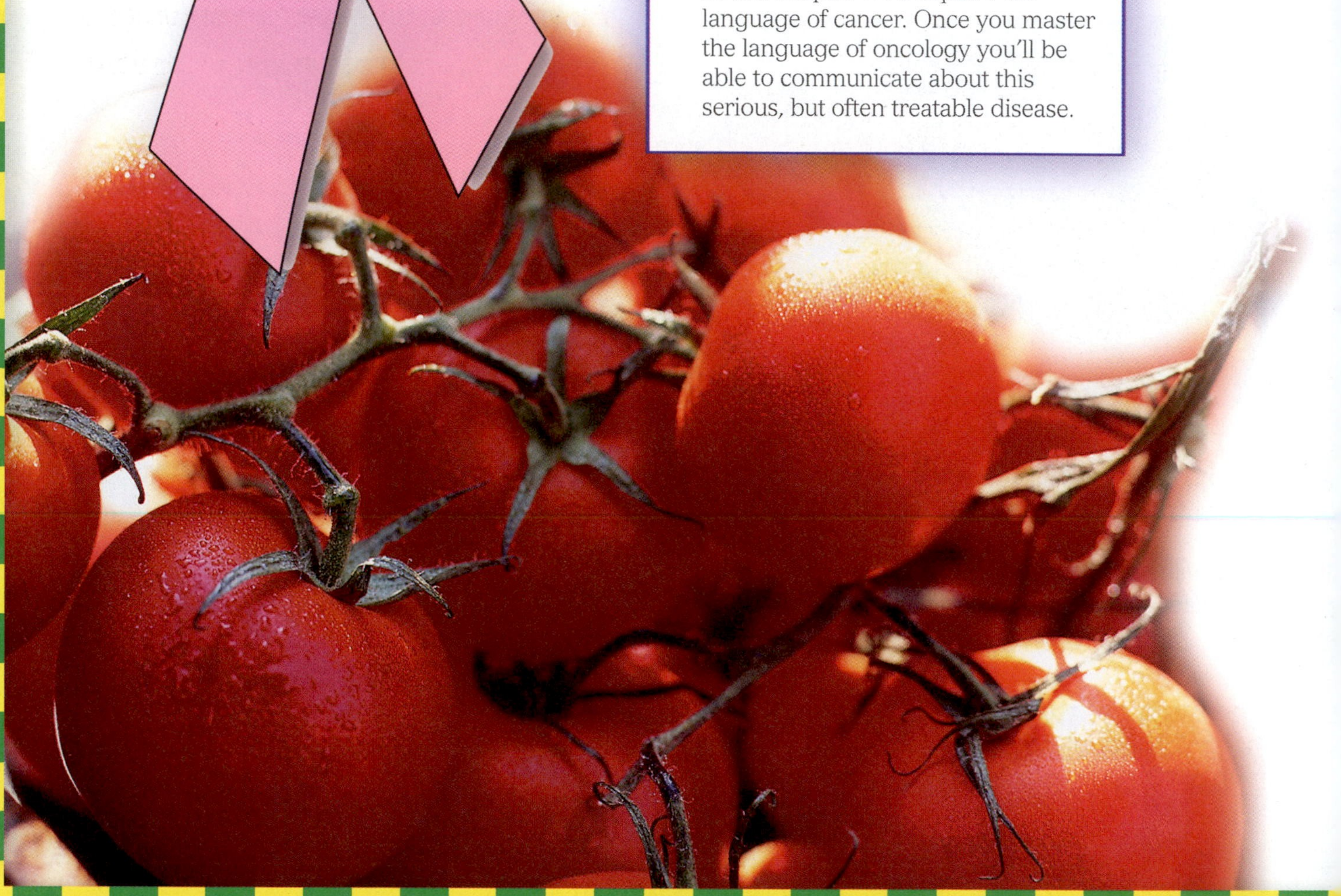

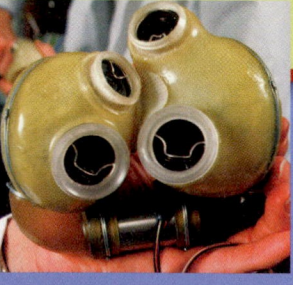

1982

Barney Clark is the first person to receive an implanted artificial heart, the Jarvik-7 created by Dr. Robert Jarvik

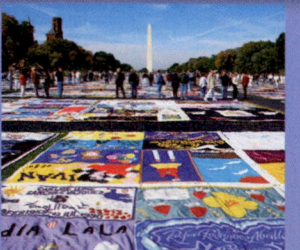

1982

The phrase acquired immunodeficiency syndrome (AIDS) is first used

1984

OPEN
PUSH
DOWN WHIL
TURNING
CLOSE TIGHTLY

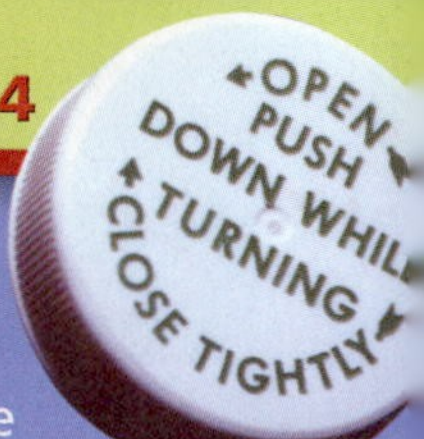

The child-proof safety cap for medicine bottles is invented

18
Oncology

Oncology (ong-KAWL-oh-jee) is the medical specialty that studies the anatomy and physiology of a cancer cell and uses diagnostic tests, medical and surgical procedures, and drugs to treat cancerous diseases.

▼ Cells are marvels of engineering, but any change in their structure or function can result in cancer.

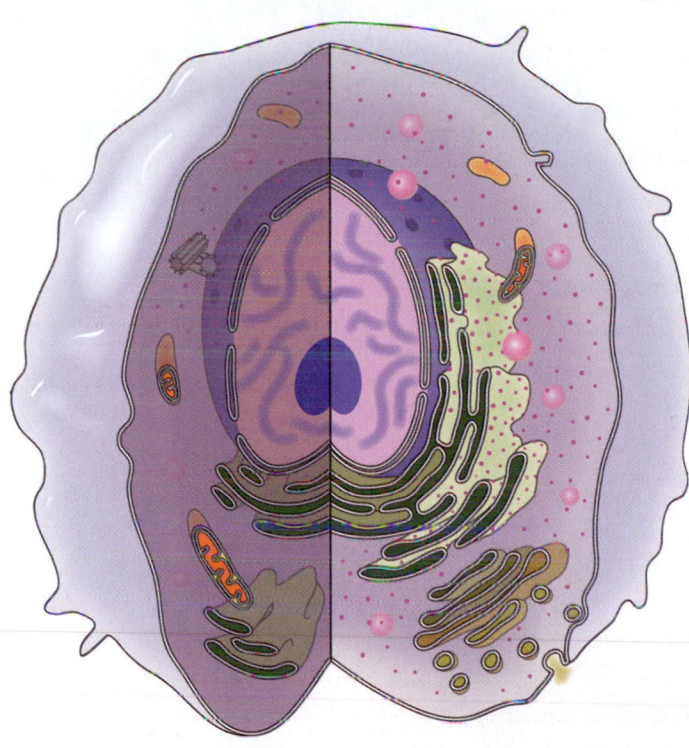

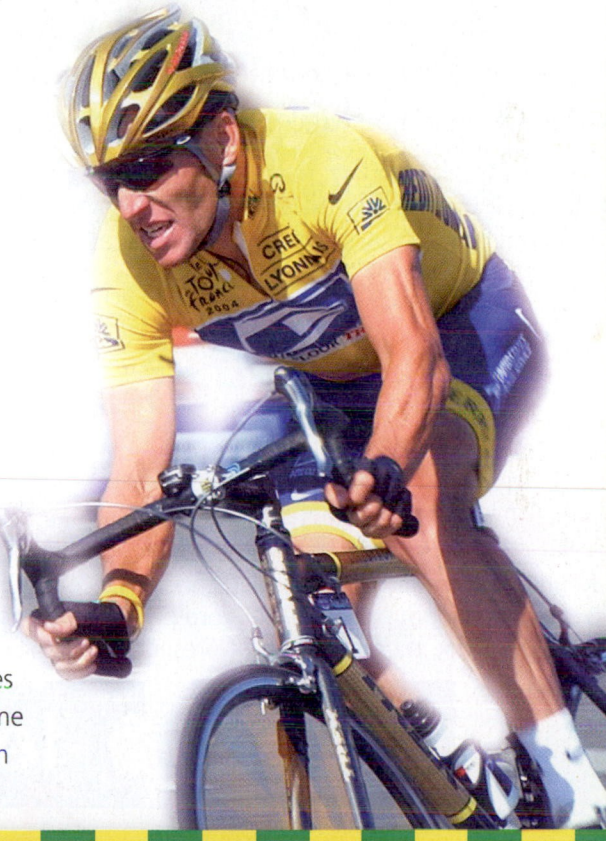

▶ Lance Armstrong overcame testicular cancer and continues to compete. He is one of the best cyclists in history.

◀ Pass the ketchup! Lycopene is an antioxidant found in tomatoes that may help reduce the risk of prostate cancer.

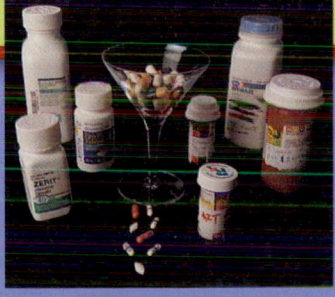

1984

AZT (Retrovir) is introduced as part of the drug "cocktail" used to treat AIDS

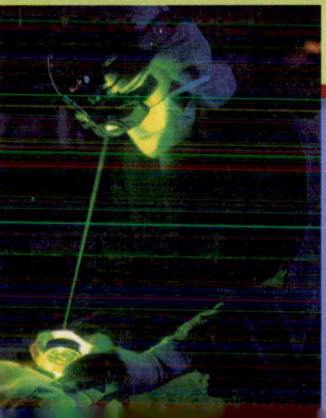

1988

Cataract surgery using a laser is first performed by Dr. Patricia Bath. She is also the first African American female physician to receive a patent for a medical device.

Measure Your Progress: Learning Objectives

After you study this chapter, you should be able to

1. Identify the structures of a cell.

2. Describe the process by which a normal cell divides and how a normal cell becomes a cancerous cell.

3. List six characteristics of cancerous cells and tumors.

4. Describe common types of cancer, laboratory and diagnostic procedures, medical and surgical procedures, and drug categories.

5. Give the medical meaning of word parts related to cancer.

6. Build cancer words from word parts and divide and define cancer words.

7. Spell and pronounce cancer words.

8. Analyze the medical content and meaning of an oncology report.

9. Dive deeper into oncology by reviewing the activities at the end of this chapter and online at Medical Terminology Interactive.

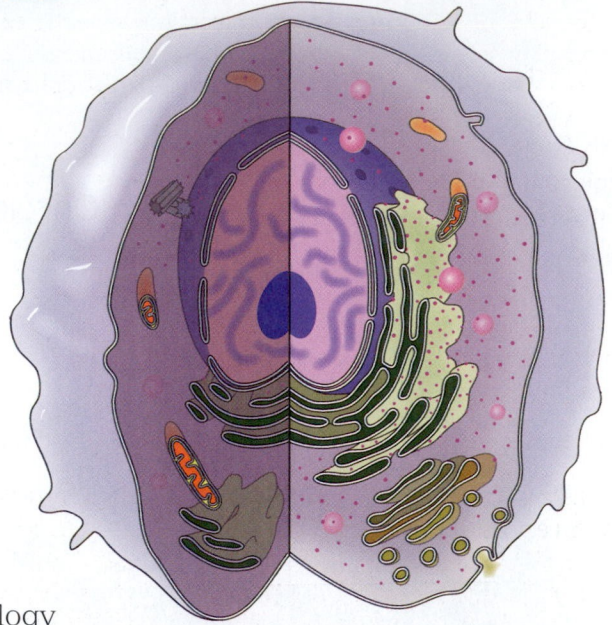

Figure 18-1 ■ **A cell.**

Each cell is a marvel of engineering, but a change in its structure or function can result in cancer.

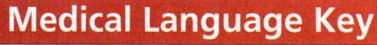

Medical Language Key

To unlock the definition of a medical word, break it into word parts. Define each word part. Put the word part meanings in order, beginning with the suffix, then the prefix (if present), then the combining form(s).

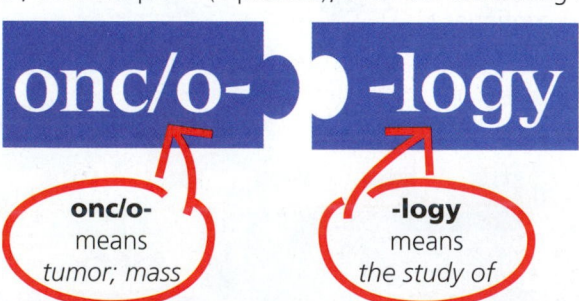

onc/o-
means
tumor; mass

-logy
means
the study of

	Word Part	Word Part Meaning
Suffix	-logy	*the study of*
Combining Form	onc/o-	*tumor; mass*

Oncology: *The study of a (cancerous) tumor or mass.*

Anatomy and Physiology

Unlike the other medical specialties you have already studied, the medical specialty of oncology is not based on a particular body system. Oncology encompasses all body systems because cancer can occur anywhere in the body. **Cancer** arises from various types of cells and tissues that often lend their names to the cancer.

Cancer begins as a single normal cell (see Figure 18-1 ■) that becomes an abnormal cell, and so we will begin our study of oncology by studying the structure and function of a normal cell.

cancer (KAN-ser)

cancerous (KAN-ser-us)
 cancer/o- *cancer*
 -ous *pertaining to*
The combining form *carcin/o-* also means *cancer.*

Anatomy Related to Oncology

Cells

A **cell** is the smallest independently functioning structure in the body that can reproduce itself by division. All cells contain certain basic structures (see Figure 18-2 ■). The **cell membrane** around the cell is a permeable barrier that protects and supports the **intracellular contents**. It allows water and nutrients to enter the cell and cellular waste products to leave the cell. It also contains ion pumps that actively bring electrolytes (sodium, potassium, and so forth) in and out of the cell.

cell (SEL)

cellular (SEL-yoo-lar)
 cellul/o- *cell*
 -ar *pertaining to*
The combining form *cyt/o-* also means *cell.*

intracellular (IN-trah-SEL-yoo-lar)
 intra- *within*
 cellul/o- *cell*
 -ar *pertaining to*

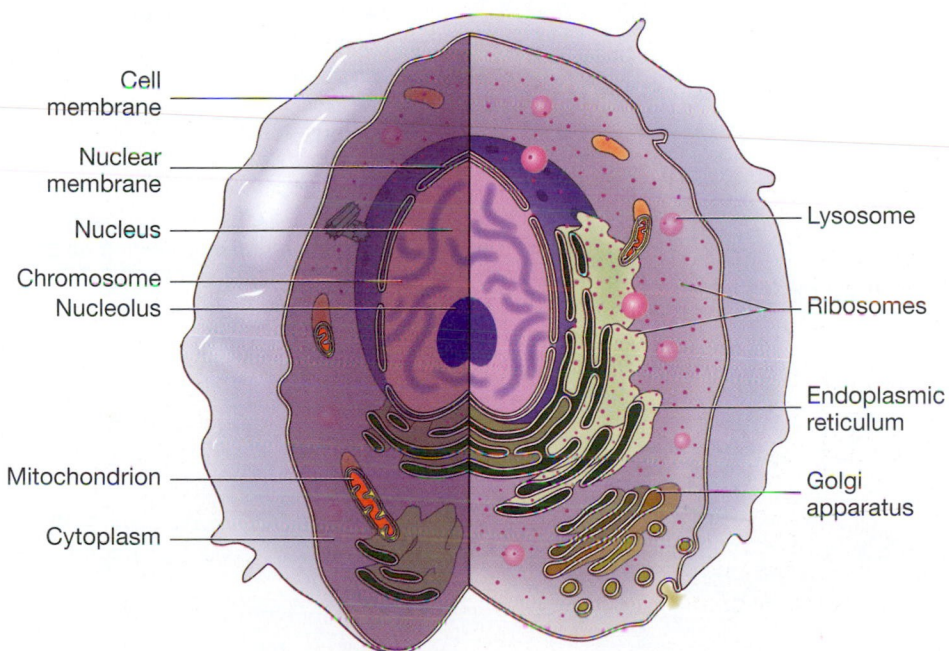

Cell membrane
Nuclear membrane
Nucleus
Chromosome
Nucleolus
Mitochondrion
Cytoplasm
Lysosome
Ribosomes
Endoplasmic reticulum
Golgi apparatus

Figure 18-2 ■ Structures of a cell.
A cell consists of many different structures, each of which plays a unique role in securing nutrients, producing energy, building proteins, fighting invading pathogens, or overseeing cellular division and other cellular activities.

The **cytoplasm** is a gel-like substance that fills the cell. The cytoplasm contains dissolved substances as well as different structures that are known as **organelles.**

- **Endoplasmic reticulum.** Network of channels throughout the cytoplasm that transports materials. It is also the site of protein, fat, and glycogen production.
- **Golgi apparatus.** Curved, stacked membranes that process and store proteins (such as hormones or enzymes) until they are released by the cell. It also makes lysosomes.
- **Lysosomes.** Small sacs that contain powerful digestive enzymes to destroy a bacterium or virus that invades the cell. When a cell dies, the lysosomes release their enzymes into the cell, and the cell is slowly dissolved.
- **Messenger RNA.** Messenger RNA (**ribonucleic acid**) duplicates the information contained in a gene and carries it to the ribosome where it is used to assemble amino acids to make a protein molecule.
- **Mitochondria.** Capsule-shaped structures with sectioned chambers that produce and store ATP, a high-energy molecule obtained from the metabolism of glucose. As needed, the mitochondria convert ATP to ADP to release energy for cellular activities.
- **Nucleus.** Large, round, centralized structure that is surrounded by a nuclear membrane. Through the action of DNA, it controls all of the activities that

WORD BUILDING

cytoplasm (SY-toh-plazm)
  cyt/o- *cell*
  -plasm *growth; formed substance*

organelle (OR-gah-NEL)
  organ/o- *organ*
  -elle *little thing*

endoplasmic (EN-doh-PLAS-mik)
  endo- *innermost; within*
  plasm/o- *plasma*
  -ic *pertaining to*

reticulum (reh-TIK-yoo-lum)

Golgi (GOHL-jee)

lysosome (LY-soh-sohm)
  lys/o- *break down; destroy*
  -some *a body*
Add words to make a complete definition of *lysosome: a body (that contains enzymes that) break down or destroy.*

ribonucleic acid
(RY-boh-noo-KLEE-ik AS-id)

mitochondrion
(MY-toh-CON-dree-on)

mitochondria (MY-toh-CON-dree-ah)
Mitochondrion is a Greek singular noun. Form the plural by changing *–on* to *–a.*

nucleus (NOO-klee-us)

nuclei (NOO-klee-eye)
Nucleus is a Latin singular noun. Form the plural by changing *-us* to *-i.* The combining form *kary/o-* also means *nucleus.*

nuclear (NOO-klee-ar)
  nucle/o- *nucleus*
  -ar *pertaining to*

take place within the cell. The **nucleolus** is a round, central region within the nucleus. It produces RNA and ribosomes. **Chromosomes** are paired structures within the nucleus. Each cell nucleus contains 23 pairs of chromosomes for a total of 46 chromosomes. In each of the 23 pairs, one of the chromosomes was inherited from the mother and the other from the father. A single chromosome is made of one long DNA (**deoxyribonucleic acid**) molecule. A DNA molecule consists of repeating pairs of amino acids sequenced along two strands that form a double helix. A **gene** is one segment of a DNA molecule that contains enough amino acid pairs to provide the information to produce one protein molecule. In a cell that is not dividing, each long DNA molecule is loosely coiled, giving the nucleus a woven, grainy appearance under the microscope. As the cell prepares to divide, each DNA molecule coils tightly, making the chromosomes visible as rod-like structures in the nucleus.

- **Ribosomes.** Granular structures in the cytoplasm and on the endoplasmic reticulum. Ribosomes contain RNA and proteins and are the site where proteins are produced.

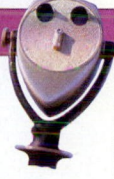

Did You Know?

Most body cells contain one nucleus. However, a mature erythrocyte (red blood cell) does not contain any nucleus, and a skeletal muscle cell contains many nuclei.

Physiology of Cellular Division and Cancer

Mitosis is the process by which a cell divides. Mitosis begins in the cell's nucleus as each chromosome makes an exact copy of itself. (The double helix of its DNA molecule splits down its length and rebuilds to form another double helix.) All of the chromosomes and their identical copies align themselves along threadlike filaments in the nucleus and then separate to opposite sides of the nucleus. Then the entire nucleus and cytoplasm split, forming two cells that are identical to the original cell.

Normal body cells divide in an orderly fashion and in response to a particular need. During childhood, growth hormone causes the body cells to divide rapidly as the child grows. During times of blood loss, the hormone erythropoietin from the kidneys stimulates stem cells in the bone marrow to divide and produce more mature erythrocytes (red blood cells). The rate of cell division is different for different types of cells. Skin cells have a high rate because they are constantly being shed from the surface of the body. In contrast, muscle cells divide less frequently. **Suppressor genes,** a group of genes in the DNA of each cell, inhibit mitosis and keep each cell from dividing excessively.

A Closer Look

The p53 gene is the most important suppressor gene. It is located on chromosome 17 in every cell. It is inactive until DNA in the cell's nucleus is damaged. Then, the p53 gene activates proteins to repair the DNA. While the DNA is being repaired, the p53 gene inhibits mitosis to decrease the chance of producing more defective cells. Because of their role in preventing the formation of cancer cells, suppressor genes are also known as tumor suppressor genes. If the DNA cannot be repaired, the p53 gene directs the cell to shut down. This is **apoptosis** or programmed cell death.

Types of damage to the DNA molecule of a chromosome include **genetic mutations** that delete genes, reverse their normal order, or break off segments of genes and insert them into other chromosomes (a process known as **translocation**).

Causes of DNA damage include carcinogens, pathogens, or heredity. Most of these factors do not immediately cause cancer. It is only after repeated damage that the cellular DNA is damaged beyond repair.

Factors that Contribute to the Development of Cancer (see Figure 18-3 ■)

1. **Carcinogens** (environmental substances)

   radiation (sunlight, x-rays, radiation therapy, nuclear weapons)

   chemicals (insecticides, dyes)

   fumes (industrial pollution, radon gas from the soil, cigarette tar and smoke, automobile exhaust)

   foreign particles that cause chronic irritation (asbestos)

   some chemotherapy drugs

   some hormone drugs

2. **Pathogens** (bacteria and viruses)

   Chronic irritation and inflammation from a bacterial or viral infection can eventually damage DNA. Examples: The human papillomavirus causes genital warts and chronic inflammation that can

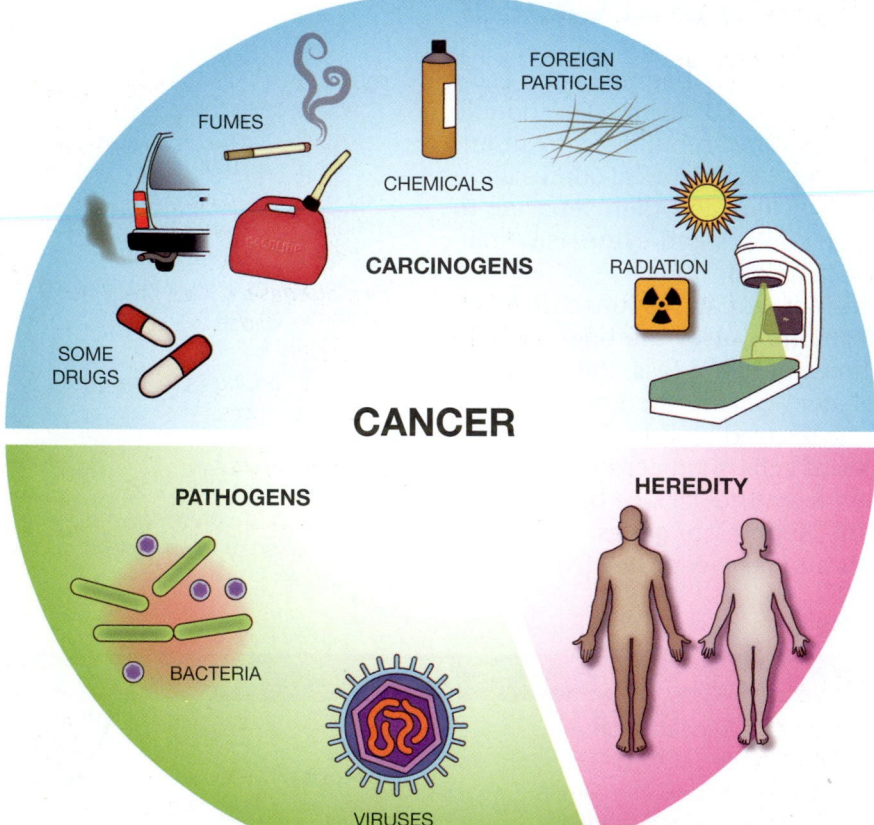

Figure 18-3 ■ **Causes of cancer.**

Cancer is caused by carcinogens in the environment, heredity, pathogens (bacteria and viruses), and oncogenes (genes within a virus).

lead to cervical cancer in women. Human immunodeficiency virus (HIV) weakens the immune response until the body is unable to destroy newly formed cancerous cells. **Oncogenes** are mutated genes in the RNA of a virus. When the virus enters and infects a normal cell, its oncogene joins with the normal cell's DNA, changing it into a cancerous cell.

Heredity. Some persons inherit damaged DNA or an oncogene from one of their parents.

If the DNA in a chromosome is damaged, and the damaged area includes the p53 gene, then the cell loses the mechanism with which to repair itself. The damage remains, and the damaged cell cannot stop itself from dividing and producing more damaged cells. More than half of cancer cells have damage to the p53 gene.

Characteristics of Cancerous Cells and Tumors

1. Cancerous cells are not part of and do not contribute to the normal structure and function of the body. Once a single cancerous cell has been produced, it stops functioning as a normal cell and takes on the characteristics of a cancerous cell.

2. Cancerous cells lack differentiation and cannot perform the specialized functions of normal cells.

3. Cancerous cells are not arranged in an orderly fashion (stacked on top of each other or all oriented in the same direction) like normal cells.

4. Cancerous cells often divide more rapidly than normal cells. Cancerous tumors often grow more quickly than normal tissue.

5. Cancerous cells can form a solid tumor. Cancerous tumors are irregular in shape and are not **encapsulated.** (Benign tumors do have a capsule).

6. A cancerous tumor releases a substance that causes blood vessels in the surrounding tissues to grow into the tumor and provide it with nutrients. This is known as **angiogenesis.** The tumor grows rapidly but often has a central core of necrosis because the blood supply is inadequate.

7. Cancerous tumors are **invasive.** They penetrate (infiltrate) the normal tissues around them, interfere with tissue functions, and destroy normal cells (see Figure 18-4 ■).

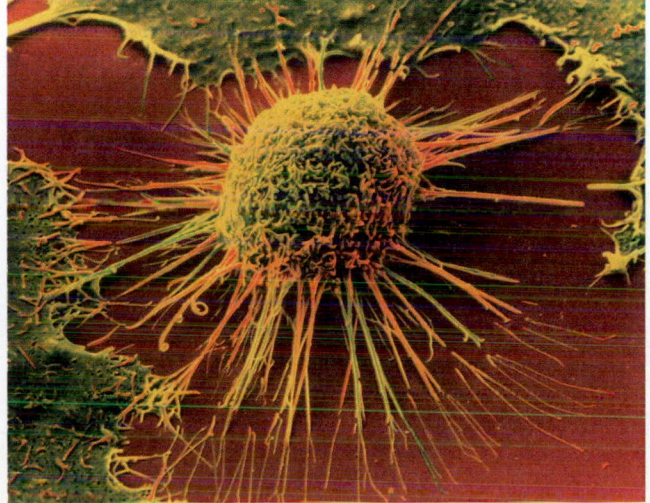

Figure 18-4 ■ Cancer cell.
This cancer cell is a carcinoma of the cervix. It has many projections of cytoplasm from the cell that infiltrate into the surrounding tissues.

WORD BUILDING

oncogene (ONG-koh-jeen)
  onc/o- *tumor; mass*
  -gene *gene*

heredity (heh-RED-ih-tee)
  hered/o- *genetic inheritance*
  -ity *state; condition*

encapsulated (en-KAP-soo-lay-ted)
  en- *in; within; inward*
  capsul/o- *capsule (enveloping structure)*
  -ated *pertaining to a condition; composed of*

angiogenesis (AN-jee-oh-JEN-eh-sis)
  angi/o- *blood vessel; lymphatic vessel*
  gen/o- *arising from; produced by*
  -esis *a process*

invasive (in-VAY-siv)
  invas/o- *to go into*
  -ive *pertaining to*

8. Cancerous cells break off from a solid tumor and move through the blood vessels and lymphatic vessels to other sites in the body. This process is known as **metastasis.** The cancerous cells **metastasize** and are characterized as being **metastatic** (see Figure 18-5 ■).

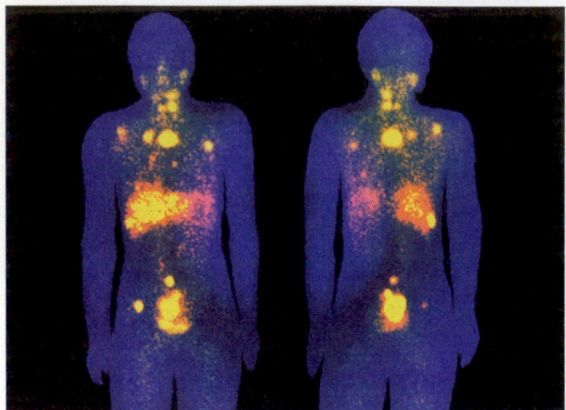

Figure 18-5 ■ **Metastases.**
These anterior and posterior views on a colorized scintigram show many areas of increased metabolism due to metastases. There are metastatic lesions in the neck, lungs, liver, and pelvic area.

9. The growth of cancerous cells and tumors cannot be easily controlled by the body. The body's defenses against cancerous cells and tumors include (1) the cell's p53 gene; (2) special lymphocytes known as NK cells (natural killer cells) that detect, engulf, and destroy cancerous cells; (3) lymph nodes that filter cancerous cells out of the lymph fluid; macrophages that engulf and destroy cancerous cells in the tissues; and (4) **tumor necrosis factor** released from lymph nodes that causes the tumor to become necrotic and die. However, the body's defenses are often overwhelmed by the cancer. Cancerous cells and tumors that are not destroyed by any of these means go on to multiply and metastasize.

A Closer Look

A human being begins as a single cell that immediately begins to divide. By the end of the first week of life, those cells begin to differentiate, migrating to various parts of the body and producing specific tissues (such as muscle or bone) with different shapes and functions. This process is known as cellular **differentiation.** Cancer cells arise from a particular type of tissue, but then lose this differentiation and revert back to an immature, embryonal, **undifferentiated** state.

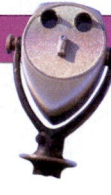

differentiation
(DIF-er-EN-shee-AA-shun)
  differentiat/o- *being distinct; specialized*
  -ion *action; condition*

undifferentiated
(un-DIF-er-EN-shee-aa-ted)
  un- *not*
  differentiat/o- *being distinct; specialized*
  -ed *pertaining to*

Did You Know?

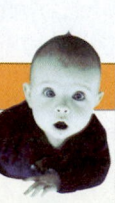

In his 1974 text *An Introduction to Drugs,* Michael C. Gerald wrote: "Cancerous cells are the anarchists of the body, for they know no law, pay no regard for the commonwealth, serve no useful function, and cause disharmony and death in their surrounds."

Vocabulary Review

Word or Phrase	Description	Combining Forms
angiogenesis	Process by which a cancerous tumor causes blood vessels in the surrounding tissues to grow into the tumor and provide it with nutrients	**angi/o-** *blood vessel; lymphatic vessel* **gen/o-** *arising from; produced by*
apoptosis	Programmed cell death in which the p53 gene directs the cell to shut down when its DNA is too damaged to be repaired	
cancer	Single abnormal cell that develops into a tumor or mass and is not encapsulated. Most grow rapidly and are invasive, growing into normal tissues around them.	**cancer/o-** *cancer* **carcin/o-** *cancer*
carcinogen	Environmental substance that can contribute to the development of cancer	**carcin/o-** *cancer*
cell	Smallest, independently functioning structure in the body that can reproduce itself by division	**cellul/o-** *cell* **cyt/o-** *cell*
cell membrane	Permeable barrier that surrounds a cell and holds in the cytoplasm. It allows water and nutrients to enter and waste products to leave the cell.	
chromosome	Paired, rodlike structures within the nucleus. Each cell contains 46 chromosomes (23 pairs).	**chrom/o-** *color*
cytoplasm	Gel-like intracellular substance. Organelles are embedded in it.	**cyt/o-** *cell*
differentiation	Process by which embryonic cells assume different shapes and function in different parts of the body	**differentiat/o-** *being distinct; specialized*
DNA	**Deoxyribonucleic acid.** Sequenced pairs of amino acids that form a double helix chain within a chromosome. One segment of DNA makes up a gene.	
encapsulated	Having a capsule or enveloping structure around it. Benign tumors have a capsule; cancerous tumors do not.	**capsul/o-** *capsule (enveloping structure)*
endoplasmic reticulum	Organelle that is a network of channels that transport materials within the cell. It is also the site of protein, fat, and glycogen production.	**plasm/o-** *plasma*
gene	An area on a chromosome that contains all the DNA information to produce one type of protein molecule	**gene/o-** *gene*
genetic mutation	Damage to the DNA molecule that deletes genes, reverses the normal order of genes, or breaks off gene segments from one chromosome and inserts them in a place on another chromosome (**translocation**)	**gene/o-** *gene* **mutat/o-** *to change* **locat/o-** *a place*
Gogli apparatus	Organelle that consists of curved, stacked membranes that process and store hormones and enzymes. It also makes lysosomes.	
heredity	Genetic inheritance passed on from the DNA of the father and mother to the child. Genetic mutations that cause cancer can be inherited.	**hered/o-** *genetic inheritance*
intracellular	Within a cell	**cellul/o-** *cell*
invasive	Characteristic of cancerous tumors. They penetrate and destroy the normal cells around them, compromising tissue functions.	**invas/o-** *to go into*
lysosome	Organelle that consists of a small sac with digestive enzymes in it. It destroys pathogens that invade the cell.	**lys/o-** *break down; destroy*

Word or Phrase	Description	Combining Forms
metastasis	Process by which cancerous cells break off from a tumor and move (**metastasize**) through the blood vessels or lymphatic vessels to other sites in the body. They are **metastatic.**	**stas/o-** *standing still; staying in one place* **stat/o-** *standing still; staying in one place*
mitochondria	Organelles that are capsule shaped and produce and store ATP and then convert it to ADP to release energy for cellular activities	
mitosis	Process of cellular division. The chromosomes duplicate, align along threadlike structures, and then migrate to either end of the nucleus as the cell divides.	**mit/o-** *threadlike structure*
nucleolus	Round, central region within the nucleus. It makes RNA and ribosomes.	
nucleus	Large, round, centralized intracellular structure that contains chromosomes and their DNA. It controls all of the cell's activities. It is surrounded by the nuclear membrane.	**nucle/o-** *nucleus* **kary/o-** *nucleus*
oncogene	Damaged and mutated genes that cause a cell to become cancerous. A virus can carry an oncogene in its RNA. Then when it enters a normal cell, the oncogene becomes incorporated into the normal cell's DNA and it becomes a cancerous cell.	**onc/o-** *tumor; mass*
organelles	Small structures in the cytoplasm that have specialized functions. They include mitochondria, ribosomes, the endoplasmic reticulum, the Golgi apparatus, and lysosomes.	**organ/o-** *organ*
pathogen	Microorganism such as a bacterium or virus that causes infection	**path/o-** *disease; suffering*
ribosomes	Granular organelles in the cytoplasm and on the endoplasmic reticulum. Ribosomes contain RNA and proteins and are the site where proteins are produced.	**rib/o-** *ribonucleic acid*
RNA	**Ribonucleic acid.** It is created in the nucleolus and stored in ribosomes. Messenger RNA duplicates DNA information in the nucleus and carries it to the ribosome.	
suppressor genes	Group of genes in the DNA of each cell that inhibits mitosis. The p53 gene is the most important suppressor gene.	**suppress/o-** *press down*
tumor necrosis factor	Substance released from lymph nodes that causes a cancerous tumor to become necrotic and die	**necr/o-** *dead cells, tissue, or body*
undifferentiated	Cancerous cells that are immature and embryonal in appearance and behavior	**differentiat/o-** *being distinct; specialized*

Labeling Exercise

Match each anatomy word or phrase to its structure and write it in the numbered box. Be sure to check your spelling. Use the Answer Key at the end of the book to check your answers.

cell membrane	endoplasmic reticulum	mitochondrion	nucleus
chromosome	Golgi apparatus	nuclear membrane	ribosomes
cytoplasm	lysosome	nucleolus	

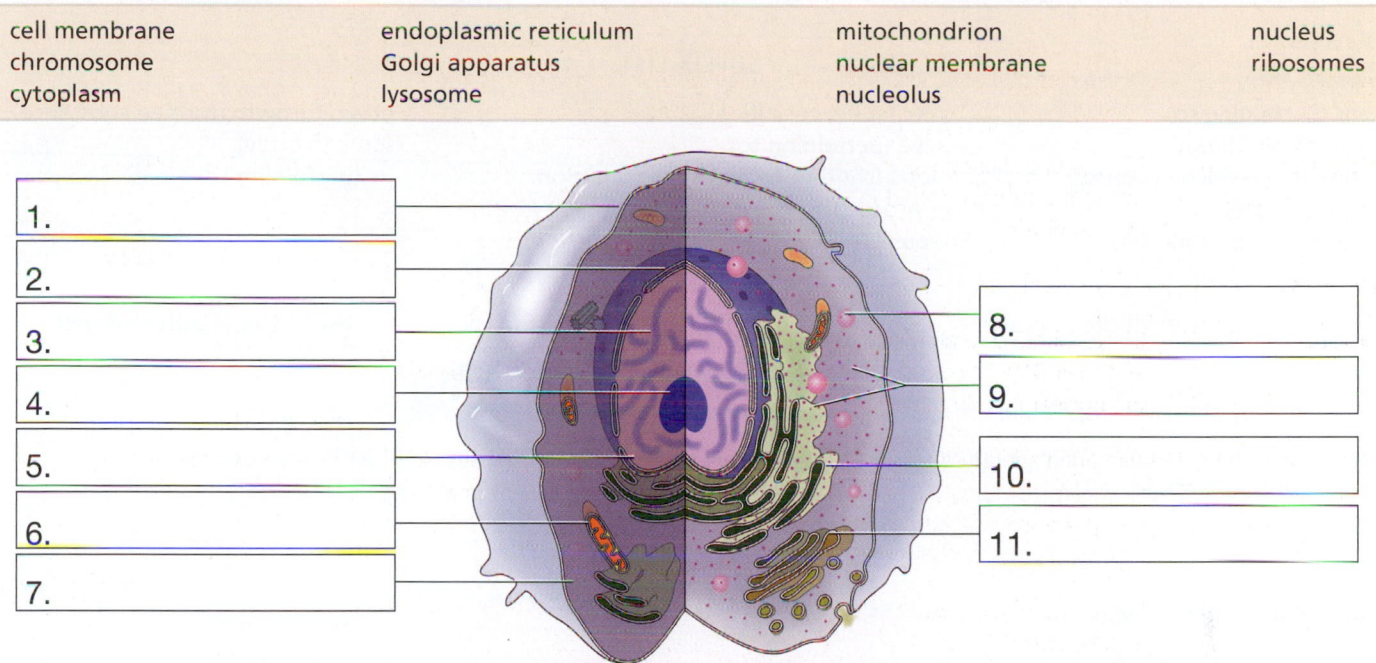

1.
2.
3.
4.
5.
6.
7.
8.
9.
10.
11.

Building Medical Words

Use the Answer Key at the end of the book to check your answers.

Combining Forms Exercise

Before you build cell and cancer words, review these combining forms. Next to each combining form, write its medical meaning. The first one has been done for you.

Combining Form	Medical Meaning	Combining Form	Medical Meaning
1. differentiat/o-	being distinct; specialized	14. locat/o-	
2. angi/o-		15. lys/o-	
3. cancer/o-		16. mit/o-	
4. capsul/o-		17. mutat/o-	
5. carcin/o-		18. necr/o-	
6. cellul/o-		19. nucle/o-	
7. chrom/o-		20. onc/o-	
8. cyt/o-		21. organ/o-	
9. gene/o-		22. path/o-	
10. gen/o-		23. plasm/o-	
11. hered/o-		24. rib/o-	
12. invas/o-		25. stas/o-	
13. kary/o-		26. stat/o-	
		27. suppress/o-	

Combining Form and Suffix Exercise

Read the definition of the medical word. Look at the combining form that is given. Select the correct suffix from the Suffix List and write it on the blank line. Then build the medical word and write it on the line. (Remember: You may need to remove the combining vowel. Always remove the hyphens and slash.) Be sure to check your spelling. The first one has been done for you.

SUFFIX LIST		
-ar (pertaining to)	-ity (state; condition)	-plasm (growth; formed substance)
-elle (little thing)	-ive (pertaining to)	-some (a body)
-gen (that which produces)	-osis (condition; abnormal condition; process)	-tic (pertaining to)
-gene (gene)		
-ion (action; condition)	-ous (pertaining to)	

Definition of the Medical Word	Combining Form	Suffix	Build the Medical Word
1. A body (that contains) ribonucleic acid	**rib/o-** **-some**		*ribosome*

(You think *a body* (-some) + *ribonucleic acid* (rib/o-). You change the order of the word parts to put the suffix last. You write *ribosome*.)

Definition of the Medical Word	Combining Form	Suffix	Build the Medical Word
2. Pertaining to cancer	cancer/o-	_____	_____
3. Condition of dead cells or tissue	necr/o-	_____	_____
4. Pertaining to go into	invas/o-	_____	_____
5. Pertaining to genes	gene/o-	_____	_____
6. Formed substance (that makes up a) cell	cyt/o-	_____	_____
7. Little thing (that is an) organ (within a cell)	organ/o-	_____	_____
8. Pertaining to a cell	cellul/o-	_____	_____
9. A body (that contains an enzyme that) breaks down and destroys	lys/o-	_____	_____
10. That which produces cancer	carcin/o-	_____	_____
11. Gene (that causes a) tumor or mass	onc/o-	_____	_____
12. State of genetic inheritance	hered/o-	_____	_____
13. Pertaining to the nucleus	nucle/o-	_____	_____
14. A (microscopic) body (that takes on) color (when stained)	chrom/o-	_____	_____
15. Action (that involves a) change	mutat/o-	_____	_____

Types of Cancer

General

Word or Phrase	Description	Word Building
anaplasia	Condition in which normal cells that are mature and differentiated become cancerous cells that are undifferentiated in appearance and behavior	**anaplasia** (AN-ah-PLAY-zee-ah) (AN-ah-PLAY-zha) **ana-** *apart from; excessive* **-plasia** *abnormal condition of growth* The ending –*plasia* contains the combining form *plas/o-* and the suffix –*ia*.
cancer	General word for any type of **cancerous** cell or tumor. There are four broad categories of cancer: carcinoma, sarcoma, leukemia, and embryonal cell carcinoma. Treatment: Chemotherapy, radiation therapy, surgery, or a combination of these, depending on the type and extent of the cancer.	**cancer** (KAN-ser) **cancerous** (KAN-ser-us)
carcinoid tumor	Slow-growing cancerous tumor that occurs mainly in the digestive tract. It does not exhibit all of the characteristics of cancer, and it seldom metastasizes. **Carcinoid syndrome** is a set of symptoms caused by the release of the hormone serotonin from a carcinoid tumor.	**carcinoid** (KAR-sih-noyd) **carcin/o-** *cancer* **-oid** *resembling*
carcinomatosis	Condition in which cancerous tumors are present at multiple sites in the body	**carcinomatosis** (KAR-sih-NOH-mah-TOH-sis) *Carcinomatosis* is a combination of *carcinomata* (the plural form of carcinoma) and the suffix *-osis* (condition; abnormal condition; process).
dysplasia	Condition of atypical cells that are abnormal in size, shape, or organization, but have not yet become cancerous (see Figure 13-19). These cells are **dysplastic.** Dysplasia is the result of chronic irritation and inflammation.	**dysplasia** (dis-PLAY-zee-ah) (dis-PLAY-zha) **dys-** *painful; difficult; abnormal* **-plasia** *abnormal condition of growth*
		dysplastic (dis-PLAS-tik) **dys-** *painful; difficult; abnormal* **plas/o-** *growth; formation* **-tic** *pertaining to* Select the correct prefix meaning to get the definition of *dysplastic*: *pertaining to abnormal growth or formation (of cells).*
lymphadenopathy	Enlarged lymph nodes. The lymph nodes trap cancerous cells that break away from the site of the original tumor. The lymph node itself then becomes a site of cancer. Chains of lymph nodes in the neck, axillae, and groin regions are common sites of lymphadenopathy (see Figure 6-19).	**lymphadenopathy** (LIM-fad-eh-NAWP-ah-thee) **lymph/o-** *lymph; lymphatic system* **aden/o-** *gland* **-pathy** *disease; suffering*

Word or Phrase	Description	Word Building
neoplasm	Any growing tissue that is not part of the normal body structure or function. **Neoplasia** is the process by which a neoplasm develops. Neoplasms are also known as **tumors.** Neoplasms are either **malignant** (cancerous) or **benign** (not cancerous). Malignant neoplasms are known as **cancer.**	**neoplasm** (NEE-oh-plazm) **ne/o-** *new* **-plasm** *growth; formed substance* **neoplasia** (NEE-oh-PLAY-zee-ah) **ne/o** *new* **-plasia** *abnormal condition of growth* **malignant** (mah-LIG-nant) **malign/o-** *intentionally causing harm; cancer* **-ant** *pertaining to* **benign** (bee-NINE)
relapse	Return of the symptoms or signs of cancer after a period of improvement or even remission	**relapse** (REE-laps)
remission	Period of time during which there are no symptoms or signs of cancer. A remission occurs after the successful treatment of cancer.	**remission** (ree-MISH-un) **remiss/o-** *send back* **-ion** *action; condition*
site of the tumor	Area where the cancerous cell first grew into a cancerous tumor is known as the **primary site.** When the tumor is still contained in that area it is said to be ***in situ.*** When the tumor spreads or metastasizes via the blood or lymphatic system to a distant part of the body, that is the **secondary site.** There is always just one primary site, but there may be several secondary sites.	***in situ*** (in SY-too)

Did You Know?

Screening examinations are extremely important in the early detection of cancer. Self-examination of the breasts or testes is performed by the patient. Other examinations, such as mammography and colonoscopy, should be performed at regular intervals by healthcare professionals.

Warning Signs of some Common Types of Cancer

The American Cancer Society uses the acronym CAUTION as a memory aid to help healthcare professionals and others remember the ways in which early cancer can present.

C   Change in bowel or bladder habits
A   A sore that does not heal
U   Unusual bleeding or discharge
T   Thickening or lump
I   Indigestion or trouble swallowing
O   Obvious changes in a wart or mole
N   Nagging cough or hoarseness

Carcinomas

Word or Phrase	Description	Word Building

adenocarcinoma	An adenocarcinoma is cancer of a gland. Adenocarcinoma of the breast occurs in the epithelial cells lining the ducts of the milk glands of the breast (see Figures 18-6 ■ and 18-7 ■). An adenocarcinoma can also occur in the ducts of the pancreas, prostate gland, or salivary glands. It is also known as **ductal cell carcinoma.** An adenocarcinoma of the ducts of the gallbladder is known as **cholangiocarcinoma.**	**adenocarcinoma**
		(AD-eh-noh-KAR-sih-NOH-mah)
		  aden/o- *gland*
		  carcin/o- *cancer*
		  -oma *tumor; mass*
		
		ductal (DUK-tal)
		  duct/o- *bring; move; a duct*
		  -al *pertaining to*
		
		cholangiocarcinoma
		(koh-LAN-jee-oh-KAR-sih-NOH-mah)
		  cholangi/o- *bile duct*
		  carcin/o- *cancer*
		  -oma *tumor; mass*

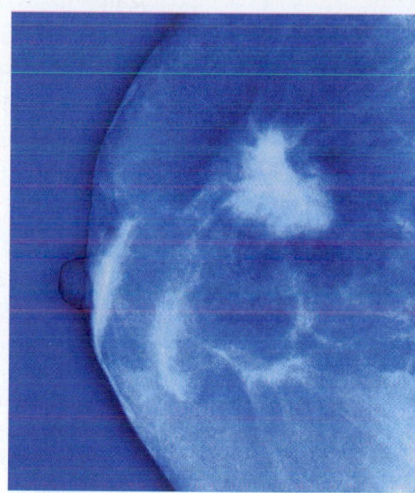

Figure 18-6 ■ Adenocarcinoma of the breast.

On a colorized mammogram, this patient has an adenocarcinoma of the breast, seen as a dense white mass in the center of the breast. Note the characteristic irregular edges of the tumor with infiltration into the surrounding breast tissue. Normal supporting fibers and lactiferous ducts in the breast are visible as individual white streaks, and the fatty tissues of the breast appear as dark blue areas.

Did You Know?

Advanced adenocarcinoma of the breast can cause dimpling of the skin of the breast as the tumor pulls on supporting tissues around the ducts. This dimpling, known by the French phrase *peau d'orange* (peel of the orange), looks like the dimpled surface of an orange (see Figure 13-21).

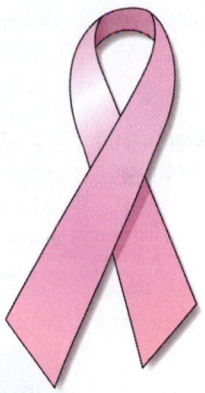

Figure 18-7 ■ The fight against breast cancer.

A pink ribbon is the universal symbol for the fight against breast cancer.

Word or Phrase	Description	Word Building

carcinoma	Cancer of epithelial cells in the skin or mucous membranes. Carcinomas grow more slowly than sarcomas, but they occur more often. Carcinomas usually metastasize via the lymphatic system.	**carcinoma** (KAR-sih-NOH-mah)
		  carcin/o- *cancer*
		  -oma *tumor; mass*

Word or Phrase	Description	Word Building
basal cell carcinoma	Cancer of the deepest layer (basal layer) of the epidermis of the skin (see Figure 18-8 ■)	**basal** (BAY-sal) **bas/o-** *base of a structure* **-al** *pertaining to*

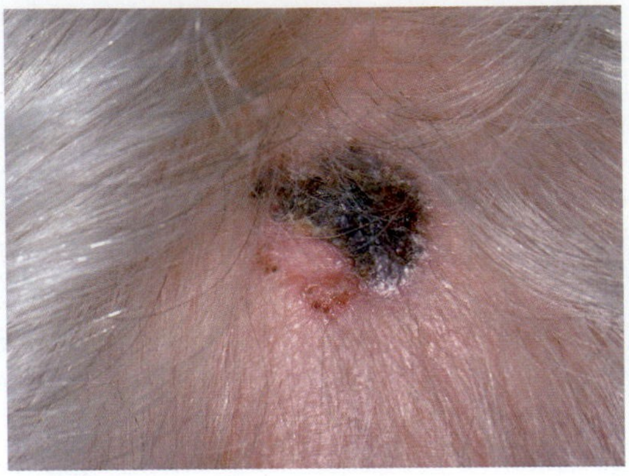

Figure 18-8 ■ Basal cell carcinoma.
This basal cell carcinoma of the skin shows a characteristic asymmetrical shape with a central ulcerated area that will become necrotic. There is crusting from oozing tissue fluid and periodic bleeding that forms a scab.

Word or Phrase	Description	Word Building
bronchogenic carcinoma	Cancer of the mucous membranes lining the bronchi of the lungs (see Figure 4-13).	**bronchogenic** (BRONG-koh-JEN-ik) **bronch/o-** *bronchus* **gen/o-** *arising from; produced by* **-ic** *pertaining to*
endometrial carcinoma	Cancer of the endometrium that lines the intrauterine cavity of the uterus	**endometrial** (EN-doh-MEE-tree-al) **endo-** *innermost; within* **metri/o-** *uterus (womb)* **-al** *pertaining to*
hepatocellular carcinoma	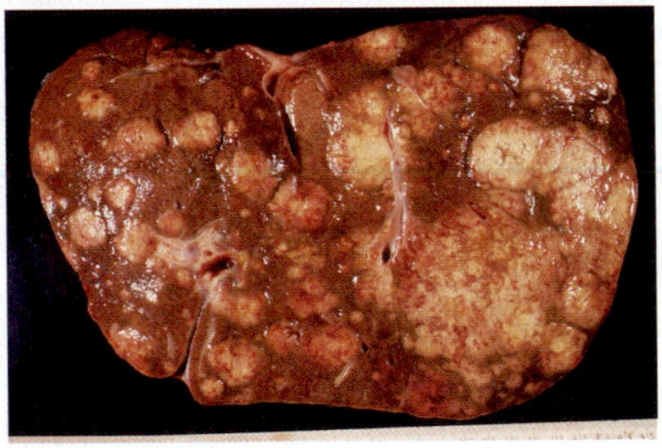 Cancer of the liver cells (see Figure 18-9 ■). It is also known as a **hepatoma**.	**hepatocellular** (HEP-ah-to-SEL-yoo-lar) **hepat/o-** *liver* **cellul/o-** *cell* **-ar** *pertaining to* **hepatoma** (HEP-ah-TOH-mah) **hepat/o-** *liver* **-oma** *tumor; mass*

Figure 18-9 ■ Hepatocellular carcinoma.
This liver was removed from a patient who died of cancer. It shows multiple tumors.

Word or Phrase	Description	Word Building
small cell carcinoma	Cancer of the epithelial cells of the lungs. These cancerous cells are small and round or oval (in contrast to large cell carcinoma, a less common type of lung cancer that has larger cancerous cells). It is also known as **oat cell carcinoma.**	
squamous cell carcinoma	Cancer of the squamous cells (top layer) of the epidermis of the skin	**squamous** (SKWAY-mus) **squam/o-** *scalelike cell* **-ous** *pertaining to*
transitional cell carcinoma	Cancer of the epithelial cells lining the urinary tract. Transitional cells are unique in that their shape transitions (changes) each time the bladder is filled with urine.	**transitional** (trans-ZIH-shun-al) **transit/o-** *change over from one to another* **-ion** *action; condition* **-al** *pertaining to*

Word or Phrase	Description	Word Building

malignant melanoma	Cancer of melanocytes (melanin pigment cells) of the skin (see Figure 7-20)	**melanoma** (MEL-ah-NOH-mah)
		  melan/o- *black*
		  -oma *tumor; mass*
		Add words to make a complete definition of *melanoma: tumor (whose color is brown or) black.*

Sarcomas

angiosarcoma	Cancer of a blood vessel or lymphatic vessel	**angiosarcoma**
		(AN-jee-oh-sar-KOH-mah)
		  angi/o- *blood vessel; lymphatic vessel*
		  sarc/o- *connective tissue*
		  -oma *tumor; mass*

astrocytoma	Cancer of an astrocyte (branching cell that supports neurons) in the cerebrum of the brain. Cancer of an immature, embryonic astrocyte is known as **glioblastoma multiforme.**	**astrocytoma** (AS-troh-sy-TOH-mah)
		  astr/o- *starlike structure*
		  cyt/o- *cell*
		  -oma *tumor; mass*
		
		glioblastoma multiforme (GLY-oh-blas-TOH-mah mul-tee-FOR-may)
		  gli/o- *cells that provide support*
		  blast/o- *immature; embryonic*
		  -oma *tumor; mass*

chondrosarcoma	Cancer of the cartilage	**chondrosarcoma**
		(CON-droh-sar-KOH-mah)
		  chondr/o- *cartilage*
		  sarc/o- *connective tissue*
		  -oma *tumor; mass*

Ewing's sarcoma	Cancer of the growth area (epiphysial plate) at the end of a bone, usually of an arm or leg	**Ewing** (YOO-ing)
Kaposi's sarcoma	Cancer of the skin and subcutaneous tissue (see Figure 18-10 ■)	**Kaposi** (KAH-poh-see)

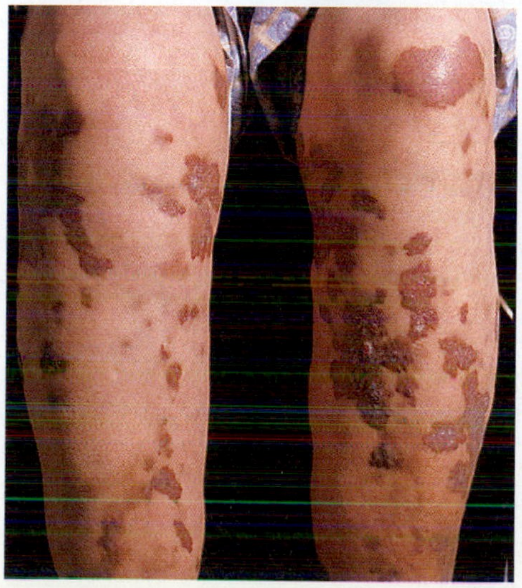

Figure 18-10 ■ Kaposi's sarcoma.
This previously rare cancer is now commonly seen in AIDS patients because of their impaired immune response. The cancer involves the skin, subcutaneous tissue, and internal organs.

Word or Phrase	Description	Word Building
leiomyosarcoma	Cancer of the smooth muscle layer in the uterus, digestive tract, bladder, or prostate gland	**leiomyosarcoma** (LIE-oh-MY-oh-sar-KOH-mah) **lei/o-** *smooth* **my/o-** *muscle* **sarc/o-** *connective tissue* **-oma** *tumor; mass*
liposarcoma	Cancer of the fatty tissue	**liposarcoma** (LIP-oh-sar-KOH-mah) **lip/o-** *lipid (fat)* **sarc/o-** *connective tissue* **-oma** *tumor; mass*
myosarcoma	Cancer of a muscle and connective tissue	**myosarcoma** (MY-oh-sar-KOH-mah) **my/o-** *muscle* **sarc/o-** *connective tissue* **-oma** *tumor; mass*
neurofibrosarcoma	Cancer of Schwann cells that produce myelin and surround the larger axons of neurons of the cranial nerves and spinal nerves	**neurofibrosarcoma** (NYOOR-oh-FY-broh-sar-KOH-mah) **neur/o-** *nerve* **fibr/o-** *fiber* **sarc/o-** *connective tissue* **-oma** *tumor; mass*
oligodendroglioma	Cancer of oligodendroglia, cells that surround the larger axons of neurons in the brain and spinal cord. They provide support and produce myelin. These cells have only a few branching structures.	**oligodendroglioma** (OH-lih-goh-DEN-droh-glee-OH-mah) **olig/o-** *scanty; few* **dendr/o-** *branching structure* **gli/o-** *cells that provide support* **-oma** *tumor; mass*
osteosarcoma	Cancer of a bone (see Figure 18-11 ■). It is also known as **osteogenic sarcoma.** 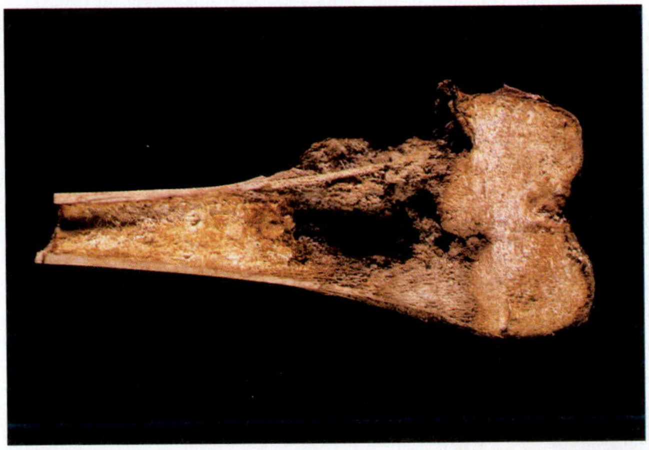 **Figure 18-11** ■ Osteosarcoma. This patient, an 11-year-old girl, had an osteosarcoma of the distal end of her femur. The tumor also spread to the soft tissues around the bone.	**osteosarcoma** (AWS-tee-oh-sar-KOH-mah) **oste/o-** *bone* **sarc/o-** *connective tissue* **-oma** *tumor; mass* **osteogenic** (AWS-tee-oh-JEN-ik) **oste/o-** *bone* **gen/o-** *arising from; produced by* **-ic** *pertaining to*

Word or Phrase	Description	Word Building
rhabdomyo-sarcoma	Cancer of a skeletal (voluntary) muscle in the arms or legs	**rhabdomyosarcoma** (RAB-doh-MY-oh-sar-KOH-mah) **rhabd/o-** *rod shaped* **my/o-** *muscle* **sarc/o-** *connective tissue* **-oma** *tumor; mass* The muscle cells in this tumor are shaped like a rod.
sarcoma	Cancer of connective tissues (cartilage, bone, tendon, ligament, aponeurosis, fascia, fat, subcutaneous tissue), muscles, or nerves. Sarcomas grow rapidly and most often show anaplasia of their cells. Sarcomas usually metastasize via the circulatory system. A **fibrosarcoma** is a cancer of a tendon, ligament, aponeurosis, or scar tissue.	**sarcoma** (sar-KOH-mah) **sarc/o-** *connective tissue* **-oma** *tumor; mass* **fibrosarcoma** (FY-broh-sar-KOH-mah) **fibr/o-** *fiber* **sarc/o-** *connective tissue* **-oma** *tumor; mass*

Cancers of the Blood and Lymphatic System

leukemia	Cancer of leukocytes (white blood cells) (see Figure 6-17). Leukemia is named according to the type of leukocyte that is the most prevalent and whether the onset of symptoms is acute or chronic. Types of leukemia include acute **myelogenous leukemia** (AML), chronic myelogenous leukemia (CML), acute **lymphocytic leukemia** (ALL), and chronic lymphocytic leukemia (CLL).	**leukemia** (loo-KEE-mee-ah) **leuk/o-** *white* **-emia** *condition of the blood; substance in the blood* **myelogenous** (MY-eh-LAW-jeh-nus) **myel/o-** *bone marrow; spinal cord; myelin* **gen/o-** *arising from; produced by* **-ous** *pertaining to* **lymphocytic** (LIM-foh-SIT-ik) **lymph/o-** *lymph; lymphatic system* **cyt/o-** *cell* **-ic** *pertaining to*
lymphoma	Cancer of a lymph node, lymphoid tissue, or T or B lymphocytes. There are two types of lymphomas. **Hodgkin's lymphoma,** the most common type, shows characteristic Reed-Sternberg cells upon biopsy (see Figure 18-12 ■). **Non-Hodgkin's lymphoma,** a group of more than 20 different lymphomas, does not have any Reed-Sternberg cells. A lymphoma that originates in a lymph node should not be confused with metastasis to a lymph node from a primary tumor located elsewhere in the body.	**lymphoma** (lim-FOH-mah) **lymph/o-** *lymph; lymphatic system* **-oma** *tumor; mass* **Hodgkin** (HAWJ-kin)

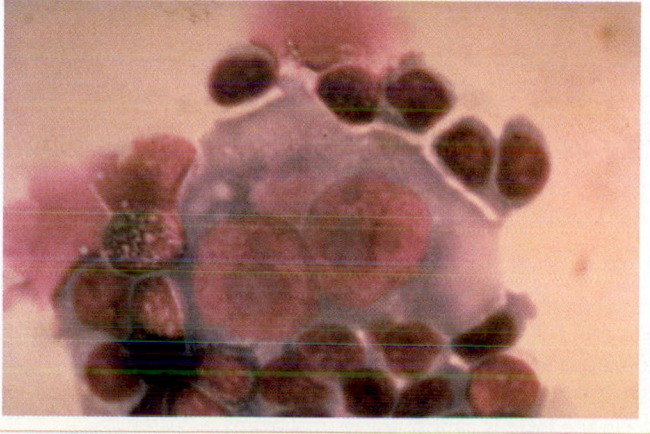

Figure 18-12 ■ Reed-Sternberg cell.
This Reed-Sternberg cell was found in the specimen of a lymph node of a patient who was then diagnosed as having Hodgkin's lymphoma. It is a large, atypical, cancerous lymphocyte. It is shown here surrounded by smaller, normal lymphocytes.

Word or Phrase	Description	Word Building
multiple myeloma	Cancer of the bone marrow. It contains malignant plasma cells. Normal plasma cells are B lymphocytes that produce antibodies (immunoglobulins) when activated by a pathogen. Malignant plasma cells produce abnormal antibodies known as Bence Jones protein. The patient's immune response is abnormal because of decreased levels of normal plasma cells and antibodies.	**myeloma** (MY-eh-LOH-mah) **myel/o-** *bone marrow; spinal cord; myelin* **-oma** *tumor; mass* Select the correct combining form meaning to get the definition of *myeloma: a tumor of the bone marrow.*

Embryonal Cell Cancer

Word or Phrase	Description	Word Building
choriocarcinoma	Cancer that develops during pregnancy. It involves the chorion, the membrane that surrounds the developing embryo and later becomes the placenta.	**choriocarcinoma** (KOH-ree-oh-KAR-sih-NOH-mah) **chori/o-** *chorion (fetal membrane)* **carcin/o-** *cancer* **-oma** *tumor; mass*
embryonal cell cancer	Cancer of an embryonal cell. It develops during childhood or adolescence. It includes choriocarcinoma, germ cell tumors, hepatoblastoma, neuroblastoma, retinoblastoma, teratoma, and Wilms' tumor.	**embryonal** (EM-bree-OH-nal) **embryon/o-** *embryo; immature form* **-al** *pertaining to*
germ cell tumor	Cancer of a germ cell, an embryonal cell in the ovary or testis. A **dysgerminoma** is cancer of an oocyte (immature cell that becomes an ovum) in the ovary. It occurs in young, adult females. A **seminoma** is cancer of a spermatoblast (immature cell that becomes a spermatozoon) in the testis. It occurs in young, adult males. **Word Alert** Germ cells have nothing to do with "germs" (bacteria, viruses). Germ cells are immature cells that "germinate" (grow or develop) into mature, specialized cells.	**dysgerminoma** (DIS-jer-mih-NOH-mah) **dys-** *painful; difficult; abnormal* **germin/o-** *embryonic tissue* **-oma** *tumor; mass* **seminoma** (SEM-ih-NOH-mah) **semin/o-** *spermatozoon; semen* **-oma** *tumor; mass*
hepatoblastoma	Cancer of an embryonal cell in the liver. It occurs in young children.	**hepatoblastoma** (HEP-ah-toh-blas-TOH-mah) **hepat/o-** *liver* **blast/o-** *immature; embryonic* **-oma** *tumor; mass*
neuroblastoma	Cancer of an embryonal nerve cell. It occurs in young children.	**neuroblastoma** (NYOOR-oh-blas-TOH-mah) **neur/o-** *nerve* **blast/o-** *immature; embryonic* **-oma** *tumor; mass*
retinoblastoma	Cancer of an embryonal cell in the retina of the eye. It occurs in young children.	**retinoblastoma** (RET-ih-noh-blas-TOH-mah) **retin/o-** *retina* **blast/o-** *immature; embryonic* **-oma** *tumor; mass*
teratoma	Cancer of the ovary or testis that contains cells from other parts of the body. In the ovary, a teratoma can be malignant but usually is in the form of a benign dermoid cyst that contains hair and sometimes even teeth. However, a teratoma in the testis is almost always malignant.	**teratoma** (TAIR-ah-TOH-mah) **terat/o-** *bizarre form* **-oma** *tumor; mass*

Word or Phrase	Description	Word Building

Wilms' tumor	Cancer of an embryonal cell of the kidney. It occurs in young children. This is also known as **nephroblastoma**.	**Wilms' tumor** (WILMZ TOO-mor)
		
		nephroblastoma
		(NEF-roh-blas-TOH-mah)
		    nephr/o- *kidney; nephron*
		    blast/o- *immature; embryonic*
		    -oma *tumor; mass*

Laboratory and Diagnostic Procedures

Cytology Tests

Word or Phrase	Description	Word Building

bone marrow aspiration	Diagnoses leukemia or lymphoma and monitors its progression. A sample of bone marrow is taken from the posterior iliac crest. The stages of cell development (stem cell to mature cell) and the numbers of cells are examined under a microscope.	**aspiration** (AS-pih-RAY-shun)
		    aspir/o- *to breathe in; to suck in*
		    -ation *a process; being or having*

exfoliative cytology	Uses cells found in secretions or cells that are scraped or washed away from the tissue. The sample is examined under a microscope to look for abnormal or cancerous cells. Examples: Pap smear of the cervix (see Figures 13-25 and 13-26), bronchial or gastric washings, sputum.	**exfoliative** (eks-FOH-lee-ah-tiv)
		
		cytology (sy-TAWL-oh-jee)
		    cyt/o- *cell*
		    -logy *the study of*

frozen section	Involves freezing a tissue specimen obtained from a biopsy. Thin slices of the specimen are stained and examined under a microscope. This procedure is done in the laboratory during the surgery so that the surgeon knows immediately whether the tissue is cancerous or not. Freezing the tissue distorts some of the cell architecture, and so a permanent section is also done using a paraffin-like substance to make the tissue firm.	
Her2/neu	Detects a gene that affects the prognosis of and treatment options for breast cancer, ovarian cancer, and bladder cancer. A tumor that is Her2/neu positive is an aggressive tumor that is resistant to hormone therapy and some chemotherapy drugs.	

karyotype	Examines the chromosomes under a microscope. A photograph of the karyotype (see Figure 18-13 ■) is then studied to look for chromosome deletions or translocations. A translocation of chromosome 9 to chromosome 22 (known as the *Philadelphia chromosome*) is diagnostic of chronic myelogenous leukemia. A translocation between chromosomes 11 and 22 causes Ewing's sarcoma.	**karyotype** (KAIR-ee-oh-type)
		    kary/o- *nucleus*
		    -type *particular kind of; a model of*

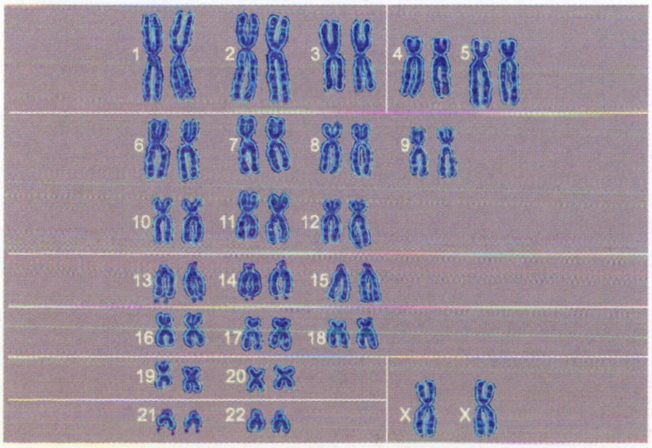

Figure 18-13 ■ **Normal karyotype.**
There are 23 pairs of chromosomes in a normal karyotype. Pairs 1–22 are shown here with pair 23 (the sex chromosomes) in the bottom right-hand corner. Two X sex chromosomes make this patient a female.

Word or Phrase	Description	Word Building
receptor assays	Cytology test that measures the number of **estrogen receptors (ER)** or **progesterone receptors (PR)** on the cell membrane of a cancer cell to determine the prognosis of and treatment options for breast cancer. A tumor with increased numbers of ER or PR receptors (known as *ER-positive* or *PR-positive*) is dependent on the estrogen (or progesterone) hormone, and so it is treated with a male hormone drug that creates the opposite hormonal environment.	**receptor** (ree-SEP-tor) **recept/o-** *receive* **-or** *person or thing that produces or does* **assay** (AS-say)

Blood Tests

Word or Phrase	Description	Word Building
alpha fetoprotein (AFP)	Detects a protein normally present in a fetus, but not in an adult. An elevated level of AFP is seen with cancer of the liver, testes, and ovaries. The higher the level, the more advanced the cancer. (An elevated level is also seen in noncancerous conditions, such as cirrhosis, hepatitis, neural tube defects, and Down syndrome.)	**alpha fetoprotein** (AL-fah FEE-toh-PRO-teen)
blood smear	A drop of blood is smeared across a glass slide and then examined under a microscope. This test is done manually to examine the characteristics of leukocytes when an automated complete blood count (CBC) done by a machine is abnormal and suggests leukemia.	
BRCA1 or BRCA2 gene	Detects the BRCA1 or BRCA2 gene, a genetic mutation that significantly increases the risk of breast cancer. The BRCA1 gene also increases the risk of ovarian cancer. This test is performed when there is a strong family history of breast or ovarian cancer. BRCA stands for **br**east **ca**ncer.	
carcinoembryonic antigen (CEA)	Detects a protein normally present in an embryo, but not in an adult. An elevated level of CEA is seen with several different cancers. The higher the level, the more advanced the cancer. (An elevated level is also seen in noncancerous conditions, such as diseases of the colon and liver or in patients who smoke.)	**carcinoembryonic** (KAR-sih-noh-EM-bree-AW-nik) **carcin/o-** *cancer* **embryon/o-** *embryo; immature form* **-ic** *pertaining to* **antigen** (AN-tih-jen)
human chorionic gonadotropin (HCG)	Detects a hormone normally present during pregnancy but not at other times. An elevated level of HCG is seen in choriocarcinoma in women and in cancer of the testes in men. (An elevated level is also seen in noncancerous conditions, such as cirrhosis, duodenal ulcer, and inflammatory bowel disease.)	**chorionic** (KOH-ree-AWN-ik) **chorion/o-** *chorion (fetal membrane)* **-ic** *pertaining to* **gonadotropin** (GOH-nad-oh-TROH-pin) **gonad/o-** *gonads (ovaries and testes)* **trop/o-** *having an affinity for; stimulating; turning* **-in** *a substance*
prostate-specific antigen (PSA)	Measures a protein in the prostate gland. An elevated level of PSA is seen in cancer of the prostate gland. The higher the level, the more advanced the cancer. Both free PSA and total PSA levels are measured.	
tumor markers	Detects antigens on the surface of cancer cells. Tumor markers are used to evaluate the extent of the cancer and the effectiveness of the treatment being given. Tumor markers include CA 15-3 and CA 27.29 (for breast cancer), CA 125 (for ovarian cancer), and CA 19-9 (for cancer of the pancreas and bile ducts). AFP, CEA, and HCG are also tumor markers.	

Urine Tests

Word or Phrase	Description	Word Building
urinalysis (UA)	Detects chemical compounds in the urine that indicate the presence of various cancers. These include Bence Jones protein (for multiple myeloma), vanillylmandelic acid (VMA) (for neuroblastoma), and 5-HIAA (for carcinoid syndrome).	**urinalysis** (yoo-rih-NAL-ih-sis)

Radiology and Nuclear Medicine Procedures

Word or Phrase	Description	Word Building
computed axial tomography (CAT, CT)	Radiologic procedure that uses x-rays to create many individual, closely spaced images or "slices" (see Figure 18-14 ■). The computer can combine these into a three-dimensional image to precisely locate a tumor or metastases. Radiopaque contrast dye can also be injected to provide more detail.	**tomography** (toh-MAWG-rah-fee) **tom/o-** cut; slice; layer **-graphy** process of recording

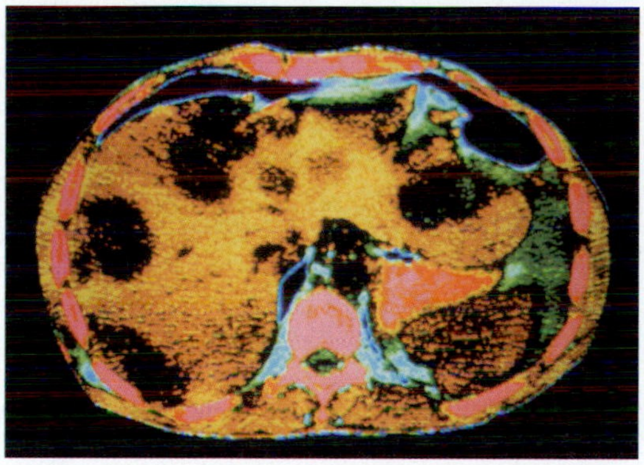

Figure 18-14 ■ CT scan.

This colorized computed tomography shows several large, dark brown areas of metastases within the dark yellow, enlarged liver. *Note:* A CT image is read as if you were standing at the feet of the patient who is lying on the CT scanner table. The patient's vertebra (pink) is at the bottom center of the image.

Word or Phrase	Description	Word Building
lymphangiography	Radiologic procedure in which a radiopaque contrast dye is injected into a lymphatic vessel. X-rays taken as the dye travels through the lymphatic vessels show enlarged lymph nodes, lymphomas, and areas of blocked lymph drainage. The x-ray image is a **lymphangiogram.**	**lymphangiography** (lim-FAN-jee-AWG-rah-fee) **lymph/o-** lymph; lymphatic system **angi/o-** blood vessel; lymphatic vessel **-graphy** process of recording **lymphangiogram** (lim-FAN-jee-oh-gram) **lymph/o-** lymph; lymphatic system **angi/o-** blood vessel; lymphatic vessel **-gram** a record or picture
magnetic resonance imaging (MRI)	Radiologic procedure that uses a magnetic field and radiowaves to align protons in the body and cause them to emit signals. MRI is a tomography that creates many individual "slice" images that the computer combines into a three-dimensional image to precisely locate a tumor or metastases. Radiopaque contrast dye can also be injected to provide more detail. An MRI scan does not use x-rays so the patient is not exposed to any radiation. Patients with extensive fibrocystic disease of the breast can be more accurately evaluated for breast cancer with an MRI scan instead of mammography.	**magnetic** (mag-NET-ik) **magnet/o-** magnet **-ic** pertaining to
mammography	Radiologic procedure that uses low-dose x-rays to produce an image of the breast to detect tumors. The breast is compressed between two flat surfaces to decrease its thickness and increase the quality of the image (see Figure 13-28). The x-ray image is a **mammogram** (see Figure 18-6).	**mammography** (mah-MAWG-rah-fee) **mamm/o-** breast **-graphy** process of recording **mammogram** (MAM-oh-gram) **mamm/o-** breast **-gram** a picture or record

Word or Phrase	Description	Word Building
scintigraphy	Nuclear medicine procedure that uses a radioactive tracer that collects in particular organs and tissues. A gamma camera scans and counts the radioactivity (gamma rays) and creates an image known as a **scintigram.** Areas of increased uptake are abnormal and can be due to infection, cancer, or metastases (see Figure 18-5).	**scintigraphy** (sin-TIG-rah-fee) **scint/i-** *point of light* **-graphy** *process of recording* **scintigram** (SIN-tih-gram) **scint/i-** *point of light* **-gram** *a record or picture*
ultrasonography	Radiologic procedure that uses ultra high-frequency sound waves to produce an image. It is used to distinguish benign, fluid-filled tumors (cysts) from solid tumors that need to be biopsied. It is used to evaluate the breasts, abdominal organs, pelvic organs, and testes. It is also known as **sonography,** and the **ultrasound** image is a **sonogram.**	**ultrasonography** (UL-trah-soh-NAWG-rah-fee) **ultra-** *beyond; higher* **son/o-** *sound* **-graphy** *process of recording* **ultrasound** (UL-trah-sound) **sonography** (soh-NAWG-rah-fee) **son/o-** *sound* **-graphy** *process of recording* **sonogram** (SAWN-oh-gram) **son/o-** *sound* **-gram** *a record or picture*

Medical, Surgical, and Radiation Therapy Procedures

Medical Procedures

Word or Phrase	Description	Word Building
bone marrow transplantation (BMT)	Medical treatment for patients with leukemia and lymphoma. Bone marrow cells are harvested from the posterior iliac crest of a matched donor. The patient is treated with high-dose chemotherapy drugs or radiation to destroy all cancerous cells (this also destroys the patient's bone marrow cells). The donor bone marrow cells, which are administered through a central intravenous line, travel through the blood and implant in the patient's bones. In 2–4 weeks, the donor marrow begins to produce normal blood cells. In **stem cell transplantation,** stem cells from the patient or from a matched donor are used. Stem cells from the umbilical cord blood of a matched donor can also be given.	**transplantation** (TRANS-plan-TAY-shun) **transplant/o-** *move something to another place* **-ation** *a process; being or having*
cryosurgery	Liquid nitrogen is sprayed or painted onto a small malignant lesion. The liquid nitrogen freezes and destroys the cancerous cells.	**cryosurgery** (KRY-oh-SER-jer-ee) **cry/o-** *cold* **surg/o-** *operative procedure* **-ery** *process of*

Word or Phrase	Description	Word Building

electrosurgery	An electrode and an electrical current is used to evaporate the intracellular contents of small, cancerous tumors on the skin. In **fulguration,** the electrode is held away from the skin and transmits the electrical current as a spark to the skin surface. In **electrodesiccation,** the electrode is touched to or inserted into the cancerous tumor.	**electrosurgery** (ee-LEK-troh-SER-jer-ee)
		  electr/o- *electricity*
		  surg/o- *operative procedure*
		  -ery *process of*
		
		fulguration (FUL-gyoo-RAY-shun)
		  fulgur/o- *spark of electricity*
		  -ation *a process; being or having*
		
		electrodesiccation
		(ee-LEK-troh-DES-ih-KAY-shun)
		  electr/o- *electricity*
		  desicc/o- *to dry up*
		  -ation *a process; being or having*

grading	Classifies cancers by how differentiated their cells appear under a microscope. Normal cells appear well differentiated and characteristic of that tissue type. Poorly differentiated or undifferentiated cancerous cells lack specialization and appear immature and embryonic. The greater the number of undifferentiated cells, the poorer the prognosis.	

insertion of a catheter to administer chemotherapy drugs	A catheter is inserted as an **intravenous line** in a vein in the arm. A **peripherally inserted central catheter** (PICC) is inserted in a vein in the arm and then threaded to the superior vena cava. An **intrathecal catheter** is inserted after a lumbar puncture is performed, and chemotherapy drugs circulate through the cerebrospinal fluid. **Intravesical chemotherapy** is administered through a catheter inserted into the bladder. The chemotherapy drug is held in the bladder for several hours and then removed. This procedure is done weekly for several weeks.	**intravenous** (IN-trah-VEE-nus)
		  intra- *within*
		  ven/o- *vein*
		  -ous *pertaining to*
		
		peripheral (peh-RIF-eh-ral)
		  peripher/o- *outer aspects*
		  -al *pertaining to*
		
		intrathecal (IN-trah-THEE-kal)
		  intra- *within*
		  thec/o- *sheath; layer of membranes*
		  -al *pertaining to*
		
		catheter (KATH-eh-ter)
		
		intravesical (IN-trah-VES-ih-kal)
		  intra- *within*
		  vesic/o- *bladder; fluid-filled sac*
		  -al *pertaining to*

staging	Classifies cancer by how far it has spread in the body. The TNM staging system is used to describe the size of the tumor and whether the tumor has spread to lymph nodes and other sites (see Table 18-1).	

Table 18-1   Classification Systems for Cancer

TNM System	
T	Size of the primary **tumor** (on a scale of T1 through T4)
N	Number of regional lymph **nodes** affected (on a scale of N1 through N4)
M	Presence or absence of **metastases** to other sites in the body (on a scale of M0 or M1)

Other Systems	
Bethesda System	Cervical cancer
CIN Classification	Cervical cancer
Clark Level	Malignant melanoma
Dukes Classification	Cancer of the colon or rectum
FIGO Staging	Ovarian cancer
Gleason Score	Adenocarcinoma of the prostate gland
Jewett Classification	Bladder carcinoma

Surgical Procedures

Word or Phrase	Description	Word Building
biopsy (Bx)	Tissue removed from a suspected cancerous tumor is sent to the pathology department for examination and diagnosis.	**biopsy** (BY-awp-see) **bi/o-** *life; living organisms; living tissue* **-opsy** *process of viewing*
core needle biopsy	A large-gauge needle is inserted into the tumor to obtain several long cores of tissue.	
excisional biopsy	An incision is made to expose the tumor, and the entire tumor is removed (excised) along with a surrounding margin of normal tissue.	**excisional** (ek-SIH-shun-al) **excis/o-** *to cut out* **-ion** *action; condition* **-al** *pertaining to*
fine-needle aspiration	A very fine needle is inserted into the tumor, and the fluid or tissue inside the tumor is aspirated into a syringe.	**aspiration** (AS-pih-RAY-shun) **aspir/o-** *to breathe in; to suck in* **-ation** *a process; being or having*
incisional biopsy	An incision is made to expose the tumor, and part (but not all) of the tumor is removed.	**incisional** (in-SIH-shun-al) **incis/o-** *to cut into* **-ion** *action; condition* **-al** *pertaining to*

Word or Phrase	Description	Word Building
optical biopsy	During an endoscopic procedure (see Figure 18-15 ■), a probe is inserted into the tumor. A laser from the probe creates a microscopic image of the cells of the tumor that can be used for diagnosis. 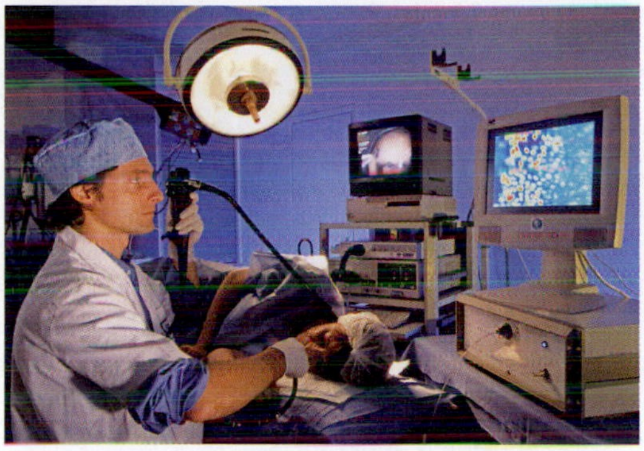 **Figure 18-15 ■ Optical biopsy.** An optical biopsy is done without ever removing tissue from the tumor. The endoscope lens creates an image of the area and displays it on a computer screen in the operating room. A laser probe passed through the endoscope creates a microscopic image of the tumor cells that is displayed on a second computer screen. The computer image is saved and studied to determine the diagnosis.	**optical** (AWP-tih-kal) **optic/o-** *lenses; properties of light* **-al** *pertaining to*
punch biopsy	Special forceps are used to grasp part of the tumor. As the forceps closes, it punches out a small, cylindrical tissue specimen. Multiple punch biopsies can be taken at one time.	
sentinel node biopsy	The sentinel lymph node, the first lymph node that receives drainage from the site of the primary tumor, is removed and examined.	**sentinel** (SEN-tih-nal)
stereotactic biopsy	Uses a CT scan to pinpoint the location of the tumor in three dimensions and guide the biopsy needle	**stereotactic** (STAIR-ee-oh-TAK-tik) **stere/o-** *three dimensions* **tact/o-** *touch* **-ic** *pertaining to*
vacuum-assisted biopsy	A probe with a cutting device is inserted through the skin and rotated around to take multiple specimens. The specimens are then suctioned out.	
debulking	Excision (removal) of part of a bulky, cancerous tumor. This reduces the size of the tumor and makes the patient more comfortable or leaves a smaller tumor that can be treated with chemotherapy or radiation therapy.	**debulk** (dee-BULK)
en bloc resection	Excision of a cancerous tumor and all surrounding structures, which are removed as one block of tissue	**en bloc** (en BLAWK) **resection** (ree-SEK-shun) **resect/o-** *to cut out; remove* **-ion** *action; condition*
endoscopy	A fiberoptic endoscope is used to examine a body cavity for signs of abnormal tissues or tumors. Grasping and cutting instruments are inserted through the endoscope to perform a biopsy. An optical biopsy can also be done at the same time (see Figure 18-15).	**endoscopy** (en-DAWS-koh-pee) **endo-** *innermost; within* **-scopy** *process of using an instrument to examine* The ending *-scopy* contains the combining form *scop/o-* and the one letter suffix *-y*.
excision of a tumor	Removal of all or part of a cancerous tumor. In a wide excision, the tumor plus a wide margin of normal tissue around it is excised.	**excision** (ek-SIH-shun) **excis/o-** *to cut out* **-ion** *action; condition*
exenteration	Excision (removal) of a cancerous tumor as well as all nearby organs. It is used to treat cancer that has metastasized throughout the abdominopelvic cavity.	**exenteration** (eks-EN-ter-AA-shun) **ex-** *out; away from* **enter/o-** *intestine* **-ation** *a process; being or having*

Word or Phrase	Description	Word Building

exploratory laparotomy	An abdominal incision is performed to widely open the abdominopelvic cavity so that it can be explored.	**exploratory** (eks-PLOR-ah-TOR-ee)
		  explorat/o- *to search out*
		  -ory *having the function of*
		
		laparotomy (LAP-ah-RAW-toh-mee)
		  lapar/o- *abdomen*
		  -tomy *process of cutting or making an incision*

insertion of a catheter or device to administer chemotherapy drugs	A **central venous catheter** (Broviac, Hickman, or Groshong catheter) is tunneled through the subcutaneous tissue in the upper chest. It is inserted into a large vein and advanced until its tip is positioned in the superior vena cava. The external end of the catheter is capped except when a chemotherapy drug is administered (see Figure 18-16 ■). An **intra-arterial catheter** is implanted in a main artery that brings blood to the organ where the cancerous tumor is located. A pump is also implanted under the skin or an externally worn portable infusion pump is used to administer regular doses of the chemotherapy drug. In **transarterial chemoembolization (TACE)**, a catheter is threaded through the femoral artery, aorta, and into the hepatic artery to deliver a one-time dose of chemotherapy to a cancerous tumor in the liver. After the drug is injected, a substance is injected to block the flow of blood and keep the drug concentrated at the site of the cancerous tumor. An **intraperitoneal catheter** is inserted into the peritoneal cavity with a capped end on the surface of the body. The chemotherapy drug is injected into the peritoneal fluid and comes in contact with the surfaces of all the organs in the abdominopelvic cavity. An **implantable port** is a metal or plastic reservoir that is placed in a pocket created in the subcutaneous tissue. The port is attached to a catheter in the superior vena cava. The chemotherapy drug is given by inserting a needle through the overlying skin and depositing the drug into the reservoir that releases the drug into the blood. An Ommaya reservoir is placed beneath the scalp with a connecting catheter placed in a ventricle in the brain, and the cerebrospinal fluid is used to circulate the chemotherapy drug. An **implantable wafer** is a dissolvable disk that contains a chemotherapy drug. It is surgically implanted in the area where a tumor has been excised.	**venous** (VEE-nus)
		  ven/o- *vein*
		  -ous *pertaining to*
		
		intra-arterial (IN-trah-ar-TEER-ee-al)
		  intra- *within*
		  arteri/o- *artery*
		  -al *pertaining to*
		
		transarterial (TRANS-ar-TEER-ee-al)
		  trans- *across; through*
		  arteri/o- *artery*
		  -al *pertaining to*
		
		chemoembolization (KEE-moh-EM-bol-ih-ZAY-shun)
		  chem/o- *chemical; drug*
		  embol/o- *embolus (occluding plug)*
		  -ization *process of making, creating, or inserting*
		
		intraperitoneal (IN-trah-PAIR-ih-toh-NEE-al)
		  intra- *within*
		  peritone/o- *peritoneum*
		  -al *pertaining to*
		
		implantable (im-PLANT-ah-bl)
		  implant/o- *placed within*
		  -able *able to be*
		
		port (PORT)

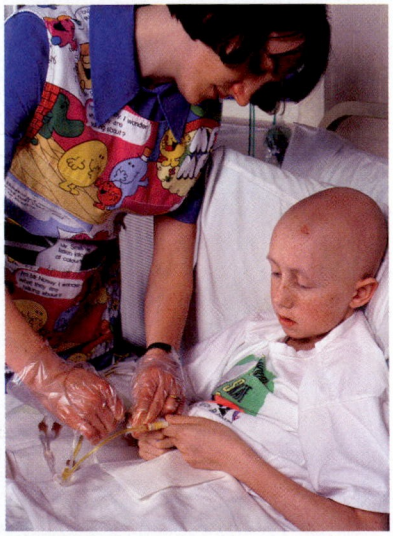

Figure 18-16 ■ **Central venous catheter.**
This young boy with leukemia has a central venous catheter. The nurse is allowing him to hold part of the tubing so that he can feel that he is participating in his treatment while she prepares to inject the chemotherapy drug. Treatment with the chemotherapy drug has already caused him to lose his hair.

Word or Phrase	Description	Word Building
lumpectomy	Excision (removal) of a small cancerous tumor without taking any surrounding tissue	**lumpectomy** (lum-PEK-toh-mee) *Lumpectomy* is a combination of the English word *lump* and the suffix *-ectomy* (surgical excision).

Word or Phrase	Description	Word Building
lymph node dissection	Procedure separating (dissecting) lymph nodes from tissue and removing several or all of the lymph nodes in a lymph node chain during extensive cancer surgery. Involved lymph nodes represent metastasis of the cancer from its original site.	**dissection** (dy-SEK-shun) **dissect/o-** *to cut apart* **-ion** *action; condition*
percutaneous radiofrequency ablation	A needle electrode is placed through the skin into a small cancerous tumor (less than 2 inches in diameter). High-frequency radiowaves (similar to microwaves) heat and kill the cancerous cells.	**percutaneous** (PER-kyoo-TAY-nee-us) **per-** *through; throughout* **cutane/o-** *skin* **-ous** *pertaining to* **ablation** (ah-BLAY-shun) **ablat/o-** *take away; destroy* **-ion** *action; condition*
radical resection	Cutting out and removing a cancerous tumor, as well as all nearby lymph nodes, soft tissue, muscle, and even bone	**radical** (RAD-ih-kal) **radic/o-** *all parts including the root* **-al** *pertaining to*

Radiation Therapy

Word or Phrase	Description	Word Building
brachytherapy	Category of radiation therapy that includes internal, interstitial, and intracavitary radiotherapy in which a radioactive substance is placed within the cancerous tumor or in tissues or in a cavity a short distance from the tumor.	**brachytherapy** (BRAK-ee-THAIR-ah-pee) **brachy-** *short* **-therapy** *treatment*
fractionation	The total dose of external beam radiation is divided into smaller doses (fractions of the total dose) that are given each day to decrease the occurrence of side effects.	**fractionation** (FRAK-shun-AA-shun)
radiotherapy	Uses one of several types of **radiation** to disrupt the DNA in cancer cells. The radiation is in the form of waves (x-rays or gamma rays) or particles (electrons, neutrons, or protons). Radiotherapy is used to treat solid tumors, as well as leukemia and lymphoma by radiating the bone marrow. Radiotherapy can be delivered from outside the body or as implants inside the body. Cancerous tumors that are readily destroyed by radiation therapy are said to be **radiosensitive**. Cancerous tumors that are not affected by radiation therapy are **radioresistant**.	**radiotherapy** (RAY-dee-oh-THAIR-ah-pee) **radi/o-** *radius (forearm bone); x-rays; radiation* **-therapy** *treatment* Select the correct combining form meaning to get the definition of *radiotherapy: treatment (using) radiation.* **radiation** (RAY-dee-AA-shun) **radi/o-** *radius (forearm bone); x-rays; radiation* **-ation** *a process; being or having* **radiosensitive** (RAY-dee-oh-SEN-sih-tiv) **radi/o-** *radius (forearm bone); x-rays; radiation* **sensit/o-** *affected by; sensitive to* **-ive** *pertaining to* **radioresistant** (RAY-dee-oh-ree-ZIS-tant) **radi/o-** *radius (forearm bone); x-rays; radiation* **resist/o-** *withstand the effect of* **-ant** *pertaining to*

Word or Phrase	Description	Word Building
conformal radiotherapy	Uses a computer to map the location of the tumor and create a three-dimensional image of the tumor. The external beam radiation is then matched to conform to the exact shape of the tumor to protect nearby vital organs.	**conformal** (con-FOR-mal) **conform/o-** *having the same scale or angle* **-al** *pertaining to*
external beam radiotherapy	Beams of radiation are generated by a machine outside the body and directed at the site of a cancerous tumor (see Figure 18-17 ■). Linear accelerators are used to increase the energy of the radiation so that it can penetrate more deeply into the body.	**external** (eks-TER-nal) **extern/o-** *outside* **-al** *pertaining to*

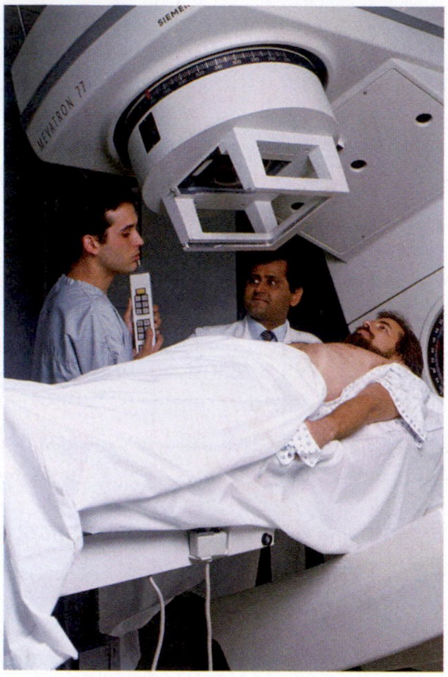

Figure 18-17 ■ External beam radiotherapy.

This patient is being prepared to receive external radiation therapy. The external beam of radiation is generated by the equipment over his head. Not all tumors can be treated with radiation therapy.

Word or Phrase	Description	Word Building
internal radiotherapy	An implant that contains a radioactive substance (such as cesium, iridium, iodine, phosphorus, or palladium that emits radiation) is implanted near the cancerous tumor	**internal** (in-TER-nal) **intern/o-** *inside* **-al** *pertaining to*
interstitial radiotherapy	Radioactive implants (needles, wires, capsules, or pellets, which are known as seeds) are inserted into the tumor or into the tissue around the cancerous tumor	**interstitial** (IN-ter-STISH-al) **interstiti/o-** *spaces within tissue* **-al** *pertaining to*
intracavitary radiotherapy	Radioactive implants are inserted into a body cavity near the cancerous tumor	**intracavitary** (IN-trah-KAV-ih-TAIR-ee) **intra-** *within* **cavit/o-** *hollow space* **-ary** *pertaining to*
intravenous radiotherapy	Radioactive iodine is given intravenously. It concentrates in the thyroid gland and releases radiation to kill cancerous cells of the thyroid gland.	**intravenous** (IN-trah-VEE-nus) **intra-** *within* **ven/o-** *vein* **-ous** *pertaining to*

Drug Categories

These categories of drugs are used to treat cancer. The most common generic and trade name drugs in each category are listed.

Category	Indication	Examples	Word Building
alkylating drugs	Break DNA strands in the cancerous cell by substituting an alkyl group for a hydrogen molecule in the DNA	busulfan (Myleran), carmustine (Gliadel), chlorambucil (Leukeran), cyclophosphamide (Cytoxan, Neosar), estramustine (Emcyt)	**alkylating** (AL-kih-LAY-ting)
antiemetic drugs	Not chemotherapy drugs. These drugs are used to treat the nausea and vomiting that are common side effects of chemotherapy.	dolasetron (Anzemet), dronabinol (Marinol), nabilone (Cesamet)	**antiemetic** (AN-tee-eh-MET-ik) **anti-** *against* **emet/o-** *to vomit* **-ic** *pertaining to*
antimetabolite drugs	Take the place of an important metabolite needed to build DNA, or they block an enzyme that produces an important metabolite. These drugs target cancerous cells that have a high rate of metabolism and cell division.	capecitabine (Xeloda), fludarabine (Fludara), fluorouracil (5-FU, Adrucil), gemcitabine (Gemzar), methotrexate (Trexall)	**antimetabolite** (AN-tee-meh-TAB-oh-lite) **anti-** *against* **metabol/o-** *change; transformation* **-ite** *thing that pertains to*
chemotherapy antibiotic drugs	Inhibit the production of DNA and RNA, and this keeps a cell from dividing	bleomycin (Blenoxane), doxorubicin (Adriamycin), epirubicin (Ellence)	**chemotherapy** (KEE-moh-THAIR-ah-pee) **chem/o-** *chemical; drug* **-therapy** *treatment* **antibiotic** (AN-tee-by-AWT-ik) **anti-** *against* **bi/o-** *life; living organisms; living tissue* **-tic** *pertaining to*

Did You Know?
Chemotherapy antibiotic drugs are not used to treat infections like regular antibiotic drugs are. Regular antibiotic drugs act on the cell wall of bacteria. Human cells do not have a cell wall and are not affected by regular antibiotic drugs. Chemotherapy antibiotic drugs do affect human cells, whether they are cancerous or normal.

Category	Indication	Examples	Word Building
chemotherapy enzyme drugs	Break down the amino acid asparagine. Normal body cells can synthesize their own supply of asparagine, but cancerous cells cannot.	asparaginase (Elspar), pegasparagase (Oncaspar)	

Clinical Connections

Pharmacology. Chemotherapy protocols use a combination of several different chemotherapy drugs that are administered together. This increases their effectiveness against cancerous cells while minimizing the side effects caused by large doses of just one drug. A **protocol** is a standardized written plan of treatment for a particular type of cancerous tumor. A protocol details which chemotherapy drugs should be given, in what order they should be given, and at what doses. Protocols are named by combining the first letter of each drug name. For example, the ABVD chemotherapy protocol for treating Hodgkin's lymphoma consists of the chemotherapy drugs Adriamycin, bleomycin, vinblastine, and dacarbazine.

Adjuvant therapy is the use of chemotherapy drugs after another type of therapy (surgery, radiation therapy) has been used as the primary treatment.

protocol (PROH-toh-kawl)

adjuvant (AD-joo-vant)
adjuv/o- *giving help or assistance*
-ant *pertaining to*

Category	Indication	Examples	Word Building
hormonal chemotherapy drugs	Produce an opposite hormonal environment from the one that the cancer needs to reproduce. For example, estrogen (a female hormone drug) is given to men with prostate cancer.	anastrozole (Arimidex), goserelin (Zoladex), letrozole (Femara), leuprolide (Eligard, Lupron), megestrol (Megace), tamoxifen (Soltamox)	**hormonal** (hor-MOH-nal) **hormon/o-** *hormone* **-al** *pertaining to*
mitosis inhibitor drugs	Cause DNA strands in the cancerous cell to break during the early stages of cell division (mitosis)	etoposide (VePesid), irinotecan (Camptosar), paclitaxel (Taxol), topotecan (Hycamtin), vinblastine (Velban)	**inhibitor** (in-HIB-ih-tor) **inhibit/o-** *block; hold back* **-or** *person or thing that produces or does*
monoclonal antibodies	Bind to specific antigens on the surface of a cancerous cell and destroy the cell. Monoclonal antibodies are created using recombinant DNA technology. A human antibody is modified so that it will bind to a specific antigen on a cancerous cell.	alemtuzumab (Campath), trastuzumab (Herceptin)	**monoclonal** (MAWN-oh-KLOH-nal) **mon/o-** *one; single* **clon/o-** *identical group derived from one* **-al** *pertaining to* **antibody** (AN-tih-BAWD-ee) *Antibody is a combination of the prefix anti- (against) and the English word body (a structure or thing).*
platinum chemotherapy drugs	Create crosslinks in the DNA strands that prevent the cancerous cell from dividing. These drugs actually contain the precious metal platinum.	carboplatin (Paraplatin), cisplatin	**platinum** (PLAT-ih-num)

Abbreviations

AFP	alpha fetoprotein	**DNA**	deoxyribonucleic acid
ALL	acute lymphocytic leukemia	**ER**	estrogen receptor
AML	acute myelogenous leukemia	**FIGO**	Federation Internationale de Gynécologie et Obstétrique
BMT	bone marrow transplantation		
BRCA	breast cancer (gene)	**5-HIAA**	5-hydroxyindoleacetic acid
Bx	biopsy	**HCG**	human chorionic gonadotropin
Ca	carcinoma, cancer	**mets**	metastases (slang)
CEA	carcinoembryonic antigen	**NK**	natural killer (cells)
chemo	chemotherapy (slang)	**PICC**	peripherally inserted central catheter
CIN	cervical intraepithelial neoplasia	**PR**	progesterone receptor
CIS	carcinoma *in situ*	**PSA**	prostate-specific antigen
CLL	chronic lymphocytic leukemia	**RNA**	ribonucleic acid
CML	chronic myelogenous leukemia	**TACE**	transarterial chemoembolization
CRT	certified radiation therapist	**TNM**	tumor, nodes, metastases
CTR	certified tumor registrar	**VMA**	vanillylmandelic acid

Word Alert

ABBREVIATIONS

Abbreviations are commonly used in all types of medical documents; however, they can mean different things to different people and their meanings can be misinterpreted. Always verify the meaning of an abbreviation.

Ca means *carcinoma* or *cancer,* but it also means *calcium.*

ER means *estrogen receptor,* but it also means *emergency room.*

Mets is slang for *metastases,* but it also means a unit of measurement that is used during cardiac treadmill stress tests to measure metabolic rate and oxygen consumption.

It's Greek to Me!

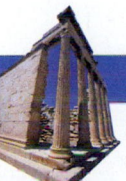

Did you notice that some words have two different combining forms? Combining forms from both Greek and Latin languages remain a part of medical language today.

Word	Greek	Latin	Medical Word Examples
cancer	carcin/o-	cancer/o-	carcinogen, cancerous
cell	cyt/o-	cellul/o-	cytoplasm, cellular
embryonic	blast/o-	germin/o-	neuroblastoma, dysgerminoma
	embryon/o-		embryonal cell carcinoma
nucleus	kary/o-	nucle/o-	karyotype, nuclear membrane

CAREER FOCUS

Meet Shah, a surgical assistant

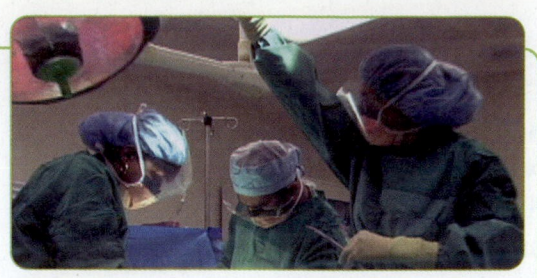

"I'm a surgical assistant. I help the doctor from the beginnning to the end of the surgery. The very best part is assisting during cesarean sections. I like that part because sometimes there's a really sick baby or mom and, after the cesarean section, the baby is okay and the mom is okay. For a cesarean section, we have 50 different instruments. Each doctor uses different ways and different instruments. I keep track of the instruments and purchase new instruments."

Surgical assistants are allied health professionals who assist surgeons in the operating room. They position and drape the patient and prepare the patient's surgical site by shaving and prepping the skin. Using sterile technique, they assist the surgeon during the operation by holding retractors, clamping or cutting tissues, and placing sutures.

Medical oncologists are physicians who specialize in treating patients with cancer. After the patient's cancer has been diagnosed, a medical oncologist assigns a grade and stage to the cancer and prescribes chemotherapy, radiation therapy, surgery, or a combination of all three, depending on the type of cancer and how advanced it is. Medical oncologists calculate the dose of the chemotherapy drugs based on the patient's body weight.

Radiation oncologists are physicians who have received additional training in using radiation therapy to treat cancer. They select the type of radiation and the most effective radiation technique for the type of cancer. They calculate the total dose of radiation to be given and then divide the dose into fractional amounts to be given each week.

surgical (SER-jih-kal)
   surg/o- *operative procedure*
   -ical *pertaining to*

medical (MED-ih-kal)
   medic/o- *physician; medicine*
   -al *pertaining to*

oncologist (ong-KAWL-oh-jist)
   onc/o- *tumor; mass*
   log/o- *word; the study of*
   -ist *one who specializes in*

radiation (RAY-dee-AA-shun)
   radi/o- *radius (forearm bone);*
      x-rays; radiation
   -ation *a process; being or having*

PEARSON
myhealthprofessionskit™ To see Shah's complete video profile, visit Medical Terminology Interactive at www.myhealthprofessionskit.com. Select this book, log in, and go to the 18th floor of Pearson General Hospital. Enter the Laboratory, and click on the computer screen.

CHAPTER REVIEW EXERCISES

Test your knowledge of the chapter by completing these review exercises. Use the Answer Key at the end of the book to check your answers.

Anatomy and Physiology

Matching Exercise

Match each word or phrase to its description.

1. chromosome

2. cytoplasm

3. gene

4. Golgi apparatus

5. lysosome

6. mitochondrion

7. ribosome

8. suppressor gene

_____ Intracellular gel-like substance

_____ Makes lysosomes and enzymes

_____ Produces energy for the cell's activities

_____ Area on a chromosome with information to build one protein molecule

_____ Site of protein synthesis

_____ 23 pairs

_____ Inhibits mitosis

_____ Becomes active when a pathogen enters the cell

True or False Exercise

Indicate whether each statement is true or false by writing T or F on the line.

1. _____ The nucleolus is an enlarged type of nucleus that is seen during cell division.

2. _____ An organelle is an intracellular structure that is embedded in the cytoplasm of a cell.

3. _____ Mitosis is the process by which a normal cell becomes cancerous.

4. _____ The gene p53 is an important suppressor gene.

5. _____ A cell has 23 pairs of chromosomes plus two sex chromosomes.

6. _____ RNA in the cell is in the shape of a double helix.

Circle Exercise

Circle the correct word from the choices given.

1. Epithelial tissues contains (**cancer, Schwann, squamous**) cells.

2. Messenger RNA carries information from the nucleus to the (**cell membrane, mitochondrion, ribosome**).

3. When a cell loses its unique, differentiated structure, this is known as (**anaplasia, apoptosis, mitosis**).

4. (**Apoptosis, Mitosis, Translocation**) is the process by which a cell duplicates itself.

Types of Cancer

True or False Exercise

Indicate whether each statement is true or false by writing T *or* F *on the line.*

1. _____ Peau d'orange is a dimpling seen in cancer of the uterus.

2. _____ Carcinomatosis shows cancerous tumors in multiple places in the body.

3. _____ A carcinoid tumor is the most serious type of cancer.

4. _____ Neoplasms are always malignant cancers.

5. _____ Carcinomas arise from connective tissues.

6. _____ Sarcomas grow rapidly and show anaplasia.

7. _____ A chondrosarcoma is a cancer of the cartilage.

8. _____ Kaposi's sarcoma most often affects patients with AIDS.

9. _____ Leukemia can be acute or chronic.

10. _____ A seminoma is an embryonal cell cancer of the breast.

Matching Exercise

Match each word or phrase to its definition.

1. adenocarcinoma

2. astrocytoma

3. cholangiocarcinoma

4. sentinal node

5. Hodgkin's lymphoma

6. leiomyosarcoma

7. lymphadenopathy

8. malignant melanoma

9. myosarcoma

10. neoplasm

11. relapse

_____ Cancer of the muscle

_____ Enlarged lymph nodes

_____ Cancer of the smooth muscle of the uterus

_____ Benign or cancerous tumor

_____ First to receive lymphatic drainage from cancer site

_____ Cancer of a starlike cell in the brain

_____ Cancer of the ducts of the gallbladder

_____ Opposite of remission

_____ Cancer of a gland

_____ Shows Reed-Sternberg cells

_____ Cancer of a melanocyte

Memory Exercise

1. Ways in which early cancer can present itself. What does each letter of this acronym stand for?

C _____

A _____

U _____

T _____

I _____

O _____

N _____

2. Define and match each abbreviation to its definition.

a. AFP _____

b. Bx _____

c. CML _____

d. ER _____

e. RNA _____

f. TNM _____

_____ Can be excisional or incisional

_____ Messenger is a type

_____ Normally present in a fetus

_____ Type of leukemia

_____ Tells how far a tumor has spread

_____ Numbers of these on the cell membrane affect the prognosis of breast cancer

Laboratory, Radiology, Surgery, and Drugs

Matching Exercise

Match each word or phrase to its description.

1. Bence Jones protein	_____ Way to stage tumor, nodes, and metastases
2. BRCA1	_____ Pap smear is an example
3. exfoliative cytology	_____ Another name for radiation therapy
4. frozen section	_____ Performed while surgery is still going on
5. Jewett classification	_____ Used to stage bladder carcinoma
6. radiotherapy	_____ Mutated gene related to breast cancer in families
7. scintigraphy	_____ Protein in the urine of patients with multiple myeloma
8. TNM	_____ Radioactive whole body bone scan to look for metastases

True or False Exercise

Indicate whether each statement is true or false by writing T or F on the line.

1. _____ A bone marrow aspiration is used to diagnose breast cancer.

2. _____ A karyotype is an x-ray that shows bony metastases.

3. _____ ER and PR assay tests tell whether the tumor is hormone dependent.

4. _____ PSA is performed to check for colon cancer.

5. _____ Grading is a procedure that removes just part of a tumor.

6. _____ A colonoscopy is done to examine the colon for tumors.

7. _____ A cancerous tumor that is radioresistant will die if treated with radiation therapy.

8. _____ Antibiotic drugs and chemotherapy antibiotic drugs can be used interchangeably to treat cancer.

Matching Exercise

Match each word or phrase to its description.

1. cryosurgery	_____ Implantable, dissolvable way to deliver a chemotherapy drug to a specific area
2. excisional biopsy	_____ Uses special forceps to remove a cylindrical tissue specimen
3. exenteration	_____ Surgery performed through a large abdominal incision
4. exploratory laparotomy	_____ Uses cold to freeze and kill cancerous tumors
5. intrathecal catheter	_____ Surgical removal of a cancerous tumor, and all the organs and surrounding tissues and muscles
6. punch biopsy	_____ Surgical procedure that removes the entire tumor
7. stereotactic biopsy	_____ Delivers a chemotherapy drug into the spinal canal
8. wafer	_____ Uses a CT scan to pinpoint the tumor location during surgery

Circle Exercise

Circle the correct word from the choices given.

1. (**Adjuvant therapy, Chemotherapy protocol, Endoscopy**) is the use of chemotherapy after radiation or surgery has been used as the primary treatment.

2. (**Endoscopy, Intravesical chemotherapy, Lymph node dissection**) is looking into a body cavity and using instruments to perform a biopsy.

3. *En bloc* resection means (**debulking part of a large tumor, excising the tumor and surrounding structures as one block of tissue, widening an area blocked by a tumor**).

4. A (**debulking, fractionation, protocol**) is a standard written plan of treatment for a particular type of cancer.

Building Medical Words

Review the Combining Forms Exercise and Combining Form and Suffix Exercise that you already completed in the anatomy section on pages 899–900.

Combining Forms Exercise

Before you build cancer words, review these additional combining forms. Next to each combining form, write its medical meaning. The first one has been done for you.

Combining Form	Medical Meaning	Combining Form	Medical Meaning
1. aden/o-	gland	16. mamm/o-	
2. bi/o-		17. melan/o-	
3. blast/o-		18. my/o-	
4. chem/o-		19. ne/o-	
5. chondr/o-		20. nephr/o-	
6. cry/o-		21. onc/o-	
7. dissect/o-		22. oste/o-	
8. excis/o-		23. radi/o-	
9. hepat/o-		24. remiss/o-	
10. incis/o-		25. resect/o-	
11. leuk/o-		26. resist/o-	
12. lip/o-		27. retin/o-	
13. log/o-		28. sarc/o-	
14. lymph/o-		29. semin/o-	
15. malign/o-		30. surg/o-	

Related Combining Forms Exercise

Write the combining forms on the line provided. (Hint: See the It's Greek to Me feature box.)

1. Two combining forms that mean *cancer*. _____

2. Two combining forms that mean *cell*. _____

3. Two combining forms that mean *nucleus*. _____

4. Three combining forms that mean *embryonic*. _____

Combining Form and Suffix Exercise

Read the definition of the medical word. Select the correct suffix from the Suffix List. Select the correct combining form from the Combining Form List. Build the medical word and write it on the line. Be sure to check your spelling. The first one has been done for you.

SUFFIX LIST	COMBINING FORM LIST	
-ant (pertaining to)	bi/o- (life; living organisms; living tissue)	malign/o- (intentionally causing harm; cancer)
-emia (condition of the blood; substance in the blood)	carcin/o- (cancer)	mamm/o- (breast)
-graphy (process of recording)	cyt/o- (cell)	melan/o- (black)
-ion (action; condition)	dissect/o- (to cut apart)	ne/o- (new)
-logy (the study of)	hepat/o- (liver)	resect/o- (to cut out; remove)
-oid (resembling)	kary/o- (nucleus)	sarc/o- (connective tissue)
-oma (tumor; mass)	leuk/o- (white)	semin/o- (spermatozoon; sperm)
-opsy (process of viewing)	lymph/o- (lymph; lymphatic system)	
-plasm (growth; formed substance)		
-type (particular kind of; a model of)		

Definition of the Medical Word

Build the Medical Word

1. Resembling a cancer   carcinoid
2. Action to cut apart (a tumor from surrounding tissue)
3. Tumor (of the testes that produce) spermatozoa
4. Tumor of the connective tissue
5. Growth or formed substance (that is) new
6. Pertaining to (something that is) intentionally causing harm (like a) cancer
7. Tumor that is cancer
8. Tumor of the liver
9. Condition of the blood (of too many) white (blood cells)
10. Process of recording the breast
11. Process of viewing living tissue
12. Action to cut out and remove (tissue)
13. The study of cells
14. Tumor of the lymphatic system
15. A model of (the chromosomes in the) nucleus
16. Tumor (of the skin whose color is brown or) black

Multiple Combining Forms and Suffix Exercise

Read the definition of the medical word. Select the correct suffix and combining forms. Then build the medical word and write it on the line. Be sure to check your spelling. The first one has been done for you.

SUFFIX LIST	COMBINING FORM LIST	
-ant (pertaining to)	aden/o- (gland)	my/o- (muscle)
-ery (process of)	angi/o- (blood vessel; lymphatic vessel)	nephr/o- (kidney; nephron)
-graphy (process of recording)	blast/o- (immature; embryonic)	onc/o- (tumor; mass)
-ist (one who specializes in)	carcin/o- (cancer)	oste/o- (bone)
-oma (tumor; mass)	chondr/o- (cartilage)	radi/o- (x-rays; radiation)
-pathy (disease; suffering)	cry/o- (cold)	resist/o- (withstand the effect of)
	hepat/o- (liver)	retin/o- (retina)
	lip/o- (lipid; fat)	sarc/o- (connective tissue)
	log/o- (word; the study of)	surg/o- (operative procedure)
	lymph/o- (lymph; lymphatic system)	

Definition of the Medical Word

Build the Medical Word

1. Tumor of the liver with immature (cells)   *hepatoblastoma*

2. Process of recording the lymph and lymphatic vessels   _____

3. Tumor of the lipid (fat) and connective tissue   _____

4. Tumor of the kidney (that has) immature, embryonic (cells)   _____

5. Process of (using) cold (to kill cancer during an) operative procedure   _____

6. Tumor of the muscle and connective tissue   _____

7. Disease (of the) lymph glands   _____

8. Tumor of a gland (that contains) cancer   _____

9. Tumor of the retina (of the eye that has) immature, embryonic (cells)   _____

10. Pertaining to (a cancer that is treated with) radiation (but) withstands the effect of it   _____

11. Tumor of the cartilage and connective tissue   _____

12. Tumor of bone and connective tissue   _____

13. One who specializes in the tumors (and) the study of (them)   _____

Abbreviations

Matching Exercise

Match each abbreviation to its description.

1. AML   _____ A cancer staging system

2. BMT   _____ Surgical procedure to remove a tissue specimen

3. Bx   _____ Treatment for leukemia

4. ER   _____ Determines if breast cancer can be treated with hormones

5. NK   _____ A way to give chemotherapy

6. PICC   _____ Cells that attack cancer cells

7. TNM   _____ A type of leukemia

Applied Skills

Medical Report Exercise

This exercise contains two pathology reports. The first is the gross description of the tissue specimen, and the second is the microscopic description of the same tissue specimen. Read both reports and answer the questions.

PATHOLOGY REPORT

PATIENT NAME: FOSTER, Virginia

HOSPITAL NUMBER: 564-542-8763

DATE OF SURGERY: November 19, 20xx

GROSS DESCRIPTION

CLINICAL HISTORY: This is a 49-year-old white female with a right breast mass. She performs occasional self-examination of her breasts. While performing this procedure 2 days ago, she noted a lump in her right breast. She was seen by her primary care physician and referred for a mammogram. Mammography and subsequent ultrasound showed a solid rather than cystic mass. She was immediately scheduled for a biopsy. She has no family history of cancer.

PREOPERATIVE DIAGNOSIS: Rule out carcinoma of the breast.

OPERATION: Needle biopsy of right breast mass.

TISSUE SPECIMEN: Right breast mass. Specimen labeled "needle biopsy, right breast" is received in gauze. It consists of a single piece of tissue measuring 1.0 × 0.1 × 0.1 cm. It is cylindrical, tannish, soft, and pliable. It is submitted in its entirety for a frozen section. Axillary lymph nodes submitted: 28.

Alfredo P. Martinez, M.D.

Alfredo P. Martinez, M.D.

APM:rrg
D: 11/19/xx
T: 11/19/xx

PATHOLOGY REPORT

PATIENT NAME: FOSTER, Virginia

HOSPITAL NUMBER: 564-542-8763

DATE OF SURGERY: November 24, 20xx

MICROSCOPIC DESCRIPTION

CLINICAL HISTORY: This is a 49-year-old white female who presented to her primary care physician with a right breast mass. Subsequent needle biopsy on 11-19-xx revealed carcinoma of the breast. She was scheduled for a right mastectomy and axillary lymph node dissection.

PREOPERATIVE DIAGNOSIS: Carcinoma of the breast.

OPERATION: Right mastectomy and axillary lymph node dissection.

TISSUE SPECIMENS: Tumor and 28 axillary lymph nodes.

MICROSCOPIC COMMENTS: Sections of the tumor reveal an invasive tumor composed of irregular nests of pleomorphic, anaplastic cells having prominent nucleoli. Some of the larger nests show central areas of necrosis. The tumor extends to an ulcerated skin surface. The margins of resection are free of tumor. A section of the nipple demonstrates tumor extending along the large lactiferous ducts. A total of 28 lymph nodes are submitted. Ten are positive for metastasis. The largest positive lymph node is 2.0 cm.

DIAGNOSIS: Infiltrating ductal carcinoma, grade 3. Metastatic carcinoma involving 10 of 28 axillary lymph nodes.

Alfredo P. Martinez, M.D.

Alfredo P. Martinez, M.D.

APM:rrg
D: 11/19/xx
T: 11/19/xx

Fact Finding Questions

1. How did the patient discover her breast mass?

_____

2. What was the first test that the doctor ordered for her to have?

_____

3. What operative procedure was performed after the mammography?

_____

4. How many of the patient's lymph nodes showed signs of cancer?

_____

5. What is anaplasia?

_____

Word Analysis Questions

1. The patient had metastasis to 10 lymph nodes. If you wanted to use the adjective form of *metastasis*, you would say, "She had cancer that was _____."

2. Divide *biopsy* into its two word parts and define each word part.

   Word Part   **Definition**

   _____   _____

   _____   _____

3. Divide *dissection* into its two word parts and define each word part.

   Word Part   **Definition**

   _____   _____

   _____   _____

4. Divide *carcinoma* into its two word parts and define each word part.

   Word Part   **Definition**

   _____   _____

   _____   _____

Critical Thinking Questions

1. Why is it important to know that the patient has no history of cancer in her family?

   _____

2. What is a frozen section and when is it performed?

   _____

3. A tumor that extends into the tissue near it is said to be _____.
   a. metastatic
   b. invasive
   c. carcinoma
   d. embryonic

4. What sentence tells you that all of the tumor was removed?

   _____

Hearing Medical Words Exercise

You hear someone speaking the medical words given below. Read each pronunciation and then write the medical word it represents. Be sure to check your spelling. The first one has been done for you.

1. AD-eh-noh-KAR-sih-NOH-mah   *adenocarcinoma*
2. KEE-moh-THAIR-ah-pee   _____
3. KRY-oh-SER-jer-ee   _____
4. HAWJ-kinz lim-FOH-mah   _____
5. LIM-fad-eh-NAWP-ah-thee   _____
6. lim-FOH-mah   _____
7. MET-ah-STAT-ik   _____
8. NEE-oh-plazm   _____
9. ong-KAWL-oh-jist   _____
10. AWS-tee-oh-sar-KOH-mah   _____

Pronunciation Exercise

Read the medical word that is given. Then review the syllables in the pronunciation. Circle the primary (main) accented syllable. The first one has been done for you.

1. cancer (kan-ser)
2. angiosarcoma (an-jee-oh-sar-koh-mah)
3. benign (bee-nine)
4. biopsy (by-awp-see)
5. carcinogen (kar-sin-oh-jen)
6. carcinoma (kar-sih-noh-mah)
7. dysplasia (dis-play-zee-ah)
8. genetic (jeh-net-ik)
9. lumpectomy (lum-pek-toh-mee)
10. metastatic (met-ah-stat-ik)

Dividing Medical Words

Separate these words into their component parts (prefix, combining form, suffix). Note: Some words do not contain all three word parts. The first one has been done for you.

Medical Word	Prefix	Combining Form	Suffix	Medical Word	Prefix	Combining Form	Suffix
1. carcinogen		carcin/o-	-gen	6. oncogene			
2. translocation				7. metastatic			
3. karyotype				8. dysplastic			
4. cytology				9. leukemia			
5. encapsulated				10. intravesical			

Multimedia Preview

Immerse yourself in a variety of activities inside Medical Terminology Interactive. Getting there is simple:

1. Click on www.myhealthprofessionskit.com.
2. Select "Medical Terminology" from the choice of disciplines.
3. First-time users must create an account using the scratch-off code on the inside front cover of this book.
4. Find this book and log in using your username and password.
5. Click on Medical Terminology Interactive.
6. Take the elevator to the 18th Floor to begin your virtual exploration of this chapter!

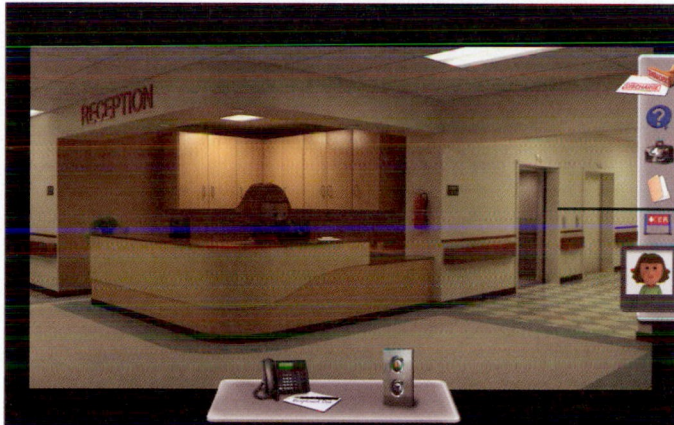 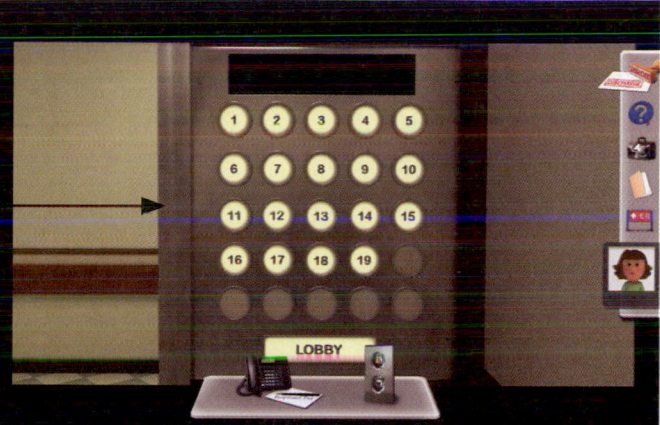

■ **Gridlock**   Are you a *Jeopardy!* Champ? Prove your quiz show smarts by clicking here to answer the medical terminology questions hidden beneath the tiles. Get them all right to clear the grid.

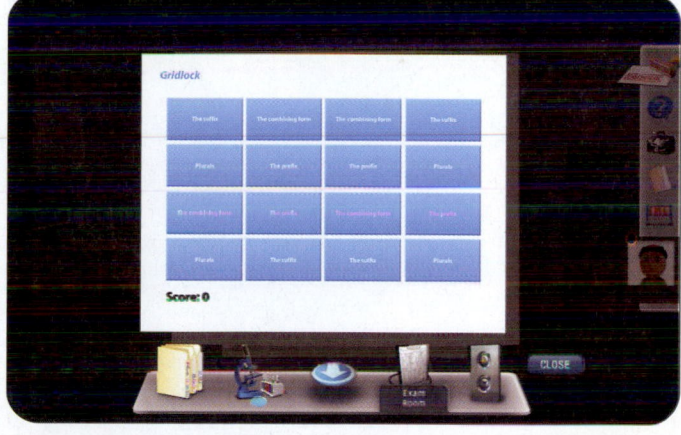

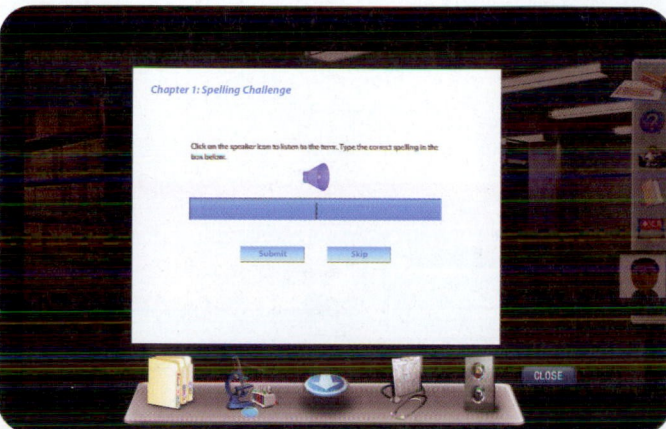

■ **Spelling Challenge**   Test your skills; listen to a pronounced medical word and then attempt to spell it correctly.

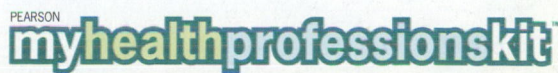

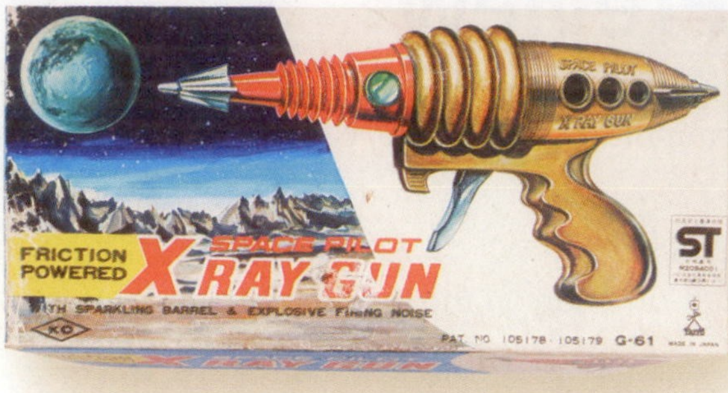

▲ While it may seem like science fiction, X-ray technology is real, and it's not kid stuff.

Dive In!

- The x-ray got its name because when it was discovered it was an unknown type of radiation—therefore called "X."
- Ultrasound often provides a clearer picture in space because low gravity allows sound waves to move with less distortion.
- If you think this is interesting, keep scanning. In this chapter we'll explore the language that describes the various processes of diagnostic imaging.
- You'll see the whole picture once you master the language of radiology!

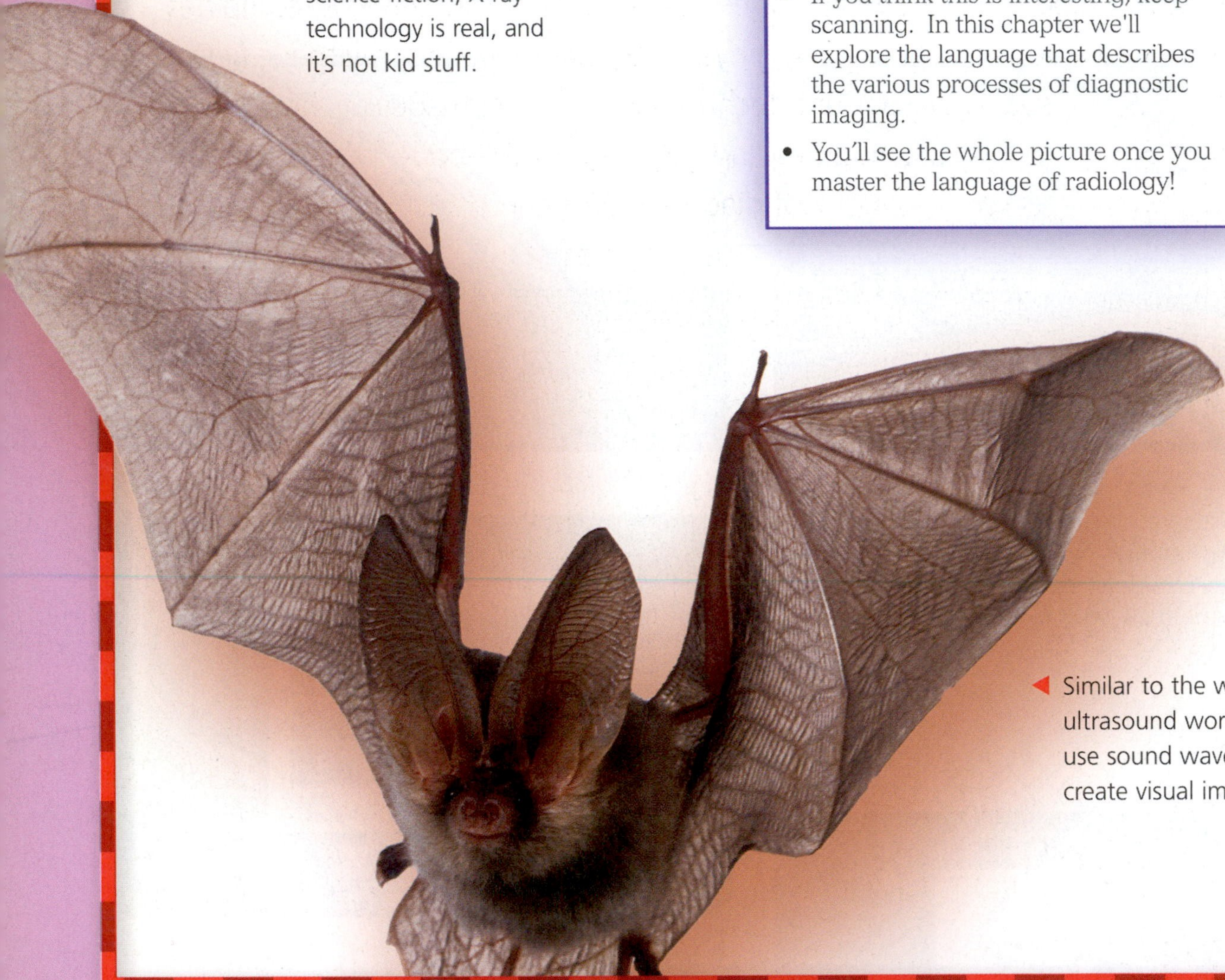

◄ Similar to the way ultrasound works, bats use sound waves to create visual images.

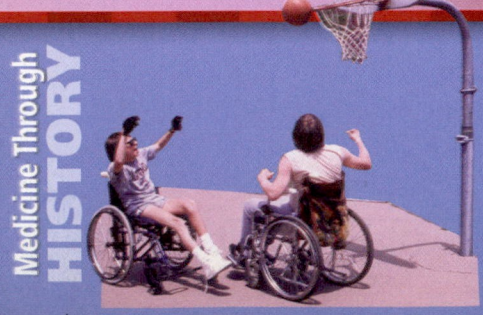

1990

The Americans with Disabilities Act (ADA) prohibits discrimination against handicapped persons

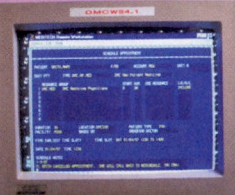

1996

The Healthcare Insurance Portability Act (HIPAA) requires that a patient's medical information be kept secure and only released to others who are caring for the patient

19
Radiology and Nuclear Medicine

Radiology (RAY-dee-AWL-oh-jee) is the medical specialty that combines the study of anatomy and physiology, energy (x-rays, magnetic fields, sound waves), and technology to create images of the internal structures and functions of the body for the purpose of diagnosis. Nuclear medicine is the medical specialty that uses radioactive substances for this same purpose.

◀ X-rays travel from the machine through the body to the plate which creates the image.

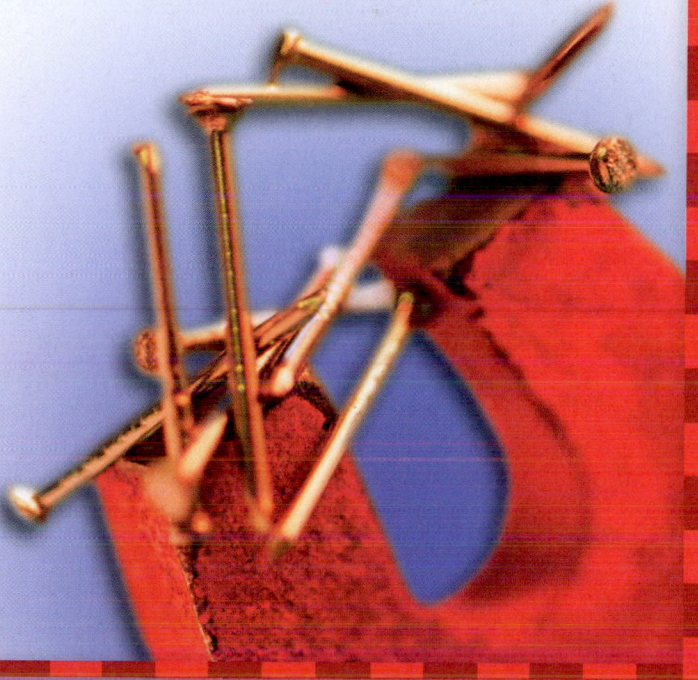

▶ Magnetic fields are used to construct diagnostic images via MRI technology.

1996

Dolly the sheep becomes the first animal to be cloned from the cells of another animal

2000

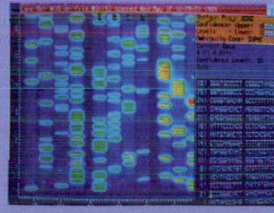

The map of the human genome is completed

2001

The first embryonic stem cell is made into a mature blood cell. This ignites a controversy over the use of embryos in stem cell research

Measure Your Progress: Learning Objectives

After you study this chapter, you should be able to

1. Describe five radiology procedures that use x-rays.

2. Describe common x-ray projections (views) and patient positions.

3. Identify common radiology procedures that use x-rays and a contrast dye.

4. Describe other radiology procedures that use a magnetic field, an electron beam, or sound waves.

5. Describe nuclear medicine procedures that use gamma rays or positrons.

6. Build radiology and nuclear medicine words from word parts and divide and define words.

7. Spell and pronounce radiology and nuclear medicine words.

8. Analyze the medical content and meaning of a radiology report.

9. Dive deeper into radiology and nuclear medicine by reviewing the activities at the end of this chapter and online at Medical Terminology Interactive.

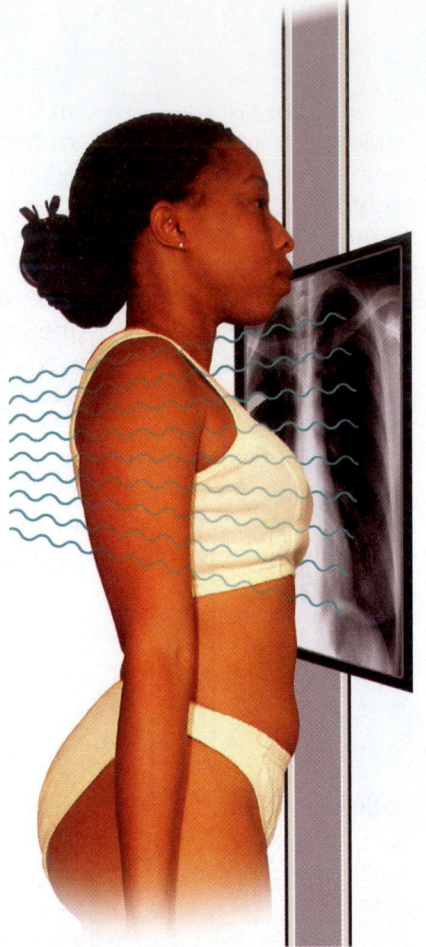

Figure 19-1 ■ **Radiography.**
Radiography is the most common subspecialty within the medical specialty of radiology.

Medical Language Key

To unlock the definition of a medical word, break it into word parts. Define each word part. Put the word part meanings in order, beginning with the suffix, then the prefix (if present), then the combining form(s).

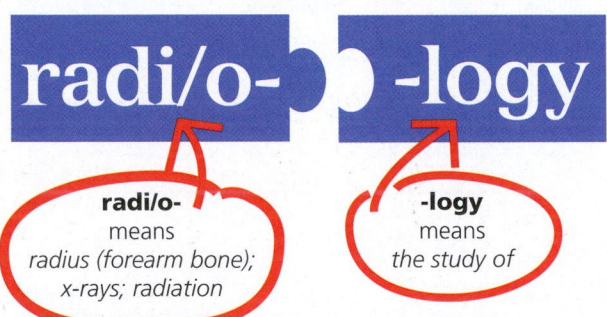

radi/o-
means
radius (forearm bone);
x-rays; radiation

-logy
means
the study of

	Word Part	Word Part Meaning
Suffix	-logy	*the study of*
Combining Form	radi/o-	*radius (forearm bone); x-rays; radiation*

Radiology: *The study of x-rays and (other imaging techniques).*

Anatomy and Physiology

The anatomy of the body can be seen in a whole new way in radiology and nuclear medicine. X-rays, contrast dyes, magnetic fields, sound waves, and radioactive substances allow us to view structures and functions within the body that are otherwise only accessible during surgery. Radiology is the medical specialty that studies x-ray and other imaging techniques (see Figure 19-1 ■). Within the medical specialty of radiology are the subspecialties of radiography, fluoroscopy, mammography, bone density testing, computerized axial tomography, magnetic resonance imaging, ultrasonography, and electron beam tomography. Nuclear medicine is the medical specialty that uses radioactive substances to produce images. These procedures are performed in the radiology and nuclear medicine department of a hospital or in an outpatient facility.

Diagnostic imaging (or medical imaging) is an all-encompassing phrase that includes radiology and nuclear medicine but also includes medical photography, microscopic imaging of pathology tissue specimens, and other types of imaging.

Radiology

Radiography

Radiography is the most common subspecialty of radiology. Radiography uses x-rays to produce a diagnostic image. **X-rays** are a form of invisible ionizing **radiation.** They are produced when a positively charged metal plate inside a vacuum tube is bombarded with a stream of electrons. X-rays have a very short wavelength and contain so much energy that they are able to pass through the body.

During radiography (or **roentgenography**), the patient is placed between the x-ray machine and a large, flat, silver x-ray plate. X-ray beams travel through the patient's body to the x-ray plate (see Figure 19-2 ■). The image created by the x-rays is in various shades of black, white, and gray that relate to the density of the various tissues. For example, air (in a body

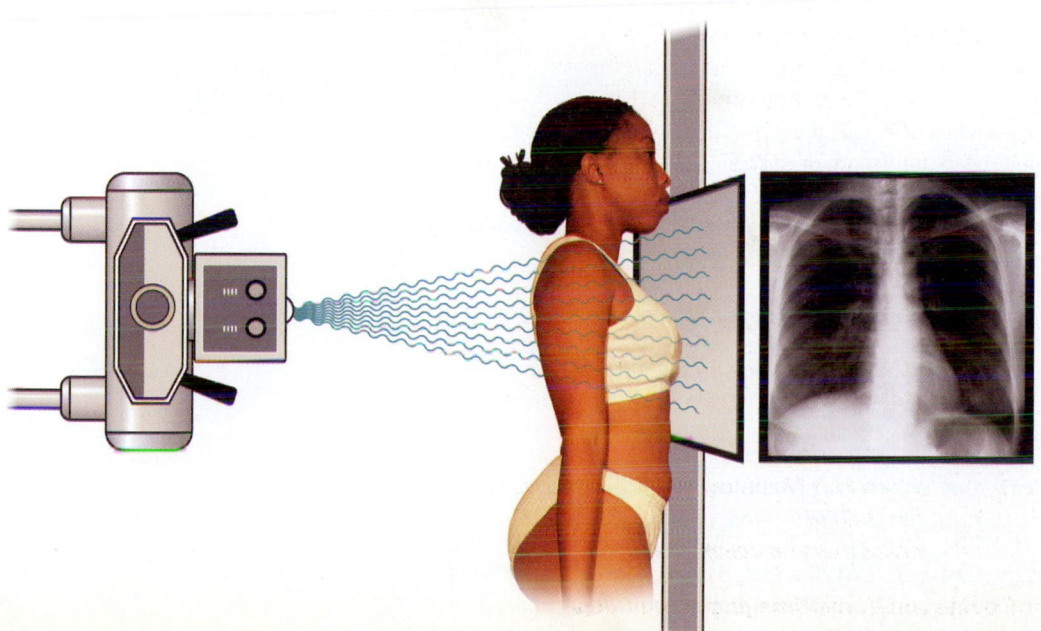

Figure 19-2 ■
Radiography.

This patient is having a PA (posteroanterior) chest x-ray. The x-ray machine projects a set of crossed lines onto the patient's back to help the technologist center the x-ray beam. The patient is asked to remain still so that the radiograph will not show motion artifact (a blurred image). The x-rays penetrate the patient's posterior chest. They exit through the patient's anterior chest, enter the x-ray plate, and create an image.

cavity or the lungs) has a low density, and x-rays pass through it, creating a nearly black area on the x-ray image; areas of low density are said to be **radiolucent.** A bone or a body organ has a high tissue density that absorbs x-rays, creating a white area on the x-ray image (see Figure 19-2); areas of high density are said to be **radiopaque.** Areas of intermediate density create various shades of gray.

The image on the x-ray plate is like the negative that is created when photographic film is exposed to light. The x-ray plate is developed with chemicals, and the positive image is printed on flexible plastic film. The radiologist views or reads the x-ray film by placing it in front of a light box (see Figure 19-3 ■). The film image is a **radiograph.** See Table 19-1 for other words and phrases related to radiography.

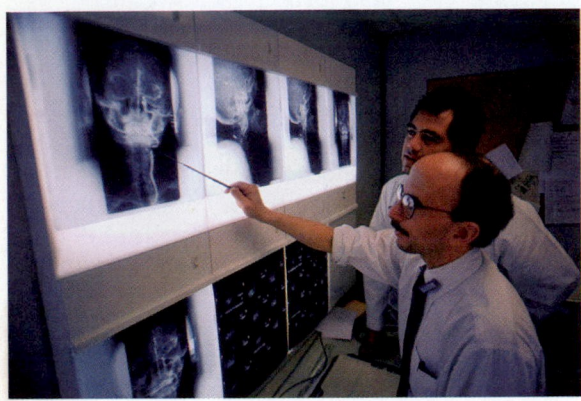

Figure 19-3 ■ Reading a radiograph.

This radiologist is viewing the patient's radiograph (a cerebral arteriogram) in consultation with another radiologist. The intense light of the light box illuminates fine details on the x-ray image.

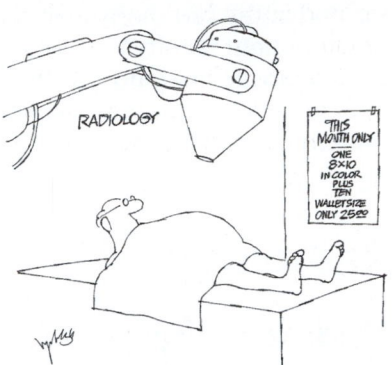

Table 19-1   Radiography Words and Phrases

Word or Phrase	Description	Word Building
film badge	A badge worn by all healthcare professionals who work in the radiology and nuclear medicine department. The badge contains a clear, unexposed piece of x-ray film that becomes progressively more opaque with cumulative exposure to radiation (x-rays, gamma rays from radioactive substances). Radiation exposure is measured in **rems. Dosimetry** is the process of measuring the amount of radiation exposure, as detected by a film badge and measured by a **dosimeter.**	**rem** (REM) *Rem is an abbreviation for roentgen-equivalent man.* **dosimetry** (doh-SIM-eh-tree) **dos/i-** *dose* **-metry** *process of measuring* **dosimeter** (doh-SIM-eh-ter) **dos/i-** *dose* **-meter** *instrument used to measure*
lead apron	Lead is an extremely dense substance that does not permit x-rays to pass through it. Lead aprons are used to shield parts of the patient's body that are not being x-rayed; they are also worn by the radiology department staff if they must be in the room with the patient while the procedure is being performed (see Figure 19-4).	
plain film	Any radiograph that is taken without the use of a radiopaque contrast dye	
portable film	Radiograph taken at the patient's bedside on the nursing unit or in the emergency department when the patient cannot be transported to the radiology department	
scout film	Preliminary x-ray that is taken to provide an initial view of an area before a radiopaque contrast dye is administered	
x-ray cassette and buckey	A cassette is the case that holds the x-ray film. A buckey is an adjustable frame that is mounted on the wall, beneath the x-ray table, or is a mobile frame on wheels. It positions and holds the x-ray cassette.	

Obtaining radiographs of different parts of the body requires the patient to be placed in different positions. These positions are known as **projections** or **views,** and each position has a standardized, fixed orientation between the patient, the x-ray cassette, and x-ray machine (see Table 19-2).

Radiography with Fluoroscopy

Fluoroscopy uses continuous x-rays to capture the motion of the internal organs as it occurs. The x-rays pass through the patient's body to a fluorescent screen that transforms the x-rays into long wavelengths of light that the eye can see as they are displayed on a TV monitor. Fluoroscopy is used to follow the movement of contrast dye during a cardiac catheterization, an angiography, an upper GI series (barium swallow) (see Figure 19-4 ■), a small-bowel follow-through, and other procedures. Individual x-ray images are taken to capture the most important aspects of the procedure. The entire fluoroscopy can be recorded on disk or videotape, a procedure known as **cineradiography.**

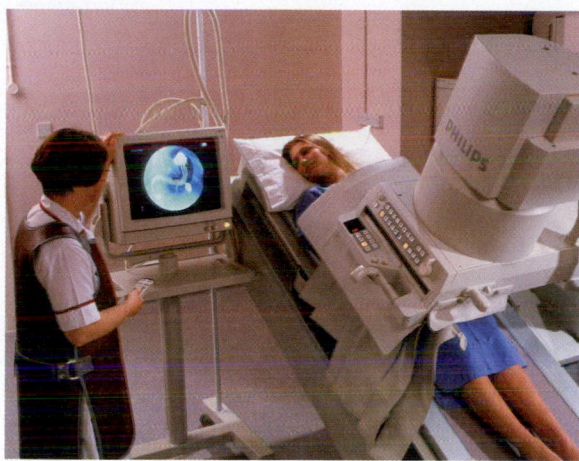

Figure 19-4 ■ Fluoroscopy.
This patient swallowed the contrast medium barium, and the tilted table allows the barium to flow through the stomach and intestine, coating and outlining them to make them visible during fluoroscopy. The radiologist has a handheld device that allows her to create selected still radiographs from the continuously moving images on the fluoroscopy screen. The radiologist is wearing a lead apron to protect her from exposure to x-rays.

WORD BUILDING

projection (proh-JEK-shun)
  project/o- *orientation*
  -ion *action; condition*

fluoroscopy (floor-AWS-koh-pee)
  fluor/o- *fluorescence*
  -scopy *process of using an instrument to examine*

cineradiography
(SIN-eh-RAY-dee-AWG-rah-fee)
  cin/e- *movement*
  radi/o- *radius (forearm bone); x-rays; radiation*
  -graphy *process of recording*

Table 19-2   Radiography Projections

Projection	Description	Word Building
PA chest x-ray (posteroanterior)	The x-ray beam enters the patient's posterior upper back, exits through the anterior chest, and enters the x-ray plate. Position: The patient is in a standing position with the chest next to the x-ray plate. Comment: This is the standard position and most common type of chest x-ray (see Figure 19-2).	**posteroanterior** (POHS-ter-oh-an-TEER-ee-or) **poster/o-** *back part* **anter/o-** *before; front part* **-ior** *pertaining to*
AP chest x-ray (anteroposterior)	The x-ray beam enters the patient's anterior chest, exits through the posterior upper back, and enters the x-ray plate. Position: The patient is in a lying position with the upper back next to the x-ray plate. Comment: This position is most often used for portable chest x-rays taken at the patient's bedside.	**anteroposterior** (AN-ter-oh-pohs-TEER-ee-or) **anter/o-** *before; front part* **poster/o-** *back part* **-ior** *pertaining to*
lateral chest x-ray	The x-ray beam enters the patient's chest from the side and exits through the chest on the other side. Position: The patient is in a standing or lying position. In a left lateral x-ray, the left side of the chest is beside the x-ray plate. Comment: It is also known as a lateral view or side view.	**lateral** (LAT-er-al) **later/o-** *side* **-al** *pertaining to*
oblique x-ray	The x-ray beam enters the body from an oblique angle, midway between anterior and lateral. Position: The patient can be standing or lying.	**oblique** (awb-LEEK)
cross-table lateral x-ray	The x-ray beam enters the patient's chest and abdomen from the side. Position: The patient is lying on the x-ray table; the x-ray plate is on one side, and the x-ray machine is on the other. Comment: The x-ray beam travels across the x-ray table.	
lateral decubitus x-ray	The x-ray beam enters the patient's chest and abdomen from the side. Position: The patient is lying on his/her side on the x-ray table, and the x-ray plate is beneath the x-ray table. Comment: For a left lateral decubitus film, the patient is lying on the left side.	**decubitus** (dee-KYOO-bih-tus)
flat plate of the abdomen	The x-ray beam enters the patient's abdomen, exits through the back, and enters the x-ray plate. Position: The patient is lying on the x-ray table, and the x-ray plate is beneath the x-ray table. Comment: *Flat plate* refers to the fact that the patient is lying down flat with the x-ray plate beneath.	
KUB	The x-ray beam enters the patient's chest and abdomen, exits through the back, and enters the x-ray plate. Position: The patient is lying on the x-ray table, and the x-ray plate is beneath the x-ray table. KUB stands for kidneys, ureters, and bladder, the organs that are x-rayed.	

Radiography with Contrast

The details on an x-ray or fluoroscopic image can be enhanced by using the contrast medium barium or an intravenous **iodinated contrast dye** to outline anatomical structures.

WORD BUILDING

iodinated (EYE-oh-dih-NAY-ted)
  iodin/o- *iodine*
  -ated *pertaining to a condition; composed of*

Word or Phrase	Description	Word Building

angiography	Contrast dye is injected to outline a blood vessel. The x-ray image is an **angiogram. In digital subtraction angiography (DSA)**, two x-ray images are obtained, without contrast dye and then with contrast dye. A computer compares the two images and digitally "subtracts" the image of the soft tissues, bones, and muscles, leaving just the image of the arteries. In **rotational angiography,** the x-ray machine moves around the area to be examined, using multiple x-rays and contrast dye. The computer creates a three-dimensional image that can be rotated and viewed from all angles. This is useful when arteries have a twisted path or when normal anatomy is distorted.
	
	In **arteriography,** contrast dye is injected into an artery to show blockage, narrowed areas, or aneurysms (see Figures 19-5 ■ and 5-17). The x-ray image is an **arteriogram. Aortography** uses contrast dye injected into the aorta, the largest artery. In **venography,** contrast dye is injected into a vein to show weakened valves and dilated walls. The x-ray image is a **venogram.**
		angiography (AN-jee-AWG-rah-fee)
		  angi/o- *blood vessel; lymphatic vessel*
		  -graphy *process of recording*
		
		angiogram (AN-jee-OH-gram)
		  angi/o- *blood vessel; lymphatic vessel*
		  -gram *a record or picture*
		
		arteriography (ar-TEER-ee-AWG-rah-fee)
		  arteri/o- *artery*
		  -graphy *process of recording*
		
		arteriogram (ar-TEER-ee-OH-gram)
		  arteri/o- *artery*
		  -gram *a record or picture*
		
		aortography (AA-or-TAWG-rah-fee)
		  aort/o- *aorta*
		  -graphy *process of recording*
		
		venography (vee-NAWG-rah-fee)
		  ven/o- *vein*
		  -graphy *process of recording*
		
		venogram (VEE-noh-gram)
		  ven/o- *vein*
		  -gram *a record or picture*

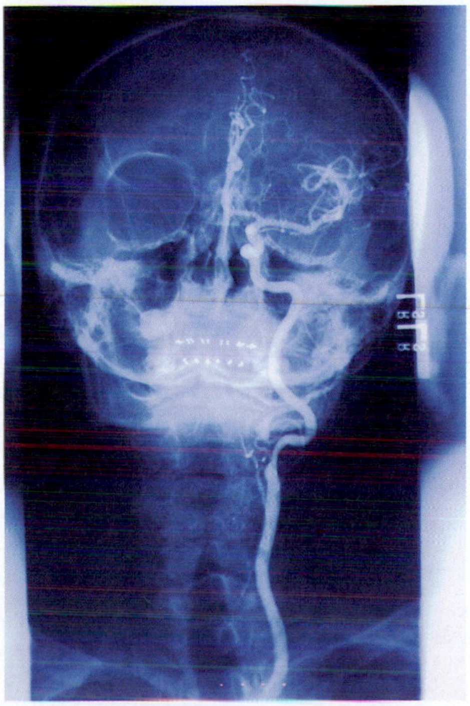

Figure 19-5 ■ Arteriogram of the left carotid artery and cerebral arteries.

This procedure is also known as a cerebral angiography or carotid arteriography. The injected dye clearly outlines the carotid artery and its many smaller branches within the cranial cavity. There is no evidence of carotid artery plaques or cerebral aneurysm.

Word or Phrase	Description	Word Building

arthrography	Contrast dye is injected into a joint. It outlines the bones, joint capsule, and soft tissue structures. The image is an **arthrogram.**	**arthrography** (ar-THRAWG-rah-fee)
		  arthr/o- *joint*
		  -graphy *process of recording*
		
		arthrogram (AR-throh-gram)
		  arthr/o- *joint*
		  -gram *a record or picture*

Word or Phrase	Description	Word Building
barium enema	Barium contrast medium is inserted into the rectum. It outlines the colon and rectum and shows tumors, polyps, or diverticula in the bowel wall (see Figure 3-24). For a **double contrast (air contrast) enema,** the barium is removed and air is instilled as a second contrast. Fluoroscopy and individual radiographs are done to document the procedure.	**barium** (BAIR-ee-um) **enema** (EN-eh-mah)

cholangiography, intravenous (IVC)	Contrast dye is injected intravenously. It travels through the blood to the liver and is then excreted with bile into the gallbladder. It outlines the gallbladder and shows thickening of the gallbladder wall and gallstones. The x-ray image is a **cholangiogram.** In **endoscopic retrograde cholangio-pancreatography,** an endoscope is passed through the mouth and into the duodenum. A catheter is passed through the endoscope, and contrast dye is injected to visualize the pancreatic duct and the common bile duct (see Figure 3-25).	**cholangiography** (KOH-lan-jee-AWG-rah-fee)
		   cholangi/o- *bile duct*
		   -graphy *process of recording*
		
		intravenous (IN-trah-VEE-nus)
		   intra- *with*
		   ven/o- *vein*
		   -ous *pertaining to*
		
		cholangiogram (koh-LAN-jee-OH-gram)
		   cholangi/o- *bile duct*
		   -gram *a record or picture*
		
		cholangiopancreatography (koh-LAN-jee-oh-PAN-kree-ah-TAWG-rah-fee)
		   cholangi/o- *bile duct*
		   pancreat/o- *pancreas*
		   -graphy *process of recording*

cholecystography, oral (OCG)	Contrast dye in a tablet form is taken orally. From the small intestine, it enters the blood, is processed by the liver, and then excreted with bile into the gallbladder. It outlines the gallbladder and shows thickening of the gallbladder wall and gallstones. The x-ray image is a **cholecystogram.**	**cholecystography** (KOH-lee-sis-TAWG-rah-fee)
		   chol/e- *bile; gall*
		   cyst/o- *bladder; fluid-filled sac; semisolid cyst*
		   -graphy *process of recording*
		
		cholecystogram (KOH-lee-SIS-toh-gram)
		   chol/e- *bile; gall*
		   cyst/o- *bladder; fluid-filled sac; semisolid cyst*
		   -gram *a record or picture*

hysterosalpingo-graphy	Contrast dye is inserted through a catheter that was passed through the vagina and into the uterus. It outlines the cavity of the uterus and the uterine tubes and shows narrowing, scarring, and blockage of the tubes. The x-ray image is a **hysterosalpingogram.**	**hysterosalpingography** (HIS-ter-oh-SAL-ping-GAWG-rah-fee)
		   hyster/o- *uterus (womb)*
		   salping/o- *uterine (fallopian) tube*
		   -graphy *process of recording*
		
		hysterosalpingogram (HIS-ter-oh-sal-PING-goh-gram)
		   hyster/o- *uterus (womb)*
		   salping/o- *uterine (fallopian) tube*
		   -gram *a record or picture*

Word or Phrase	Description	Word Building
lymphangiography	Contrast dye is injected into a lymphatic vessel. It outlines the vessel and shows enlarged lymph nodes, lymphomas, and blockages of lymphatic drainage. The x-ray image is a **lymphangiogram.**	**lymphangiography** (lim-FAN-jee-AWG-rah-fee) **lymph/o-** *lymph; lymphatic system* **angi/o-** *blood vessel; lymphatic vessel* **-graphy** *process of recording* **lymphangiogram** (lim-FAN-jee-OH-gram) **lymph/o-** *lymph; lymphatic system* **angi/o-** *blood vessel; lymphatic vessel* **-gram** *a record or picture*
myelography	Contrast dye is injected into the subarachnoid space of the spine at the level of the L3 and L4 vertebrae. It outlines the spinal cavity, spinal nerves, nerve roots, intervertebral disks, and shows tumors and herniated disks. The x-ray image is a **myelogram.** Because a myelogram can have the side effect of a severe headache, a CT scan or MRI scan of the spine is often performed instead.	**myelography** (MY-eh-LAWG-rah-fee) **myel/o-** *bone marrow; spinal cord; myelin* **-graphy** *process of recording* **myelogram** (MY-eh-LOH-gram) **myel/o-** *bone marrow; spinal cord; myelin* **-gram** *a record or picture*
pyelography	In an **intravenous pyelography,** contrast dye is injected into a vein and is excreted in the urine by the kidneys. It outlines the urinary tract and shows narrowing, blockage, and stones (see Figure 11-18). It is also known as an **excretory urography.** In **retrograde pyelography,** a cystoscopy is performed, and contrast dye is injected through a catheter into each ureter. The x-ray image is a **pyelogram** or **urogram.**	**pyelography** (PY-eh-LAWG-rah-fee) **pyel/o-** *renal pelvis* **-graphy** *process of recording* **excretory** (EKS-kreh-TOH-ree) **excret/o-** *removing from the body* **-ory** *having the function of* **urography** (yoo-RAWG-rah-fee) **ur/o-** *urine; urinary system* **-graphy** *process of recording* **retrograde** (RET-roh-grayd) **retro-** *behind; backward* **-grade** *pertaining to going* **pyelogram** (PY-eh-LOH-gram) **pyel/o-** *renal pelvis* **-gram** *a record or picture*
upper gastro-intestinal series (UGI)	Barium contrast medium as a liquid is swallowed. It outlines the esophagus and stomach to show ulcers and blockage. This is also known as a **barium swallow.** A **small-bowel follow-through** follows the barium as it outlines the small intestine. To evaluate a patient's ability to swallow, liquid barium is mixed with crackers and swallowed (a barium meal).	**gastrointestinal** (GAS-troh-in-TES-tin-al) **gastr/o-** *stomach* **intestin/o-** *intestine* **-al** *pertaining to*

Mammography

Mammography uses x-rays to create an image of the breast (see Figure 13-28). The breast is compressed to lessen its thickness and improve the quality of the image. Mammography is used to detect areas of microcalcifications, infection, cysts, and tumors, many of which cannot be felt on a breast examination. The image is a **mammogram** (see Figure 18-6). **Xeromammography** uses a special x-ray plate that is processed with dry chemicals, and the image, a **xeromammogram,** is printed on paper rather than x-ray film.

WORD BUILDING

mammography (mah-MAWG-rah-fee) **mamm/o-** *breast* **-graphy** *process of recording*

mammogram (MAM-oh-gram) **mamm/o-** *breast* **-gram** *a record or picture*

Bone Density Testing

A bone density test uses x-rays to measure the bone mineral density (BMD) and determine if demineralization (from osteoporosis) has occurred. This is also known as **bone densitometry.** The heel or wrist bone can be tested, but the hip and spine bones give the most accurate results (see Figure 8-26).

There are two types of bone density tests: DEXA (or DXA) scan and quantitative computerized tomography (QCT). A **DEXA scan** (dual-energy x-ray absorptiometry) uses two (dual) x-ray beams with different energy levels to create a two-dimensional image. This scan can detect as little as a 1 percent loss of bone. **Quantitative computerized tomography (QCT)** uses x-rays and a CT scan (described in the next section) to create a three-dimensional image. QCT is able to take separate density measurements for the different areas within a bone.

Computerized Axial Tomography

Computerized axial tomography (CAT) or **computerized tomography (CT)** uses x-rays and a computer to create an image. The patient lies on a narrow bed inside the CT scanner. The x-ray emitter moves in a circle around the patient, while the x-ray detector moves along the opposite side of the circle. The paths of the x-ray emitter and detector are oriented along one of the imaginary planes of the body: coronal, sagittal, or transverse (see Figure 19-6 ■). The computer analyzes and creates a two-dimensional

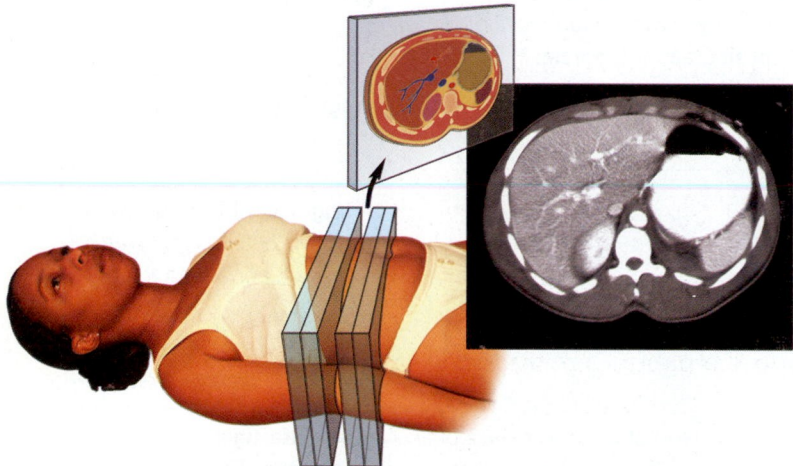

VENTRAL

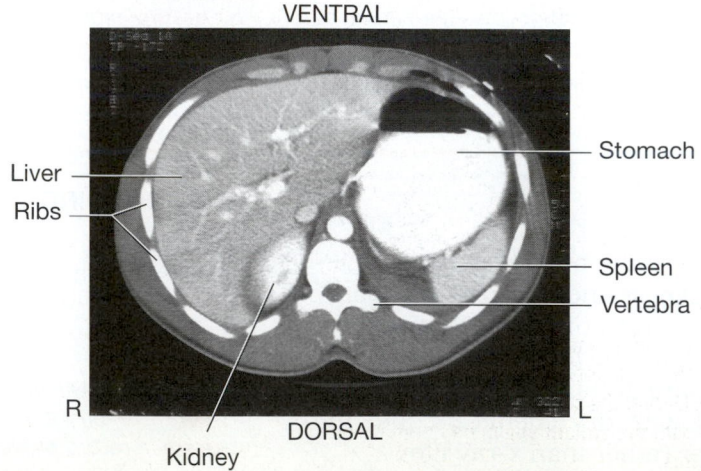

Liver
Ribs
Stomach
Spleen
Vertebra

R   L

DORSAL

Kidney

Figure 19-6 ■ Computerized axial tomography (CAT) of the abdomen taken in the transverse plane.

The radiologist reads a CT scan image as if he were standing at the patient's feet while she is lying in the scanner. This CT scan image shows the liver on the left, which is actually the patient's right side when viewed from her feet. Only one kidney is visible in this "slice" because the other kidney is positioned lower in the body (a normal occurrence) and will appear in subsequent "slices" (images).

image or "slice" of that part of the body. Then the x-ray emitter and detector move a short distance (about 20 mm) proximally or distally and begin the process again to create another image or "slice." The radiologist views each of these individual images; together they make up a three-dimensional view of the area. Computerized tomography shows all types of tissues, but soft tissues are particularly clear (see Figures 11-12, 16-13, and 18-14). Computerized tomography is also known as a scan because the machine scans (moves across) the body. A multidetector-row CT scanner (MDCT) has an area of x-ray detectors (not just a row), and it can quickly scan multiple "slices" simultaneously. A spiral CT scan moves the patient's bed through the scanner as the x-ray emitter rotates around the patient. This produces a spiral image; this procedure is 10 times faster than a regular CT scan. When a CT scan is used to guide the insertion of a needle (for a biopsy), this is known as **interventional radiology.**

A contrast dye can be injected intravenously or into a body cavity to produce an enhanced CT image. A CT scan that uses no contrast dye is said to be unenhanced. Often two sets of images are obtained, one set before contrast dye is given and another set after contrast dye is given. These are known as precontrast and postcontrast images.

WORD BUILDING

interventional (IN-ter-VEN-shun-al)
  inter- *between*
  vent/o- *a coming*
  -ion *action; condition*
  -al *pertaining to*

Clinical Connections

Obstetrics (Chapter 13). Pregnant women are generally advised to avoid x-rays. However, sometimes x-rays are necessary. Although an exposure of 5000 mrems has been shown to cause a risk of fetal deformity, most x-rays involve significantly less radiation, as shown below. The abbreviation mrem stands for microrem (one-thousandth of a rem).

dental x-ray	1 mrem
mammography	2 mrems
chest x-ray (two views)	8 mrems
CT scan	1,000 mrems

Magnetic Resonance Imaging

Magnetic resonance imaging (MRI) uses a scanner and a strong magnetic field (see Figure 19-7 ■) to align protons in the atoms of the patient's body. Then high-frequency radiowaves are sent through the patient's body. The

magnetic (mag-NET-ik)
  magnet/o- *magnet*
  -ic *pertaining to*

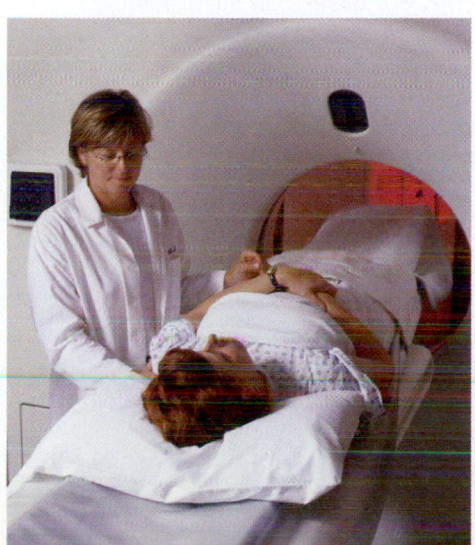

Figure 19-7 ■ MRI scan.
This radiologic technologist is positioning the patient before the bed slides into the MRI scanner. During the scan, the technologist is in contact with the patient via an intercom inside the scanner.

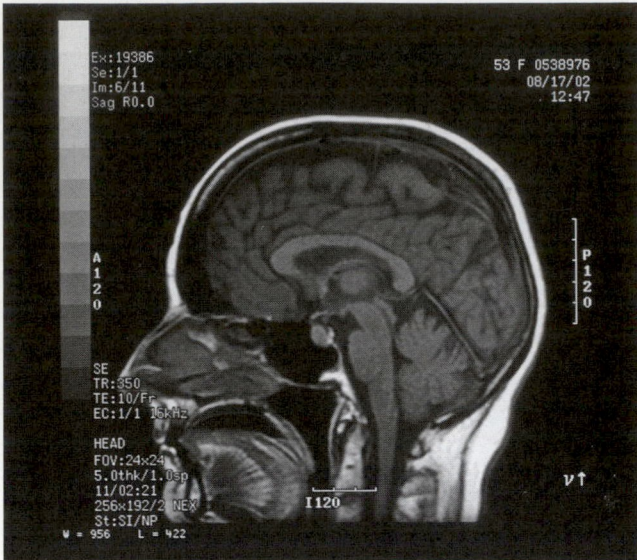

Figure 19-8 ■ MRI of the head.
This MRI image was created along the midsagittal plane that divides the right half from the left half of the head. This is just one of many thin "slices" that were individually imaged. The computer then merges the individual images into a three-dimensional image.

protons absorb the radiowaves and then emit signals. The signals, which vary according to the type of tissue, are used to create an image. Like a CT scan, magnetic resonance imaging is a type of tomography that creates many individual "slice" images. The patient lies in a scanner, and an emitter and detector rotate in a circle around the patient to create a two-dimensional image (see Figure 19-8 ■). The computer then combines these into a three-dimensional image. An MRI scan does not use x-rays so the patient is not exposed to any radiation. An open MRI is performed on a modified MRI scanner that is not enclosed on all sides. Open MRI is ideal for pediatric, older adult, claustrophobic, anxious, or extremely obese patients. Magnetic resonance imaging is the best procedure for showing soft tissues, blood vessels, intervertebral disks, muscles, nerves, organs, tumors, and areas of infection. **Gadolinium,** a metallic element that responds to a magnetic field, can be injected intravenously during magnetic resonance angiography (MRA) or into a body cavity to produce an enhanced MRI image. An unenhanced MRI uses no gadolinium. See the Did You Know? feature box on page 947 for a list of metal items that are contraindicated during an MRI scan.

Ultrasonography

Ultrasonography or **sonography** uses pulses of inaudible, ultra high-frequency sound waves to create an image. A handheld **ultrasound transducer** that emits sound waves is held against the skin over the organ or structure to be imaged (see Figure 5-25). A conducting gel on the skin optimizes transmission of the sound waves. The transducer is moved back and forth to view the organ or structure from different angles. Alternately, an **ultrasound probe** can be placed inside a body cavity. Sound waves from either a transducer or probe are reflected from the internal structures as echoes. The echoes are changed into electrical signals and analyzed by a computer. The strongest echoes produce the brightest areas on the ultrasound image. The ultrasound image is a **sonogram.** Ultrasonography can produce several different types of images (see Table 19-3). Ultrasonography can be used to guide the insertion of a needle for a biopsy or for amniocentesis (see Figure 13-27).

WORD BUILDING

gadolinium (GAD-oh-LIN-ee-um)

ultrasonography
(UL-trah-soh-NAWG-rah-fee)
　ultra- *beyond; higher*
　son/o- *sound*
　-graphy *process of recording*

sonography (soh-NAWG-rah-fee)
　son/o- *sound*
　-graphy *process of recording*

ultrasound (UL-trah-sound)

transducer (trans-DOO-ser)
　trans- *across; through*
　duc/o- *bring; move*
　-er *person or thing that produces or does*

sonogram (SAWN-oh-gram)
　son/o- *sound*
　-gram *a record or picture*

Did You Know?

Patients who undergo an MRI scan must sign a consent form that describes what types of metal items can or cannot be subjected to the magnetic field. You might be surprised to see which items are contraindicated and which things are allowed.

Contraindicated Items

- All metal objects that are not permanently attached to the body. These include glasses, watches, jewelry, hairpins, metal false teeth, artificial limbs, and clothing with metal zippers, buttons, or snaps. These objects respond to the magnetic field and can be forcefully pulled into the scanner, causing damage to the scanner.
- Nose rings, lip rings, tongue studs, pierced earrings, and other piercings must be removed or they could be forcefully pulled into the scanner, causing damage to the patient's tissues.
- Implanted devices such as pacemakers, pacing wires, some heart valves, aneurysm clips, cochlear implants, some penile implants, artificial eyes, and some intrauterine devices may be moved by the magnetic field, causing internal tissue damage.
- Hearing aids, some pacemakers, TENS units, and insulin pumps can have their working parts damaged by the magnetic field.
- Metal workers, gunshot victims, or military personnel with shrapnel injuries are presumed to have metal fragments in their tissues and should not undergo MRI scans.
- Transdermal patches that deliver heart, pain, contraceptive, or smoking cessation drugs must be removed because some contain a small metal wire that can cause burns to the skin.
- Metallic eye shadow may cause the eyelids to flutter as they are pulled and then released by the magnetic field.

Allowed Items

- Permanent metal dental work such as crowns are allowed because they will not detach, although they may produce artifact (an unwanted image) on the MRI image.
- Artificial metal or ceramic prostheses in joints and orthopedic hardware (screws, nails, plates, and rods).

Table 19-3   Types of Ultrasonography

Type	Description
Two-dimensional	Provides a two-dimensional image in various shades of gray. It is also known as a grayscale ultrasonography or B scan.
Three-dimensional	Provides a three-dimensional image. In addition to signals sent by the transducer or probe, a position sensor relays information that the computer uses to generate an image in three dimensions. The computer also colorizes the image in shades of brown.
Four-dimensional	Provides a three-dimensional, computer-colorized image that is continuously moving. The computer updates the ultrasound image on the screen as it receives new signals from the transducer or probe and position sensor. It is also known as real-time ultrasonography.

Ultrasonography is used to differentiate solid tumors and stones from fluid-filled cysts of the breast, gallbladder, kidney, ovary, or uterus (see Figure 11-19). It can be used to assess the internal structures of the eye. It can provide images of a fetus in the uterus (see Figure 13-29), and the fetal parts can be measured to estimate the gestational age and the mother's due date.

Echocardiography   **Echocardiography** uses ultra high-frequency sound waves to show real-time, moving images of the heart during contraction and relaxation (see Figure 19-9 ■). The ultrasound image, which is viewed on a TV monitor or as individual still images, is an **echocardiogram**.

WORD BUILDING

echocardiography
(EK-oh-KAR-dee-AWG-rah-fee)
  ech/o- *echo (sound wave)*
  cardi/o- *heart*
  -graphy *process of recording*

echocardiogram
(EK-oh-KAR-dee-oh-gram)
  ech/o *echo (sound wave)*
  cardi/o- *heart*
  -gram *a record or picture*

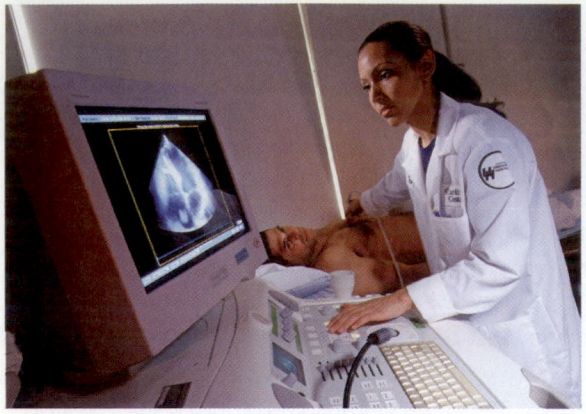

Figure 19-9 ■
Echocardiography.
This patient is having an echocardiography. The ultrasound technician is holding a transducer that produces sound waves. These bounce off the structures of the heart as echoes that the computer displays on the monitor screen.

WORD BUILDING

Transesophageal echocardiography (TEE) may be ordered when a standard echocardiogram cannot produce a good-quality image. During a TEE, the patient swallows an endoscope that contains a tiny sound wave–emitting transducer at its tip. The tip is positioned in the esophagus directly behind the heart.

transesophageal
(TRANS-ee-SAWF-ah-JEE-al)
trans- *across; through*
esophag/o- *esophagus*
-eal *pertaining to*

Doppler Ultrasonography

Doppler ultrasonography uses ultra high-frequency sound waves and Doppler technology to produce the audible sound of blood flowing through an artery. The transducer emits and then collects reflected sound waves. If the artery is patent, a loud "swish . . . swish . . . swish" will be heard as the blood is pumped through the artery. If the artery is blocked, little or no sound will be heard. Doppler technology is also used in automatic blood pressure machines that give a digital readout of the blood pressure and in fetal monitors that, when placed on the mother's abdomen, make the heartbeat of the fetus audible.

Doppler (DAWP-ler)

Color flow duplex ultrasonography combines a two-dimensional ultrasound image and Doppler technology to create an ultrasound image that shows anatomy as well as colors that correlate to the velocity, direction, and turbulence of the blood flow in that area. It is used to image the coronary arteries, carotid arteries, or arteries of the legs.

duplex (DOO-pleks)

Unlike many types of radiologic procedures, ultrasonography does not expose the patient to harmful radiation (see Table 19-4).

Table 19-4 Radiologic Procedures and Exposure to Radiation

Source	Radiologic Procedure	Exposure to Radiation
X-rays	Radiography (plain films or with contrast)	Yes
	Fluoroscopy	Yes
	Mammography, xeromammography	Yes
	Bone density testing	Yes
	Computerized tomography (CT scan)	Yes
Electron beam	Electron beam tomography (usually combined with CT scan)	Yes
Radiowaves and magnetic field	Magnetic resonance imaging (MRI scan)	No
Ultra high-frequency sound waves	Ultrasonography	No
	Echocardiography	No
	Doppler ultrasonography	No

Electron Beam Tomography

Electron beam tomography (EBT) uses a beam of electrons and a computer to create an image. EBT is also known as a full body scan, although only the area from the shoulders to the upper legs is actually scanned. These scans are being marketed directly to consumers and do not need to be ordered by a physician. They are considered screening tests, not diagnostic tests. The Virtual Physical and the Virtual Colonoscopy use a spiral CT scan combined with an EBT scan to produce a detailed three-dimensional image. The Virtual Physical is able to reveal small areas of plaque in the coronary arteries, early signs of emphysema in the lungs, and early stages of cancer. The Virtual Colonoscopy produces results that are as reliable as those of a colonoscopy, but it costs only about one-third as much.

Nuclear Medicine

Nuclear medicine is the medical specialty that uses **radioactive** substances to create an image of the internal structures and function of the body. When a radioactive substance decays, it produces alpha particles, beta particles, gamma rays, positrons, or other subatomic particles that are a form of radiation. Radioactive substances that produce gamma rays or positrons are used for nuclear medicine imaging. *Note:* Radioactive substances that produce alpha and beta particles are used in radiation therapy to destroy cancerous cells (discussed in "Oncology," Chapter 18).

Radiopharmaceuticals are man-made or naturally occurring radioactive substances that have been processed and measured so that they can be given as a drug dose. They are administered intravenously, except for radioactive gases, which are administered by inhalation. Radiopharmaceuticals are also known as **tracers** because their presence in a particular area of the body can be traced by the gamma rays they produce. The radiopharmaceuticals used in nuclear medicine imaging have short half-lives of a few hours to a few days. This means that the patient is exposed to a minimal amount of radiation. The length of time it takes for half of the atoms in a radioactive substance to decay (emit gamma rays or positrons) and become stable is the **half-life.**

WORD BUILDING

electron (ee-LEK-tron)
electr/o- *electricity*
-on *a substance; structure*

nuclear (NOO-klee-er)
nucle/o- *nucleus (of an atom)*
-ar *pertaining to*

radioactive (RAY-dee-oh-AK-tiv)
radi/o- *radius (forearm bone);*
x-rays; radiation
act/o- *action*
-ive *pertaining to*

radiopharmaceutical
(RAY-dee-oh-FAR-mah-SOO-tik-al)
radi/o- *radius (forearm bone);*
x-rays; radiation
pharmaceutic/o- *medicine; drug*
-al *pertaining to*

tracer (TRAY-ser)
trac/o- *visible path*
-er *person or thing that produces*
or does

Did You Know?

In 1898, while working with uranium, Polish physicist Marie Curie and her husband, French physicist Pierre Curie, discovered the radioactive chemical element radium and coined the word *radioactivity.* They were awarded the Nobel Prize in physics. This was the first time a woman had won the Nobel Prize. Marie Curie's subsequent work with radium also earned her a Nobel Prize in chemistry, making her the first person to ever receive a Nobel Prize in two disciplines. The Curies often had severe radiation burns from handling radium or carrying it their pockets. Marie Curie died in 1934, from leukemia or aplastic anemia, most likely from long-term exposure to radiation. Her oldest daughter, Irene Joliot-Curie, discovered how to produce radioactive elements artificially. She was awarded the Nobel Prize in chemistry 1 year after her mother's death.

Nuclear Medicine Procedures That Use Gamma Rays

Radiopharmaceutical drugs that emit gamma rays include gallium-67, indium-111, iodine-123 and iodine-131, krypton-81m, technetium-99m, thallium-201, and xenon-133 (see Table 19-5).

After a radiopharmaceutical drug is administered, a gamma scintillation camera scans the area. When a gamma ray from the radioactive radiopharmaceutical drug enters the scintillation camera, it strikes a crystal structure, the crystal emits a flash of visible light (a photon), and a computer compiles the flashes of light into a two-dimensional image. This is known as **scintigraphy.** It is also known as a **scintiscan** because the scintillation camera moves back and forth (scanning) across the body. The image is a **scintigram.**

Areas of increased uptake on a scintigram are known as "hot spots," and areas of decreased uptake are known as "cold spots." When the blood flow (perfusion) to an organ is being studied, areas of decreased uptake are known as filling defects.

WORD BUILDING

scintigraphy (sin-TIG-rah-fee)
  scint/i- *point of light*
  -graphy *process of recording*

scintiscan (SIN-tih-skan)

scintigram (SIN-tih-gram)
  scint/i- *point of light*
  -gram *a record or picture*

Table 19-5   Radiopharmaceutical Drugs That Emit Gamma Rays

Radiopharmaceutical	Description	Word Building
gallium-67	Intravenous drug used to detect inflammation, infection, and benign and cancerous tumors. Gallium is a soft, silvery metal that is a liquid at room temperature.	gallium (GAL-ee-um)
indium-111	Intravenous drug used to look for cancerous tumors. Indium-111 is combined with a hormone that is attracted to cancerous cells of the endocrine system, or it is combined with a monoclonal antibody that is attracted to cancerous cells of the ovary or colon. Indium is a soft, silvery metal.	indium (IN-dee-um)
iodine-123 and iodine-131	Intravenous drug used to image the thyroid gland. Iodine is a purple-black, shiny crystalline solid that is a trace element in the soil.	iodine (EYE-oh-dine)
krypton-81m	Inhaled gas used to image the lung. It is also used in krypton lasers in surgery. Krypton is a colorless, odorless gas that is present in trace amounts in the atmosphere.	krypton (KRIP-tawn)
technetium-99m	Intravenous drug used to image many different areas of the body. It is the most common radiopharmaceutical used in nuclear imaging. Technetium is a silvery gray metal.	technetium (tek-NEE-shee-um)
thallium-201	Intravenous drug used to image the heart. Thallium is a gray metal that is so soft it can be cut with a knife.	thallium (THAL-ee-um)
xenon-133	Inhaled gas used to image the lungs. Xenon is a colorless, odorless gas that is present in trace amounts in the atmosphere.	xenon (ZEE-nawn)

Bone scintigraphy is used to detect areas of increased uptake related to arthritis, fracture, osteomyelitis, cancerous tumors of the bone, or areas of bony metastasis.

Cholescintigraphy or a **HIDA scan** is used to detect areas of decreased uptake related to cystic duct obstruction and acute cholecystitis. HIDA stands for hydroxyiminodiacetic acid, a molecule that carries the radiopharmaceutical drug to the liver.

A liver-spleen scan is used to detect areas of decreased uptake that indicate nonfunctioning tissue due to inflammation, infection, benign tumors, or cancer in the liver or spleen.

cholescintigraphy
(KOH-lee-sin-TIG-rah-fee)
  chol/e- *bile; gall*
  scint/i- *point of light*
  -graphy *process of recording*

A **MUGA (multiple-gated acquisition) scan** is used to detect how well the heart walls move as they contract. It also calculates the ejection fraction (how much blood the ventricle can pump out in one contraction). The ejection fraction is the most accurate predictor of overall heart function. The gamma camera is coordinated (gated) with the patient's EKG. This procedure is also known as a **nuclear ventriculogram** or a **gated blood pool scan**. A **SPECT (single-photon emission computed tomography) scan** is a MUGA scan of the heart in which the gamma camera moves in a circle around the patient to create individual images as "slices" of the heart (tomography).

An **OncoScint scan** is used to detect areas of increased activity that are metastases from a cancerous tumor's primary site in the colon or ovary. OncoScint is the trade name for the combination of indium-111 and a monoclonal antibody that binds to receptors on those cancerous cells. A **ProstaScint scan** does the same thing for metastases from prostate cancer.

A thyroid scan is used to detect areas of increased activity that indicate a hyperfunctioning, benign thyroid nodule or goiter or decreased activity that indicate a cyst or cancerous tumor of the thyroid (see Figure 19-10 ■). It is also known as a radioactive iodine uptake (RAIU) and thyroid scan.

A **ventilation-perfusion scan (V/Q)** is a two-part test that uses two radioactive substances, one that is inhaled and one that is given intravenously. It is used to detect areas of decreased uptake that indicate poor air flow, pneumonia, atelectasis, or a pleural effusion. Areas of decreased uptake on the perfusion scan indicate poor blood flow to the lung tissues. It is also known as a **lung scan**. The *Q* stands for quotient.

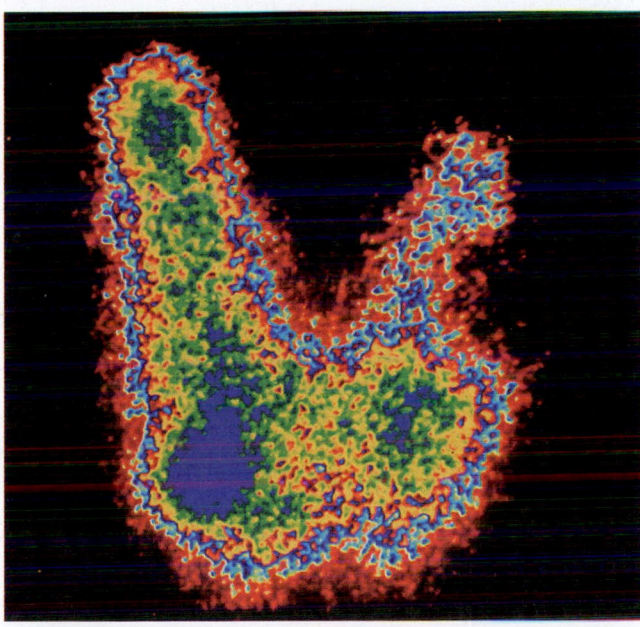

Figure 19-10 ■ Thyroid scan.
The radiopharmaceutical drug technetium-99m outlines the size and shape of the thyroid gland. At the same time, the radiopharmaceutical drug iodine-123 is taken up by the thyroid gland cells and shows their rate of metabolism. This scan shows a blue "cold spot" in the right lower lobe of the thyroid gland where the cells are not taking up iodine. This could be a cyst or a cancerous tumor. (Remember, the patient's right side is on your left side when you view the scan image.)

WORD BUILDING

MUGA (MUH-gah)

ventriculogram
(ven-TRIK-yoo-LOH-gram)
   ventricul/o- *ventricle (lower heart chamber; chamber in the brain)*
   -gram *a record or picture*

SPECT (SPEKT)

OncoScint (AWN-koh-sint)

ProstaScint (PRAW-stah-sint)

ventilation (VEN-tih-LAY-shun)
   ventilat/o- *movement of air*
   -ion *action; condition*

perfusion (per-FYOO-shun)
   per- *through; throughout*
   fus/o- *pouring*
   -ion *action; condition*

Nuclear Medicine Procedures That Use Positrons

A positron is a positively charged particle that has the same mass as an electron, but the opposite charge. Radioactive substances that emit positrons are used in **positron emission tomography (PET)**. Like a CT scan or an MRI scan, a PET scan is a tomography that produces individual images of the body in "slices." However, unlike CT and MRI scans that produce images of the anatomy of an organ, a PET scan produces images of the physiology and metabolism of an organ. PET scans are of particular value in identifying areas of cancer (because cancerous cells have a higher metabolic rate than normal cells). They also show areas of ischemia in the heart (because ischemic cells have poor blood flow and a lower metabolic rate than normal cells). PET scans also show areas of abnormally increased or decreased metabolism in the brains of patients with Alzheimer's disease (see Figures 10-15 and 10-16), Parkinson's disease, epilepsy, and schizophrenia.

WORD BUILDING

positron (PAWZ-ih-trawn)

tomography (toh-MAWG-rah-fee)
  tom/o- *cut; slice; layer*
  -graphy *process of recording*

A Closer Look

A cyclotron (subatomic particle accelerator) is needed to produce a radioactive substance that emits positrons. The half-life of radioactive substances that emit positrons is very brief (a few minutes in length). Therefore the cyclotron must be at the hospital where the PET scan is performed. A cyclotron, however, is a large, expensive piece of equipment, so PET scans are only available in the largest hospitals. For a PET scan, a positron-emitting radioactive substance is combined with glucose molecules and injected intravenously. The higher the rate of metabolism in a cell, the more glucose is consumed and the more radioactive substance that is carried into the cell. As the radioactive substance decays, it releases a positron. Almost immediately the positron collides with a nearby electron. The collision simultaneously produces two gamma rays that move in opposite directions from each other. A special circular gamma camera is set so that it only records simultaneously produced gamma rays. A computer traces the rays back to identify where they originated in an organ. This then becomes a point on the PET scan image.

Vocabulary Review

Word or Phrase	Description	Combining Forms
angiography	Procedure that uses x-rays and a contrast dye injected into a blood vessel to create an image. The image is an **angiogram**. Special types of angiography include **digital subtraction angiography, rotational angiography,** and **magnetic resonance angiography (MRA).**	**angi/o-** blood vessel; lymphatic vessel
anteroposterior	Pertaining to going from the front to the back, as in the path of x-rays during an AP chest x-ray	**anter/o-** before; front part **poster/o-** back part
aortography	Procedure that uses x-rays and a contrast dye injected into the aorta to create an image	**aort/o-** aorta
arteriography	Procedure that uses x-rays and a contrast dye injected into an artery to create an image. The image is an **arteriogram.**	**arteri/o-** artery
arthrography	Procedure that uses x-rays and a contrast dye injected into a joint to create an image. The image is an **arthrogram.**	**arthr/o-** joint
barium	Contrast medium made of small, chalky particles suspended in a liquid. It is swallowed (upper GI series, barium swallow) or inserted in the rectum and colon (barium enema).	
barium enema	Procedure that uses x-rays, fluoroscopy, and barium contrast medium inserted in the rectum to create an image of the colon. A **double contrast enema** uses barium and then air as a second contrast medium.	
bone density testing	Procedure that uses x-rays to measure the bone mineral density. This is also known as **bone densitometry.** The two types are a DEXA scan and quantitative computerized tomography (QCT).	**densit/o-** density
cholangiography, intravenous (IVC)	Procedure that uses x-rays and a contrast dye injected intravenously to create an image of the gallbladder. The image is a **cholangiogram.**	**cholangi/o-** bile duct **ven/o-** vein
cholangio-pancreatography, endoscopic retrograde (ERCP)	Procedure that uses an endoscope passed through the mouth, a catheter, and contrast dye to create an image of the common bile duct and pancreatic duct	**cholangi/o-** bile duct **pancreat/o-** pancreas
cholecystography	Procedure that uses x-rays and a contrast dye taken orally to create an image of the gallbladder. The image is a **cholecystogram.**	**chol/e-** bile; gall **cyst/o-** bladder; fluid-filled sac; semisolid cyst
cholescintigraphy	Nuclear medicine procedure that uses scintigraphy and a radiopharmaceutical drug attached to a carrier molecule (HIDA) to create an image of the gallbladder. HIDA stands for hydroxyiminodiacetic acid. It is also known as a **HIDA scan.**	**chol/e-** bile; gall **scint/i-** point of light

Word or Phrase	Description	Combining Forms
computerized axial tomography (CAT)	Procedure that uses x-rays controlled by a computer; the x-ray source moves around the body axis of a patient inside the CT scanner. The scan can be done with or without contrast dye. It produces individual images as "slices," as well as a composite three-dimensional view. It is also known as **computerized tomography (CT).** A multidetector-row CT scanner (MDCT) has an area (not just a row) of x-ray detectors and can scan multiple "slices" simultaneously. During a spiral CT scan, the patient's bed moves through the scanner while the x-ray beam rotates around it, creating a spiral.	**axi/o-** *axis* **tom/o-** *cut; slice; layer*
decubitus	Lying down position; on the back, as in a position for a radiograph	
DEXA scan	Type of bone density test that uses two x-ray beams at two different energy levels. It is also known as dual-energy x-ray absorptiometry or a DXA scan.	
diagnostic imaging	Includes radiology and nuclear medicine, as well as medical photography, microscopic imaging of pathology tissue specimens, etc.	**gnos/o-** *knowledge*
Doppler ultrasonography	Procedure that uses ultra high-frequency sound waves emitted by an ultrasound transducer placed over an artery and Doppler technology to create an audible sound of blood flow through an artery. **Color flow duplex ultrasonography** uses ultrasonography and Doppler technology to create an ultrasound image with colors that reflect the velocity, direction, and turbulence of blood in an artery or vein.	**son/o-** *sound*
dosimetry	Process of measuring the amount of radiation exposure as detected by a film badge and measured by a **dosimeter**	**dos/i-** *dose*
echocardiography	Procedure that uses ultra high-frequency sound waves emitted by an ultrasound transducer placed on the chest. (Alternatively, a tiny transducer is swallowed and positioned in the esophagus behind the heart for **transesophageal echocardiography**). The sound waves bounce off the contracting and relaxing heart, creating echoes that are seen as an image on the computer. The image is an **echocardiogram.**	**ech/o-** *echo (sound wave)* **cardi/o-** *heart* **esophag/o-** *esophagus*
electron beam tomography (EBT)	Procedure that uses an electron beam and a spiral CT scan to create an image. It is also known as a full body scan. These scans are marketed directly to consumers and do not need to be ordered by a physician. They are considered screening tests, not diagnostic tests. Examples: The Virtual Physical and the Virtual Colonoscopy.	**electr/o-** *electricity* **tom/o-** *cut; slice; layer*
enhanced	Radiography, CT scan, or MRI scan that uses a contrast dye or contrast medium to enhance anatomical details. If none is used, the image is said to be **unenhanced.**	
film badge	Badge worn by healthcare professionals who work in radiology and nuclear medicine. It holds an unexposed piece of x-ray film that detects the amount of exposure to x-rays and gamma rays from radioactive substances.	
flat plate of the abdomen	The x-ray beam enters the patient's abdomen and then enters the x-ray plate. The patient is lying down flat on the x-ray table with the x-ray plate beneath the x-ray table.	
fluoroscopy	Procedure that uses continuous x-rays to capture the motion of internal organs after the administration of a contrast medium or contrast dye. A fluorescent screen acts like a TV monitor to display a series of changing images. **Cineradiography** permanently records a fluoroscopy on disk or videotape.	**fluor/o-** *fluorescence* **cin/e-** *movement* **radi/o-** *radius (forearm bone); x-rays; radiation*

Word or Phrase	Description	Combining Forms
gadolinium	Contrast medium used in MRI scans. It is a metallic element that responds to a magnetic field.	
gallium-67	Radioactive radiopharmaceutical drug that is given intravenously. It emits gamma rays and is used in nuclear medicine.	
gamma ray	Form of radiation emitted from a radioactive substance. It is also known as a **photon.**	
half-life	Length of time it takes for half of the atoms in a radioactive substance to decay (emit gamma rays or positrons) and become stable	
hysterosalpingo-graphy	Procedure that uses x-rays and a contrast dye inserted into the uterus to create an image of the uterus and uterine tubes. The image is a **hysterosalpingogram.**	**hyster/o-** *uterus (womb)* **salping/o-** *uterine (fallopian) tube*
indium-111	Radioactive radiopharmaceutical drug that is given intravenously. It emits gamma rays and is used in nuclear medicine.	
interventional radiology	Uses CT, MRI, or ultrasonography to guide the insertion of a needle for a biopsy or for another procedure (such as an amniocentesis)	**vent/o-** *a coming*
iodinated contrast dye	Contrast dye that contains iodine and is radiopaque. It is used during radiography, fluoroscopy, and CT scans.	**iodin/o-** *iodine*
iodine-123 and iodine-131	Radioactive radiopharmaceutical drug that is given intravenously. It emits gamma rays and is used in nuclear medicine.	
krypton-81m	Radioactive radiopharmaceutical drug that is inhaled as a gas. It emits gamma rays and is used in nuclear medicine.	
KUB	X-ray of the kidneys, ureters, and bladder	
lateral	Pertaining to the side, as in the path of x-rays during a lateral chest x-ray. In a **cross-table lateral x-ray,** the patient is lying on the x-ray table with the x-ray plate on one side and the x-ray machine on the other, and the x-ray beam travels across the x-ray table. In a **lateral decubitus x-ray,** the patient is lying on his/her side on the x-ray table and the x-ray plate is beneath the x-ray table.	**later/o-** *side*
lead apron	Shielding apron worn by radiologic personnel to protect themselves from radiation exposure. A lead apron is also used to shield parts of the patient's body that are not being x-rayed.	
lymphangiography	Procedure that uses x-rays and a contrast dye injected into a lymphatic vessel to create an image of lymph nodes and lymphatic drainage. The image is a **lymphangiogram.**	**lymph/o-** *lymph; lymphatic system* **angi/o-** *blood vessel; lymphatic vessel*
magnetic resonance imaging (MRI)	Procedure that uses a magnetic field and radiowaves to align the protons in atoms and then cause them to vibrate and emit energy as a signal. It produces individual images as "slices" through the body, as well as a composite three-dimensional view. The metallic contrast medium gadolinium can be used to produce an enhanced image.	**magnet/o-** *magnet*
mammography	Procedure that uses x-rays to create an image of the breast. The image is a **mammogram. Xeromammography** uses a special plate and dry chemicals to create an image on paper. This image is a **xeromammogram.**	**mamm/o-** *breast* **xer/o-** *dry*

Word or Phrase	Description	Combining Forms
MUGA scan	Nuclear medicine procedure that uses scintigraphy and a radiopharmaceutical drug to create an image of the blood in the heart. The gamma camera is coordinated (gated) with the patient's EKG. It is used to calculate the ejection fraction of the heart. MUGA stands for multiple-gated acquisition. It is also known as a **nuclear ventriculogram** or a **gated blood pool scan.**	**ventricul/o-** *ventricle (lower heart chamber; chamber in the brain)*
myelography	Procedure that uses x-rays and a contrast dye inserted through a catheter into the subarachnoid space of the spine to create an image of the spinal cavity, spine, and spinal nerves. The image is a **myelogram.**	**myel/o-** *bone marrow; spinal cord; myelin*
nuclear medicine	Medical specialty that uses radioactive substances to create an image of the internal structures of the body	**nucle/o-** *nucleus (of an atom)*
oblique	On a slant or angle midway between anterior and lateral, as in the path of x-rays during an oblique x-ray	
OncoScint scan	Nuclear medicine procedure that uses scintigraphy and a radiopharmaceutical drug to create an image of metastases from cancer of the colon or ovary. The drug is attached to a monoclonal antibody that binds to receptors on the cancerous cells. The drug (indium-111) plus the monoclonal antibody is the trade name drug OncoScint.	
PET scan	Nuclear medicine procedure that uses a radioactive radiopharmaceutical drug combined with glucose molecules. The glucose is taken up by cells with active metabolism. The radiopharmaceutical drug emits positrons that then become two gamma rays traveling in opposite directions. A circular gamma scintillation camera detects the gamma rays and creates an image that shows cellular metabolism. PET stands for **positron emission tomography.**	**tom/o-** *cut; slice; layer*
plain film	Radiograph obtained without the use of a contrast medium or contrast dye	
portable film	Radiograph obtained at the bedside or in the emergency department with a portable x-ray machine because the patient cannot be transported to the radiology department	
posteroanterior	Pertaining to going from the back to the front, as in the path of x-rays during a PA chest x-ray	**poster/o-** *back part* **anter/o-** *before; front part*
projection	Standardized, fixed orientation between the position of the patient, the x-ray cassette, and the x-ray machine that determines the direction in which the x-ray beam travels through the patient. It is also known as a **view.**	**project/o-** *orientation*
ProstaScint scan	Nuclear medicine procedure that uses scintigraphy and a radiopharmaceutical drug to create an image of metastases from prostate cancer. The drug is attached to a monoclonal antibody that binds to receptors on cancerous cells. The drug (indium-111) plus the monoclonal antibody is the trade name drug ProstaScint.	
pyelography	Procedure that uses x-rays and a contrast dye injected intravenously (intravenous pyelography) or instilled into the bladder (retrograde pyelography) to create an image of the kidneys, ureters, bladder, and urethra. It is also known as **excretory urography. Retrograde pyelography** uses a cystoscope and catheter to inject contrast dye into the ureters. The image is a **pyelogram** or **urogram.**	**pyel/o-** *renal pelvis* **excret/o-** *removing from the body* **ur/o-** *urine; urinary system*
quantitative computerized tomography (QCT)	Type of bone density test that uses x-rays and a CT scan to create a three-dimensional image to measure the bone density of different areas of a bone	**quantitat/o-** *quantity or amount* **tom/o-** *cut; slice; layer*

Word or Phrase	Description	Combining Forms
radioactive substance	Substance that produces gamma rays or positrons as it decays and its atoms change from an unstable to a stable state. It is used to create images in nuclear medicine.	**radi/o-** *radius (forearm bone); x-rays; radiation* **act/o-** *action*
radiography	Procedure that uses x-rays, fluoroscopy, and/or contrast dye to create an image of the internal structures of the body. The image is a **radiograph.** This is also known as **roentgenography.**	**radi/o-** *radius (forearm bone); x-rays; radiation* **roentgen/o-** *x-rays; radiation*
radiology	Medical specialty that uses energy (x-rays, magnetic fields, sound waves, or an electron beam) and technology to create images of internal body structures	**radi/o-** *radius (forearm bone); x-rays; radiation*
radiolucent	Areas of low density tissue (such as an air-filled cavity) that allow x-rays to pass through and create a black area on a radiograph	**radi/o-** *radius (forearm bone); x-rays; radiation* **luc/o-** *clear*
radiopaque	Areas of high-density tissue (such as bone) that do not allow x-rays to pass through, and this creates a white area on a radiograph.	**radi/o-** *radius (forearm bone); x-rays; radiation*
radio-pharmaceutical	Naturally occurring or man-made radioactive substance that has been processed and measured to be given as a drug in nuclear medicine. It is also known as a **tracer.** Radiopharmaceuticals include gallium-67, indium-111, iodine-123, iodine-131, krypton-81m, technetium-99m, thalium-201, and xenon-133.	**pharmaceutic/o-** *medicine; drug* **trac/o-** *visible path*
rem	Unit of measurement for radiation exposure. Rem stands for roentgen-equivalent man.	
scintigraphy	Nuclear medicine procedure that uses a radioactive radiopharmaceutical drug as a tracer. It emits gamma rays that enter a gamma scintillation camera, interact with a crystal, and produce a flash of light. It is also known as a **scintiscan.** The image is a **scintigram.**	**scint/i-** *point of light*
scout film	Radiograph obtained to provide a preliminary view of an area before a contrast medium or contrast dye is given	
SPECT scan	Nuclear medicine procedure that is a MUGA scan of the heart in which the gamma scintillation camera moves around the patient to create images in "slices." The computer compiles the individual images into one three-dimensional image. SPECT stands for single-photon emission computed tomography.	**tom/o-** *cut; slice; layer*
technetium-99m	Radioactive radiopharmaceutical drug that is given intravenously. It emits gamma rays and is used in nuclear medicine.	
thallium-201	Radioactive radiopharmaceutical drug that is given intravenously. It emits gamma rays and is used in nuclear medicine.	
ultrasonography (US)	Procedure that uses ultra high-frequency sound waves emitted by an **ultrasound transducer** placed on the skin. (Alternatively, an **ultrasound probe** is inserted vaginally or rectally to create images of the internal pelvic organs.) The sound waves bounce off organs, creating echoes that are changed into an image by a computer. This is also known as **sonography,** and the image is a **sonogram.** A gray-scale ultrasonography (B scan) creates a two-dimensional image in shades of gray. A three-dimensional ultrasound uses a position sensor to add another dimension and the computer also colorizes the image in shades of brown. Real-time ultrasonography creates a three-dimensional, colorized image that shows motion.	**son/o-** *sound* **duc/o-** *bring; move*

Word or Phrase	Description	Combining Forms
upper gastrointestinal (UGI) series	Fluoroscopic procedure that uses x-rays and barium contrast medium that is swallowed to create an image of the esophagus, stomach, and duodenum. It is also known as a **barium swallow.** A **small-bowel follow-through** follows the barium as it outlines the small intestine.	**gastr/o-** *stomach* **intestin/o-** *intestine*
venography	Procedure that uses x-rays and a contrast dye injected into a vein to create an image of the vein. The image is as a **venogram.**	**ven/o-** *vein*
ventilation-perfusion (V/Q) scan	Nuclear medicine procedure that uses scintigraphy and an inhaled radiopharmaceutical drug to create an image of the lungs. It is also known as a **lung scan.**	**ventilat/o-** *movement of air* **fus/o-** *pouring*
x-rays	Form of invisible ionizing **radiation.** They have a short wavelength that can pass through the body.	**radi/o-** *radius (forearm bone); x-rays; radiation*
x-ray cassette	Case that holds the x-ray film. It is mounted on a **buckey,** an adjustable frame on the wall, beneath the x-ray table, or on a mobile frame on wheels.	
xenon-133	Radioactive radiopharmaceutical drug that is inhaled as a gas. It emits gamma rays and is used in nuclear medicine.	

Abbreviations

AP	anteroposterior	**MRA**	magnetic resonance angiography
Ba	barium	**MRI**	magnetic resonance imaging
BE	barium enema	**MUGA**	multiple-gated acquisition (scan)
CAT	computerized axial tomography	**PA**	posteroanterior
CT	computerized tomography	**PET**	positron emission tomography
CXR	chest x-ray	**QCT**	quantitative computerized tomography
DEXA, DXA	dual energy x-ray absorptiometry	**R, r**	roentgen (unit of exposure to x-rays or gamma rays)
		rad	radiation absorbed dose
DSA	digital subtraction angiography	**RAIU**	radioactive iodine uptake
EBT	electron beam tomography	**rem**	roentgen-equivalent man
ERCP	endoscopic retrograde cholangiopancreatography	**RRT**	registered radiologic technologist
HIDA	hydroxyiminodiacetic acid	**SPECT**	single-photon emission computed tomography
IVC	intravenous cholangiography	**TEE**	transesophageal echocardiography
IVP	intravenous pyelography	**UGI**	upper gastrointestinal (GI) series
KUB	kidneys, ureters, bladder	**US**	ultrasound
Lat	lateral	**V/Q**	ventilation-perfusion (scan)

CAREER FOCUS

Meet Jennifer, a radiologic technologist

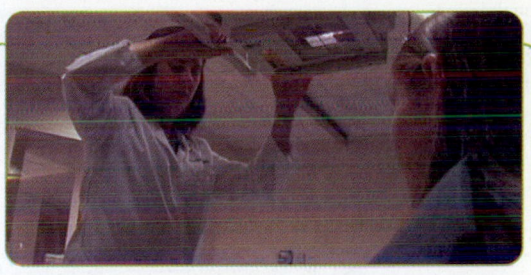

"I became an x-ray technologist because I wanted to work in a profession where I worked with all different patients. You get to work in the emergency room; you get to work doing procedures alongside a physician, dealing with acutely ill patients. You also get to go to the operating room. We also deal with outpatients. We not only do routine x-rays, but we're also involved in minor procedures, along with assisting the radiologists during upper GIs, barium enemas, etc. You're not in any single area all the time, and it's just very nice to see every aspect of the hospital. We use medical terminology every day in our profession. When reading the requisitions that are sent over from the doctors' offices or notifying nurses if we have questions about a patient's exam, we need to use appropriate medical terminology."

Radiologic technologists are allied health professionals who perform and document a variety of radiologic procedures and assist the physician during radiologic procedures in the radiology and nuclear medicine department in a hospital or in a diagnostic imaging outpatient facility.

Radiologists are physicians who practice in the medical specialty of radiology. They view and interpret the results of radiologic procedures to diagnose conditions of all body systems. Nuclear medicine physicians practice in the medical specialty of nuclear medicine. They view and interpret the results of nuclear medicine procedures.

radiologic (RAY-dee-oh-LAWJ-ik)
radi/o- *radius (forearm bone); x-rays; radiation*
log/o- *word; the study of*
-ic *pertaining to*

technologist (tek-NAWL-oh-jist)
techn/o- *technical skill*
log/o- *word; the study of*
-ist *one who specializes in*

radiologist (RAY-dee-AWL-oh-jist)
radi/o- *radius (forearm bone); x-rays; radiation*
log/o- *word; the study of*
-ist *one who specializes in*

PEARSON myhealthprofessionskit To see Jennifer's complete video profile, visit Medical Terminology Interactive at www.myhealthprofessionskit.com. Select this book, log in, and go to the 19th floor of Pearson General Hospital. Enter the Laboratory, and click on the computer screen.

CHAPTER REVIEW EXERCISES

Test your knowledge of the chapter by completing these review exercises. Use the Answer Key at the end of the book to check your answers.

Diagnostic Imaging Procedures

Matching Exercise

Match each word or phrase to its description.

1. arthrography
2. fluoroscopy
3. gamma scintillation camera
4. krypton-81m
5. portable film
6. OncoScint scan
7. radiolucent
8. radiopharmaceutical
9. MRI
10. V/Q scan

_____ Pertaining to an area of low density on a radiograph

_____ Uses a continuous x-ray and a TV monitor

_____ Uses a magnetic field and radiowaves

_____ Contrast dye is injected into a joint

_____ Radioactive substance measured to be given as a drug dose

_____ Radiopharmaceutical drug that is inhaled as a gas and used in nuclear medicine

_____ Detects gamma rays from radioactive substances

_____ Used to detect metastases from colon or ovary cancer

_____ Ventilation-perfusion scan of the lungs

_____ Radiograph performed somewhere other than the radiology department

Circle Exercise

Circle the correct word from the choices given.

1. A (**plain, portable, scout**) film is a preliminary radiograph taken before contrast dye is given.
2. A spiral scan is one type of a/an (**CT, MRI, PET**) scan.
3. The Virtual Physical uses what technology? (**arteriography, EBT, MRI**)
4. During all of these procedures, the patient is exposed to radiation, *except* during a/an (**CT scan, mammography, MRI scan**).
5. During a (**MUGA, PET, SPECT**) scan, the ejection fraction of the heart can be calculated.

Recall and List Exercise

List 10 metal items that might be on or inside a patient that should not be subjected to an MRI scan.

1. _____
2. _____
3. _____
4. _____
5. _____
6. _____
7. _____
8. _____
9. _____
10. _____

Fill in the Blank Exercise

Fill in the blank with the correct word from the word list.

Doppler	film badge	gadolinium	half-life	light box	PA (posteroanterior)

1. The radiologist uses a _____ to view radiographs.

2. A _____ chest x-ray is the most common type of chest x-ray.

3. Every person in radiology must wear a _____ to detect exposure to radiation.

4. _____ is a metallic element that is used in MRI scans because it responds to a magnetic field.

5. The _____ effect states that a sound wave generated by an object will change pitch as the object moves toward or away from the observer.

6. The _____ is the length of time it takes for half of the atoms in an amount of a radioactive substance to decay and become stable.

True or False Exercise

Indicate whether each statement is true or false by writing T or F on the line.

1. _____ Postcontrast images are taken after the injection of contrast dye.

2. _____ Both radiology and nuclear medicine use radioactive substances to create images of the internal structures of the body.

3. _____ The process of measuring the amount of radiation exposure is known as densitometry.

4. _____ Using a CT scan to guide the placement of a needle for biopsy is known as interventional radiology.

5. _____ Fluoroscopy is used during a bone densitometry test.

6. _____ IVC and OCG are both types of radiologic procedures that use contrast dye to view the gallbladder.

7. _____ Ultrasonography uses ultra high-frequency sound waves generated by a transducer or a probe.

8. _____ A PET scan detects positrons and shows areas of cellular metabolism.

9. _____ Iodinated contrast dye contains iodine.

10. _____ The contrast medium barium is used during SPECT scans.

Multiple Choice Exercise

Circle the correct answer from the choices given.

1. Roentgenography is the same thing as _____.
   a. IVP
   b. radiography
   c. KUB
   d. tomography

2. All of the following procedures use x-rays *except* _____.
   a. mammography
   b. cross-table lateral
   c. KUB
   d. ultrasonography

3. When standard echocardiography cannot produce a good-quality image, the physician may order a _____.
   a. KUB
   b. TEE
   c. MRI
   d. DSA

4. PET scans are useful in detecting or studying _____.
   a. cancerous cells
   b. Alzheimer's disease
   c. schizophrenia
   d. all of the above

Matching Exercise

Match each word or phrase to its description.

1. barium swallow
2. B scan
3. bone densitometry
4. cineradiography
5. enhanced
6. filling defect
7. HIDA scan
8. pyelography
9. radiopharmaceutical
10. ultrasonography
11. xeromammogram

_____ Fluoroscopy captured on disk or videotape

_____ Breast image from x-rays captured on paper rather than on film

_____ DEXA scan and QCT

_____ Any procedure that uses a contrast dye

_____ Another name for urography

_____ Upper GI series

_____ Another name for sonography

_____ Two-dimensional, gray-scale ultrasound

_____ Drug that acts as a tracer in the body

_____ Area of decreased uptake in an organ on a perfusion scan

_____ Another name for cholescintigraphy

Building Medical Words

Combining Forms Exercise

Before you build radiologic words, review these combining forms. Next to each combining form, write its medical meaning. The first one has been done for you.

Combining Form	Medical Meaning	Combining Form	Medical Meaning
1. act/o-	*action*	23. gnos/o-	
2. angi/o-		24. hyster/o-	
3. anter/o-		25. intestin/o-	
4. aort/o-		26. iodin/o-	
5. arteri/o-		27. later/o-	
6. arthr/o-		28. log/o-	
7. axi/o-		29. luc/o-	
8. cardi/o-		30. lymph/o-	
9. cholangi/o-		31. magne/to-	
10. chol/e-		32. mamm/o-	
11. cin/e-		33. myel/o-	
12. cyst/o-		34. nucle/o-	
13. densit/o-		35. pancreat/o-	
14. dos/i-		36. pharmaceutic/o-	
15. duc/o-		37. poster/o-	
16. ech/o-		38. project/o-	
17. electr/o-		39. pyel/o-	
18. esophag/o-		40. quantitat/o-	
19. excret/o-		41. rad/io-	
20. fluor/o-		42. roentgen/o-	
21. fus/o-		43. salping/o-	
22. gastr/o-		44. scint/i-	

(continued)

Combining Form	Medical Meaning		Combining Form	Medical Meaning
45. son/o-	_____		50. ven/o-	_____
46. techn/o-	_____		51. ventilat/o-	_____
47. tom/o-	_____		52. vent/o-	_____
48. trac/o-	_____		53. ventricul/o-	_____
49. ur/o-	_____		54. xer/o-	_____

Combining Form and Suffix Exercise

Read the definition of the medical word. Select the correct suffix from the Suffix List. Select the correct combining form from the Combining Form List. Build the medical word and write it on the line. Be sure to check your spelling. The first one has been done for you.

SUFFIX LIST	COMBINING FORM LIST	
-al (pertaining to)	angi/o- (blood vessel; lymphatic vessel)	nucle/o- (nucleus)
-ar (pertaining to)	arteri/o- (artery)	pyel/o- (renal pelvis)
-ated (pertaining to a condition; composed of)	arthr/o- (joint)	radi/o- (radius; x-rays; radiation)
-er (person or thing that produces or does)	axi/o- (axis)	scint/i- (point of light)
-gram (a record or picture)	cholangi/o- (bile duct)	son/o- (sound)
-graphy (process of recording)	densit/o- (density)	tom/o- (cut; slice; layer)
-meter (instrument used to measure)	dos/i- (dose)	trac/o- (visible path)
-metry (process of measuring)	fluor/o- (fluorescence)	ur/o- (urine)
-scopy (process of using an instrument to examine)	iodin/o- (iodine)	ven/o- (vein)
	mamm/o- (breast)	

Definition of the Medical Word

1. Pertaining to the nucleus (of an atom)
2. Process of recording (an image of a) blood vessel
3. (Contrast dye that is) composed of iodine
4. Process of recording x-rays
5. A record or picture of the breast
6. Process of recording (an image of a) cut, slice, or layer
7. Process of using an instrument to examine fluorescence
8. A record or picture of an artery
9. Pertaining to an axis
10. Process of recording sound
11. Process of recording (the image of a) joint
12. Process of measuring a dose (of radiation)
13. Process of recording (the image of a) vein
14. Process of recording a point of light
15. Thing that produces or does a visible path
16. A record or picture of sound
17. A record or picture of (structures that contain) urine
18. Process of recording (an image of a) breast
19. Process of measuring the density
20. Instrument used to measure a dose (of radiation)
21. A record or picture of the renal pelvis
22. Process of recording the bile duct

Build the Medical Word

1. nuclear
2. _____
3. _____
4. _____
5. _____
6. _____
7. _____
8. _____
9. _____
10. _____
11. _____
12. _____
13. _____
14. _____
15. _____
16. _____
17. _____
18. _____
19. _____
20. _____
21. _____
22. _____

Multiple Combining Forms and Suffix Exercise

Read the definition of the medical word. Select the correct suffix and combining forms. Then build the medical word and write it on the line. Be sure to check your spelling. The first one has been done for you.

SUFFIX LIST	COMBINING FORM LIST	
-al (pertaining to)	angi/o- (blood vessel; lymphatic vessel)	lymph/o- (lymph; lymphatic system)
-gram (a record or picture)	anter/o- (before; front part)	mamm/o- (breast)
-graphy (process of recording)	cardi/o- (heart)	pharmaceutic/o- (medicine; drug)
-ior (pertaining to)	chol/e- (bile; gall)	poster/o- (back part)
-ist (one who specializes in)	cin/e- (movement)	radi/o- (x-rays; radiation)
	cyst/o- (bladder; fluid-filled sac)	salping/o- (uterine tube)
	ech/o- (echo; sound wave)	techn/o- (technical skill)
	hyster/o- (uterus)	xer/o- (dry)
	log/o- (word; the study of)	

Definition of the Medical Word

Build the Medical Word

1. Pertaining to the back and the front

   posteroanterior

2. Process of recording the gallbladder

3. A record or picture of the uterus and uterine tubes

4. Process of recording movement (during an) x-ray

5. A record or picture of lymph and a lymphatic vessel

6. A record or picture (processed with) dry (chemical) of the breast

7. A record or picture of echoes (sound waves reflected from) the heart

8. Pertaining to radiation from a medicine or drug

9. One who specializes in technical skill in the study of (radiology)

Abbreviations

Abbreviation Exercise

Write the definition for each abbreviation.

1. US _____

2. PET _____

3. BE _____

4. CXR _____

5. SPECT _____

6. MUGA _____

7. CAT _____

8. IVP _____

Applied Skills

Medical Report Exercise

This exercise contains three radiologic and nuclear medicine reports. Read each report and answer the questions.

RADIOLOGY REPORT

PATIENT NAME: BENTLEY, Jean

HOSPITAL NUMBER: 327-01-1982

DATE OF X-RAY: November 19, 20xx

PORTABLE PELVIS

Portable AP study of the right pelvis and hip in surgery shows the femoral part of the prosthesis to now be in place and in a normal relationship with the acetabular prosthesis. A total hip replacement prosthesis is also noted to be in place on the left.

Daniel P. Raddick, M.D.

Daniel P. Raddick, M.D.

DPR:apt
D: 11/19/xx
T: 11/19/xx

Fact Finding Questions

1. What does the abbreviation AP stand for? _____

2. What one word and one phrase tell you that this x-ray was not taken in the radiology department?

   _____   _____

3. Where did the radiologic technologist have to go to take this x-ray? _____

4. When this x-ray was taken, the patient was undergoing a total hip replacement in which hip?   **Right**   **Left**

5. Define *prosthesis*. _____

RADIOLOGY REPORT

PATIENT NAME: ADAMS, Bryce

HOSPITAL NUMBER: 11-98-64370

DATE OF X-RAY: November 19, 20xx

AIR CONTRAST BARIUM ENEMA

PROCEDURE

Under fluoroscopic control, the barium was allowed to flow in a retrograde manner to fill the cecum. Using a double-contrast technique, multiple films were obtained. Several small diverticula are noted. There is also some displacement of the small bowel. A soft tissue density is seen within the lower abdomen. No mucosal ulcerations or polypoid lesions are identified.

IMPRESSION

Barium and air contrast study shows displacement of the small bowel with a tissue density. This is suggestive of a pelvic mass. No evidence of polypoid lesions is seen in the colon.

Robert C. Johnson, M.D.

Robert C. Johnson, M.D.

RCJ:smt
D: 11/19/xx
T: 11/19/xx

Fact Finding Questions

1. What type of radiologic procedure was done?

    a. KUB

    b. flat plate of the abdomen

    c. fluoroscopy

2. Name the two types of contrast that were used for this procedure.

    _____

    _____

3. In addition to watching the procedure on a TV monitor, how many radiographs (films) were taken?

    _____

4. Divide *fluoroscopic* into its three word parts and define each word part.

    Word Part   **Definition**

    _____   _____

    _____   _____

    _____   _____

NUCLEAR MEDICINE REPORT

PATIENT NAME: MATHESON, Latrise

HOSPITAL NUMBER: 901156-48376

DATE OF X-RAY: November 19, 20xx

RADIOACTIVE IODINE UPTAKE
The patient was given an oral capsule containing 100 microcuries of I-123, and uptake by the thyroid gland was measured at 6 hours and 24 hours. The 6-hour uptake was 5.5% (normal 4–12%). The 24-hour uptake was 14.0% (normal 7–24%).

THYROID SCAN
Fifteen minutes after the intravenous injection of 10 millicuries of technetium-99m, views of the thyroid gland were performed. The thyroid gland was in a normal position in the neck. The overall size of the gland was within normal limits, and there was uniform uptake throughout both the right and left lobes.

IMPRESSION
1.   Normal thyroid radioiodine uptake.
2.   Normal thyroid scan.

Victoria J. Evans, M.D.

Victoria J. Evans, M.D.

VJE:mja
D: 11/19/xx
T: 11/19/xx

Fact Finding Questions

1. What are the names and atomic numbers of the two radiopharmaceuticals given in this procedure?

   _____

   _____

2. What are the two units of measurement for the doses of these radiopharmaceuticals?

   _____

   _____

3. What is the range of normal values for the 24-hour uptake? _____

4. How was the radioactive iodine administered? _____

5. How was the radioactive technetium-99m administered? _____

6. Divide *radioactive* into its three word parts and define each word part.

   Word Part   **Definition**

   _____   _____

   _____   _____

   _____   _____

7. What phrase tells you that there was an equal amount of radioactive tracer present in all parts of the thyroid gland?

   _____

Hearing Medical Words Exercise

You hear someone speaking the medical words given below. Read each pronunciation and then write the medical word it represents. Be sure to check your spelling. The first one has been done for you.

1. BAIR-ee-um   <u>barium</u>

2. ar-TEER-ee-OH-gram   _____

3. KOH-lee-SIS-toh-gram   _____

4. DEN-sih-TAWM-eh-tree   _____

5. EK-oh-KAR-dee-OH-gram _____

6. HIS-ter-oh-sal-PING-goh-gram _____

7. lim-FAN-jee-OH-gram   _____

8. SAWN-oh-gram   _____

9. toh-MAWG-rah-fee   _____

10. ZEER-oh-mah-MAWG-rah-fee _____

Pronunciation Exercise

Read the medical word that is given. Then review the syllables in the pronunciation. Circle the primary (main) accented syllable. The first one has been done for you.

1. angiography (an-jee-awg-rah-fee)

2. arthrogram (ar-throh-gram)

3. arthrography (ar-thrawg-rah-fee)

4. dosimeter (doh-sim-eh-ter)

5. fluoroscopy (floor-aws-koh-pee)

6. lymphangiogram (lim-fan-jee-oh-gram)

7. mammogram (mam-oh-gram)

8. mammography (mah-mawg-rah-fee)

9. tomography (toh-mawg-rah-fee)

10. venogram (vee-noh-gram)

Multimedia Preview

Immerse yourself in a variety of activities inside Medical Terminology Interactive. Getting there is simple:

1. Click on www.myhealthprofessionskit.com.
2. Select "Medical Terminology" from the choice of disciplines.
3. First-time users must create an account using the scratch-off code on the inside front cover of this book.
4. Find this book and log in using your username and password.
5. Click on Medical Terminology Interactive.
6. Take the elevator to the 19th Floor to begin your virtual exploration of this chapter!

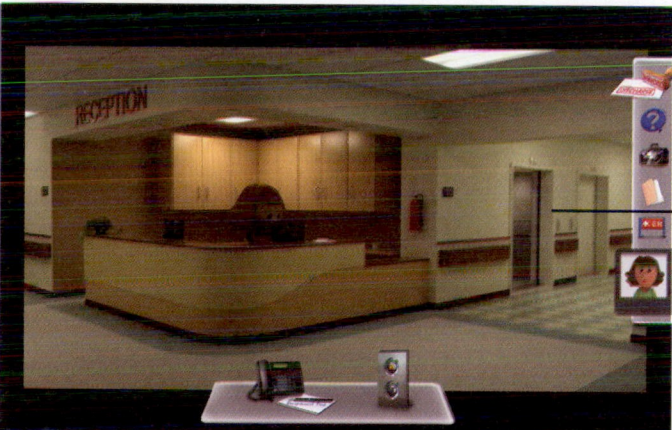 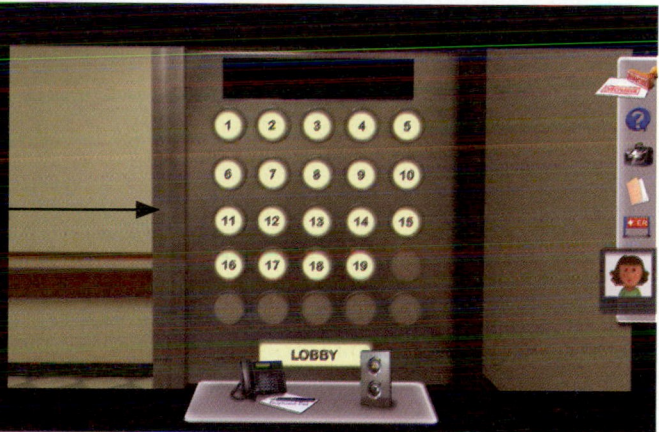

■ **Speedway** Take a ride on the Medical Terminology superhighway. Choose a set of wheels and steer your way toward mastery by choosing the correct lanes. How fast can you accumulate 15 correct answers? Start your engines!

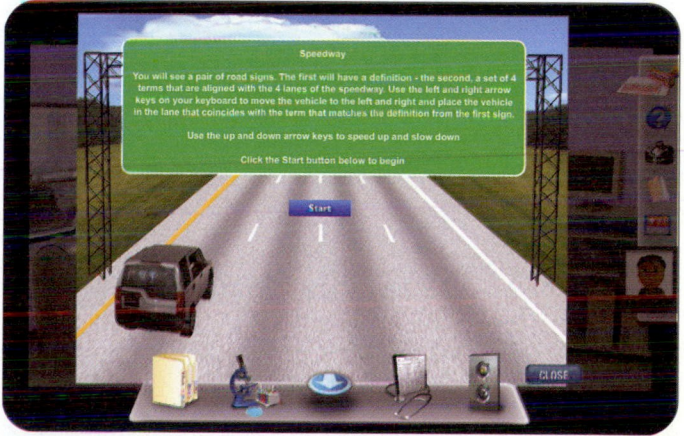

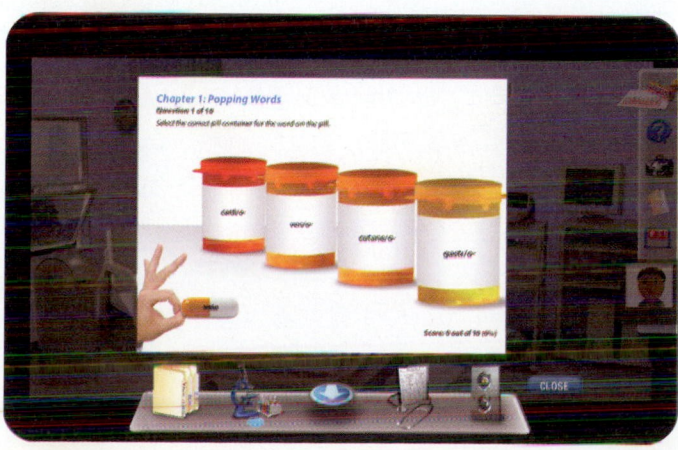

■ **Popping Words** Popping pills won't help you study, but popping words might do the trick. Test your knowledge by launching the term pill into the correct container. Ready, aim, fire!

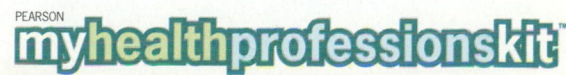

Appendix A
GLOSSARY OF MEDICAL WORD PARTS
COMBINING FORMS, PREFIXES, AND SUFFIXES

A

a-	prefix	away from; without
ab-	prefix	away from
abdomin/o-	combining form	abdomen
ablat/o-	combining form	take away; destroy
-able	suffix	able to be
abort/o-	combining form	stop prematurely
abras/o-	combining form	scrape off
absorpt/o-	combining form	absorb; take in
-ac	suffix	pertaining to
access/o-	combining form	supplemental or contributing part
accommod/o-	combining form	to adapt
acetabul/o-	combining form	acetabulum (hip socket)
acid/o-	combining form	acid (low pH)
acous/o-	combining form	hearing; sound
acr/o-	combining form	extremity; highest point
acromi/o-	combining form	acromion
actin/o-	combining form	rays of the sun
act/o-	combining form	action
acu/o-	combining form	needle; sharpness
ad-	prefix	toward
-ad	suffix	toward; in the direction of
addict/o-	combining form	surrender to; be controlled by
-ade	suffix	action; process
aden/o-	combining form	gland
adenoid/o-	combining form	adenoids
adhes/o-	combining form	to stick to
adip/o-	combining form	fat
adjuv/o-	combining form	giving help or assistance
adnex/o-	combining form	accessory connecting parts
adolesc/o-	combining form	the beginning of being an adult
adrenal/o-	combining form	adrenal gland
adren/o-	combining form	adrenal gland
affect/o-	combining form	state of mind; mood; to have an influence on
affer/o-	combining form	bring toward the center
agglutin/o-	combining form	clumping; sticking
aggreg/o-	combining form	crowding together
ag/o-	combining form	to lead to
agon/o-	combining form	causing action
agor/a-	combining form	open area or space

-al	suffix	pertaining to
albin/o-	combining form	white
albumin/o-	combining form	albumin
alges/o-	combining form	sensation of pain
-algia	combination combining form and suffix	painful condition
alg/o-	combining form	pain
align/o-	combining form	arranged in a straight line
aliment/o-	combining form	food; nourishment
-alis	suffix	pertaining to
alkal/o-	combining form	base (high pH)
allerg/o-	combining form	allergy
all/o-	combining form	other; strange
alopec/o-	combining form	bald
alveol/o-	combining form	alveolus (air sac)
ambly/o-	combining form	dimness
ambulat/o-	combining form	walking
amnes/o-	combining form	forgetfulness
amni/o-	combining form	amnion (fetal membrane)
-amnios	suffix	amniotic fluid
amputat/o-	combining form	to cut off
amput/o-	combining form	to cut off
amygdal/o-	combining form	almond shape
amyl/o-	combining form	carbohydrate; starch
an-	prefix	without; not
-an	suffix	pertaining to
ana-	prefix	apart from; excessive
anabol/o-	combining form	building up
analy/o-	combining form	to separate
anastom/o-	combining form	create an opening between two structures
-ance	suffix	state of
ancill/o-	combining form	servant; accessory
-ancy	suffix	state of
andr/o-	combining form	male
aneurysm/o-	combining form	aneurysm (dilation)
angin/o-	combining form	angina
angi/o-	combining form	blood vessel; lymphatic vessel
anis/o-	combining form	unequal
ankyl/o-	combining form	fused together; stiff
an/o-	combining form	anus
ant-	prefix	against

-ant	suffix	pertaining to
antagon/o-	combining form	oppose or work against
ante-	prefix	forward; before
anter/o-	combining form	before; front part
anthrac/o-	combining form	coal
anti-	prefix	against
anxi/o-	combining form	fear; worry
aort/o-	combining form	aorta
apher/o-	combining form	withdrawal
aphth/o-	combining form	ulcer
apic/o-	combining form	apex (tip)
apo-	prefix	away from
appendic/o-	combining form	appendix
appendicul/o-	combining form	limb; small attached part
append/o-	combining form	small structure hanging from a larger structure; appendix
appercept/o-	combining form	fully perceived
aque/o-	combining form	watery substance
-ar	suffix	pertaining to
arachn/o-	combining form	spider; spider web
-arche	suffix	a beginning
areol/o-	combining form	small area around the nipple
-arian	suffix	pertaining to a person
-aris	suffix	pertaining to
arteri/o-	combining form	artery
arteriol/o-	combining form	arteriole
arter/o-	combining form	artery
arthr/o-	combining form	joint
articul/o-	combining form	joint
-ary	suffix	pertaining to
asbest/o-	combining form	asbestos
ascit/o-	combining form	ascites
-ase	suffix	enzyme
aspir/o-	combining form	to breathe in; to suck in
asthen/o-	combining form	lack of strength
asthm/o-	combining form	asthma
astr/o-	combining form	starlike structure
-ate	suffix	composed of; pertaining to
-ated	suffix	pertaining to a condition; composed of
atel/o-	combining form	incomplete
ather/o-	combining form	soft, fatty substance
atheromat/o-	combining form	fatty deposit or mass
athet/o-	combining form	without position or place
-atic	suffix	pertaining to
-ation	suffix	a process; being or having
-ative	suffix	pertaining to
-ator	suffix	person or thing that produces or does
-atory	suffix	pertaining to

atri/o-	combining form	atrium (upper heart chamber)
attenu/o-	combining form	weakened
-ature	suffix	system composed of
audi/o-	combining form	the sense of hearing
audit/o-	combining form	the sense of hearing
augment/o-	combining form	increase in size or degree
aur/i-	combining form	ear
auricul/o-	combining form	ear
auscult/o-	combining form	listening
aut/o-	combining form	self
autonom/o-	combining form	independent; self-governing
axill/o-	combining form	axilla (armpit)
axi/o-	combining form	axis

B

bacteri/o-	combining form	bacterium
balan/o-	combining form	glans penis
bar/o-	combining form	weight
basil/o-	combining form	base of an organ
bas/o-	combining form	base of a structure; basic (alkaline)
behav/o-	combining form	activity; manner of acting
bi-	prefix	two
bili/o-	combining form	bile; gall
bilirubin/o-	combining form	bilirubin
bi/o-	combining form	life; living organisms; living tissue
-blast	suffix	immature cell
blast/o-	combining form	immature; embryonic
blephar/o-	combining form	eyelid
-body	suffix	a structure or thing
botul/o-	combining form	sausage
brachi/o-	combining form	arm
brachy-	prefix	short
brady-	prefix	slow
bronchi/o-	combining form	bronchus
bronchiol/o-	combining form	bronchiole
bronch/o-	combining form	bronchus
brux/o-	combining form	to grind the teeth
buccinat/o-	combining form	cheek
bucc/o-	combining form	cheek
bulb/o-	combining form	like a bulb
bunion/o-	combining form	bunion
burs/o-	combining form	bursa

C

cac/o-	combining form	bad; poor
calcane/o-	combining form	calcaneus (heel bone)
calc/i-	combining form	calcium

calcific/o-	combining form	hard from calcium
calci/o-	combining form	calcium
calc/o-	combining form	calcium
calcul/o-	combining form	stone
calic/o-	combining form	calix
cali/o-	combining form	calix
calor/o-	combining form	heat
cancell/o-	combining form	lattice structure
cancer/o-	combining form	cancer
candid/o-	combining form	*Candida* (a yeast)
can/o-	combining form	resembling a dog
capill/o-	combining form	hairlike structure; capillary
capn/o-	combining form	carbon dioxide
capsul/o-	combining form	capsule (enveloping structure)
carb/o-	combining form	carbon atoms
carbox/y-	combining form	carbon monoxide
carcin/o-	combining form	cancer
card/i-	combining form	heart
cardi/o-	combining form	heart
cari/o-	combining form	caries (tooth decay)
carot/o-	combining form	stupor; sleep
carp/o-	combining form	wrist
cartilagin/o-	combining form	cartilage
cata-	prefix	down
catabol/o-	combining form	breaking down
catheter/o-	combining form	catheter
caud/o-	combining form	tail (tail bone)
caus/o-	combining form	burning
cavit/o-	combining form	hollow space
cav/o-	combining form	hollow space
cec/o-	combining form	cecum (first part of large intestine)
-cele	suffix	hernia
celi/o-	combining form	abdomen
cellul/o-	combining form	cell
-centesis	suffix	procedure to puncture
centr/o-	combining form	center; dominant part
cephal/o-	combining form	head
-cephalus	suffix	head
-ceps	suffix	head
-cere	suffix	waxy substance
cerebell/o-	combining form	cerebellum (posterior part of the brain)
cerebr/o-	combining form	cerebrum (largest part of the brain)
cervic/o-	combining form	neck; cervix
cheil/o-	combining form	lip
chem/o-	combining form	chemical; drug
chez/o-	combining form	to pass feces
chir/o-	combining form	hand

chlor/o-	combining form	chloride
cholangi/o-	combining form	bile duct
chol/e-	combining form	bile; gall
cholecyst/o-	combining form	gallbladder
choledoch/o-	combining form	common bile duct
cholesterol/o-	combining form	cholesterol
chol/o-	combining form	bile; gall
chondr/o-	combining form	cartilage
chori/o-	combining form	chorion (fetal membrane)
chorion/o-	combining form	chorion (fetal membrane)
choroid/o-	combining form	choroid (middle layer around the eye)
chrom/o-	combining form	color
chron/o-	combining form	time
cid/o-	combining form	killing
cili/o-	combining form	hairlike structure
cin/e-	combining form	movement
cingul/o-	combining form	structure that surrounds
circa-	prefix	about
circulat/o-	combining form	movement in a circular route
circul/o-	combining form	circle
circum-	prefix	around
cirrh/o-	combining form	yellow
cis/o-	combining form	to cut
-clast	suffix	cell that breaks down substances
claudicat/o-	combining form	limping pain
claustr/o-	combining form	enclosed space
clavicul/o-	combining form	clavicle (collar bone)
clav/o-	combining form	clavicle (collar bone)
-cle	suffix	small thing
cleid/o-	combining form	clavicle (collar bone)
clinic/o-	combining form	medicine
clon/o-	combining form	identical group derived from one; rapid contracting and relaxing
-clonus	suffix	condition of rapid contracting and relaxing
-cnemius	suffix	leg
coagul/o-	combining form	clotting
coarct/o-	combining form	pressed together
cocc/o-	combining form	spherical bacterium
-coccus	suffix	spherical bacterium
coccyg/o-	combining form	coccyx (tail bone)
cochle/o-	combining form	cochlea (of the inner ear)
cognit/o-	combining form	thinking
coit/o-	combining form	sexual intercourse
coll/a-	combining form	fibers that hold together
-collis	suffix	condition of the neck
col/o-	combining form	colon (part of large intestine)

colon/o-	combining form	colon (part of large intestine)
colp/o-	combining form	vagina
comat/o-	combining form	unconsciousness
comminut/o-	combining form	break into small pieces
communicat/o-	combining form	impart; transmit
communic/o-	combining form	impart; transmit
compens/o-	combining form	counterbalance; compensate
compress/o-	combining form	press together
compromis/o-	combining form	exposed to danger
compuls/o-	combining form	drive or compel
con-	prefix	with
concept/o-	combining form	to conceive or form
concuss/o-	combining form	violent shaking or jarring
conduct/o-	combining form	carrying; conveying
conform/o-	combining form	having the same scale or angle
congenit/o-	combining form	present at birth
congest/o-	combining form	accumulation of fluid
coni/o-	combining form	dust
conjug/o-	combining form	joined together
conjunctiv/o-	combining form	conjunctiva
con/o-	combining form	cone
constip/o-	combining form	compacted feces
constrict/o-	combining form	drawn together; narrowed
construct/o-	combining form	to build
contin/o-	combining form	hold together
contra-	prefix	against
contract/o-	combining form	pull together
contus/o-	combining form	bruising
converg/o-	combining form	coming together
convuls/o-	combining form	seizure
copr/o-	combining form	feces; stool
corne/o-	combining form	cornea (of the eye)
cor/o-	combining form	pupil (of the eye)
coron/o-	combining form	structure that encircles like a crown
corpor/o-	combining form	body
cortic/o-	combining form	cortex (outer region)
cosmet/o-	combining form	attractive; adorned
cost/o-	combining form	rib
crani/o-	combining form	cranium (skull)
-crasia	suffix	a mixing
-crine	suffix	thing that secretes
crin/o-	combining form	secrete
-crit	suffix	separation of
cry/o-	combining form	cold
crypt/o-	combining form	hidden
cubit/o-	combining form	elbow
culd/o-	combining form	cul-de-sac
cusp/o-	combining form	projection; point

cutane/o-	combining form	skin
cut/i-	combining form	skin
cyan/o-	combining form	blue
cycl/o-	combining form	ciliary body of the eye; circle; cycle
cyst/o-	combining form	bladder; fluid-filled sac; semisolid cyst
-cyte	suffix	cell
cyt/o-	combining form	cell

D

dacry/o-	combining form	lacrimal sac; tears
dactyl/o-	combining form	finger or toe
-dactyly	suffix	condition of fingers or toes
de-	prefix	reversal of; without
dec/i-	combining form	one tenth
decidu/o-	combining form	falling off
defici/o-	combining form	lacking; inadequate
degluti/o-	combining form	swallowing
delt/o-	combining form	triangle
delus/o-	combining form	false belief
dem/o-	combining form	people; population
dendr/o-	combining form	branching structure
densit/o-	combining form	density
dent/i-	combining form	tooth
dentit/o-	combining form	eruption of teeth
dent/o-	combining form	tooth
depend/o-	combining form	to hang onto
depress/o-	combining form	press down
derm/a-	combining form	skin
-derma	suffix	skin
dermat/o-	combining form	skin
derm/o-	combining form	skin
desicc/o-	combining form	to dry up
-desis	suffix	procedure to fuse together
dextr/o-	combining form	right; sugar
di-	prefix	two
dia-	prefix	complete; completely through
diabet/o-	combining form	diabetes
diaphore/o-	combining form	sweating
diaphragmat/o-	combining form	diaphragm
diaphys/o-	combining form	shaft of a bone
diastol/o-	combining form	dilating
-didymis	suffix	testes (twin structures)
didym/o-	combining form	testes (twin structures)
dietet/o-	combining form	foods; diet
diet/o-	combining form	foods; diet
differentiat/o-	combining form	being distinct; specialized
different/o-	combining form	being distinct; different

digest/o-	combining form	break down food; digest
digit/o-	combining form	digit (finger or toe)
dilat/o-	combining form	dilate; widen
dipl/o-	combining form	double
dips/o-	combining form	thirst
dis-	prefix	away from
disk/o-	combining form	disk
dissect/o-	combining form	to cut apart
dissemin/o-	combining form	widely scattered throughout the body
distent/o-	combining form	distended; stretched
dist/o-	combining form	away from the center or point of origin
diverticul/o-	combining form	diverticulum
donat/o-	combining form	give as a gift
dors/o-	combining form	back; dorsum
-dose	suffix	measured quantity
dos/i-	combining form	dose
-drome	suffix	a running
duc/o-	combining form	bring; move
-duct	suffix	duct (tube)
duct/o-	combining form	bring; move; a duct
du/o-	combining form	two
duoden/o-	combining form	duodenum (first part of small intestine)
dur/o-	combining form	dura mater
dynam/o-	combining form	power; movement
dyn/o-	combining form	pain
dys-	prefix	painful; difficult; abnormal

E

e-	prefix	without; not
-eal	suffix	pertaining to
ec-	prefix	out; outward
ecchym/o-	combining form	blood in the tissues
ech/o-	combining form	echo (sound wave)
eclamps/o-	combining form	a seizure
-ectasis	suffix	condition of dilation
ectat/o-	combining form	dilation
ecto-	prefix	outermost; outside
-ectomy	suffix	surgical excision
ectop/o-	combining form	outside of a place
-ed	suffix	pertaining to
-edema	suffix	swelling
edentul/o-	combining form	without teeth
-ee	suffix	person who is the object of an action
efface/o-	combining form	do away with; obliterate
effer/o-	combining form	go out from the center

effus/o-	combining form	a pouring out
ejaculat/o-	combining form	to expel suddenly
-elasma	suffix	platelike structure
elast/o-	combining form	flexing; stretching
electr/o-	combining form	electricity
-elle	suffix	little thing
em-	prefix	in
-ema	suffix	condition
emaci/o-	combining form	to make thin
embol/o-	combining form	embolus (occluding plug)
embryon/o-	combining form	embryo; immature form
-emesis	suffix	condition of vomiting
emet/o-	combining form	to vomit
-emia	suffix	condition of the blood; substance in the blood
-emic	suffix	pertaining to a condition of the blood or a substance in the blood
emiss/o-	combining form	to send out
emot/o-	combining form	moving; stirring up
emulsific/o-	combining form	droplets of fat suspended in a liquid; particles suspended in a solution
en-	prefix	in; within; inward
-ence	suffix	state of
encephal/o-	combining form	brain
-encephaly	suffix	condition of the brain
-ency	suffix	condition of being
endo-	prefix	innermost; within
-ent	suffix	pertaining to
enter/o-	combining form	intestine
-entery	suffix	condition of the intestine
enucle/o-	combining form	to remove the main part
enur/o-	combining form	to urinate
-eon	suffix	one who performs
eosin/o-	combining form	eosin (red acidic dye)
ependym/o-	combining form	cellular lining
epi-	prefix	upon; above
epilept/o-	combining form	seizure
epiphys/o-	combining form	growth area at the end of a long bone
episi/o-	combining form	vulva (female external genitalia)
-er	suffix	person or thing that produces or does
erect/o-	combining form	to stand up
erg/o-	combining form	activity; work
-ergy	suffix	activity; process of working
erupt/o-	combining form	breaking out
-ery	suffix	process of
erythemat/o-	combining form	redness

erythr/o-	combining form	red
-esis	suffix	a process
es/o-	combining form	inward
esophag/o-	combining form	esophagus
esthes/o-	combining form	sensation; feeling
esthet/o-	combining form	sensation; feeling
estr/a-	combining form	female
estr/o-	combining form	female
ethm/o-	combining form	sieve
-etic	suffix	pertaining to
eti/o-	combining form	cause of disease
-ety	suffix	condition; state
etym/o-	combining form	word origin
eu-	prefix	normal; good
ex-	prefix	out; away from
exacerb/o-	combining form	increase; provoke
excis/o-	combining form	to cut out
excori/o-	combining form	to take out skin
excret/o-	combining form	removing from the body
exhibit/o-	combining form	showing
ex/o-	combining form	away from; external; outward
explorat/o-	combining form	to search out
express/o-	combining form	communicate
extens/o-	combining form	straightening
extern/o-	combining form	outside
extra-	prefix	outside of
extrins/o-	combining form	on the outside
exud/o-	combining form	oozing fluid

fiss/o-	combining form	splitting
fixat/o-	combining form	to make stable or still
flatul/o-	combining form	flatus (gas)
flex/o-	combining form	bending
fluor/o-	combining form	fluorescence
-flux	suffix	flow
foc/o-	combining form	point of activity
foli/o-	combining form	leaf
follicul/o-	combining form	follicle (small sac)
foramin/o-	combining form	foramen (opening into a cavity or channel)
forens/o-	combining form	court proceedings in criminal law
-form	suffix	having the form of
format/o-	combining form	structure; arrangement
fove/o-	combining form	small, depressed area
fract/o-	combining form	break up
fratern/o-	combining form	close association or relationship
-frice	suffix	thing that produces friction
front/o-	combining form	front
fruct/o-	combining form	fruit
fulgur/o-	combining form	spark of electricity
fund/o-	combining form	fundus (part farthest from the opening)
fundu/o-	combining form	fundus (part farthest from the opening)
fung/o-	combining form	fungus
fus/o-	combining form	pouring

F

faci/o-	combining form	face
factiti/o-	combining form	artificial; made up
fallopi/o-	combining form	uterine (fallopian) tube
fasci/o-	combining form	fascia
fec/a-	combining form	feces; stool
fec/o-	combining form	feces; stool
femor/o-	combining form	femur (thigh bone)
fer/o-	combining form	to bear
ferrit/o-	combining form	iron
ferr/o-	combining form	iron
fertil/o-	combining form	able to conceive a child
fet/o-	combining form	fetus
fibrill/o-	combining form	muscle fiber; nerve fiber
fibrin/o-	combining form	fibrin
fibr/o-	combining form	fiber
fibul/o-	combining form	fibula (lower leg bone)
filtrat/o-	combining form	filtering; straining
filtr/o-	combining form	filter

G

galact/o-	combining form	milk
ganglion/o-	combining form	ganglion
gangren/o-	combining form	gangrene
gastr/o-	combining form	stomach
gemin/o-	combining form	set or group
-gen	suffix	that which produces
-gene	suffix	gene
gene/o-	combining form	gene
gener/o-	combining form	production; creation
genit/o-	combining form	genitalia
gen/o-	combining form	arising from; produced by
germin/o-	combining form	embryonic tissue
ger/o-	combining form	old age
gestat/o-	combining form	from conception to birth
gest/o-	combining form	from conception to birth
gigant/o-	combining form	giant
gingiv/o-	combining form	gums
glandul/o-	combining form	gland

glen/o-	combining form	socket of a joint
-glia	suffix	cells that provide support
gli/o-	combining form	cells that provide support
glob/o-	combining form	shaped like a globe; comprehensive
globul/o-	combining form	shaped like a globe
glomerul/o-	combining form	glomerulus
gloss/o-	combining form	tongue
glott/o-	combining form	glottis (of the larynx)
gluc/o-	combining form	glucose (sugar)
glycer/o-	combining form	glycerol (sugar alcohol)
glyc/o-	combining form	glucose (sugar)
glycos/o-	combining form	glucose (sugar)
gnos/o-	combining form	knowledge
gonad/o-	combining form	gonads (ovaries and testes)
goni/o-	combining form	angle
gon/o-	combining form	seed (ovum or spermatozoon)
-grade	suffix	pertaining to going
-graft	suffix	tissue for implant or transplant
-gram	suffix	a record or picture
granul/o-	combining form	granule
-graph	suffix	instrument used to record
graph/o-	combining form	record
-graphy	suffix	process of recording
-gravida	suffix	pregnancy
gustat/o-	combining form	the sense of taste
gynec/o-	combining form	female; woman

H

habilitat/o-	combining form	give ability
halit/o-	combining form	breath
hallucin/o-	combining form	imagined perception
hal/o-	combining form	breathe
hebe/o-	combining form	youth
hec/o-	combining form	habitual condition of the body
hedon/o-	combining form	pleasure
helic/o-	combining form	a coil
hemat/o-	combining form	blood
hemi-	prefix	one half
hem/o-	combining form	blood
hemoglobin/o-	combining form	hemoglobin
hemorrh/o-	combining form	a flowing of blood
hemorrhoid/o-	combining form	hemorrhoid
hepat/o-	combining form	liver
heredit/o-	combining form	genetic inheritance
hered/o-	combining form	genetic inheritance
herni/o-	combining form	hernia
heter/o-	combining form	other

hex/o-	combining form	habitual condition of the body
hiat/o-	combining form	gap; opening
hidr/o-	combining form	sweat
hil/o-	combining form	hilum (indentation in an organ)
hirsut/o-	combining form	hairy
histi/o-	combining form	tissue
home/o-	combining form	same
hom/i-	combining form	man
hormon/o-	combining form	hormone
humer/o-	combining form	humerus (upper arm bone)
hyal/o-	combining form	clear, glasslike substance
hydatidi/o-	combining form	fluid-filled vesicles
hydr/o-	combining form	water; fluid
hygien/o-	combining form	health
hy/o-	combining form	U-shaped structure
hyper-	prefix	above; more than normal
hypn/o-	combining form	sleep
hypo-	prefix	below; deficient
hypophys/o-	combining form	pituitary gland
hyster/o-	combining form	uterus (womb)

I

-ia	suffix	condition; state; thing
-iac	suffix	pertaining to
-ial	suffix	pertaining to
-ian	suffix	pertaining to
-ias	suffix	condition
-iasis	suffix	state of; process of
-iatic	suffix	pertaining to a state or process
iatr/o-	combining form	physician; medical treatment
-iatry	suffix	medical treatment
-ic	suffix	pertaining to
-ical	suffix	pertaining to
-ice	suffix	state; quality
-ician	suffix	skilled professional or expert
-ics	suffix	knowledge; practice
icter/o-	combining form	jaundice
ict/o-	combining form	seizure
-id	suffix	resembling; source or origin
-ide	suffix	chemically modified structure
idi/o-	combining form	unknown; individual
-ie	suffix	a thing
-il	suffix	a thing
-ile	suffix	pertaining to
ile/o-	combining form	ileum (third part of small intestine)
ili/o-	combining form	ilium (hip bone)
illus/o-	combining form	false perception

im-	prefix	not
-immune	suffix	immune response
immun/o-	combining form	immune response
impact/o-	combining form	wedged in
implant/o-	combining form	placed within
in-	prefix	in; within; not
-in	suffix	a substance
incarcer/o-	combining form	to imprison
incis/o-	combining form	to cut into
incud/o-	combining form	incus (anvil-shaped bone)
induct/o-	combining form	a leading in
-ine	suffix	thing pertaining to
infarct/o-	combining form	area of dead tissue
infect/o-	combining form	disease within
infer/o-	combining form	below
inflammat/o-	combining form	redness and warmth
infra-	prefix	below; beneath
-ing	suffix	doing
inguin/o-	combining form	groin
inhibit/o-	combining form	block; hold back
inject/o-	combining form	insert; put in
insemin/o-	combining form	plant a seed
insert/o-	combining form	to put in; introduce
inspect/o-	combining form	looking at
insulin/o-	combining form	insulin
insul/o-	combining form	island
integument/o-	combining form	skin
integu/o-	combining form	to cover
inter-	prefix	between
intern/o-	combining form	inside
interstiti/o-	combining form	spaces within tissue
intestin/o-	combining form	intestine
intra-	prefix	within
intrins/o-	combining form	on the inside
intussuscep/o-	combining form	to receive within
invas/o-	combining form	to go into
involut/o-	combining form	enlarged organ returns to normal size
iodin/o-	combining form	iodine
iod/o-	combining form	iodine
-ion	suffix	action; condition
-ior	suffix	pertaining to
-ious	suffix	pertaining to
irid/o-	combining form	iris (colored part of the eye)
ir/o-	combining form	iris (colored part of the eye)
ischi/o-	combining form	ischium (hip bone)
isch/o-	combining form	keep back; block
-ism	suffix	process; disease from a specific cause

-ist	suffix	one who specializes in
-istic	suffix	pertaining to
-istry	suffix	process related to the specialty of
-isy	suffix	condition of inflammation or infection
-ite	suffix	thing that pertains to
-itian	suffix	a skilled professional or expert
-itic	suffix	pertaining to
-ition	suffix	condition of having
-itis	suffix	inflammation of; infection of
-ity	suffix	state; condition
-ium	suffix	a chemical element; a structure
-ive	suffix	pertaining to
-ix	suffix	a thing
-ization	suffix	process of making, creating, or inserting
-ize	suffix	affecting in a particular way
-izer	suffix	thing that affects in a particular way

J

jaund/o-	combining form	yellow
jejun/o-	combining form	jejunum (middle part of small intestine)
jugul/o-	combining form	jugular (throat)

K

kal/i-	combining form	potassium
kary/o-	combining form	nucleus
kel/o-	combining form	tumor
kerat/o-	combining form	cornea (of the eye); hard, fibrous protein
ket/o-	combining form	ketones
keton/o-	combining form	ketones
kilo-	prefix	one thousand
-kine	suffix	movement
-kinesis	suffix	condition of movement
kines/o-	combining form	movement
kin/o-	combining form	movement
klept/o-	combining form	to steal
kyph/o-	combining form	bent; humpbacked

L

labi/o-	combining form	lip; labium
laborat/o-	combining form	workplace; testing place
labyrinth/o-	combining form	labyrinth (of the inner ear)
lacer/o-	combining form	a tearing
lacrim/o-	combining form	tears

lact/i-	combining form	milk
lact/o-	combining form	milk
-lalia	suffix	abnormal condition of talk
lamin/o-	combining form	lamina (flat area on the vertebra)
lapar/o-	combining form	abdomen
laryng/o-	combining form	larynx (voice box)
later/o-	combining form	side
lei/o-	combining form	smooth
lenticul/o-	combining form	lens (of the eye)
lent/o-	combining form	lens (of the eye)
-lepsy	suffix	seizure
leuk/o-	combining form	white
lev/o-	combining form	left
lex/o-	combining form	word
ligament/o-	combining form	ligament
ligat/o-	combining form	to tie up; to bind
limb/o-	combining form	edge; border
lingu/o-	combining form	tongue
lipid/o-	combining form	lipid (fat)
lip/o-	combining form	lipid (fat)
-listhesis		see -olisthesis
-lith	suffix	stone
lith/o-	combining form	stone
lob/o-	combining form	lobe of an organ
locat/o-	combining form	a place
loc/o-	combining form	in one place
log/o-	combining form	word; the study of
-logy	suffix	the study of
lord/o-	combining form	swayback
luc/o-	combining form	clear
lumb/o-	combining form	lower back; area between the ribs and pelvis
lumin/o-	combining form	lumen (opening)
lun/o-	combining form	moon
-ly	suffix	going toward
lymph/o-	combining form	lymph; lymphatic system
ly/o-	combining form	break down; destroy
-lysis	combining form	process of breaking down or destroying
lys/o-	combining form	break down; destroy
-lyte	suffix	dissolved substance

M

macr/o-	combining form	large
macul/o-	combining form	small area or spot
magnet/o-	combining form	magnet
mal-	prefix	bad; inadequate

-malacia	combination combining form and suffix	condition of softening
malac/o-	combining form	softening
malign/o-	combining form	intentionally causing harm; cancer
malle/o-	combining form	malleus (hammer-shaped bone)
malleol/o-	combining form	malleolus
mamm/a-	combining form	breast
mamm/o-	combining form	breast
mandibul/o-	combining form	mandible (lower jaw)
-mania	combination combining form and suffix	condition of frenzy
man/o-	combining form	thin; frenzy
manu/o-	combining form	hand
masset/o-	combining form	chewing
mastic/o-	combining form	chewing
mast/o-	combining form	breast; mastoid process
mastoid/o-	combining form	mastoid process
matur/o-	combining form	mature
maxill/o-	combining form	maxilla (upper jaw)
mediastin/o-	combining form	mediastinum
medic/o-	combining form	physician; medicine
medi/o-	combining form	middle
medull/o-	combining form	medulla (inner region)
meg/a-	combining form	large
megal/o-	combining form	large
-megaly	suffix	enlargement
melan/o-	combining form	black
melen/o-	combining form	black
meningi/o-	combining form	meninges
mening/o-	combining form	meninges
menisc/o-	combining form	meniscus (crescent-shaped cartilage)
men/o-	combining form	month
menstru/o-	combining form	monthly discharge of blood
-ment	suffix	action; state
ment/o-	combining form	mind; chin
mesenter/o-	combining form	mesentery
mesi/o-	combining form	middle
meso-	prefix	middle
meta-	prefix	after; subsequent to; transition; change
metabol/o-	combining form	change; transformation
-meter	suffix	instrument used to measure
metri/o-	combining form	uterus (womb)
metr/o-	combining form	measurement; uterus (womb)
-metry	suffix	process of measuring

micr/o-	combining form	one millionth; small
micturi/o-	combining form	making urine
mid-	prefix	middle
-mileusis	suffix	process of carving
mineral/o-	combining form	mineral; electrolyte
mi/o-	combining form	narrowing
mit/o-	combining form	threadlike structure
mitr/o-	combining form	structure like a miter (tall hat with two points)
mitt/o-	combining form	to send
mon/o-	combining form	one; single
morbid/o-	combining form	disease
morb/o-	combining form	disease
morph/o-	combining form	shape
mort/o-	combining form	death
motil/o-	combining form	movement
mot/o-	combining form	movement
-motor	suffix	thing that produces movement
muc/o-	combining form	mucus
mucos/o-	combining form	mucous membrane
mult/i-	combining form	many
muscul/o-	combining form	muscle
mutat/o-	combining form	to change
myc/o-	combining form	fungus
mydr/o-	combining form	widening
myelin/o-	combining form	myelin
myel/o-	combining form	bone marrow; spinal cord; myelin
my/o-	combining form	muscle
myop/o-	combining form	near
myos/o-	combining form	muscle
myring/o-	combining form	tympanic membrane (eardrum)
myx/o-	combining form	mucus-like substance

N

narc/o-	combining form	stupor; sleep
nas/o-	combining form	nose
-nate	suffix	thing that is born
nat/o-	combining form	birth
necr/o-	combining form	dead cells, tissue, or body
ne/o-	combining form	new
nephr/o-	combining form	kidney; nephron
nerv/o-	combining form	nerve
neur/o-	combining form	nerve
neutr/o-	combining form	not taking part
nid/o-	combining form	nest; focus
-nine	suffix	pertaining to a single chemical substance
noct/o-	combining form	night

nocturn/o-	combining form	night
nod/o-	combining form	node (knob of tissue)
nodul/o-	combining form	small, knobby mass
non-	prefix	not
norm/o-	combining form	normal; usual
nosocomi/o-	combining form	hospital
nuch/o-	combining form	neck
nucle/o-	combining form	nucleus (of a cell or an atom)
null/i-	combining form	none
nutri/o-	combining form	nourishment
nutriti/o-	combining form	nourishment

O

obes/o-	combining form	fat
obsess/o-	combining form	besieged by thoughts
obstetr/o-	combining form	pregnancy and childbirth
obstip/o-	combining form	severe constipation
obstruct/o-	combining form	blocked by a barrier
occipit/o-	combining form	occiput (back of the head)
occlus/o-	combining form	close against
ocul/o-	combining form	eye
odont/o-	combining form	tooth
odyn/o-	combining form	pain
-oid	suffix	resembling
-ol	suffix	chemical substance
-ole	suffix	small thing
olfact/o-	combining form	the sense of smell
olig/o-	combining form	scanty; few
olisthe/o-	combining form	slipping
-olisthesis	combination combining form and suffix	abnormal condition with slipping
-oma	suffix	tumor; mass
-omatosis	combination combining form and suffix	abnormal condition of multiple tumors or masses
oment/o-	combining form	omentum
om/o-	combining form	tumor; mass
omphal/o-	combining form	umbilicus; navel
-on	suffix	a substance; structure
onc/o-	combining form	tumor; mass
-one	suffix	chemical substance
onych/o-	combining form	nail (fingernail or toenail)
o/o-	combining form	ovum (egg)
oophor/o-	combining form	ovary
operat/o-	combining form	perform a procedure; surgery
ophidi/o-	combining form	snake
ophthalm/o-	combining form	eye
-opia	suffix	condition of vision

opportun/o-	combining form	well timed; taking advantage of an opportunity
oppos/o-	combining form	forceful resistance
-opsy	suffix	process of viewing
optic/o-	combining form	lenses; properties of light
opt/o-	combining form	eye; vision
-or	suffix	person or thing that produces or does
orbicul/o-	combining form	small circle
orbit/o-	combining form	orbit (eye socket)
orchi/o-	combining form	testis
orch/o-	combining form	testis
orex/o-	combining form	appetite
organ/o-	combining form	organ
or/o-	combining form	mouth
orth/o-	combining form	straight
-ory	suffix	having the function of
-ose	suffix	full of
-osing	suffix	condition of doing
-osis	suffix	condition; abnormal condition; process
osm/o-	combining form	the sense of smell
osse/o-	combining form	bone
ossicul/o-	combining form	ossicle (little bone)
ossificat/o-	combining form	changing into bone
oste/o-	combining form	bone
ot/o-	combining form	ear
-ous	suffix	pertaining to
ovari/o-	combining form	ovary
ov/i-	combining form	ovum (egg)
ov/o-	combining form	ovum (egg)
ovul/o-	combining form	ovum (egg)
ox/i-	combining form	oxygen
ox/o-	combining form	oxygen
ox/y-	combining form	oxygen; quick

P

palat/o-	combining form	palate
palliat/o-	combining form	reduce the severity of
palpat/o-	combining form	touching; feeling
palpit/o-	combining form	to throb
pan-	prefix	all
pancreat/o-	combining form	pancreas
papill/o-	combining form	elevated structure
par-	prefix	beside
para-	prefix	beside; apart from; two parts of a pair; abnormal
parenchym/o-	combining form	parenchyma (functional cells of an organ)

-paresis	suffix	condition of weakness
pareun/o-	combining form	sexual intercourse
pariet/o-	combining form	wall of a cavity
par/o-	combining form	birth
paroxysm/o-	combining form	sudden, sharp attack
part/o-	combining form	childbirth
-partum	suffix	childbirth
parturit/o-	combining form	to be in labor
patell/o-	combining form	patella (kneecap)
-path	suffix	disease; suffering
pathet/o-	combining form	suffering
path/o-	combining form	disease; suffering
-pathy	suffix	disease; suffering
pat/o-	combining form	to be open
-pause	suffix	cessation
paus/o-	combining form	cessation
pect/o-	combining form	stiff
pector/o-	combining form	chest
pedicul/o-	combining form	lice
ped/o-	combining form	child
pelv/i-	combining form	pelvis (hip bone; renal pelvis)
pelv/o-	combining form	pelvis (hip bone; renal pelvis)
pendul/o-	combining form	hanging down
-penia	suffix	condition of deficiency
pen/o-	combining form	penis
pepsin/o-	combining form	pepsin
peps/o-	combining form	digestion
pept/o-	combining form	digestion
per-	prefix	through; throughout
percuss/o-	combining form	tapping
perfor/o-	combining form	to have an opening
peri-	prefix	around
perine/o-	combining form	perineum
peripher/o-	combining form	outer aspects
peritone/o-	combining form	peritoneum
periton/o-	combining form	peritoneum
perone/o-	combining form	fibula (lower leg bone)
person/o-	combining form	person
petechi/o-	combining form	petechiae
-pexy	suffix	process of surgically fixing in place
phac/o-	combining form	lens (of the eye)
-phage	suffix	thing that eats
-phagia	combination combining form and suffix	abnormal condition of eating and swallowing
phag/o-	combining form	eating; swallowing
phak/o-	combining form	lens (of the eye)
phalang/o-	combining form	phalanx (finger or toe)

pharmaceutic/o-	combining form	medicine; drug
pharmac/o-	combining form	medicine; drug
pharyng/o-	combining form	pharynx (throat)
-pharynx	suffix	pharynx (throat)
-phasia	combination combining form and suffix	abnormal condition of speech
phas/o-	combining form	speech
phe/o-	combining form	gray
-phil	suffix	attraction to; fondness for
-phile	suffix	person who is attracted to or is fond of
phil/o-	combining form	attraction to; fondness for
phim/o-	combining form	closed tight
phleb/o-	combining form	vein
phob/o-	combining form	fear; avoidance
phor/o-	combining form	to bear; to carry; range
phosph/o-	combining form	phosphorus
phot/o-	combining form	light
phren/o-	combining form	diaphragm; mind
phylact/o-	combining form	guarding; protecting
-phylaxis	suffix	condition of guarding or protecting
-phyma	suffix	tumor; growth
physic/o-	combining form	body
physi/o-	combining form	physical function
-physis	suffix	state of growing
phys/o-	combining form	inflate; distend; grow
-phyte	suffix	growth
pigment/o-	combining form	pigment
pil/o-	combining form	hair
pituitar/o-	combining form	pituitary gland
pituit/o-	combining form	pituitary gland
placent/o-	combining form	placenta
plak/o-	combining form	plaque
-plant	suffix	procedure to transfer or graft
-plasia	combination combining form and suffix	abnormal condition of growth
-plasm	suffix	growth; formed substance
plasm/o-	combining form	plasma
plas/o-	combining form	growth; formation
plast/o-	combining form	growth; formation
-plasty	suffix	process of reshaping by surgery
-plegia	combination combining form and suffix	condition of paralysis
pleg/o-	combining form	paralysis
pleur/o-	combining form	pleura (lung membrane)
-plex	suffix	parts

-pnea	suffix	breathing
pne/o-	combining form	breathing
pneum/o-	combining form	lung; air
pneumon/o-	combining form	lung; air
pod/o-	combining form	foot
-poiesis	suffix	condition of formation
-poietin	suffix	a substance that forms
poikil/o-	combining form	irregular
polar/o-	combining form	positive or negative state
pol/o-	combining form	pole
poly-	prefix	many; much
polyp/o-	combining form	polyp
poplite/o-	combining form	back of the knee
por/o-	combining form	small openings; pores
port/o-	combining form	point of entry
post-	prefix	after; behind
poster/o-	combining form	back part
potent/o-	combining form	being capable of doing
pract/o-	combining form	medical practice
pre-	prefix	before; in front of
pregn/o-	combining form	being with child
presby/o-	combining form	old age
press/o-	combining form	pressure
preventat/o-	combining form	prevent
prevent/o-	combining form	prevent
priap/o-	combining form	persistent erection
prim/i-	combining form	first
pro-	prefix	before
-probe	suffix	rodlike instrument
proct/o-	combining form	rectum and anus
product/o-	combining form	produce
project/o-	combining form	orientation
pronat/o-	combining form	face down
prostat/o-	combining form	prostate gland
prosthet/o-	combining form	artificial part
protein/o-	combining form	protein
proxim/o-	combining form	near the center or point of origin
prurit/o-	combining form	itching
psor/o-	combining form	itching
psych/o-	combining form	mind
-ptosis	suffix	state of prolapse; drooping; falling
-ptysis	suffix	abnormal condition of coughing up
puber/o-	combining form	growing up
pub/o-	combining form	pubis (hip bone)
pulmon/o-	combining form	lung
pulsat/o-	combining form	rhythmic throbbing

punct/o-	combining form	hole; perforation
pupill/o-	combining form	pupil (of the eye)
purul/o-	combining form	pus
pyel/o-	combining form	renal pelvis
pylor/o-	combining form	pylorus
py/o-	combining form	pus
pyret/o-	combining form	fever
pyr/o-	combining form	fire; burning

Q

quadri-	prefix	four
quantitat/o-	combining form	quantity or amount

R

radic/o-	combining form	all parts, including the root
radicul/o-	combining form	spinal nerve root
radi/o-	combining form	radius (forearm bone); x-rays; radiation
rap/o-	combining form	to seize and drag away
re-	prefix	again and again; backward; unable to
react/o-	combining form	reverse movement
recept/o-	combining form	receive
recess/o-	combining form	to move back
rect/o-	combining form	rectum
recuper/o-	combining form	recover
reduct/o-	combining form	to bring back; decrease
refract/o-	combining form	bend; deflect
regurgitat/o-	combining form	flow backward
relax/o-	combining form	relax
remiss/o-	combining form	send back
ren/o-	combining form	kidney
repress/o-	combining form	press back
resect/o-	combining form	to cut out; remove
resist/o-	combining form	withstand the effect of
resuscit/o-	combining form	revive; raise up again
retard/o-	combining form	slow down; delay
retent/o-	combining form	keep; hold back
reticul/o-	combining form	small network
retin/o-	combining form	retina (of the eye)
retro-	prefix	behind; backward
rex/o-		see *orex/o-*
rhabd/o-	combining form	rod shaped
rheumat/o-	combining form	watery discharge
rhin/o-	combining form	nose
rhiz/o-	combining form	spinal nerve root
rhythm/o-	combining form	rhythm

rhytid/o-	combining form	wrinkle
rib/o-	combining form	ribonucleic acid
roentgen/o-	combining form	x-rays; radiation
rotat/o-	combining form	rotate
-rrhage	suffix	excessive flow or discharge
rrhag/o-	combining form	excessive flow or discharge
-rrhaphy	suffix	procedure of suturing
-rrhea	suffix	flow; discharge
rrhe/o-	combining form	flow; discharge
rrhythm/o-	combining form	rhythm
-rubin	suffix	red substance
rub/o-	combining form	red
rug/o-	combining form	ruga (fold)

S

sacchar/o-	combining form	sugar
sacr/o-	combining form	sacrum
sagitt/o-	combining form	going from front to back
saliv/o-	combining form	saliva
salping/o-	combining form	uterine (fallopian) tube
-salpinx	suffix	uterine (fallopian) tube
saphen/o-	combining form	clearly visible
sarc/o-	combining form	connective tissue
satur/o-	combining form	filled up
scal/o-	combining form	series of graduated steps
scaph/o-	combining form	boat shaped
scapul/o-	combining form	scapula (shoulder blade)
schiz/o-	combining form	split
scient/o-	combining form	science; knowledge
scint/i-	combining form	point of light
scintill/o-	combining form	point of light
scler/o-	combining form	hard; sclera (white of the eye)
scoli/o-	combining form	curved; crooked
-scope	suffix	instrument used to examine
scop/o-	combining form	examine with an instrument
-scopy	suffix	process of using an instrument to examine
scot/o-	combining form	darkness
script/o-	combining form	write
scrot/o-	combining form	a bag; scrotum
sebace/o-	combining form	sebum (oil)
seb/o-	combining form	sebum (oil)
secret/o-	combining form	produce; secrete
sect/o-	combining form	to cut
sedat/o-	combining form	to calm agitation
semi-	prefix	half; partly
semin/i-	combining form	spermatozoon; sperm
semin/o-	combining form	spermatozoon; sperm

sen/o-	combining form	old age
sensitiv/o-	combining form	affected by; sensitive to
sensit/o-	combining form	affected by; sensitive to
sens/o-	combining form	sensation
sensor/i-	combining form	sensory
septic/o-	combining form	infection
sept/o-	combining form	septum (dividing wall)
ser/o-	combining form	serum of the blood; serumlike fluid
sex/o-	combining form	sex
sial/o-	combining form	saliva; salivary gland
sigmoid/o-	combining form	sigmoid colon
-sin	suffix	a substance
sin/o-	combining form	hollow cavity; channel
sinus/o-	combining form	sinus
-sis	suffix	process; condition; abnormal condition
skelet/o-	combining form	skeleton
soci/o-	combining form	human beings; community
somat/o-	combining form	body
-some	suffix	a body
somn/o-	combining form	sleep
som/o-	combining form	a body
son/o-	combining form	sound
sorb/o-	combining form	to suck up
spad/o-	combining form	tear; opening
-spasm	suffix	sudden, involuntary muscle contraction
spasm/o-	combining form	spasm
spasmod/o-	combining form	spasm
spast/o-	combining form	spasm
spermat/o-	combining form	spermatozoon; sperm
sperm/o-	combining form	spermatozoon; sperm
sphen/o-	combining form	wedge shape
sphenoid/o-	combining form	sphenoid bone; sphenoid sinus
-sphere	suffix	sphere; ball
spher/o-	combining form	sphere; ball
sphincter/o-	combining form	sphincter
sphygm/o-	combining form	pulse
spin/o-	combining form	spine; backbone
spir/o-	combining form	breathe; a coil
splen/o-	combining form	spleen
spondyl/o-	combining form	vertebra
squam/o-	combining form	scalelike cell
stal/o-	combining form	contraction
-stalsis	combination combining form and suffix	process of contraction
staped/o-	combining form	stapes (stirrup-shaped bone)

-stasis	suffix	condition of standing still; staying in one place
stas/o-	combining form	standing still; staying in one place
stat/o-	combining form	standing still; staying in one place
steat/o-	combining form	fat
sten/o-	combining form	narrowness; constriction
stere/o-	combining form	three dimensions
stern/o-	combining form	sternum (breast bone)
-steroid	suffix	steroid
steroid/o-	combining form	steroid
-sterol	suffix	lipid-containing compound
steth/o-	combining form	chest
sthen/o-	combining form	strength
stigmat/o-	combining form	point; mark
stimul/o-	combining form	exciting; strengthening
stomat/o-	combining form	mouth
stom/o-	combining form	surgically created opening or mouth
-stomy	suffix	surgically created opening
strangul/o-	combining form	to constrict
strept/o-	combining form	curved
stress/o-	combining form	disturbing stimulus
styl/o-	combining form	stake
sub-	prefix	below; underneath; less than
sucr/o-	combining form	sugar (cane sugar)
suct/o-	combining form	to suck
sudor/i-	combining form	sweat
su/i-	combining form	self
super-	prefix	above; beyond
superfici/o-	combining form	on or near the surface
super/o-	combining form	above
supinat/o-	combining form	lying on the back
supposit/o-	combining form	placed beneath
suppress/o-	combining form	press down
suppur/o-	combining form	pus formation
supra-	prefix	above
surg/o-	combining form	operative procedure
suspens/o-	combining form	hanging
sym-	prefix	together; with
symptomat/o-	combining form	collection of symptoms
syn-	prefix	together
syncop/o-	combining form	fainting
synovi/o-	combining form	synovium (membrane)
synov/o-	combining form	synovium (membrane)
system/o-	combining form	the body as a whole
-systole	suffix	contraction
systol/o-	combining form	contracting

T

Term	Type	Definition
tachy-	prefix	fast
tact/o-	combining form	touch
tampon/o-	combining form	stop up
tard/o-	combining form	late; slow
tars/o-	combining form	ankle
tax/o-	combining form	coordination
techn/o-	combining form	technical skill
tele/o-	combining form	distance
tempor/o-	combining form	temple (side of the head)
tendin/o-	combining form	tendon
tendon/o-	combining form	tendon
ten/o-	combining form	tendon
tens/o-	combining form	pressure; tension
terat/o-	combining form	bizarre form
termin/o-	combining form	end; boundary
testicul/o-	combining form	testis; testicle
test/o-	combining form	testis; testicle
tetr/a-	combining form	four
thalam/o-	combining form	thalamus
thanat/o-	combining form	death
thec/o-	combining form	sheath; layer of membranes
theli/o-	combining form	cellular layer
then/o-	combining form	thumb
therapeut/o-	combining form	therapy; treatment
therap/o-	combining form	treatment
-therapy	suffix	treatment
therm/o-	combining form	heat
thorac/o-	combining form	thorax (chest)
-thorax	suffix	thorax (chest)
thromb/o-	combining form	thrombus (blood clot)
thym/o-	combining form	thymus; rage
thyr/o-	combining form	shield-shaped structure (thyroid gland)
thyroid/o-	combining form	thyroid gland
tibi/o-	combining form	tibia (shin bone)
-tic	suffix	pertaining to
till/o-	combining form	pull out
-tion	suffix	a process; being or having
toc/o-	combining form	labor and childbirth
toler/o-	combining form	to become accustomed to
-tome	suffix	instrument used to cut; area with distinct edges
tom/o-	combining form	cut; slice; layer
-tomy	suffix	process of cutting or making an incision
ton/o-	combining form	pressure; tone
tonsill/o-	combining form	tonsil

Term	Type	Definition
-tope	suffix	place; position
topic/o-	combining form	a specific area
-tor	suffix	person or thing that produces or does
tort/i-	combining form	twisted position
-tous	suffix	pertaining to
toxic/o-	combining form	poison; toxin
tox/o-	combining form	poison
trabecul/o-	combining form	trabecula (mesh)
trache/o-	combining form	trachea (windpipe)
trac/o-	combining form	visible path
tract/o-	combining form	pulling
tranquil/o-	combining form	calm
trans-	prefix	across; through
transit/o-	combining form	change over from one thing to another
transmitt/o-	combining form	to send across or through
transplant/o-	combining form	move something to another place
traumat/o-	combining form	injury
tremul/o-	combining form	shaking
-tresia	suffix	opening or hole
tri-	prefix	three
trich/o-	combining form	hair
triglycerid/o-	combining form	triglyceride
-tripsy	suffix	process of crushing
-triptor	suffix	thing that crushes
trochanter/o-	combining form	trochanter
trochle/o-	combining form	structure shaped like a pulley
-tron	suffix	instrument
troph/o-	combining form	development
-trophy	suffix	process of development
trop/o-	combining form	having an affinity for; stimulating; turning
tubercul/o-	combining form	nodule; tuberculosis
tuber/o-	combining form	nodule
tuberos/o-	combining form	knoblike projection
tub/o-	combining form	tube
tubul/o-	combining form	tube; small tube
turbin/o-	combining form	scroll-like structure; turbinate
tuss/o-	combining form	cough
-ty	suffix	quality or state
tympan/o-	combining form	tympanic membrane (eardrum)
-type	suffix	particular kind of; a model of

U

Term	Type	Definition
-ual	suffix	pertaining to
-ula	suffix	small thing

-ular	suffix	pertaining to a small thing
ulcerat/o-	combining form	ulcer
-ule	suffix	small thing
uln/o-	combining form	ulna (forearm bone)
ultra-	prefix	beyond; higher
-um	suffix	a structure; period of time
umbilic/o-	combining form	umbilicus; navel
un-	prefix	not
ungu/o-	combining form	nail (fingernail or toenail)
uni-	prefix	single; not paired
-ure	suffix	system; result of
ureter/o-	combining form	ureter
urethr/o-	combining form	urethra
urin/o-	combining form	urine; urinary system
ur/o-	combining form	urine; urinary system
-us	suffix	thing; condition
uter/o-	combining form	uterus (womb)
uve/o-	combining form	uvea (of the eye)

V

vaccin/o-	combining form	giving a vaccine
vagin/o-	combining form	vagina
vag/o-	combining form	wandering; vagus nerve
valv/o-	combining form	valve
valvul/o-	combining form	valve
varic/o-	combining form	varix; varicose vein
vascul/o-	combining form	blood vessel
vas/o-	combining form	blood vessel; vas deferens
vegetat/o-	combining form	growth
veget/o-	combining form	vegetable
venere/o-	combining form	sexual intercourse
ven/i-	combining form	vein
ven/o-	combining form	vein
ventilat/o-	combining form	movement of air
ventil/o-	combining form	movement of air

vent/o-	combining form	a coming
ventricul/o-	combining form	ventricle (lower heart chamber; chamber in the brain)
ventr/o-	combining form	front; abdomen
verd/o-	combining form	green
-verse	suffix	to travel; to turn
vers/o-	combining form	to travel; to turn
vertebr/o-	combining form	vertebra
vert/o-	combining form	to travel; to turn
vesic/o-	combining form	bladder; fluid-filled sac
vesicul/o-	combining form	bladder; fluid-filled sac
vestibul/o-	combining form	vestibule (entrance)
vest/o-	combining form	to dress
viril/o-	combining form	masculine
vir/o-	combining form	virus
viscer/o-	combining form	large internal organs
viscos/o-	combining form	thickness
vis/o-	combining form	sight; vision
vitre/o-	combining form	transparent substance; vitreous humor
voc/o-	combining form	voice
volunt/o-	combining form	done of one's own free will
vuls/o-	combining from	to tear
vulv/o-	combining form	vulva

X–Y

xanth/o-	combining form	yellow
xen/o-	combining form	foreign
xer/o-	combining form	dry
xiph/o-	combining form	sword

Z

-zoon	suffix	animal; living thing
zygomat/o-	combining form	zygoma (cheekbone)

Appendix B
GLOSSARY OF MEDICAL ABBREVIATIONS

* An asterisk beside an abbreviation means it is included (or may be included in the future) on a list compiled by the Joint Commission on Accreditation of Healthcare Organizations (JCAHO). The JCAHO list contains abbreviations that have been the cause of errors. These abbreviations should not be used, and the JCAHO's National Safety Goal states that these abbreviations also must appear on a healthcare facility's "Do Not Use" list. This is a short list because it is the minimum required by JCAHO to obtain facility accreditation. However, because these abbreviations are still used by some healthcare providers, they are included here.

■ A square beside an abbreviation means it is from a more comprehensive list of abbreviations that should not be used, as compiled by the Institute for Safe Medication Practices (ISMP).

5-HIAA	5-hydroxyindoleacetic acid

A

A	blood type A in the ABO blood group
A&O	alert and oriented
A&P	anatomy and physiology; auscultation and percussion
AAA	abdominal aortic aneurysm
AB	blood type AB in the ABO blood group
AB, Ab	abortion
ABD	abdomen
ABG	arterial blood gases
ABR	auditory brainstem response
ACE	angiotensin-converting enzyme
Ach	acetylcholine
ACS	acute coronary syndrome
ACT	activated clotting time
ACTH	adrenocorticotropic hormone
AD, A.D.*■	right ear (Latin, auris dextra)
ADA	American Dental Association; American Diabetes Association; American Dietetic Association; Americans with Disabilities Act
ADD	attention deficit disorder
ADH	antidiuretic hormone
ADHD	attention-deficit hyperactivity disorder
ADLs	activities of daily living
AED	automatic external defibrillator
AFB	acid-fast bacillus
A fib	atrial fibrillation
AFP	alpha fetoprotein
AGA	appropriate for gestational age
AI	aortic insufficiency; apical impulse; artificial insemination; artificial intelligence
AICD	automatic implantable cardiac defibrillator; automatic implantable cardioverter-defibrillator
AIDS	acquired immunodeficiency syndrome
AKA	above-the-knee amputation
alk phos	alkaline phosphatase
ALL	acute lymphocytic leukemia

ALP	alkaline phosphatase
ALS	amyotrophic lateral sclerosis
ALT	alanine aminotransferase
AMI	acute myocardial infarction
AML	acute myelogenous leukemia
ANS	autonomic nervous system
AP	anteroposterior
ARDS	acute respiratory distress syndrome; adult respiratory distress syndrome
ARF	acute renal failure; acute respiratory failure; acute rheumatic fever
ARM	artificial rupture of membranes
ARMD	age-related macular degeneration
AS	aortic stenosis
AS, A.S.*■	left ear (Latin, auris sinister)
ASC	ambulatory surgery center
ASC-H	atypical squamous cells, cannot exclude HSIL
ASC-US	atypical squamous cells of undetermined significance
ASCVD	arteriosclerotic cardiovascular disease
ASD	atrial septal defect
ASHD	arteriosclerotic heart disease
ASIS	anterior-superior iliac spine
AST	aspartate aminotransferase
ATN	acute tubular necrosis
AU, A.U.*■	both ears (Latin, auris unitas); each ear (Latin, auris uterque)
AV	atrioventricular
AVM	arteriovenous malformation

B

B	blood type B in the ABO blood group
Ba	barium
BAEP	brainstem auditory evoked potential
BAER	brainstem auditory evoked response
bagged	manually ventilated with an Ambu bag (slang)
baso	basophil (slang)
BBT	basal body temperature

BDI	Beck Depression Inventory
BE	barium enema; base excess (in the blood)
BKA	below-the-knee amputation
BM	bowel movement
BMD	bone mineral density
BMT	bone marrow transplantation
BOM	bilateral otitis media
BP	blood pressure
BPD	biparietal diameter (of the fetal head)
BPH	benign prostatic hypertrophy
BPM, bpm	beats per minute
BPP	biophysical profile
BRBPR	bright red blood per rectum
BRCA	breast cancer (gene)
BS	bowel sounds; breath sounds
BSE	breast self-examination
BSO	bilateral salpingo-oophorectomy
BUN	blood urea nitrogen
Bx	biopsy

C

C&S	culture and sensitivity
C1–C7	cervical vertebrae 1–7
Ca	cancer; carcinoma
Ca, Ca++	calcium
CABG	coronary artery bypass graft ("cabbage" slang)
CAD	coronary artery disease
CAPD	continuous ambulatory peritoneal dialysis
CAT	computerized axial tomography
cath	catheterize; catheterization (slang)
CBC	complete blood count
CBD	common bile duct
CBT	cognitive-behavioral therapy
CC	chief complaint
cc*■	cubic centimeter (measure of volume)
CCPD	continuous cycling peritoneal dialysis
CCU	coronary care unit
CDC	Centers for Disease Control
CDCP	Centers for Disease Control and Prevention
CDE	certified diabetes educator
CDH	congenital dislocation of the hip
CEA	carcinoembryonic antigen
CF	cystic fibrosis
chemo	chemotherapy (slang)
CHF	congestive heart failure
CIN	cervical intraepithelial neoplasia (grading system on Pap smear)
CIS	carcinoma *in situ*

CK	conductive keratoplasty; creatine kinase
CKD	chronic kidney disease
CK-MB	creatine kinase–MB band
Cl, Cl⁻	chloride
CLL	chronic lymphocytic leukemia
CLO	*Campylobacter*-like organism
CML	chronic myelogenous leukemia
cmm	cubic millimeter
CN1–CN12	cranial nerves 1–12
CNM	certified nurse midwife
CNS	central nervous system
CO	carbon monoxide
CO₂	carbon dioxide
COMT	catechol-*O*-methyltransferase
COPD	chronic obstructive pulmonary disease
COTA	certified occupational therapy assistant
CP	cardiopulmonary; cerebral palsy
CPAP	continuous positive airway pressure
CPD	cephalopelvic disproportion
CPK-MB	creatine phosphokinase–MB band
CPK-MM	creatine phosphokinase-MM
CPR	cardiopulmonary resuscitation; computerized patient record
CRF	cardiac risk factors; chronic renal failure
CRNA	certified registered nurse anesthetist
CRP	C-reactive protein
CRPS	chronic regional pain syndrome; complex regional pain syndrome
CRT	certified radiation therapist
CS	cesarean section ("C-section" slang)
CSF	cerebrospinal fluid
CT	computerized tomography
CTD	cumulative trauma disorder
CTR	certified tumor registrar
CTS	carpal tunnel syndrome
CV	cardiovascular
CVA	cerebrovascular accident
CVS	chorionic villus sampling
CXR	chest x-ray
cysto	cystoscopy (slang)

D

D/C*■	discharge; discontinue
D&C	dilation and curettage
dB, db	decibel
D.C.	Doctor of Chiropracty (or Chiropractic Medicine)
D.D.S.	Doctor of Dental Surgery
derm	dermatology (slang)

DEXA, DXA	dual energy x-ray absorptiometry
DI	diabetes insipidus
DIC	disseminated intravascular coagulation
diff	differential count of WBCs (slang)
DIP	distal interphalangeal (joint)
DJD	degenerative joint disease
DKA	diabetic ketoacidosis
DM	diabetes mellitus
DNA	deoxyribonucleic acid
D.O.	Doctor of Osteopathy (or Osteopathic Medicine)
DOE	dyspnea on exertion
D.P.M.	Doctor of Podiatry (or Podiatric Medicine)
Dr.	doctor
DRE	digital rectal examination
DS	discharge summary
DSA	digital subtraction angiography
DSM-IV	*Diagnostic and Statistical Manual of Mental Disorders*, 4th edition
DT	delirium tremens
DTR	deep tendon reflex
DUB	dysfunctional uterine bleeding
DVT	deep venous thrombosis
Dx	diagnosis
DXA	dual energy x-ray absorptiometry

E

EAC	external auditory canal
EBT	electron beam tomography
EBV	Epstein-Barr virus
ECCE	extracapsular cataract extraction
ECG	electrocardiogram; electrocardiography
echo	echocardiogram; echocardiography (slang)
ECT	electroconvulsive therapy
ECV	external cephalic version
ED	emergency department; erectile dysfunction
EDB	estimated date of birth
EDC	estimated date of confinement; extensor digitorum communis
EEG	electroencephalogram; electroencephalography
EGA	estimated gestational age
EGD	esophagogastroduodenoscopy
EHR	electronic health record
EKG	electrocardiogram; electrocardiography
ELISA	enzyme-linked immunosorbent assay
EMB	endometrial biopsy
EMG	electromyogram; electromyography
END	electroneurodiagnostic (technician)
ENT	ears, nose, and throat
eo	eosinophil (slang)

EOM	extraocular movements; extraocular muscles
EOMI	extraocular muscles intact
epi	epithelial cell (in a urine specimen); epinephrine (slang)
EPO	erythropoietin
EPR	electronic patient record
EPS	electrophysiologic study
ER	emergency room; estrogen receptor
ERCP	endoscopic retrograde cholangiopancreatography
ESRD	end-stage renal disease
ESWL	extracorporeal shock wave lithotripsy
ESWT	extracorporeal shock wave therapy
ET	endotracheal
ETOH	ethyl alcohol; ethanol (liquor)
ETT	endotracheal tube

F

FBS	fasting blood sugar
Fe	ferritin (iron)
FEV_1	forced expiratory volume (in one second)
FHR	fetal heart rate
fib	fibula (slang)
FIGO	Federation Internationale de Gynécologie et Obstétrique (scoring system)
FiO_2	fraction (percentage) of inspired oxygen
FOBT	fecal occult blood test
FSH	follicle-stimulating hormone
FTI	free thyroxine index
FVC	forced vital capacity
Fx	fracture

G

G	gravida; gauge (of a needle)
G/TPAL	see *G* and *TPAL*
GC	gonococcus (*Neisseria gonorrhoeae*)
GCS	Glasgow Coma Scale (or Score)
G-CSF	granulocyte colony-stimulating factor
GDM	gestational diabetes mellitus
GERD	gastroesophageal reflux disease
GGT	gamma-glutamyl transpeptidase
GH	growth hormone
GI	gastrointestinal
GIFT	gamete intrafallopian transfer
GM-CSF	granulocyte-macrophage colony-stimulating factor
GTT	glucose tolerance test
GU	genitourinary; gonococcal urethritis
GVHD	graft-versus-host disease
GYN	gynecology

H

H&H	hemoglobin and hematocrit
H&P	history and physical examination
HAV	hepatitis A virus
Hb	hemoglobin
HbA$_{1C}$	hemoglobin A$_{1C}$
HbCO	carboxyhemoglobin
HBV	hepatitis B virus
HCG, hCG	human chorionic gonadotropin
HCO$_3^-$	bicarbonate
HCT	hematocrit
HCV	hepatitis C virus
HDL	high-density lipoprotein
HEENT	head, eyes, ears, nose, and throat
Hg	mercury
Hgb	hemoglobin
HIDA	hydroxyiminodiacetic acid
HIPAA	Health Insurance Portability and Accountability Act
HIV	human immunodeficiency virus
HLA	human leukocyte antigen
HMD	hyaline membrane disease
HNP	herniated nucleus pulposus
hpf	high-power field
HPI	history of present illness
HPV	human papillomavirus
HRT	hormone replacement therapy
HSG	hysterosalpingogram; hysterosalpingography
HSIL	high-grade squamous intraepithelial lesion
HSV	herpes simplex virus
HTN	hypertension
Hx	history
Hz	hertz

I

I&D	incision and drainage
I&O	intake and output
IBD	inflammatory bowel disease
IBS	irritable bowel syndrome
ICCE	intracapsular cataract extraction
ICD-9	*International Classification of Diseases,* 9th edition
ICP	intracranial pressure
ICSI	intracytoplasmic sperm injection
IDDM	insulin-dependent diabetes mellitus
IgA	immunoglobulin A
IgD	immunoglobulin D
IgE	immunoglobulin E
IgG	immunoglobulin G
IgM	immunoglobulin M

IM	intramuscular
INR	international normalized ratio
IOL	intraocular lens
IOP	intraocular pressure
IRS	insulin resistance syndrome
IUGR	intrauterine growth retardation
IVC	intravenous cholangiogram; intravenous cholangiography
IVF	*in vitro* fertilization
IVP	intravenous pyelogram; intravenous pyelography

J

JOD	juvenile onset diabetes (mellitus)
JVD	jugular venous distention

K

K, K$^+$	potassium
KS	Kaposi's sarcoma
KUB	kidneys, ureters, bladder

L

L&D	labor and delivery
L/S	lecithin/sphingomyelin (ratio)
L1–L5	lumbar vertebrae 1–5
LA	left atrium
LASIK	laser-assisted *in situ* keratomileusis
Lat	lateral
LBBB	left bundle branch block
LDH	lactic dehydrogenase
LDL	low-density lipoprotein
LEEP	loop electrocautery excision procedure
LES	lower esophageal sphincter
LFTs	liver function tests
LGA	large for gestational age
LH	luteinizing hormone
LLE	left lower extremity
LLL	left lower lobe (of the lung)
LLQ	left lower quadrant (of the abdomen)
LMP	last menstrual period
LP	lumbar puncture
LPN	licensed practical nurse
LSD	lysergic acid diethylamide (a street drug)
LSIL	low-grade squamous intraepithelial lesion
LTK	laser thermal keratoplasty
LUE	left upper extremity
LUL	left upper lobe (of the lung)
LUQ	left upper quadrant (of the abdomen)
LV	left ventricle

LVAD	left ventricular assist device
LVH	left ventricular hypertrophy
lymph	lymphocyte (slang)

M

MAO	monoamine oxidase
MCH	mean cell hemoglobin
MCHC	mean cell hemoglobin concentration
MCP	metacarpophalangeal (joint)
MCV	mean cell volume
M.D.	Doctor of Medicine
MD	muscular dystrophy
MDCT	multidetector-row computerized tomography
MDI	metered-dose inhaler
mets	metastases (slang); unit of measurement during cardiac treadmill stress test
MI	myocardial infarction
mL	milliliter (measure of volume)
mm Hg	millimeters of mercury
mm³	cubic millimeter
MMSE	mini mental status examination
mono	monocyte (slang); mononucleosis (slang)
MR	mitral regurgitation
MRA	magnetic resonance angiography
MRI	magnetic resonance imaging
MS*■	magnesium sulfate; morphine sulfate; multiple sclerosis
MSH	melanocyte-stimulating hormone
MUGA	multiple-gated acquisition (scan)
MVP	mitral valve prolapse

N

N&V	nausea and vomiting
Na, Na⁺	sodium
NB	newborn
NCS	nerve conduction study
NG	nasogastric
NICU	neonatal intensive care unit ("NIK-yoo"); neurologic intensive care unit ("NIK-yoo")
NIDDM	non-insulin-dependent diabetes mellitus
NK	natural killer (cell)
NP	nurse practitioner
NPH	neutral protamine Hagedorn (type of insulin); normal pressure hydrocephalus
NPO (n.p.o.)	nothing by mouth (Latin, *nil per os*)
NSAID	nonsteroidal anti-inflammatory drug
NSR	normal sinus rhythm
NST	nonstress test
NSVD	normal spontaneous vaginal delivery

O

O	blood type O in the ABO blood group
O&P	ova and parasites
O₂	oxygen
OA	osteoarthritis
OB	obstetrics
OCD	obsessive–compulsive disorder
OCG	oral cholecystogram; oral cholecystography
OCP	oral contraceptive pill
OD	overdose
OD, O.D.*■	right eye (Latin, *oculus dexter*)
O.D.	Doctor of Optometry
OGTT	oral glucose tolerance test
OOB	out of bed
ORIF	open reduction and internal fixation
ortho	orthopedics (slang)
OS, O.S.*■	left eye (Latin, *oculus sinister*)
OSHA	Occupational Safety and Health Administration
OT	occupational therapy; occupational therapist
OU, O.U.*■	both eyes (Latin, *oculus unitas*); each eye (Latin, *oculus uterque*)

P

P	para; phosphorus; pulse
PA	physician's assistant; posteroanterior
PAC	premature atrial contraction
PACU	postanesthesia recovery room ("PAK-yoo")
PAD	peripheral artery disease
Pap	Papanicolaou (smear or test)
PAP	prostatic acid phosphatase
PCO₂, pCO₂	partial pressure of carbon dioxide
PCP	phencyclidine (angel dust, a street drug); *Pneumocystis carinii* pneumonia; primary care physician
PD	prism diopter
PDA	patent ductus arteriosus
PDT	photodynamic therapy
PE	physical examination; pressure-equalizing (tube); pulmonary embolus
PEG	percutaneous endoscopic gastrostomy
PEJ	percutaneous endoscopic jejunostomy
PERRL	pupils equal, round, and reactive to light
PERRLA	pupils equal, round, reactive to light and accommodation
PET	positron emission tomography
PFT	pulmonary function test
pH	potential of hydrogen (acidity or alkalinity)
Pharm. D.	Doctor of Pharmacy

PICC	peripherally inserted central catheter
PICU	pediatric intensive care unit ("PIK-yoo")
PID	pelvic inflammatory disease
PIP	proximal interphalangeal (joint)
PM&R	physical medicine and rehabilitation
PMDD	premenstrual dysphoric disorder
PMH	past medical history
PMI	point of maximum impulse
PMN	polymorphonucleated (leukocyte)
PMS	premenstrual syndrome
PND	paroxysmal noctural dyspnea; postnasal drip; postnasal drainage
PO, p.o.	by mouth (Latin, *per os*)
PO$_2$, pO$_2$	partial pressure of oxygen
poly	polymorphonucleated leukocyte (slang)
PPD	protein purified derivative (TB test); packs per day (of cigarettes)
PR	progesterone receptor
PRBCs	packed red blood cells
PRK	photorefractive keratectomy
PRN, p.r.n.	as needed (Latin, *pro re nata*)
pro time	prothrombin time (slang)
PROM	passive range of motion; premature rupture of membranes
PSA	prostate-specific antigen
Psy, Psych	psychiatry (slang), psychology (slang)
PT	physical therapist; physical therapy; prothrombin time
PTC	percutaneous transhepatic cholangiography
PTCA	percutaneous transluminal coronary angioplasty
PTSD	posttraumatic stress disorder
PTT	partial thromboplastin time
PUD	peptic ulcer disease
PUVA	psoralen (drug) and ultraviolet A (light therapy)
PVC	premature ventricular contraction
PVD	peripheral vascular disease

Q

QCT	quantitative computerized tomography

R

R, r	roentgen (unit of exposure to x-rays or gamma rays)
RA	rheumatoid arthritis; right atrium; room air (no supplemental oxygen)
rad	radiation absorbed dose
RAIU	radioactive iodine uptake
RAST	radioallergosorbent test
RBBB	right bundle branch block

RBC	red blood cell
RDS	respiratory distress syndrome
rehab	rehabilitation (slang)
rem	roentgen-equivalent man
REM	rapid eye movement
RFA	radiofrequency (catheter) ablation
RIA	radioimmunoassay
RICE	rest, ice, compression, elevation
RIND	reversible ischemic neurologic deficit
RLE	right lower extremity
RLL	right lower lobe (of the lung)
RLQ	right lower quadrant (of the abdomen)
RML	right middle lobe (of the lung)
RN	registered nurse
RNA	ribonucleic acid
RNV	radionuclide ventriculography
R/O	rule out
ROM	range of motion; rupture of membranes
ROP	retinopathy of prematurity
ROS	review of systems
RP	retinitis pigmentosa
RPR	rapid plasma reagin (test)
RRT	registered radiologic technologist; registered respiratory therapist
RSI	repetitive strain injury
RUE	right upper extremity
RUL	right upper lobe (of the lung)
RUQ	right upper quadrant (of the abdomen)
RV	right ventricle

S

S1	first sacral vertebra
S$_1$–S$_4$	heart sounds 1–4
SA	sinoatrial
SAB	spontaneous abortion
SAD	seasonal affective disorder
SARS	severe acute respiratory syndrome
SBE	subacute bacterial endocarditis
SCC	squamous cell carcinoma
SCI	spinal cord injury
seg	segmented neutrophil (slang)
SG	specific gravity
SGA	small for gestational age
SGOT	serum glutamic-oxaloacetic transaminase
SGPT	serum glutamic-pyruvic transaminase
SIADH	syndrome of inappropriate ADH
SICU	surgical intensive care unit ("SIK-yoo")
SIDS	sudden infant death syndrome

SLE	systemic lupus erythematosus
SMA	sequential multichannel analysis
SMAC	sequential multichannel analysis with computer
SNF	skilled nursing facility ("sniff")
SOB	shortness of breath
SOM	serous otitis media
SPECT	single-photon emission computerized tomography
sp gr, SG	specific gravity
SQ*■	subcutaneous
SSEP	somatosensory evoked potential
SSER	somatosensory evoked response
SSRI	selective serotonin reuptake inhibitor
STD	sexually transmitted disease
subcu	subcutaneous
subQ■	subcutaneous
SVT	supraventricular tachycardia
Sx	symptoms

T

T&A	tonsillectomy and adenoidectomy
T1–T12	thoracic vertebrae 1–12
T_3, T3■	triiodothyronine
T_4	thyroxine
T_7	free thyroxine index (FTI)
TAB	therapeutic abortion
TACE	transarterial chemoembolization
TAH-BSO	total abdominal hysterectomy and bilateral salpingo-oophorectomy
TAT	Thematic Apperception Test
TB	tuberculosis
TEE	transesophageal echocardiogram; transesophageal echocardiography
TENS	transcutaneous electrical nerve stimulation (unit)
TFT	thyroid function test
THR	total hip replacement
TIA	transient ischemic attack
tib	tibia (slang)
TIBC	total iron-binding capacity
tib-fib	tibia and fibula (slang)
TM	tympanic membrane
TMJ	temporomandibular joint
TNF	tumor necrosis factor
TNM	tumor, nodes, metastases
TnT	troponin T
TNTC	too numerous to count

TPA	tissue plasminogen activator (drug)
TPAL	term newborns, premature newborns, abortions, living children
TPR	temperature, pulse, and respiration
trach	tracheostomy (slang)
TRAM	transverse rectus abdominis muscle (flap)
TRUS	transrectal ultrasound
TSE	testicular self-examination
TSH	thyroid-stimulating hormone
TURBT	transurethral resection of bladder tumor
TURP	transurethral resection of the prostate
TVH	total vaginal hysterectomy
Tx	treatment
TXM	type and crossmatch (slang)

U

UA	urinalysis
UGI	upper gastrointestinal (series)
URI	upper respiratory infection
US	ultrasound
UTI	urinary tract infection

V

V fib	ventricular fibrillation (slang)
V tach	ventricular tachycardia (slang)
V/Q	ventilation-perfusion (scan)
VBAC	vaginal birth after ceserean section ("V-back")
VCUG	voiding cystourethrogram; voiding cystourethrography
VD	venereal disease
VDRL	Venereal Disease Research Laboratory (test)
VEP	visual evoked potential
VER	visual evoked response
VF	visual field
VLDL	very low-density lipoprotein
VMA	vanillylmandelic acid
VS	vital signs
VSD	ventricular septal defect

W

WBC	white blood cell

Z

ZIFT	zygote intrafallopian transfer

Answer Key

Chapter 1   The Structure of Medical Language

CHAPTER REVIEW EXERCISES

Matching Exercise (p. 27)

2, 1, 1, 2, 3, 1

True or False Exercise (p. 27)

1. F 2. F 3. F 4. T 5. F 6. T 7. F 8. T

Fill in the Blank Exercise (p. 27)

1. a. combining form
   b. suffix
   c. prefix
2. a. reading
   b. listening
   c. thinking, analyzing, and understanding
   d. writing (or typing) and spelling
   e. speaking and pronouncing
3. a. cutane/o-, derm/o-
   b. intestin/o-, enter/o-
   c. psych/o-, ment/o-
4. a. hyper-
   b. sub-
   c. post-

Latin and Greek Singular and Plural Nouns Exercise (p. 28)

1. vertebrae
2. bursae
3. petechiae
4. rugae
5. bronchi
6. alveoli
7. thrombi
8. nuclei
9. bacteria
10. hila
11. diverticula
12. labia
13. ova
14. testes
15. diagnoses
16. irides
17. epididymides
18. phalanges
19. carcinomata
20. leiomyomata
21. ganglia
22. mitochondria

BUILDING MEDICAL WORDS

Word Parts Exercise (pp. 28–29)

1. P — away from; without
2. CF — abdomen
3. S — pertaining to
4. S — pertaining to
5. P — without; not
6. P — against
7. CF — small structure hanging from a larger structure; appendix
8. S — pertaining to
9. CF — artery
10. CF — joint
11. S — pertaining to
12. S — a process; being or having
13. P — two
14. CF — life; living organisms; living tissue
15. P — slow
16. CF — heart
17. CF — heart
18. CF — gallbladder
19. CF — colon
20. CF — colon
21. CF — rib
22. CF — skin
23. P — reversal of; without
24. CF — skin
25. CF — break down food; digest
26. P — painful; difficult; abnormal
27. S — surgical excision
28. P — innermost; within
29. CF — intestine
30. P — upon; above
31. CF — sensation; feeling
32. P — normal; good
33. CF — stomach
34. CF — set or group
35. S — a record or picture
36. S — process of recording
37. P — one half
38. CF — blood
39. CF — liver
40. P — above; more than normal
41. P — below; deficient
42. CF — uterus (womb)
43. S — condition; state; thing
44. S — medical treatment
45. S — pertaining to
46. S — pertaining to
47. P — between
48. CF — intestine
49. P — within
50. S — action; condition
51. S — process; disease from a specific cause
52. S — one who specializes in
53. S — inflammation of; infection of
54. S — pertaining to
55. CF — abdomen
56. CF — larynx (voice box)
57. CF — side
58. S — the study of
59. S — process of breaking down or destroying
60. P — bad; inadequate
61. CF — breast
62. S — enlargement
63. CF — monthly discharge of blood
64. CF — mind; chin
65. S — process of measuring
66. P — one; single
67. CF — muscle
68. CF — nose
69. CF — nerve
70. CF — nucleus
71. CF — nourishment
72. S — tumor; mass
73. S — condition; abnormal condition; process
74. S — pertaining to
75. S — disease; suffering
76. CF — pelvis
77. P — around
78. CF — eating; swallowing
79. CF — paralysis
80. CF — lung; air
81. P — many; much
82. P — after; behind
83. P — before; in front of
84. CF — mind
85. P — four
86. P — again and again; backward; unable to
87. S — instrument used to examine
88. S — process of using an instrument to examine
89. CF — spermatozoon; sperm
90. CF — breathe; a coil
91. S — surgically created opening
92. P — below; underneath; less than

93. P   fast
94. CF   pressure; tension
95. CF   treatment
96. S   treatment
97. CF   thyroid gland
98. S   process of cutting or making an incision
99. CF   tonsil
100. CF   trachea (windpipe)
101. P   across; through
102. P   three
103. CF   urine; urinary system
104. CF   uterus (womb)
105. CF   vagina
106. CF   vein

Meaning of a Word Part Exercise (p. 30)

1. poly-   polyneuritis
2. arthr/o-   arthropathy (or arthritis)
3. -logy   etymology (or cardiology)
4. -ectomy   appendectomy (or tonsillectomy)
5. brady-   bradycardia
6. tonsill/o-   tonsillitis
7. muscul/o-   muscular
8. ven/o-   venous (or intravenous)
9. -ism   hypothyroidism (or euthyroidism)
10. pneumon/o- pneumonia
11. -itis   tonsillitis (or arthritis or polyneuritis or laryngitis)
12. sub-   subcutaneous
13. -megaly   cardiomegaly
14. -pathy   arthropathy (or polyneuropathy)
15. gastr/o-   gastric (or gastroscopy or esophagogastroduodenoscopy)
16. esthes/o-   anesthesia
17. -scopy   gastroscopy (or esophagogastroduodenoscopy)

Analyze and Define Medical Words Exercise (pp. 30–32)

1. -ac   cardi/o-
   pertaining to   heart
   pertaining to the heart
2. -ic   hepat/o-
   pertaining to   liver
   pertaining to the liver
3. -itis   laryng/o-
   inflammation of; infection of   larynx (voice box)
   inflammation or infection of the larynx (voice box)
4. -ectomy   tonsill/o-
   surgical excision   tonsil
   surgical excision of the tonsil(s)
5. -logy   neur/o-
   the study of   nerve
   the study of the nerve(s)
6. -logy   psych/o-
   the study of   mind
   the study of the mind
7. -ia   pneumon/o-
   condition; state; thing   lung; air
   condition of the lung
8. -itis   arthr/o-
   inflammation of; infection of   joint
   inflammation of the joint
9. -scopy   gastr/o-
   using an instrument to examine   stomach
   using an instrument to examine the stomach
10. -pathy   poly-   neur/o-
    disease; suffering   many; much   nerve
    disease of many nerve(s)
11. -ia   an-   esthes/o-
    condition; state; thing   without; not   sensation; feeling
    condition without sensation or feeling
12. -ous   sub-   cutane/o-
    pertaining to   below;   skin
                                underneath;
                                less than
    pertaining to below or underneath the skin
13. -ia   tachy-   card/i-
    condition; state; thing   fast   heart
    condition of a fast heart (rate)

14. -ous   intra-   ven/o-
    pertaining to   within   vein
    pertaining to within the vein
15. -al   intra-   nas/o-
    pertaining to   within   nose
    pertaining to within the nose
16. -al   endo-   trache/o-
    pertaining to   innermost; within   trachea (windpipe)
    pertaining to within the trachea (windpipe)

Combining Form and Suffix Exercise (p. 33)

1. cardiac   9. urinary
2. digestive   10. urination
3. intestinal   11. arthropathy
4. appendectomy   12. cardiology
5. neuroma   13. cardiomegaly
6. pneumonia   14. colonoscope
7. therapist   15. hemolysis
8. tonsillitis

Prefix Exercise (p. 33)

1. hyper-   thyroidism   hyperthyroidism
2. poly-   uria   polyuria
3. epi-   gastric   epigastric
4. an-   uria   anuria
5. intra-   muscular   intramuscular
6. tachy-   cardia   tachycardia
7. post-   nasal   postnasal
8. dys-   uria   dysuria

Matching Exercise (p. 34)

4, 8, 12, 6, 5, 9, 2, 10, 1, 11, 3, 7

Word Analysis Exercise (p. 34)

1. -scopy   process of using an instrument to examine
   esophag/o-   esophagus
   gastr/o-   stomach
   duoden/o-   duodenum
   Process of using an instrument to examine the esophagus, stomach, and duodenum
2. -logy   the study of
   ot/o-   ear
   rhin/o-   nose
   laryng/o-   larynx (voice box)
   The study of the ear(s), nose, (throat), and larynx.

THE MEDICAL RECORD

True or False Exercise (p. 34)

1. T 2. F 3. T 4. F 5. F

Critical Thinking Questions (p. 35)

1. a. healthcare professionals can access the same record at the same time
   b. the record cannot be lost or damaged (because there is always a back-up electronic copy)
   c. it takes only seconds to retrieve a patient's past medical records (because the record is stored in computer that is on-site or can be accessed electronically in a remote location)
2. a. immunizations
   b. routine physical exams
   c. limit sun exposure and apply sunscreen
      (Other answers: have smoke detectors in the home, use seat belts, do monthly self-examination of the breasts or testicles, secure firearms kept in the home)
3. a. electronic medical record (EMR)
   b. electronic patient record (EPR)
   c. electronic health record (HER)

ABBREVIATIONS

Abbreviation Exercise (p. 35)

1. computerized patient record (or cardiopulmonary resuscitation)
2. discharge summary
3. chief complaint
4. history and physical (examination)
5. diagnosis
6. review of systems

APPLIED SKILLS

Circle Exercise (p. 35)

1. phalanx
2. testis
3. vertebrae
4. gastric
5. tonsillitis
6. bacteria
7. cardiac
8. appendectomy
9. urinary
10. psychiatrist

Spelling Exercise (p. 36)

1. cardiac
2. appendectomy
3. subcutaneous
4. laryngitis
5. mammography
6. psychiatry
7. tachycardia
8. tonsillitis
9. urination
10. venous

Hearing Medical Words Exercise (p. 36)

1. cardiac
2. appendectomy
3. urination
4. psychotherapy
5. intravenous
6. neurology
7. tonsillitis
8. uterine
9. subcutaneous
10. pneumonia

Pronunciation Exercise (p. 36)

1. kar
2. nair
3. tray
4. mus
5. kawl
6. pat
7. meg
8. mawg
9. koh
10. raw

Chapter 2   The Body in Health and Disease

ANATOMY AND PHYSIOLOGY

Labeling Exercise (pp. 60–61)

Exercise A

1. posterior (dorsal), 2. anterior (ventral), 3. medial, 4. lateral, 5. proximal, 6. distal

Exercise B

1. cranial cavity, 2. spinal cavity, 3. thoracic cavity, 4. diaphragm, 5. abdominal cavity, 6. pelvic cavity

Exercise C

1. cardiovascular system, 2. cardiology, 3. integumentary system, 4. dermatology, 5. urinary system, 6. urology, 7. gastrointestinal system, 8. gastroenterology

BUILDING MEDICAL WORDS

Combining Forms Exercise (pp. 62–63)

1. back; dorsum
2. abdomen
3. before; front part
4. heart
5. tail (tail bone)
6. hollow space
7. head
8. cartilage
9. structure that encircles like a crown
10. cranium (skull)
11. secrete
12. tooth
13. skin
14. foods; diet
15. away from the center or point of origin
16. intestine
17. outside
18. front
19. stomach
20. genitalia
21. old age
22. female; woman
23. blood
24. physician; medical treatment
25. ilium (hip bone)
26. immune response
27. below
28. groin
29. skin
30. inside
31. intestine
32. larynx (voice box)
33. side
34. lower back; area between the ribs and pelvis
35. lymph; lymphatic system
36. large
37. physician; medicine
38. middle
39. one millionth; small
40. muscle
41. birth
42. new
43. nerve
44. nerve
45. nucleus (of an atom)
46. pregnancy and childbirth
47. tumor; mass
48. eye
49. straight
50. ear
51. child
52. pelvis (hip bone; renal pelvis)
53. medicine; drug
54. physical function
55. back part
56. produce
57. near the center or point of origin
58. mind
59. lung
60. radius (forearm bone); x-rays; radiation
61. going from front to back
62. examine with an instrument
63. skeleton
64. spine; backbone
65. breathe; a coil
66. above
67. thorax (chest)
68. cut; slice; layer
69. umbilicus; navel
70. urine; urinary system
71. urine; urinary system
72. blood vessel
73. front; abdomen
74. to travel; to turn
75. large internal organs

Combining Form and Suffix Exercise (pp. 63–64)

1. -al — abdominal
2. -logy — physiology
3. -ar — lumbar
4. -ad — cephalad
5. -al — distal
6. -ic — thoracic
7. -al — cranial
8. -ior — posterior
9. -logy — dermatology
10. -atic — lymphatic
11. -al — lateral
12. -al — internal
13. -logy — cardiology
14. -ics — obstetrics
15. -logy — urology
16. -logy — pulmonology
17. -logy — ophthalmology
18. -ary — integumentary
19. -logy — gynecology
20. -iatry — psychiatry
21. -ous — nervous
22. -ary — urinary
23. -logy — oncology
24. -ior — anterior
25. -al — inguinal

26. -ity	cavity
27. -logy	hematology
28. -istry	dentistry
29. -logy	neurology
30. -ar	muscular
31. -al	medial
32. -ior	superior
33. -logy	cardiology
34. -logy	pharmacology
35. -ics	dietetics
36. -logy	radiology
37. -al	visceral

Prefix Exercise (p. 64)

1. endo-	endocrine
2. ana-	anatomical
3. mid-	midsagittal
4. hypo-	hypochondriac
5. re-	respiratory
6. epi-	epigastric
7. re-	reproductive

BUILDING MEDICAL WORDS
Combining Forms Exercise (p. 75)

1. end; boundary
2. walking
3. servant; accessory
4. listening
5. time
6. impart; transmit
7. present at birth
8. cause of disease
9. increase; provoke
10. break up
11. production; creation
12. arising from; produced by
13. knowledge
14. give ability
15. genetic inheritance
16. physician; medical treatment
17. unknown; individual
18. disease within
19. looking at
20. word; the study of
21. physician; medicine
22. new
23. hospital
24. nourishment
25. reduce the severity of
26. touching; feeling
27. disease; suffering
28. tapping
29. body
30. growth; formation
31. prevent
32. recover
33. send back
34. operative procedure
35. collection of symptoms
36. technical skill
37. therapy; treatment
38. treatment

Combining Form and Suffix Exercise (p. 76)

1. -ion	inspection
2. -al	terminal
3. -ist	therapist
4. -eon	surgeon
5. -ive	palliative
6. -ician	technician
7. -ary	hereditary
8. -gen	pathogen
9. -logy	symptomatology
10. -ion	palpation
11. -ation	auscultation

12. -ious	infectious
13. -ic	therapeutic
14. -ery	surgery
15. -ion	percussion
16. -ic	chronic
17. -al	congenital
18. -logy	etiology

Prefix Exercise (p. 77)

1. dia-	diagnosis
2. de-	degenerative
3. a-	asymptomatic
4. pro-	prognosis
5. re-	refractory

CHAPTER REVIEW EXERCISES
THE BODY IN HEALTH AND DISEASE
Matching Exercise (p. 79)

7, 5, 1, 9, 4, 2, 6, 8, 3

Circle Exercise (p. 79)

1. blood
2. thoracic
3. cells
4. gastroenterology
5. anatomical
6. anterior
7. thoracic
8. respiratory
9. distal

True or False Exercise (pp. 79–80)

1. T 2. F 3. F 4. T 5. F 6. T 7. T 8. T 9. T 10. F

HEALTHCARE PROFESSIONALS AND HEALTHCARE SETTINGS
Circle Exercise (p. 80)

1. physician's office
2. etiology
3. refractory
4. remission
5. hereditary

Fill in the Blank Exercise (p. 80)

1. subacute
2. palpation
3. auscultation
4. syndrome
5. idiopathic
6. symptomatology
7. clinic

True or False Exercise (p. 80)

1. F 2. T 3. T 4. F 5. T 6. F 7. F 8. F

BUILDING MEDICAL WORDS
Matching Exercise (p. 81)

13, 12, 7, 9, 6, 4, 16, 10, 17, 2, 15, 11, 14, 1, 5, 8, 3

Word Parts Exercise (pp. 81–82)

1. neurology
2. anterior
3. microscope
4. neoplastic
5. cardiology
6. pathogen
7. superior
8. thoracic
9. congenital
10. internal
11. dermatology
12. auscultation
13. symptomatic
14. dietetics

Dividing Medical Words (p. 82)

1. ana-	tom/o-	-ical
2.	nosocomi/o-	-al
3.	cephal/o-	-ad
4. endo-	crin/o-	-logy
5.	gynec/o-	-logy
6. de-	gener/o-	-ative
7.	ophthalm/o-	-logy
8. a-	symptomat/o-	-ic
9.	poster/o-	-ior
10. re-	product/o-	-ive
11.	thorac/o-	-ic
12.	urin/o-	-ary

ABBREVIATIONS

Matching Exercise (p. 82)

4, 5, 6, 11, 1, 8, 2, 3, 10, 9, 7

APPLIED SKILLS

Fill in the Blank Exercise (p. 83)

1. gynecology
2. obstetrics
3. otolaryngology
4. neurology
5. dermatology
6. pulmonology
7. neonatology
8. radiology
9. orthopedics

Proofreading and Spelling Exercise (p. 83)

1. anatomical
2. posteriorly
3. thoracic
4. cavity
5. cardiovascular
6. ophthalmology
7. otolaryngology
8. pulmonology
9. gynecology
10. physiology

English and Medical Word Equivalents Exercise (p. 83)

1. anterior or ventral
2. posterior or dorsal
3. lateral
4. medial (or midsagittal)
5. supine (or dorsal supine)
6. prone
7. superior
8. inferior
9. cephalad
10. caudad

Hearing Medical Words Exercise (p. 84)

1. disease
2. ambulatory
3. cardiovascular
4. degenerative
5. epigastric
6. exacerbation
7. hereditary
8. hospice
9. integumentary
10. neoplastic
11. palliative
12. pediatrics
13. prognosis
14. therapeutic

Pronunciation Exercise (p. 84)

1. teer
2. tawm
3. tay
4. jen
5. nawl
6. at
7. path
8. noh
9. fish
10. nawl

Chapter 3   Gastroenterology

ANATOMY AND PHYSIOLOGY

Labeling Exercise (pp. 101-102)

First Exercise

1. oral cavity, 2. tongue, 3. teeth, 4. submandibular gland, 5. sublingual gland, 6. parotid gland, 7. pharynx, 8. esophagus

Second Exercise

1. esophagus, 2. lower esophageal sphincter, 3. pancreas, 4. pyloric sphincter, 5. pylorus, 6. duodenum, 7. rugae, 8. fundus, 9. cardia, 10. body of stomach, 11. omoentum

Third Exercise

1. liver, 2. gallbladder, 3. pancreas, 4. duodenum, 5. ascending colon, 6. transverse colon, 7. descending colon, 8. cecum, 9. appendix, 10. rectum, 11. sphincter, anal, 12. stomach, 13. jejunum, 14. ileum, 15. sigmoid colon, 16. anus

BUILDING MEDICAL WORDS

Combining Forms Exercise (p. 103)

1. water; fluid
2. abdomen
3. absorb; take in
4. food; nourishment
5. carbohydrate; starch
6. anus
7. appendix
8. small structure hanging from a larger structure; appendix
9. bile; gall
10. cecum (first part of large intestine)
11. abdomen
12. to pass feces
13. chloride

14. bile duct
15. bile; gall
16. gallbladder
17. common bile duct
18. colon (part of large intestine)
19. colon (part of large intestine)
20. swallowing
21. break down food; digest
22. duodenum (first part of small intestine)
23. droplets of fat suspended in a liquid
24. intestine
25. esophagus
26. feces; stool
27. feces; stool
28. stomach
29. tongue
30. the sense of taste
31. liver
32. ileum (third part of small intestine)
33. intestine
34. jejunum (middle part of small intestine)
35. movement
36. milk
37. abdomen
38. tongue
39. lipid (fat)
40. mandible (lower jaw)
41. chewing
42. mouth
43. ear
44. pancreas
45. pelvis (hip bone; renal pelvis)
46. digestion
47. pepsin
48. peritoneum
49. peritoneum
50. pharynx (throat)
51. rectum and anus
52. pylorus
53. rectum
54. saliva
55. saliva; salivary gland
56. sigmoid colon
57. contraction
58. mouth

Combining Form and Suffix Exercise (p. 104)

1. -al — intestinal
2. -ic — gastric
3. -cyte — hepatocyte
4. -al — oral
5. -ary — salivary
6. -ion — digestion
7. -ation — mastication
8. -al — rectal
9. -ase — lipase
10. -eal — appendiceal
11. -ary — alimentary
12. -ic — colonic
13. -ive — digestive
14. -eal — esophageal
15. -gen — pepsinogen
16. -ic — pancreatic
17. -ary — biliary
18. -al — duodenal
19. -ory — gustatory
20. -eal — pharyngeal
21. -in — gastrin
22. -ic — pyloric
23. -al — jejun/o-
24. -ac — celiac
25. -al — fecal
26. -ion — absorption
27. -ase — lactase
28. -ation — emulsification
29. -al — peritoneal

Prefix Exercise (p. 105)

1. sub-   submandibular
2. peri-   peristalsis
3. meso-   mesenteric
4. de-   defecation
5. sub-   sublingual

Multiple Combining Forms and Suffix Exercise (p. 105)

1. hydr/o   chlor/o   -ic   hydrochloric
2. gastr/o   intestin/o   -al   gastrointestinal
3. abdomin/o   pelv/o   -ic   abdominopelvic
4. gastr/o   enter/o   -logy   gastroenterology
5. cholecyst/o kin/o   -in   cholecystokinin

CHAPTER REVIEW EXERCISES

ANATOMY AND PHYSIOLOGY

Matching Exercise (p. 134)

7, 9, 12, 1, 11, 13, 10, 6, 4, 5, 3, 8, 2

Circle Exercise (p. 134)

1. duodenum
2. defecation
3. cardia
4. salivary gland
5. hydrochloric acid
6. sigmoid
7. bile

True or False Exercise (pp. 134–135)

1. T 2. T 3. F 4. T 5. F 6. T 7. F 8. F 9. F 10. T

Sequencing Exercise (p. 135)

1. oral cavity
2. pharynx
3. esophagus
4. stomach
5. duodenum
6. jejunum
7. ileum
8. cecum
9. colon
10. rectum
11. anus

DISEASES AND CONDITIONS

Matching Exercise (p. 135)

13, 9, 2, 6, 7, 8, 12, 1, 11, 5, 3, 4, 10

True or False (p. 136)

1. T 2. F 3. T 4. F 5. F 6. T 7. T

LABORATORY, RADIOLOGY, SURGERY, AND DRUGS

Fill in the Blank Exercise (p. 136)

1. stoma, 2. antiemetic, 3. albumin, 4. ova and parasites, 5. cholangiography, 6. sonogram, 7. barium swallow, 8. nasogastric tube, 9. herniorrhaphy, 10. laxative

Circle Exercise (p. 136)

1. liver transplantation
2. sonogram
3. cholecystectomy
4. colostomy
5. obesity
6. SGPT
7. CLO
8. laparotomy
9. gastrectomy

BUILDING MEDICAL WORDS

Combining Forms Exercise (p. 137)

1. create an opening between two structures
2. lip
3. yellow
4. compacted feces
5. hold together
6. diverticulum
7. to vomit
8. blood
9. hemorrhoid
10. hernia
11. gap; opening
12. groin
13. to receive within
14. yellow
15. stone
16. word; the study of
17. severe constipation
18. blocked by a barrier
19. umbilicus; navel
20. appetite
21. digestion
22. to have an opening
23. eating; swallowing
24. polyp
25. fire; burning
26. flow backward
27. rotate
28. spleen
29. fat
30. umbilicus; navel

Related Combining Forms Exercise (p. 137)

1. steat/o-, lip/o-
2. enter/o-, intestin/o-
3. gloss/o-, lingu/o-
4. celi/o-, abdomen/o-, lapar/o-, or ventr/o-
5. cholangi/o-, bili/o-, choledoch/o-

Dividing Medical Words (p. 137)

1. an-   orex/o-   -ia
2.   append/o-   -ectomy
3.   mesenter/o- -ic
4. dys-   phag/o-   -ia
5.   hemat/o-   -emesis
6.   hepat/o-   -megaly
7.   herni/o-   -rrhaphy
8. sub-   lingu/o-   -al

Combining Form and Suffix Exercise (pp. 138–139)

1. constipation
2. gastritis
3. hematemesis
4. hepatomegaly
5. appendicitis
6. enteropathy
7. cholecystectomy
8. diverticulosis
9. laparotomy
10. hepatitis
11. polypectomy
12. hepatoma
13. appendectomy
14. herniorrhaphy
15. sigmoidoscopy
16. cholecystitis
17. anastomosis
18. glossitis
19. colostomy
20. laparoscope
21. hemorrhoidectomy
22. rectocele
23. sialolith
24. cirrhosis
25. cholangiogram

Prefix Exercise (p. 139)

1. in-   indigestion
2. an-   anorexia
3. dys-   dyspepsia
4. mal-   malrotation
5. sub-   sublingual
6. poly-   polyphagia
7. anti-   antiemetic
8. dys-   dysphagia
9. im-   imperforate
10. in-   incontinence

Multiple Combining Forms and Suffix Exercise (p. 140)

1. bilirubin
2. esophagogastroduodenoscopy
3. gastroenteritis
4. hepatosplenomegaly
5. nasogastric
6. hematochezia
7. colorectal
8. gastroenterologist
9. choledocholithotomy
10. laparoscopy

ABBREVIATIONS

Matching Exercise (p. 140)

13, 1, 3, 4, 8, 5, 6, 2, 11, 7, 12, 9, 10

APPLIED SKILLS

Adjective Spelling Exercise (p. 141)

1. abdominal
2. oral
3. pharyngeal
4. esophageal
5. gastric
6. pyloric
7. duodenal
8. jejunal
9. cecal
10. appendiceal
11. colonic
12. rectal
13. anal
14. peritoneal
15. hepatic
16. pancreatic

Proofreading and Spelling Exercise (p. 141)

1. gastroenterology
2. pharynx
3. esophagus
4. diverticula
5. hemorrhoids
6. cholelithiasis
7. lumen
8. polyps
9. rectocele
10. albumin

English and Medical Word Equivalents Exercise (p. 141)

1. abdomen
2. umbilicus or navel
3. intestine
4. defecation or feces or stool
5. mastication
6. flatus
7. pyrosis
8. dyspepsia
9. oral cavity
10. hemorrhoids
11. deglutition
12. pharynx
13. emesis

You Write the Medical Report (p. 142)

1. anorexia
2. colostomy
3. gastroenteritis
4. constipation, obstipation
5. colonoscopy
6. gastroenterologist
7. esophageal, hematemesis, cirrhosis, ascites
8. pyrosis (or gastritis), flatus
9. cholecystitis, cholecystectomy
10. dysphagia

Word Analysis Questions (p. 144)

1. gastric
2. appendic/o- (appendix), -itis (inflammation of; infection of)
3. fec/a- (feces; stool), -lith (stone)
4. In the right upper quadrant
5. N&V

Fact Finding Questions (pp. 144–145)

1. antacid
2. emesis
3. the colon
4. wormlike
5. appendectomy
6. acute appendicitis

Critical Thinking Questions (p. 145)

1. pyrosis
2. gastroenteritis
3. in the appendix
4. peritonitis
5. The physician presses on the right lower quadrant of the abdomen and then quickly removes the hand and releases the pressure, causing severe rebound pain in a patient with appendicitis.
6. liver
7. pancreas

On the Job Challenge Exercise (p. 145)

1. condition (caused by) air that is swallowed (excessively)
2. process of (air being) brought up (from the stomach), belching
3. painful straining to have a stool
4. hiccups
5. a rumbling sound due to gas in the intestines

Hearing Medical Words Exercise (p. 146)

1. anorexia
2. ascites
3. cholecystitis
4. cirrhosis
5. colostomy
6. gastroenteritis
7. herniorrhaphy
8. laparotomy
9. nasogastric
10. sigmoidoscopy

Pronunciation Exercise (p. 146)

1. gas
2. sy
3. tek
4. fay
5. awl
6. tes
7. pat
8. ty
9. meg
10. stal

Chapter 4   Pulmonology

ANATOMY AND PHYSIOLOGY

Labeling Exercise (p. 161)

First exercise

1. larynx, 2. bronchus, 3. cluster of alveoli, 4. bronchioles, 5. diaphragm, 6. nasal cavity, 7. pharynx, 8. trachea, 9. apex of lung, 10. rib, 11. sternum, 12. lower lobe of lung

Second exercise

1. bronchiole, 2. cluster of alveoli, 3. carbon dioxide, 4. oxygen, 5. capillary wall, 6. red blood cell

BUILDING MEDICAL WORDS

Combining Forms Exercise (p. 162)

1. alveolus (air sac)
2. bronchus
3. bronchiole
4. bronchus
5. carbon dioxide
6. heart
7. cell
8. rib
9. diaphragm
10. arising from; produced by
11. shaped like a globe; comprehensive
12. glottis (of the larynx)
13. breathe
14. blood
15. hilum (indentation in an organ)
16. larynx (voice box)
17. lobe of an organ
18. change; transformation
19. mucus
20. mucous membrane
21. nose
22. mouth
23. oxygen
24. oxygen
25. oxygen; quick
26. wall of a cavity
27. chest
28. pharynx (throat)
29. diaphragm; mind
30. pleura (lung membrane)
31. breathing
32. lung; air
33. lung; air
34. lung
35. septum (dividing wall)
36. breathe; a coil
37. chest
38. thorax (chest)
39. trachea (windpipe)
40. scroll-like structure; turbinate
41. movement of air
42. large internal organs

Combining Form and Suffix Exercise (p. 163)

1.	-ar	alveolar
2.	-al	nasal
3.	-al	tracheal
4.	-ary	pulmonary
5.	-ic	phrenic
6.	-ole	bronchiole
7.	-ic	thoracic
8.	-ar	lobar
9.	-logy	pulmonology
10.	-ation	ventilation
11.	-ism	metabolism
12.	-al	bronchial
13.	-ar	bronchiolar
14.	-eal	laryngeal
15.	-al	mucosal
16.	-ic	diaphragmatic
17.	-eal	pharyngeal

Prefix Exercise (p. 164)

1. in-	inspiration
2. inter-	intercostal
3. re-	respiration
4. epi-	epiglottic
5. ex-	exhalation
6. re-	respiratory

Multiple Combining Forms and Suffix Exercise (p. 164)

1. cardi/o-	pulmon/o-	-ary	cardiopulmonary
2. ox/y-	gen/o-	-ated	oxygenated
3. bronch/o-	pulmon/o-	-ary	bronchopulmonary
4. hem/o-	glob/o-	-in	hemoglobin

CHAPTER REVIEW EXERCISES

ANATOMY AND PHYSIOLOGY

Matching Exercise (p. 189)

6, 11, 2, 3, 5, 7, 8, 9, 1, 10, 4

Circle Exercise (p. 189)

1. lobe
2. bronchioles
3. hilum
4. parenchyma
5. epiglottis
6. surfactant
7. phrenic nerve

True or False Exercise (p. 189)

1. T, 2. F, 3. T, 4. F, 5. F, 6. T, 7. T, 8. F

DISEASES AND CONDITIONS

Matching Exercise (p. 190)

3, 6, 4, 1, 2, 7, 8, 5

True or False Exercise (p. 190)

1. T, 2. T, 3. F, 4. T, 5. T, 6. F, 7. T, 8. T, 9. F

Fill in the Blank Exercise (p. 190)

1. bronchopneumonia
2. status asthmaticus
3. wheezing
4. cystic fibrosis
5. tachypnea
6. Legionnaire's disease
7. carcinoma
8. pulmonary edema
9. tuberculosis

LABORATORY, RADIOLOGY, SURGERY, AND DRUGS

Matching Exercise (p. 191)

6, 2, 8, 1, 3, 7, 4, 9, 5

Circle Exercise (p. 191)

1. lung
2. nasal cannula
3. carboxyhemoglobin
4. productive coughs

Dividing Medical Words (p. 191)

1. in-	hal/o-	-ation	
2.	pharyng/o-	-eal	
3. re-	spir/o-	-atory	
4.	hem/o-	-ptysis	
5. circum-	or/o-	-al	
6.	bronchi/o-	-ectasis	
7. pan-	lob/o-	-ar	
8.	pneum/o-	-thorax	

BUILDING MEDICAL WORDS

Combining Forms Exercise (p. 192)

1. gland
2. coal
3. to breathe in; to suck in
4. asthma
5. incomplete
6. listening
7. carbon monoxide
8. cancer
9. spherical bacterium
10. dust
11. blue
12. dilate; widen
13. embolus (occluding plug)
14. word; the study of
15. blocked by a barrier
16. tapping
17. pus
18. pus
19. to cut out; remove
20. revive; raise up again
21. treatment
22. nodule; tuberculosis
23. nodule
24. cough

Multiple Combining Forms and Suffix Exercise (p. 192)

1. cardiothoracic
2. adenocarcinoma
3. bronchodilator
4. bronchopneumonia
5. pneumococcal
6. carboxyhemoglobin
7. pulmonologist

Combining Form and Suffix Exercise (pp. 193–194)

1. asthmatic
2. bronchitis
3. pyothorax
4. auscultation
5. cyanosis
6. tracheostomy
7. hemoptysis
8. pneumonectomy
9. stethoscope
10. bronchospasm
11. bronchiectasis
12. oximeter
13. ventilator
14. laryngoscope
15. pleurisy
16. pneumonia
17. anthracosis
18. thoracotomy
19. bronchoscopy
20. lobectomy
21. therapist
22. pneumothorax
23. hemothorax
24. spirometer
25. resuscitation
26. oximetry
27. thoracocentesis
28. orthopnea

Related Combining Forms Exercise (p. 194)

1. spir/o-, hal/o-, pne/o-
2. thorac/o-, steth/o-, pector/o-
3. pneum/o-, pulmon/o-, pneumon/o-

Prefix Exercise (p. 194)

1. in-	intubation
2. dys-	dyspneic
3. pan-	panlobar
4. hyper-	hypercapnia
5. anti-	antitussive
6. tachy-	tachypneic
7. an-	anoxia
8. em-	empyemia
9. endo-	endotracheal
10. ex-	expectorant

ABBREVIATIONS

Matching Exercise (p. 195)

7, 2, 5, 8, 1, 4, 6, 3

APPLIED SKILLS

Plural Noun and Adjective Spelling Exercise (p. 195)

1.	nasal
2. alveoli	alveolar
3.	anoxic
4. apices	
5.	apneic
6.	asthmatic
7. bronchi	bronchial
8.	cyanotic
9.	diaphragmatic
10. hila	hilar
11.	laryngeal
12. lungs	pulmonary
13.	mucosal
14.	pharyngeal
15.	pleural
16.	tachypneic
17.	thoracic
18.	tracheal

English and Medical Word Equivalents Exercise (p. 195)

1. pharynx
2. anthracosis
3. thorax
4. atelectasis
5. sudden infant death syndrome
6. influenza
7. dyspnea
8. pharynx
9. larynx
10. trachea

Word Analysis Questions (p. 197)

1. shortness of breath; SOB
2. dyspneic
3. bronch/o-   bronchus
   -scopy   process of using an instrument to examine
4. cyan/o-   blue
   -osis   condition; abnormal condition; process
5. a. culture and sensitivity
   b. chronic obstructive pulmonary disease
   c. left lower lobe

Fact Finding Questions (p. 197)

1. anthracosis
2. bronchoscopy with a biopsy
3. appendectomy
4. consolidative changes, density in LLL, patchy infiltrates, atelectasis

Critical Thinking Questions (p. 197)

1. fever
2. barrel chest
3. auscultation
4. right-sided pneumonia
5. 44 pack-years

On the Job Challenge Exercise (p. 198)

1. fibrosis
2. syndrome
3. Search under the noun in a medical phrase, not the adjective.

Hearing Medical Words (p. 198)

1. anoxia
2. asthmatic
3. auscultation
4. bronchoscopy
5. emphysema
6. hemoptysis
7. laryngeal
8. lobectomy
9. pneumothorax
10. tracheostomy

Pronunciation Exercise (p. 198)

1. ky
2. pul
3. noh
4. moh
5. ray
6. ras
7. tray
8. aws

Chapter 5   Cardiology

ANATOMY AND PHYSIOLOGY

Labeling Exercise (pp. 220–221)

First exercise

1. right pulmonary artery, 2. ascending aorta, 3. superior vena cava, 4. aortic valve, 5. pulmonary trunk, 6. right atrium, 7. tricuspid valve, 8. inferior vena cava, 9. chordae tendinae, 10. right ventricle, 11. aortic arch, 12. left pulmonary artery, 13. pulmonary valve, 14. left pulmonary veins, 15. left atrium, 16. mitral valve, 17. left ventricle, 18. interventricular septum, 19. apex of heart

Second exercise

1. atrioventricular node, 2. sinoatrial node, 3. right atrium, 4. bundle of His, 5. bundle branches, 6. right ventricle, 7. left atrium, 8. left ventricle, 9. Purkinje fibers

Third exercise

1. coronary artery, 2. abdominal aorta, 3. carotid artery, 4. subclavian artery, 5. axillary artery, 6. brachial artery, 7. thoracic aorta, 8. renal artery, 9. ulnar artery, 10. radial artery, 11. iliac artery, 12. femoral artery, 13. popliteal artery, 14. tibial artery 15. peroneal artery

BUILDING MEDICAL WORDS

Combining Forms Exercise (p. 222)

1. axilla (armpit)
2. abdomen
3. blood vessel; lymphatic vessel
4. aorta
5. apex (tip)
6. artery
7. arteriole
8. artery
9. atrium (upper heart chamber)
10. arm
11. hairlike structure; capillary
12. heart
13. heart
14. stupor; sleep
15. movement in a circular route
16. clavicle (collar bone)
17. carrying; conveying
18. drawn together; narrowed
19. structure that encircles like a crown
20. projection; point
21. dilating
22. dilate; widen
23. outside of a place
24. femur (thigh bone)
25. break up
26. ilium (hip bone)
27. jugular (throat)
28. mediastinum
29. structure like a miter (tall hat with two points)
30. muscle
31. wall of a cavity
32. fibula (lower leg bone)
33. vein
34. positive or negative state
35. back of the knee
36. point of entry
37. lung
38. radius (forearm bone); x-rays; radiation
39. kidney
40. clearly visible
41. septum (dividing wall)
42. hollow cavity; channel
43. the body as a whole
44. contracting
45. cellular layer
46. thorax (chest)
47. tibia (shin bone)
48. ulna (forearm bone)
49. valve
50. valve
51. blood vessel
52. blood vessel; vas deferens
53. vein
54. ventricle (lower heart chamber; chamber in the brain)
55. large internal organs

Combining Form and Suffix Exercise (p. 223)

1. -ic   thoracic
2. -al   arterial
3. -ar   valvular
4. -ion   circulation
5. -ac   cardiac
6. -ary   capillary
7. -ous   venous
8. -ic   systemic
9. -al   artrial
10. -al   brachial
11. -ole   arteriole
12. -ous   saphenous
13. -ic   aortic
14. -ature   vasculature
15. -ic   systolic
16. -ory   circulatory
17. -ar   ventricular
18. -ule   venule

Multiple Combining Forms and Suffix Exercise (p. 224)

1. vas/o-   dilat/o-   vasodilation
2. cardi/o-   pulmon/o-   cardiopulmonary
3. cardi/o-   vascul/o-   cardiovascular
4. sin/o-   atri/o-   sinoatrial
5. vas/o-   constrict/o-   vasoconstriction
6. my/o-   cardi/o-   myocardial
7. atri/o-   ventricul/o-   atrioventricular

CHAPTER REVIEW EXERCISES
ANATOMY AND PHYSIOLOGY
Matching Exercise (p. 253)

9, 8, 6, 2, 4, 1, 5, 3, 7, 10

True or False Exercise (p. 253)

1. F, 2. T, 3. F, 4. F, 5. F, 6. F, 7. T, 8. T, 9. F, 10. T, 11. T, 12. T, 13. T

Sequencing Exercise (p. 254)

1. right atrium
2. tricuspid valve
3. right ventricle
4. pulmonary valve, pulmonary trunk, and pulmonary arteries
5. lungs
6. pulmonary veins
7. left atrium
8. mitral valve
9. left ventricle
10. aortic valve and aorta
11. arteries and arterioles
12. capillaries
13. venules and veins
14. superior and inferior venae cavae

Circle Exercise (p. 254)

1. aorta
2. heart valves
3. auscultation
4. foramen ovale
5. jugular
6. SA node

DISEASES AND CONDITIONS
Matching Exercise (p. 255)

6, 9, 1, 3, 8, 2, 5, 4, 7, 10

Circle Exercise (p. 255)

1. bradycardia
2. stenosis
3. aneurysm
4. patent foramen ovalve

True or False Exercise (p. 255)

1. F, 2. T, 3. T, 4. T, 5. F, 6. F, 7. T, 8. F, 9. T, 10. T

LABORATORY, RADIOLOGY, SURGERY, AND DRUGS
Laboratory Test Exercise (p. 256)

PANELS AND PROFILES		TESTS	
968T	✓ Lipid Panel	19687W	Bilirubin (Direct)
315F	Electrolyte Panel	265F	HBsAg
10256F	Hepatic Function Panel	51870R	HB Core Antibody
10165F	Basic Metabolic Panel	1012F	✓ Cardio CRP
10231A	Comprehensive Metabolic Panel	23242E	GGT
10306F	Hepatitis Panel, Acute	28852E	Protein, Total
182Aaa	Obstetric Panel	141A	CBC Hemogram
18T	Chem-Screen Panel (Basic)	21105R	hCG, Qualitative, Serum
554T	Chem-Screen Panel (Basic with HDL)	10321A	ANA
7971A	Chem-Screen Panel (Basic with HDL, TIBC)	80185	✓ Cardio CRP with Lipid Profile
TESTS		26F	PT with INR
56713E	Lead, Blood	232Aaa	UA, Dipstick
2782A	Antibody Screen	42A	CBC with Diff
3556F	Iron, TIBC	20867W	✓ HDL Cholesterol
20933E	✓ Cholesterol	31732E	PTT
3084111E	Uric Acid	34F	UA, Dipstick and Microscopic
53348W	Rubella Antibody	20396R	CEA
27771E	Phosphate	45443E	Hematocrit
2111600E	Creatinine	28571E	PSA, Total
29868W	Testosterone, Total	66902E	WBC count
9704F	Creatinine Clearance	20750E	Chloride
19752E	Bilirubin (Total)	7187W	Hemoglobin
30536Rrr	T3, Total	4259T	HIV-1 Antibody
687T	Protein Electrophoresis	45484R	Hemoglobin A1c
3563444R	✓ Digoxin	67868R	Alk Phosphatase
15214R	Glucose, 2-Hour Postprandial	24984R	Iron
30502E	T3, Uptake	28512E	Sodium
7773E	Platelet Count	17426R	ALT
39685R	Dilantin (phenytoin)	**MICROBIOLOGY**	
30494R	✓ Triglycerides	112680E	Group A Beta Strep Culture, Throat
26013E	Magnesium	5827W	Group B Beta Strep Culture, Genitals
15586R	Glucose, Fasting	49932E	Chlamydia, Endocervix/Urethra
30237W	T4, Free	6007W	Culture, Blood
28233E	Potassium	2692E	Culture, Genitals
19208W	AST	2649T	Culture, HSV
30163E	TSH	612A	Culture, Sputum
22764R	Ferritin	6262E	Culture, Throat
20008W	Calcium	6304R	Culture, Urine
54726F	Occult Blood, Stool	50286R	Gonococcus, Endocervix/Urethra
51839W	HAV Antibody, Total	6643E	Gram Stain
430A	Blood Group and Rh Type	**STOOL PATHOGENS**	
28399W	Progesterone	10045F	Culture, Stool
30262E	T4, Total	4475F	Culture, Campylobacter
20289W	Carbon Dioxide	10018T	Culture, Salmonella
1156F	RPR	86140A	E. coli Toxins
30940E	Urea Nitrogen	1099T	Ova and Parasites
17417W	Albumin	**VENIPUNCTURE**	
28423E	Prolactin	63180	Venipuncture

True or False Exercise (p. 256)

1. F, 2. T, 3. T, 4. F, 5. F

BUILDING MEDICAL WORDS
Combining Forms Exercise (p. 257)

1. angina
2. aneurysm (dilation)
3. soft, fatty substance
4. listening
5. cholesterol
6. limping pain
7. echo (sound wave)
8. electricity
9. muscle fiber; nerve fiber
10. set or group
11. unknown; individual
12. area of dead tissue
13. keep back; block
14. lipid (fat)
15. lumen (opening)
16. break down; destroy
17. thin; frenzy
18. dead cells, tissue, or body
19. to throb
20. disease; suffering
21. to be open
22. rhythm
23. hard; sclera (white of the eye)
24. pulse
25. narrowness; constriction
26. distance
27. pressure; tension
28. thrombus (blood clot)
29. varix; varicose vein
30. to travel; to turn

Related Combining Forms Exercise (p. 257)

1. angi/o-, vas/o-, vascul/o-
2. card/i-, cardi/o-
3. phleb/o-, ven/o-

Dividing Medical Words (p. 257)

1.		circulat/o-	-ion
2.	de-	polar/o-	-ization
3.		ischm/o-	-emia
4.	endo-	card/i-	-itis
5.	a-	rrhythm/o-	-ia
6.	brady-	card/i-	-ia
7.		aneurym/o-	-al
8.	hyper-	lipid/o-	-emia
9.		angi/o-	-plasty
10.	trans-	lumin/o-	-al

Combining Form and Suffix Exercise (p. 258)

1. necrotic
2. cardiomegaly
3. atheroma
4. claudication
5. aneurysmectomy
6. stenosis
7. infarction
8. angioplasty
9. auscultation
10. sclerotherapy
11. telemetry
12. phlebitis
13. patent
14. fibrillation
15. angiography
16. valvulotome
17. palpitation
18. arteriogram
19. valvuloplasty
20. stethoscope

Prefix Exercise (p. 259)

1. hyper-   hypercholesterolemia
2. tachy-   tachycardic
3. hyper-   hypertension
4. bi-   bigeminal
5. peri-   pericardiocentesis
6. trans-   transluminal
7. brady-   bradycardia
8. hyper-   hyperlipidemia
9. supra-   supraventricular
10. a-   arrhythmia
11. peri-   pericarditis
12. endo-   endarterectomy
13. hypo-   hypotensive
14. endo-   endocarditis
15. tri-   trigeminal

Multiple Combining Forms and Suffix Exercise (p. 260)

1. arteriosclerosis
2. myocardial
3. echocardiography
4. thrombolytic
5. atherosclerosis
6. electrocardiography
7. thrombophlebitis
8. cardiomyopathy
9. sphygmomanometer
10. idiopathic
11. cardioversion

ABBREVIATIONS
Matching Exercise (p. 260)
10, 6, 3, 2, 4, 9, 7, 5, 8, 1

APPLIED SKILLS
Plural Noun and Adjective Spelling Exercise (p. 261)

1.		pericardial
2.	arteries	arterial
3.	atria	atrial
4.	ventricles	ventricular
5.		septal
6.		myocardial
7.	valves	valvular
8.		aortic
9.	veins	venous
10.		cardiac
11.	arteries	arterial

Proofreading and Spelling Exercise (p. 261)
1. sphygmomanometer
2. carotid
3. atheromatous
4. arrhythmia
5. tachycardia
6. digitalis
7. angioplasty
8. myocardial
9. infarction
10. cardiomegaly

You Write the Medical Report (pp. 261–262)
1. angina pectoris, diaphoresis
2. tachycardia, cardioversion, palpitations, electrocardiography
3. atherosclerosis, claudication, necrotic
4. hypertension, diuretic

Word Analysis Questions (p. 263)
1. HTN
2. hypertensive
3. a. congestive heart failure
   b. creatine kinase, MB bands
   c. cardiopulmonary resuscitation
   d. left ventricular hypertrophy
4. vascul/o-   -ar
   blood vessel   pertaining to
5. cardi/o-   -megaly
   heart   enlargement
6. pertaining to two sides, pertaining to being without logical thought or language, pertaining to being in a stupor (unawareness like sleep)

Fact Finding Questions (p. 263)
1. 70–80 beats per minute
2. a. congestive heart failure (CHF)
   b. diabetes mellitus, type 2
3. cardiac arrest
4. troponin, CK-MB
5. asystole

Critical Thinking Questions (p. 264)
1. right
2. left
3. congestive heart failure
4. fluid retention from congestive heart failure

Hearing Medical Words Exercise (p. 264)
1. cardiac
2. aneurysm
3. cardiothoracic
4. myocardium
5. coronary artery
6. vasoconstriction
7. cardiomegaly
8. arrhythmia
9. atherosclerosis
10. echocardiogram
11. angioplasty
12. sphygmomanometer

Pronunciation Exercise (p. 264)
1. kar
2. kor
3. lay
4. pul
5. dy
6. kar, fark
7. lay
8. roh
9. tay
10. an

Chapter 6   Hematology and Immunology
ANATOMY AND PHYSIOLOGY
Labeling Exercise (pp. 288–289)
First exercise

1. eosinophil, 2. neutrophil, 3. lymphocyte, 4. basophil, 5. monocyte,

Second exercise

1. cervical lymph nodes, 2. axillary lymph nodes, 3. mediastinal lymph nodes, 4. celiac lymph nodes, 5. appendix and Peyer's patches, 6. inguinal lymph nodes, 7. tonsils and adenoids, 8. thymus, 9. spleen, 10. mesenteric lymph nodes, 11. red bone marrow

BUILDING MEDICAL WORDS
Combining Forms Exercise (p. 290)
1. crowding together
2. base of a structure; basic (alkaline)
3. clotting
4. cell
5. electricity
6. eosin (red acidic dye)
7. red
8. fibrin
9. fiber
10. shaped like a globe; comprehensive
11. shaped like a globe
12. granule
13. blood
14. blood
15. immune response
16. nucleus
17. white
18. lymph; lymphatic system
19. large
20. large
21. one; single
22. shape
23. bone marrow; spinal cord; myelin
24. not taking part
25. normal; usual
26. nucleus (of a cell or an atom)
27. oxygen
28. disease; suffering
29. eating; swallowing
30. plasma
31. growth; formation
32. small network
33. spleen
34. press down
35. thrombus (blood clot)
36. thymus; rage
37. poison

Combining Form and Suffix Exercise (p. 291)

1.	-poiesis	hematopoiesis
2.	-cyte	leukocyte
3.	-ation	coagulation
4.	-ic	splenic
5.	-cyte	phagocyte
6.	-oid	lymphoid
7.	-logy	hematology
8.	-poietin	erythropoietin
9.	-phil	eosinophil
10.	-gen	pathogen
11.	-cyte	thrombocyte
12.	-blast	myeloblast
13.	-lyte	electrolyte
14.	-ity	immunity
15.	-ation	aggregation
16.	-atic	lymphatic
17.	-cyte	granulocyte
18.	-cyte	erythrocyte
19.	-phil	basophil
20.	-phage	macrophage

Prefix Exercise (p. 292)

1. endo-   endotoxin
2. a-   agranulocyte
3. poly-   polymorphonuclear
4. pro-   prothrombin

Multiple Combining Forms and Suffix Exercise (p. 292)

1. cyt/o-   tox/o-   -ic   cytotoxic
2. thromb/o-   plast/o-   -in   thromboplastin
3. meg/a-   kary/o-   -cyte   megakaryocyte
4. immun/o-   globul/o-   -in   immunoglobulin
5. phag/o-   cyt/o-   -osis   phagocytosis

CHAPTER REVIEW EXERCISES

ANATOMY AND PHYSIOLOGY

Matching Exercise (p. 312)

6, 15, 16, 12, 9, 4, 13, 8, 5, 14, 11, 7, 3, 1, 10, 2

True or False Exercise (p. 312)

1. T, 2. T, 3. F, 4. F, 5. F, 6. F, 7. T, 8. F, 9. T, 10. F

Circle Exercise (p. 313)

1. blood   5. electrolytes
2. red blood cells   6. IgA
3. fibrin   7. heme
4. pathogens   8. aggregation

Multiple Choice Exercise (p. 313)

1. d   3. d
2. b   4. c

Fill in the Blank Exercise (p. 313)

1. A, B, AB, O
2. neutrophils, eosinophils, basophils
3. (Pick any three) segmented neutrophil, segmenter, seg, polymorphonuclear leukocyte, PMN, poly
4. thymus, spleen

Matching Exercise (p. 314)

7, 4, 3, 5, 8, 9, 6, 10, 2, 1

DISEASES AND CONDITIONS

Matching Exercise (p. 314)

5, 4, 8, 10, 13, 14, 7, 6, 12, 11, 2, 1, 3, 15, 9

True or False Exercise (p. 314)

1. F, 2. T, 3. F, 4. T, 5. T, 6. F, 7. F, 8. F, 9. T, 10. T

Multiple Choice Exercise (p. 315)

1. a   3. d
2. b   4. c

LABORATORY, RADIOLOGY, SURGERY, AND DRUGS

Circle Exercise (p. 315)

1. ferritin level   5. electrophoresis
2. iliac crest   6. CD4 count
3. MCV   7. thrombolytic
4. INR

Matching Exercise (p. 315)

4, 1, 7, 3, 10, 6, 8, 5, 2, 9

BUILDING MEDICAL WORDS

Combining Forms Exercise (p. 316)

1. blood vessel; lymphatic vessel
2. gland
3. clumping; sticking
4. other; strange
5. unequal
6. weakened
7. self
8. life; living organisms; living tissue
9. calcium
10. color
11. lacking; inadequate
12. to cut apart
13. embolus (occluding plug)
14. to cut out

15. iron
16. pouring
17. other
18. unknown; individual
19. word; the study of
20. break down; destroy
21. large
22. one millionth; small
23. shape
24. attraction to; fondness for
25. vein
26. irregular
27. hole; perforation
28. infection
29. giving a vaccine
30. vein

Prefix Exercise (p. 316)

1. a-   aplastic
2. hypo-   hypochromic
3. pan-   pancytopenia
4. trans-   transfusion
5. anti-   anticoagulant
6. hyper-   hypercalcemia
7. intra-   intravascular

Related Combining Forms Exercise (p. 317)

1. cyt/o-, cellul/o-
2. kary/o-, nucle/o-
3. phleb/o-, ven/o-

Combining Form and Suffix Exercise (pp. 317–318)

1. microcyte   11. myeloma
2. hemorrhage   12. phlebotomy
3. leukemia   13. vaccination
4. hemolysis   14. splenectomy
5. coagulopathy   15. lymphedema
6. embolism   16. autoimmune
7. lymphoma   17. agglutination
8. septicemia   18. splenomegaly
9. morphology   19. thymoma
10. thrombosis   20. attenuated

Multiple Combining Forms and Suffix Exercise (p. 318)

1. poikilocytosis   8. electrophoresis
2. hemophilia   9. thrombolytic
3. lymphadenopathy   10. lymphangiography
4. mononucleosis   11. anisocytosis
5. normocytic   12. venipuncture
6. thrombocytopenia   13. hematologist
7. immunodeficiency

ABBREVIATIONS

Matching Exercise (p. 319)

5, 8, 11, 6, 1, 9, 3, 2, 7, 4, 10

APPLIED SKILLS

Fact Finding Questions (pp. 319–320)

1. complete blood count
2. m/cmm
3. millions per milliliter
4. platelets
5. one thousand

Fact Finding Questions (p. 321)

1. b
2. Candida albicans in the mouth (leukoplakia), wasting syndrome
3. 500, 100, 500
4. Retrovir, Epivir, Sustiva
5. CD4 count
6. The lymph nodes are enlarged (cervical lymphadenopathy)

Critical Thinking Questions (p. 321)

1. intravenous heroin use
2. c
3. Because Pneumocystis jiroveci pneumonia is an opportunistic infection
   and this qualifies for a change from a diagnosis of HIV to a diagnosis of
   AIDS. Also, oral or esophageal candidiasis (the patient had oral candidiasis) qualifies for change to a diagnosis of AIDS.

4. a. weight loss
   b. weight 128 pounds
   c. wasting of the extremities

Hearing Medical Words Exercise (p. 322)

1. anemia
2. autoimmune
3. embolism
4. hematologist
5. hemorrhage
6. immunoglobulin
7. leukemia
8. lymphangiogram
9. mononucleosis
10. phlebotomy

Pronunciation Exercise (p. 322)

1. loo
2. rith
3. sin
4. fat
5. lay
6. path
7. see
8. fil
9. baw
10. nek

Chapter 7   Dermatology

ANATOMY AND PHYSIOLOGY

Labeling Exercise (p. 335)

First Exercise

1. hair shaft, 2. pore, 3. sebaceous gland, 4. hair follicle, 5. duct of sweat gland, 6. vein, 7. artery, 8. nerve, 9. sweat gland, 10. epidermis, 11. dermis, 12. subcutaneous tissue

Second Exercise

1. nail root, 2. cuticle, 3. lunula, 4. nail plate, 5. nail bed

BUILDING MEDICAL WORDS

Combining Forms Exercise (p. 336)

1. follicle (small sac)
2. fat
3. other; strange
4. base of a structure; basic (alkaline)
5. fibers that hold together
6. skin
7. skin
8. skin
9. skin
10. skin
11. sweating
12. flexing; stretching
13. to stand up
14. activity; work
15. away from; external; outward
16. to bear
17. leaf
18. sweat
19. skin
20. to cover
21. cornea (of the eye); hard, fibrous protein
22. lipid (fat)
23. in one place
24. moon
25. black
26. nail (fingernail or toenail)
27. guarding; protecting
28. hair
29. sebum (oil)
30. sebum (oil)
31. affected by; sensitive to
32. breathe; a coil
33. sweat
34. the body as a whole
35. cellular layer
36. hair
37. nail (fingernail or toenail)

Combining Form and Suffix Exercise (p. 337)

1. -in   elastin
2. -al   ungual
3. -tome   dermatome
4. -in   keratin
5. -gen   collagen

6. -ose   adipose
7. -cyte   melanocyte
8. -ous   cutaneous
9. -ous   sebaceous
10. -cyte   lipocyte
11. -ary   integumentary
12. -ula   lunula
13. -ment   integument

Prefix Exercise (p. 337)

1. ex-   exfoliation
2. epi-   epidermal
3. sub-   subcutaneous
4. per-   perspiration

CHAPTER REVIEW EXERCISES

ANATOMY AND PHYSIOLOGY

Matching Exercise (p. 363)

6, 3, 8, 5, 4, 7, 1, 2, 9

Circle Exercise (p. 363)

1. nail bed
2. keratin
3. hair
4. exfoliation
5. dermatome
6. nail

True or False Exercise (p. 363)

1. T, 2. F, 3. T, 4. F, 5. T, 6. T

DISEASES AND CONDITIONS

Circle Exercise (p. 364)

1. fissue
2. macule
3. cyst

Matching Exercise (p. 364)

5, 9, 1, 10, 12, 3, 11, 2, 4, 6, 8, 7

True or False Exercise (p. 364)

1. F, 2. F, 3. T, 4. T, 5. F, 6. F, 7. T

Circle Exercise (p. 365)

1. flat
2. pustule
3. excoriation
4. eschar
5. feet
6. cellulitis
7. xanthoma
8. ringworm

Matching Exercise (p. 365)

5, 6, 8, 1, 7, 2, 9, 3, 4

LABORATORY, RADIOLOGY, SURGERY, AND DRUGS

Matching Exercise (p. 365)

4, 5, 2, 3, 1, 7, 6

Circle Exercise (p. 366)

1. debridement
2. curettage
3. intradermal
4. rhytidectomy
5. incisional biopsy
6. incision and drainage
7. antifungal drugs

BUILDING MEDICAL WORDS

Combining Forms Exercise (p. 366)

1. scrape off
2. bald
3. self
4. life; living organisms; living tissue
5. eyelid
6. bruising
7. cold

8. blue
9. redness
10. sensation; feeling
11. to cut out
12. oozing fluid
13. spark of electricity
14. fungus
15. blood
16. sweat
17. tumor
18. a tearing
19. intentionally causing harm; cancer
20. fungus
21. dead cells, tissue, or body
22. new
23. lice
24. pigment
25. growth; formation
26. itching
27. itching
28. wrinkle
29. connective tissue
30. dry

Related Combining Forms Exercise (p. 366)

1. lip/o-, adip/o-
2. onych/o-, ungu/o-
3. trich/o-, hirsut/o-, pil/o-
4. diaphor/o-, hidr/o-, sudor/i-
5. derm/a-, derm/o-, dermat/o-, cutane/o-, cut/i-, integument/o-

Combining Form and Suffix Exercise (pp. 367–368)

1. dermatoplasty
2. hematoma
3. xeroderma
4. onychomycosis
5. abrasion
6. melanoma
7. cyanosis
8. dermatitis
9. pruritic
10. lipoma
11. neoplasm
12. erythematous
13. necrotic
14. pediculosis
15. keloid
16. contusion
17. exudate
18. fulguration
19. biopsy
20. lipectomy
21. dermatome
22. blepharoplasty
23. rhytidectomy
24. autograft

Prefix Exercise (p. 368)

1. anti-   antifungal
2. dys-   dysplastic
3. an-   anesthesia
4. de-   depigmentation
5. an-   anhidrosis
6. intra-   intradermal
7. pre-   premalignant
8. anti-   antipruritic

ABBREVIATIONS

Matching Exercise (p. 368)

4, 6, 1, 3, 5, 7, 2

APPLIED SKILLS

Plural Noun and Adjective Spelling (p. 369)

1. follicles   follicular
2.   cutaneous (or integumentary)
3.   epidermal
4.   dermal
5. nails   ungual
6.   epithelial
7. vesicles   vesicular
8.   pruritic
9.   cyanotic
10.   erythematous
11.   icteric
12.   necrotic
13.   gangrenous
14. verrucae
15. malignancies   malignant
16. keratoses   keratotic
17.   psoriatic
18.   diaphoretic
19. comedones

English and Medical Word Equivalents Exercise (p. 369)

1. eczema
2. senile lentigo
3. alopecia
4. decubitus
5. furuncle (or abscess)
6. abrasion
7. urticaria
8. pediculosis
9. scabies
10. nevus (or birthmark)
11. tinea
12. papilloma
13. verruca

Word Analysis Questions (p. 371)

1. cellul/o-   cell
   -itis   inflammation of; infection of
2. erythematous

Fact Finding Questions (p. 371)

1. pruritus
2. erythematous
3. welts
4. integumentary
5. drug reaction

Critical Thinking Skills (p. 371)

1. itchy scalp, wheals, welts, hives on the chest
2. erythema nodosum

On the Job Challenge Exercise (p. 372)

1. Condition of (pieces of) the nail (fingernails or toenails) being eaten; biting the nails
2. Abnormal condition of the nail (fingernail or toenail) being hidden; ingrown nail
3. Condition of the hair (being) pulled out (from the head)

Hearing Medical Words Exercise (p. 372)

1. acne vulgaris
2. anaphylaxis
3. blepharoplasty
4. cryosurgery
5. cyanosis
6. debridement
7. dermatologist
8. erythematous
9. pruritus
10. psoriasis

Pronunciation Exercise (p. 372)

1. bray
2. ad
3. pee
4. by
5. ly
6. toh
7. lip
8. nee
9. ry
10. tay

Chapter 8   Orthopedics (Skeletal)

ANATOMY AND PHYSIOLOGY

Labeling Exercise (pp. 396–397)

First Exercise

1. temporal bone, 2. frontal bone, 3. sphenoid bone, 4. lacrimal bone, 5. nasal bone, 6. ethmoid bone, 7. zygomatic bone, 8. maxilla, 9. mandible, 10. coronal suture, 11. parietal bone, 12. occipital bone

Second Exercise

1. tarsal bones, 2. metatarsal bones, 3. phalanges, 4. tibia, 5. talus, 6. calcaneus

Third Exercise

1. clavicle, 2. glenoid fossa, 3. humerus, 4. xiphoid process, 5. costal cartilage, 6. radius, 7. ulna, 8. carpal bones, 9. phalanges, 10. metacarpal bones, 11. patella, 12. fibula, 13. tibia, 14. rib, 15. manubrium, 16. scapula, 17. sternum, 18. vertebra, 19. ilium, 20. sacrum, 21. coccyx, 22. pubis or pubic bone, 23. ischium, 24. femur

BUILDING MEDICAL WORDS

Combining Forms Exercise (p. 398)

1. acetabulum (hip socket)
2. limb; small attached part
3. joint
4. joint
5. calcaneus (heel bone)
6. wrist
7. cartilage
8. neck; cervix

9. cartilage
10. clavicle (collar bone)
11. rib
12. cranium (skull)
13. finger or toe
14. shaft of a bone
15. growth area at the end of a long bone
16. sieve
17. femur (thigh bone)
18. fibula (lower leg bone)
19. front
20. socket of a joint
21. humerus (upper arm bone)
22. U-shaped structure
23. ilium (hip bone)
24. ischium (hip bone)
25. tears
26. ligament
27. lower back; area between the ribs and pelvix
28. mandible (lower jaw)
29. breast; mastoid process
30. maxilla (upper jaw)
31. nose
32. occiput (back of the head)
33. bone
34. changing into bone
35. bone
36. palate
37. wall of a cavity
38. patella (kneecap)
39. pelvis (hip bone; renal pelvis)
40. fibula (lower leg bone)
41. phalanx (finger or toe)
42. pubis (hip bone)
43. radius (forearm bone); x-rays; radiation
44. sacrum
45. scapula (shoulder blade)
46. skeleton
47. wedge shape
48. spine; backbone
49. vertebra
50. sternum (breast bone)
51. synovium (membrane)
52. ankle
53. temple (side of the head)
54. thorax (chest)
55. tibia (shin bone)
56. ulna (forearm bone)
57. vertebra
58. sword

Combining Form and Suffix Exercise (p. 399)

1. -al — cranial
2. -ic — thoracic
3. -al — costal
4. -ar — mandibular
5. -ous — ligamentous
6. -ic — pelvic
7. -eal — phalangeal
8. -ous — osseous
9. -ation — articulation
10. -clast — osteoclast
11. -al — vertebral
12. -ar — lumbar
13. -ar — ulnar
14. -ar — fibular
15. -ion — ossification
16. -oid — ethmoid
17. -al — sternal
18. -al — cervical
19. -ar — clavicular
20. -al — humeral
21. -ic — pubic
22. -al — carpal
23. -ar — patellar
24. -cyte — osteocyte

CHAPTER REVIEW EXERCISES
ANATOMY AND PHYSIOLOGY
Matching Exercise (p. 417)
12, 4, 11, 9, 18, 17, 15, 8, 6, 13, 3, 14, 1, 10, 2, 16, 5, 7

Circle Exercise (p. 417)
1. humerus
2. ossification
3. ilium
4. osteocytes
5. ankle
6. medial epicondyle
7. elbow
8. peroneal
9. clavicle

True or False Exercise (p. 418)
1. T, 2. T, 3. F, 4. T, 5. T, 6. T

DISEASES AND CONDITIONS
True or False Exercise (p. 418)
1. T, 2. T, 3. F, 4. F, 5. T, 6. F, 7. T, 8. F, 9. F

Matching Exercise (p. 418)
6, 8, 7, 2, 9, 1, 5, 3, 4

Circle Exercise (pp. 418–419)
1. osteomyelitis
2. avascular necrosis
3. demineralization
4. hemarthrosis
5. pectus excavatum
6. vertebrae
7. comminuted

LABORATORY, RADIOLOGY, SURGERY, AND DRUGS
Circle Exercise (p. 419)
1. goniometer
2. prosthesis
3. arthrodesis
4. rheumatoid arthritis
5. a blood test
6. bone densitometry
7. arthrography
8. orthosis
9. allograft
10. rheumatoid factor

BUILDING MEDICAL WORDS
Combining Forms Exercise (p. 419)
1. pain
2. sensation of pain
3. arranged in a straight line
4. to cut off
5. to cut off
6. bunion
7. break into small pieces
8. present at birth
9. right; sugar
10. disk
11. break up
12. production; creation
13. angle
14. blood
15. bent; humpbacked
16. left
17. a place
18. swayback
19. softening
20. mineral; electrolyte
21. bone marrow; spinal cord; myelin
22. straight
23. disease; suffering
24. child
25. body
26. small openings; pores
27. artificial part
28. connective tissue
29. curved; crooked
30. blood vessel

Related Combining Forms Exercise (p. 420)

1. oste/o-, osse/o-
2. chondr/o-, cartilagin/o-
3. arthr/o-, articul/o-
4. spondyl/o-, vertebr/o-
5. perone/o-, fibul/o-

Combining Form and Suffix Exercise (p. 420)

1. arthropathy
2. chondroma
3. kyphosis
4. arthritis
5. congenital
6. densitometry
7. osteoma
8. prosthetic
9. goniometer
10. bunionectomy
11. arthrodesis
12. arthroscope
13. amputee
14. comminuted
15. spondylolisthesis
16. lordosis

Prefix Exercise (p. 421)

1. a-   avascular
2. de-   demineralization
3. intra-   intra-articular
4. dis-   dislocation
5. mal-   malalignment
6. de-   degenerative
7. an-   analgesic

Multiple Combining Forms and Suffix Exercise (p. 421)

1. levoscoliosis
2. chondromalacia
3. osteoporosis
4. orthopedics
5. hemarthrosis
6. dextroscoliosis
7. arthralgia
8. osteomyelitis
9. osteosarcoma

Dividing Medical Words (p. 422)

1.		oste/o-	-cyte
2.	inter-	vertebr/o-	-al
3.	meta-	tars/o-	-al
4.		phalang/o-	-eal
5.		densit/o-	-metry
6.	a-	vascul/o-	-ar
7.		scoli/o-	-osis
8.	mal-	align/o-	-ment
9.		arthr/o-	-graphy
10.	de-	mineral/o-	-ization

Test Yourself (p. 422)

1. immature cell in the bone. Osteoblasts form new bone or rebuild bone.
2. cell that breaks down substances (bone). Osteoclasts break down old or damaged areas of bone.
3. cell in the bone. Osteocytes maintain and monitor the mineral content of the bone.
4. growth of bone. An osteophyte is new bone that forms abnormally, sometimes as a sharp bone spur that causes pain.

Osteophyte is the word that is not related.

ABBREVIATIONS

Matching Exercise (p. 422)

3, 6, 5, 2, 7, 1, 4

APPLIED SKILLS

Plural Noun and Adjective Spelling Exercise (p. 423)

1.		cranial
2.		mandibular
3.		thoracic
4.	ribs	costal
5.	vertebrae	vertebral
6.	phalanges	phalangeal
7.		ilial
8.	fibulae	fibular
9.	patellae	patellar
10.	scapulae	scapular

English and Medical Word Equivalents Exercise (p. 423)

1. cranium
2. zygoma (or zygomatic bone)
3. fontanel
4. maxilla (or maxillary bone)
5. mandible
6. scapula
7. sternum
8. clavicle
9. olecranon
10. phalanx (or ray or digit)
11. coccyx
12. femur
13. patella
14. tibia
15. calcaneus
16. kyphosis
17. lordosis
18. genu varum
19. genu valgum
20. talipes equinovarus
21. osteophyte
22. hallux

Word Analysis Questions (pp. 424–425)

1. dextr/o-   right; sugar
   Scoli/o-   curved; crooked
   -osis   condition; abnormal condition; process
2. True
3. orth/o-   straight
   Ped/o-   child
   -ist   one who specializes in

Fact Finding Questions (p. 425)

1. tibia
2. right leg
3. vertebrae
4. L

Critical Thinking Questions (p. 425)

1. to the right
2. nonsteroidal anti-inflammatory drugs; decrease inflammation and pain
3. the number of degrees of curvature of the dextroscoliosis

On the Job Challenge Exercise (p. 425)

1. A fracture whose pieces do not break through the overlying skin
2. Medical procedure in which manual manipulation of a displaced fracture is performed so that the bone ends go back into normal alignment without the need for surgery
3. A fracture whose pieces do break through the overlying skin
4. Surgical procedure to treat a complicated fracture. An incision is made at the fracture site, the fracture is reduced (realigned), and an internal fixation procedure is done using screws, nails, or plates to hold the fracture fragments in correct anatomical alignment.

Hearing Medical Words Exercise (p. 425)

1. arthritis
2. arthralgia
3. chondroma
4. comminuted fracture
5. dextroscoliosis
6. musculoskeletal
7. orthopedist
8. osteoporosis
9. phalanx
10. prosthesis

Pronunciation Exercise (p. 426)

1. tay
2. thrall
3. thraws
4. laj
5. throh
6. hyoo
7. foh
8. dib
9. kar
10. thry

Chapter 9 Orthopedics (Muscular)

ANATOMY AND PHYSIOLOGY

Labeling Exercise (pp. 448–449)

First Exercise

1. rotation, 2. flexion and adduction, 3. slight flexion, 4. flexion, 5. abduction and extension

Second Exercise

1. temporalis muscle, 2. masseter muscle, 3. trapezius muscle, 4. deltoid muscle, 5. triceps brachii muscle, 6. biceps brachii muscle, 7. brachioradialis muscle, 8. gluteus maximus muscle, 9. gastrocnemius muscle, 10. peroneus longus muscle, 11. frontalis muscle, 12. sternocleidomastoid muscle, 13. trapezius muscle, 14. latissimus dorsi muscle, 15. rectus abdominis muscle, 16. rectus femoris muscle, 17. tibialis anterior muscle

BUILDING MEDICAL WORDS

Combining Forms Exercise (p. 450)

1. done of one's own free will
2. abdomen
3. before; front part
4. arm
5. cheek
6. bursa
7. clavicle (collar bone)
8. pull together
9. rib
10. triangle
11. bring; move; a duct
12. straightening
13. outside
14. fascia
15. fiber
16. bending
17. front
18. stomach
19. to put in; introduce
20. inside
21. chewing
22. breast; mastoid process
23. muscle
24. muscle
25. muscle
26. nerve
27. small circle
28. chest
29. fibula (lower leg bone)
30. face down
31. radius (forearm bone); x-rays; radiation
32. rotate
33. skeleton
34. sternum (breast bone)
35. lying on the back
36. temple (side of the head)
37. tendon
38. tendon
39. tendon
40. thumb
41. tibia (shin bone)
42. to send across or through
43. development
44. to travel; to turn
45. to travel; to turn

Combining Form and Suffix Exercise (p. 451)

1.	-or	rotator
2.	-ous	tendinous
3.	-ar	muscular
4.	-ion	flexion
5.	-al	fascial
6.	-ature	musculature
7.	-oid	deltoid
8.	-ary	voluntary
9.	-er	masseter
10.	-aris	orbicularis
11.	-alis	pectoralis
12.	-ion	supination
13.	-ion	contraction

CHAPTER REVIEW EXERICSES

ANATOMY AND PHYSIOLOGY

Fill in the Blank Exercise (p. 466)

1. gastrocnemius muscle
2. pectoralis major muscle
3. deltoid muscle
4. latissimus dorsi muscle
5. rectus femoris muscle
6. sternocleidomastoid muscle
7. biceps brachii muscle
8. tibialis anterior muscle
9. rectus abdominis muscle
10. trapezius muscle
11. masseter muscle
12. gluteus maximus muscle
13. biceps femoris muscle

Circle Exercise (p. 466)

1. origin
2. aponeurosis
3. musculature
4. striated
5. big toe
6. deltoid
7. tri-

Matching Exercise (p. 467)

11, 5, 1, 9, 4, 8, 6, 10, 2, 7, 3, 12

Recall and Describe Exercise (p. 467)

1. Moving the arm away from the midline of the body
2. Straightening the knee joint and extending the leg
3. Turning the palm of the hand posteriorly or downward
4. Moving the head from side to side around its axis (the neck and spine)
5. Bending the knee joint to decrease the angle between the upper and lower leg
6. Pointing the toes upward

DISEASES AND CONDITIONS

Matching Exercise (p. 467)

8, 2, 4, 7, 9, 6, 5, 1, 3

True or False Exercise (p. 468)

1. F, 2. T, 3. F, 4. T, 5. F, 6. F, 7. T, 8. T, 9. T, 10. F

Circle Exercise (p. 468)

1. ataxia
2. tendon
3. athetoid
4. avulsion
5. Dupuytren's
6. rhabdomyosarcoma

LABORATORY, SURGERY, AND DRUGS

Multiple Choice (p. 468)

1. a
2. c
3. a
4. b
5. b

Circle Exercise (p. 469)

1. fibromyalgia
2. passive
3. thymectomy
4. incisional biopsy

BUILDING MEDICAL WORDS

Combining Forms Exercise (p. 469)

1. sensation of pain
2. pain
3. lack of strength
4. without position or place
5. hand
6. bruising
7. skin
8. electricity
9. ganglion
10. give ability
11. physician; medical treatment
12. inflammation of; infection of
13. movement
14. foot
15. rod shaped
16. synovium (membrane)
17. coordination
18. treatment
19. twisted position
20. to tear

Dividing Medical Words (p. 469)

1. ab-	duct/o-	-ion
2. a-	troph/o-	-ic
3. brady-	kines/o-	-ia
4.	delt/o-	-oid
5.	fasci/o-	-al
6.	gastr/o-	-cnemius
7.	myos/o-	-itis
8.	ganglion/o-	-ectomy
9. re-	habilitat/o-	-ion
10.	ten/o-	-rrhaphy

Combining Form and Suffix Exercise (p. 470)

1. fasciectomy
2. myopathy
3. inflammation
4. contracture
5. fasciitis
6. athetoid
7. fasciotomy
8. contusion
9. myoclonus
10. myositis
11. tenorrhaphy
12. tendonitis
13. gangionectomy
14. myorrhaphy
15. bursitis
16. torticollis

Prefix Exercise (p. 471)

1. re-	rehabilitation
2. intra-	intramuscular
3. brady-	bradykinesia
4. a-	ataxia
5. hyper-	hyperextension
6. inter-	intercostal
7. a-	atrophic
8. poly-	polymyalgia
9. a-	avulsion
10. dys-	dyskinesia
11. poly-	polymyositis
12. an-	analgesic

Multiple Combining Forms and Suffix Exercise (pp. 471–472)

1. musculoskeletal
2. brachioradialis
3. neuromuscular
4. dermatomyositis
5. fibromyalgia
6. electromyography
7. rhabdomyoma
8. tenosynovitis
9. podiatrist

ABBREVIATIONS

Define and Match Exercise (p. 472)

1. electromyography
2. activities of daily living
3. nonsteroidal anti-inflammatory drug
4. right upper extremity
5. occupational therapy (or occupational therapist)
6. muscular dystrophy
7. intramuscular

1, 4, 5, 6, 2, 7, 3

APPLIED SKILLS

Proofreading and Spelling Exercise (p. 472)

1. orthopedics
2. tendon
3. fascia
4. rectus
5. fibromyalgia
6. bursitis
7. ganglion
8. biopsy
9. dystrophy
10. tenorrhaphy

English and Medical Words Equivalents Exercise (p. 472)

1. bursitis
2. atrophy
3. torticollis
4. strain
5. hyperextension-hyperflexion injury
6. contusion
7. medial epicondylitis
8. lateral epicondylitis

Word Analysis Exercise (p. 474)

1. my/o-	muscle
	-pathy	disease; suffering
2. eti/o-	cause of disease
	-logy	the study of
3. bi/o-	life; living organisms; living tissue
	-opsy	process of viewing

4. Glutaraldehyde is a solution that is used as a tissue fixative for examination under a microscope. A protocol is a detailed plan of a procedure.

Fact Finding Questions (p. 475)

1. muscle biopsy x 3
2. right quadriceps
3. anterior upper leg
4. 3
5. climbing stairs; getting up from a chair or bed
6. red-tan
7. myopathy of undetermined etiology

Critical Thinking Skills (p. 475)

1. b
2. b

On the Job Challenge (p. 475)

1. musculus
2. No
3. muscles (muscle or musculus)

Hearing Medical Words Exercise (p. 476)

1. bursa
2. atrophy
3. bradykinesia
4. electromyography
5. fascial
6. gastrocnemius muscle
7. myalgia
8. podiatrist
9. rehabilitation
10. tenorrhapy

Pronunciation Exercise (p. 476)

1. duc	5. per
2. at	6. mus
3. ky	7. skel
4. al	8. mas

Chapter 10   Neurology

ANATOMY AND PHYSIOLOGY

Labeling Exercise (pp. 501–502)

First Exercise

1. frontal lobe, 2. temporal lobe, 3. parietal lobe, 4. occipital lobe, 5. cerebellum

Second Exercise

1. cranium, 2. dura mater, 3. arachnoid, 4. subarachnoid space, 5. pia mater, 6. gray matter of the cerebrum (cortex), 7. white matter of the cerebrum

Third Exercise

1. cerebrum, 2. sulcus, 3. gyrus, 4. thalamus, 5. midbrain, 6. pons, 7. medulla oblongata, 8. corpus callosum, 9. lateral ventricle, 10. hypothalamus, 11. fourth ventricle, 12. cerebellum

BUILDING MEDICAL WORDS

Combining Forms Exercise (p. 503)

1. set or group
2. supplemental or contributing part
3. bring toward the center
4. spider; spider web
5. starlike structure
6. the sense of hearing
7. independent; self-governing
8. hollow space
9. cerebellum (posterior part of the brain)
10. cerebrum (largest part of the brain)
11. cochlea (of the inner ear)
12. cortex (outer region)

13. cranium (skull)
14. cell
15. branching structure
16. back; dorsum
17. dura mater
18. go out from the center
19. brain
20. cellular lining
21. sensation; feeling
22. sensation; feeling
23. face
24. splitting
25. front
26. tongue
27. the sense of taste
28. meninges
29. meninges
30. one millionth; small
31. movement
32. myelin
33. bone marrow; spinal cord; myelin
34. nerve
35. nerve
36. occiput (back of the head)
37. eye
38. the sense of smell
39. scanty; few
40. eye; vision
41. wall of a cavity
42. suffering
43. outer aspects
44. pharynx (throat)
45. spinal nerve root
46. receive
47. spinal nerve root
48. sensation
49. body
50. spine; backbone
51. temple (side of the head)
52. thalamus
53. to send across or through
54. structure shaped like a pulley
55. wandering; vagus nerve
56. ventricle (lower heart chamber; chamber in the brain)
57. front; abdomen
58. vestibule (entrance)
59. sight; vision

Combining Form and Suffix Exercise (p. 504)

1. -ic   somatic
2. -al   cerebral
3. -al   cranial
4. -ous   nervous
5. -ory   auditory
6. -ar   ventricular
7. -oid   arachnoid
8. -eal   meningeal
9. -cyte   astrocyte
10. -al   spinal
11. -ite   dendrite
12. -ent   efferent
13. -ure   fissure
14. -al   peripheral
15. -ic   thalamic
16. -ory   sensory
17. -or   receptor
18. -ated   myelinated
19. -ic   autonomic
20. -on   neuron
21. -al   temporal
22. -ory   olfactory
23. -ar   cerebellar
24. -glia   neuroglia
25. -al   dural
26. -al   occipital

Prefix Exercise (p. 505)

1. sym-   sympathetic
2. hypo-   hypothalamus
3. epi-   epidural
4. sub-   subarachnoid
5. hemi-   hemisphere
6. tri-   trigeminal
7. hypo-   hypoglossal

CHAPTER REVIEW EXERCISES
ANATOMY AND PHYSIOLOGY

Matching Exercise (p. 533)

7, 15, 9, 12, 11, 4, 2, 1, 14, 13, 8, 6, 5, 10, 3

Circle Exercise (p. 533)

1. cerebrum
2. nose
3. pia mater
4. neuron
5. left hemisphere of the cerebrum
6. below
7. oculomotor
8. acetylcholine

True or False Exercise (p. 534)

1. F, 2. T, 3. F, 4. F, 5. T, 6. T, 7. T, 8. T

Fill in the Blank Exercise (p. 534)

1. dura mater, arachnoid, pia mater
2. gyri, sulci
3. hemisphere
4. ependymal
5. hypothalamus

Multiple Choice Exercise (p. 534)

1. c
2. a
3. d

DISEASES AND CONDITIONS

True or False Exercise (p. 535)

1. T, 2. F, 3. F, 4. T, 5. T, 6. F, 7. T, 8. T

Circle Exercise (p. 535)

1. shingles
2. aura
3. subdural hematoma
4. Parkinson's disease
5. paresthesias

Fill in the Blank Exercise (p. 535)

1. multiple sclerosis
2. concussion
3. narcolepsy
4. hydrocephalus
5. status epilepticus
6. amnesia
7. sciatica
8. mental retardation
9. nuchal rigidity
10. aphasia
11. syncope

Multiple Choice Exercise (p. 536)

1. b
2. d
3. d
4. c

LABORATORY, RADIOLOGY, SURGERY, DRUGS

True or False Exercise (p. 536)

1. T, 2. T, 3. F, 4. F, 5. T, 6. T, 7. F

Matching Exercise (p. 536)

9, 2, 7, 1, 3, 4, 5, 8, 6

Fill in the Blank Exercise (p. 537)

1. corticosteroid drug
2. myelography
3. alpha fetoprotein
4. rhizotomy
5. EEG
6. PET scan
7. polysomnography
8. spinal tap

BUILDING MEDICAL WORDS

Combining Forms Exercise (p. 537)

1. pain
2. life; living organisms; living tissue
3. burning
4. head
5. identical group derived from one; rapid contracting and relaxing
6. unconsciousness
7. violent shaking or jarring
8. seizure
9. cell

10. disk
11. electricity
12. seizure
13. fiber
14. blood
15. water; fluid
16. seizure
17. area of dead tissue
18. word
19. word; the study of
20. mind; chin
21. stupor; sleep
22. speech
23. fear; avoidance
24. light
25. paralysis
26. sleep
27. operative procedure
28. fainting
29. pressure; tone
30. blood vessel

Related Combining Forms Exercise (p. 538)

1. psych/o-, ment/o-
2. neur/o-, nerv/o-
3. rhiz/o-, radicul/o-
4. esthes/o-, sens/o-
5. myel/o-, spin/o-
6. epilept/o-, convuls/o-, ict/o-

Combining Form and Suffix Exercise (pp. 538–539)

1. mental
2. epileptic
3. hematoma
4. neuritis
5. biopsy
6. craniotomy
7. meningitis
8. narcolepsy
9. hydrocephalus
10. clonic
11. concussion
12. ependymoma
13. infarction
14. myelography
15. neuropathy
16. rhizotomy
17. convulsion
18. encephalitis
19. comatose
20. glioma
21. syncopal
22. meningocele
23. radiculopathy
24. neuroma
25. disectomy

Prefix Exercise (p. 539)

1. intra-   intraventricular
2. de-   dementia
3. post-   postictal
4. an-   anesthesia
5. poly-   polyneuritis
6. anti-   anticonvulsant
7. dys-   dyslexic
8. intra-   intracranial
9. a-   aphasia
10. hemi-   hemiplegic
11. sub-   subdural
12. quadri-   quadriplegia
13. poly-   polysomnography
14. hyper-   hyperesthesia
15. dys-   dysphasia

Multiple Combining Forms and Suffix Exercise (p. 540)

1. neurologic
2. photophobia
3. myelomeningocele
4. causalgia
5. neurofibromatosis
6. electroencephalogram
7. neuralgia
8. neurosurgery
9. cerebrovascular
10. astrocytoma
11. cephalagia

ABBREVIATIONS
Matching Exercise (p. 540)

6, 2, 1, 8, 7, 3, 5, 4

APPLIED SKILLS
Proofreading and Spelling Exercise (p. 541)

1. neurosurgery
2. hematoma
3. meningioma
4. cerebrovascular
5. infarct
6. cephalagia
7. paralyzed
8. hemiplegia
9. epilepsy
10. polyneuritis

Word Analysis Questions (p. 542)

1. neur/o-   nerve
   log/o-   word; the study of
   -ic   pertaining to
2. par-   beside
   Esthes/o-   sensation; feeling
   -ia   condition; state; thing
3. VER
4. arteri/o-   artery
   -graphy   process of recording

Fact Finding Questions (p. 543)

1. paresthesias of the fingers
2. multiple sclerosis, transient ischemic attack, cerebrospinal fluid
3. light touch, pinprick, vibration, position, 2-point discrimination
4. a. current and recent presidents, b. oriented x3 (knows name, date, and where she is), c. count back by serial 7s
5. Romberg
6. paresthesias
7. blockage of the artery
8. cerebrospinal fluid

Critical Thinking Questions (p, 543)

1. c
2. lumbar puncture (or spinal tap)
3. coordination
4. alteration in memory
5. multiple sclerosis

Dividing Medical Words (p. 544)

1. a-   phas/o-   -ia
2. de-   ment/o-   -ia
3. epi-   dur/o-   -al
4. hypo-   thalam/o-   -ic
5. intra-   crani/o-   -al
6.   meningi/o-   -oma
7.   narc/o-   -lepsy
8.   neur/o-   -glia
9. post-   ict/o-   -al
10. sub-   dur/o-   -al

Hearing Medical Words Exercise (p. 544)

1. seizure
2. cephalalgia
3. craniotomy
4. hemiplegia
5. migraine
6. intracranial
7. occipital
8. syncope
9. meningitis
10. comatose

Pronunciation Exercise (p. 544)

1. ner
2. thee
3. fay
4. toh
5. sef
6. in
7. nin
8. ral
9. at
10. sin

Chapter 11   Urology

ANATOMY AND PHYSIOLOGY

Labeling Exercise (pp. 560–561)

First Exercise

1. renal pyramid, 2. renal pelvis, 3. major calix, 4. minor calix, 5. ureter, 6. renal cortex, 7. hilum

Second Exercise

1. ureter, 2. urinary bladder, 3. penis, 4. urethra, 5. urethral meatus, 6. external urinary sphincter, 7. kidney, 8. prostate gland

Third Exercise

1. glomerular capsule, 2. glomerulus, 3. renal artery, 4. proximal convoluted tubule, 5. nephron loop, 6. distal convoluted tubule, 7. collecting duct

BUILDING MEDICAL WORDS

Combining Forms Exercise (pp. 561–562)

1. absorb; take in
2. calix
3. calix
4. cortex (outer region)
5. bladder; fluid-filled sac; semisolid cyst
6. away from the center or point of origin
7. electricity
8. to urinate
9. red
10. removing from the body
11. filtering; straining
12. filter
13. genitalia
14. glomerulus
15. hilum (indentation in an organ)
16. making urine
17. mucous membrane
18. kidney; nephron
19. pelvis (hip bone; renal pelvis)
20. penis
21. peritoneum
22. prostate gland
23. near the center or point of origin
24. renal pelvis
25. kidney
26. tube
27. tube; small tube
28. ureter
29. urethra
30. urine; urinary system
31. urine; urinary system
32. bladder; fluid-filled sac

Combining Form and Suffix Exercise (p. 562)

1. -al   mucosal
2. -ation   urination
3. -eal   caliceal
4. -al   renal
5. -al   vesical
6. -ic   prostatic
7. -ar   glomerular
8. -ule   tubule
9. -ory   excretory
10. -ate   filtrate
11. -ary   urinary
12. -ar   hilar
13. -al   ureteral
14. -ile   penile
15. -al   urethral
16. -lyte   electrolyte
17. -tion   micturition
18. -poietin   erythropoietin

CHAPTER REVIEW EXERCISES

ANATOMY AND PHYSIOLOGY

Unscramble and Match Exercise (p. 585)

1. bladder
2. kidneys
3. hilum
4. tubule
5. sphincter
6. rugae
7. glomerulus
8. meatus
9. prostate
10. ureter
11. calix
12. medulla
13. urethra

11, 4, 8, 12, 7, 2, 5, 13, 1, 9, 11, 3, 6

Sequencing Exercise (p. 585)

1. renal artery
2. glomerulus (or glomerular capsule)
3. glomerular capsule (or glomerulus)
4. proximal convoluted tubule
5. nephron loop
6. distal convoluted tubule
7. collecting duct
8. calix
9. renal pelvis
10. ureter
11. bladder
12. urethra
13. urethral meatus

DISEASES AND CONDITIONS

Matching Exercise (p. 586)

3, 8, 2, 6, 9, 1, 4, 10, 7, 5

Antonyms Exercise (p. 586)

1. chronic
2. anuria
3. hypospadias
4. occult blood in the urine
5. incontinence

Synonyms Exercise (p. 586)

1. proteinuria
2. vesicocele
3. bedwetting
4. frank blood
5. Wilms' tumor

True or False Exercise (p. 586)

1. T, 2. T, 3. F, 4. F, 5. F, 6. T, 7. F, 8. F, 9. T, 10. T, 11. T

LABORATORY, RADIOLOGY, SURGERY, AND DRUGS

Laboratory Test Exercise (p. 587)

PANELS AND PROFILES		TESTS	
968T	Lipid Panel	19687W	Bilirubin (Direct)
315F	Electrolyte Panel	265F	HBsAg
10256F	Hepatic Function Panel	51870R	HB Core Antibody
10165F	Basic Metabolic Panel	1012F	Cardio CRP
10231A	Comprehensive Metabolic Panel	23242E	GGT
10306F	Hepatitis Panel, Acute	28852E	Protein, Total
182Aaa	Obstetric Panel	141A	CBC Hemogram
18T	Chem-Screen Panel (Basic)	21105R	hCG, Qualitative, Serum
654T	Chem-Screen Panel (Basic with HDL)	10321A	ANA
7971A	Chem-Screen Panel (Basic with HDL, TIBC)	80185	Cardio CRP with Lipid Profile
TESTS		26F	PT with INR
56713E	Lead, Blood	232Aaa	UA, Dipstick
2782A	Antibody Screen	42A	CBC with Diff
3556F	Iron, TIBC	20067W	HDL Cholesterol
20933E	Cholesterol	31732E	PTT
3084111E ✓	Uric Acid	34F ✓	UA, Dipstick and Microscopic
53348W	Rubella Antibody	20396R	CEA
27771E	Phosphate	45443E	Hematocrit
2111600E ✓	Creatinine	28571E	PSA, Total
29868W	Testosterone, Total	66902E	WBC count
9704F ✓	Creatinine Clearance	20750E	Chloride
19752E	Bilirubin (Total)	7187W	Hemoglobin
30536Rrr	T3, Total	4259T	HIV-1 Antibody
687T	Protein Electrophoresis	45484R	Hemoglobin A1c
3563444R	Digoxin	67868R	Alk Phosphatase
15214R	Glucose, 2-Hour Postprandial	24984R	Iron
30502E	T3, Uptake	28512E	Sodium
7773E	Platelet Count	1742bH	ALT
39685R	Dilantin (phenytoin)	MICROBIOLOGY	
30494R	Triglycerides	112680E	Group A Beta Strep Culture, Throat
26013E	Magnesium	5827W	Group B Beta Strep Culture, Genitals
15586R	Glucose, Fasting	49932E	Chlamydia, Endocervix/Urethra
30237W	T4, Free	6007W	Culture, Blood
28233E	Potassium	2692E	Culture, Genitals
1920BW	AST	2649T	Culture, HSV
30163E	TSH	612A	Culture, Sputum
22764R	Ferritin	6262E	Culture, Throat
20008W	Calcium	6304R ✓	Culture, Urine
54726F	Occult Blood, Stool	50286R ✓	Gonococcus, Endocervix/Urethra
51839W	HAV Antibody, Total	6643E	Gram Stain
430A	Blood Group and Rh Type	STOOL PATHOGENS	
28399W	Progesterone	10045F	Culture, Stool
30262E	T4, Total	4475F	Culture, Campylobacter
20209W	Carbon Dioxide	10018T	Culture, Salmonella
1156F	RPR	86140A	E. coli Toxins
30940E ✓	Urea Nitrogen	1099T	Ova and Parasites
17417W ✓	Albumin	VENIPUNCTURE	
28423E	Prolactin	63180	Venipuncture

Circle Exercise (p. 588)

1. sound waves
2. IVP
3. nephrectomy
4. shunt
5. UA
6. dialysis
7. contrast dye

Multiple Choice Exercise (p. 588)

1. c
2. d
3. a

BUILDING MEDICAL WORDS

Combining Forms Exercise (pp. 588–589)

1. albumin
2. walking
3. bacterium
4. immature; embryonic
5. stone
6. catheter
7. time
8. arising from; produced by
9. glucose (sugar)
10. blood
11. blood
12. clear, glasslike substance
13. potassium
14. ketones
15. stone
16. word; the study of
17. nerve
18. night
19. scanty; few
20. protein
21. pubis (hip bone)
22. pus
23. keep; hold back
24. hard; sclera (white of the eye)
25. tear; opening
26. spasm
27. cut; slice; layer
28. poison
29. move something to another place
30. vagina

Related Combining Forms Exercise (p. 589)

1. cyst/o-, vesic/o-
2. nephr/o-, ren/o-
3. lith/o-, calcul/o-
4. enur/o-, micturi/o-, urin/o-
5. pyel/o-, pelv/o-

Combining Form and Suffix Exercise (p. 589)

1. urethritis
2. nephroptosis
3. pyelography
4. urinometer
5. cystitis
6. caliectasis
7. nephropathy
8. nephrectomy
9. cystoscopy
10. cystocele
11. urogram
12. catheterization
13. lithotripsy
14. cystometry
15. nephropexy

Prefix Exercise (p. 590)

1. hypo-   hypokalemia
2. dys-   dysuria
3. poly-   polycystic
4. trans-   transurethral
5. an-   anuria
6. supra-   suprapubic
7. poly-   polyuria
8. anti-   antispasmodic
9. epi-   epispadias

Multiple Combining Forms and Suffix Exercise (pp. 590–591)

1. lithogenesis
2. nephrolithotomy
3. glomerulosclerosis
4. pyelonephritis
5. nephroblastoma
6. pyuria
7. nephrolithiasis
8. genitourinary
9. hematuria
10. nephrotomography
11. glycosuria
12. vesicovaginal
13. oliguria
14. nephrologist
15. ketonuria
16. nephrotoxic
17. nocturia

ABBREVIATIONS

Define and Match Exercise (p. 591)

1. blood urea nitrogen
2. cubic centimeter
3. chronic renal failure
4. culture and sensitivity
5. extracorporeal shock wave lithotripsy
6. intake and output

7. intravenous pyelography (or pyelogram)
8. potassium
9. kidneys, ureters, bladder
10. too numerous to count
11. urinalysis
12. white blood cell

7, 4, 3, 12, 9, 2, 10, 1, 6, 11, 8, 5

APPLIED SKILLS

Plural Noun and Adjective Spelling Exercise (p. 591)

1. cortices   cortical
2. glomeruli   glomerular
3. hila   hilar
4. kidneys   renal
5. medullae
6. pelves   pelvic
7. tubules   tubular
8. ureters   ureteral
9.   urethral
10.   urinary

Word Analysis Questions (p. 593)

1. ur/o-   urine; urinary system
   log/o-   word; the study of
   -ist   one who specializes in
2. supra-   above
   pub/o-   pubis (pubic bone)
   -ic   pertaining to
3. hemat/o-   blood
   ur/o-   urine; urinary system
   -ia   condition; state; thing
4. anti-   against
   bi/o-   life; living organisms; living tissue
   -tic   pertaining to
5. kidneys, ureters, bladder; intravenous
6. UTI

Fact Finding Questions (p. 593)

1. clean-catch urine
2. to acidify the urine to decrease the growth of bacteria
3. a spasm of the smooth muscle of the ureter or bladder as the kidney stone's jagged edges scrape the mucosa; pain located above the pubic bone
4. catheterized specimen
5. The patient was given a urine strainer to strain her urine to catch a kidney stone that could be sent to the lab for analysis.

Critical Thinking Questions (p. 593)

1. Because it can be assumed that the patient did not have appendicitis and that the pain was from another source.
2. Because it can be assumed that the patient was not pregnant and that the pain was from another source.
3. Her pulse, respirations, and blood pressure were elevated in response to the renal colic pain. Her temperature was not elevated because she did not have an infection.
4. The vaginal examination revealed no discharge or tenderness so there was no infection or other abnormality there.
5. The kidney stone scraping the mucosa and causing bleeding as it passed through the urinary system.

On the Job Challenge Exercise (p. 594)

a slow and painful discharge of urine because of spasms of the bladder and urethra

Hearing Medical Words Exercise (p. 594)

1. catheter
2. calculus
3. cystitis
4. cystoscopy
5. dysuria
6. glomerulonephritis
7. hemodialysis
8. lithotripsy
9. nocturia
10. pyelonephritis

Pronunciation Exercise (p. 594)

1. nay
2. at
3. taws
4. eks
5. mair
6. tyoo
7. frek
8. yoo
9. fry
10. rawl

Chapter 12   Male Reproductive Medicine

ANATOMY AND PHYSIOLOGY

Labeling Exercise (p. 608)
1. vas deferens
2. prostate gland
3. corpus cavernosum of the penis
4. penile urethra
5. glans penis
6. seminal vesicle
7. ejaculatory duct
8. bulbourethral gland
9. epididymis
10. testis
11. scrotum

BUILDING MEDICAL WORDS

Combining Forms Exercise (p. 609)
1. the beginning of being an adult
2. glans penis
3. like a bulb
4. sexual intercourse
5. testes (twin structures)
6. to expel suddenly
7. to stand up
8. to bear
9. genitalia
10. arising from; produced by
11. seed (ovum or spermatozoon)
12. groin
13. spaces within tissue
14. threadlike structure
15. testis
16. testis
17. sexual intercourse
18. penis
19. perineum
20. produce
21. prostate gland
22. growing up
23. a bag; scrotum
24. spermatozoon; sperm
25. spermatozoon; sperm
26. spermatozoon; sperm
27. spermatozoon; sperm
28. testis; testicle
29. testis; testicle
30. tube
31. urethra
32. urine; urinary system
33. urine; urinary system
34. blood vessel; vas deferens
35. sexual intercourse

Combining Form and Suffix Exercise (p. 610)
1. -al perineal
2. -al scrotal
3. -ty puberty
4. -cyte spermatocyte
5. -ule tubule
6. -ion erection
7. -ence adolescence
8. -al genital
9. -ar testicular
10. -ile penile
11. -ic prostatic
12. -ory ejaculatory
13. -al inguinal

CHAPTER REVIEW EXERCISES

ANATOMY AND PHYSIOLOGY

Fill in the Blank Exercise (p. 624)
1. spermatogenesis
2. genitals
3. testes
4. perineum
5. lumen
6. sperm
7. epididymis
8. interstitial
9. spermatic cord
10. spermatocytes
11. flagellum
12. testosterone
13. ductus deferens
14. ejaculatory duct
15. prostate gland
16. prepuce

True or False Exercise (p. 624)
1. F, 2. F, 3. T, 4. F, 5. F, 6. T, 7. T, 8. T, 9. F

Circle Exercise (p. 625)
1. scrotum
2. epididymis
3. seminiferous tubules
4. ejaculatory duct
5. meiosis

Sequencing Exercise (p. 625)
1. seminiferous tubules, 2. epididymis, 3. vas deferens, 4. ejaculatory duct, 5. prostatic urethra, 6. urethra in the penis, 7. urethral meatus

DISEASES AND CONDITIONS

Matching Exercise (p. 625)
12, 9, 7, 10, 11, 4, 1, 2, 5, 3, 8, 6

Circle Exercise (pp. 625–626)
1. breasts
2. balanitis
3. oligospermia
4. dyspareunia
5. syphilis
6. retrovirus
7. phimosis
8. sexual intercourse
9. phimosis
10. human immunodeficiency virus

LABORATORY, RADIOLOGY, SURGERY, AND DRUGS

Circle Exercise (p. 626)
1. sperm count
2. testicular self-examination
3. orchiopexy
4. gonorrhea
5. erectile dysfunction
6. female hormone

Fill in the Blank Exercise (p. 626)
1. varicocelectomy
2. morphology
3. acid phosphatase
4. ultrasonography
5. digital rectal exam
6. resectoscope
7. vasovasostomy
8. circumcision

BUILDING MEDICAL WORDS

Related Combining Forms Exercise (p. 626)
1. balan/o-, pen/o-
2. pareun/o-, venere/o-, coito/o-
3. didym/o-, test/o-, orchi/o-, testicul/o-, orch/o-

Combining Forms Exercise (p. 627)
1. to breathe in; to suck in
2. take away; destroy
3. male
4. life; living organisms; living tissue
5. cancer
6. to cut
7. hidden
8. lacking; inadequate
9. able to conceive a child
10. female; woman
11. immune response
12. to cut into
13. workplace; testing place
14. intentionally causing harm; cancer
15. breast; mastoid process
16. shape
17. movement
18. scanty; few
19. closed tight
20. persistent erection
21. to cut out; remove
22. science; knowledge
23. sound
24. development
25. urethra
26. varix; varicose vein

Prefix Exercise (p. 627)
1. trans- transurethral
2. dys- dyspareunia
3. ultra- ultrasonography
4. a- aspermia
5. circum- circumcision
6. re- reproductive
7. post- postcoital
8. epi- epididymitis
9. in- infertility

Combining Form and Suffix Exercise (p. 628)
1. motility
2. vasectomy
3. cancerous
4. varicocele
5. seminoma
6. orchitis
7. morphology
8. prostatectomy
9. orchiopexy
10. malignancy
11. balanitis
12. androgen
13. biopsy
14. resectoscope

15. venereal
16. orchiectomy
17. prostatitis

18. priapism
19. phimosis

Multiple Combining Forms and Suffix Exercise (p. 629)

1. immunodeficiency
2. genitourinary
3. vasovasostomy
4. gynecomastia
5. spermatogenesis
6. cryptorchism
7. oligospermia

ABBREVIATIONS

Definition Exercise (p. 629)

1. benign prostatic hypertrophy
2. erectile dysfunction
3. gonococcus (or gonorrhea)
4. herpes simplex virus
5. prostate-specific antigen
6. sexually transmitted disease
7. transurethral resection of the prostate
8. venereal disease

APPLIED SKILLS

Plural Noun and Adjective Spelling Exercise (p. 630)

1. tubules — tubular
2. testicles — testicular
3. — perineal
4. spermatozoa
5. epididymides
6. — prostatic
7. — penile

Proofreading and Spelling Exercise (p. 630)

1. glans
2. perineal
3. scrotum
4. spermatozoa
5. inguinal
6. epididymis
7. gametes
8. deferens
9. seminal
10. prostate

English and Medical Word Equivalents Exercise (p. 630)

1. seminoma
2. dyspareunia
3. erectile dysfunction
4. venereal disease
5. cryptorchism (or cryptorchidism)
6. condylomata acuminata
7. benign prostatic hypertrophy

Dividing Medical Words (p. 630)

1. dys- — pareun/o- — -ia
2. — venere/o- — -al
3. circum- — cis/o- — -ion
4. — testicul/o- — -ar
5. a- — sperm/o- — -ia
6. — priap/o- — -ism
7. re- — product/o- — -ive
8. post- — coit/o- — -al

Word Analysis Questions (p. 632)

1. orchi/o- — testis
   -pexy — process of surgically fixing in place
2. b

Fact Finding Questions (p. 632)

1. back
2. scrotum, testes, epididymides, penis, urethra
3. suprapubic skin on the left side; scrotum (scrotal incision)
4. True
5. under the skin
6. left orchiopexy

Critical Thinking Questions (p. 632)

1. before
2. spermatic cord

Hearing Medical Words (p. 632)

1. perineum
2. balanitis
3. chancre
4. dyspareunia
5. epididymis
6. gonorrhea

7. orchitis
8. prostatectomy
9. seminoma
10. syphilis

Pronunciation Exercise (p. 632)

1. pyoo
2. sper
3. lay
4. rek
5. tay
6. mas
7. til
8. ek
9. tik
10. neer

Chapter 13   Gynecology and Obstetrics

ANATOMY AND PHYSIOLOGY

Labeling Exercise (p. 659)

First Exercise

1. mons pubis, 2. labia majora, 3. clitoris, 4. urethral meatus, 5. vaginal introitus, 6. labia minora, 7. vulva, 8. perineum, 9. anus

Second Exercise

1. round ligament, 2. uterine tube, 3. ovarian ligament, 4. broad ligament, 5. intrauterine cavity, 6. endometrium, 7. myometrium, 8. perimetrium, 9. cervical canal, 10. cervical os, 11. infundibulum, 12. lumen of uterine tube, 13. ovary, 14. follicle at time of ovulation, 15. ovum, 16. fimbriae, 17. uterine fundus, 18. corpus of uterus, 19. uterine cervix, 20. vagina

BUILDING MEDICAL WORDS

Combining Forms Exercise (pp. 660–661)

1. seed (spermatozoon or ovum)
2. extremity; highest point
3. accessory connecting parts
4. amnion (fetal membrane)
5. small area around the nipple
6. head
7. neck; cervix
8. chorion (fetal membrane)
9. vagina
10. to conceive or form
11. pull together
12. cul-de-sac
13. blue
14. dilate; widen
15. do away with; obliterate
16. embryo; immature form
17. vulva (female external genitalia)
18. female
19. female
20. uterine (fallopian) tube
21. to bear
22. able to conceive a child
23. fetus
24. bending
25. close association or relationship
26. fundus (part farthest from the opening)
27. milk
28. genitalia
29. arising from; produced by
30. from conception to birth
31. gonads (ovaries and testes)
32. female; woman
33. uterus (womb)
34. enlarged organ returns to normal size
35. keep back; block
36. lip; labium
37. milk
38. milk
39. lobe of an organ
40. breast
41. breast
42. breast; mastoid process
43. month
44. monthly discharge of blood
45. uterus (womb)
46. measurement; uterus (womb)
47. muscle
48. birth

49. new
50. ovum (egg)
51. ovary
52. ovary
53. ovum (egg)
54. ovum (egg)
55. ovum (egg)
56. oxygen; quick
57. birth
58. childbirth
59. to be in labor
60. perineum
61. placenta
62. being with child
63. produce
64. uterine (fallopian) tube
65. produce; secrete
66. contraction
67. labor and childbirth
68. having an affinity for; stimulating; turning
69. umbilicus; navel
70. urethra
71. urine; urinary system
72. urine; urinary system
73. uterus (womb)
74. vagina
75. vulva

Combining Form and Suffix Exercise (pp. 661–662)

1. -al   fundal
2. -ary   mammary
3. -ine   uterine
4. -cyte   oocyte
5. -an   ovarian
6. -ar   areolar
7. -ation   ovulation
8. -arche   menarche
9. -al   cervical
10. -ation   menstruation
11. -tic   amniotic
12. -ation   lactation
13. -al   adnexal
14. -al   fetal
15. -ion   conception
16. -ant   pregnant
17. -ic   embryonic
18. -duct   oviduct
19. -al   vaginal
20. -al   labial
21. -ancy   pregnancy
22. -ization   fertilization
23. -al   perineal
24. -nate   neonate
25. -al   placental
26. -ion   involution
27. -ar   vulvar
28. -ment   effacement
29. -ion   gestation

Prefix Exercise (p. 662)

1. pre-   prenatal
2. intra-   intrauterine
3. re-   reproductive
4. ante-   anteflexion
5. peri-   perimetrium
6. post-   postnatal
7. endo-   endometrium
8. tri-   trimester

Multiple Combining Forms and Suffix Exercise (p. 663)

1. lact/i-   fer/o-   -ous   lactiferous
2. my/o-   metri/o- -um   myometrium
3. o/o-   gen/o-   -esis oogenesis
4. ne/o-   nat/o-   -al   neonatal
5. ox/y-   toc/o-   -in   oxytocin
6. acr/o-   cyan/o-   -osis acrocyanosis
7. genit/o- urin/o-   -ary   genitourinary

CHAPTER REVIEW EXERCISES
ANATOMY AND PHYSIOLOGY
Matching Exercise (p. 694)

3, 6, 3, 1, 4, 5, 6, 5, 7, 8, 3, 7, 1, 2, 6

True or False Exercise (p. 694)

1. T, 2. F, 3. T, 4. F, 5. T, 6. F, 7. T, 8. F, 9. F, 10. F, 11. F, 12. T, 13. F

Fill in the Blank Exercise (p. 695)

1. zygote
2. fertilization
3. presenting part
4. amnion
5. gamete
6. placenta
7. umbilical cord
8. embryo
9. fetus
10. gestation
11. trimester
12. engagement
13. false labor

Sequencing Exercise (p. 695)

1. engagement
2. dilation and effacement
3. crowning
4. birth of the newborn
5. placenta delivered
6. involution

Matching Exercise (p. 695)

7, 4, 9, 8, 5, 3, 6, 1, 2

DISEASES AND CONDITIONS
Matching Exercise (p. 696)

7, 3, 1, 9, 5, 4, 6, 2, 8

Circle Exercise (p. 696)

1. breasts
2. amenorrhea
3. ovarian
4. endometriosis
5. candidiasis
6. myometritis
7. hemosalpinx
8. breast
9. prolapsed cord
10. jaundice
11. dyspareunia

Matching Exercise (p. 696)

1, 3, 5, 8, 4, 7, 6, 2

LABORATORY, RADIOLOGY, SURGERY, AND DRUGS
True or False Exercise (p. 697)

1. F, 2. F, 3. F, 4. T, 5. F, 6. F, 7. F, 8. T, 9. T, 10. T

Matching Exercise (p. 697)

8, 1, 6, 4, 2, 3, 10, 9, 7, 5

Multiple Choice Exercise (p. 697)

1. d
2. d
3. b
4. a

BUILDING MEDICAL WORDS
Combining Forms Exercise (p. 698)

1. take away; destroy
2. stop prematurely
3. cancer
4. head
5. cone
6. cold
7. bladder; fluid-filled sac; semisolid cyst
8. a seizure
9. outside of a place
10. blood
11. fluid-filled vesicles
12. water; fluid
13. abdomen
14. smooth
15. white
16. hand
17. many
18. neck
19. none
20. pregnancy and childbirth
21. scanty; few
22. child
23. pelvis (hip bone; renal pelvis)
24. growth; formation
25. first
26. pus
27. rectum
28. excessive flow or discharge
29. operative procedure
30. dry

Related Combining Form Exercise (p. 698)

1. par/o-, nat/o-
2. oophor/o-, ovari/o-
3. colp/o-, vagin/o-
4. episi/o-, vulv/o-
5. mast/o-, mamm/a-, mamm/o-
6. gynec/o-, estr/a-, estr/o-
7. o/o-, ov/i-, ov/o-, ovul/o-
8. hyster/o-, uter/o-, metri/o-, metr/o-

Combining Form and Suffix Exercise (pp. 699–700)

1. nuchal
2. galactorrhea
3. salpingitis
4. menopause
5. cystocele
6. mastopexy
7. vaginitis
8. leukorrhea
9. cryoprobe
10. primigravida
11. laparoscope
12. ectopic
13. episiotomy
14. hemosalpinx
15. mastitis
16. hydatidiform
17. rectocele
18. salpingectomy
19. colposcopy
20. amniocentesis
21. conization
22. mastectomy
23. culdoscopy
24. pyosalpinx
25. colporrhaphy
26. abortion
27. hysterectomy
28. mammography
29. mammoplasty
30. oophorectomy

Prefix Exercise (p. 700)

1. dys-   dysplasia
2. pre-   premenstrual
3. poly-   polycystic
4. dys-   dysmenorrhea
5. endo-   endometriosis
6. hyper-   hyperemesis
7. bi-   bimanual
8. trans-   transvaginal
9. pre-   preeclampsia
10. dys-   dyspareunia
11. an-   anovulation
12. dys-   dystocia

Multiple Combining Forms and Suffix Exercise (p. 701)

1. pyometritis
2. leiomyoma
3. cephalopelvic
4. oligohydramnios
5. multiparous
6. hysterosalpingogram
7. cryosurgery
8. salpingo-oophorectomy
9. oligomenorrhea
10. menorrhagia

ABBREVIATIONS

Matching Exercise (pp. 701–702)

5, 10, 8, 12, 11, 13, 3, 7, 9, 4, 6, 1, 14, 2

APPLIED SKILLS

Plural Noun and Adjective Spelling Exercise (p. 702)

1. areolae   areolar
2.   amniotic
3. breasts   mammary
4.   cervical
5. fetuses   fetal
6. ovaries   ovarian
7. ova
8.   perineal
9.   placental
10.   umbilical
11.   uterine
12.   vaginal

Proofreading and Spelling Exercise (p. 702)

1. gynecologic
2. dyspareunia
3. uterus
4. uterine
5. obstetrical
6. primigravida
7. amniocentesis
8. cesarean
9. hysterectomy
10. oophorectomy

English and Medical Word Equivalents Exercise (p. 703)

1. mammary glands
2. placenta
3. neonate
4. amniotic sac (or amnion)
5. Braxton Hicks contractions
6. tubal ligation
7. fontanel
8. uterus
9. hyperemesis gravidarum

You Write the Medical Report (p. 703)

1. failure of lactation
2. hysterectomy, salpingo-oophorectomy
3. leucorrhea, antifungal
4. engagement, EDB (or EDC)
5. infertility, salpingitis, polycystic, dyspareunia, laparoscopy, endometriosis
6. menarche, dysmenorrheal, oligomenorrhea, menopause

Word Analysis Questions (p. 705)

1. a. appropriate for gestational age
   b. estimated date of birth
   c. estimated gestational age
   d. neonatal intensive care unit
   e. spontaneous abortion
2. gestational
3. gestat/o-   from conception to birth
   -ion   action; condition
   -al   pertaining to
4. pre-   before; in front of
   nat/o-   birth
   -al   pertaining to
5. NSVD

Fact Finding Questions (p. 705)

1. breech
2. version
3. 0 number of term births, 0 number of premature births, 1 abortion (spontaneous), 0 number of living children
4. molding
5. Yes
6. The anterior fontanel or soft spot is a soft area on the top of the head. There is also a smaller posterior fontanel at the back of the head.
7. A chest x-ray

Critical Thinking Questions (p. 705)

1. Mother's temperature was 103.2 degrees and she was started on an antibiotic drug. The newborn's temperature was 101.2
2. fetal distress

Dividing Medical Words (p. 706)

1.   menstru/o-   -ation
2. pre-   nat/o-   -al
3.   ne/o-   -nate
4. an-   ovul/o-   -ation
5. poly-   cyst/o-   -ic
6. dys-   men/o-   -rrhea
7.   lact/o-   -ation
8. post-   part/o-   -um
9. retro-   vers/o-   -ion
10.   cyst/o-   -cele

Hearing Medical Words Exercise (p. 706)

1. biopsy
2. menarche
3. mammography
4. lactation
5. amniocentesis
6. cystocele
7. dyspareunia
8. episiotomy

Pronunciation Exercise (p. 706)

1. men
2. laws
3. mam
4. vair
5. yoo
6. ree
7. jy
8. tek

Chapter 14 Endocrinology

ANATOMY AND PHYSIOLOGY

Labeling Exercise (p. 725)

First Exercise

1. thyroid gland, 2. parathyroid glands, 3. pancreas, 4. adrenal gland,
5. ovary, 6. pineal body, 7. hypothalamus, 8. pituitary gland, 9. thymus,
10. testis

Second Exercise

1. thyroid cartilage of the larynx, 2. right lobe of the thyroid gland,
3. isthmus of the thyroid gland, 4. trachea, 5. tracheal cartilage, 6. left
lobe of the thyroid gland, 7. parathyroid glands

BUILDING MEDICAL WORDS

Combining Forms Exercise (p. 726)

1. ovary
2. gland
3. adrenal gland
4. adrenal gland
5. to lead to
6. male
7. oppose; work against
8. before; front part
9. calcium
10. calcium
11. cortex (outer region)
12. secrete
13. activity; work
14. female
15. female
16. milk
17. gland
18. glucose (sugar)
19. glucose (sugar)
20. glucose (sugar)
21. gonads (ovaries and testes)
22. same
23. hormone
24. pituitary gland
25. block; hold back
26. insulin
27. island
28. iodine
29. milk
30. black
31. mineral; electrolyte
32. nerve
33. oxygen; quick
34. pancreas
35. pituitary gland
36. pituitary gland
37. receive
38. kidney
39. body
40. standing still; staying in one place
41. exciting; strengthening
42. testis; testicle
43. testis; testicle
44. thalamus
45. thymus; rage
46. shield-shaped structure (thyroid gland)
47. thyroid gland
48. labor and childbirth
49. pressure; tone
50. having an affinity for; stimulating; turning
51. urine; urinary system
52. masculine

Combining Form and Suffix Exercise (p. 727)

1. -ic   thymic
2. -al   hormonal
3. -gen   androgen
4. -an   ovarian
5. -stasis homeostasis
6. -ation stimulation
7. -oid   thyroid
8. -ic   pancreatic
9. -ar   testicular
10. -or   receptor
11. -ism   antagonism

Prefix Exercise (p. 727)

1. hypo-   hypophysial
2. eu-   euthyroidism
3. para-   parathyroid
4. hypo-   hypothalamic
5. pro-   prolactin
6. syn-   synergism
7. ad-   adrenal

CHAPTER REVIEW EXERCISES

ANATOMY AND PHYSIOLOGY

Location Exercise (p. 748)

1. in the center of the brain, on top of the brainstem, below the thalamus
2. within the brain, in the bony sella turcica of the sphenoid bone, at the end of the stalk of the hypothalamus
3. between the two lobes of the thalamus
4. in the neck on either side of the trachea and across its anterior surface
5. on the posterior surface of the thyroid gland
6. posterior to the sternum within the mediastinum of the thoracic cavity
7. posterior to the stomach
8. draped over the superior end of each kidney
9. in the pelvic cavity
10. in the scrotum

Unscramble and Match Exercise (p. 748)

1. insulin
2. aldosterone
3. TSH
4. oxytocin
5. ACTH
6. glucagon
7. ADH
8. epinephrine
9. testosterone
10. prolactin
11. melatonin
12. estradiol
13. thyroxine

3, 5, 10; 4, 7; 11; 13; 1; 2; 8; 9; 12

Circle Exercise (pp. 748–749)

1. testis
2. ovary
3. parathyroid glands
4. adrenal gland
5. thymus

DISEASES AND CONDITIONS

Matching Exercise (p. 749)

4, 8, 2, 7, 9, 3, 5, 1, 6

True or False Exercise (p. 749)

1. T, 2. F, 3. F, 4. F, 5. F, 6. T, 7. F

LABORATORY, RADIOLOGY, SURGERY, AND DRUGS

Circle Exercise (p. 749)

1. virilism
2. thyroid scan
3. diabetes insipidus
4. glycosylated hemoglobin
5. thyroid gland
6. calcium
7. estradiol

Matching Exercise (p. 750)

6, 4, 1, 2, 3, 5

Laboratory Test Exercise (p. 750)

PANELS AND PROFILES			TESTS	
06BT	Lipid Panel	19687W	Bilirubin (Direct)	
315F ✓	Electrolyte Panel	265F	HBsAg	
10256F	Hepatic Function Panel	51870R	HB Core Antibody	
10165F	Basic Metabolic Panel	1012F	Cardio CRP	
10231A	Comprehensive Metabolic Panel	23242E ✓	GGT	
10306F	Hepatitis Panel, Acute	28852E	Protein, Total	
182Aaa	Obstetric Panel	141A	CBC Hemogram	
18T	Chem-Screen Panel (Basic)	21105R	hCG, Qualitative, Serum	
554T	Chem-Screen Panel (Basic with HDL)	10321A	ANA	
7971A	Chem-Screen Panel (Basic with HDL, TIBC)	80185	Cardio CRP with Lipid Profile	
	TESTS	26F	PT with INR	
56713E	Lead, Blood	232Aaa	UA, Dipstick	
2782A	Antibody Screen	42A	CBC with Diff	
3556F	Iron, TIBC	20867W	HDL Cholesterol	
20933E	Cholesterol	31732E	PTT	
3084111E	Uric Acid	34F	UA, Dipstick and Microscopic	
53348W	Rubella Antibody	20396R	CEA	
27771E	Phosphate	45443E	Hematocrit	
2111600E	Creatinine	28571E	PSA, Total	
29868W	Testosterone, Total	66902E	WBC count	
9704F	Creatinine Clearance	20750E	Chloride	
19752E	Bilirubin (Total)	71187W	Hemoglobin	
30536Rtr ✓	T3, Total	4259T	HIV-1 Antibody	
687T	Protein Electrophoresis	45484R	Hemoglobin A1c	
3563444R	Digoxin	67868R	Alk Phosphatase	
15214R	Glucose, 2-Hour Postprandial	24984R	Iron	
30502E	T3, Uptake	28512E ✓	Sodium	
7773E	Platelet Count	17426R	ALT	
39685R	Dilantin (phenytoin)		MICROBIOLOGY	
30494R	Triglycerides	112680E	Group A Beta Strep Culture, Throat	
26013E	Magnesium	5827W	Group B Beta Strep Culture, Genitals	
15586R ✓	Glucose, Fasting	49003E	Chlamydia, Endocervix/Urethra	
30237W	T4, Free	6007W	Culture, Blood	
28233E ✓	Potassium	2692E	Culture, Genitals	
19208W	AST	2649T	Culture, HSV	
30163E ✓	TSH	612A	Culture, Sputum	
22764R	Ferritin	6262E	Culture, Throat	
20008W	Calcium	6304R	Culture, Urine	
54726F	Occult Blood, Stool	50286R	Gonococcus, Endocervix/Urethra	
51839W	HAV Antibody, Total	6643E	Gram Stain	
430A	Blood Group and Rh Type		STOOL PATHOGENS	
28399W	Progesterone	10045F	Culture, Stool	
30262E ✓	T4, Total	4475F	Culture, Campylobacter	
20280W	Carbon Dioxide	10018T	Culture, Salmonella	
1156F	RPR	86140A	E. coli Toxins	
30940E	Urea Nitrogen	1099T	Ova and Parasites	
17417W	Albumin		VENIPUNCTURE	
28423E	Prolactin	63180	Venipuncture	

BUILDING MEDICAL WORDS

Combining Forms Exercise (p. 751)

1. acid (low pH)
2. extremity; highest point
3. color
4. cell
5. people; population
6. right; sugar
7. diabetes
8. thirst
9. able to conceive a child
10. genitalia
11. from conception to birth
12. giant
13. female; woman
14. hairy
15. ketones
16. breast; mastoid process
17. month
18. many
19. mucus-like substance
20. kidney; nephron
21. nerve
22. node (knob of tissue)
23. small, knobby mass
24. eating swallowing
25. gray
26. retina (of the eye)
27. sphenoid bone; sphenoid sinus
28. poison; toxin
29. poison
30. urine; urinary system

Multiple Combining Forms and Suffix Exercise (p. 751)

1. multinodular
2. ketoacidosis
3. adrenogenital
4. pheochromocytoma
5. gynecomastia
6. glycosuria

Combining Form and Suffix Exercise (p. 752)

1. toxic
2. nodular
3. hypophysectomy
4. thyroiditis
5. adenoma
6. adrenalectomy
7. diabetic
8. thyromegaly
9. hirsutism
10. galactorrhea
11. myxedema
12. thyroidectomy
13. gigantism
14. acromegaly
15. virilism
16. thymectomy

Prefix Exercise (p. 753)

1. hyper- — hypercalcemia
2. hypo- — hypoglycemia
3. in- — infertility
4. hyper- — hyperthyroidism
5. en- — endemic
6. poly- — polyuria
7. para- — parathyroidectomy
8. anti- — antidiabetic
9. hyper- — hyperglycemia
10. trans- — transsphenoidal

ABBREVIATIONS

Abbreviation Exercise (p. 753)

1. IDDM
2. TFTs
3. FBS
4. DKA
5. ADA
6. HbA1c
7. SAD
8. CDE
9. IRS
10. T3

APPLIED SKILLS

Plural Noun and Adjective Spelling Exercise (p. 754)

1. — hypophysial
2. adenomata — adenomatous
3. cortices — cortical
4. glands — glandular
5. hormones — hormonal
6. — hypothalamic
7. ovaries — ovarian
8. — pancreatic
9. testes — testicular
10. — thymic

Proofreading and Spelling Exercise (p. 754)

1. endocrinology
2. pituitary
3. mellitus
4. glucose
5. medulla
6. pheochromocytoma
7. thyroidectomy
8. exophthalmos
9. thyromegaly
10. galactorrhea

Word Analysis Questions (p. 755)

1. endo- — innermost; within
   crin/o- — secrete
   log/o- — word; the study of
   -ist — one who specializes in
2. hypo- — below; deficient
   pituitar/o- — pituitary gland
   -ism — process; disease from a specific cause
3. TSH

Fact Finding Questions (p. 756)

1. ophthalmologist, endocrinologist
2. testosterone (patches), thyroid replacement hormone (Synthroid)
3. antidiuretic hormone; follicle-stimulating hormone; luteinizing hormone
4. hypothyroidism

Critical Thinking Questions (p. 756)

1. MRI of the brain
2. pituitary gland (surgical removal of an adenoma)
3. thyroid hormone replacement (Synthroid)

Hearing Medical Words Exercise (p. 756)

1. diabetes
2. adenoma
3. glandular
4. hyperglycemia
5. infertility
6. synergism
7. thyroidectomy

Pronunciation Exercise (p. 756)

1. hor
2. vair
3. kor
4. bet
5. nawl
6. stay
7. too

Chapter 15   Ophthalmology

ANATOMY AND PHYSIOLOGY

Labeling Exercise (p. 773)

First Exercise

1. lacrimal gland, 2. lacrimal ducts, 3. iris, 4. sclera, 5. pupil, 6. limbus, 7. lacrimal sac, 8. caruncle, 9. nasolacrimal duct

Second Exercise

1. sclera, 2. ciliary body, 3. conjunctivae, 4. suspensory ligaments, 5. cornea, 6. pupil, 7. iris, 8. lens, 9. choroid, 10. retina, 11. optic disk, 12. optic nerve, 13. fovea, 14. macula, 15. posterior cavity

BUILDING MEDICAL WORDS

Combining Forms Exercise (p. 774)

1. to adapt
2. before; front part
3. watery substance
4. eyelid
5. capsule (enveloping structure)
6. hollow space
7. choroid (middle layer around the eye)
8. hairlike structure
9. conjunctiva
10. cornea (of the eye)
11. pupil (of the eye)
12. ciliary body of the eye; circle; cycle
13. lacrimal sac; tears
14. small, depressed area
15. fundus (part farthest from the opening)
16. fundus (part farthest from the opening)
17. below
18. iris (colored part of the eye)
19. iris (colored part of the eye)
20. cornea (of the eye); hard, fibrous protein
21. tears
22. side
23. lens (of the eye)
24. lens (of the eye)
25. small area of spot
26. middle
27. narrowing
28. widening
29. nose
30. eye
31. eye
32. eye; vision
33. lens (of the eye)
34. lens (of the eye)
35. back part
36. pupil (of the eye)
37. retina (of the eye)
38. hard, sclera (white of the eye)
39. examine with an instrument
40. three dimensions
41. above
42. trabecula (mesh)
43. uvea (of the eye)
44. sight; vision
45. transparent substance; vitreous humor

Combining Form and Suffix Exercise (p. 775)

1. -al — corneal
2. -al — retinal
3. -ual — visual
4. -ual — pupillary
5. -al — scleral
6. -iasis — mydriasis
7. -ic — optic
8. -ous — aqueous
9. -ar — macular
10. -al — lacrimal
11. -ion — vision
12. -ation — accommodation
13. -al — conjunctival
14. -osis — miosis

CHAPTER REVIEW EXERCISES
ANATOMY AND PHYSIOLOGY
Matching Exercise (p. 794)

8, 3, 9, 11, 5, 7, 10, 4, 12, 1, 2, 6

Circle Exercise (p. 794)

1. iris
2. caruncle
3. sclera
4. optic disk
5. cones
6. II

True or False Exercise (p. 794)

1. F, 2. F, 3. T, 4. T, 5. T, 6. F, 7. T

Sequencing Exercise (p. 795)

1. light rays from an object, 2. conjunctiva, 3. cornea, 4. pupil, 5. lens, 6. vitreous humor, 7. fovea of the retina, 8. vitreous humor

DISEASES AND CONDITIONS
Circle Exercise (p. 795)

1. nystagmus
2. hyperthyroidism
3. glaucoma
4. floaters
5. hyperopia

Matching Exercise (p. 795)

7, 4, 3, 8, 6, 1, 2, 5

LABORATORY, RADIOLOGY, SURGERY, AND DRUGS
True or False Exercise (p. 795)

1. T, 2. T, 3. T, 4. F

Fill in the Blank Exercise (p. 796)

1. peripheral vision
2. ophthalmoscope
3. accommodation
4. conjugate gaze
5. penlight
6. convergence
7. tonometry
8. photocoagulation
9. retinopexy
10. phorometer
11. angiogram
12. Ishihara
13. trabeculoplasty
14. Snellen
15. phacoemulsification

BUILDING MEDICAL WORDS
Combining Forms Exercise (pp. 796–797)

1. dimness
2. unequal
3. immature; embryonic
4. clotting
5. joined together
6. coming together
7. cold
8. bladder; fluid-filled sac; semisolid cyst
9. double
10. particles suspended in a solution
11. to remove the main part
12. inward
13. away from; external; outward
14. angle
15. jaundice
16. measurement
17. one millionth; small
18. near
19. new
20. elevated structure
21. fear; avoidance
22. to bear; to carry; range
23. light
24. paralysis
25. old age
26. darkness
27. pressure; tone
28. having an affinity for; stimulating; turning
29. blood vessel
30. dry

Related Combining Forms Exercise (p. 797)

1. kerat/o-, corne/o-
2. ophthalm/o-, ocul/o-
3. cor/o-, pupill/o-
4. opt/o-, vis/o-
5. phac/o-, phak/o-, lent/o-, lenticul/o-

Combining Form and Suffix Exercise (pp. 797–798)

1. conjunctivitis
2. retinopathy
3. blepharitis
4. diplopia
5. presbyopia
6. trabeculoplasty
7. gonioscopy
8. iritis
9. blepharoptosis
10. keratectomy
11. convergence
12. enucleation
13. cryotherapy
14. tonometer
15. funduscopy
16. retinopexy
17. blepharoplasty
18. keratomileusis

Prefix Exercise (p. 798)

1. en-   entropion
2. a-   aphakia
3. extra-   extracapsular
4. dys-   dysconjugate
5. an-   anicteric
6. intra-   intraocular
7. hemi-   hemianopia
8. retro-   retrolental
9. ec-   ectropion

Multiple Combining Forms and Suffix Exercise (p. 799)

1. esotropia
2. anisocoria
3. microkeratome
4. photophobia
5. retinoblastoma
6. photocoagulation
7. cycloplegia
8. dacryocystitis
9. phakoemulsification
10. xerophthalmia
11. optometrist

ABBREVIATIONS
Matching Exercise (p. 799)

7, 6, 1, 8, 3, 2, 4, 5

Word Analysis Questions (p. 801)

1. funduscopic
2. intra-   within
   ocul/o-   eye
   -ar   pertaining to
3. an-   without; not
   icter/o-   jaundice
   -ic   pertaining to

Fact Finding Questions (p. 801)

1. the fundus (retina)
2. myopia
3. large floaters in her visual field, blurred vision at close range
4. False. It is just scar tissue.
5. pupils equal, round, and reactive to light
6. O.D.

Critical Thinking Questions (p. 801)

1. blepharitis
2. sclera (or the white of the eye)
3. glaucoma
4. because of her mild exophthalmos bilaterally

Proofreading and Spelling Exercise (p. 802)

1. visual
2. aqueous
3. conjunctiva
4. sclera
5. macula
6. mydriasis
7. cataract
8. blepharoptosis
9. funduscopic
10. ophthalmology

Hearing Medical Words Exercise (p. 802)

1. amblyopia
2. cataract
3. cycloplegia
4. myopia
5. ophthalmologist
6. optician
7. presbyopia
8. strabismus
9. tonometer
10. vitreous humor

Pronunciation Exercise (p. 802)

1. ty (or junk)
2. fay
3. vy
4. ploh
5. koh
6. mak
7. tawm
8. kay
9. pek
10. biz

Chapter 16 Otolaryngology

ANATOMY AND PHYSIOLOGY

Labeling Exercise (pp. 818–819)

First Exercise

1. temporal bone, 2. malleus, 3. incus, 4. stapes, 5. tympanic membrane, 6. external auditory canal, 7. mastoid bone, 8. round window, 9. eustachian tube, 10. semicircular canals, 11. oval window, 12. vestibular branch of the vestibulocochlear nerve, 13. cochlear branch of the vestibulocochlear nerve, 14. cochlea, 15. vestibule

Second Exercise

1. sphenoid bone, 2. entrance to eustachian tube, 3. adenoids, 4. soft palate, 5. nasopharynx, 6. uvula, 7. palatine tonsil, 8. lingual tonsil 9. oropharynx, 10. epiglottis, 11. laryngopharynx, 12. esophagus, 13. frontal sinus, 14. turbinates or conchae, 15. nasal cavity, 16. hard palate, 17. oral cavity, 18. tongue, 19. mandible, 20. larynx, 21. trachea

BUILDING MEDICAL WORDS

Combining Forms Exercise (p. 820)

1. hearing; sound
2. gland
3. adenoids
4. the sense of hearing
5. the sense of hearing
6. ear
7. ear
8. cheek
9. hollow space
10. lip
11. circle
12. cochlea (of the inner ear)
13. back; dorsum
14. sieve
15. outside
16. front
17. tongue
18. glottis (of the larynx)
19. incus (anvil-shaped bone)
20. below
21. lip; labium
22. labyrinth (of the inner ear)
23. larynx (voice box)
24. tongue
25. malleus (hammer-shaped bone)
26. mandible (lower jaw)
27. breast; mastoid process
28. mastoid process
29. maxilla (upper jaw)
30. mind; chin
31. mucous membrane
32. tympanic membrane (eardrum)
33. nose
34. mouth
35. bone
36. ossicle (little bone)
37. ear
38. palate
39. pharynx (throat)
40. nose
41. septum (dividing wall)
42. sinus
43. wedge shape
44. stapes (stirrup-shaped bone)
45. above
46. temple (side of the head)
47. tonsil
48. scroll-like structure; turbinate
49. tympanic membrane (eardrum)
50. vestibule (entrance)
51. voice

Combining Form and Suffix Exercise (p. 821)

1. -al   palatal
2. -al   nasal
3. -ory   audiory
4. -ic   tympanic
5. -al   septal
6. -ate   turbinate
7. -ar   tonsillar
8. -al   buccal
9. -ial   stapedial
10. -oid   ethmoid
11. -eal   pharyngeal
12. -al   glossal
13. -pharynx   nasopharynx
14. -oid   adenoid
15. -al   lingual
16. -al   mucosal
17. -ar   auricular
18. -al   oral
19. -ar   ossicular
20. -cle   auricle
21. -oid   mastoid
22. -eal   laryngeal

CHAPTER REVIEW EXERCISES

ANATOMY AND PHYSIOLOGY

Matching Exercise (p. 839)

5, 12, 16; 6, 7, 11, 14; 3, 13, 18; 2, 8; 4, 9, 17; 1, 10, 15

True or False Exercise (p. 839)

1. T, 2. F, 3. T, 4. T, 5. T, 6. F, 7. F. 8. T

Sequencing Exercise (p. 839)

1. external auditory canal, 2. tympanic membrane, 3. malleus, 4. incus, 5. stapes, 6. oval window, 7. vestibule, 8. cochlea, 9. vestibulocochlear nerve, 10. auditory cortex of the brain

DISEASES AND CONDITIONS

True or False Exercise (p. 840)

1. F, 2. F, 3. T, 4. F, 5. F, 6. F, 7. F, 8. T

Matching Exercise (p. 840)

1, 9, 8, 7, 4, 3, 5, 2, 10, 6

LABORATORY, RADIOLOGY, SURGERY, AND DRUGS

Fill in the Blank Exercise (pp. 840–841)

1. Rinne test
2. antitussive
3. CT scan
4. rhinoplasty
5. culture
6. otoscopy
7. antihistamine
8. audiometry
9. cochlear implant
10. cheiloplasty

BUILDING MEDICAL WORDS

Combining Forms Exercise (p. 841)

1. pain
2. allergy
3. accumulation of fluid
4. a pouring out
5. blood
6. side
7. white
8. word; the study of
9. lymph; lymphatic system
10. nerve
11. the sense of smell
12. plaque
13. polyp
14. old age
15. hard; sclera (white of the eye)
16. examine with an instrument
17. sensory
18. serum of the blood; serumlike fluid
19. pus formation
20. cough

Related Combining Forms Exercise (p. 841)

1. ot/o-, aur/i-, auricul/o-
2. tympan/o-, myring/o-
3. cheil/o-, labi/o-
4. rhin/o-, nas/o-
5. gloss/o-, lingu/o-
6. acous/o-, audi/o-, audit/o-

Combining Form and Suffix Exercise (pp. 842–843)

1. acoustic
2. neuroma
3. labyrinthitis
4. serous
5. rhinorrhea
6. tympanometry
7. tonsillitis
8. otoscope
9. rhinophyma
10. otitis
11. suppurative
12. laryngectomy
13. septoplasty
14. polypectomy
15. myringotome
16. pharyngitis
17. otorrhea
18. glossitis
19. cheiloplasty
20. tympanotomy
21. glossectomy
22. audiogram
23. laryngitis
24. otoscopy
25. rhinoplasty
26. tonsillectomy
27. rhinitis
28. tympanostomy
29. allergic
30. otoplasty

Prefix Exercise (p. 843)

1. bi-   bilateral
2. anti-   antitussive
3. post-   postnasal
4. an-   anosmia
5. de-   decongestant
6. endo-   endoscopic
7. pan-   pansinusitis

Multiple Combining Forms and Suffix Exercise (pp. 843–844)

1. sensorineural
2. otalgia
3. lymphadenopathy
4. leukoplakia
5. otosclerosis
6. temporomandibular
7. otorhinolaryngologist
8. audiologist

APPLIED SKILLS

Word Analysis Questions (pp. 844–845)

1. sinus/o-   sinus
   -itis   inflammation of; infection of
2. bi-   two
   later/o-   side
   -al   pertaining to
3. tympanic membranes

Fact Finding Questions (p. 845)

1. severe pain and pressure over her right cheekbone and right forehead
2. palpation of the forehead and cheekbone areas bilaterally
3. sinusitis
4. amoxicillin

Critical Thinking Questions (p. 845)

1. Assessment
2. frontal sinuses and maxillary sinuses
3. O.U.
4. Increased fever, severe pain and pressure in the sinuses, increasing fatigue, dizziness, pain in the ears

English and Medical Word Equivalents Exercise (p. 845)

1. external auditory canal
2. tympanic membrane
3. cerumen
4. malleus
5. incus
6. stapes
7. naris
8. pharynx
9. larynx
10. allergic rhinitis
11. upper respiratory infection (URI)
12. anakusis
13. epistasis
14. otalgia
15. pharyngitis
16. tinnitus

On the Job Challenge (p. 845)

inflammation of the nose (mucous membranes) due to excessive topical nasal medicines

Hearing Medical Words Exercise (p. 846)

1. adenoids
2. audiologist
3. cheiloplasty
4. cholesteatoma
5. epistaxis
6. eustachian tube
7. laryngitis
8. myringotomy
9. sinusitis
10. tonsillar

Pronunciation Exercise (p. 846)

1. koh
2. aw
3. rik
4. roo
5. tim
6. rin
7. tal
8. nay
9. dib
10. tawn

ABBREVIATIONS

Matching Exercise (p. 846)

6, 7, 5, 2, 4, 1, 3

Chapter 17   Psychiatry

ANATOMY AND PHYSIOLOGY

BUILDING MEDICAL WORDS

Combining Forms Exercise (p. 856)

1. almond shape
2. state of mind; mood; to have an influence on
3. structure that surrounds
4. moving; stirring up
5. edge; border
6. nerve
7. to send across or through

Combining Form and Suffix Exercise (p. 856)

1. -oid   amygdaloid
2. -ic   limbic
3. -ion   emotion
4. -ive   affective

CHAPTER REVIEW EXERCISES

ANATOMY AND PHYSIOLOGY

Matching Exercise (p. 877)

6, 4, 1, 5, 1, 2, 3, 1

True or False Exercise (p. 877)

1. F, 2. T, 3. F, 4. T, 5. F, 6. T, 7. T

Matching Exercise (p. 877)

1, 4, 5; 3; 2; 1; 2; 1, 4

MENTAL DISORDERS AND CONDITIONS

Circle Exercise (p. 878)

1. panic
2. bulimia
3. delirium tremens
4. before
5. echolalia
6. mood disorders
7. depression
8. bipolar disorder
9. Munchausen by proxy
10. histrionic

Matching Exercise (p. 878)

6, 10, 1, 11, 5, 12, 13, 8, 4, 2, 3, 7, 9, 15, 14

True or False Exercise (p. 878)

1. T, 2. F, 3. F, 4. T, 5. F, 6. F, 7. T, 8. T

Matching Exercise (p. 879)

4, 8, 5, 7, 3, 2, 1, 6

DIAGNOSTIC PROCEDURES, THERAPIES, AND DRUGS

True or False Exercise (p. 879)

1. T, 2. F, 3. T, 4. T, 5. F, 6. F, 7. F, 8. T, 9. T, 10. T

Matching Exercise (p. 879)

7, 3, 2, 5, 4, 1, 6

BUILDING MEDICAL WORDS

Combining Forms Exercise (p. 880)

1. extremity; highest point
2. surrender to; be controlled by
3. open air or space
4. forgetfulness
5. fear; worry
6. spider; spider web
7. self
8. killing
9. enclosed space
10. thinking
11. drive; compel
12. feces; stool
13. false belief
14. press down
15. artificial; made up
16. imagined perception
17. pleasure
18. man
19. sleep
20. physician; medical treatment
21. to steal
22. word; the study of
23. thin; frenzy
24. mind; chin
25. one millionth; small
26. shape
27. new
28. besieged by thoughts
29. snake
30. child
31. attraction to; fondness for
32. fear; avoidance
33. diaphragm; mind
34. pole
35. mind
36. fire; burning
37. to seize and drag away
38. split
39. sex
40. human beings; community
41. body
42. disturbing stimulus

43. self
44. death
45. therapy; treatment
46. pull out
47. calm
48. injury
49. hair
50. foreign

Combining Form and Suffix Exercise (p. 881)

1. compulsion
2. stressor
3. hypnosis
4. social
5. cognitive
6. delusion
7. hallucinogen
8. addiction
9. psychotherapy
10. pedophile
11. factitious
12. coprolalia
13. autism
14. anxiety
15. obsession
16. pyromania
17. affective
18. rapist
19. therapeutic
20. kleptomania

Prefix Exercise (p. 882)

1. dys-   dysmorphic
2. de-   dementia
3. post-   posttraumatic
4. bi-   bipolar
5. an-   anhedonia
6. anti-   antisocial
7. trans-   transvestism

Multiple Combining Forms and Suffix Exercise (pp. 882–883)

1. microphobia
2. acrophobia
3. claustrophobia
4. schizophrenia
5. suicidal
6. agoraphobia
7. arachnophobia
8. trichotillomania
9. psychiatric
10. neologism
11. ophidiophobia
12. thanatophobia
13. homicidal
14. xenophobia

ABBREVIATIONS

Matching Exercise (p. 883)

5, 4, 3, 1, 9, 7, 6, 8, 2

APPLIED SKILLS

Proofreading and Spelling Exercise (p. 883)

1. psychiatry
2. affect
3. dopamine
4. serotonin
5. dysthymia
6. suicide
7. homicidal
8. schizophrenic
9. personality
10. paranoia
11. narcissistic
12. addiction
13. therapeutic
14. milieu

Word Analysis Questions (p. 885)

1. psych/o-   mind
   soci/o-   human beings; community
   -al   pertaining to
2. factiti/o-   artificial; made up
   -ous   pertaining to
3. hom/i-   man
   cid/o-   killing
   -al   pertaining to
4. suicidal

Fact Finding Questions (p. 885)

1. A factitious disorder is a mental illness characterized by physical or psychological symptoms and signs that are consciously made up (fabricated) by the patient and that the patient knows are not true. Patients pretend to be sick (often with symptoms that are difficult to evaluate) or even make themselves sick because of a desire to be cared for.
2. a. She has little contact with her ex-husband, even though they were just divorced.
   b. She is experiencing difficulties with her finances.
   c. Her oldest son is experiencing difficulties in his schoolwork and was recently given a speeding ticket.
3. She has been taking Cymbalta 20 mg P.O. at bedtime, as prescribed by you; however, she has also obtained a prescription for a tricyclic antidepressant drug from another physician and is taking this as well as Ambien for sleep.

Critical Thinking Questions (p. 886)

1. bipolar disorder
2. A delusion is a continued false belief concerning events of everyday life. These beliefs are fixed and unchanging despite the efforts of others to persuade or evidence showing the contrary. A hallucination is also a false belief, but it is a false impression of vision, smell, sound, taste, or touch.
3. delusions of persecution or paranoia

Hearing Medical Words Exercise (p. 886)

1. addiction
2. anxiety
3. delusion
4. detoxification
5. euphoria
6. kleptomania
7. milieu
8. paranoia
9. psychiatrist
10. schizophrenic

Pronunciation Exercise (p. 886)

1. pan
2. kawg
3. leer
4. nay
5. noh
6. foh
7. ky
8. pyoo

Chapter 18   Oncology

ANATOMY AND PHYSIOLOGY

Labeling Exercise (p. 899)

1. cell membrane, 2. nuclear membrane, 3. chromosome, 4. nucleolus, 5. nucleus, 6. mitochondrion, 7. cytoplasm, 8. lysosome, 9. ribosomes, 10. endoplasmic reticulum, 11. Golgi apparatus

BUILDING MEDICAL WORDS

Combining Form and Suffix Exercise (p. 900)

1. being distinct; specialized
2. blood vessel; lymphatic vessel
3. cancer
4. capsule (enveloping structure)
5. cancer
6. cell
7. color
8. cell
9. gene
10. arising from; produced by
11. genetic inheritance
12. to go into
13. nucleus
14. a place
15. break down; destroy
16. threadlike structure
17. to change
18. dead cells, tissue, or body
19. nucleus (of a cell)
20. tumor; mass
21. organ
22. disease; suffering
23. plasma
24. ribonucleic acid
25. standing still; staying in one place
26. standing still; staying in one place
27. press down

Combining Form and Suffix Exercise (p. 900)

1. -some   ribosome
2. -ous   cancerous
3. -osis   necrosis
4. -ive   invasive
5. -tic   genetic
6. -plasm   cytoplasm
7. -elle   organelle
8. -ar   cellular
9. -some   lysosome
10. -gen   carcinogen
11. -gene   oncogene
12. -ity   heredity
13. -ar   nuclear
14. -some   chromosome
15. -ion   mutation

CHAPTER REVIEW EXERCISES

ANATOMY AND PHYSIOLOGY

Matching Exercise (p. 923)

2, 4, 6, 3, 7, 1, 8, 5

True or False Exercise (p. 923)

1. F, 2. T, 3. F, 4. T, 5. F, 6. F

Circle Exercise (p. 923)

1. squamous
2. ribosome
3. anaplasia
4. mitosis

TYPES OF CANCER

True or False Exercise (p. 924)

1. F, 2. T, 3. F, 4. F, 5. F, 6. T, 7. T, 8. T, 9. T, 10. F

Matching Exercise (p. 924)

9, 7, 6, 10, 4, 2, 3, 11, 1, 5, 8

Memory Exercise (p. 924)

1. C: Change in bowel or bladder habits, A: a sore that does not heal, U: unusual bleeding or discharge, T: thickening or lump, I: indigestion or trouble swallowing, O: obvious changes in a wart or mole, N: nagging cough or hoarseness.

2.
alpha fetoprotein	b
biopsy	e
chronic myelogenous leukemia	a
estrogen receptor	c
ribonucleic acid	f
tumor, nodes, metastases	a

LABORATORY, RADIOLOGY, SURGERY, AND DRUGS

Matching Exercise (p. 925)

8, 3, 6, 4, 5, 2, 1, 7

True or False Exercise (p. 925)

1. F, 2. F, 3. T, 4. F, 5. F, 6. T, 7. F, 8. F

Matching Exercise (p. 925)

8, 6, 4, 1, 3, 2, 5, 7

Circle Exercise (p. 925)

1. adjuvant therapy
2. endoscopy
3. excising the tumor and surrounding structures as one block of tissue
4. protocol

BUILDING MEDICAL WORDS

Combining Forms Exercise (p. 926)

1. gland
2. life; living organisms, living tissue
3. immature; embryonic
4. chemical; drug
5. cartilage
6. cold
7. to cut apart
8. to cut out
9. liver
10. to cut into
11. white
12. lipid (fat)
13. word; the study of
14. lymph; lymphatic system
15. intentionally causing harm; cancer
16. breast; mastoid process
17. black
18. muscle
19. new
20. kidney; nephron
21. tumor; mass
22. bone
23. radius (forearm bone); x-rays; radiation
24. send back
25. to cut out; remove
26. withstand the effect of
27. retina (of the eye)
28. connective tissue
29. spermatozoon; sperm
30. operative procedure

Related Combining Forms Exercise (p. 926)

1. carcin/o-, cancer/o-
2. cyt/o-, cellul/o-
3. kary/o-, nucle/o-
4. blast/o-, germin/o-, embryon/o-

Combining Form and Suffix Exercise (p. 927)

1. carcinoid
2. dissection
3. seminoma
4. sarcoma
5. neoplasm
6. malignant
7. carcinoma
8. hepatoma
9. leukemia
10. mammography
11. biopsy
12. resection
13. cytology
14. lymphoma
15. karyotype
16. melanoma

Multiple Combining Forms and Suffix Exercise (p. 928)

1. hepatoblastoma
2. lymphangiography
3. liposarcoma
4. nephroblastoma
5. cryosurgery
6. myosarcoma
7. lymphadenopathy
8. adenocarcinoma
9. retinoblastoma
10. radioresistant
11. chondrosarcoma
12. osteosarcoma
13. oncologist

ABBREVIATIONS

Matching Exercise (p. 928)

7, 3, 2, 4, 6, 5, 1

Fact Finding Questions (p. 930)

1. During a breast self-examination two days ago
2. mammography (or mammogram)
3. needle biopsy of the right breast mass
4. metastatic carcinoma involving 10 of 28 axillary lymph nodes
5. normal cells that are mature and differentiated become cancerous cells that are undifferentiated in appearance and behavior

Word Analysis Questions (p. 931)

1. metastatic
2. bi/o-   life; living organisms; living tissue
   -opsy   process of viewing
3. dissect/o-   to cut apart
   -ion   action; condition
4. carcin/o-   cancer
   -oma   tumor; mass

Critical Thinking Questions (p. 931)

1. Because some breast cancers have a hereditary component. If there is a strong family history of breast cancer, a test for the BRCA1 or BRCA2 gene is performed.
2. A frozen section involves freezing a tissue specimen obtained from a biopsy. Thin slices of the specimen are stained and examined under the microscope. A frozen section is performed during surgery so that the surgeon knows immediately whether the tissue is cancerous or not.
3. b
4. The margins of resection are free of tumor

Hearing Medical Words Exercise (p. 931)

1. adenocarcinoma
2. chemotherapy
3. cryosurgery
4. Hodgkin's lymphoma
5. lymphadenopathy
6. lymphoma
7. metastatic
8. neoplasm
9. oncologist
10. osteosarcoma

Pronunciation Exercise (p. 932)

1. kan
2. koh
3. nine
4. by
5. sin
6. noh
7. play
8. net
9. pek
10. stat

Dividing Medical Words (p. 932)

1.	carcin/o-	-gen
2. trans-	locat/o-	-ation
3.	kary/o-	-type
4.	cyt/o-	-logy
5. en-	capsul/o-	-ated
6.	onc/o-	-gene
7. meta-	stat/o-	-ic
8. dys-	plast/o-	-ic
9.	leuk/o-	-emia
10. intra-	vesic/o-	-al

Chapter 19   Radiology and Nuclear Medicine

CHAPTER REVIEW EXERCISES

DIAGNOSTIC IMAGING PROCEDURES

Matching Exercise (p. 960)

7, 2, 9, 1, 8, 4, 3, 6, 10, 5

Circle Exercise (p. 960)

1. scout
2. CT
3. EBT
4. MRI scan
5. MUGA

Recall and List Exercise (p. 960)

Any 10 of these are correct answers: glasses, watches, jewelry, hairpins, metal false teeth, artificial limbs, clothing with metal zippers, metal buttons, or snaps, nose rings, lip rings, tongue studs, pierced earrings, implanted pacemakers or pacing wires, some heart valves, aneurysm clips, cochlear implants, some penile implants, artificial eyes, some intrauterine devices, hearing aids, TENS units, insulin pumps, persons who are metal workers, persons who are gunshot victims, persons who are military personnel, transdermal patches, metallic eye shadow.

Fill in the Blank Exercise (p. 961)

1. light box
2. PA (posteroanterior)
3. film badge
4. gadolinium
5. Doppler
6. half-life

True or False Exercise (p. 961)

1. T, 2. F, 3. F, 4. T, 5. F, 6. T, 7. T, 8. T, 9. T, 10. F

Multiple Choice Exercise (p. 961)

1. b
2. d
3. b
4. d

Matching Exercise (p. 962)

4, 11, 3, 5, 8, 1, 10, 2, 9, 6, 7

BUILDING MEDICAL WORDS

Combining Forms Exercise (pp. 962–963)

1. action
2. blood vessel; lymphatic vessel
3. before; front part
4. aorta
5. artery
6. joint
7. axis
8. heart
9. bile duct
10. bile; gall
11. movement
12. bladder; fluid-filled sac; semisolid cyst
13. density
14. dose
15. bring; move
16. echo (soundwave)
17. electricity
18. esophagus
19. removing from the body
20. fluorescence
21. pouring
22. stomach
23. knowledge
24. uterus (womb)
25. intestine
26. iodine
27. side
28. word; the study of
29. clear
30. lymph; lymphatic system
31. magnet
32. breast
33. bone marrow; spinal cord; myelin
34. nucleus (of an atom)
35. pancreas
36. medicine; drug
37. back part
38. orientation
39. renal pelvis
40. quantity of amount
41. radius (forearm bone); x-rays; radiation
42. x-rays; radiation
43. uterine (fallopian) tube
44. point of light
45. sound
46. technical skill
47. cut; slice; layer
48. visible path
49. urine; urinary system
50. vein
51. movement of air
52. a coming
53. ventricle (lower heart chamber; chamber in the brain)
54. dry

Combining Form and Suffix Exercise (p. 963)

1. nuclear
2. angiography
3. iodinated
4. radiography
5. mammogram
6. tomography
7. fluoroscopy
8. arteriogram
9. axial
10. sonography
11. arthrography
12. dosimetry
13. venography
14. scintigraphy
15. tracer
16. sonogram
17. urogram
18. mammography
19. densitometry
20. dosimeter
21. pyelogram
22. cholangiography

Multiple Combining Forms and Suffix Exercise (p. 964)

1. posteroanterior
2. cholecystography
3. hysterosalpingogram
4. cineradiography
5. lymphangiogram
6. xeromammogram
7. echocardiogram
8. radiopharmaceutical
9. technologist

ABBREVIATIONS

Abbreviation Exercise (p. 964)

1. ultrasound
2. positron emission tomography
3. barium enema
4. chest x-ray
5. single-photon emission computed tomography
6. multiple-gated acquisition (scan)
7. computerized axial tomography
8. intravenous pyelography

APPLIED SKILLS

Fact Finding Questions (p. 965)

1. anteroposterior
2. portable, in surgery
3. operating room
4. right
5. An orthopedic device such as an artificial joint.

Fact Finding Questions (p. 966)

1. c
2. barium, air
3. multiple
4. fluor/o-   fluorescence
   scop/o-   examine with an instrument
   -ic   pertaining to

Fact Finding Questions (p. 967)

1. iodine-123 (I-123), technetium-99m
2. microcuries, millicuries
3. 7–24%
4. oral capsule
5. intravenous injection
6. radi/o-   radius (forearm bone); x-rays; radiation
   act/o-   action
   -ive   pertaining to
7. uniform uptake throughout both the right and left lobes

Hearing Medical Words Exercise (p. 968)

1. barium
2. arteriogram
3. cholecystogram
4. densitometry
5. echocardiogram
6. hysterosalpingogram
7. lymphangiogram
8. sonogram
9. tomography
10. xeromammography

Pronunciation Exercise (p. 968)

1. awg
2. ar
3. thrawg
4. sim
5. aws
6. fan
7. mam
8. mawg
9. mawg
10. vee

Photo Credits

Feature boxes throughout the text: *Dive In!:* Three Images/Getty Images, Inc—Lifesize Royalty Free; *Medical Language Key:* Spike Mafford/Getty Images, Inc.—Photodisc-Royalty Free; *Clinical Connections:* Corbis Royalty Free; *Word Alert:* Getty Images/Digital Vision; *A Closer Look:* Jupiter Images—Thinkstock Images Royalty Free; *Did You Know?:* Getty Images—Photodisc-Royalty Free; *Across the Life Span:* Getty Images—Photodisc-Royalty Free; *It's Greek to Me!:* Jupiter Images—PictureArts Corporation/Brand X Pictures-Royalty Free.

p. 2: *medical records folder labels:* F. Schussler/PhotoLink/Getty Images—Photodisc-Royalty Free; *paramedic with radio:* Keith Brofsky/Getty Images—Photodisc-Royalty Free; *two pharmacologists:* Alvis Upitis/Jupiter Images—PictureArts Corporation/Brand X Pictures-Royalty Free; *Chinese boy:* Dover Publications, Inc., Clip Art book #318; *Hippocrates:* Dover Publications, Inc.; *Black Death:* Ben Stahl/Pearson Education PH School Division; **p. 3:** *doctor and child:* Jupiter Images—PictureArts Corporation/Brand X Pictures-Royalty Free; *puzzle pieces:* EyeWire Collection/Getty Images—Photodisc-Royalty Free; *girl brushing teeth:* PhotoDisc/Getty Images; *Ambroïse Paré:* Brian Warling/International Museum of Surgical Science, Chicago, IL; **p. 4:** EyeWire Collection/Getty Images—Photodisc-Royalty Free; **p. 5:** Keith Brofsky/Getty Images—Photodisc-Royalty Free; **p. 6:** Jose Pelaez/CORBIS-NY; **p. 23:** Michael Donne/Photo Researchers, Inc.; **p. 26:** Dan Frank/Pearson Education/PH College; **p. 32:** Nathan Eldridge/Pearson Education.

p. 38: *woman with saw:* Donna Day/Getty Images Inc.—Stone Allstock; *Andreas Vesalius:* Dover Publications, Inc.; *lab technician using a microscope:* PhotoDisc/Getty Images; **p. 39:** *hospital sign:* S. Meltzer/PhotoLink/Getty Images—Photodisc-Royalty Free; *kiwifruit:* Ian O'Leary © Dorling Kindersley; *William Harvey:* Dover Publications, Inc.; *child with thermometer:* Jim Corwin/Stock Connection; **p. 43:** DR Unique/Custom Medical Stock Photo, Inc.; **p. 49:** *microscope:* Custom Medical Stock Photo, Inc.; *heart muscle:* Michael Abbey/Photo Researchers, Inc.; **p. 67:** *inspection:* S. O'Brien/Custom Medical Stock Photo, Inc.; *palpation:* Michal Heron/Pearson Education/PH College; *ausculation:* Corbis RF; *percussion:* Michal Heron/Pearson Education/PH College; **p. 71:** Andy Levin/Photo Researchers, Inc.; **p. 78:** Dan Frank/Pearson Education.

p. 86: *apple:* FoodPix/Getty Images, Inc.; *orange:* PhotoDisc/Getty Images; *Benjamin Franklin:* Bettmann/CORBIS; **p. 87:** *baby eating spaghetti:* Nancy Ney/Getty Images/Digital Vision; *Edward Jenner:* Mary Evans Picture Library/Photo Researchers, Inc.; *poppy:* © Dorling Kindersley; **p. 95:** Robert W. Ginn/PhotoEdit Inc.; **p. 107:** *(top)* Centers for Disease Control and Prevention (CDC); *(bottom)* David M. Martin, M.D./Photo Researchers, Inc.; **p. 109:** David M. Martin, M.D./Photo Researchers, Inc.; **p. 111:** David M. Martin, M.D./Photo Researchers, Inc.; **p. 113:** Staats/Custom Medical Stock Photo, Inc.; **p. 115:** From Rudolph, A.M., Hoffman, J.I.E., & Rudolph, C.D. (Eds.). (1991). Rudolph's *Pediatrics.* (19th ed., p. 1040) Stamford, CT: Appleton & Lange; **p. 116:** Custom Medical Stock Photo, Inc.; **p. 117:** Arthur Glauberman/Photo Researchers, Inc.; **p. 118:** PhotoDisc/Getty Images; **p. 119:** *(top)* Dr. M.A. Ansary/Photo Researchers, Inc.; *(bottom)* GCa/Photo Researchers, Inc.; **p. 120:** Custom Medical Stock Photo, Inc.; **p. 123:** Custom Medical Stock Photo, Inc.; **p. 126:** Pearson Education/PH College; **p. 127:** Geoff Tompkinson/Photo Researchers, Inc.; **p. 128:** Pearson Education/PH College; **p. 129:** BSIP/Phototake NYC; **p. 133:** Dan Frank/Pearson Education.

p. 148: *bubbles:* Lawrence Lawry/Getty Images, Inc.—Photodisc-Royalty Free; *man and boy balloons:* Stockbyte/Getty Images; *stethoscope:* Nancy R. Cohen/PhotoDisc/Getty Images; *blood transfusion:* Dover Publications, Inc.; **p. 149:** *boy with balloon:* Rotner, Shelley/Omni—Photo Communications, Inc.; *Dorthea Dix:* Dover Publications, Inc.; *general anesthesia:* Dover Publications, Inc.; *medical insignia:* U.S. Army Photograph; **p. 155:** Jim Corwin/Photo Researchers, Inc.; **p. 165:** *(top)* Mednet/Phototake NYC; *(bottom)* © Dorling Kindersley; **p. 168:** *(left)* Pearson Education/PH College; *(right)* Hattie Young/Photo Researchers, Inc.; **p. 170:** *(left)* James Stevenson/Photo Researchers, Inc.; *(right)* St. Bartholomew's Hospital/Photo Researchers, Inc.; **p. 171:** Custom Medical Stock Photo, Inc.; **p. 177:** O'Brien/Custom Medical Stock Photo, Inc.; **p. 178:** *(top)* BSIP/Phototake NYC; *(bottom)* Science Heritage/Custom Medical Stock Photo, Inc.; **p. 180:** Michal Heron/Pearson Education/PH College; **p. 182:** *(left)* © Ray Kemp/911 Imaging; *(right)* Pearson Education/PH College; **p. 184:** ©Jenny Thomas/Pearson Education; **p. 185:** Custom Medical Stock Photo, Inc.; **p. 188:** Dan Frank/Pearson Education.

p. 200: *tin man:* Picture Desk, Inc./Kobal Collection; *red water pump:* Omni—Photo Communications, Inc.; *valentine candy:* EyeWire Collection/Getty Images—Photodisc-Royalty Free; *Elizabeth Blackwell's office:* EMG Education Management Group; *Pfizer Pharmaceutical:* Registered Trademark of Pfizer Inc. Reproduced with Permission.; **p. 201:** *ophthalmoscope:* Keith Brofsky/PhotoDisc/Getty Images; *syringe:* Dover Publications, Inc; **p. 214:** John Garrett © Dorling Kindersley; **p. 226:** Antonia Reeve/Photo Researchers, Inc.; **p. 228:** Abrahas/Custom Medical Stock Photo, Inc.; **p. 231:** Michael English, M.D./Custom Medical Stock Photo; **p. 232:** *(top)* SIU BioMed/Custom Medical Stock Photo, Inc.; *(bottom)* C. Abrahams, M.D./Custom Medical Stock Photo; **p. 235:** SPL/Photo Researchers, Inc.; **p. 237:** *(top)* Fotopic/Miles Simons/Phototake NYC; *(bottom)* Jupiter Images—PictureArts Corporation/Brand X Pictures-Royalty Free; **p. 240:** *(top)* Custom Medical Stock Photo, Inc.; *(bottom)* Matt Meadows/Science Photo Library/Photo Researchers, Inc.; **p. 242:** Pearson Education/PH College; **p. 243:** Michal Heron/Pearson Education/PH College; **p. 245:** F. Schussler/PhotoDisc/Getty Images; **p. 246:** *(left)* English/Custom Medical Stock Photo, Inc.; *(right)* Alvis Upitis/Jupiter Images—PictureArts Corporation/Brand X Pictures-Royalty Free; **p. 247:** Custom Medical Stock Photo, Inc.; **p. 252:** Dan Frank/Pearson Education.

p. 266: *test tubes:* C. Sherburne/PhotoLink/PhotoDisc/Getty Images; *mosquito:* Noah Poritz/Photo Researchers, Inc.; *microscopic organisms:* Centers for Disease Control and Prevention (CDC); *Snellen eye chart:* National Library of Medicine; *WWI ambulance:* Jerry Young © Dorling Kindersley; **p. 267:** *highway:* Kimball Andrew Schmidt/Stock Connection; *peapod:* © Dorling Kindersley; *horse and buggy:* David Gillingwater © Dorling Kindersley; **p. 271:** Andrew Syred/Photo Researchers, Inc.; **p. 276:** Shout Pictures/Custom Medical Stock Photo, Inc.; **p. 277:** Susumu Nishinaga/Photo Researchers, Inc.; **p. 294:** *(top)* Joaquin Carrillo Farga/Photo Researchers, Inc.; *(bottom)* Eye of Science/Photo Researchers, Inc.; **p. 296:** *(top)* Chris Bjornberg/Photo Researchers, Inc.; *(bottom)* S. Meltzer/PhotoDisc/Getty Images; **p. 297:** Peres/Custom Medical Stock Photo, Inc.; **p. 299:** Custom Medical Stock Photo, Inc.; **p. 302:** Alvis Upitis/Jupiter Images—PictureArts Corporation/Brand X Pictures-Royalty Free; **p. 305:** Getty Images—Photodisc-Royalty Free; **p. 307:** Dr. Yorgos Nikas/Photo Researchers, Inc.; **p. 311:** Dan Frank/Pearson Education.

p. 324: *Red Cross:* Eileen Tweedy/Picture Desk, Inc./Kobal Collection; *Louis Pasteur:* The Bridgeman Art Library International; **p. 325:** *girl:* © Dorling Kindersley; *man with beard:* JUDITH HADEN/DanitaDelimont.com; *henna on hand:* Colin Anderson/Getty Images—Photodisc-Royalty Free; *The Starry Night:* Digital Image © The Museum of Modern Art/Licensed by SCALA/Art Resource, NY; *Johns Hopkins:* Ron Solomon/Stock Connection; **p. 341:** *(top)* Meyer/Custom Medical Stock Photo, Inc.; *(bottom)* © Custom Medical Stock Photo; **p. 342:** Logical Images, Inc.; **p. 343:** *(top)* Custom Medical Stock Photo, Inc.; *(bottom)* Custom Medical Stock Photo, Inc.; **p. 344:** Gill/Custom Medical Stock Photo, Inc.; **p. 345:** SPL/Photo Researchers, Inc.; **p. 346:** Custom Medical Stock Photo, Inc.; **p. 349:** ISM/Phototake NYC; **p. 350:** *(top)* Zeva Oelbaum/Peter Arnold, Inc.; *(bottom)* NMSB/Custom Medical Stock Photo, Inc.; **p. 351:** *Clinical Dermatology: A Color Guide to Diagnosis and Therapy,* 2nd ed., by T.P. Habif, 1990, St. Louis: Mosby Year Book, **p. 353:** Logical Images/Custom Medical Stock Photo, Inc.; **p. 354:** SIU/Photo Researchers, Inc.; **p. 355:** Suzanne Dunn/The Image Works; **p. 356:** AJ Photo/Photo Researchers, Inc.; **p. 358:** James King-Holmes/D. Mercer/Photo Researchers, Inc.; **p. 359:** Courtesy Martin R. Eichelberger, M.D., Children's National Medical Center, Washington, DC; **p. 362:** Dan Frank/Pearson Education.

p. 374: *house:* Don Farrall/Light-Works Studio/Getty Images, Inc.—PhotoDisc; *nitroglycerin factory:* Science Photo Library/Photo Researchers, Inc.; *Freud:* Image Works/Mary Evans Picture Library Ltd; **p. 375:** *boy with cast:* SW Productions/PhotoDisc/Getty Images; *Marie Curie:* The Granger Collection, New York; *pill bottle:* PhotoLink/PhotoDisc/Getty Images *ambulance:* Dover Publications, Inc. **p. 379:** Reprinted from McMinn's *Color Atlas of Human Anatomy,* 2/E. McMinn, Hutchings, *Human Anatomy,* 19,46,66,71,78,127,237,238. Copyright 2002, with permission from Elsevier.; **p. 382:** *(top)* Reprinted from McMinn's *Color Atlas of Human Anatomy,* 2/E. McMinn, Hutchings, *Human Anatomy,* 19,46,66,71,78,127,237,238. Copyright 2002, with permission from Elsevier.; *(bottom)* Dover Publications, Inc.; **p. 384:** David W. Harbaugh/Pearson Education; **p. 401:** Scott Camazine/Photo Researchers, Inc.; **p. 404:** *(top)* ESRF-CREATIS/Phanie Agency/Photo Researchers, Inc.;*(bottom)* Dr. P. Marazzi/Photo Researchers, Inc.; **p. 405:** Princess Margaret Rose Orthopaedic Hospital, Edinburgh, Scotland/Science Photo Library/Photo Researchers, Inc.; **p. 406:** Custom Medical Stock Photo, Inc.; **p. 407:** Custom Medical Stock Photo, Inc.; **p. 408:** *(top)* NMSB/Custom Medical Stock Photo, Inc.;*(bottom)* Shea, MD/Custom Medical Stock Photo, Inc.; **p. 409:** Yoav Levy/Phototake NYC; **p. 410:** *(left)* Steinmark/Custom Medical Stock Photo, Inc.; *(right)* PhotoDisc/Getty Images; *(bottom)* Patrick Watson/Pearson Education/PH College; **p. 411:** Jupiter Images—PictureArts Corporation; **p. 412:** Custom Medical Stock Photo, Inc.; **p. 413:** *(top)* James Cavallini/Photo Researchers, Inc.; *(bottom)* Mauro Fermariello/Photo Researchers, Inc.; **p. 416:** Dan Frank/Pearson Education.

p. 428: *high-jumper:* Hans Deryk/AP/Wide World Photos; *sphygmomanometer:* Jack Star/PhotoLink/PhotoDisc/Getty Images; *mosquito:* Noah Poritz/Photo Researchers, Inc.; **p. 429:** *ball of yarn:* Pearson Learning Photo Studio; *apple:* Dover Publications, Inc.; *sickle cell:* Eye of Science/Photo Researchers, Inc.; *drug box:* Dover Publications, Inc.; **p. 434:** *top (left)* Rubberball/Getty Images Inc—Rubberball-Royalty Free; *top (right)* Mark Andersen/Rubberball/Getty Images Inc—Rubberball-Royalty Free; *bottom (right)* Anthony Saint James/Getty Images—Photodisc-Royalty Free; **p. 438:** Reprinted from McMinn's *Color Atlas of Human Anatomy,* 2/E. McMinn, Hutchings, *Human Anatomy,* 19,46,66,71,78,127,237,238. Copyright 2002, with permission from Elsevier.; **p. 441:** Pearson Education/PH College; **p. 448:** Glaser & Associates/Custom Medical Stock Photo, Inc., **p. 452:** Michal Heron/Pearson Education/PH College; **p. 453:** Pearson Education/PH College; **p. 457:** Dr. P. Marazzi/Photo Researchers, Inc.; **p. 459:** *(top)* Glaser & Associates/Custom Medical Stock Photo, Inc.; *(bottom)* PhotoAlto/Ale Ventura/Getty Images Royalty Free—PhotoAlto; **p. 460:** Jupiter Images—PictureArts Corporation; **p. 463:** Elena Dorfman/Pearson Education/PH College; **p. 465:** Dan Frank/Pearson Education.

p. 478: *carrots:* Dover Publications, Inc., Clip Art book #318; *surgery bubble:* Alvis Upitis/Brand X Pictures/Jupiter Images; *chest x-ray:* Dick Luria/Photo Researchers, Inc.; **p. 479:** *circuit board:* Ryan McVay/Photodisc Green/Getty Images—Photodisc-Royalty Free; *Stephen Hawking:* The Scotsman/CORBIS-NY; *policeman:* Getty Images; **p. 482:** Reprinted from McMinn's *Color Atlas of Human Anatomy,* 2/E. McMinn, Hutchings, *Human Anatomy,* 19,46,66,71,78,127,237,238. Copyright 2002, with permission from Elsevier.; **p. 483:** Reprinted from McMinn's *Color Atlas of Human Anatomy,* 2/E. McMinn, Hutchings, *Human Anatomy,* 19,46,66,71,78,127,237,238. Copyright 2002, with permission from Elsevier.; **p. 484:** Pearson Education/PH College; **p. 507:** Simon Fraser/Photo Researchers, Inc.; **p. 509:** Michal Heron/Pearson Education/PH College; **p. 510:** HENNY RAY ABRAMS/AFP/Getty Images; **p. 511:** *(left)* Science Photo Library/Custom Medical Stock Photo, Inc.; *(right)* Science Photo Library/Custom Medical Stock Photo, Inc.; **p. 512:** *(top)* PhotoLink/Getty Images—Photodisc-Royalty Free; *(bottom)* Will & Deni McIntyre/Photo Researchers, Inc.; **p. 513** Yoav Levy/Phototake NYC; **p. 514:** Shout Pictures/Custom Medical Stock Photo, Inc.; **p. 515:** Barts Medical Library/Phototake NYC; **p. 516:** *(top)* AP Wide World Photos; *(bottom)* JPD/Custom Medical Stock Photo, Inc.; **p. 519:** NIH/Phototake NYC; **p. 522:** Used with permission from Pfizer Inc. All rights reserved.; **p. 523:** Corbis RF; **p. 524:** Phanie/Photo Researchers, Inc.; **p. 526:** Pearson Education/PH College; **p. 527:** Peres/Custom Medical Stock Photo, Inc.; **p. 528:** Vanstrum/Custom Medical Stock Photo, Inc.; **p. 532:** Dan Frank/Pearson Education.

p. 546: *asparagus:* Ian O'Leary © Dorling Kindersley; *F.D.R.:* The Granger Collection, New York; **p. 547:** *hose:* Ryan McVay/Getty Images, Inc.—Photodisc-Royalty Free; *syringe with drug:* Jack Star/PhotoLink/PhotoDisc/Getty Images; **p. 550:** Reprinted from McMinn's *Color Atlas of Human Anatomy,* 2/E. McMinn, Hutchings, *Human Anatomy,* 19,46,66,71,78,127,237,238. Copyright 2002, with permission from Elsevier.; **p. 555:** Richard Hutchings/PhotoEdit Inc.; **p. 563:** Custom Medical Stock Photo, Inc.; **p. 564:** Dr. E. Walker/Science Photo Library/Photo Researchers, Inc.; **p. 565:** *(top)* Custom Medical Stock Photo, Inc.; *(bottom)* Simon Fraser/Freeman Hospital/Photo Researchers, Inc.; **p. 566:** Courtesy Chiang Mai University, The Faculty of Medicine, www.med.cmu.ac.th; **p. 571:** Birn/Custom Medical Stock Photo, Inc.; **p. 572:** Faye Norman/Photo Researchers, Inc.; **p. 574:** CNRI/Photo Researchers, Inc.; **p. 575:** Custom Medical Stock Photo, Inc.; **p. 578:** Michal Heron/Pearson Education/PH College; **p. 579:** Custom Medical Stock Photo, Inc.; **p. 580:** Visuals Unlimited; **p. 584:** Dan Frank/Pearson Education.

p. 596: *egg and sperm:* D. Phillips/Photo Researchers, Inc.; *contacts:* David Buffington/PhotoDisc/Getty Images; *March of Dimes:* March of Dimes Birth Defects Foundation; **p. 597:** *rooster:* DON HEBERT/Getty Images, Inc.—Taxi; *monkey:* AP Wide World Photos; *penicillin:* Andrew McClenaghan/Photo Researchers, Inc.; *vacuum tube:* Keith Brofsky/PhotoDisc/Getty Images; **p. 611:** Custom Medical Stock Photo, Inc.; **p. 614:** *(left)* Biophoto Associates/Photo Researchers, Inc.; *(right)* Kenneth E. Greer/Visuals Unlimited; **p. 616:** John Walsh/Photo Researchers, Inc.; **p. 620:** Custom Medical Stock Photo, Inc.; **p. 623:** Dan Frank/Pearson Education.

p. 634: *seedling:* STEFAN MOKRZECKI/Photolibrary.com; *Pap test:* CORBIS-NY; **p. 635:** *bird egg:* BananaStock/Robert Harding World Imagery; *smoking ad:* The Granger Collection; *prescription:* PhotoLink/PhotoDisc/Getty Images; **p. 647:** D. Phillips/Photo Researchers, Inc.; **p. 648:** *(top)* Photo Lennart Nilson/Albert Bonniers Forlag; *(bottom)* CNRI/Photo Researchers, Inc.; **p. 665:** *(top)* Z. Binor/Custom Medical Stock Photo, Inc.; *(bottom)* CNRI/Photo Researchers, Inc.; **p. 668:** SPL/Photo Researchers, Inc.; **p. 670:** CNRI/Phototake NYC; **p. 671:** Vince Michaels/Getty Images Inc.—Stone Allstock; **p. 677:** Neuromedical Systems, Inc.; **p. 679:** Yoav Levy/Phototake NYC; **p. 680:** Getty Images—Photodisc-Royalty Free; **p. 681:** GE Medical Systems/Photo Researchers, Inc.; **p. 682:** Simon Fraser/Science Photo Library/Photo Researchers, Inc.; **p. 683:** Keith Brofsky/PhotoDisc/Getty Images; **p. 685:** Zephyr/Photo Researchers, Inc.; **p. 686:** David M. Grossman/Phototake NYC; **p. 688:** Getty Images—Photodisc-Royalty Free; **p. 693:** Dan Frank/Pearson Education.

p. 708: *Robinson:* Culver Pictures, Inc.; *Kennedy:* Ted Streshinsky/CORBIS-NY; *Devers:* Koji Sasahara/AP Wide World Photos; *control panel:* Jeff Sherman/Getty Images, Inc.—Taxi; *pacemaker:* English/Custom Medical Stock Photo, Inc.; *heart-lung machine:* Maximilian Stock Ltd./Photo Researchers, Inc.; *Salk:* Getty Images/Time Life Pictures; **p. 709:** *rollercoaster:* Alan Thornton/Getty Images Inc—Stone Allstock; *CPR:* Corbis RF; *chromosomes:* L. Willatt/East Anglian Regional Genetics Service/Photo Researchers, Inc.; **p. 729:** *(top)* CORBIS-NY; *(bottom)* NMSB/Custom Medical Stock Photo, Inc.; **p. 731** Custom Medical Stock Photo, Inc.; **p. 732:** *(top)* Marka/Custom Medical Stock Photo, Inc.; *(bottom)* Pearson Education/PH College; **p. 735:** David W. Harbaugh/Pearson Education; **p. 738:** Biophoto Associates/Science Source/Photo Researchers, Inc.; **p. 741:** Pearson Education/PH College; **p. 743:** Custom Medical Stock Photo, Inc.; **p. 745:** *(left)* Custom Medical Stock Photo, Inc.; *(right)* SIU BioMed/Custom Medical Stock Photo, Inc.; **p. 747:** Dan Frank/Pearson Education.

p. 758: *lenses:* JOHN WILKES/Getty Images, Inc.—Taxi; *contact to eye:* Jon Feingersh; *oral contraceptive:* © Dorling Kindersley; *breast implant:* Keith Brofsky/PhotoDisc/Getty Images; *DNA helix:* M. Freeman/PhotoDisc/Getty Images; **p. 759:** *camera:* © Judith Miller/Dorling Kindersley/Collectors Cameras; *kissing:* Charles Gatewood/Pearson Education/PH College; *elderly:* Larry Mulvehill/Corbis RF; **p. 776:** Science Photo Library/Photo Researchers, Inc.; **p. 777:** Barbara Galati/Phototake NYC; **p. 778:** James Stevenson/Photo Researchers, Inc.; **p. 779:** NMSB/Custom Medical Stock Photo, Inc.; **p. 780:** Western Ophthalmic Hospital/Photo Researchers, Inc.; **p. 785:** REGGIE PARKER/Getty Images, Inc.—Taxi; **p. 786:** Custom Medical Stock Photo, Inc.; **p. 787:** *(top)* Custom Medical Stock Photo, Inc.; *(bottom)* Marka/Custom Medical Stock Photo, Inc.; **p. 788:** National Library of Medicine **p. 789:** Geoff Tompkinson/Photo Researchers, Inc.; **p. 790:** *(top)* Courtesy of National Eye Institute; *(bottom)* Chris Barry/Phototake NYC; **p. 793:** Dan Frank/Pearson Education.

p. 804: *skunk:* Digital Zoo/Getty Images/Digital Vision; *aspartame:* Martin Bond/Photo Researchers, Inc.; *cigarettes:* Jonathan A. Meyers/Stock Connection; *Barnard:* Getty Images Inc.—Hulton Archive Photos; **p. 805:** *drums:* Silver Burdett Ginn; *911:* D. Falconer/PhotoDisc/Getty Images; *helicopter:* PhotoDisc/Getty Images; *mammogram:* Keith Brofsky/PhotoDisc/Getty Images; **p. 808:** Pearson Education/PH College; **p. 824:** ISM/Phototake NYC; **p. 826:** ISM/Phototake NYC; **p. 827:** *(top)* Courtesy of Dr. Elizabeth Peterson; *(bottom)* Caliendo/Custom Medical Stock Photo, Inc.; **p. 828:** *(top)* Caliendo/Custom Medical Stock Photo, Inc.; *(bottom)* Dr. P. Marazzi/Photo Researchers, Inc.; **p. 829:** ISM/Phototake NYC; **p. 830:** *(top)* Phanie/Photo Researchers, Inc.; *(bottom)* Pearson Education/PH College; **p. 832:** *(top)* David W. Harbaugh/Pearson Education; *(bottom)* Saturn Stills/Photo Researchers, Inc.; **p. 838:** Dan Frank/Pearson Education.

p. 848: *staircase:* Peter Adams/Photolibrary.com; *Valium:* Getty Digital Vision; **p. 849:** *MRI:* Jupiter Images—PictureArts Corporation; *Brown:* Getty Images Inc—Hulton Archive Photos; *nicotine patch:* Corbis/Pearson Education/PH College; **p. 857:** John Greim/Photo Researchers, Inc.; **p. 859:** NMSB/Custom Medical Stock Photo, Inc.; **p. 863:** Will Hart; **p. 873:** Kramer/Custom Medical Stock Photo, Inc.; **p. 876:** Dan Frank/Pearson Education.

p. 888: *tomatoes:* Ian O'Leary © Dorling Kindersley; *Jarvik heart:* Hank Morgan/Photo Researchers, Inc.; *AIDS quilt:* Corbis RF; *safety cap:* S. Meltzer/PhotoLink/PhotoDisc/Getty Images; **p. 889:** *Armstrong:* Peter Dejong/AP Wide World Photos; *AZT:* Jana Birchum; *Bath:* Joe McNally Photography; **p. 895:** Quest/Photo Researchers, Inc.; **p. 896:** Collection CNRI/Phototake NYC; **p. 903:** Zephyr/Photo Researchers, Inc.; **p. 904:** *(top)* Logical Images, Inc.; *(bottom)* CNRI/Photo Researchers, Inc.; **p. 905:** Zeva Oelbaum/Peter Arnold, Inc.; **p. 906:** Siebert/Custom Medical Stock Photo, Inc.; **p. 907:** NYU Franklin Research Fund/Phototake NYC; **p. 909:** Cavallini/Custom Medical Stock Photo, Inc.; **p. 911:** GCa/Photo Researchers, Inc.; **p. 915:** Photo Researchers, Inc.; **p. 916:** © Simon Fraser, Photo Researchers, Inc.; **p. 918:** Custom Medical Stock Photo, Inc.; **p. 922:** Dan Frank/Pearson Education.

p. 934: *toy gun:* © Judith Miller/Dorling Kindersley/Huxtins; *bat:* Frank Greenaway © Dorling Kindersley; *basketball:* PhotoLink/PhotoDisc/Getty Images; *HIPPA:* Brian Warling/Pearson Education/PH College; **p. 935:** *magnet:* Llu's Real/AGE Fotostock America, Inc.; *Dolly:* AP Wide World Photos; *human genome:* PETER MENZEL/Stock Boston; *stem cell:* Dr. Yorgos Nikas/Photo Researchers, Inc.; **p. 938:** *(left)* Corbis RF; *(right)* David W. Harbaugh/Pearson Education; **p. 939:** Geoff Tompkinson/Photo Researchers, Inc.; **p. 941:** Corbis RF; **p. 945:** Jupiter Images—PictureArts Corporation; **p. 946:** DR Unique/Custom Medical Stock Photo, Inc.; **p. 948:** Yoav Levy/Phototake NYC; **p. 951:** Custom Medical Stock Photo, Inc.; **p. 959:** Dan Frank/Pearson Education.

Index